Textbook of Orthodontics

Textbook of
Orthodontics

Sandeep Goyal
BDS, MDS, MBA, PGDBA, MPH
Former Professor
Department of Orthodontics and Dentofacial Orthopedics
ITS-CDSR, Murad Nagar, Ghaziabad, UP

Edited by
Sonia Goyal BDS, MDS
Former Associate Professor
Department of Oral and Maxillofacial Surgery
ITS-CDSR, Murad Nagar, Ghaziabad, UP

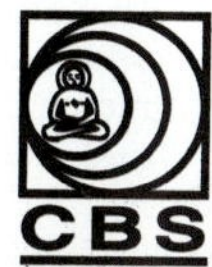

CBS Publishers & Distributors Pvt Ltd
New Delhi • Bengaluru • Chennai • Kochi • Mumbai • Pune
Hyderabad • Kolkata • Nagpur • Patna • Vijayawada

Disclaimer

Science and technology are constantly changing fields. New research and experience broaden the scope of information and knowledge. The authors have tried their best in giving information available to them while preparing the material for this book. Although, all efforts have been made to ensure optimum accuracy of the material, yet it is quite possible some errors might have been left uncorrected. The publisher, printer and authors will not be held responsible for any inadvertent errors or inaccuracies.

Textbook of
Orthodontics

ISBN: 978-81-239-2465-6

First Edition: 2015

Published by Satish Kumar Jain and produced by Varun Jain for
CBS Publishers & Distributors Pvt Ltd
4819/XI Prahlad Street, 24 Ansari Road, Daryaganj, New Delhi 110 002, India.
Ph: 23289259, 23266861, 23266867 Fax: 011-23243014 Website: www.cbspd.com
e-mail: delhi@cbspd.com; cbspubs@airtelmail.in.

Corporate Office: 204 FIE, Industrial Area, Patparganj, Delhi 110 092
Ph: 4934 4934 Fax: 4934 4935 e-mail: publishing@cbspd.com; publicity@cbspd.com

Branches

- **Bengaluru:** Seema House 2975, 17th Cross, K.R. Road, Banasankari 2nd Stage, Bengaluru 560 070, Karnataka
  Ph: +91-80-26771678/79 Fax: +91-80-26771680 e-mail: bangalore@cbspd.com
- **Chennai:** No. 7, Subbaraya Street, Shenoy Nagar, Chennai 600 030, Tamil Nadu
  Ph: +91-44-26680620, 26681266 Fax: +91-44-42032115 e-mail: chennai@cbspd.com
- **Kochi:** 36/14 Kalluvilakam, Lissie Hospital Road, Kochi 682 018, Kerala
  Ph: +91-484-4059061-65 Fax: +91-484-4059065 e-mail: kochi@cbspd.com
- **Mumbai:** 83-C, Dr E Moses Road, Worli, Mumbai-400018, Maharashtra
  Ph: +91-22-24902340/41 Fax: +91-22-24902342 e-mail: mumbai@cbspd.com
- **Pune:** Bhuruk Prestige, Sr. No. 52/12/2+1+3/2 Narhe, Haveli (Near Katraj-Dehu Road Bypass), Pune 411 041, Maharashtra
  Ph: +91-20-64704058-59, 32392277 Fax: +91-20-24300160 e-mail: pune@cbspd.com

Representatives

- **Hyderabad** 0-9885175004
- **Nagpur** 0-9021734563
- **Kolkata** 0-9831437309, 0-9051152362
- **Patna** 0-9334159340
- **Vijayawada** 0-9000660880

Printed At : Goyal Offset Printers

to
my family
and
my teachers

Preface

The *Textbook of* ***Orthodontics*** has been written to simplify the understanding of the orthodontic concepts for the students at undergraduate level. The undergraduate students find themselves helpless when the subjects of orthodontics and the growth of craniofacial skeleton are discussed. An attempt has been made to explain the concepts in a simple language. A lacuna was also observed about the understanding by the students about the development of dentition and we have tried to explain this in the simplest possible terms.

This book will also help the students to diagnose an orthodontic problem and classify its severity, so that they are able to either manage the condition or to guide the patient for comprehensive management by the orthodontist.

During the last 2–3 decades, a number of new concepts have been introduced in the field of orthodontics. In this book, we have briefly incorporated some of them, especially early treatment, lasers, microimplants, white spot lesions, evidence-based dentistry, etc. to keep students abreast with the latest knowledge, but due to lack of space we are not able to explain them in details. Our most efforts were concentrated on the clinical aspects of the orthodontic conditions and their development, because practically these concepts are to be learnt and understood by the students for their clinical practice.

We are grateful to our friends whose wishes, suggestions and contributions are of immense value to this book. Also, the tireless effort of the staff of CBS Publishers & Distributors, New Delhi, to bring the book in its present form is commendable. At the end of the book, we have also incorporated a list of books and/or articles for further reading, if more information is sought by the reader.

No compilation is devoid of drawbacks and mistakes. Therefore, we request our readers to provide their constructive and encouraging responses. Their valuable suggestions will help for further improvement of this book.

Sandeep Goyal

Sonia Goyal

e-mail: goyalsandeep2000@rediffmail.com

Acknowledgements

I bow my head to the Almighty and my Guru Ji for providing me the strength to take this task.

I sincerely thank my teacher, Prof DN Kapoor (former, Professor and Head, Department of Orthodontics, and Dean, Faculty of Dental Sciences, KGMC, Lucknow; and Principal and Director, Kothiwal Dental College, Moradabad), whose immense and valuable guidance, persistent efforts and continuous inspiration have helped me in achieving this goal. His critical thinking, constructive criticism, discipline and his fatherly attitude towards every student always inspired me during my postgraduation days, and left a long-lasting effect on me.

My teachers, Prof VP Sharma, and Prof Pradeep Tandon, had always been on my side to help me at every moment of need, and their immense guidance during my postgraduation at King George's Medical College, Lucknow, helped me to get knowledge of orthodontics. My teachers have always been an immense source of inspiration to me and their influence will be there throughout my life.

I cannot forget to acknowledge my teacher, Late Dr VK Grover, Ex-Principal, Govt. Dental College, Rohtak, who gave me the first idea what orthodontics is, and guided me well for undergraduate practical and theoretical training.

I wish to thank my teacher Dr Prof Sanjay Tewari, Principal, Pt BD Sharma Govt. Dental College, Rohtak, who taught me during my undergraduation and influenced me by his sheer dedication to his work and dentistry. He always motivated me directly and indirectly and has always guided me for all my endeavors. I also thank Dr Sandhya Maheshwari, Professor of Orthodontics, Aligarh Muslim University, for her teaching and guidance at Rohtak. I wish to give special words of thanks to Dr Sanjay Mittal, who always selflessly guided me during my learning phases of the orthodontic problems and their solutions at Govt. Dental College, Rohtak.

I thank my parents and all my family members and especially my kids without whose support and blessings I had not been able to complete this book.

I thank my seniors (Dr GK Singh, Dr Bagga, Dr Mona, Dr TP Chaturvedi, Dr Gera, Dr Gujar, Dr Priyank Rai, Dr Deepa, Dr Seema Sheoran, Dr Mridula, to name a few), my batch mates (Dr Pradeep Raghav, Dr Shyaka, Dr Abha, Dr Deepali) and the juniors (Dr Sanjeev, Dr Deepak, Dr Rekha and others) and my friends (Dr Arti, Dr Gopal K Kataria, Dr Shruti Mittal), and the UG and PG students whom I taught for their help and wishes, the contributions and suggestions.

I wish to thank Dr Kamal Kapoor, from ITS-CDSR, who provided me many pictures of his pre-clinical exercise work to be incorporated in the book, and Dr Prajeesh Padmanabhan for his constant support.

I appreciate the immense efforts put in place by the staff of CBS Publishers & Distributors, New Delhi, to bring out the book in its present form. The nice art work by their artists and the arrangement of text in the manuscript have added value to the presentation of the book. I wish to thank Mr YN Arjuna for his constant advice.

Last but not the least, I wish to thank all those the names whom I could not incorporate here, but who have in one way or the other helped me in compiling this book.

Sandeep Goyal

Contents

1

Introduction to Orthodontics

INTRODUCTION

The word "orthodontics" is derived from Greek words "orthos" meaning normal, correct, or straight and 'odontos' meaning teeth. Orthodontics deals with correction or improving the position of teeth and correcting any malocclusion. It should be remembered that malocclusion is not a pathology/disease but is simply a variation in the normal position of teeth. The term orthodontics was first coined by LeFoulon. In the past, the orthodontics was perceived to be related to the correction of irregular teeth only. But the recent era has witnessed comprehensive expansion of the scope of orthodontics and thereby elaborate understanding of the term. With the advent of knowledge, it has been proved that it is limited not only to the teeth, but also to the bones of face and surrounding craniofacial tissues. So, the concept of dentofacial orthopedics has born. The continuous research has helped to refine the clinical skills and knowledge, and consideration of soft tissues and smile of the patient in diagnosis and treatment planning.

DEFINITION OF ORTHODONTICS

It is the branch of dentistry which deals with the study of growth and development of craniofacial complex, the occlusion and dentition, facial harmony and balance, prevention, interception and correction of malrelationship of jaws and teeth and achievement of harmonious relationship and balance. It includes all preventive, interceptive and corrective procedures to bring teeth and jaws in harmonious relation with each other and with the face of the individual, to establish normal occlusion and pleasing facial esthetics. Various definitions have been put forward in an attempt to define orthodontics.

British Society of Orthodontics in 1922 defined it as "Orthodontics includes the study of growth and development of the jaws and face particularly, and the body generally, as influencing the position of the teeth, the study of the action and the reaction of internal and external influences on the development, and the prevention and correction of arrested and perverted development".

American Association of Orthodontists (1996) adopted a more comprehensive definition in 1996. It defined orthodontics as "the area of dentistry concerned with the supervision, guidance and correction of the growing and mature dentofacial structures, including those conditions that require movement of teeth or correction of malrelationship and malformations of related structures by the application of forces and/or the stimulation and redirection of the functional forces within the craniofacial complex".

HISTORY OF ORTHODONTICS

Crowded and irregular teeth have been a problem for many individuals since antiquity. Dental anomalies and malocclusion have been found in human skulls from Neanderthal era of around 50,000–60,000 years ago.

Hippocrates discussed dental irregularities in his books as early as 460–377 BC. Celsus (25 BC–50 AD) was the first person to suggest treatment of irregular tooth with the help of finger pressure. Pliny (23–79 AD) suggested first mechanical method for treatment of irregular teeth.

Kniesel (1836) advocated the use of removable appliance, and also introduced impression trays. Pierre Fauchard (1928) gave Bandelette expansion arch to orthodontics. Norman Kingsley (1879) introduced bite plane and occipital anchorage. John Nutting Farrar (1839–1913) was the first person to write exclusively for orthodontics. In 1888, he wrote "treatise on irregularities of teeth and their correction".

The term "orthodontia" was given by LeFoulon (1839), while the term "orthodontics" was given by Murray. Orthodontics as a specialty emerged at the turn of 20th century with the efforts of Angle, who has been rightly called as **"Father of Modern Orthodontics"**. Angle (1899) described **classification** of malocclusion based on relation of permanent first molars, which is still relevant and widely used today. He described his concept of occlusion based on the **line of occlusion**. With continued research, he refined his work and contributed to the profession various fixed appliances to treat the malocclusions. He gave pin and tube appliance, ribbon arch appliance and then **the edgewise appliance** to the profession.

Angle (1921–27) introduced various modification of fixed appliances for treatment of malocclusion ultimately designing "edgewise appliance" for 3D control of teeth. All the systems present today are the modification of his original design, e.g. Andrew's SWA, Roth's PEA and MBT. Even Begg's appliance is a modified ribbon arch appliance designed by Angle. Edward H Angle, the father of modern orthodontics, gave the concept of line of occlusion.

Broadbent and Hoffrath's introduction of **cephalometry** (1941) started a new era in the practice and study of orthodontics, which helped us to quantify the growth and treatment changes. It proved to be a powerful tool for various researches to unfold the mystery of growth and development of craniofacial complex. Initially it was an art only, the dentist used to evaluate the face and teeth from an artist's eyes only, but with the subsequent researches, it was proved to be a science also, as it included biological tissues of bones, teeth and their supporting structures.

The main practice of US based orthodontists was mainly concerned with teeth and their correction, while in the parallel era, European orthodontists were using removable appliances and myofunctional appliances, mainly directed to correct the skeletal malrelationship of the jaws. So, the concept of dentofacial orthopedics has its roots in Europe. Field of molecular biology and genetics gives us increased understanding and appreciation of the complexity of orthodontics tooth movement.

Various modifications and development of materials have influenced the way nowadays the orthodontic treatment is done. Due to availability of tooth colored braces and wires; invisible/lingual braces; invisalign; shape memory wires, etc. more patients including adults have started opting for orthodontic treatment now due to inherent comfort and esthetics. It has involved 3D imaging, CBCT, etc. for research studies, diagnosis and treatment planning. Computers have got the roots in every walk of orthodontics now ranging from data storage, diagnosis, treatment planning, surgical planning, and fabrication of the appliances for treatment, e.g. invisalign. History of orthodontics is very vast, as the modern orthodontics can be traced to at least 125 years back, but the details are beyond the scope of this book.

GOALS OF ORTHODONTICS

Goals of orthodontics include improvement of function, esthetics, stability and health of dentofacial tissues. It can be best described as **Jackson's triad**, i.e. functional efficiency, esthetic harmony, and structural balance.

Functional Efficiency

Dentocraniofacial structures are involved in a number of functions, e.g. mastication, swallowing, respiration and speech. The normal interrelationship of various structures is important for smooth functioning. Any disturbance in the relationship, e.g. disturbed muscular equilibrium, disturbed occlusion, etc. leads to various habits/abnormal forces on the dentofacial and other related structures.

Esthetic Harmony

Esthetic/facial beauty is one of the foremost desires of any individual. Orthodontics helps to achieve the balanced, pleasing soft tissue structure in relation to underlying skeletal structures. Many malocclusions lead to poor esthetics and thus affect the person's psychological status. Orthodontics helps to improve the esthetics and thus the self-confidence of the person.

Structural Balance

Factors causing disturbances of equilibrium of various forces lead to changes in adjacent structures. Thus by removing such causes, a structural balance can be achieved. All the structures, e.g. teeth, bone, soft tissues, etc. should be in prefect harmony and balance to achieve the optimal function and esthetics. It also helps in achieving stable orthodontic results.

Sequelae of Malocclusion

Irregular teeth and disturbed functions may lead to pathological changes in the supporting tissues, further aggravating the health of dentofacial tissues. Some of the problems can be as follows:

- Poor facial appearance and negative psychosocial impact
- Abnormal functioning of the tissues
- Loss of soft tissues, gingival recession, etc.
- Risk of caries development
- Risk of development of periodontal diseases
- Abnormal growth and musculoskeletal patterns
- Risk of trauma to the teeth, TMJ, etc.
- Impaired speech.

Needs for Orthodontic Treatment

Generally, there are three main reasons for doing orthodontic treatment:

1. To improve esthetics/dentofacial appearance
2. To correct the occlusal function of the teeth
3. To improve the health of the teeth and periodontium by eliminating faulty occlusion.

Dentofacial Appearance

Psychosocial and esthetic needs are one of the most important causes leading to orthodontic treatment. Well-aligned teeth and a pleasing smile carry a positive status, and help to boost confidence. People with irregular teeth refrain from laughing in public. A poor dental appearance may have broad psychosocial effects. So, the orthodontic treatment improves the psychosocial condition of the patients.

Occlusal Function

Harmonious function of orofacial tissues is very important for the overall health of associated tissues. Some of the abnormal functions associated with malocclusion can be as follows.

- Difficulty in mastication
- Severe malocclusion may make adaptive alterations in swallowing, thus disturbing neuromuscular equilibrium of the dental and facial structures.
- Difficulty in producing certain sounds, therefore speech therapy may be required, e.g. in cleft lip and palate patients.
- Greater incidence of temporomandibular disorders (TMDs). Improper occlusion of teeth leads to faulty mastication and may cause to temporomandibular joint (TMJ) dysfunction. However, the association with TMJ dysfunction and malocclusion has not been proved as yet.

Dental Health

Overall dental health is of paramount importance for the longevity of the dental and supporting mechanism. There is a positive relationship of malocclusion to injury and dental disease.

- Due to crowding, teeth are difficult to clean, that leads to tooth decay and periodontal diseases. There is no strong connection between irregular teeth and dental caries or periodontal disease, if the person is able to maintain the oral hygiene. Although straight teeth may be easier to clean, a proper oral hygiene helps in preventing gingivitis and periodontitis.
- Other conditions which may cause long-term problems, e.g. anterior crossbite with an associated mandibular displacement leads to attrition of teeth, gingival recession, mobility of teeth, abnormal growth, etc.
- More prominent upper incisors are more prone to trauma. Reduction of large overjet minimises the risk of trauma to front teeth and improves esthetics and psychosocial benefits also, e.g. in Angle's class II division 1 cases.
- Deep overbite lead to gingival trauma and recession, e.g. on palatal side of upper incisors in class II division 1, and labial of lower incisors in class II division 2 cases. If it continues, there is a risk of early loss of the lower incisors.
- Trauma from occlusion: Abnormal stresses are transferred to supporting structures and TMJ, leading to chronic problems.

In order to assess the need for orthodontic treatment, various indices have been developed. **Index of orthodontic treatment need (IOTN)** ranks the malocclusion, in order, from worst to best. It has two parts, an esthetic component and a dental health component. The esthetic component is evaluated by comparing the patient's condition with a series of 10 photographs ranging from most to least attractive. The dental health component has a series of occlusal traits that could affect the long-term dental health. Various features are graded from 1–5 (least severe—worst). The worst feature of patient's malocclusion is matched to the list and an appropriate score is allotted. IOTN is a useful guide in prioritising treatment and determining treatment needs, but it does not consider the degree of treatment difficulty.

Branches of Orthodontics

Orthodontics is a very vast field, since it has a long history of more than 125 years. It has evolved various treatment procedures to correct myriad of malocclusion conditions over the years. For simplification, these procedures can be divided into following mentioned branches. However, it should be understood that these treatment options are not limited to that branch and the age of the patients, but are generally overlapping and thus can be used at any stage of treatment as deemed necessary by the clinicians.

Orthodontics can be divided into following branches:

Few years back, the orthodontics used to have four branches, but clinical needs and demands led to evolution of 5th branch also.

1. Preventive orthodontics
2. Interceptive orthodontics
3. Corrective orthodontics
4. Surgical orthodontics
5. Adjunctive orthodontics/adult orthodontics.

They can be defined as follows for a proper understanding of the terms, as defined by Graber.

Preventive Orthodontics

It may be defined as "the actions taken to preserve the integrity of what appears to be normal occlusion at a specific time". These actions are generally undertaken during primary dentition period.

Interceptive Orthodontics

"It involves the procedures used to recognize and eliminate or reduce their severity the potential developing irregularities and malpositions in the developing dentofacial complex". These actions are undertaken during mixed dentition period especially growth phase.

Corrective Orthodontics

It recognizes the existence of malocclusion and thus certain procedures are used to reduce or eliminate the problem and associated sequelae.

Surgical Orthodontics

It involves the surgical procedures used for assisting the clinicians during orthodontic treatment. It can be divided into:

Major surgical procedures: These are the procedures which are used to treat major skeletal discrepancies, e.g. correction of cleft lip and palate, cosmetic surgeries, surgical assisted RME, and orthognathic surgeries, etc.

Minor surgical procedures: These procedures are used to assist the clinician during the fixed orthodontic treatment, e.g. it includes extractions for making spaces, exposure of impacted teeth for bonding and alignment in the arches, frenectomy, gingival contouring, laser surgeries, fixing of microimplants for anchorage, periodontal surgeries and grafting, transplantation of teeth, etc.

Adjunctive Orthodontics

These are the procedures carried out to facilitate other dental procedures necessary to control other dental diseases and restore function and facilitate maintenance of oral hygiene. Thus in adult/older age groups, who have oral health problems and hence need orthodontic treatment as a part of an extensive/elaborate dental treatment plan, the adjunctive orthodontic procedures are used, e.g. uprighting of migrated/tilted teeth in extraction spaces of long standing duration to facilitate proper FPD formation or implant placement, extrusion of fractured teeth for restoration with post and core, closure of spaces in migrated teeth, etc.

Conclusion

Orthodontics being the first specialty of dentistry has blossomed in a vast field with continued research and work contributed by great clinicians. The face is now considered from a three-dimensional perspective, even adding the fourth dimension in the form of "time", to assess and treat the patients. Skeletal, dental and soft tissues are given their due consideration during diagnosis and treatment planning. Consideration of smile of patient and soft tissue relation has evolved with continued work and has influenced the orthodontic treatment. Correction of skeletal malrelationship during active period of growth can be accomplished by myofunctional appliances and dentofacial orthopedic appliances. With the advent of latest materials and invisible braces, the thinking of the patients towards orthodontics has greatly modified and many adult patients are now opting for the orthodontic treatment. The use of microimplants has redefined the concept of anchorage during orthodontic treatment. The adjunctive orthodontic procedures have helped to achieve a better occlusion for the restoration of the remaining dentition and increasing the life of the remaining dentition and associated structures.

2

General Concepts of Growth

INTRODUCTION

A balanced facial growth is a complex process involving growth of the maxilla, mandible, dental and cranial tissues. Growth of craniofacial complex has always been a perplexing topic for most of the students of orthodontics. However, the study of growth is very important for every student of orthodontics, because he has to deal with normalizing the relations of jaws and teeth in relation to each other for a stable and successful orthodontic treatment. Without the knowledge of concepts of growth, a proper and timely treatment cannot be given to the patient.

DEFINITIONS OF GROWTH (Table 2.1)

Various definitions proposed are:

- Growth may be defined as the normal change in the amount of living substance.
- Growth refers to increase in size according to **Todd**.
- Growth usually refers to an increase in size and number as defined by **Proffit**.
- **Huxley** defines it as self-multiplication of living substance.
- **Moss** defined growth as "change in any morphological parameter which is measurable".
- According to **Krogmann**, it is the increase in size, change in proportion and progressive maturity.

Development

- It is a progress towards maturity, as described by **Todd**.
- **Enlow** defined "development as a maturational process involving progressive differentiation at the cellular and tissue levels". However, the maturity comes due to combination of differentiation and translocation of different tissues and attainment of their specific functions and locations. Thus, **development is a combination of** growth + differentiation + translocation.

Differentiation can be defined as a change from generalized cell to a specialized kind, i.e. a change in quality.

Table 2.1: Differences between growth and development

Growth	*Development*
It is an increase in size	It is progress towards maturity.
It is an anatomic phenomenon	It is a physiologic and behavioral phenomenon.
It leads to change in form or proportions, and size.	It includes the changes occurring during the life of the person.
It is quantitative, and units of measurements are cm/year or kg/month, etc.	It is not quantitative, but it is combination of different processes, i.e. growth + differentiation + translocation.

Importance of Growth and Development to Orthodontist

- Proper knowledge of growth and development of craniofacial skeleton is of paramount importance for an orthodontist for proper treatment planning, and guidance of occlusion.
- It helps to identify the etiology of malocclusion.
- It gives an idea of health and nutrition status of children.
- Knowledge of growth helps in devising the norms and hence comparison of growth among individuals and races. It also helps in treatment planning.
- It helps in identification of any abnormal occlusal development at an earlier stage, which can then be timely intercepted to avoid further severity in future.
- Use of growth spurts helps to provide appropriate treatment at the appropriate time.
- It helps in surgical planning in case of severe skeletal problems.
- Growth pattern and timing helps in planning of retention regime.

Factors Affecting the Growth

Since growth of body generally and craniofacial complex particularly, is a long process, there are a number of factors which affect the timing, rate and character of growth. These are heredity, nutritional status, effects of prenatal and postnatal illness or diseases, race, socioeconomic status, exercise, psychological status, climate, secular trends, family size and birth order, health of mother during pregnancy, etc.

Heredity

It is the most important factor affecting growth. Genes play a major role in the rate of growth, height and weight, size of body parts and onset of growth, and growth spurts.

Nutritional Status

Nutrition plays very important role before and after birth. Lack of nutrition affects size and proportions of body parts, texture of tissues, etc. Long-standing malnutrition can lead to permanent deformity, while if malnutrition can be controlled early, then children can catch up the growth, e.g. low birth weight babies if given proper care and nutrition gain weight and growth similar to the normal birth weight babies.

Effect of Illness and Drugs

Prolonged illnesses and drug therapy affect the growth severely leading to permanent defects.

Race

Since different races have different genetic make-up, the growth status differs for different races. It also affects the size and proportions of body parts.

Socioeconomic Status and Family Size and Birth Order

SE status and family size have an inter link and these factors also affect the growth of children. Poor people with large families are not able to provide proper nutrition to every member, thus their growth is affected negatively. Poor families also have to work hard to make ends meet, and their education status is also low.

Climate

It may have a direct little effect on growth of babies. Extreme hot conditions lead to decreased appetite and hence lesser nutrition. Thus, it may affect the adipose tissue content and weight of the children.

Psychological Problems

Affected children do not take proper nutrition and care of themselves. Stress lead to reduction of growth hormone secretion and more production of steroids, which may retard growth.

Exercise

Since it affects the muscle mass and density of bones, the regular light exercises, e.g.

cycling, running, gymnastics, etc. can influence the growth of body. However, strenuous exercises like weightlifting, etc. at an early age can negatively affect the growth.

PRINCIPLES OF GROWTH

1. Pattern
2. Variability
3. Timing.

Pattern

Pattern in growth represents proportionality. It refers not just to a set of proportional relationships at a point in time but to change in these proportional relationships over time. The physical arrangement of the body at any one time is a pattern of spatially proportioned parts.

Variability

Variability of growth is the law of nature. Number 2 individuals grow in the same pattern. It can be expressed quantitatively as the range of differences found in a large population of individuals of similar age, sex, socioeconomic background and race. Variability is expressed quantitatively in terms of deviations from the usual pattern. Variations in response to environment cause increasing differences among similar individuals with time.

How to Evaluate Variability?

It can be done by comparing a given child relative to peers on a standard growth chart, which is also known as **Wetzel's grids** (Fig. 2.1). Here, height and weight of the child is plotted against the age over a period of time. The resultant curve is compared to the average normal curve. There are different curves in the graph chart based on the percentiles, e.g. 10th, 25th, 50th, 60th, 75th, 90th percentiles. The child should follow the same percentile curve during growth. But, any drastic variation of the child's curve indicates unexpected growth change and it should be evaluated for any abnormal growth. These charts can be used in two ways to determine where the growth is normal or abnormal.

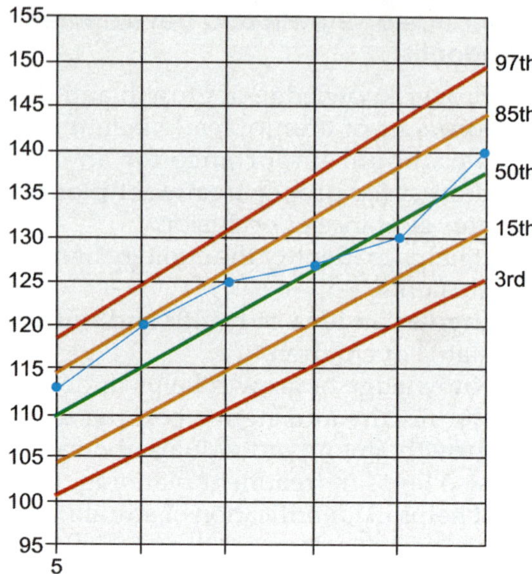

Fig. 2.1: Schematic chart showing different growth percentiles. Blue line shows the average 50th percentile. Children growing below 50th percentile are slow/late growing, while above 50th percentiles are early/fast growing.

1. The location of an individual relative to the group can be established.
2. Growth charts can be used to follow a child over time to evaluate whether there is an unexpected change in growth pattern

Timing

Timing variations are seen in different individuals. It is the occurrence of similar events at different times for different individuals. It occurs due to different body build, sexual differences, and growth spurts. Variations in growth and development because of timing are particularly evident in human adolescence. The timing of developmental events is largely under genetic control, yet it is affected by the environment. It is one of the factors for variablity in growth. Timing variations arise because biologic clock of different individuals is different. It is influenced by factors like genetics, sex, physique, environmental influences, etc.

Physique

Body build can be of three types, which show different timings of growth. Ectomorphic individuals are late-maturers and grow for a longer time. Mesomorphics follow average growth period, while the endomorphics are early maturers, and show faster growth completion.

Sexual Difference (Fig. 2.2)

In girls, there is early onset of menarche, and thus growth completes before boys. Onset of menarche in girls indicates that most of the growth has completed. In boys, the puberty comes late and thus they grow for a longer period.

BASIC CONCEPTS OF GROWTH

Since growth is a natural process, it follows certain basic principles. These can be summarised as follows:

- Concept of normality
- Growth rhythm
- Growth spurts
- Cephalocaudal gradient of growth
- Differential growth of tissues as explained by Scammon's growth curve.

Concept of Normality

Since the concept of ideal growth cannot be applied to every individual, a concept of normality has been suggested. According to it, normal is what is usually occurring and is expected. Also, what is normal for one age group may not be normal for the other age group.

Growth Rhythm

Growth is not a constant, steady and uniform process, i.e. growth rate of one year is not the same as for other year. Rather, it is a rhythmic process, i.e. certain period shows a rapid growth while other periods show slow growth.

Growth Spurts

Growth does not occur at a uniform rate throughout the life. There are certain periods of growth when a sudden acceleration of growth occurs. This sudden increase of growth is called the growth spurt. It may be due to changes in levels of hormones. The timing of spurts differs in boys and girls. According to Graber, there are at least 2–3 peaks of growth spurts in the children, as shown in Table 2.2.

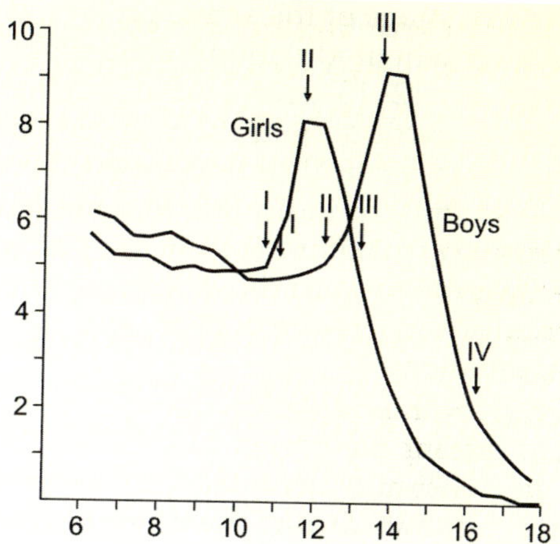

Fig. 2.2: Growth curves of boys and girls. Note that the girls complete their growth before boys. Most girls are in end stage of their pubertal growth spurt, when the boys are starting their pubertal growth spurt *(Adapted from Enlow's)*.

Table 2.2: Growth spurts

	Female	*Male*
1st peak (infantile/ childhood)	3 years	3 years
2nd peak (juvenile)	6–7 years	7–9 years
3rd peak (prepubertal)	11–12 years	13–15 years

There exist growth timing differences between boys and girls. Boys generally show 3 peaks, while the girls show only 2 peaks. Very few girls show mixed dentition period growth spurt, but all show pubertal growth spurt. Females mature earlier (2–3 years earlier) than males, so early treatment is more critical in girls than in boys.

Clinical Importance

The functional therapy should be started earlier in girls, around the age of 10–11 years to take advantage of the active growth, while in boys, growth modulation treatment can be delayed till 12–13 years. Also during the pubertal growth period, there is directional change from vertical to horizontal. Peak of growth spurt is the indication that the growth is occurring at maximum rate at this particular time. The growth spurt show three periods, i.e. a period of acceleration, a peak, and a period of deceleration.

The growth modulation therapy should be started during the period of acceleration, so that the maximum advantage can be taken of the active growth during **peak height velocity** (PHV).

Clinical significance: Knowledge of growth spurts and the growth status of the patient is very important to plan the treatment with functional and orthopaedic appliances. The treatment instituted during periods of rapid growth leads to skeletal changes, better and stable results. If missed, the option left is surgical correction, which should only be given after the periods of growth are over, at least after 18 years of age.

Differential Growth (Figs 2.3a and b)

Growth of body is not the same throughout life. Different organs and tissues grow at different rates at different times. This phenomenon is termed as differential growth. There are two basic concepts helping to understand the differential growth.

1. Scammon's curve of differential growth
2. Cephalocaudal gradient of growth.

Scammon's Curve of Differential Growth

The body tissues can be broadly divided into four types viz. general, neural, lymphoid and genital tissues. Not all the tissue system of the body grow at the same rate. These tissues grow at different rates at different times.

Neural Tissues

Growth of neural tissues is very fast during first few years of childhood. At the age of 7–8 years, the brain is nearly 95% of its adult

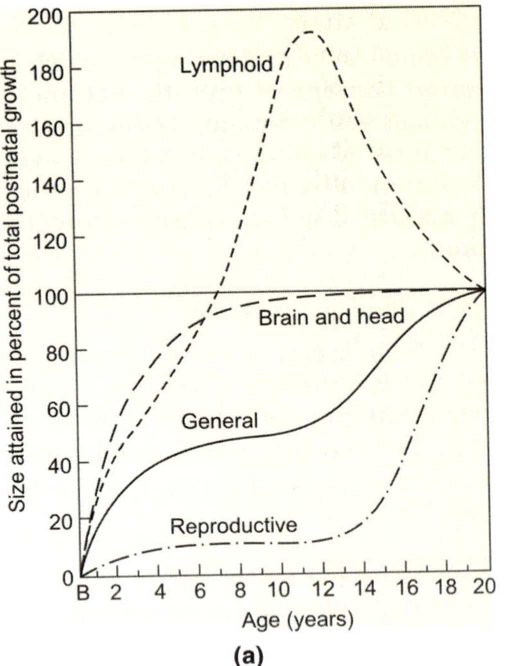

(a)

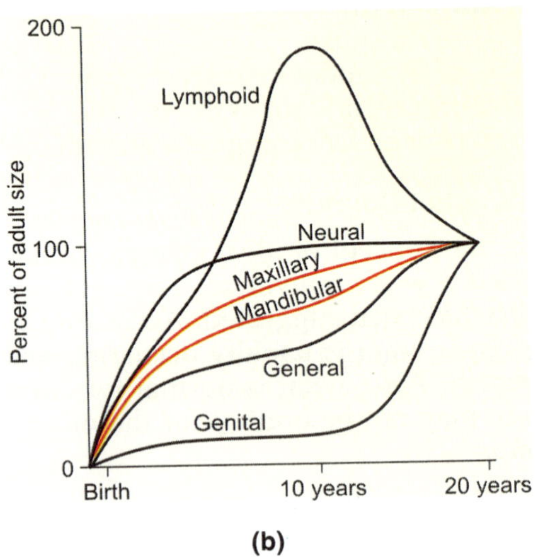

(b)

Figs 2.3a and b: Scammon's growth curve of different tissues of body. Note that lymphoid tissues grow to 200% by 11–12 years of age and then start regressing; while the reproductive tissues start growing only at around 12–14 years of age during the pubertal growth spurt. General tissues grow steadily as S-shaped growth curve, the jaws follow general tissue growth curves. Growth of nervous tissue is mostly complete by 6 years of age *(Adapted from Graber's).*

size. The size of cranium depends on brain growth, and attains its approx adult size by that age. As can be seen below that at birth, cranium is 55–60% of adult size, at 4–7 years, it is 94% of adult size, while at 8–13 years, it is 98% of adult size. So after 7 years of age, there is very little increase in the size of the cranium (Fig. 2.4).

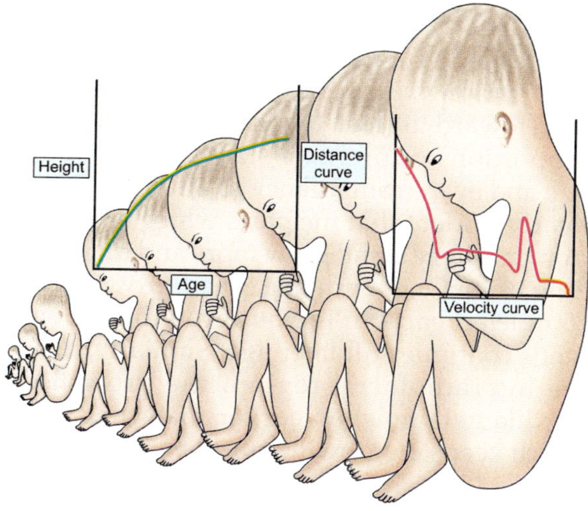

Fig. 2.4: Growth of a baby from intrauterine phase till birth, and related proportions of the body.

Lymphoid Tissues

It includes the thymus, pharyngeal and tonsillar adenoids, lymph nodes and intestinal lymphatic masses. Lymphoid tissues proliferate rapidly far beyond the adult amount in late childhood. They grow most rapidly in late childhood and attain 200% of the adult size by approx. 10 years of age. They provide resistance to infections to the children. Then they undergo involution at the time when growth of genital tissues accelerates rapidly. They start regressing to attain normal adult size by 18 years of age.

General and Visceral Tissues of Body (Fig. 2.5)

These are general tissue of the body which include the external dimensions of the body, muscles, bones, etc. maxilla and mandible also follow general tissue growth curve. Growth curve of these tissues follows an S-shaped curve. There is a rapid growth in 2–3 years age, then a slowdown of growth rate in 3–10 years of age, and again a rapid phase of growth between 11 and 15 years at the time of puberty, gradually slowing and terminating at 18–20 years of age. It has been observed that even upto 45 years and more, there are growth changes in maxilla and mandible.

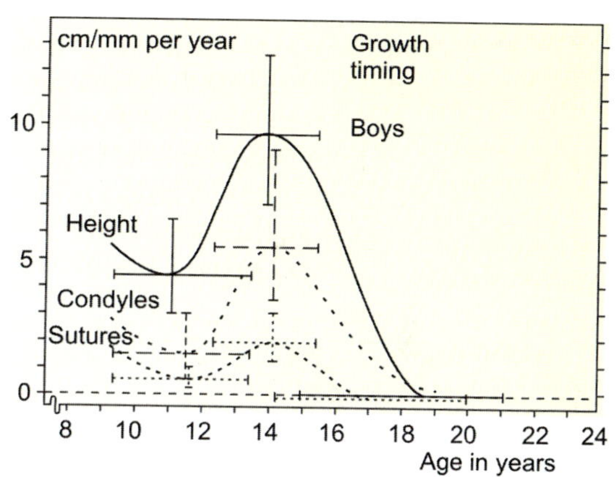

Fig. 2.5: Growth curves of sutures, condyle and height of an individual. Note that all these curves are almost parallel to each other, i.e. follow the same pattern of general tissues growth at almost the same age, the only difference is the quantity of growth *(Adapted from Graber's)*.

Genital Tissues

These are primary sex organs, testes, ovaries, etc. Growth of genital tissues is very slow upto 10–12 years of age. They have just grown upto approx 10–15% by that age of 10 years. It starts increasing at around 12 years of age during period of puberty, and reaches the peak at 20 years of age. Puberty occurs 2–3 years earlier in girls than boys. After this, the growth ceases. Pubertal changes are evident by appearance of secondary sexual characteristics, e.g. in girls, development of breasts, appearance of axillary and pubic hair, change in voice, etc. Pubertal changes evident in boys are development of testes, appearance of facial, axillary and pubic hair, change in hoarseness of voice, increase in the size of penis, prominence of Adam's apple, increase in height and weight, etc.

Cephalocaudal Gradient of Growth

As the name suggests, it means there exists a gradient or axis of increasing growth from head toward the feet. If you compare the body proportions of prenatal size, and postnatal size and even from infancy to adulthood, it is clearly evident that the parts which are away from pituitary gland grow more and till a later time of life, e.g. with age, head growth gets completed early in life but growth of lower limbs continues till later age. Similarly, if we see in craniofacial region, the growth of maxilla gets finished earlier than mandible which keeps on growing till 18 years of age.

Head Size (Figs 2.6 and 2.7)

Head is approx. 50% size of body at around 3 months of IU life. At birth, the head is approx. 30% size of body, while at adult age, it is approx. 12% size of body. It occurs due to the fact that body and esp lower limbs grow more than the head. Lower limb grow fast and attain approx 50% size of total body by adult age.

In head region, the cranium is larger at birth than the face (8 times than the face), while with continued growth, face grows faster than cranium, and at adult age, the proportion is approx 1:1. Face literally comes out from beneath the cranium. Also, the mandible grows more and for a longer time than maxilla, (mandible being caudal to maxilla). Therefore, the treatment to maxilla is to be given at earlier age than to mandible, e.g. treatment for the correction maxillary deficiency by reverse face mask is started at around 8–9 years of age, while for mandibular retrognathism, the functional appliance therapy is started at around 11–12 years of age.

Order of Growth Completion

Growth is a 3D phenomenon, the order of growth completion is different in different planes. In cranium, width completes first, followed by height and depth (WHD). In face also, there is a definite sequence in which growth is "completed" in the three planes of space in both the maxilla and mandible. Growth in width is completed first, then growth in length / depth, and finally growth in height (WDH). Growth of width of both jaws, including dental arches, is completed before adolescent growth spurt and it is affected

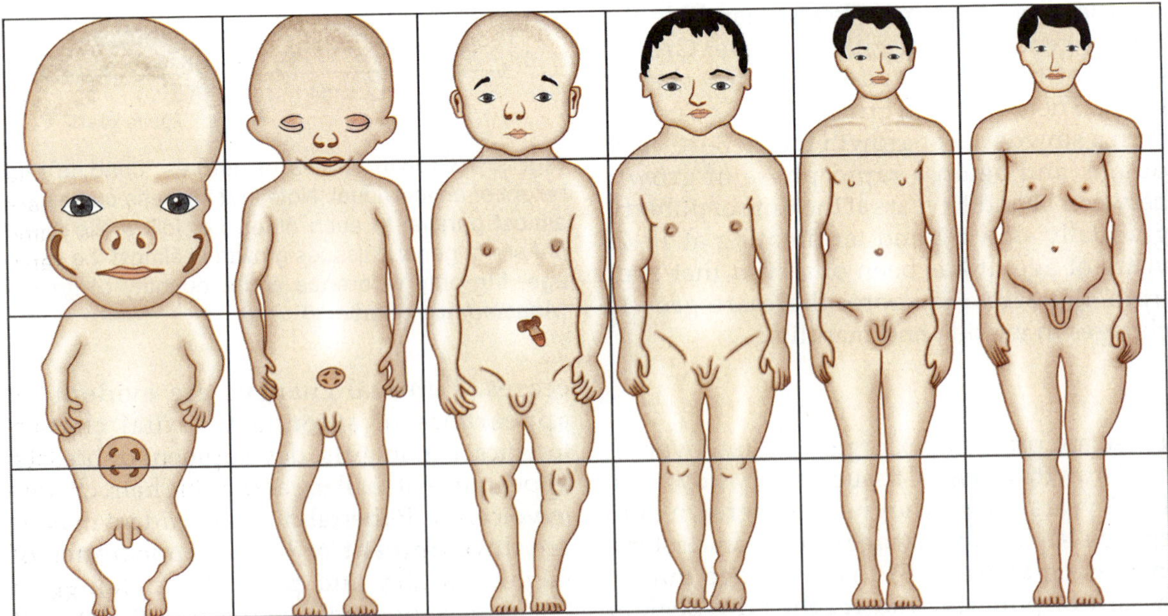

Fig. 2.6: Proportional relation of especially head and rest of the body, and how it changes during growth till adulthood.

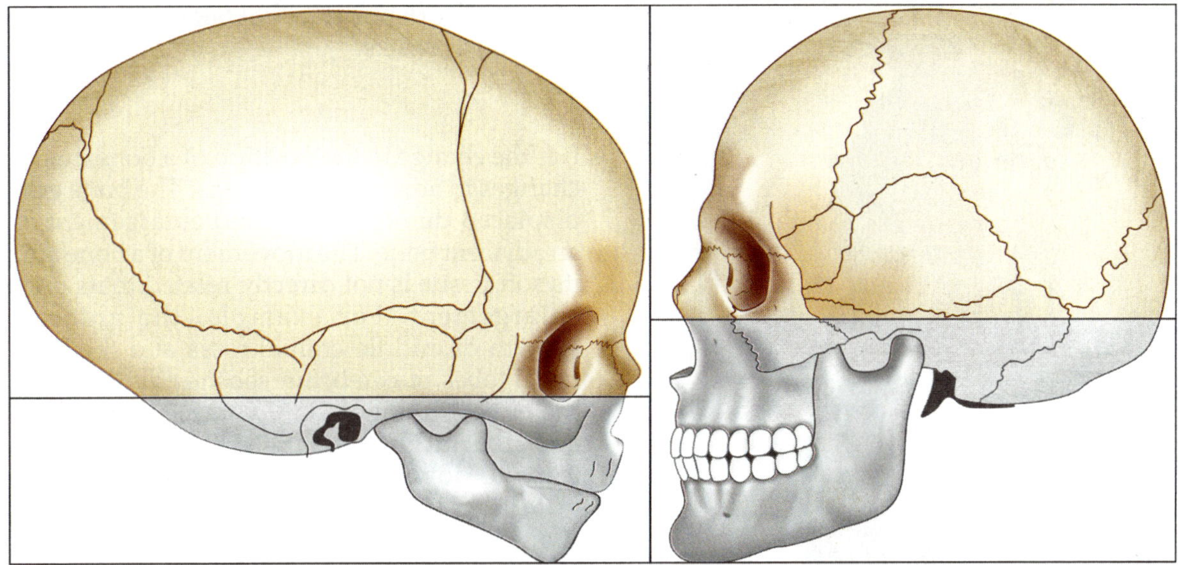

Fig. 2.7: Proportion of sizes of the face with cranium: in infant (1:8) and in the adult (1:2).

minimally by the ensuing adolescent growth changes (approx. age 9–12 years). Intercanine width of mandible gets completed by 9 years of age, while in maxilla, it grows upto 18 years in males, and upto 12 years in females. Intercanine width in upper and lower jaws increase most at the time of canine eruption. Also, arch width is more likely to decrease than increase after age 12. However, in the posterior region, as the jaws grow in length posteriorly, their width also increases. In maxilla, width across second molars, and in the region of tuberosity increases. In mandible, both molar and bicondylar widths show small increases until the end of growth in depth/length.

Growth in length and height of both jaws continues through the period of puberty. In females, the maxilla grows slowly downward and forward to the age 14–15 years, and then tends to grow slightly straight forward. In both sexes, growth in vertical height of the face continues longer than length, with the late vertical growth more in mandible than maxilla.

ENLOW'S CONCEPTS OF GROWTH

1. Drift
2. Displacement
3. Differentiation
4. Remodeling
5. Growth spurts
6. Growth field
7. Growth site
8. Growth center
9. Relocation
10. Counterpart system
11. "V" principle.

Cortical Drift

It is the growth movement of bone due to remodeling of its own tissues. Drift is seen with remodeling enlargement. It is produced by deposition of new bone on one side of the cortical plate, while resorption occurs on the opposite side. It occurs in the direction of bone deposition.

Displacement (Figs 2.8a and b)

It is the movement of whole bone as a unit. It is due to pull or push of different soft tissues and bone tissues as they all continue to enlarge. It is of two types:

Primary or Active Displacement (Table 2.3)

Changes in position and form of bone occur due to inherent growth of the bone itself. The

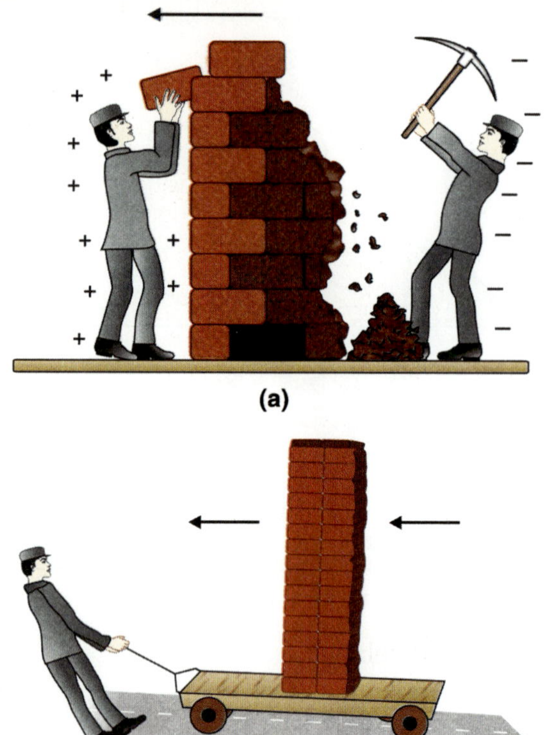

Figs 2.8a and b: During growth, the displacement of a bone may occur by two means: It can grow (cortical drift) by selective deposition and resorption/remodeling of the bone (a), or it gets displaced from one position to another (translocation) (b) under the influence of bone remodeling at a distant site.

bone gets displaced due to the growth of its own parts, e.g. growth at maxillary tuberosity pushes maxilla anteriorly. Similarly, growth at condylar cartilage causes mandible to grow forward. The whole bone is displaced in opposite directions and the amount of primary displacement exactly equals the amount of new bone deposition that takes place within articular contacts.

Secondary or Passive Displacement

It is the change in the position of a bone due to changes in adjacent bony areas. The bone gets displaced due to growth and enlargement of an adjacent bone. The movement of a bone and its soft tissue is not directly related to its own enlargement. For example, the anterior growth of middle cranial fossa and the temporal lobes of cerebrum secondarily displace the entire nasomaxillary complex anteriorly and inferiorly. Also growth of cranial base leads to downward and forward shifting of maxilla.

Translocation

It is passive growth, as the term suggests that there is change in the location of the bone. It depends on capsular matrix and is known as displacement of the bone. **Primary growth** is a combination of actual **translation** (passive growth) and remodeling of bones.

Transformation

It is the active growth. As the term suggests, there is change in the form of the bone. It occurs by remodeling, i.e. apposition and resorption of bone. It is a local change and occurs under the influence of periosteal matrix. **Secondary growth** is a combination of **transformation** (periosteal) + sutural growth.

Remodeling (Fig. 2.9)

It is defined as the selective bone apposition by osteoblasts and resorption by osteoclasts

Table 2.3: Differences between primary and secondary displacements

Primary displacement	*Secondary displacement*
It is the movement of bone as it enlarges itself.	It is the movement of bone due to enlargement of adjacent or distant bones.
Growth remodeling occurs to maintain contact with the adjacent bones.	
It may occur in either direction of bone resorption or deposition.	

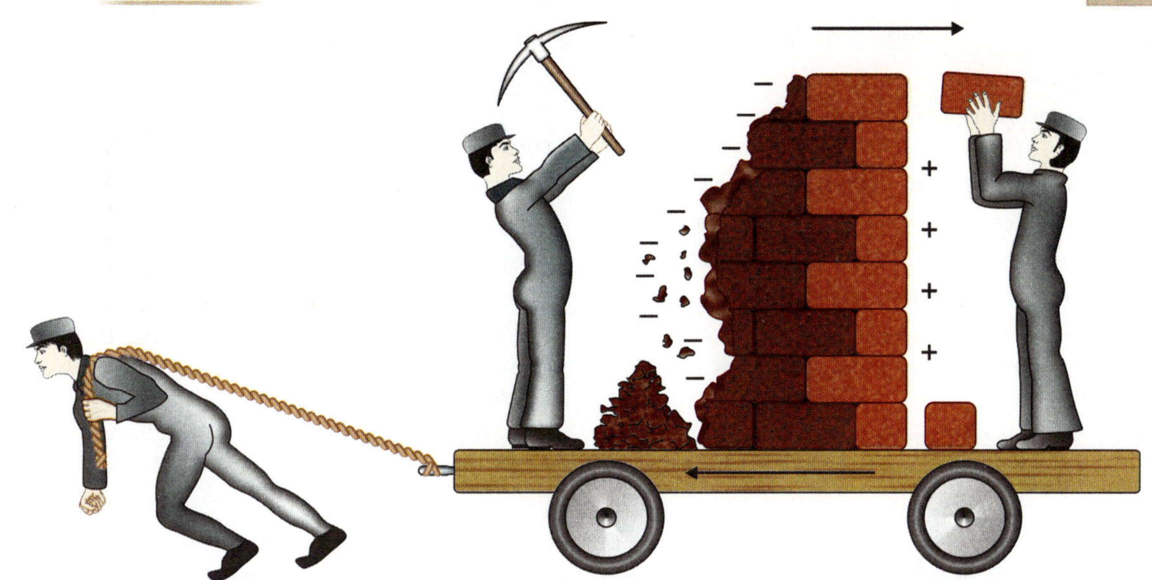

Fig. 2.9: Remodeling of the bone being depicted by apposition (+) and resorption (–), and the arrow shows that adjacent bone is being translated in the opposite direction to that of bone apposition.

resulting in differential changes and alterations in the size and morphology of bone as per needs. Bone does **not** grow by a generalized deposition on its outer surfaces and resorption on its inner surfaces. The bone must remodel during growth because its **regional parts** must become **moved**. The sequential movement of component parts as a bone enlarges is termed **relocation**.

Remodeling helps to sequentially **relocate** parts of whole bone to allow for overall enlargement. It progressively **shapes** the bone to accommodate its various functions, and provides **progressive adaptation** of parts of bones to each other and to the functional demand; and to the intrinsic and extrinsic changes in conditions. It also helps in changing the **size** of different parts and whole bone.

Fields of Remodeling

Resorptive and depository **fields** of growth are present in different areas of the outer and inner surfaces of a bone. The growth movement of the bone **follows** in the direction of the resultant of these two fields. Remodeling helps in maintaining the form of a whole bone while providing for its enlargement at the same time. Remodeling is carried out by osteogenic, i.e. periosteal **membranes** and other surrounding tissues.

Growth Fields

Growth fields are the irregular patterns on inside and outside surfaces of every bone comprised of various soft tissue osteogenic membranes and cartilages. The genetic program for bone growth is not contained in the hard tissue, but in the bone's investing soft tissues. The varying activities of these fields produce bones of irregular shapes. All individuals have different facial pattern due to differences in the **pattern** of the fields of resorption and deposition, and differential **rates** and **amounts** of deposition and resorption throughout each field.

Growth Center (Table 2.4)

The locations at which independent (genetically controlled) growth occurs are called growth centers, e.g. synchondroses, epiphyseal plates, etc.

Growth Site

A site where actual growth or its effect occurs, but that is not genetically controlled, e.g.

Table 2.4: Differences between growth site and growth centers

Growth site	*Growth centre*
It is any location where growth takes place.	It is the site where genetically controlled growth occurs.
All growth sites are not the growth centers.	All growth centers are the growth sites also.
They do not control overall growth of bone.	They control overall bone growth
They do not have independent growth potential.	They have independent growth potential.
When transplanted on other sites, they do not grow.	When transplanted, they can grow independently.
They are affected by external influences markedly.	They are mainly affected by functional needs.
They do not lead to growth of whole bone, but only some part of the bone.	They lead to growth of major parts of the bone.

sutures of the maxilla and the cranium. All centers of growth also are sites, but the reverse is not true.

Relocation

According to Enlow, it is the progressive, sequential movement of component parts (change in the location) as a bone enlarges. The maxillary arch and palate, move downward due to remodeling. Bone deposition occurs on the downward-facing oral surface, together with resorption from the superior facing nasal surface of the palate, resulting in a downward relocation of the whole palate and the maxillary arch. Because of the relocation process, the inferior nasal region of the adult occupies an area where the bony maxillary arch used to be located during earlier childhood age, resulting in a downward relocation of the whole palate and the maxillary arch.

Enlow's Expanding V-principle

Many bones / parts of the bone have V-shape pattern of the growth, which occurs toward wider ends of the V due to selective apposition and resorption.

Enlow's Counterpart Principle (Fig. 2.10)

It states that the growth of any given facial or cranial part relates specifically to other structural and geometric counterparts in face and cranium. There exist different counterparts for different bone components, e.g. counterpart of maxilla is mandible. Upper alveolar bone is counterpart of lower alveolar bone.

Neurotrophism

It is a nonimpulse transmitting neural function which involves axoplasmic transport and provides for long-term interaction between neurons and innervated tissues, which homeostatically regulates the morphological, compositional and functional integrity of these tissues. In simple words, it can be said that a vital nerve supply is essential to muscle functioning, which is then essential for growth of the bone. A vital neural stimulus is essential for soft tissue and bone growth. If nerve supply is cut off or damaged, the corresponding muscles get paralyzed. This leads to atrophy of muscles and soft tissues and hence the growth of bone does not occur properly, e.g. in poliomyelitis.

METHODS TO STUDY GROWTH

Why Growth is Studied?

Growth and development are very important aspects of one's life, and the knowledge of proper pattern and timing of growth is important. The growth of child is followed by the pediatrician from the beginning, which is an indicator of the normal development of the

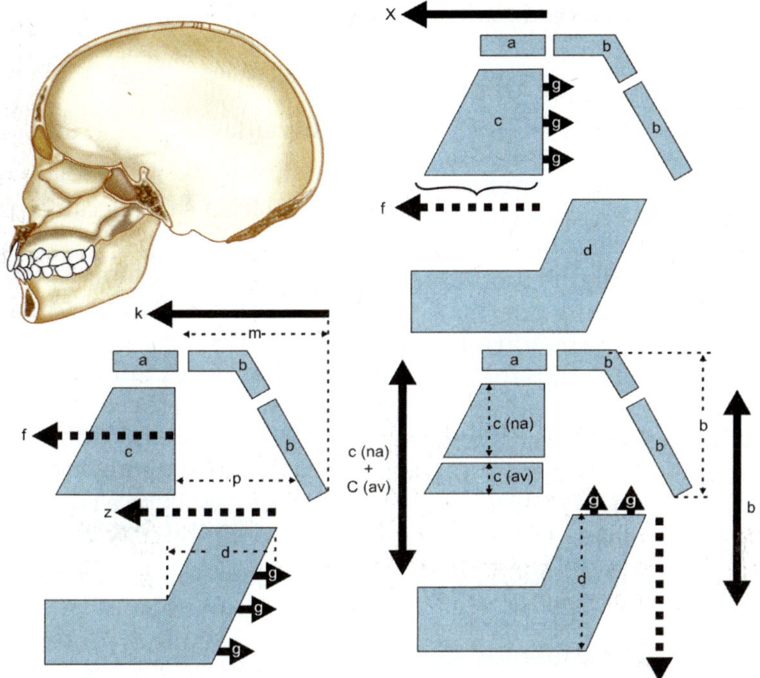

Fig. 2.10: Various counterparts of cranial base, maxilla and mandible, and direction of growth movements, as described by Enlow in his counterpart principle of growth *(Adapted from Enlow's)*.

child. An infant's growth is regularly monitored by noting his skull perimeter, weight and the height, which is plotted on the growth charts. Any deviation of the pattern of growth should warn the clinician for any abnormal growth. Growth is studied for the following purposes.

1. To assess the health and nutrition of children.
2. To compare the growth of an individual with the norms of the growth to find out any deviation and timely interception.
3. In orthodontics, prediction of both the time and amount of active growth in the craniofacial complex, i.e. the maturational status helps in diagnosis, treatment planning and eventual outcome of orthodontic treatment.

The physical growth can be studied as:

1. Analysis of measured data
2. Measurement approaches
3. Experimental approaches.

Analysis of Measured Data

After obtaining the various parameters of the growth, the data is analyzed statistically to derive the scientific evidence. The growth data can be collected either as a longitudinal study or as a cross-sectional study.

Methods of Gathering Growth Data

Data for growth can be collected in three different ways:

1. Longitudinal studies
2. Cross-sectional studies
3. Semilongitudinal studies.

Longitudinal Studies

Here, the data is collected from the same group of individuals over a long period of time by taking repeated measurements at frequent, uniform intervals. So, it is a long-term study.

Advantages of longitudinal studies: These are:

- It provides a pure data of the group.
- It provides lots of information from a relatively small number of individuals.
- Specific developmental events of the same individuals can be studied over a period of time.
- Longitudinal data highlights individual variations caused by timing effects.
- It also helps to compare variations among the individuals within the study group.
- Exact data of sequence of events expected to occur during a life-time of an individual is obtained, and thus comparisons are easy to make.

Disadvantages: The disadvantages of this type of study are:

- It requires a very long time to study same group of subjects/individuals at different times to obtain the results.
- Smaller number of subjects are involved in the study.
- Some participants may loose interest or go away from that area of study, or fall out of the study, thus affecting the results.
- It needs a prolonged maintenance of data.
- It is costly.

Some of the famous longitudinal growth studies are:

- Bolton brush growth study
- Burlington growth study
- Michigan growth study
- Denver child growth study
- Iowa child welfare study.

Cross-sectional Studies

Cross-sectional study is the simplest form of study, where the subjects of different ages, malocclusion, etc. can be studied at the same time. The subjects are studied only once to obtain the data, and they are not required to be followed for a long time. Data can be gathered within short span of time. So, it is the examination of a group or more groups at the same time. They are also known as prevalence studies.

Advantages:

- It is quicker and less costly.
- A larger sample can be used to obtain the data.
- Due to large sample, the statistical analysis is easier. The results are also more sensitive.
- Chances of fall out of subjects are minimal, since these individuals are studied only once and do not require to be followed for a longer time.
- Studies can be easily repeated and modified by the new researcher.

Its disadvantages are that the fluctuations of growth pattern of individuals cannot be recorded. Details of growth pattern cannot be found by these studies.

Over Lapping or Semilongitudinal Data

They involve both methods, i.e. longitudinal and cross-sectional methods to take advantages of each. Different groups are made based on different age ranges, malocclusion types, etc. and each group is studied longitudinally for the same time period (but for a shorter period than the pure longitudinal study).

Advantages:

- Advantages of cross-sectional and longitudinal studies get incorporated.
- Chance of fall-out of subjects is minimized, so data gathered becomes more reliable.
- It is easy and less expensive than longitudinal study.

Graphic Interpretation and Presentation of Growth Data

The measured data can be presented graphically either using a distance curve or a velocity curve.

Distance curve (cumulative curve): In this curve, growth can be plotted in height or weight recorded at various ages. It indicates the distance the child has traversed along the growth path. For example, if the height of an individual is plotted against the age, this distance curve is indicating the height attained by the individual as the age progress.

Velocity curve (incremental curve): It indicates the rate of growth of a child over a period. For example, if the height gain per year is plotted against the age, increments of height can be seen every year.

TYPES OF GROWTH DATA

There are a number of ways to study the growth.

1. Opinion

Opinion is an individual interpretation, based on experience of a person. They are crudest form of knowledge without any scientific evidence. They should not be used when better data are available. They can be biased guess and cannot be applied reliably on the population. There exists no quantification and statistical evidence of such information, and thus cannot be applied for comparison purpose.

2. Observations

They are useful for studying "all or none-phenomenon", e.g. congenital absence of teeth. Their use is also limited as more quantitative data are not possible and thus not reliable for comparison purpose. It also does not have any scientific basis, and can be a form of personal bias. It cannot be applied on whole population or race.

3. Ratings and Rankings

When certain data is difficult to quantify, then they are compared to standard conventional ratings scales. These scales can be based on stages, forms, patterns or standard colored charts, e.g. tooth shape, facial forms. **Ratings** make use of comparisons with conventional accepted scales. **Rankings** arrange the data, in an ordered sequence based on the value.

4. Quantitative Measurements

A scientific approach for studying the growth should be based on accurate measurements, which can be evaluated statistically. It should be repeatable by other workers, without the introduction of errors. It is very important to express an idea or a fact as a meaningful quantity. Various methods to quantify measurements are as follows:

1. **Direct data:** It is derived from direct measurements taken on living person or on a cadaver by means of calipers, scales, measuring tapes and other measuring devices.
2. **Indirect growth measurements:** This data is taken from images or reproductions of the actual persons, for example, measurements made from photographs, dental cast and cephalograms.
3. **Derived data:** Derived data is obtained by comparing two measurements taken at two different times or from two different samples, e.g. when we say that the person's mandible grew 3 mm between ages 7 and 10 years, the 3 mm has not actually been measured. Rather, the mandibular length at 7 years has been subtracted from that at 10 years and the increment thus derived is assumed to represent growth.

According to kind of growth: Growth data can be classified as:

- **Size change:** Changes in size during growth are easily recognized and measured in many ways, e.g. weight (mass), height (length) and width (thickness).
- **Proportional change:** Parts of the body change in relationship with one another during growth.
- **Functional change:** Tissues and organs undergo changes in functional capabilities during the growth process.
- **Compositional change:** Growth involves changes in composition of parts of the body.

Another way to classify growth is:

1. **Prenatal growth:** Is characterized by the rapid increase in cell number and fast growth rates.
2. **Postnatal growth:** It lasts for about first 20 years of life and is characterized by differential growth rates, growth spurts, and increasing maturation of tissues.

Biologic Maturity Indicators

During growth, certain signs can be assessed which give a fair idea of the growth status and maturation of the individual. They help to find out the approximate age of the person, which helps in determining the treatment plan for that person. Some of them are as follows.

Chronologic age: It is calculated from the time of birth of the individual till present. But it has poor correlation with growth status.

Morphologic age: It is based on the height attainment. The data is plotted on the height-age curve, and compared with the norms. It gives an idea where the person stands on the curve.

Dental age: Stage of development and age of eruption of teeth is noted, which is compared with the norms.

Another way to determine the dental age is to note the stages of crown calcification to root completion using X-rays of the unerupted and developing teeth. It can be compared to Hellman's stages or Demirijan stages of dental development. However, dental age is not an accurate predictor of the growth status of the child. The children with small dental age may have advanced skeletal age and fast-growing status, and vice versa.

Sexual age: It refers to the development of secondary sex characteristics. Growth of genital tissues occurs in the last as described by Scammon. This type of indicator is useful only for adolescent growth.

Skeletal age: It is also called the biologic age. It is the state of the bone development. Certain stages are achieved during growth, which indicate the exact position of the growth status of the individual. It is the best method for determining growth status. Many methods have been widely discussed in the literature.

MEASUREMENT APPROACHES

Various methods are used to acquire the growth data. Some are as follows:

1. Craniometry

It is the measurement of skull. It is one of the first methods used to measure size of the bones. The measurements are taken directly from dried skulls. It is used to study the skeletal remains found during excavations. This method formed the basis of the science of anthropology.

Advantage: Precise measurements can be made on the skulls.

Disadvantage: It can only be used on the bones, and cannot be reliably applied on the living persons. Also, the midline structures cannot be reliably measured by this method. It can be used for cross-sectional studies only.

2. Anthropometry

It is used to make direct measurements on living subjects on soft tissue landmarks lying directly over the established bony landmarks. But, it cannot be used to measure midline and intracranial structures.

The results of craniometry and anthropometry vary because of the thickness of the soft tissue overlying the bone. This method can be applied for longitudinal studies, because serial/longitudinal measurements can be made on the same growing individual and the actual amount of growth can thus be evaluated. It helps to generate the data regarding amount and pattern of the growth of the person. Faraka's anthropological data provides the longitudinal changes of human facial proportions.

CEPHALOMETRIC RADIOGRAPHY

Standardized cephalograms can be used for cross-sectional and longitudinal studies.

These radiographs are taken at specific time intervals, e.g. 12–18 months gap, which are then superimposed on each other to compare and measure the growth changes. **Brodie** in 1941 did first cephalometrics longitudinal growth study of human males from the age of third month to the eighth year of life. The orthodontic literature is replete with a number of growth studies.

Advantages

The advantages of craniometry and anthropometry are incorporated in cephalometry. Direct measurements of soft and hard tissues can be done on radiographs. It also allows the longitudinal study since serial views of same person can be taken without sacrificing him. It also allows to gather linear and angular measurements of craniofacial tissues.

Disadvantage

Radiographs give a two-dimensional representation of a three-dimensional structure. It may be difficult to reproduce the same head position and magnification every time. Left and right sides of the craniofacial skeleton do not overlap properly, thus representing as the double-image. A magnification factor is introduced during image production, so correction is needed to obtain exact data.

THREE-DIMENSIONAL (3D) IMAGING

Nowadays, 3D methods, e.g. CT scan, MRI, CBCT, etc., are available to obtain the exact measurements and volumes. Invention of digitiser has simplified the data processing and measurement. The software also help to plan the treatment showing the tooth movements, surgical corrections and the changes in soft tissue morphology with the treatment.

Computed axial tomography [(CAT) scan/ CT] allows 3D reconstruction of craniofacial structures. It allows linear and volumetric measurements. But, it is very costly. MRI is used for soft tissue analysis which is used to study changes brought about by functional appliances, especially in TMJ studies.

IMPRESSIONS AND CASTS

Models are made by taking impression of the anatomical structures. They can be used to compare with models made at later stages. Thus they can be used for longitudinal studies. In orthodontics, it can be used to study dental arch changes in length, width and height, and dental eruption status, and treatment changes.

PHOTOGRAPHS

Photographs should be taken under standardised, controlled conditions with the subjects placed against a graduated grid, which can be duplicated in future also. They are also used for various study purposes. Photos become permanent records and can be helpful in longitudinal studies. But, this method cannot be used for measurements of growth of bones since only soft tissue landmarks are available. For specific studies, the photos can be magnified and standardized as a cephalogram, which can be compared with each other (photocephalometry). It is very helpful in planning orthognathic surgeries.

OCCLUSOGRAM

An occlusogram is a 1:1 reproduction of occlusal surfaces of plaster models on a sheet of acetate tracing paper. A central groove cut into the backs of both models can be used to orient upper tracing to lower tracing.

Methods to Make an Occlusogram

Useful and accurate occlusograms can be made in a variety of ways.

- The most primitive technique for making accurate 1:1 occlusal reproductions is to trace the occlusal surfaces of the teeth onto a clear one-eight plastic sheet that is secured against the dental cast. Head of the viewer should be perpendicular to the cast, and head must no move while tracing both sides of the model. With practice, highly accurate tracings can be made with inexpensive materials.
- Another technique is the use of a xerox machine to copy the occlusal surfaces of

the dental casts. The images are quite clear, but approx. upto 10% magnification gets introduced depending on the machine used, so clinical accuracy may be seriously undermined with this technique.

- Burstone developed an occlusogram camera. It is a sophisticated method of producing 1:1 occlusal reproductions of dental casts, and requires expensive equipment.

Clinical Significance of Occlusograms

They can be used for many purposes like:

- They are the records on paper or in digital form stored in computer. So, they act as permanent records, and do not occupying any storage space.
- They can be obtained as longitudinal records and thus can be used for research purposes.
- They can be used for measuring the TSALD.
- They help in the evaluation of treatment plan and treatment results.
- They act as template for making individualized arch forms.
- They can be easily digitised and stored in computers.

FINITE ELEMENT METHOD

This method subdivides the structure into numerous two-dimensional (2D) and 3D elements termed as finite elements. It analyzes the size and shape changes occurring during growth in each of these elements individually, as well as the overall body. A growing head is subdivided by a series of imaginary lines (2D) or plane surfaces (3D). Each line is connected at each end to at least one other line, the points of connection are called nodes. In 3D case, the planes are bounded by straight lines that extend from one node to another. The lines and planes subdivide the skull or a head into a series of finite elements.

Each finite element is analyzed for elongations (growth strains) along the principle axis, and changes in the direction of principle axis. As a result of growth, the finite element is said to become strained (is said to grow, deformed or transformed). The data obtained is analyzed through computer software to determine the growth pattern and changes.

EXPERIMENTAL APPROACHES

Certain experimental approaches have been used to study growth, some of which are discussed below.

Vital Staining

Certain dyes which have affinity to bind with mineralizing tissues are injected, which remain in the bone and can be detected later after the animal is dead.

Belchier in 1736 discovered the staining of bones of animals fed on madder plants. **Duhamel** (1742) demonstrated that only newly formed bone was stained by madder. **John Hunter** observed that the bones of pigs fed on textile waste were stained and that the acting agent was a dye called alizarin. **Alizarin** reacts strongly with calcium at sites of bone calcification. Since these are the sites of active skeletal growth, the dye marks the location at which active growth occurs. Bone remodels rapidly and area from which bone has been removed also can be identified as the vital stained material gets removed from these locations. Examples of other dyes are trypan blue, lead acetate, tetracycline, xylenol orange, calcein green, porcion dyes, fluorochrome and sodium fluoride, etc.

Alizarin Red Injections

Vital staining of calcifying substances can be done by 2% alizarin red dye given IV. Ground sections are prepared for microscopic studies under reflected light, because acid decalcification leads to loss of staining. Ground sections (25–50 μm thick) show sharp red lines in the stained areas. The disadvantage of this method is that the animal has to be sacrificed for the study. Also as the resorption leads to removal of stained bone, vital staining gives incomplete data on the pattern of bone formation.

Chelating Agents

They form chelates with calcium and get selectively concentrated in mineralized areas of bone tissue, being greatest at sites of active bone formation. **Tetracycline** binds to calcium at growth sites in the same way as alizarin. These methods are very difficult to use in humans as the study can only be conducted after the individual has died.

Radioactive Tracers

Radioactive metabolites get incorporated in the tissues and their location can be detected by detecting the radioactivity. The gamma emitting isotope ^{99m}Tc can be used to detect areas of rapid bone growth in humans. Since it does not need the animal or individual to be sacrificed, and thus is useful to study human growth. It has been found to be more useful in diagnosis of localized growth problems than for studies on growth patterns. Radioactivity in experimental animal is detected by **autoradiography**, where a film emulsion is placed over the tissues and then is exposed in the dark by the radiation. The film is developed to observe the growth areas. Commonly used labels are tritiated thymidine labeling of cells synthesizing DNA and tritiated proline for labeling newly formed bone matrix. Thymidine gets incorporated into DNA and gets replicated with cell multiplication. So that labeled nuclei are those of cells who have undergone mitosis. Proline is a major constituent of collagen and thus gets incorporated in collagen being synthesized. Some other radioisotopes used are **sodium, technitium, calcium, strontium, fluorine, chlorine, iodine, carbon, plutonium, uranium, americium, and gallium.**

Lead Acetate

Most of the vital stains get lost when the tissue is decalcified. Thus, their use is limited to macroscopic observations or preparation of ground section. But, the lead acetate can be used as a vital stain as it is not lost when sample preparation is done for studies. Bones and teeth can be decalcified in an acid saturated with hydrogen sulphide (H_2S) which leads to the formation of insoluble lead sulphide. These are seen as radiopaque dark bands under the microscope in the bone trabaculae beneath the epiphyseal cartilage. These trabaculations have maximum concentration of lead.

Positron Emission Tomography (PET)

It is the technique where a PET is injected into target organ. The positron combines with electron resulting in two gamma rays emission, which is detected by PET camera which tells the position and concentration of radioisotope. Organ malfunction can be indicated, if isotope is partially taken up (cold spot), or taken in excess (hot spot).

NATURAL MARKERS OF BONE GROWTH

Certain features are present in the long bones which persist and remain unchanged in position over years during the period of growth. They are clearly visible on radiographs and serve as useful markers for measurement and study of bone growth. These features are called natural markers, e.g.:

1. Transverse Lines of Arrested Growth

These lines are seen as radiopaque lines on radiographs. They are also known as **Harris lines of arrested growth**. These are a layer of thicker and denser bony trabeculae running mainly in horizontal direction. These are formed due to disturbed equilibrium between the rate of chondrogenesis and of osteogenesis at the end of growing bone. Acute diseases or other problems lead to a temporary arrest in growth of epiphyseal cartilage, but the osteoblastic activity in the marrow continues. This osteoblastic growth diverges laterally and spreads under the surface of cartilage matrix, leading to the formation of horizontally running trabaculae. It appears as a transverse line in metaphysis region on the radiograph and eventually may get shifted into diaphysis with continuous bone growth. Later on, the normal bone formation continues when the epiphyseal cartilage resumes its normal rate of proliferation.

2. Notches in the Base of Second and Fifth Metacarpal Bones

Notches usually begin during infancy or early childhood in second and fifth metacarpals. With continuous growth, they finally fuse with the shaft and disappear about one year before the onset of puberty. The position of these notches, especially its apex, remains stationary throughout the development period, which can be shown by superimposing serial radiographs. These notches serve as markers for measuring the amount of bone growth between the ends of metacarpals.

3. Nutrient Canals

Nutrient canals are used as reference points to measure proportional growth between the ends of diaphysis of long bones in adult humans, as suggested by Digby. According to him, nutrient artery located in this canal is always directed toward initial site of ossification. This point is determined by a theoretical projection of nutrient canal to intersect the central axis of medullary cavity. The bone growth from each end can then be measured as a distance from the point of intersection to the ends of the shaft.

IMPLANT RADIOGRAPHY

Bjork in 1969 developed the technique of inserting inert and biocompatible metal pins in certain areas of facial and jaw bones, which served as radiographic reference markers for longitudinal growth study. Serial cephalograms are superimposed on these implanted pins. It allows precise observation of both, the change in the position of bone relative to another and changes in the external contours of bone.

Bjork's Implant Method to Study Facial Growth

Small pins of materials, like **gold, silver, dental silver amalgam, stainless steel, vitallium, and hard tantalum**, are placed in certain areas of bones under local anesthesia, with the help of a special instrument. The pins size is approx. 1.5 mm in length and 0.5 mm in diameter. No surgical exposure is required. The pins position in the bone does not change due to remodeling process occurring at the bone surface or by erupting teeth. These pins can be used to study amount of bone growth by measuring the change in the distance between the implants and the outer borders of the bone.

Site of Placement of Implants in Maxilla (Fig. 2.11)

1. Before the eruption of permanent incisors, the pins can be inserted in hard palate behind deciduous canines, near the median plane of face.
2. After the permanent central incisors have erupted, the implant is inserted below ANS on each side of median suture, at the level of root apices without touching them. They are useful to assess the growth of face in sagittal and transverse planes.
3. Two implants are placed on each side in the zygomatic process of maxilla, lateral to alveolar process, which help to measure the growth in maxillary width.
4. Implants can also be placed at the border between hard palate and alveolar process medial to the first molar.

Site of Placement of Implants in Mandible (Fig. 2.11)

Usually five or six pins are inserted in four areas as follows:

1. Pins are placed on the anterior aspect of symphysis in midline below the tooth germs or root tips.
2. Two pins are inserted on right side of mandibular body, one under the first premolar and other under the second premolar or the first molar, beneath their germs or root apices.
3. One pin is placed on external aspect of right ramus, at the level of occlusal surfaces of molars, as far behind the

oblique line as possible. This pin may gradually get exposed by resorption of anterior ramal border and may need a replacement.

4. In a latest technique, one or two pins are also inserted in the mandibular base on left side, under the second premolar or first molar. Smaller pins are used on right side and larger on left side, so that the two sides can be readily recognized on the radiographs.

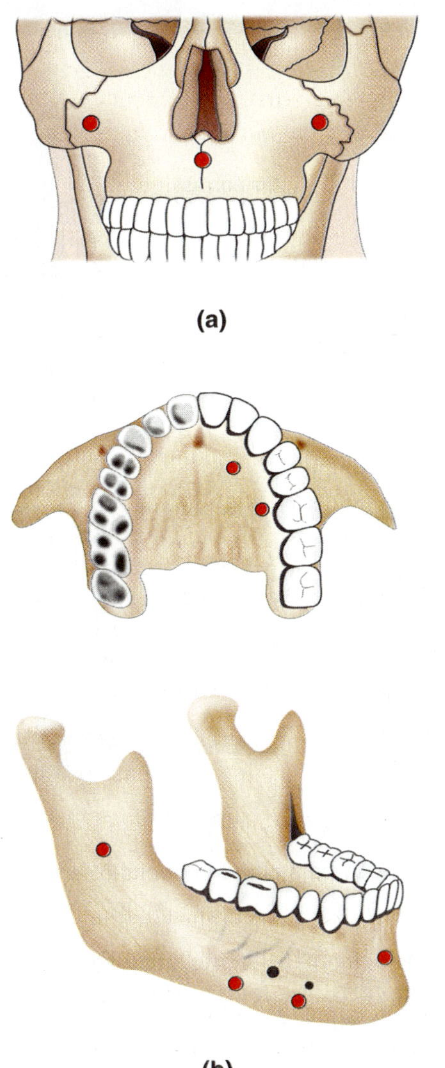

Figs 2.11a and b: Site of placement of implants for growth studies of upper and lower jaws.

MECHANISM OF BONE GROWTH

Osteogenesis

The process of bone formation is called osteogenesis. It is of two types: (1) endochondral bone formation and (2) intramembranous bone formation.

Endochondral Bone Formation (Figs 2.12a to d)

The bone is not formed directly from the cartilage, it invades the cartilage and replaces it. The bone formation is preceded by the formation of a cartilaginous framework, which provides support to the forming bone. This cartilage gets subsequently replaced by the bone. The cartilage grows both, interstitially by the cellular division of chondrocytes; and appositionally, by the activity of chondrogenic membrane. As Moyers has explained, the endochondral bone formation is a form of morphogenetic adaptation which leads to continuous bone formation in the areas of high compression.

Following steps are followed during this process:

- Mesenchymal cells get condensed at the site of bone formation. It becomes the cartilage when some cells get differentiated into chondroblasts, and lay down the hyaline cartilage framework.
- This cartilage is surrounded by a membrane called perichondrium, which provides the osteogenic cells, separated by intercellular substance.
- Cartilage cells secrete the matrix, which gets calcified under the influence of enzyme alkaline phosphatase. It leads to the loss of nutritional supply to cartilage cells, leading to their death. Thus, the empty spaces called as primary areolae are formed. Further with advanced disintegration, it gets reduced to the bars and creation of larger empty spaces called secondary areolae.
- The blood vessels and osteogenic cells from perichondrium invade this disintegrating cartilaginous matrix. The osteogenic cells become osteoblasts and

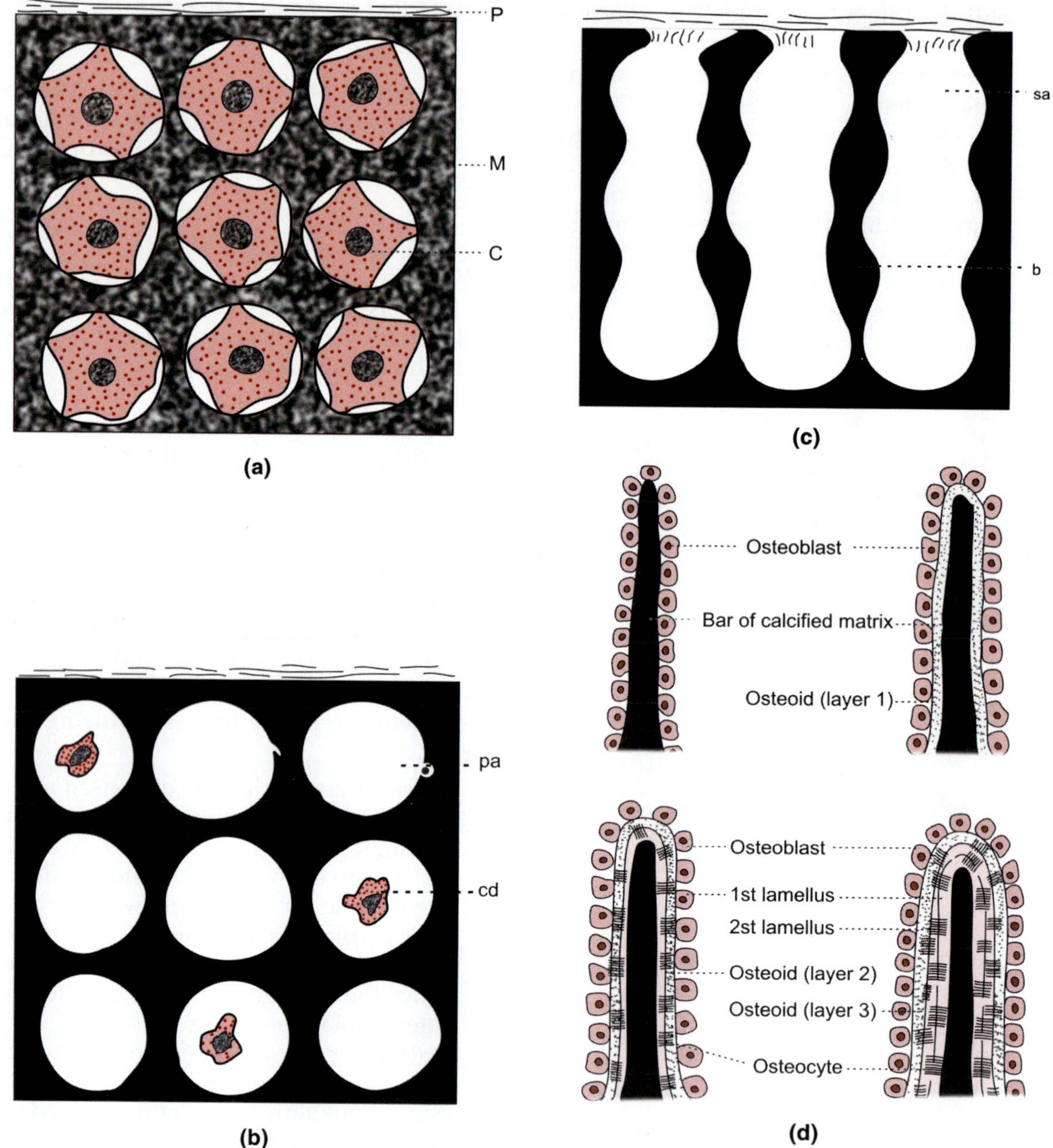

Figs 2.12a to d: Stages of endochondral osteogenesis. Details can be studied in books of embryology.

line these calcified bars. They start secreting the layers of unmineralized osteoid. With the growth of the osteoid, they start moving outward. This osteoid gets calcified to form a **lamella**. Then, another layer of osteoid is secreted to form new lamella. This process goes on.

In endochondral bone growth, the zone of reserved cartilage feeds new cells in the zone of cell division. Cells in this zone undergo rapid cell division and form the columns of chondrocytes. It leads to elongation of the bone. Further, these daughter cells undergo hypertrophy, and the calcification of the matrix occurs. It leads to cut-off of nutrition and disintegration of cells.

This calcified matrix gets partially resorbed by invading vascular channels, which also carry osteoblast cells, which deposit the osteoids on the remnants of cartilage. With further growth, these osteoids get calcified, and a new layer of osteoids is laid down and so on. It leads to lengthening of the bone. In synchondrosis, the bone proliferates on both sides of the cartilaginous plate, leading to lengthening of the cranial base bones.

Intramembranous Bone Formation (Fig. 2.13)

Here, the bone formation is not preceded by the formation of cartilaginous matrix. The bone is directly laid down in a fibrous membrane. The bone is formed as follows:

- Undifferentiated mesenchymal cells become condensed at the site of bone formation. Cells lay down the bundles of collagen fibers leading to formation of a membrane.
- Some cells change in osteoblasts, which secrete osteoid around the collagen fibers. This osteoid gets calcified to form lamella. The original blood vessels remain near the forming trabeculae.
- The osteoblasts move away from this lamella and lay another layer of osteoid, which gets calcified to form new lamella. In this process, some cells get entrapped between two lamellae and become osteocytes. Blood vessels also become enclosed in fine cancellous spaces, which also have osteoblast, fibers, and connective tissue cells.
- Bone tissue laid down by periosteum, endosteum, PD membrane, sutures are all intramembranous type of bone formation. This is a more rapid type of bone formation.

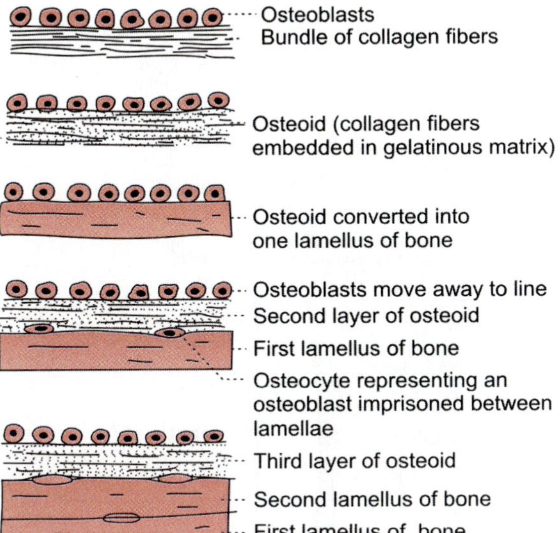

Fig. 2.13: Steps in intramembranous development and growth of the bone.

PRIMARY AND SECONDARY CARTILAGES

Primary Cartilage (Fig. 2.14)

Primary cartilage is derived from the primordial cartilage. It has an intrinsic growth potential, and can grow independently if transplanted to other sites. Primary cartilage is the tissue which has the capacity to grow from within (interstitial growth) and hence the growth is 3D. It is identical to the growth-plate cartilage of long bones. It has genetic predisposition for growth, and acts as an autonomous tissue for growth. Here, the chondroblasts divide and synthesize intercellular matrix, the chondroblasts are surrounded by cartilagenous matrix. In **primary cartilages,** the cartilaginous matrix isolates the dividing chondroblasts from local factors which are able to restrain or stimulate the cartilage growth rate, so the growth of primary cartilages is not affected by the external influences. These cells are arranged in a columnar fashion. They are not influenced by local factors, e.g. environment, etc. They act as the genetic pacemakers of growth. **Examples** of primary cartilages are spheno-occipital and other synchondrosis, nasal septal cartilage, and epiphyseal cartilages of long bones.

Secondary Cartilage (Fig. 2.15)

It does not have an intrinsic growth potential, and its growth is influenced by external

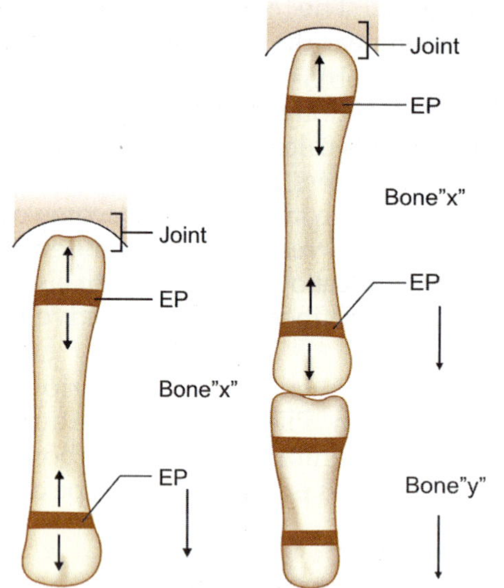

Fig. 2.14: With growth of epiphyseal plate (EP), the length of the bone increases.

influences, local and environmental factors. There is no intercellular matrix and the prechondroblasts are not surrounded by cartilaginous matrix. The cells arranged in haphazard manner. They show peripheral growth only, and help in regional adaptive growth only. In **secondary cartilages,** the dividing cells are not surrounded by the cartilaginous matrix and thus not isolated from the influence of local factors. Secondary cartilages are coronoid, condylar, angular and those in some craniofacial sutures.

GROWTH ROTATION

Growth of jaws is not uniform, but some directional movements occur within and on the surface of the jaws due to bone remodeling, etc. which change the orientation of bone. These changes are termed as rotations. Pattern of growth rotation depends on the growth pattern of face, and it affects the facial heights, profile, anchorage requirements, treatment planning, and extraction decisions. For simplicity, here is described following types of rotation especially in mandible:

Forward Rotation

It is seen in horizontal growth patterns. The posterior growth is greater than anterior growth. The increase in posterior facial height is more than anterior facial height, and it leads to an anticlockwise rotation of mandible in an upward and forward direction. It thrusts the mandible in the upper arch, and leads to development of deep bite (both skeletal and dental nature). Other features are prominent chin, short face height, pursing of lips, straight profile, etc. The masticatory muscles in such cases are stronger. Such cases should be treated by nonextraction method as far as possible, since space closure and anchorage

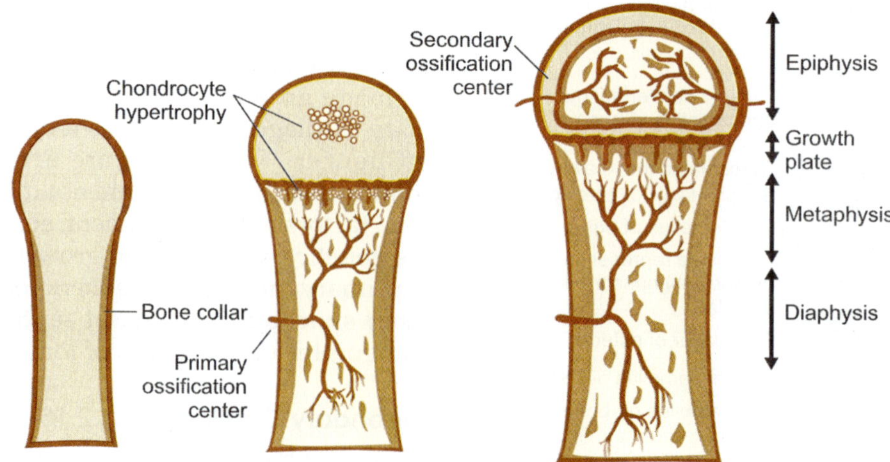

Fig. 2.15: Endochondral growth of a long bone with the help of epiphyseal plates.

loss is difficult. Extreme forward rotation leads to short face syndrome.

Backward Rotation

It occurs in vertical growth patterns. Here, the posterior growth is less than the anterior growth. The increase in posterior facial height is less than anterior facial height, and it leads to a clockwise rotation of mandible in a downward and backward direction. It rotates the mandible away from the upper arch, leads to development of open bite (which may be both skeletal and dental nature). Other features are deficient chin, increased face height, long face, incompetent lips, convex profile, etc. The masticatory muscles in such cases are weaker. Such cases generally need extraction of teeth for treatment. The anchorage requirements are more in these cases, since there are more chances of anchorage loss. Extreme backward rotation leads to long face syndrome.

If increase in anterior and posterior heights of mandible is proportionate, there is no abnormal rotation. Normally, the growth of posterior facial height keeps pace with the growth of anterior facial height. Growth of alveolar processes and eruption of teeth adapt to the growth in intermaxillary space so that a normal occlusion is established and maintained during growth. Mandibular growth rotation is due to an imbalance of growth in anterior and posterior heights.

Effect of condylar growth: These rotations depend on condylar growth. If condylar growth is greater than dentoalveolar growth in molar area, the mandible rotates anticlockwise and results in more horizontal shifting of chin and more increase in ramal and posterior facial height. It leads to deep bite and the extremes of this condition causes closed bites. Also, upward and forward/clockwise growth of condyle leads to upward and forward rotational displacement of mandible.

If the vertical growth in the molar region is greater than at the condyles, the mandible rotates clockwise and results in less horizontal change of chin and more increase in anterior facial height. Extremes of this condition cause open bites. An upward and backward/anticlockwise growth of condyle in turn causes a downward and backward mandibular/clockwise displacement.

Forward rotation can occur in the following three ways:

Type I: In this type (the one that is usually considered), there is upward and forward rotation of mandible about a center of rotation in TMJ of each side. It leads to development of deep bite. Lower dental arch gets thrust into the upper, resulting in decreased anterior facial height.

Type II: Forward rotation of mandible occurs around a center located at incisal edges of lower anterior teeth. It is due to a combination of marked increase of posterior face height and normal increase in the anterior face height. The posterior part of mandible then rotates away from the maxilla.

Type III: Here, the anterior face height increase is more than posterior face height increase. Center of rotation is present in the dental arch at the level of premolars.

STRUCTURAL SIGNS OF GROWTH ROTATION

Bjork has given following seven signs showing growth rotations:

1. Inclination of condylar head
2. Curvature of mandibular canal
3. Shape of lower border of mandible
4. Inclination of symphysis
5. Interincisal angle
6. Interpremolar angle
7. Anterior lower facial height.

In forward rotation: The following characteristics of mandible are seen:

- There is upward and forward rotation of mandible.
- The ramus is long and wide.
- The mandibular symphysis is thick and wide.
- The height of body of the mandible is more.

- A predisposition to the deep bite occurs in the case of horizontal growth type.
- Mandibular plane and gonial angle are reduced.

In **vertical rotation** of mandible, the following characteristics are seen:

- There is downward and backward rotation.
- The ramus is short and narrow.
- The mandibular symphysis is thin and elongated.
- The height of the body of mandible is smaller.
- A predisposition to the open bite occurs in the case of vertical growth type.
- Increased MP and gonial angles.

Classification of rotation of maxilla in relation to the anterior cranial base: According to Schwarz, the inclination angle records the rotation of maxillary base to the anterior cranial base, i.e. to the N-Se line.

- Normal inclination = 85°
- Anteinclination = >85°
- Retroinclination = <85°.

In anterior rotation of maxilla, (anteinclination), the angle between the palatal plane and the PN-perpendicular plane is increased. The anteinclination of the maxilla is correlated with anterior rotation of the jaw bases, and results in labial positioning of the upper anterior teeth. There is a reduced overbite and the labially tipped upper anterior teeth.

In posterior rotation of maxilla (retroclination), the inclination angle is decreased. In this type of maxillary displacement, the jaw bases are translated posteriorly and the axial inclination of the upper incisors appears to be tipped lingually. There is increased overbite and the lingually tipped upper anterior teeth.

INTERACTION BETWEEN JAW ROTATION AND TOOTH ERUPTION

Growth of mandible away from maxilla creates a space into which the teeth erupt. Movement of teeth relative to cranial base occurs by a combination of translocation and true eruption. The path of eruption of maxillary teeth is downward and somewhat forward. The eruption of mandibular teeth is upward and somewhat forward. In normal growth, the maxilla rotates a few degrees forward, tipping the incisors forward, while the backward rotation directs them posteriorly. The normal internal rotation of the mandible carries it upward and forward, which alters the eruption path of incisors, tending to direct them more posteriorly. Because of uprighting of incisors, the molars migrate further mesially during growth than do the incisors and lead to a decrease in arch length, and thus development of incisal crowding.

Growth pattern: It is the basic pattern of growth of craniofacial complex of an individual. Three types of growth patterns have been described, i.e. vertical, horizontal and average.

1. **Average growth pattern:** Here, maxillary and mandible grow in unison. Here, there is normal height of face, and their AP skeletal relation is normal.
2. **Vertical pattern:** Here, face height increases more than normal. Anterior height of face is more than posterior face height. There is D and B rotation of mandible.
3. **Horizontal growth pattern:** Here, face height is less than normal. Mandibular-growth is in U and F direction, the chin and gonial region are prominent.

These have been discussed further in subsequent chapters of anchorage, cephalometrics, etc.

3

Theories of Craniofacial Growth

INTRODUCTION

Many concepts of craniofacial growth have been proposed by various researchers based on their findings, experiments and experience. Any of these theories is not able to explain the growth completely, and hence the current understanding of growth is explained by a combination of different growth concepts. Here is the brief discussion of various growth theories.

GENETIC THEORY

It was one of the earliest theories of growth and it was proposed by Brodie. According to it, the growth is preplanned and is influenced by the genetic make-up of the individual. Genes were considered as the primary driving force of craniofacial growth. Morphological traits residing in genes are transmitted through generations as described by Mendel's laws of inheritance.

REMODELING THEORY OF CRANIOFACIAL GROWTH

Brash in 1930s described the remodeling theory of craniofacial growth. According to it, the craniofacial growth occurs exclusively by selective addition and resorption of bone at its surfaces, while sutures and the cartilages of the craniofacial skeleton have little or no role in the growth of the craniofacial skeleton. The main features of this theory were:

1. Bone grows appositionally at surfaces,
2. Jaws' growth is characterized by bone deposition at posterior surfaces of maxilla and mandible, described as **"Hunterian" growth of the jaws**, and
3. Cranial vault growth occurs by bone deposition on the ectocranial surface and bone resorption on endocranial surface.

SUTURAL THEORY

This was proposed by Weinmann and Sicher in 1940s. According to this theory, the connective tissue and cartilaginous joints of craniofacial skeleton are the **principal growth sites,** capable of intrinsic, genetically regulated, primary growth of bone, like epiphyses of long bones. **According to Sicher** "the primary event in sutural growth is the proliferation of the connective tissue present in sutures between two bones. It creates space for appositional growth at the borders of two bones to fill in".

There occurs an expansile proliferative growth of connective tissue in sutures present between bones, which force the bones of vault away from each other leading to the growth of cranial vault. Thus, it indicated that the sutural growth is primary determinant of adult skull form.

Similarly, growth in circummaxillary sutures leads to downward and forward growth of maxilla. Growth of facial bones especially maxilla, occurs mainly at sutures, which are paired, parallel and obliquely oriented between cranial base and the maxilla. Connective tissue in sutures of both the nasomaxillary complex and cranial vault produced forces which separated the bones, similar to the growth at synchondroses in cranial base and epiphyseal plates of long bones. Growth at these sutures pushes nasomaxillary complex downward and forward. It helps to grow the face in unison with mandible.

According to this concept, the sutures between the membranous bones of cranium and jaws are the growth centers, along with the sites of endochondral ossification in cranial base and at mandibular condyle. Sicher stated that cartilage of mandible grew both interstitially and appositionally. The translation of maxilla in downward and forward direction, therefore, was the result of pressure created by growth of the sutures. Growth was considered to be due to expression of a genetic program at all these sites. Thus, this theory also supports the concept of genetic theory.

Contradictory points: Some points were against this theory. If sutures have a genetic potential to grow, then the growth at the sutures should occur largely independent of any factor, and it will not be possible to change the expression of growth at the sutures very much. But, it is now clear that sutures and the periosteal tissues are not the primary determinants of craniofacial growth. The following opposing points disapproving sutural growth as the sole principal method of craniofacial growth were raised:

1. **Transplantation experiment:** When a part of suture was transplanted in another location, no growth was seen. It indicated that the sutures do not have an innate growth potential.
2. In nonoperated cleft palate cases, the growth still occurs almost normally, despite the absence of midpalatal suture.
3. Cranial abnormalities, like microcephaly and hydrocephaly, also disapprove about the intrinsic potential of sutures.
4. Growth at sutures responds to outside influences, e.g. abnormal compressive forces applied on cranium in some races lead to distortion of the cranium. Otherwise, if cranial or facial bones are pulled apart mechanically at the sutures, the new bone fills in, and bones become larger.
5. Experiments proved that sutures are secondary sites of bone growth. They are highly responsive to the growth of cranial vault contents, i.e. brain, and also to functional and orthopedic forces applied on the growing maxillary complex.

THE CARTILAGINOUS THEORY

It is also called as The Nasal Septum Theory, proposed by Scott in 1950s. He emphasized the role of cartilages as having the primary intrinsic growth potential. According to this theory, sutures play little or no direct role in craniofacial growth. Sutures are secondary and compensatory sites of bone formation and growth.

According to Scott, nasal septal cartilage is most active primary site for midface growth upto 3–4 years of age. The downward and forward growth of nasal septal cartilage, which is buttressed against the cranial base, "moves" the midface in a downward and forward direction, giving an effect of midface literally coming out from below the cranial base. It causes the separation of circum-maxillary sutures, where the bone filling occurs via secondary, compensatory sutural bone growth.

The cranial base synchondroses are analogs to epiphyseal plates of long bones, which grows in both directions, leading to cranial base growth. The mandible can also be considered as a bent long bone, and the condylar cartilage is considered equivalent to epiphyseal plates of long bones, whose growth leads to downward and forward growth of mandible. Condylar cartilage acts similar to cranial base and nasal septal cartilages, and is the primary growth center of the mandible. It grows in a upward and backward direction abutting against the cranial base and thus "pushes" mandible in a downward and forward direction.

Two types of experiments were performed:

1. Transplanting cartilage experiments
2. Removing cartilage experiments

Transplanting Experiments

They demonstrated that not all skeletal cartilages act in the same way when transplanted:

1. Epiphyseal plate of long bone continues to grow when transplanted in a new location, which indicates that these cartilages have innate growth potential.
2. Cartilages from spheno-occipital synchondrosis when transplanted show growth but the growth was not that much. It may be due to the fact that it is very difficult to obtain cartilage from the cranial base, especially at early age, when the cartilage is actively growing.
3. Nasal septal cartilage was found to grow nearly as well as epiphyseal plate cartilage, showing innate growth potential.
4. Little or no growth was observed with transplantation of the mandibular condylar cartilage.

Removing Cartilages

It was considered that if removing a cartilage stops or diminishes growth, then it is an important center for growth.

1. In animal experiments, removal of a part of nasal septum cartilage caused a considerable deficiency in midface growth. But, it was thought that the surgery and the accompanying interference with blood supply to the area leads to deficient growth, and not the loss of cartilage. Still, the loss of midfacial growth in animals helped to conclude that the septal cartilage does have some innate growth potential.
2. Humans having leprosy where the nasal cartilage is also gets affected show deficient midface.
3. Trauma to nasal septum, e.g. during CLP repair also leads to deficient midface growth.

FUNCTIONAL MATRIX CONCEPT

Melvin Moss in 1960s described a new concept of craniofacial growth, the functional matrix hypothesis. According to it, the growth and maintenance of skeletal tissues is always secondary, compensatory and obligatory response to the functions of related soft tissues or functioning spaces. The previously described **genomic paradigm** considered the craniofacial growth as primarily genetically predetermined. Moss's concept paved the way of a new concept known as the **functional paradigm**. It emphasized that craniofacial growth is influenced by the functional forces acting on bone. It can be said that "the soft tissue acts, while hard tissue reacts" according to this concept. The functional paradigm supported and evolved the myofunctional orthopedic techniques to correct a developing malocclusion. Myofunctional appliances activate the muscles and increase the oral cavity space, leading to growth modification based on functional matrix concept.

According to this concept, heredity and genes only help in initiating the process of development, and have little significant role in further growth of craniofacial skeleton. Later on, it grows in direct response to its extrinsic, epigenetic environment. Bones and cartilage lack primary growth determination, but respond to intrinsic growth of associated tissues termed as **functional matrices.** Each functional matrix performs an individual necessary function, like respiration, mastication, speech, vision, hearing, speech, olfaction, etc. while the skeletal tissues support and protect the associated functional matrices. So, the concept of functional cranial components was introduced to explain the growth. **Functional cranial components** (FCC) have two elements:

1. A functional matrix (FM)
2. An associated skeletal unit (SU).

The functional matrix is all the soft tissues and spaces that perform a given function.

The SU is the bony structure which supports the functional matrix. Individual bones can be called as macroskeletal unit, and may have a number of overlapping SU, the microskeletal units, and each such SU supports a function.

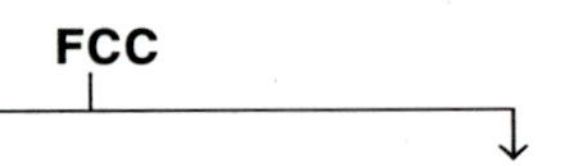

Functional matrix

Periosteal matrix

Capsular matrix

↓

1. Neurocranial capsule
2. Orofacial capsule

Skeletal unit

1. Macroskeletal unit
2. Microskeletal unit

FCC = FM + SU
FM = capsular matrix and periosteal matrix
Capsular matrix = neurocranial capsule and orofacial capsule.
Skeletal unit = macroskeletal + microskeletal units.

Fig. 3.1: Diagrammatic representation of FCC.

THE ROLE OF THE FUNCTIONAL MATRIX

According to this concept, there exists an influence of functions on craniofacial growth. Head is responsible for several vital functions and the craniofacial structures respond to the changing requirements for those functions. Craniofacial growth is the culmination of changes in the "capsular matrices", leading to changes in position of bones (**translation**), and the "periosteal matrices", causing more local changes in the size and shape of the skeleton (**remodeling**). Mainly two capsular matrices in craniofacial region have been described, i.e. neurocranial capsule, which is controlled by the growing brain, and the orofacial capsular matrix which is concerned with orofacial functions, e.g. respiration, deglutition, mastication and speech. Any alteration in size and shape of individual bones of the calvaria are under the influence of the periosteal matrices, e.g. a periosteal matrix such as muscles and tendons act directly upon an SU via periosteum, resulting in bone apposition and resorption.

Functional Matrix (Fig. 3.1)

It consists of muscles, glands, neurovascular bundles, teeth and functional spaces. There are two types of functional matrices, i.e. the capsular matrices and the periosteal matrix.

The Capsular Matrices

The capsular matrices are those soft tissues, organs and spaces which cover a bigger anatomical complex. They act on their associated SU indirectly and passively and lead to their secondary passive **translation** in space. Thus, they cause a change in location/position and size of the associated bones. They do not lead to bone remodeling directly. When there is expansion of capsular matrix, the changes in the corresponding bones occur which are embedded in that capsular matrix.

There are two capsular matrices in craniofacial complex, i.e. neurocranial, and the orofacial. Neurocranial is the capsular matrix having brain, globes of eyes, etc. and it consists of SCALP, and dura mater. Orofacial matrix has spaces such as the nasopharynx, oropharynx and associated structures and it is having skin and mucosa as the covering. Each of these capsules acts as an envelope containing the functional cranial components, i.e. SU and the related functional matrix (Table 3.1).

The Periosteal Matrix (Fig. 3.2)

It is directly in contact with the bones, and is influenced by the direct attachments of muscles, ligaments and tendon. It acts actively and directly on the related skeletal

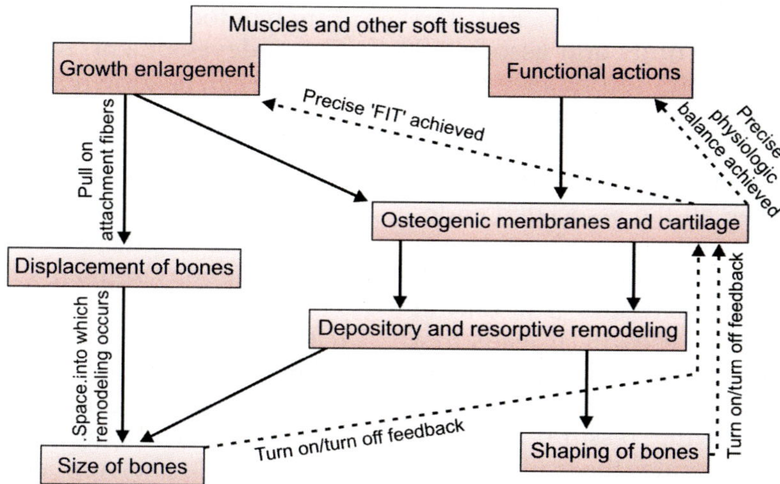

Fig. 3.2: Showing the functional matrix aspect of the growth that how the action of soft tissues activates the remodeling and growth of bones.

Adapted from Enlow, D.H.: Structural and functional " balance" during craniofacial growth. In: *Orthodontics: State of the Art, Essence of the Science.* Ed. by L.W. Graber, St. Louis, C.V. Mosby, 1986).

units. The periosteal matrix corresponds to the immediate local environment, typically muscles, blood vessels, and nerves. Changes in functional demands lead to a secondary and compensatory transformation change of the size and shape of the bone, which occurs due to remodeling of related bony tissue (Table 3.1).

Skeletal Units

All skeletal tissues associated with a single function are called the skeletal unit. It may be having bone, cartilage and tendons and ligament. SUs are of two types:

1. Macroskeletal units
2. Microskeletal units.

Change in size and shape of macroskeletal units, i.e. the neurocranium and maxillo-mandibular complex are primarily due to expansion of associated capsular matrices. According to functional matrix hypothesis, the craniofacial skeleton does not primarily grow to expand the soft tissues, organs and

Table 3.1: Differences between capsular and periosteal matrices

Capsular matrix	*Periosteal matrix*
It encloses a bigger anatomical space or tissues.	It acts locally on the associated bones.
It leads to growth by translation of bones.	It leads to transformation of the bones.
It acts indirectly and passively on the associated bones.	It acts directly and actively on associated skeletal elements.
It leads to a change in location of the bone.	It leads to a change in the shape or form of the bone by remodelling.
It does not lead to a direct remodeling of the bones.	It leads to direct remodeling of the bone.
It acts on the bones from a distance, as they cover a wider tissue area.	It corresponds to immediate local area.

spaces of the functional matrix. But, the translation of skeletal units and associated local bone growth occurs secondarily to the growth of associated functional and capsular matrices.

As the capsular matrix and its associated spaces expand, then all the associated endochondral and intramembranous skeletal units grow to support the increased physiologic spaces. Thus, the skeletal tissues grow only in response to soft tissue growth. It leads to a **passive translation** of skeletal components in space, e.g. growth of cranial vault is in a direct response to brain growth. Pressure exerted by the growing brain separates the cranial bones at the sutures, and new bone passively fills in at these sites.

Microskeletal unit supports an individual functional matrix. Maxilla and mandible consist of many microskeletal units, e.g. mandible has the corpus, ramal, coronoid, condyle, alveolar, gonial, angular microskeltal units. Maxilla has alveolar, sinus, orbital, basal, palatal microskeletal units. They all grow from the stimulation they receive from their individual functional matrices, e.g. teeth for alveolar growth, temporalis muscle for coronoid growth, masseter-medial pterygoid complex for angular/gonial growth of mandible, eyes for orbital growth, etc.

Natural Evidences

1. In cases of smaller sized brain, the cranium is also very small, leading to **microcephaly**.
2. On the other hand, in **hydrocephaly,** the reabsorption of CSF is impeded, leading to an increase in intracranial volume and enormous increased size of cranial vault. Accumulated CSF also leads to underdevelopment of brain and mental retardation.
3. Similarly, an enlarged eye or a small eye causes a corresponding change in the orbital cavity, eye being the functional matrix.
4. Teeth act as functional matrix for alveolar bone. Congenital absence, non-eruption of tooth, extraction of tooth leads to non-development/resoprtion of bone.
5. Bone can be grown at surgically created sites by **distraction osteogenesis, as** Ilizarov discovered in the 1950s. Cuts were made through the cortex of a long bone of the limbs, the arm or leg then could be lengthened by tension to separate the bony segments, and stretching of the soft tissues.
6. Strenuous physical exercises especially during active late growth stage lead to stretch of the muscles and hence the growth of chest cage, shoulders, etc. and the whole skeleton, as seen in athletes and body-builders.

VAN LIMBORGH'S THEORY

He proposed a multifactorial theory in 1970s to describe the growth of craniofacial complex. According to him, any of previous theories viz genetic, sutural, cartilage, and functional matrix theory was not completely able to describe the growth. So, he proposed his theory which had salient feature of all other theories. According to this theory, primary intrinsic stimulation of growth is present in cartilage and periosteum, while the secondary factors are the local feedback and inner communication mechanisms between cells and tissues.

He described that genetic, epigenetic and environmental factors in following five combinations. **Genetic factors** are directly inherited from parents and directly influence the growth of skeleton. **Epigenetic factors** are the factors which are genetically determined but they indirectly influence the growth by acting on associated structures. They can be local or general factors. **Environmental factors** do not have any genetic link, but affect the growth when come into play during active phase of growth (Fig. 3.3 and Table 3.2).

a. **Intrinsic genetic factors:** They are the factors which directly control the growth of skeletal units.
b. **Local epigenetic factors:** These factors are genetically determined, but control

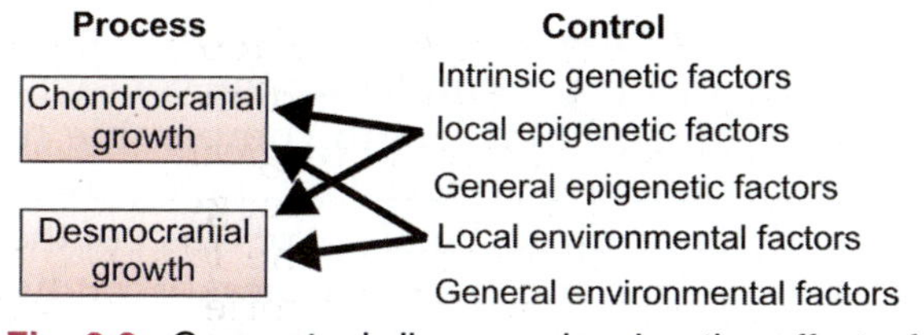

Fig. 3.3: Conceptual diagram showing the effect of different factors which affect the growth of different parts of cranium.

the growth of local/adjacent structures like eye, brain, etc. which then affect the growth of bones.

c. **General epigenetic factors:** These factors also influence the growth and are released from the distant structures, e.g. hormones.

d. **Local environmental factors:** These are non-genetic factors in the local environment, e.g. habits, abnormal muscle function, etc.

e. **General environmental factors:** These are non-genetic factors which have a generalised influence on the growth, e.g. nutrition, etc.

The overall growth of craniofacial skeleton is a culmination of the effects of these factors. The essential elements of the hypothesis are:

a. Cartilaginous parts of skull are primary growth centers, because of inherent direct genetic influence.
b. **Growth of cranial base** at synchondroses, i.e. the endochondral ossification is controlled by intrinsic genetic factors.
c. **Growth of cranial vault** follows the intramembranous bone growth in sutures and periosteum **which is controlled by few intrinsic genetic factors, but mainly by the local epigenetic factors.**
d. Sutural growth is influenced by cartilaginous growth and growth of other head structures.
e. Extent of periosteal bone growth largely depends on local tissues and growth of adjacent structures.
f. The intramembranous bone formation is also influenced by local environmental factors.

In a nut shell, the **chondrocranial growth** (cranial base) is mainly controlled by intrinsic genetic factors, with little influence of general epigenetic and environmental factors. Desmocranial growth (cranial vault) is mainly affected by local epigenetic and environmental factors, with some intrinsic genetic factors, and little influence of general epigenetic and environmental factors.

Table 3.2: Description of genetic and epigenetic factors

Factors	*Description*
Intrinsic genetic factors	These are those factors inherent to craniofacial tissues and directly affect the growth. They are determined genetically and have the major influence on growth.
Local epigenetic factors, influence the capsular matrix	These are the genetically determined influences which originate from the adjacent structures, i.e. brain, eyes, etc. These are not directly inherent in the craniofacial tissues, but they influence the growth of these tissues.
General epigenetic factors	These are also the genetically determined influences which originate from the distant structures, e.g. hormones, etc. These are not directly inherent in the craniofacial tissues, but they influence the growth of these tissues.
Local environmental factors, influence the periosteal matrices	These are the local, nongenetic influences coming from external environments, e.g. exercise, muscular forces, local external pressure, etc.
General environmental factors	These are the general influences which originate from the external environment, e.g. food, oxygen supply, etc.

SERVOSYSTEM THEORY OF CRANIOFACIAL GROWTH

This theory was proposed by Petrovic, et al in 1974. According to it, the craniofacial growth is controlled by a series of changes occurring in craniofacial skeleton and dentition, which in-turn start a **feedback mechanism**, to stimulate further growth changes to occur.

The **extrinsic and intrinsic hormonal factors** influence the cartilage growth. It has following two principal factors:

1. The hormones regulate growth of mid-face and anterior cranial base, which then provides a feedback influence via the occlusion
2. There is rate-limiting effect of midfacial growth on the growth of mandible.

STH-somatomedian complex influences the growth of primary cartilages in a cybernetic manner of command, while the growth of secondary cartilage is affected by direct and indirect effects on cell multiplication. According to Taber's Medical Dictionary, cybernetics is "the science of control and communication in biological, electronic and mechanical systems. This includes analysis of feedback mechanism that serves to govern or modify the actions of various systems".

It was demonstrated that condylar growth is highly adaptive and responsive to both extrinsic systemic factors and local biomechanical and functional factors, while the growth of primary cartilages of craniofacial complex, such as the cranial base and nasal septum, was influenced significantly less by local epigenetic factors.

As the midface grows in a downward and forward direction under the primary influence of cartilaginous cranial base and nasal septum, and mediated by hormones, the upper arch occupies a slightly more anterior position. It leads to a minute discrepancy between upper and lower dental arches. It generates a feedback signal and the proprioceptors present in PDL and TMJ activate **lateral pterygoid muscle** and other muscles of mastication, allowing the mandible to adjust to optimal occlusal position. It directly acts on condylar cartilage stimulating the condylar growth. Mandibular length comparable to maxillary length is achieved through growth of condylar cartilage. Finally, the effect of the muscle function and responsiveness of condylar cartilage is influenced both directly and indirectly by hormonal factors. This cycle works continuously as long as the midface-upper dental arch continues to grow with minute discrepancy with lower arch which provides feedback signals.

It shows that condylar growth and growth of the sutures may be affected directly and indirectly by systemic hormones, but growth of these structures is clearly more adaptive and compensatory to extrinsic factors, like local function and growth of other areas of the craniofacial complex.

In a nutshell, this theory puts more emphasis on mandibular growth. Anterior growth of the midface results in a slight change in occlusal relation between upper and lower dentitions. This change is perceived by proprioceptors which then trigger and activate the mandibular protruding muscles which help to reposition the mandible anteriorly. This muscle activity and the mandibular protrusion in presence of appropriate hormonal factors stimulate growth at the mandibular condyle.

THE LOGARITHMIC GROWTH OF THE HUMAN MANDIBLE (MOSS, 1970)

This concept of mandibular growth is based on the functional matrix involving mandibular nerve and the neural arc extending from foramen ovale to mandibular foramen to mental foramen and its corresponding skeletal unit. During growth, the size and angular relationship of these three foramina and the size and position of mandibular canal change along a logarithmic curve. This method can help to predict the direction, but not the amount, of mandibular growth. Mandibular growth consists of two integrated phenomena. The first is an active transformation of size due to the periosteal functional matrices, and the second is the passive translation of macroskeletal units to the primary expansion of capsular matrices of oronasal functioning spaces.

Gnomonic Growth and Logarithmic Spiral

Moss and Salentijn analyzed relationship of the foramina of skull and mandible through which the inferior alveolar nerve passes. They determined that the orofacial capsule, which is responsible for mandibular growth, creates a **gnomonic growth pattern**. Gnomonic growth is a process characterized by an increase in size without a shape change. This gnomonic growth is described by the **logarithmic curve**. According to this curve, the growth of mandible occurs along a logarithmic spiral/arc of inferior alveolar nerve passing along an arc from foramen ovale, to mandibular foramen to mental foramen. It can also be called as on **unloaded nerve concept** (Fig. 3.4).

Ricketts also indicated that growth of the mandible is associated with an arc. He introduced a number of gnomonic figures that are related to three branches of trigeminal nerve, i.e. ophthalmic, maxillary, and inferior dental nerves. Ricketts considered these nerves very important in growth. Thus, he combined neurotrophic concept and Moss and Salentijn logarithmic curve of mandibular growth. He introduced the concept of Fibonacci series to describe the growth of mandible.

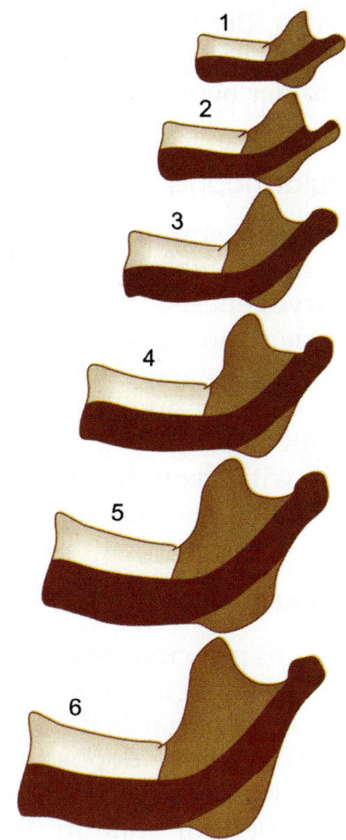

Fig. 3.4: Different parts of mandible, i.e. nervous, muscular, and dentoalveolar parts which grow in unison but are affected by different functional matrices for growth. Also note the unloaded nerve concept area of growth being influenced by inferior alveolar nerve track.

NEUROTROPHIC PROCESS IN THE OROFACIAL GROWTH (MOSS, 1971)

Neurotrophism is the phenomenon of transmitting the stimulus through axoplasm, which leads to interactions between neurons and innervated tissues and thus regulates the morphological and functional integrity of those tissues. There are three general categories:

- Neuroepithelial
- Neurovisceral
- Neuromuscular.

Neuroepithelial Trophism

It suggests that the mitosis and synthesis of epithelial tissues is controlled through neural function related to that particular tissue. Neurotrophic substances are released by nerve synapses which stimulate mitotic activity. If these substances are deficient, then there is abnormal/deficient growth of the tissues because there is no stimulation, e.g. growth of taste buds depends on the presence of intact innervations. If innervation of taste buds is cut off, then they degenerate.

Neurovisceral Trophism

Salivary glands and other viscera are trophically regulated, at least partially. Experiments have shown an increase and decrease of mature salivary glands is under trophic influence. Also, the normal rate of growth, expressed in part as regulation of cell number and size, is under neurotrophic control.

Neuromuscular Trophism

An active nervous stimulation is needed for the growth and development of muscles. During embryogenesis, the development of skeletal muscle requires motor neuron innervations at myoblast stage. If innervation is not established, further myogenesis does not occur. The developing mytomes carry their nerve supply with them. If the nerve supply gets damaged, the muscular atrophy occurs.

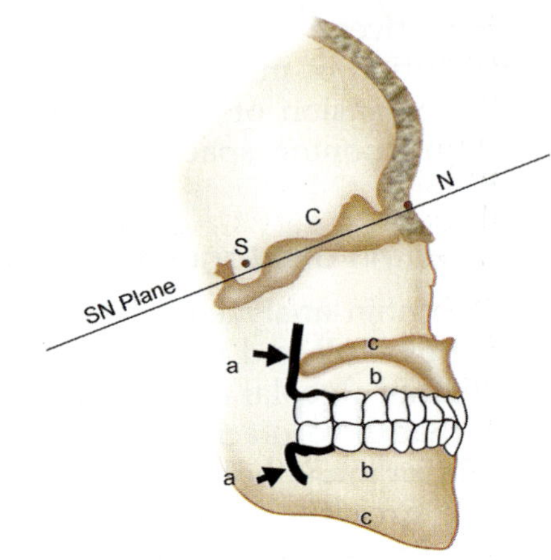

Fig. 3.5: The SN plane. Also a, b, c are the respective counterparts of maxilla and mandible.

ENLOW'S EXPANDING V-PRINCIPLE

According to this principle, many facial bones or parts of bones grow in a V-shaped pattern. The growth occurs towards the wider end of V, due to selective bone deposition and resorption. Increase in the size and the simultaneous movement of bone in the shape of expanding-V is called as expanding-V principal. It is seen in maxilla, zygomatic bone, palate, coronoid, angle region of mandible, etc.

ENLOW'S COUNTERPART PRINCIPLE (Fig. 3.5)

According to this theory, structural counterparts exist in the craniofacial region, and the growth of one part of the craniofacial skeleton relates specifically to its geometrical counterpart in the region. Balanced growth can only occur if one part and its counterpart grow in unison, in the same manner and direction. In simple words, it can be said that the growth of one part depends on the growth of its counterpart, as all the parts of craniofacial complex are interconnected. Any disturbance of the growth leads to the malrelationships. This imbalance can be generated by disturbance in the amount, time and direction of growth between the counterparts.

Thus there exist the regional relationships throughout the face and cranium. An equivalent/parallel growth occurring between each regional part and its counterpart leads to a balanced growth in that region. Any difference in respective amounts or directions of growth between parts and counterparts leads to an imbalanced growth. Each regional growth change occurs due to two processes, i.e. remodeling (deposition and resorption) and displacement.

For example, anterior cranial fossa and the palate are counterparts. Also the palate and maxillary apical base are counterparts. Maxillary arch is a counterpart of mandibular arch. With the posterior growth of maxillary tuberosity, the whole maxilla moves anteriorly. Body of the mandible is a structural counterpart of the body of maxilla. So to keep pace with the growth of maxillary body, there is resorption at the anterior border of ramus and bone deposition on posterior border, leading to a corresponding elongation of the mandibular body. Also, the whole mandible is displaced anteriorly as the maxilla is carried anteriorly. To keep pace, the condyle grows posteriorly to come in vicinity with the glenoid fossa. In summary, the increment of backward growth at maxillary tuberosity is equivalent to the amount of forward displacement by maxilla (displacement), which in turn is equivalent to the amount of growth of mandibular body. Also the remodeling on anterior part of ramus and amount of body-lengthening equals to backward growth of posterior part of ramus.

Pharyngeal space lies below the middle cranial fossa, and is laterally covered by ramus. Thus, ramus is a structural counterpart of middle cranial fossa. The middle cranial fossa, mandibular ramus [ramus bridges the pharyngeal space below middle cranial fossa (MCF)], and zygomatic arch (it bridges both the cranial fossa and the ramus) are all respective counterparts. Growth of MCF leads to increase in dimensions of pharyngeal space, ramus, and the transverse width of mandible in the inter-ramus region.

Floor of anterior cranial fossa and forehead grow in anterior direction by deposition on ectocranial site and resorption from endocranial side. Thus, the nasomaxillary complex is displaced anteriorly. Vertical lengthening of nasomaxillary complex occurs by resorption on superior (nasal) side and deposition on inferior side of palate with downward movement of whole palate. It leads to vertical enlargement of nasal and nasopharyngeal regions. These part—counterpart combinations provide an effective way to evaluate the growth and inter-relationships of all structural components of craniofacial complex.

There exist certain counterparts in craniofacial region as follows:

1. Nasomaxillary complex is related to anterior cranial fossa. It is attached to anterior cranial base (SN plane). Growth of anterior cranial base leads to displacement of nasomaxillary complex also esp in upward and forward direction.
2. Horizontal size of pharyngeal space is related to the size of middle cranial fossa. Pharyngeal space lies below the middle cranial fossa.
3. Middle cranial fossa, sagittal dimension of pharyngeal space and ramal width are counterparts, in sagittal dimension.
4. Maxillary and mandibular basal arches are counterparts.
5. Maxillary base and mandibular corpus are counterparts.
6. Maxillary tuberosity and mandibular lingual tuberosity are counterparts.
7. Upper and lower alveolar processes.

THE FUNCTIONAL MATRIX HYPOTHESIS REVISITED

It was introduced by Moss in 1990s. Three concepts of his original functional matrix theory are of particular importance for growth which are:

1. The growth and development of craniofacial skeleton and subsequent change in size, shape and location are secondary, compensatory and mechanically obligatory responses to the demands of related soft tissues and functional spaces.
2. FMH described two functional matrices, i.e. periosteal and capsular. Periosteal matrix is responsible for active growth processes on the surfaces of bones.
3. Epigenetic extraskeletal factors are primary cause of all secondary responses of skeletal tissues and organs.

FMH revisited theory deals only with the responses to periosteal matrices. It describes molecular and cellular processes underlying the active skeletal growth processes of deposition, resorption and maintenance. It includes **two concepts**:

- Cellular mechanotransduction, and
- Bone cells function multicellularly as a connected cellular network (CCN).

Mechanotransduction

All vital cells respond to external stimuli by mechanotransduction, and thus an intracellular signal is generated. This signal is transmitted through multiple cells through CCN leading to bone adaptation. It translates the information content of a periosteal matrix stimulus into a skeletal unit cell to activate the osteocytic genome. Osteocytes and osteoblasts react by this stimulus reception, transduction and signal transmission. By the interconnected chain at molecular level, the periosteal functional matrix activity regulates the activity of bone cells. With the change in muscular demands, the active bone growth process leads to the adaptation of the form of related skeletal unit to new functional demands.

The genomic thesis: Epigenetic factors control the morphogenesis of bones. Genome contains all the information necessary to regulate formation and transcription of mRNA, and regulates all of the intracellular and intercellular processes of morphogenesis. So "all (phenotype) features are ultimately determined by the DNA sequence of the genome".

The epigenetic antithesis: It rejects the genomic thesis. **Epigenetics** refer to the series of interactions among cells and cell products, which leads to morphogenesis and differentiation. Periosteal matrices are under epigenetic control. Mechanical loads and function significantly control growth, development, and maintenance of structural and physiological features of musculoskeletal structures.

A resolving synthesis: It is a combination of both genomic thesis and epigenetic antithesis. It states that morphogenesis is regulated by both genomic and epigenetic processes and mechanisms. No one alone is sufficient for growth, and both of them integrate to provide necessary stimuli for growth and development. Genomic factors are intrinsic and prior causes, while the epigenetic factors are extrinsic and proximate causes.

DEVELOPMENTAL MOLECULAR BIOLOGY AND ITS EFFECT ON GROWTH KNOWLEDGE

With the increased knowledge of the role of regulatory genes of growth and development, the viewpoint about the development of craniofacial complex has changed dramatically. **Homeobox gene**, or **Hox gene**, has been found to be the main gene responsible for growth. There are many genetically-encoded regulatory factors having strong effect on morphogenesis and prenatal development of craniofacial complex. These factors show epigenetic influence also, influencing the interaction of cells and entire organisms with environmental factors. Also, the morphogenesis, prenatal and postnatal growth can be modified by certain factors, but it cannot be guaranteed as a predictable, controlled, and clinically effective way.

These gene products do not determine growth and specific form, but they provide factors affecting the receptivity and responsiveness of cells to intrinsic and extrinsic stimuli. Through the understanding of molecular principles and regulatory mechanisms of craniofacial morphogenesis, it may become possible to target specific genes to regulate or redirect the abnormal growth of parts of craniofacial complex for orthodontic growth modification in near future.

Clinical Significance

Various treatment approaches in orthodontics are based on the sound knowledge of growth and development of craniofacial complex. Knowledge of sound principles of growth and the normal data on growth timings, pattern, status and the facial morphology is essential. It is compared with that of a particular patient to find out the deviations, and the etiology of the problem is determined, to decide the treatment plan. By redirecting and controlling the growth with orthopaedic interventions, it is possible to reduce the severity or to correct the dentofacial abnormalities.

ORTHODONTICS, RACE, AND THE CONCEPT OF FACIAL TYPE

According to Angle and his many followers, the goal of the treatment of malocclusion was to place teeth in the most harmonious position possible for a given facial type, thus compensating for an unchangeable facial form. But, Brodie stated that facial growth "cannot be changed by treatment. The teeth and the alveolar process constitute the only area of the face whose change may be expected or induced". Thus, the primary role of the orthodontist was to treat a malocclusion by moving teeth into a more harmonious position relative to the facial type, facial growth could not be affected by orthodontic treatment.

However, foramen rotundum present in sphenoid bone [which opens in pterygomaxillary fissure (PTM)] is considered as the stable centre of craniofacial growth. Original pattern of skeleton is constant and **stationary**

biologic center lies in the body of sphenoid bone. In both maxilla and mandible, growth in width is completed first, then growth in length, and finally growth in height.

Areas of the growth that are primarily under the control of heredity, are referred to as growth centers. Locations at which active skeletal growth occurs as a secondary, compensatory effect are the growth sites. Growth sites do not have direct genetic influence and are influenced by other factors, such as the primary growth centers and the environment. Sutures and periosteum are the adaptive growth sites.

- Cranium: Chondrocranium (cranial base) + desmocranium (cranial vault) + splanchocranium (lower face).
- Neurocranium: Chondrocranium (cranial base) + desmocranium (cranial vault) (cranium).

4

Prenatal Growth of Craniofacial Region

INTRODUCTION

The development of an individual has been divided in prenatal and postnatal periods. Prenatal period is a dynamic phase of development which starts with fertilization of ovum which gets implanted in the uterine wall. Here extensive cell multiplication, differentiation and organization occur to form different body tissues and organs of the body. During this period, there is around 5,000-fold increase of height, as compared to only three-fold increase of height after birth till adulthood.

PRENATAL GROWTH PHASES

The prenatal life is broadly classified into the following three phases:

1. Period of ovum (from fertilization to the 14th day)
2. Period of embryo (from 14th day to 56th day)
3. Period of foetus (56th day to birth)

Period of Ovum

This period extends to approx. 2 weeks from the time of fertilization. During this period, from the single cell stage of fertilized ovum to the cleavage of ovum and then implantation of the fertilized ovum to intrauterine wall occurs.

Period of Embryo

It extends from 14th to 56th day. This is the period of most rapid growth and cellular differentiation, and their allocation of the functions occurs. It is one of the most crucial periods of development, since during this period, major parts of craniofacial region develop. Any disturbance during this period may lead to development of craniofacial defects.

Period of Fetus (Fig. 4.1)

It extends from 56th day till birth. During this period, an accelerated growth of craniofacial structures and other body parts occurs resulting in their increased size and change in proportion.

Embryologic development: After fertilization and implantation, rapid multiplication and cellular differentiation take place. There is extreme activity at cephalic end of notochord, which gives rise to brain. Five pharyngeal arches develop on either side in the region of future head and neck, which give rise to various components of face. During development, various processes and formation of different parts is going on simultaneously. Growth of the craniofacial complex can be studied in following parts, i.e. cranial base, cranial vault, maxilla, mandible, and palate.

CRANIUM: DEVELOPMENT OF THE SKULL

The bones of skull can be divided into the **viscerocranium** which supports the nasal passages, oral cavity and the pharynx and forms the face, and the **neurocranium** which surrounds the brain. The neurocranium can be subdivided into the cranial base/**chondrocranium** and the calvaria (cranial vault/**desmocranium**). Cranial base is chondrocranium (cartilages), cranial vault is desmocranium (flat bone), and cranium is

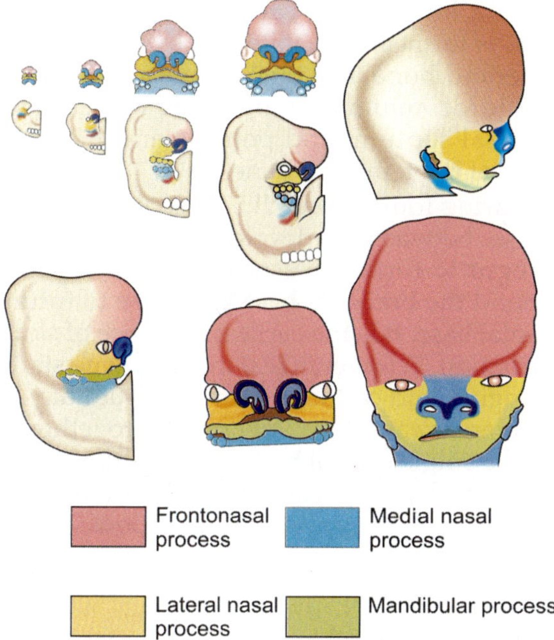

Fig. 4.1: Prenatal development of various facial structures.

neurocranium (having neural tissues, neurocranial capsule). The bones of the skull base are formed mainly by endochondral ossification and the cartilaginous joints between the bones are called **synchondroses**. The bones of cranial vault and face are primarily formed by intramembranous ossification. The skull is formed from the mesenchymal connective tissue around the developing brain.

Development of skull is considered in two parts:

1. Development of neurocranium, i.e. calvaria and base of the skull. It is derived mainly from occipital somites and somitomeres.
2. Development of viscerocranium, which includes the facial skeleton and the associated structures. The viscerocranium is derived from neural crest ectoderm. Both of these parts have some structures formed by endochondral ossification (cartilaginous component) and some structures formed by intramembranous ossification.

The size and growth of cranial vault primarily depends on growing brain which applies pressures on the sutures between bones, thus creating gaps. These gaps are filled by intermembranous bone formation in these sutures. The brain thus acts as a "functional matrix" for neurocranial bone growth. The head circumference is regularly measured by the paediatricians when they see the child during first 2 years of age, since it is a good indicator of brain growth. Considerable brain growth is mostly seen during first 5 years of life, after which there is slow growth. There is rapid increase of head circumference during 1st year, reaching an average of 46 cm, and then it slows down, at approx 49 cm at 2 years and only 50 cm at 3 years. Between 3 years and adulthood, the increase is only about 6 cm. Abnormal external forces if applied during development of cranial vault, can distort cranial morphology as can be seen in some tribes. Since brain is a functional matrix of cranial vault growth, a large skull with thinned out and expanded plates of cranial vault bones is seen in hydrocephalus. Similarly, in microcephalics, a small skull is seen.

Growth of the bones of cranial vault occurs by combination of:

1. Sutural growth
2. Surface remodeling
3. Outward displacement/thrust of bones by the expanding brain.

Sutural growth is predominant during 4 years of life due to expanding brain; after that the surface remodeling is the main method of growth. The calvarial bones of the newborn have single lamina, and do not have diploe. But from about 4 years of age, compaction of cancellous trabeculae leads to the formation of inner and outer tables of cranial vault bones. Remodeling of inner table is influenced primarily by brain growth, the outer table is more responsive to extracranial muscular influence. Inner side shows resorption, while the outer side shows bone deposition, thereby increasing the intracranial volume.

The bones of cranial vault develop by the intramembranous ossification of mesenchyme, e.g. the superior part of frontal, parietal and occipital bones. Large gaps called **fontanelles** are present at the corners between these bones which fuse within first year of birth. There are six fontanelles, i.e. as the anterior, posterior, posterolateral and anterolateral fontanelles, in relation to the corners of the two parietal bones. Sutures, also called **syndesmoses**, are also present in between the bones. They are fibrous joints comprising of sheets of dense connective tissue. The sutures and fontanelles help in molding the shape of skull during birth when the fetus passes through the birth canal.

During formation of frontal sinus, the separation of inner and outer tables of frontal bone occurs. However, the remodeling of only the external plate occurs during **frontal sinus pneumatization**, as the internal plate becomes stable at 6–7 years of age. It is because internal plate is much influenced by the growing brain which slows down extremely at this age. Since the inner aspect of frontal bone is stable, it can be used as a stable (X-ray) reference point during growth studies after 7 years age.

Viscerocranium includes the facial skeleton, which arises from pharyngeal arches. It also has two parts, (1) the cartilaginous viscerocranium which includes the middle ear ossicles, the styloid process of the temporal bone and (2) the hyoid bone, and the laryngeal cartilages. And the membranous viscerocranium includes the maxilla, zygomatic bones, the squamous temporal bones, and the mandible. These bones form by intramembranous ossification except for the mandibular condyle and the midline of the chin.

The Cranial Base (Chondrocranium)

The cartilaginous neurocranium, i.e. cranial base is also called as **chondrocranium**. It consists of several cartilages which fuse and undergo endochondral ossification to give rise to the cranial base. The junctions between two bones are called **synchondroses** as they contain intervening cartilage. The occipital bone is formed first, followed by the body of sphenoid bone and then the ethmoid bone. Chondrocranium also forms the vomer bone of nasal septum, and petrous and mastoid parts of the temporal bone.

During fourth week IU, mesenchyme condenses between the developing brain and the foregut to form the ectomeningeal capsule around the brain. Its base gives rise to future cranial base. It is the earliest evidence of skull formation. Ectomeningeal mesenchyme starts changing into cartilage at around 40th day in different areas which later on fuse together to form a single cranial base, which is the beginning of chondrocranium. These chondrification centers appear in four regions, which are (Fig. 4.2):

- Parachordal
- Hypophyseal
- Nasal
- Otic.

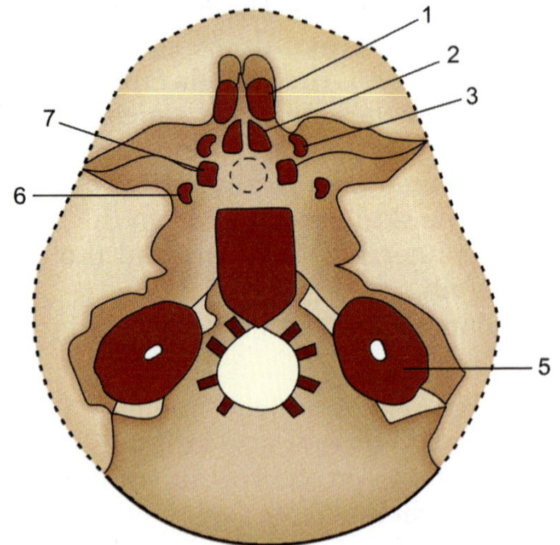

Fig. 4.2: Various cartilaginous areas in the base of skull in prenatal period.

Parachordal Chondrification

The centers forming around the cranial end of notochord are called parachordal cartilages.

Hypophyseal Cartilages

At the level of oropharyngeal membrane, the hypophyseal pouch gives rise to anterior lobe of pituitary gland. On either side, the post-sphenoid cartilages appear which fuse together and form posterior body of sphenoid bone. Cranial to pituitary gland, two cartilages develop and fuse to form anterior part of sphenoid bone.

Presphenoid cartilage gives rise to a vertical plate called mesethmoid cartilage, which forms the perpendicular plate of ethmoid bone and crista galli. **Mesethmoid cartilage** is very important for the growth of middle third of face. On the lateral side of pituitary gland, the chondrification centers appear which form the greater and lesser wings of sphenoid bone. So, sphenoid bone, ethmoid bone and crista galli are endochondral bones.

Nasal Cartilages

A nasal capsule develops around nasal sense organs which chondrifies and gets fused to cartilages of cranial base.

Otic Cartilages

A capsule forms around the vestibule-cochlear sense organs. It chondrifies and ossifies to form mastoid and petrous parts of temporal bone. It also fuses with cranial base.

These separate areas of chondrification in cranial base later on fuse together to form a single cranial base. Since the neurovascular bundles are forming simultaneously, they are housed in the different foramina and canals in the cranial base, giving rise to many ridges in the cranial base. Thus, the internal and external aspects of cranial base are quite irregular.

Cranial base is mostly cartilaginous and bones of cranial base are formed both by endochondral and intramembranous ossification, mostly by endochondral ossification. The growth of the bones in midline where synchondroses are present, e.g. cribriform plate of ethmoid, the presphenoid, the basisphenoid, and the basioccipital bones, contributes to the growth of cranial base. Postnatal growth in the **spheno-occipital synchondrosis** is the major contributor to growth of the cranial base. In addition to proliferative synchondroal growth, the cranial base undergoes selective remodeling by resorption and deposition.

Occipital and temporal bones develop by both endochondral and intramembranous ossification, by multiple ossification centers. Squamous part and tympanic part ossify by intramembranous method, while petrous and styloid process develop by endochondral method. Ethmoid bone develops only by endochondral method by three centers, one forming part of anerior cranial base and two lateral centers forming nasal capsule. Sphenoid bone also develops by both endochondral and intramembranous ossification, by multiple ossification centers. Anterior and posterior parts of body of sphenoid, lesser wing and medial pterygoid plate develop by endochondral ossification, greater wing and lateral pterygoid plate develop by intramembranous ossification.

Cranial Base Angulation/Flexure (Fig. 4.3)

The chondrocranium is a junction between the neurocranial and facial skeletons. Cranial base is relatively stable during growth as most of the growth gets completed by 5–6 years of age. It can be used as a reference plane for future comparison of growth. The cranial base of a newborn child is smaller than the cranial vault, i.e. desmocranium, due to rapid brain growth of the fetus, since the brain growth controls the cranial vault growth (cephalocaudal gradient). Thus, the cranial vault extends beyond the base laterally and posteriorly. Initially, during embryonic development, the cranial base is straight, but with proliferation of mesenchyme in brain region of notochord, the cranial base starts angulating. Initially, the foramen magnum is vertical and hence the spinal cord is horizontal. Spinal cord becomes vertically oriented with growth, as the human are bipedal and stand erect. It is different than other mammals, in which the spinal cord is horizontal, and their visual axis is also parallel to the spinal cord. In humans, the spinal cord is vertical and the visual axis is perpendicular to the spinal cord. The angle between anterior and middle cranial base is more obtuse initially, i.e. approximately 150° in the 4-week-old embryo. It gets reduced to 130° in the 7–8 weeks IU, and to 115–120° at 10 weeks IU. This flexure also helps to increase the capacity of the cranium.

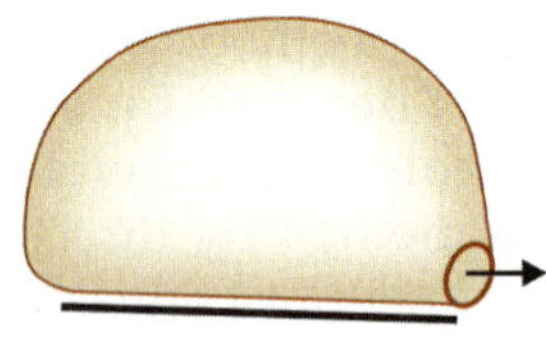

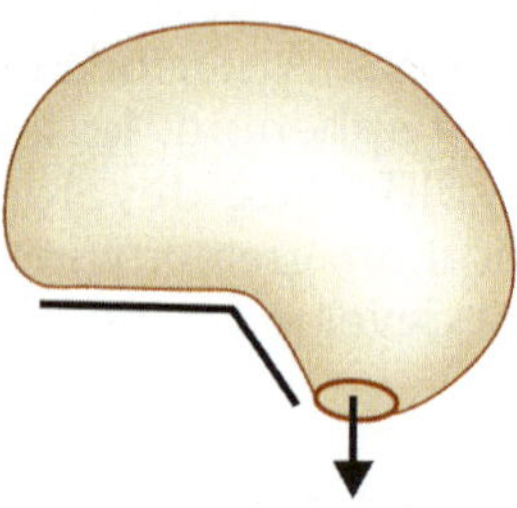

Fig. 4.3: Orientation of the foramen magnum and relation to visual axis. In first figure, the foramen magnum is opening posteriorly, thus directing the spinal cord horizontally. It is seen in animals, where spinal cord is parallel to their visual axis. In human, the foramen magnum is opening inferiorly, thus directing the spinal cord vertically, spinal cord is perpendicular to their visual axis.

DEVELOPMENT OF THE FACIAL SKELETON

(Figs 4.4a to e)

The face may be divided into thirds (the upper, middle, and lower) corresponding to frontonasal, maxillary and mandibular processes, respectively.

- The upper third/frontal region of the face is predominantly influenced by neurocranial growth and it follows neural growth curve. It grows most rapidly with the growth of frontal lobes of brain, with the frontal bone of calvaria primarily responsible for the forehead.
- Growth of middle and lower thirds is slow, and follows the growth of general body tissues (somatic growth curve). The bones of face develop by intramembranous ossification in the neural crest mesenchyme of embryonic processes.

The middle third of face is the most complex part, which is influenced partly by cranial base and the nasal extension of upper third and part of masticatory apparatus (including maxillary dentition). The lower third of face completes masticatory apparatus, being composed of mandible and dentition.

Ossification centers: A primary intramembranous ossification center appears for each maxilla in 7th week, at the termination of infraorbital nerve in the region of future infraorbital foramen. Secondary ossification centers for zygomatic, orbitonasal, nasopalatine, and intermaxillary bones appear and fuse rapidly with primary centers. Single ossification centers appear for each of the zygomatic bones and the squamous portions of the temporal bones in 8th week IU. Single intramembranous ossification centers appear for the mandible in the area of future mental foramen.

Development of face: It occurs between 4 and 8 weeks IU. After 8 weeks, slow facial development occurs, which involves changes in facial proportions and relative positions of parts of face. Facial development occurs from five processes, i.e. 1 frontonasal, 2 maxillary, and 2 mandibular processes. Maxillary and mandibular processes arise from first pharyngeal arch.

The fusion of the mandibular processes in the midline is one of the first events in formation of facial structures, and it forms the chin and lower lip. Ectodermal cells thicken to form nasal placodes in inferolateral portion of the frontonasal process. The medial nasal processes and lateral nasal processes arise by the mesenchymal proliferation along the periphery of the nasal placodes. Mesenchymal connective tissue in the maxillary processes proliferates, so the maxillary processes

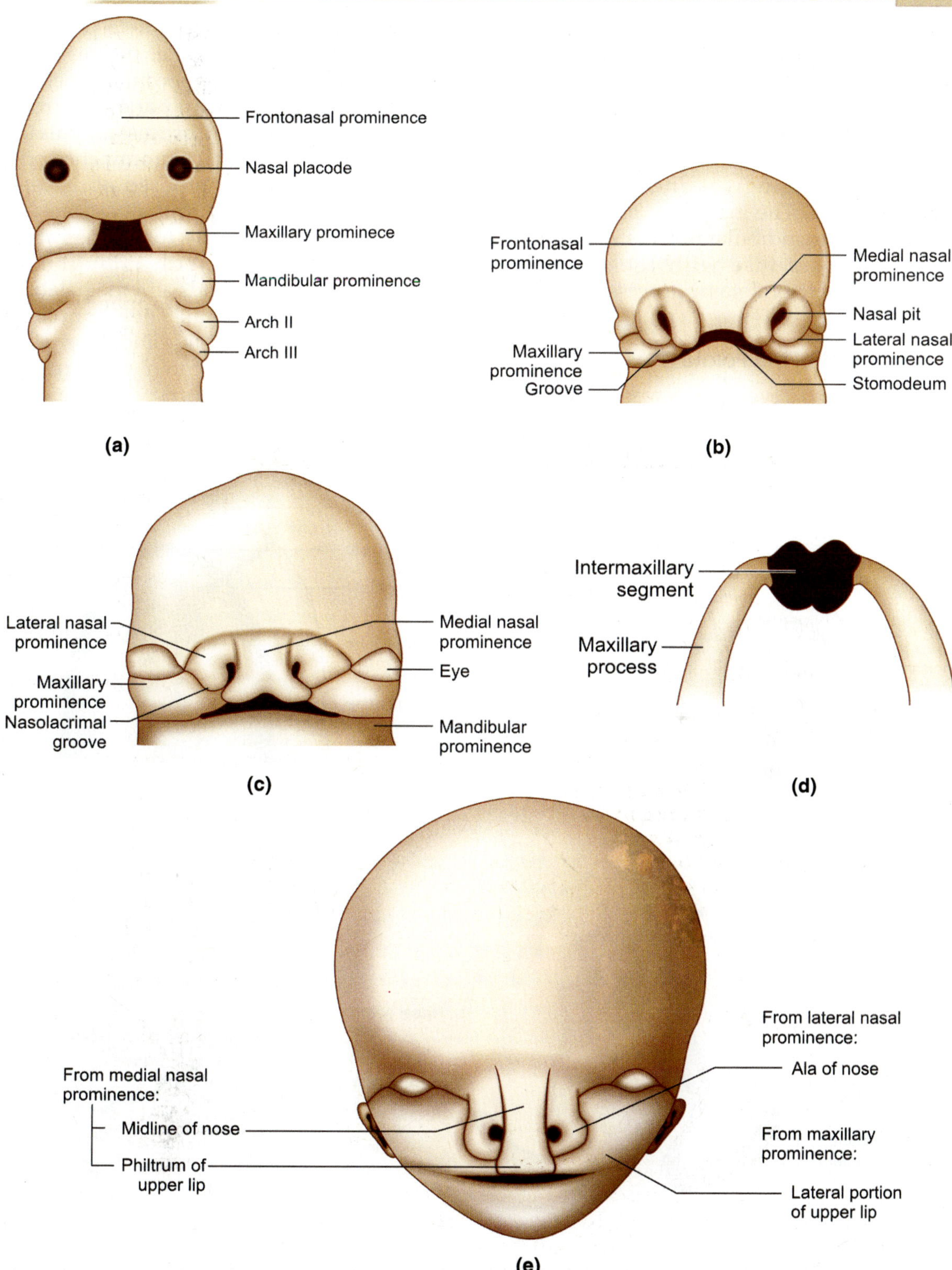

Figs 4.4a to e: Embryonic development of various parts of the face.

enlarge and start moving medially toward each other and toward the medial nasal processes. The medial nasal processes also move toward each other, and fuse in midline with each other and with frontonasal process, and give rise to philtrum, four incisors, alveolar bone, gingiva, and premaxilla/ primary palate. The maxillary process fuses laterally with mandibular process. The medial nasal processes fuse with the maxillary processes and lateral nasal processes.

Development of the Palate (Figs 4.5a to d)

Palate begins to develop in 6 week. The most critical period during palatal development is between 6 and 8 weeks. Complete palate is formed of two structures, i.e. the primary palate (premaxilla) and the secondary palate. Primary palate arises from a portion of frontonasal and medial nasal processes. Palatal shelves arise from maxillary prominence one on each side, and are composed of mesenchymal connective tissue. Initially, they are oriented vertically because tongue is interposed between them. With mandibular growth, the tongue descends and the palatine shelves become horizontal. They approach one another and fuse in the midline to form the secondary palate. Incisive foramen is present at the junction of the primary palate and lateral palatine shelves. The lateral palatine

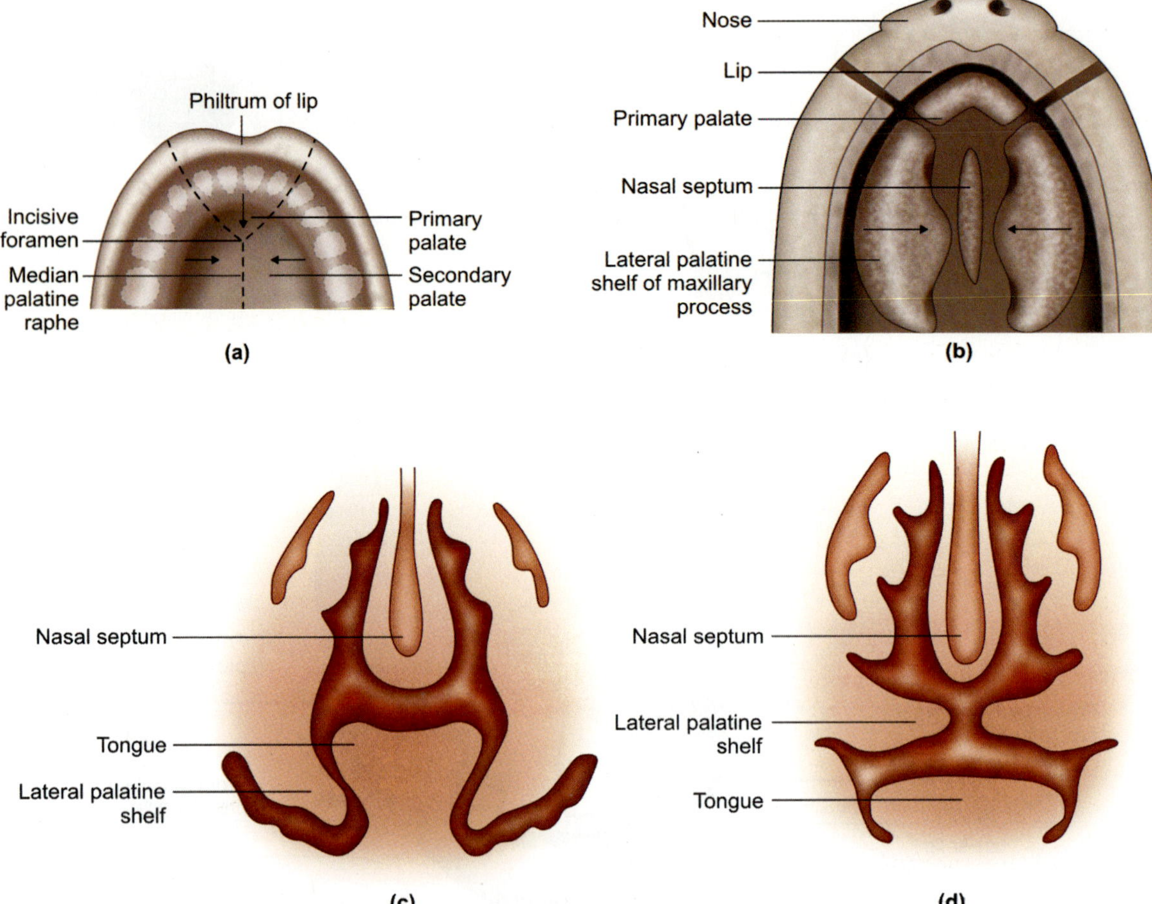

Figs 4.5a to d: Prenatal development of palate. Note medial outgrowths occurring form the palatal shelves in hard palate region, while there is downward growth of nasal septal process.

shelves also fuse with primary palate and nasal septum, thus separating oral and nasal cavities. The secondary palate ossifies partially and gives rise to hard and soft palate posterior to the incisive foramen. It occurs from 8 weeks IU and is an intramembranous type of ossification.

Pathogenesis of Cleft Lip and Cleft Palate

Cleft lip and palate occur due to failure of fusion of the processes discussed above. Cleft lip occurs due to failure of fusion of medial nasal process with maxillary process. Cleft lip may be unilateral or bilateral and may be complete or partial, and can extend into the alveolar process and nostrils. Cleft palate develops due to failure of fusion of the lateral palatine shelves with each other, with the nasal septum, or with the primary palate. Incomplete penetration of mesoderm during fusion of palatal shelves can give rise to a submucous cleft palate. Thus, cleft lip and alveolus (primary palate) occurs between the 4th and the 8th week IU, while clefts of the hard and soft palate (secondary palate) occurs between 8th and 12th weeks. Any disturbance which occurs during formation of lip, if it extends during formation of palate, may lead to CLP. First trimester of pregnancy is crucial because of rapid growth and differentiation of cells and is very sensitive to drugs, radiations, alcohol, etc. Disturbances in cellular multiplication and differentiation during this stage give rise to congenital conditions.

THE MAXILLA

A primary intramembranous ossification center appears for each maxilla at eighth week IU at the termination of the infraorbital nerve. Secondary cartilages appear at the end of the eighth week IU in the regions of the zygomatic and alveolar processes that rapidly ossify and fuse with the primary intramembranous center. Two further intramembranous premaxillary centres appear anteriorly on each side in the 8th week IU and rapidly fuse with the primary maxillary center. Single ossification centers appear for each of the zygomatic bones and the squamous portions of the temporal bones in the eighth week IU.

PRENATAL DEVELOPMENT OF MANDIBLE (Figs 4.6a to c)

The first structure to develop in the region of lower jaw is the mandibular division of trigeminal nerve. Then, ectomesenchymal condensation occurs forming first (mandibular) pharyngeal arch. The presence of nerve is a prerequisite for inducing osteogenesis by neurotrophic influence.

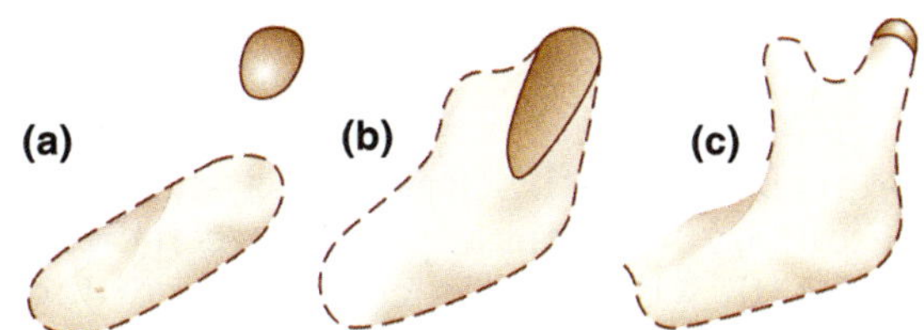

Figs 4.6a to c: Embryonic development of the mandible. Cartilage in condylar region gets converted to the secondary cartilage cap on the head of condyle, while most of the mandible is made by intramembranous growth.

Mandible develops by intramembranous ossification lateral to Meckel's cartilage of the first (mandibular) pharyngeal arch. Meckel's C only acts as a scaffold around which intramembranous bone formation occurs, but does not directly contribute to mandibular formation (Fig. 4.7). Meckel's cartilage lacks the enzyme phosphatase found in ossifying cartilages, thus its ossification does not occur. A single ossification center for each half of mandible arises in the region of future mental foramen, i.e. where the bifurcation of inferior

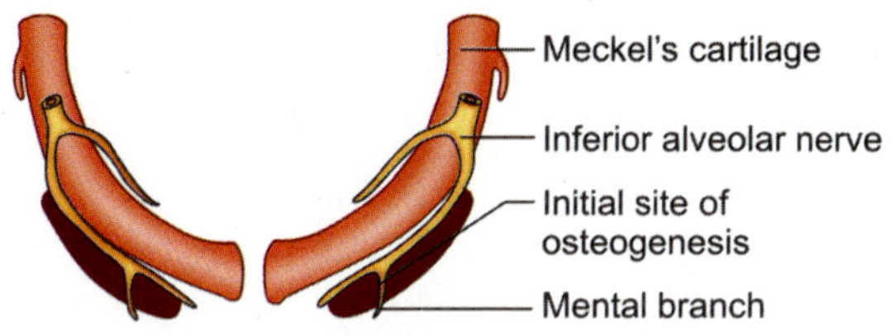

Fig. 4.7: Embryonic development of mandible, with Meckel's cartilage just acting as a scaphold around which intramembranous mandibular development takes place. Initial site of ossification is near the future mental foramen.

alveolar nerve and artery into mental and incisive branches occurs, at around 6th week IU. During the 8–12 weeks IU, there is marked acceleration of mandibular growth. The spread of the intramembranous ossification dorsally and ventrally forms the body and ramus of mandible. Almost all of Meckel's cartilage disappears by 24th week IU. Ossification stops dorsally at a point which becomes the mandibular lingula. The dorsal end of Meckel's cartilage gives rise to ligaments (the sphenomandibular and anterior malleolar ligaments) which are attached at lingula, and two auditory ossicles, (i.e. malleus and incus). The third ossicle (stapes) is derived primarily from cartilage of second pharyngeal arch (Reichert's cartilage). Secondary cartilages appear between the 10th and 14th weeks IU in condylar, coronoid process, and mental protuberance regions. This condylar cartilage forms the future condyle, is a secondary cartilage, i.e. it does not have its intrinsic growth potential, but can grow under the influence of soft tissue and other forces. Cartilage cells differentiate from its centre, and condylar head increases by interstitial and appositional growth. It is also important for the growth of ramus and body of the mandible, by leading to passive displacement of these structures.

By middle of fetal life, much of the condylar cartilage gets replaced by bone, but its upper end persists, which acts as articular cartilage, contributing to further growth of condyle and mandible. Changes in mandibular position and form are related to the direction and amount of condylar growth. The condylar growth rate peaks between 12½ and 14 years of age, and normally ceases at about 20 years of age.

Condylar C develops initially as a separate area and fuses with the mandibular body at normally at 4 weeks IU life.

5

Postnatal Growth

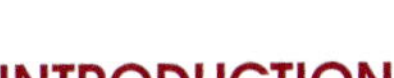

INTRODUCTION

Relative movement of different skeletal parts is one of the important phenomena during growth. The growth of different bones is interrelated. The facial skeleton is attached to cranial base and thus there is a strong chondrocranial influence on facial growth. Literally, the face comes out from beneath the cranial base.

Craniofacial complex growth can be studied under four areas:

1. The cranial vault, desmocranium
2. The cranial base, chondrocranium
3. The nasomaxillary complex
4. The mandible, splanchnocranium

THE CRANIAL VAULT (Figs 5.1a to c)

Cranial vault is formed by flat bones, like parietal, frontal, temporal and occipital bones. These are membranous bones, which are connected with sutures, i.e. the coronal, lambdoid, interparietal, parietosphenoidal and parietotemporal sutures. The growth occurs through "fill in" ossification of the proliferating connective tissue in these sutures. The growth in cranial vault occurs due to enlarging brain. At birth, approx. 65% brain growth is completed. During first 5 years of age, upto 90% of brain growth is achieved and hence of the cranial vault. Rest of the growth occurs till adulthood at a very slow pace. It follows a neural growth curve.

At birth, the fontanelles exist between the bones of cranial vault, which help in molding of skull when the fetus passes through the birth canal. These wide fontanelles close within the first year of life by bony apposition. These fontanelles are important during initial life of an infant, as they help the pediatricians to know the status of health and hydration status of the child (Fig. 5.2).

Surface of cranial vault undergoes immense periosteal activity with selective resorption on inner surfaces of the bones. It provides space for the growing brain. Bony apposition occurs on both internal and external tables of bones which helps in increasing their thickness (Fig. 5.3).

Sutures present between the bones of cranial vault separate with ensuing growth of brain, thus creating the gap between the bones. The ends of bones act like the epiphyseal plates and try to approach each other and thus sutural growth ensues. Thus the expanding brain keeps on accommodating by expansion of cranial cavity (Fig. 5.4). These sutures remain viable for many years, with increasing interdigitation with age. At birth, the frontal bone is in two parts separated by metopic suture which gets closed very early in life. Also, there is no frontal sinus at birth. With further growth, the external and internal cortical plates of frontal bone start separating at around 3–4 years of age (Fig. 5.5). Pneumatization occurs as the spongy bone between the external plates is gradually replaced by the developing frontal sinus, which runs upto puberty and even into adulthood. This growth of frontal bone also leads to forward migration of the maxilla. Height of the brain case increases due to sutural growth especially at parietal sutures, along with the occipital, temporal, and sphenoidal sutures (Figs 5.6 and 5.7).

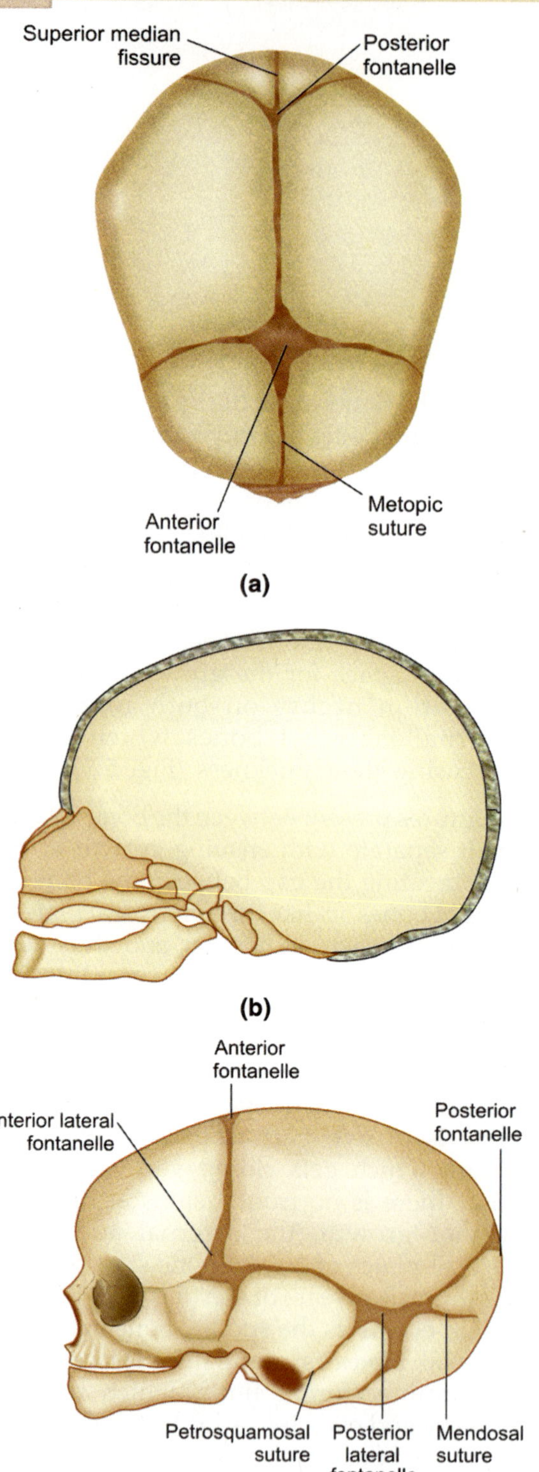

Figs 5.1a to c: Skull of an infant, depicting the various fontanelles.

The Role of Primary Cartilage during Growth

Primary cartilage develops directly from the embryonic neural crest cells (NCC), and has the capacity to grow from within (interstitial growth). It has a genetic potential of growth. Primary cartilages first appear in head during fifth week IU, which coalesce together by eighth week IU, into a cartilaginous mass known as chondrocranium. It forms the adult cranial base and nasal and otic structures. Interstitial growth and expansion of primary cartilage of cranial base especially the spheno-occipital synchondrosis, and nose, etc. influences the position of maxilla by causing **passive displacement** in a downward and forward direction. By mid-childhood, most primary cartilage gets converted to bone by endochondral osteogenesis.

THE CRANIAL BASE

The cranial base is the part of cranium which supports the brain. It can be divided in three parts, i.e. anterior, middle and posterior cranial base. Unlike cranial vault, it is not completely dependent on brain growth, but has some intrinsic growth potential. The three bones in cranial base are basioccipital, sphenoid and ethmoid bones, which are formed by endochondral ossification, especially in the midline, while the bones in the lateral parts of cranial base have sutures interposed between them. The bones of cranial base are separated by synchondroses in midline. **Synchondroses** can be defined as the type of interbony joints having portions of cartilage in them. These are primary cartilage and thus have an intrinsic growth potential. They are important growth sites for the cranial base, and are arranged in upward and backward direction, so that the growth in them causes upward and forward growth of cranial base.

Following synchondroses are found in the cranial base (Figs 5.8 and 5.9):

- Spheno-occipital
- Sphenoethmoidal
- Intersphenoidal
- Intraoccipital.

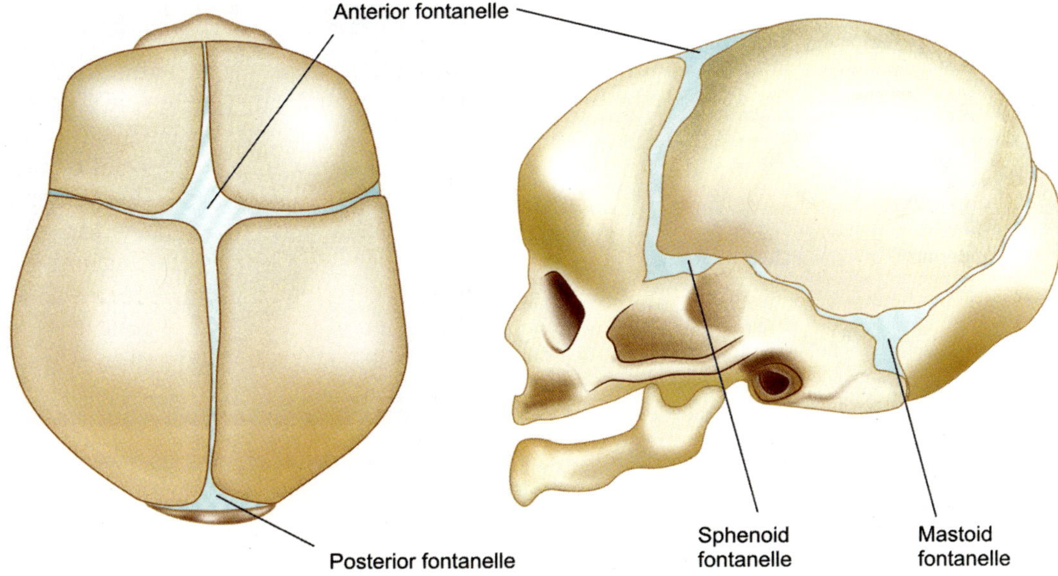

Fig. 5.2: The fontanelles in the skull of an infant.

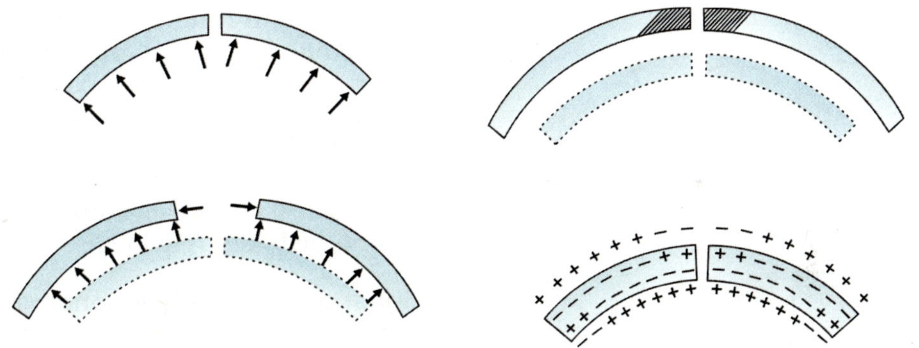

Fig. 5.3: Remodeling of bones in cranial vault and sutural growth. It also shows the increase in thickness of cranial bone due to remodeling of diploe.

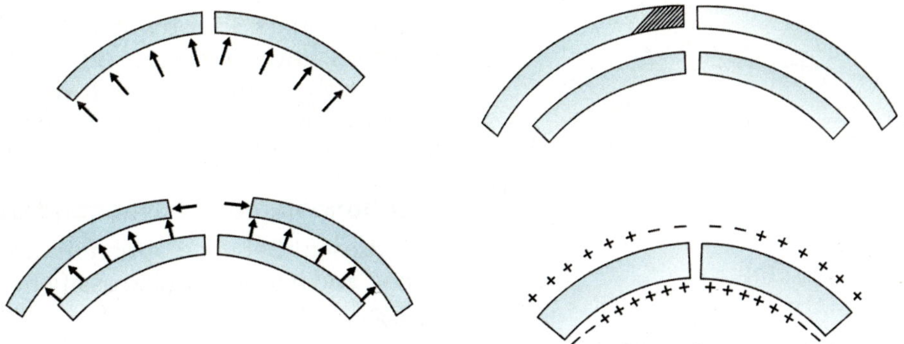

Fig. 5.4: Growth of cranial vault and sutural growth. Arrows in first figure show the expanding brain which separates the cranial sutures. Remodeling helps to fill the gap and the surface of bones also adapt to the growing nervous tissue in the skull.

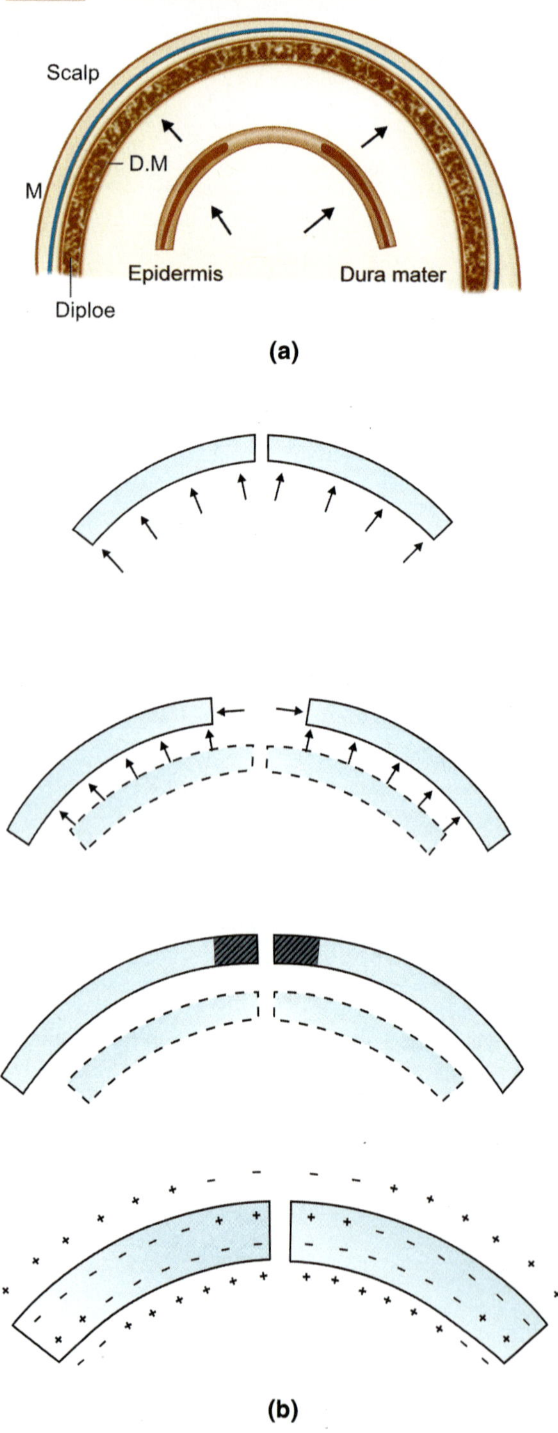

Fig. 5.5: Growth of cranial cavity with the growing brain which occurs by remodeling of cranial bones and sutural growth between cranial vault bones through intramembranous ossification.

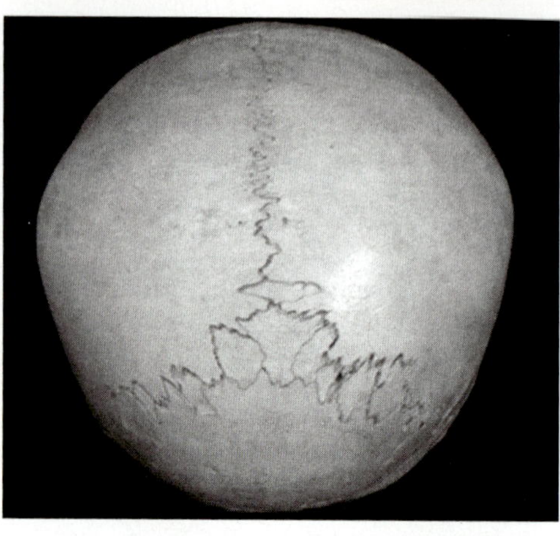

Fig. 5.6: Cranial suture system as seen from top of the cranial vault.

Synchondrosis can be viewed as a joint having two epiphyseal plates facing each other, and bone growth occurring at both sides, and increasing the length of bones (Fig. 5.10). So, it can be said that the growth here is **compression adapted bone growth**, while in sutures, the growth occurs by tension created in the sutural area when the bones there are pulled apart by the muscles and brain growth. Bony remodeling occurs on endosteal and periosteal surfaces leading to increase in width of the bones (Fig. 5.11).

a. Spheno-occipital Synchondrosis (Figs 5.12 and 5.13)

It lies between sphenoid and occipital bones. It is the principal growth site of cranial base and remains active upto 12–15 years of age. It becomes ossified at around 20 years of age. Its orientation is in upward and backward direction, and thus the direction of growth in it is upward and forward. It thus carries the anterior part of cranium in U and F direction (Figs 5.14 and 5.15).

b. Sphenoethmoidal Synchondrosis

It is present between sphenoid and ethmoid bones, and it is believed to ossify by 5–25 years of age.

c. Intersphenoidal Synchondrosis

It lies between two parts of sphenoid bone and gets ossified at birth.

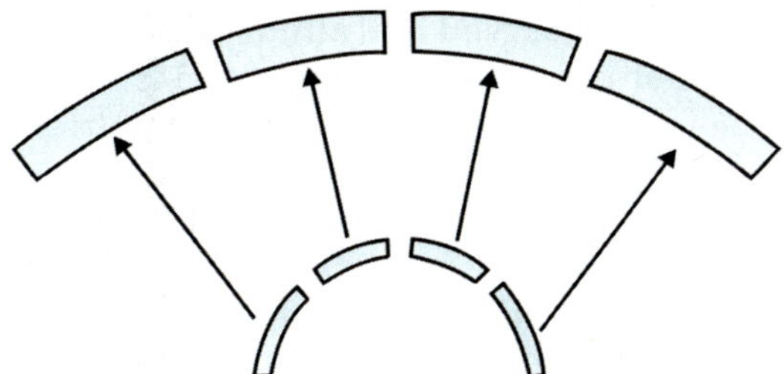

Fig. 5.7: With increased size of cranial cavity and outward movement of cranial bones during growth, the curvature of cranial bones decreases and they become more flatter. It can be explained mathematically also, as when the radius of a circle increases, its perimeter also increases, and the segments in the circle become more flatter.

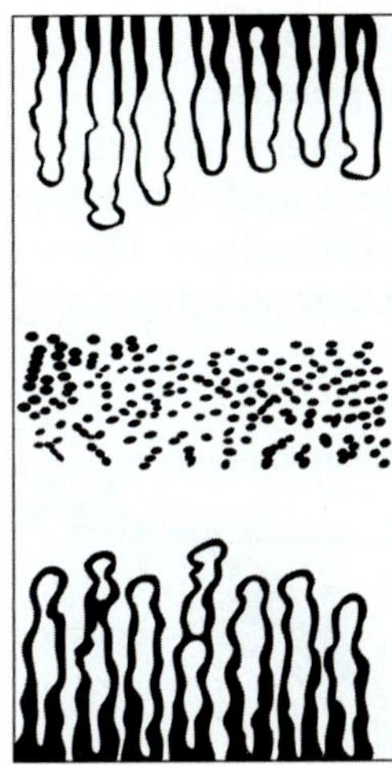

Fig. 5.10: Cross-section showing that epiphyseal cartilage helps in growth of bone in both the directions in synchondroses.

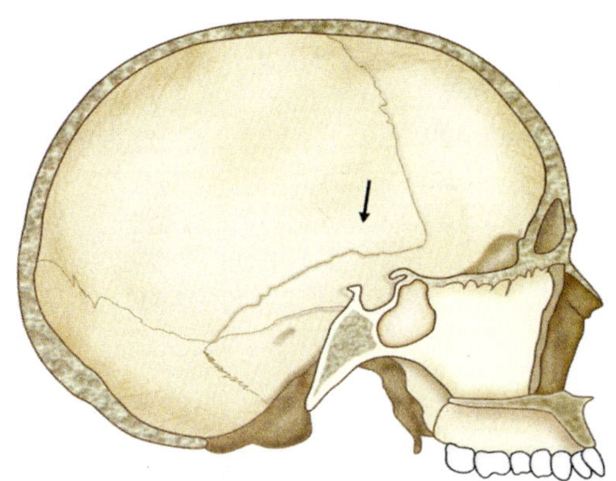

Fig. 5.8: Intracranial structures from lateral view.

d. Intraoccipital Synchondrosis

It ossifies by 3–5 years of age.

Bone remodeling in cranial base: There are various foramina, canals and ridges in the cranial base. They house nerves and vessels. As the brain and hence the cranial cavity grows, internal remodelling occurs till they achieve a final position.

Sutural growth in cranial base: Some of the sutures present in cranial base are:

a. Sphenofrontal
b. Shenoethmoidal
c. Frontotemporal

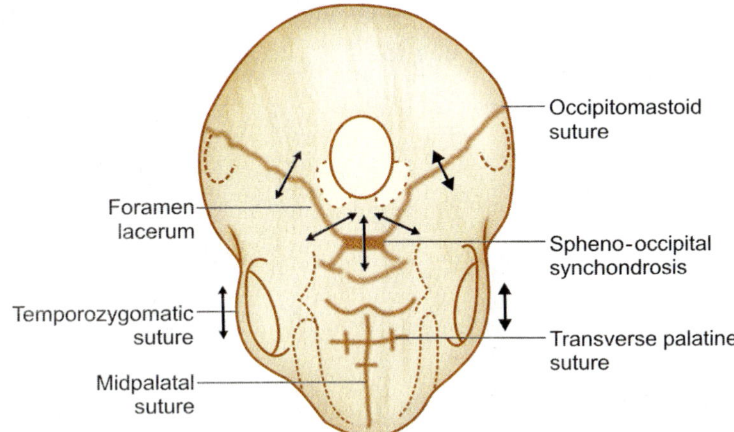

Fig. 5.9: Diagram of the inside base of skull showing different sutures and synchondrosis which are helpful during growth.

d. Frontoethmoid

e. Frontozygomatic

Growth in these sutures occurs due to expanding brain and is mainly membranous type of bone formation. These are generally present in the lateral part of the cranial base.

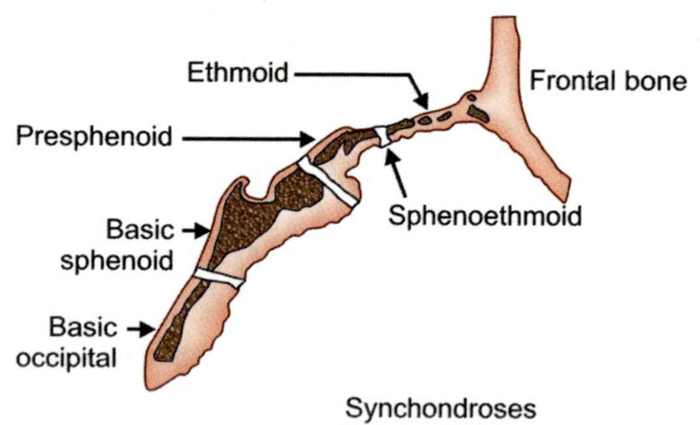

Fig. 5.11: Cross-section of cranial base showing different synchondroses which help in endochondral ossification of the cranial base and also the translational growth of nasomaxillary–mandibular complex.

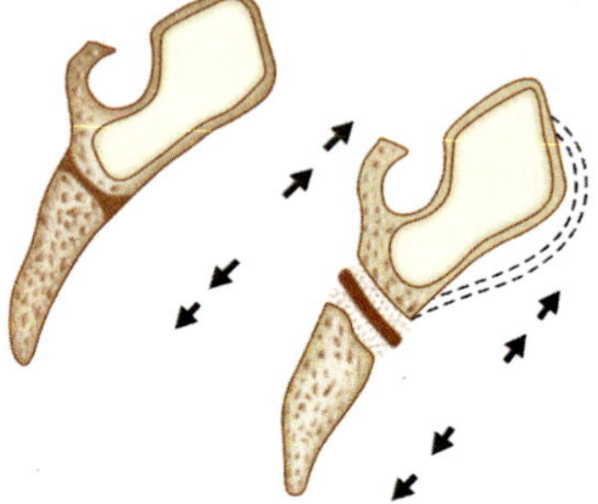

Fig. 5.12: Growth of middle cranial fossa due to growth at spheno-occipital synchondrosis.

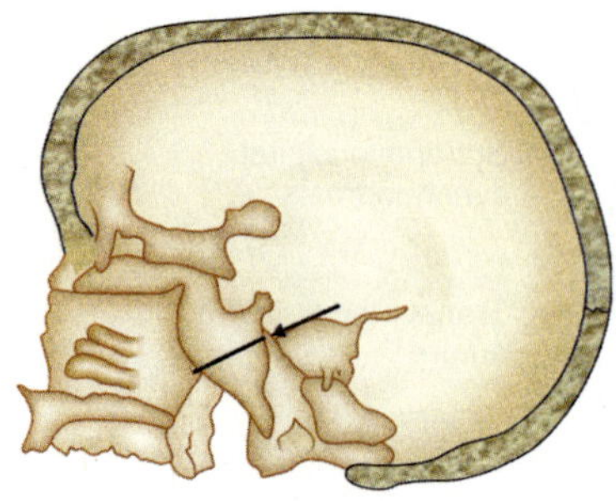

Fig. 5.13: Spheno-occipital synchondrosis from a lateral view of skull.

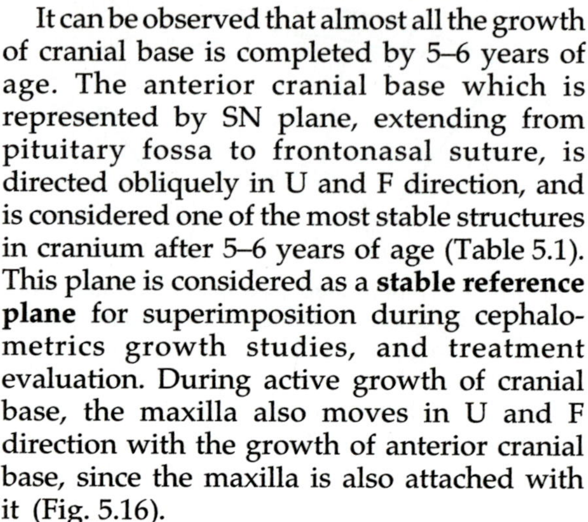

It can be observed that almost all the growth of cranial base is completed by 5–6 years of age. The anterior cranial base which is represented by SN plane, extending from pituitary fossa to frontonasal suture, is directed obliquely in U and F direction, and is considered one of the most stable structures in cranium after 5–6 years of age (Table 5.1). This plane is considered as a **stable reference plane** for superimposition during cephalometrics growth studies, and treatment evaluation. During active growth of cranial base, the maxilla also moves in U and F direction with the growth of anterior cranial base, since the maxilla is also attached with it (Fig. 5.16).

Table 5.1: Timing of growth of cranial base

At birth	*55–60%*
4–7 years age	Upto 94%
8–13 years age	Upto 98%

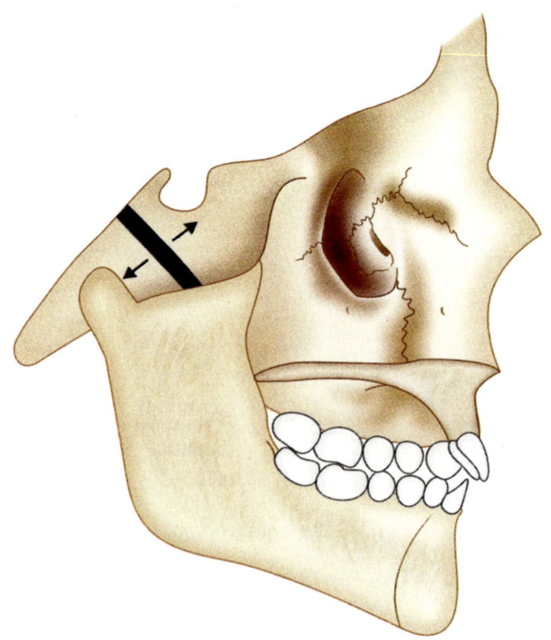

Fig. 5.14: Spheno-occipital synchondrosis is the main site of cranial base growth, and its growth also leads to translatory growth of maxilla and mandible.

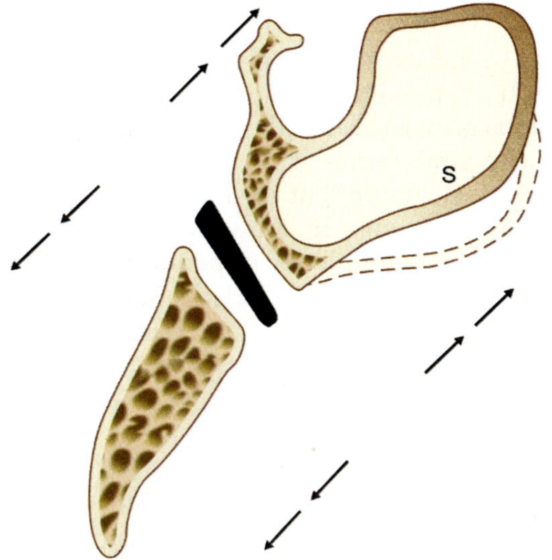

Fig. 5.15: Cartilaginous growth at spheno-occipital synchondrosis leads to growth of cranial base in both F and B directions.

and time, following cephalocaudal gradient of growth. Cephalocaudal gradient of growth means that the parts away from cranium start their main growth late and keep on growing for a longer period as compared to the parts towards cranial end, e.g. cranium finishes its growth before maxilla, and maxilla finishes its growth before mandible. By this differential growth and cephalocaudal gradient of growth, the face literally emerges from beneath the cranium. The upper face/maxilla, under the influence of cranial base inclination (which moves U and F), moves upwards and forwards, while the lower face/mandible moves downwards and forwards (due to growth at condylar region in U and B direction), thus an "expanding V" is observed in the face.

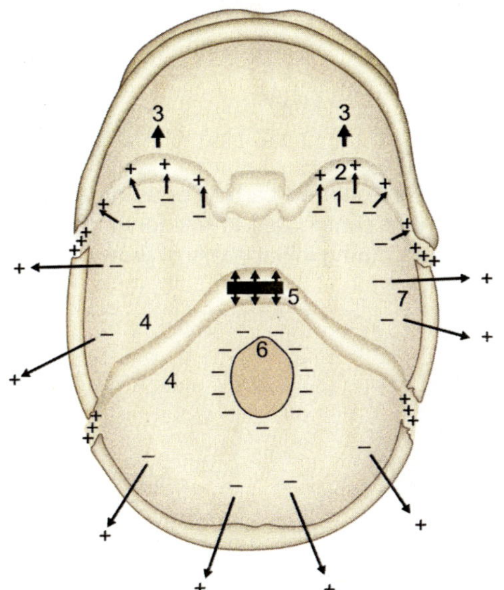

Fig. 5.16: Sutural growth and bony remodeling at sites 1–4, 6,7; while at site 5, there is sphenooccipital synchondrosis, where endochondral growth occurs.

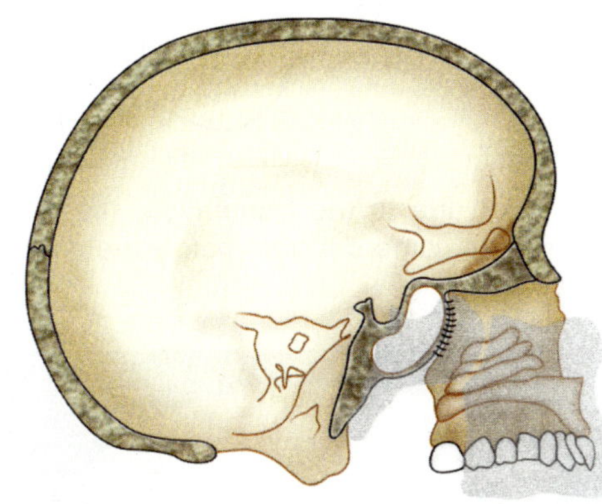

Fig. 5.17: Growth of the nasomaxillary complex as it emerges from beneath the cranium. There also occurs the translocation of maxilla due to growth in spheno-occipital synchondrosis.

THE NASOMAXILLARY COMPLEX (NMC)

(Fig. 5.17)

As depicted by Scammon, the growth of the cranium (neural tissues) and facial skeleton (general tissues) progress at different rates

Growth of nasomaxillary complex takes place by two phenomena:

1. Displacement, i.e. shift in the position of the maxillary complex. It is of two types: (a) primary and (b) secondary displacements.
2. Sutural growth and surface remodeling; leading to enlargement of the complex itself.

Basic Maxillary Unit (Figs 5.18 and 5.19)

Basic maxillary unit is the infraorbital neurovascular triad, and the maxillary basal bone serves as a protection mechanism for this nerve bundle. It provides a neurotrophic influence and maintains a constancy of the basal maxillary skeletal unit. It has been discussed in prenatal growth of maxilla, the ossification of maxilla starts in the area of future infraorbital foramen.

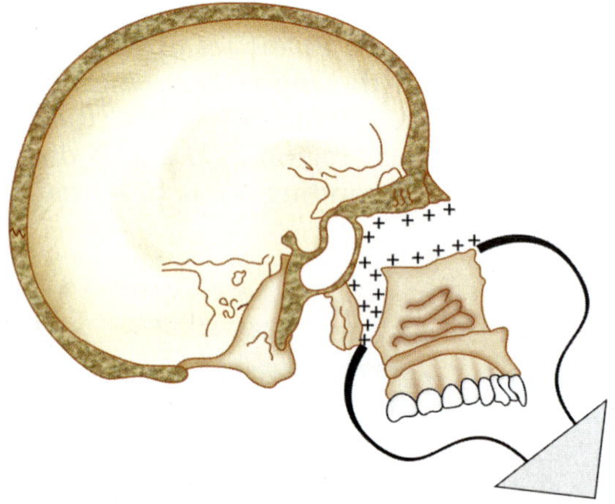

Fig. 5.18: That due to the translation, the whole maxilla seems to come out from below the cranium as a whole.

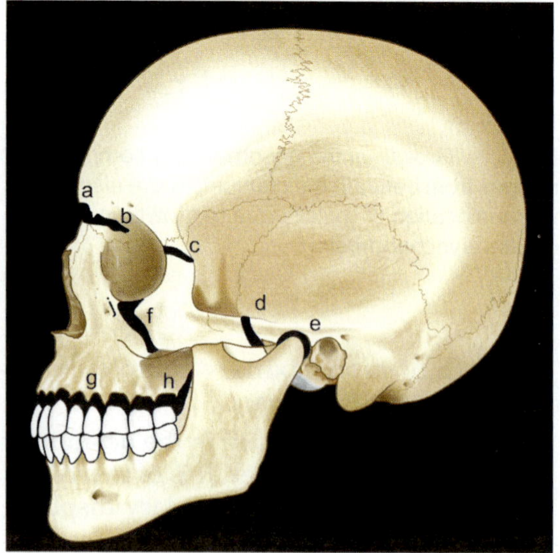

Fig. 5.19: Sites of bone remodeling in the circummaxillary complex, condylar, and maxillary dentoalveolar region.

Role of Nasal Cartilage

Nasal septal cartilage is also required for the growth of maxilla. Any deficiency in cartilaginous growth also leads to deficient maxilla. Experimental removal of nasal cartilage in animals has shown that the maxilla grows but remains deficient. It shows that maxillary growth is not completely dependent on nasal cartilage (Figs 5.20 and 5.21).

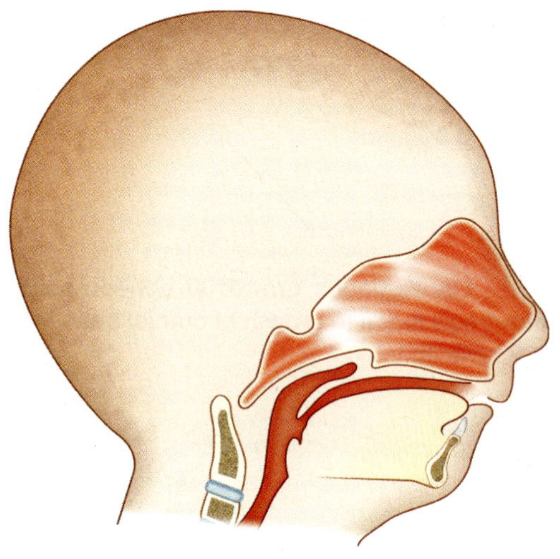

Fig. 5.20: Red-colored cartilaginous part of cranionasal segment contributes to the forward growth of face and jaws during initial years of growth of a child.

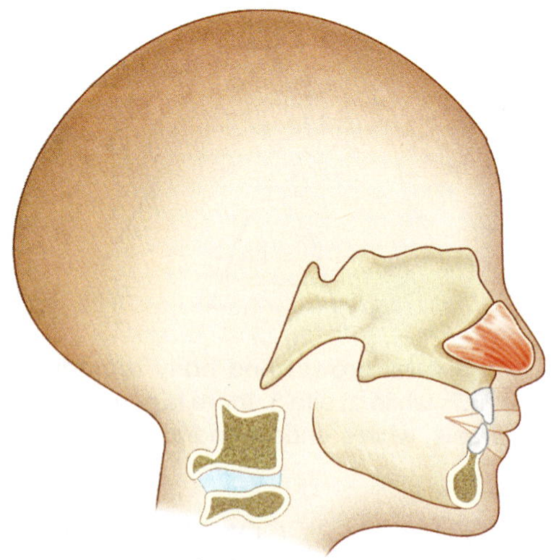

Fig. 5.21: Later on, whole cartilage is ossified leaving a smaller part of nasal septum which contributes minimal to any growth except some slow nasal growth till 14–16 years of age.

Role of Functional Matrix

The functional matrices play an important role in maxillary growth causing passive displacement. Growth of nasal cavity occurs with increased requirement of respiration. The passive movements of bones is brought about by the expansion of orofacial capsule, and thus the facial bones are passively carried outward (downward, forward, and laterally) by the primary expansion of the involved orofacial functional matrices (e.g. orbital, nasal, oral matrices), e.g. growth of the eyeball is required for development of orbital cavity.

(a) Displacement (Fig. 5.22)

Since the maxillary complex is attached to cranial base, any growth of cranial base has a strong influence on maxillary position. Achondroplasia cranial base growth is due to endochondral osteogenesis and is primarily cartilaginous. In achondroplasia, there is deficient cartilagenous bone growth in the body, and thus the body height of the patient does not increase properly due to improper cartilaginous growth in epiphysis and diaphysis. Also the length of cranial base does not increase and thus the maxillary displacement does not occur. Maxilla remains deficient in achondroplasia and leads to skeletal class III relation due to maxillary deficiency.

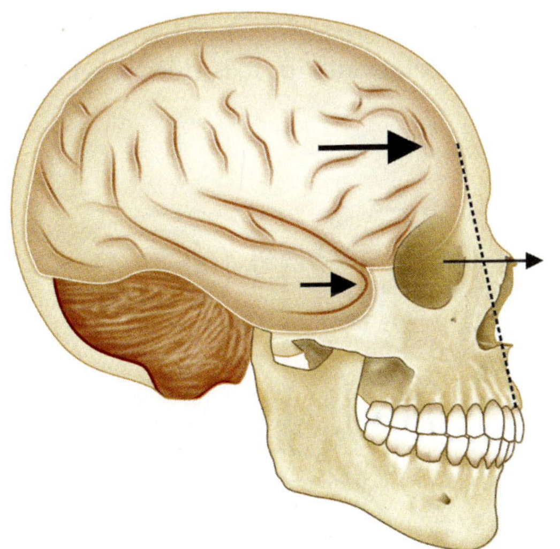

Fig. 5.22: With increased growth of neurocranial tissue in forward direction, there is also the translation of maxilla in anterior direction.

Secondary Displacement

With cranial base growth esp during first 5 years of life, the NMC observes a passive or secondary displacement. It is called secondary **or passive displacement** because the bone, (i.e. maxilla) gets displaced due to growth and enlargement of an **adjacent bone,** (i.e. cranial base). And the actual enlargement of the bone itself is not directly involved. With the almost completion of growth of cranial base at 5–6 years age, the other mechanisms of maxillary growth come into play.

Maxilla is also displaced with the growth of cartilaginous mesethmoid (nasal capsule and nasal septum), which grows actively after 4–5 years of age, and leads to separation of external and internal cortices of frontal bone. It leads to initiation of formation of the frontal sinus.

Translation of maxilla also occurs with the growth of frontal bone since it is also attached to frontal bone. The growth of frontal bone due to expanding brain, upto 3–4 years of age influences the position of maxilla by displacing it anteriorly. Maxilla is attached to external cortex of frontal bone, and thus it is also displaced anteriorly with frontal sinus pneumatization, which can go upto puberty and late adulthood.

Primary Displacement

Growth of maxillary tuberosity occurs in posterior direction, but it is resisted by stable cranium distally and cannot grow in distal direction, thus the maxilla is pushed in a forward direction. Since the growth is occurring in bone itself causing displacement, it is called primary displacement.

Elongation of maxilla: It occurs by a downward push of maxilla by rapidly-growing brain and the ocular contents till 4 years of age. At the same time, maxilla is pulled down by the muscular [soft palate, tongue, mandibular subluxation (MS)] and other soft tissue attachment and occlusal function. Growth of nasal septum also helps in elongation of maxilla. After 3–4 years, the brain growth slows down, so maxilla is mainly under the influence of downward pull of soft tissues. The bone remodeling of palatal and nasal floor and orbital floor comes into play for further growth changes.

(b) Sutural Growth of Maxilla (Figs 5.23 and 5.24)

Maxilla is attached to cranium and other bones with a number of sutures, which are oriented obliquely and almost parallel to each other, in an upward and forward direction, leading to growth of maxilla in D and F direction. These sutures are:

a. Frontonasal suture
b. Frontomaxillary suture
c. Pterygopalatine
d. Zygomaticotemporal
e. Zygomaticomaxillary
f. Mid-palatine suture.

The growth or activation of soft tissue envelop and functional matrix around maxilla, creates separation and tension in the surrounding sutural system and the maxilla moves in a D and F direction. The bone filling takes place in the sutures, leading to increase in size of bone. Thus, the sutural growth is **secondary growth**. The mid-palatine suture lies in between two halves of maxilla and is oriented in a sagittal direction. Growth in this region helps to increase the transverse dimension of the maxillary complex, nasal cavity and face.

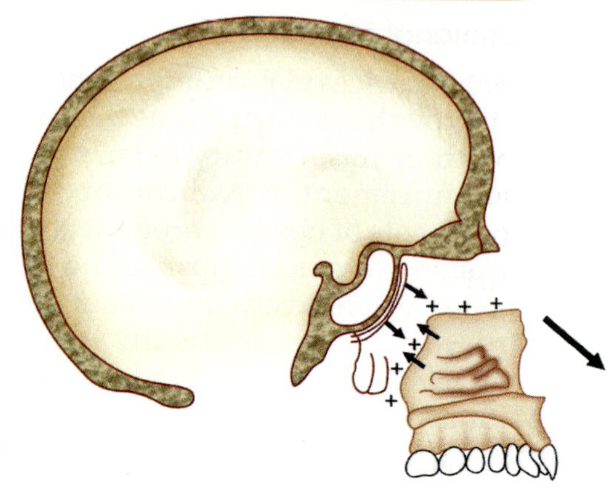

Fig. 5.24: + and - show remodeling taking place in the circummaxillary sutures, which leads to translocation of whole maxillary complex in a downward and forward direction as shown by bigger arrow. Maxilla moves D and F due to the oblique orientation of the suture in U and F direction.

(c) Bony Remodeling of the Maxilla (Figs 5.25 to 5.28)

Apart from the primary and secondary displacements of maxilla and sutural growth, massive bone remodeling occurs on maxilla, which helps in changing the shape, size, and functional relationship. It is described as **the**

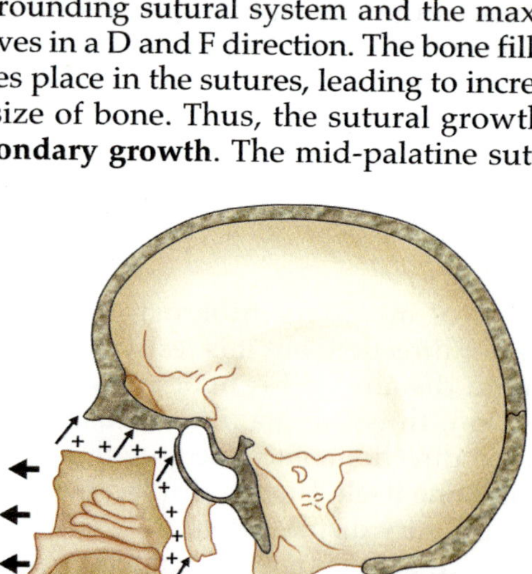

Fig. 5.23: Remodeling in circummaxillary sutures leads to displacement of maxilla in downward and forward direction.

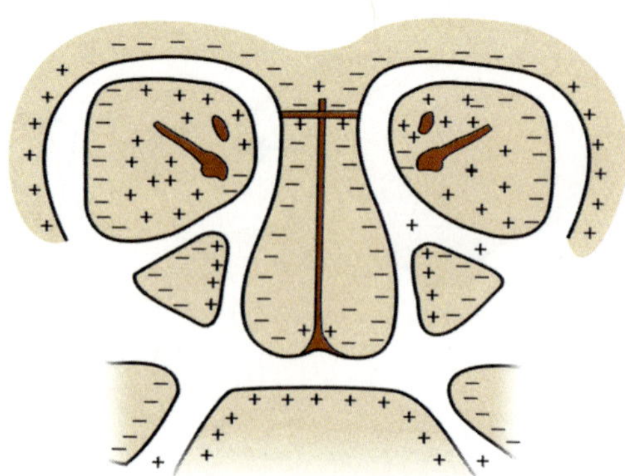

Fig. 5.25: Remodeling of bone in maxilla, nasal cavity, orbital cavity and the palate.

principle of "area relocation". Specific local areas come to occupy new actual positions, as the entire bone enlarges. Enlow has described bone growth as the **"expanding-V principle"**. Bony remodeling in maxilla can be seen in the following area (Figs 5.26 and 5.27):

a. **Maxillary tuberosity:** Bone deposition occurs in maxillary tuberosity areas, and thus displaces maxilla in forward direction. It thus creates space for eruption of permanent molars, and lengthens the dental arch.
b. **Dentoalveolar growth:** Erupting teeth act as functional matrices of the dento-alveolar growth. Bone deposition occurs on free borders of alveolar process and lateral surface of alveolus. The teeth erupt in occlusal, mesial and lateral direction. It helps to increase the height of maxillary bone, and width of dental arch. It also increases the depth of palate. Compensatory remodeling changes take place on lingual aspect of the dental arches.
c. **Hard palate:** Bone deposition occurs on the roof of oral cavity, while bone resorption occurs on the floor of nasal cavity. The bone is also deposited on the lateral aspect and resorbed from the mesial aspect in the dental arch region. It leads to an expanding-V, thereby increasing the width of dental arch and face.

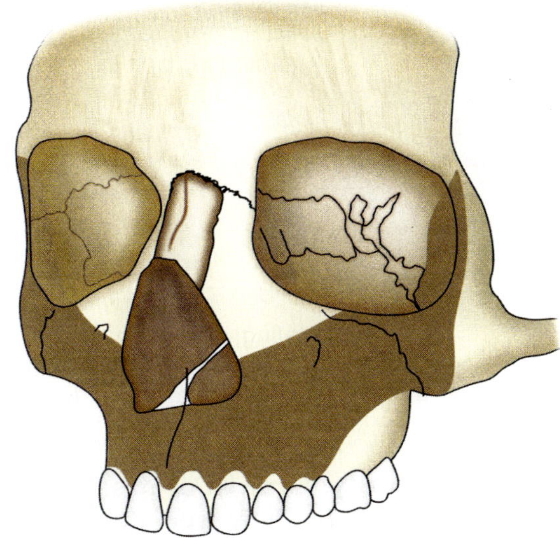

Fig. 5.27: The remodeling areas of nasomaxillary and orbital complex

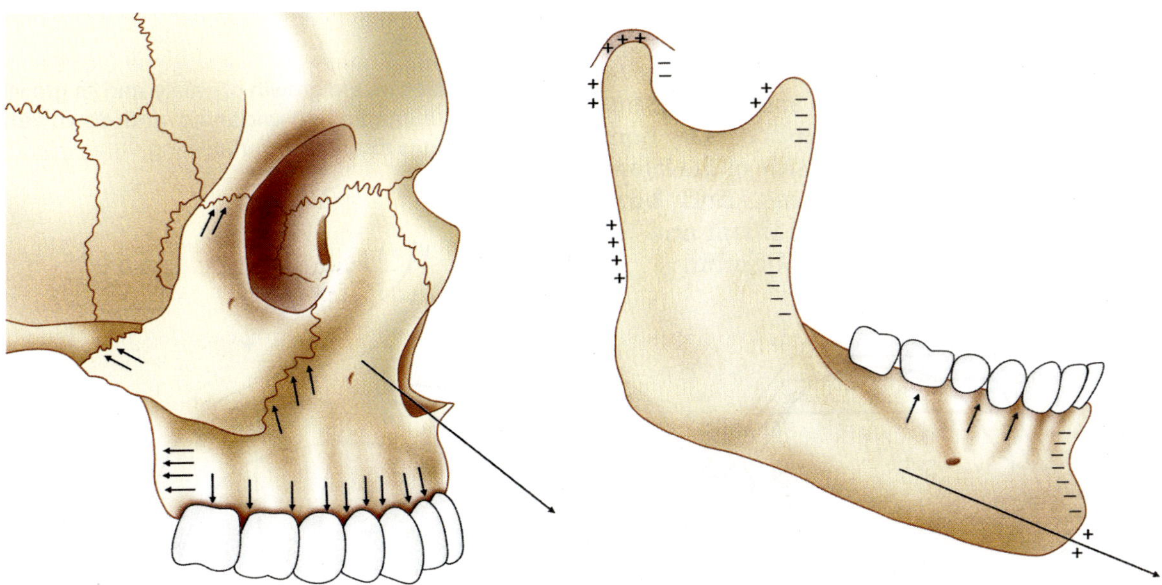

Fig. 5.26: Remodeling on the surfaces of jaws and the circummaxillary sutures contributing to growth of jaws.

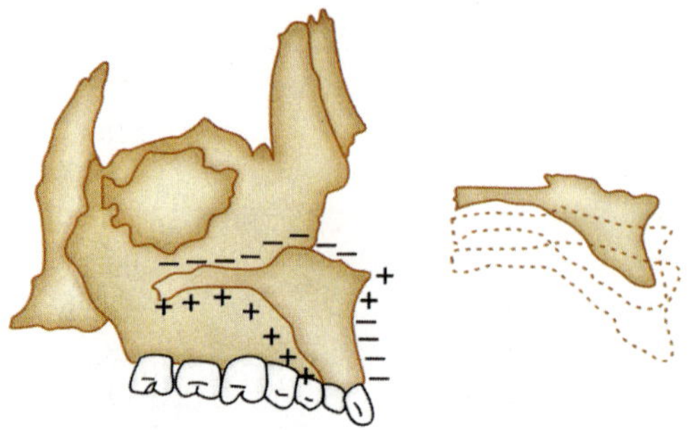

Fig. 5.28: Bony remodeling and bone growth of maxilla and palate from lateral view, and displacement of parts of maxilla in a downward and forward direction.

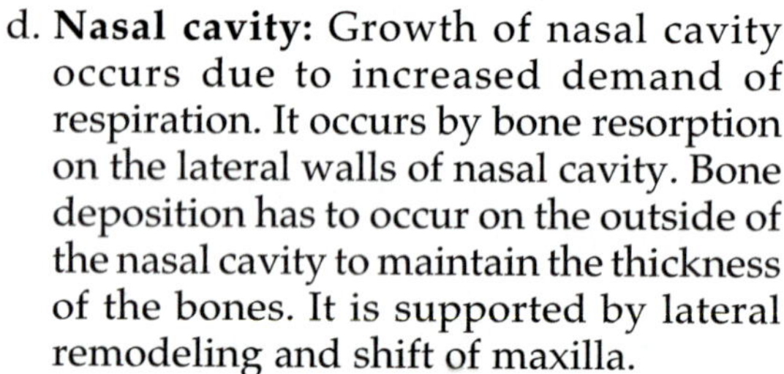

d. **Nasal cavity:** Growth of nasal cavity occurs due to increased demand of respiration. It occurs by bone resorption on the lateral walls of nasal cavity. Bone deposition has to occur on the outside of the nasal cavity to maintain the thickness of the bones. It is supported by lateral remodeling and shift of maxilla.

   Bone resorption occurs on the floor of nasal cavity (which is formed by the hard palate), while deposition occurs on the inferior surface of palate. It helps to increase the height of the nasal cavity. It helps to increase the maxillary height (Figs 5.29 to 5.31).

e. **Orbital rim:** Since nasal cavity is expanding, the orbits and its contents need to shift laterally. It occurs by bone resorption on the inner side of the lateral surface of orbital rims, and bone deposition on the medial rim and the outer side of lateral rims of orbit.

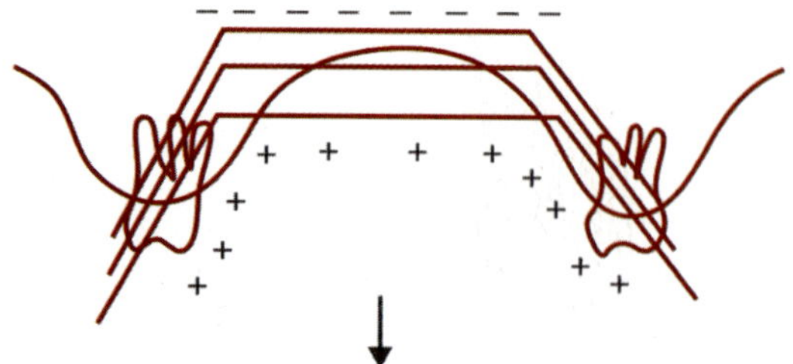

Fig. 5.29: Downward and outward remodeling of palate in a V-shape as described by Enlow.

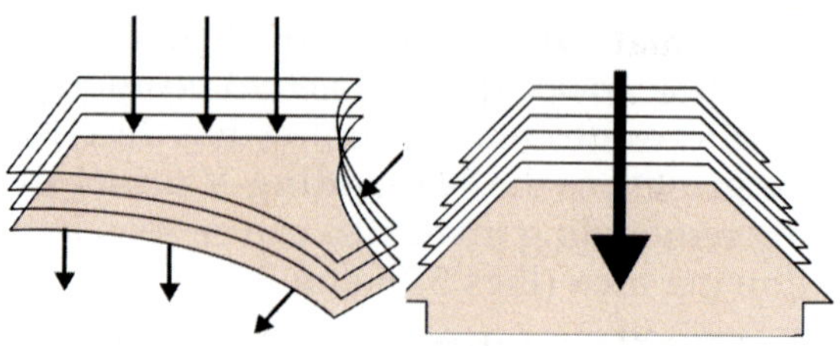

Fig. 5.30: Transverse, downward and forward growth of palate in consonance with Enlow's V-principle.

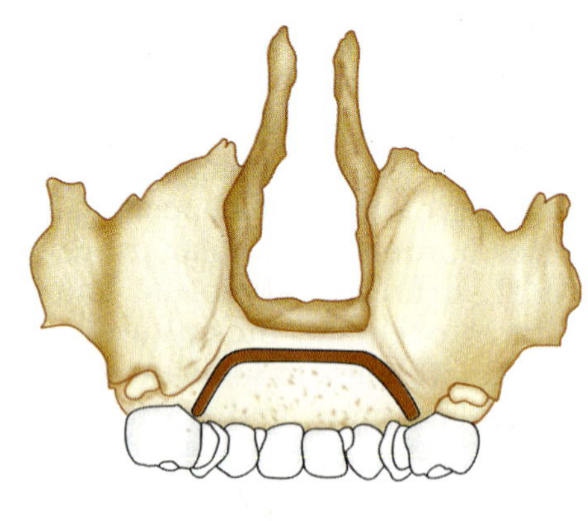

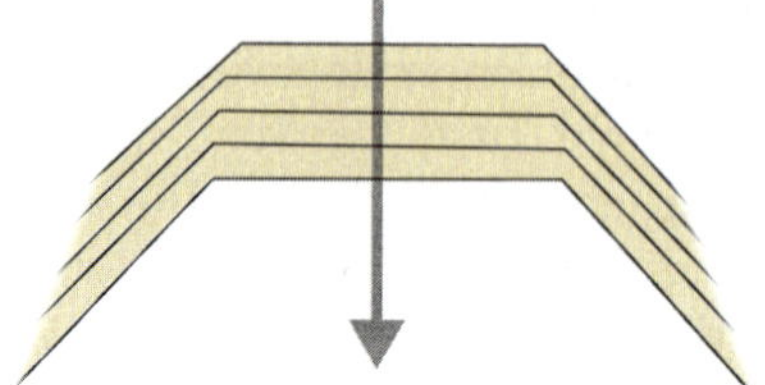

Fig. 5.31: Downward growth of palate and its growth in V-pattern leading to widening and downward transposition with ensuing remodeling.

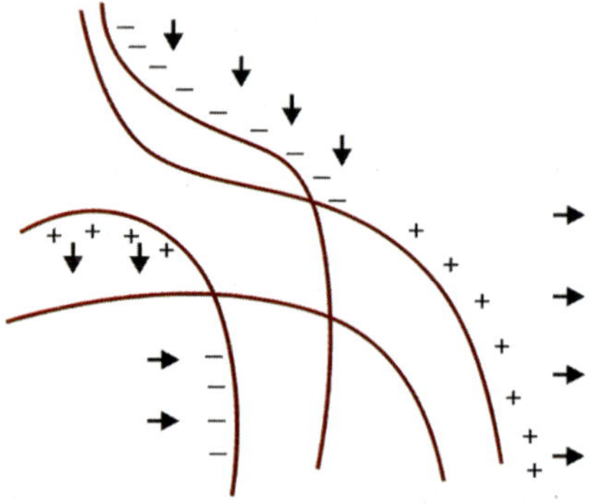

Fig. 5.32: Bone remodeling at zygomatic arch, moving it outward and backward.

f. **Zygomatic arch:** Bone resorption occurs on the anterior surface of zygomatic arch, while bone is deposited on its posterior surface. Thus, zygomatic arch moves posteriorly.

Width of the face increases by the bone deposition on lateral surface of zygomatic arch and resorption on the medial surface of arch. Alongwith, the width of maxilla increases by growth of midpalatal suture (Fig. 5.32).

g. **ANS and labial cortices:** Bone is deposited on ANS, thus making it prominent. Bone resorption occurs on labial surface of labial cortex, and the compensatory bone deposition occurs on the periosteal surface of lingual cortex, and endosteal surface of labial cortex to maintain the thickness (Fig. 5.33).

h. **Maxillary sinus:** Except mesial wall, all other walls see bone resorption, thus increasing the size of sinus. Depth of sinus increases with pneumatization, and floor of sinus comes to lie at a lower level than the nasal floor. Thus, any infection of sinus has a problem with automatic drainage through the sinus opening in lateral nasal wall. It requires a Caldwell-Luc opening in canine fossa to drain the sinus. Maxillary sinus is the **largest** of all the paranasal sinuses, it is also called as **antrum of highmore. It is the** first to develop in the body at the 4th months IU age. It opens in the middle meatus near the roof rather than the floor, so the drainage is difficult. These sinuses enlarge rapidly at 6–7 years age and then after the puberty. **Functions of sinuses are** to lighten the skull, to warm up the inspired air; to add **resonance** to the voice.

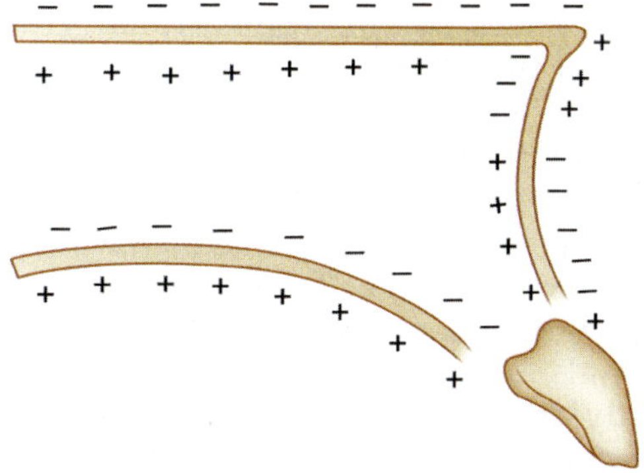

Fig. 5.33: Bone remodeling in floor of nasal cavity; oral surface of hard palate; and labial alveolar plate and ANS.

i. **Increase in width:** In the transverse direction, bone deposition occurs on the free ends of alveolar processes which increase the dental arch width. Also, the buccal segments move downward and outward, as the maxilla itself is moving downward and forward, following the principle of expanding "V".

POSTNATAL GROWTH OF MANDIBLE (Fig. 5.34)

Mandible is a U-shaped bone having condylar cartilage at each end. So, it has an endochondral growth mechanism at the ends and an intramembranous growth mechanism in the shaft, just like the long bones (Fig. 5.35). As has been discussed, only a small percentage of mandible is "endochondrally" developed, while the greater portion develops intramembrously. Growth and shape changes in the areas of muscle attachment and teeth insertion are controlled more by muscle function and eruption of teeth through bony remodeling. It follows the general growth curve and cephalocaudal gradient of growth, thus its growth continues beyond the maxillary growth.

Prenatally, the mandible ossifies by **two ossification centers,** one each in the area of future mental foramen, (appear in 6 week IU) lateral to Meckel's cartilage, ossification stops at a point, which later becomes lingula. Meckel's cartilage is the cartilage of first pharyngeal arch, and thus carries the nerve supply of the first arch, i.e. the 5th nerve. It acts

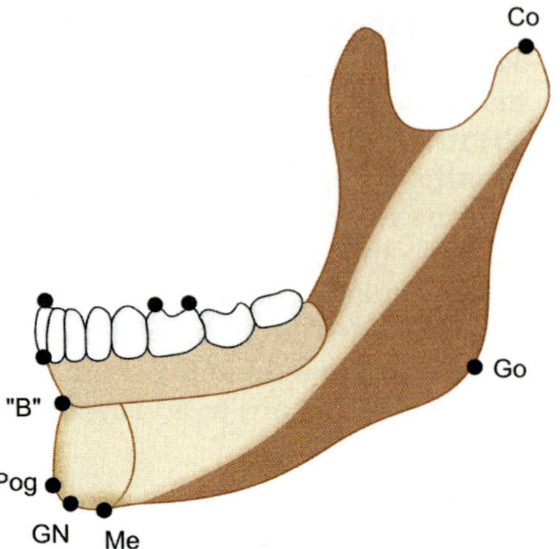

Fig. 5.34: Various functional areas on mandibular surface, where muscular attachments affect the mandibular remodeling.

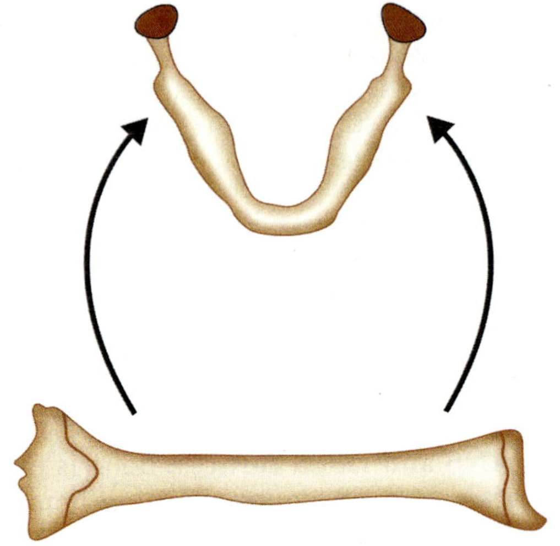

Fig. 5.35: Essentially, the mandible is like a straight bone which has been bent in middle, and has potential of growth at both ends.

only as a template, around which the mandibular development takes place mainly by intramembranous ossification. Meckel's cartilage does not itself contribute to any growth of the mandible, so mandible is not formed by endochondral ossification. It regresses with time and forms malleus, incus, mental ossicles, spine of sphenoid bone, anterior ligament of malleus and sphenomandibular ligament. Three secondary cartilages, i.e. condylar, coronoid, and symphyseal cartilages also appear.

Coronoid cartilage appears at 4 months IU, forms coronoid process and anterior ramal border, and disappears before birth.

Two symphyseal cartilages appear between two ends of Meckel's cartilage, then undergo endochondral ossification and disappear within first year of life.

Role of condylar cartilage: Condylar cartilage appears at around 12 weeks IU, occupying almost all of the developing ramus, and by 20 weeks IU, it undergoes endochondral ossification, leaving only a thin cap over the condylar head. Thus mandible is formed by both methods of ossifications. Mandible is a membrane bone which shows remodeling over all surfaces. Condylar cartilage is not a primary cartilage like in costochondral junctions, epiphyseal plates or synchondrosis. Primary cartilages have intrinsic growth potential, but the condylar cartilage is a secondary cartilage. Condylar cartilage is a secondary cartilage, (it does not develop from embryonic primary cartilages). Previously, it was considered the primary "growth center", controlling its growth. Cartilage is present as it is also a stress bearing joint (Figs 5.36a to d).

The condylar cartilage is a fibrocartilage, it has distinct collagen fibers and is affected by the environmental factors also during growth. The hyaline cartilage of the condyle is covered by a dense and thick fibrous connective tissue layer. Thus the condyle not only increases by the interstitial growth, but also by the increase in thickness by the appositional growth beneath the connective tissues covering it. Other hyaline cartilages of the body have indistinct collagen fibers and growth is affected by the epigenetic factors.

Transplantation experiments have shown that condylar cartilage does not grow in new sites. Removal of condyles in experimental animals shows the diminished size of condylar area but the rest of the mandible grows by remodeling. Experimental injection of **papain**, which interferes with chondrogenesis, also leads to deficient condylar growth but a normal remodeling. Though the

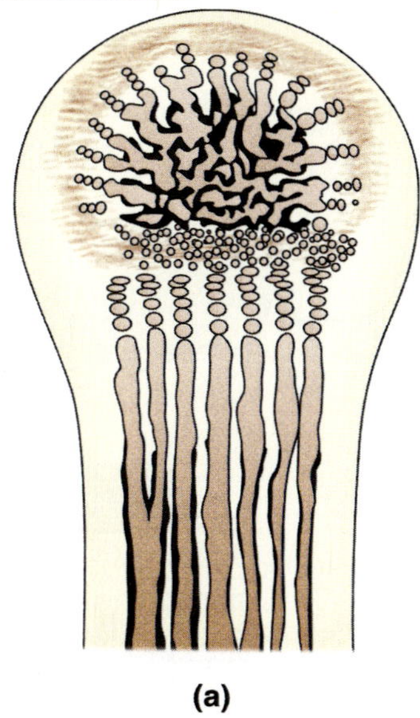

(a)

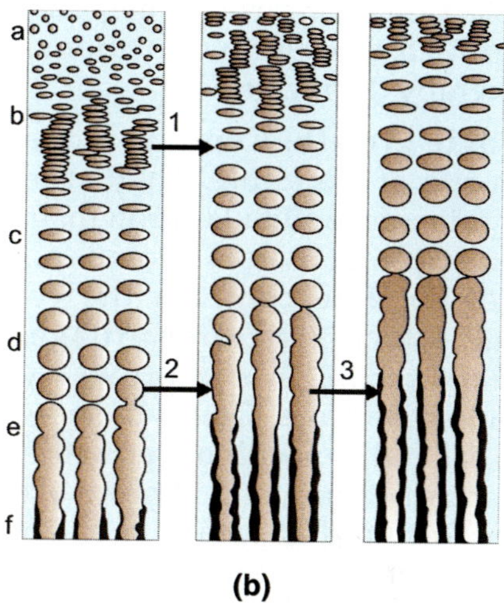

(b)

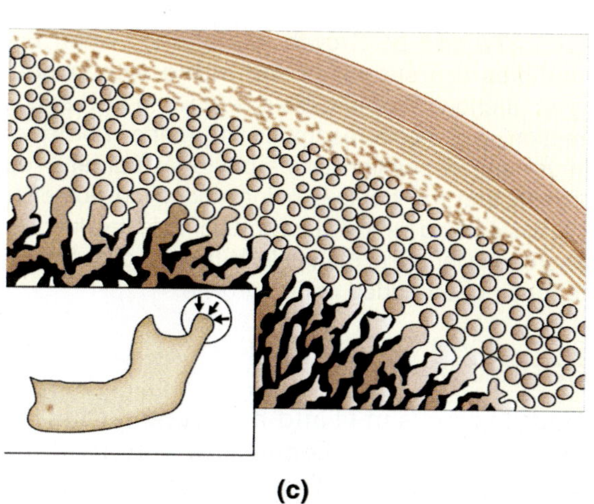

(c)

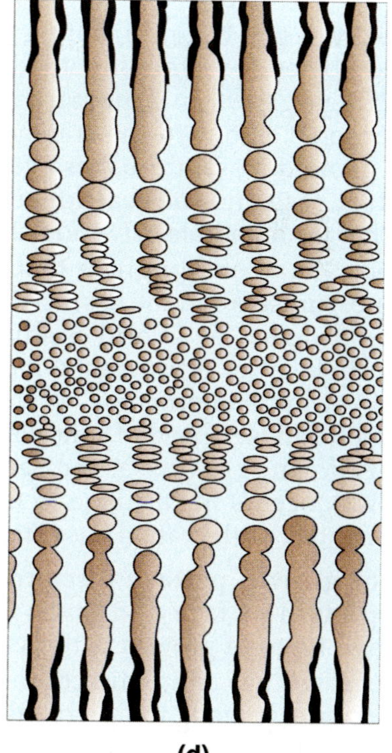

(d)

Figs 5.36a to d: Schematic diagram of endochondral ossification. Inset shows mandibular condyle which grows endochondrally, as it is having a secondary cartilage. C represents the growth cartilage of the mandibular condyle. A zone of prechondrocyte proliferation occurs just beneath a covering the layer of fibrous capsule on mandibular condyle.

condylar cartilage is a secondary cartilage, it probably plays some role in translation of the mandible. Condylar cartilage helps in mandibular growth during myofunctional appliances therapy during growth.

Condyle growth: Condyle is the major growth site of mandible. They are not the primary site of mandibular growth, but have secondary, compensatory growth potential. Head of condyle contains the condylar cartilage, which is a **fibrocartilage.** It is a secondary cartilage, and grows by proliferation of cartilage. **Condyle** shows **both interstitial and appositional growth.** Peak of condylar growth is at 12–14 years age and it ceases at around 20 years age. Condylar fractures in infants, if not managed timely, may lead to ankylosis of TMJ and mandibular growth restriction.

There are two schools of thought regarding condylar growth (Figs 5.37a and b):

1. Initially, it was believed that the condyle grows by endochondral method. As the cartilage grows in a posterosuperior direction, i.e. toward the cranial base in the glenoid fossa, it pushes against the cranial base and the reactionary thrust pushes the mandible in D and F direction.
2. Other school of thought is that the soft tissues, muscle and the orofacial capsule growth leads to D and F shifting of mandible away from cranial base, i.e. a **carry away phenomenon.** As the gap is created between head of condyle and the roof of condylar fossa, the secondary growth occurs in cartilage to maintain the contact with cranial base (Fig. 5.38).

Role of growth pattern of condyles on growth pattern of face and jaws: Condyle follows two types of growth patterns:

1. If it grows in U and B direction, i.e. anticlockwise, it leads to a vertical growth pattern of mandible, by causing a downward and backward movement of mandible.
2. If it grows in U and F direction, i.e. clockwise, then it leads to horizontal growth of the mandible (Figs 5.39a and b).

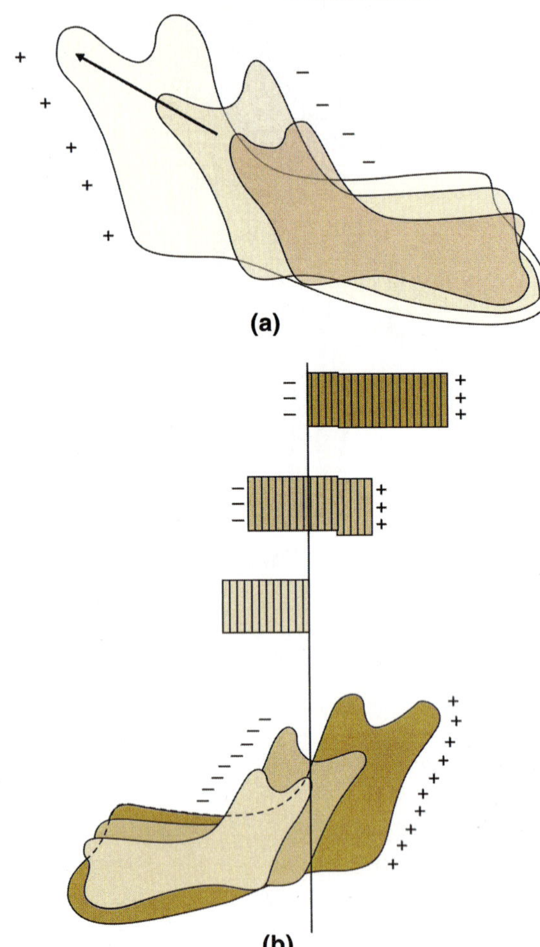

Figs 5.37a and b: Growth of mandible when the mandibles are superimposed in the symphyseal region. It shows that mandible is growing in U and B direction, with bone resorption in anterior border of ramus, and deposition on its posterior border. You can see that the bone is being added on posterior side, while being removed on anterior side and leading to increased length of mandible. Whole length of ramal width has been added during growth.

SCOTT'S CONCEPT

Condyle grows in U and B direction, thus the mandible moves in D and F direction, along an arc, which runs from foramen ovale to mandibular foramen to mental foramen (unloaded nerve concept). According to him, the mandible has three basic parts, i.e. basal/tubular, muscular and alveolar. The basal part is tube-like which is the central foundation of

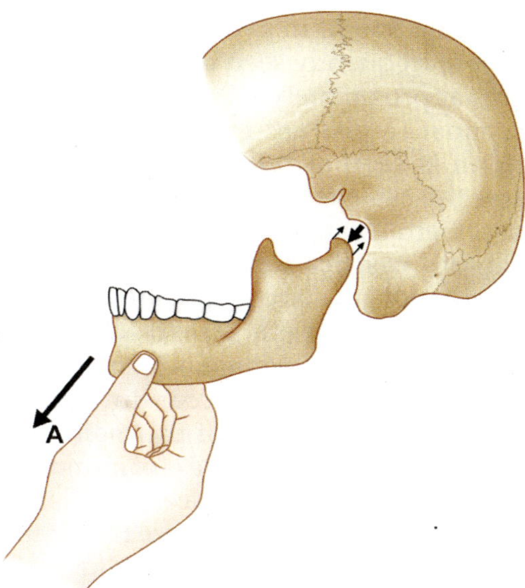

Fig. 5.38: Mandible translocates/grows in a downward and forward direction under the influence of upward and backward growth of condyle.

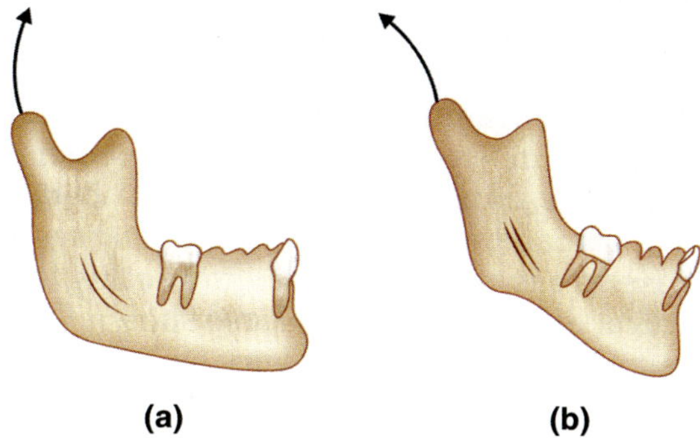

Fig. 5.39: It shows the direction of mandibular growth: (a) Arrow showing U and F direction leads to a horizontal growth of mandible, (b) while U and B arrow shows the vertical growth of mandible.

mandible, running from the condyle to the symphysis (Fig. 5.40). Basal tubular part protects mandibular nerve (**unloaded nerve concept**) and follows a logarithmic spiral in its D and F growth. The most constant portion of mandible is the arc from foramen ovale to mandibular foramen to mental foramen. It follows the arc followed by mandibular nerve. The muscular portion (gonial angle, ramus and the coronoid process) is under the influence of the masseter, medial pterygoid and temporalis muscle. Alveolar bone exists to hold the teeth and it is gradually resorbed in the event of tooth loss.

Microskeletal Units of Mandible

According to functional matrix theory of Moss, the mandible acts as a macroskeletal unit, and is composed of many microskeletal units. They are corpus of mandible, condyle, coronoid, angular part, dentoalveolar unit. Their growth is influenced by their functional matrices. Thus, the growth of mandible is a summation

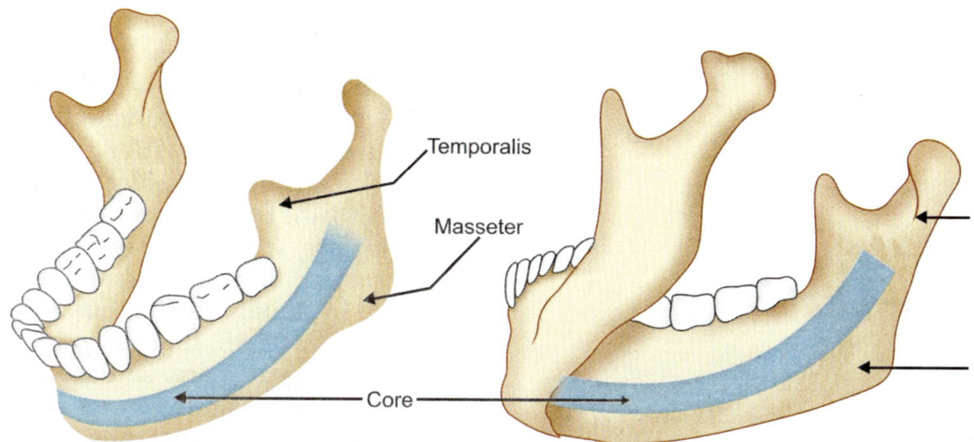

Fig. 5.40: Unloaded nerve concept of mandibular growth: the blue core shows the track of inferior alveolar nerve and canal in mandible around which the growth takes place.

of growth of these units. The coronoid process is under the influence of temporalis. The gonial angle is influenced by medial pterygoid muscle on inner side, and part of masseter on outer side. Muscle attachments on certain areas of mandible act as soft tissue matrices for those areas and help in remodeling and cortical drift. Experiments have shown that if the muscles are removed very early or if the nerves and vessels serving these muscles are severed, then there is deficiency of growth in those areas. The alveolar process is under the influence of the dentition. If tooth is absent, ankylosed, or extracted; the alveolar process in that area will remain deficient. Condyle has lateral pterygoid muscle attached. The masticatory muscles and other suprahyoid and infrahyoid muscles influence various functions of oral cavity and influence the mandibular position and growth. The soft-tissue development carries the mandible forward and downward, while condylar growth by endochondral growth mechanism fills in the resultant space to maintain contact with the articular fossa. It cannot be achieved by intramembranous growth (Fig. 5.41).

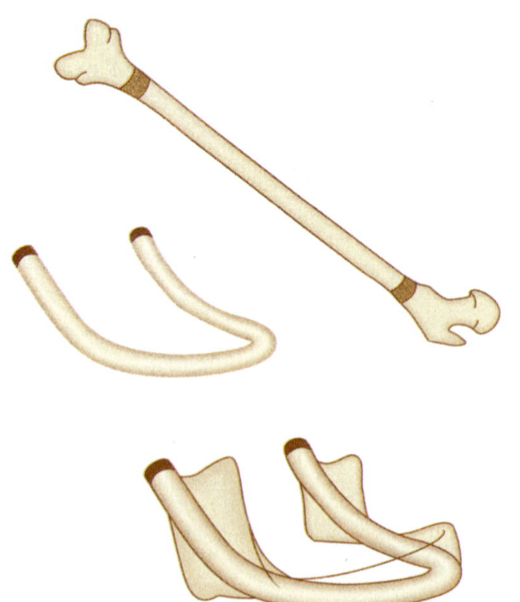

Fig. 5.41: Different areas of bone remodeling on the surface of mandible.

Timing: Spurts in mandibular dimensions are more frequently seen in boys than girls. It occurs approximately 1½ years earlier in girls. The most important spurt in mandibular growth is seen at puberty, generally seen before the peak height velocity. Almost all the first pubertal spurts are observed after ulnar-sesamoid ossification and before onset of menstruation, the two developmental events, used to predict skeletal growth spurts.

In contrast to maxilla, both endochondral and periosteal activities occur during growth of mandible. Two rami of the mandible are quite short at birth. Condyle is of minimal size, and the articular eminences are flat. This morphology is important, since the infant has to bring the mandible forward during suckling. Two halves of mandible are separated in the midline by a thin cartilage known as the symphyseal cartilage, which gets replaced by bone within first year of life, and the two halves of mandible fuse. Since there is no suture in the mandible, it is very difficult to expand by orthodontic means. Any change in width of mandible, after the first year of life is mainly due to bone remodelling at posterior border in an expanding "V" pattern. The rami diverge outward from below upward following expanding-V-principle of Enlow. Also the additive growth at coronoid notch, coronoid process and condyle increases the interramal distance (Figs 5.42 to 5.44).

Growth of Ramus

Bone resorption occurs on anterior border, and deposition on the posterior border of ramus, which helps to maintain the width of the ramus. It also provides the space for erupting molars by increasing the dental arch length. Also, the bone deposition occurs on its lateral surface, while bone resorption on the medial surface, thus increasing the width of mandible in ramal area. It thus follows the expanding-V pattern. It helps to increase the size of pharyngeal space, and accommodates the increased muscular mass attached to ramus. Functional influences are seen in growth of mandible. In Neanderthal man, the jaws were broad and big as they used to eat coarse food, which activated the muscles and helped in more growth of mandible. But due to change in dietary habits to softer diet, the growth of mandible is not that much. It has led to impaction of third molars also due to less space. Vertical ramal growth provides space vertically due to condylar growth and it provides space in which both upper and lower alveolar bones grow as the teeth erupt.

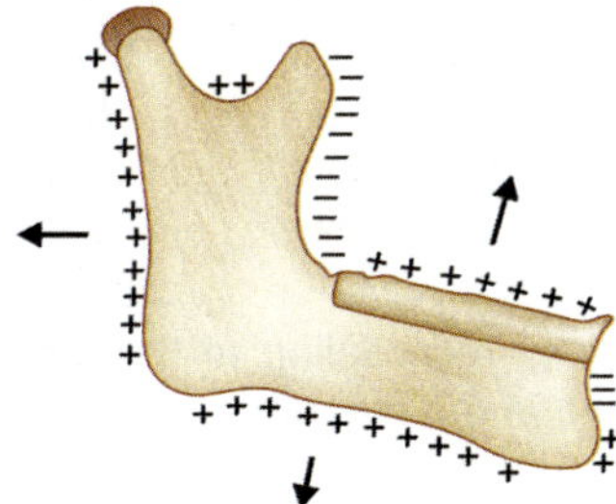

Fig. 5.42: Bone remodeling at various borders of mandible.

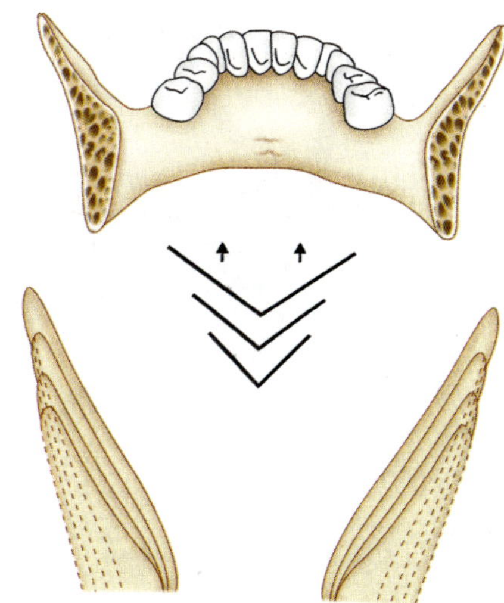

Fig. 5.43: V-shape growth of posterior region of mandible

Body or Corpus of Mandible (Fig. 5.45)

With the above discussed ramal remodelling, the length of mandibular body increases, increasing the dental arch length and providing space for permanent molars. On the lateral side of body, deposition occurs, while on the inner side resorption occurs and thus the width increases in accordance with Enlow's V-principle. It helps to accommodate the increasing bulk of soft tissues of tongue, muscles of floor of mouth, etc. The gonial angle, i.e. between ramus and mandibular body, is more in infants. With remodeling, this angle decreases to 130° in adults.

Angle of Mandible (Fig. 5.46)

Bone resorption occurs on lingual side of angle of mandible at the posteroinferior aspect and the deposition on the anterosuperior aspect. On buccal side, the bone is deposited on the posteroinferior part, while resorption on the anterosuperior part. It helps to maintain the thickness of the bone and relocates the angular part, resulting in the flaring of angle of mandible, again in consonance of the V-principle.

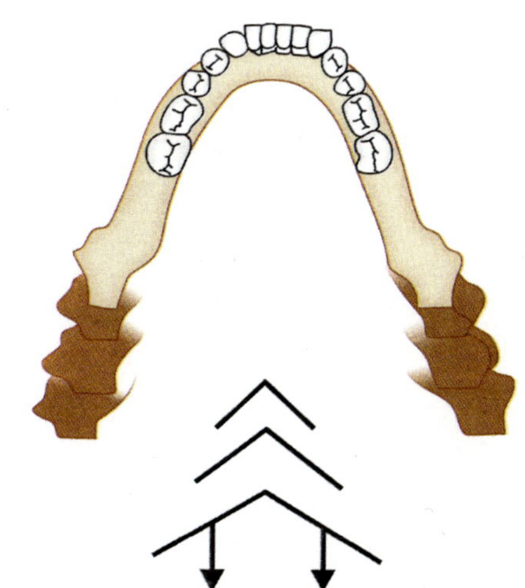

Fig. 5.44: Mandibular growth and widening from top view according to Enlow's V-principle of growth, with remodeling in coronoid areas.

The Lingual Tuberosity (Fig. 5.47)

It is the counterpart of maxillary tuberosity and forms the boundary of body and ramus of mandible. Bone deposits on the posterior face of tuberosity so it is relocated posteriorly. There is bone resorption on the anterior aspect, and also just below it, which leads to its prominence. Thus a depression is also created below the lingual tuberosity which is called lingual fossa.

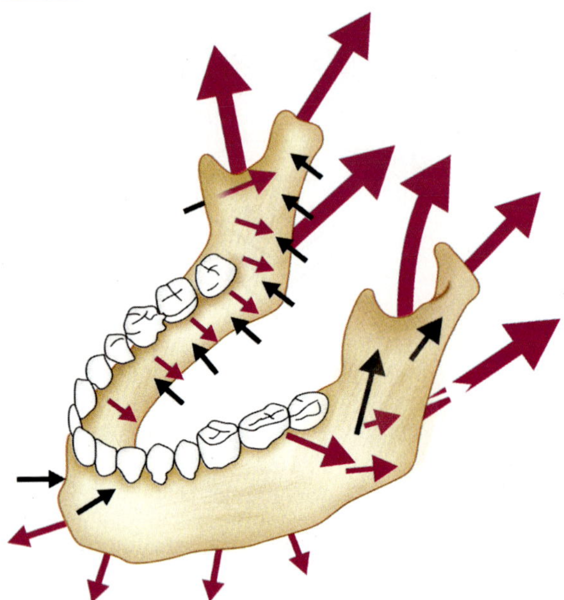

Fig. 5.45: Bone remodeling on the mandibular surface and thus change in dimension and shape of mandible.

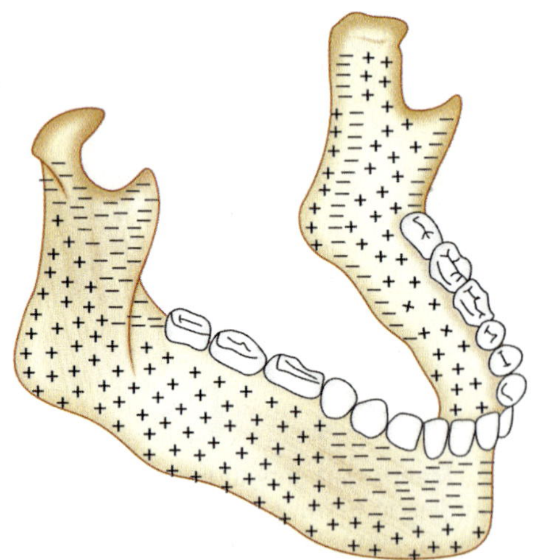

Fig. 5.46: Bone remodeling at various surfaces of mandible.

Alveolar Processes

They house the teeth and develop when teeth erupt, as the teeth are their functional matrices. The teeth erupt in occlusal, and mesial direction. Alveolar processes of the mandible grows upward and outward to accommodate the permanent teeth. As the teeth erupt, the alveolar bone is added to increase the height and width of alveolar process. If teeth is embedded, or impacted, the alveolar bone growth is deficient there. Also, after extraction, the level of alveolar bone decreases due to resorption of bone.

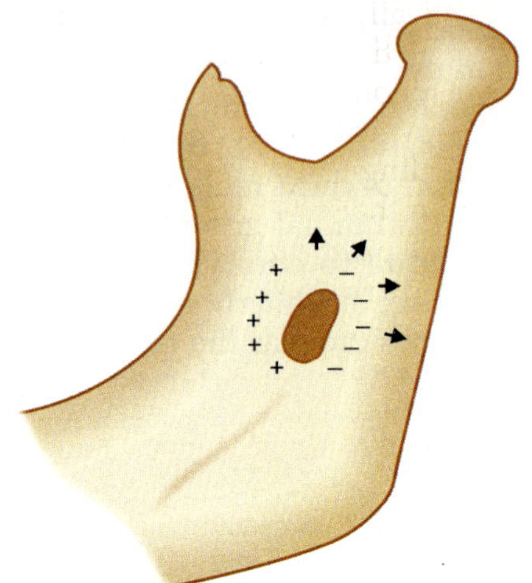

Fig. 5.47: Bony remodeling at the entry of inferior alveolar nerve in the mandible.

Chin: At birth, chin is very small, but its growth occurs with age. Its growth and form is also influenced by sex, genetics, racial and ethnicity. Bone resorption occurs in the area just above the chin and below the labial alveolar process, while deposition occurs on the prominence of chin button. It leads to increase prominence of the chin and a concavity develops above it. Bone apposition at symphysis seems to be the last change in shape during the growing period, especially in males, which occurs between 16 and 25 years of age. It gives a new shape to the symphysis in males, while it is less apparent in females. It gives rise to strong chin in males and soft chin in females.

The chin is formed in part of the mental ossicles from accessory cartilages and the ventral end of Meckel's cartilage and develops almost as independent unit of mandible. Sex differences in chin becomes significant only at adolescence, due to development of mental protuberance and tubercles. Large chins are characteristically masculine. The chin may be influenced by the functional forces exerted by lateral pterygoids, which while pulling the mandible forward, indirectly stress the mental symphyseal lingual region by the inward pull of muscles in that area.

The mental protuberance is formed by bony deposition during childhood. It gets prominent by bone resorption in the supramental alveolar region, creating the supramental concavity which is known as "point B" in cephalometrics terms. At birth, the mandible tends to be retrognathic to maxilla and a convex profile is seen. This retrognathic condition is normally corrected early in postnatal life by rapid mandibular growth and forward displacement.

Coronoid Process (Fig. 5.48)

Coronoid process develops from coronoid cartilage in the mandible and provides attachment to temporalis muscle. Its growth is under the influence of this muscle. At birth, the height of condyle and coronoid process is small. There is shallow sigmoid notch. With further remodeling, the depth of notch increases, along with the height of condyle and coronoid processes. Its growth follows expanding-V principle by remodeling (Fig. 5.49).

Differences Between Infants and Adults (Figs 5.50 and 5.51)

1. In infants, since the condyles are inclined almost horizontally, thus the condylar growth leads to an increase in length of mandible rather than its height.

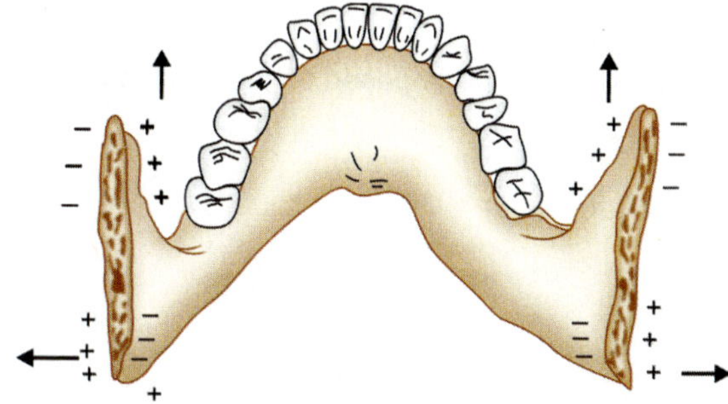

Fig. 5.48: Remodeling at gonial region and coronoid process of mandible, and growth in V-pattern.

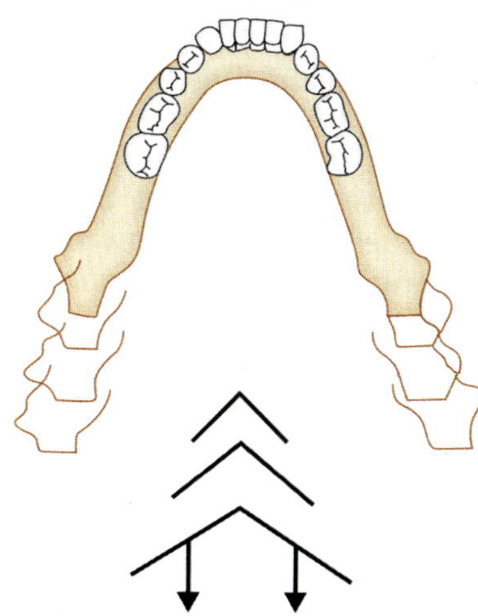

Fig. 5.49: V-shape growth of mandible, especially at condyle and coronoid regions.

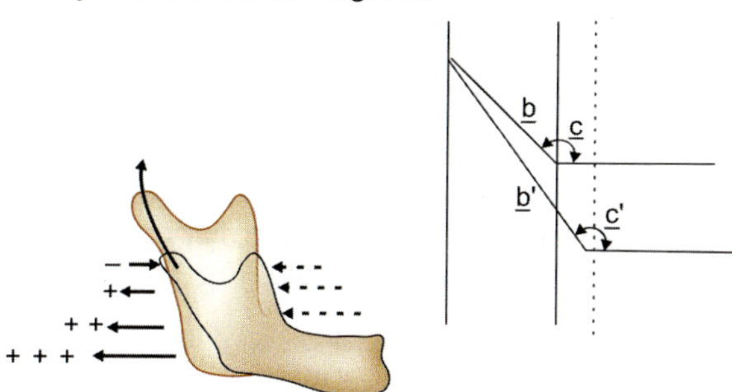

Fig. 5.50: Closure of gonial angle and posterior movement of gonial region of mandible with ensuing bony remodeling and growth. There occurs bone resorption at anterior border, and bone deposition on posterior border of ramus.

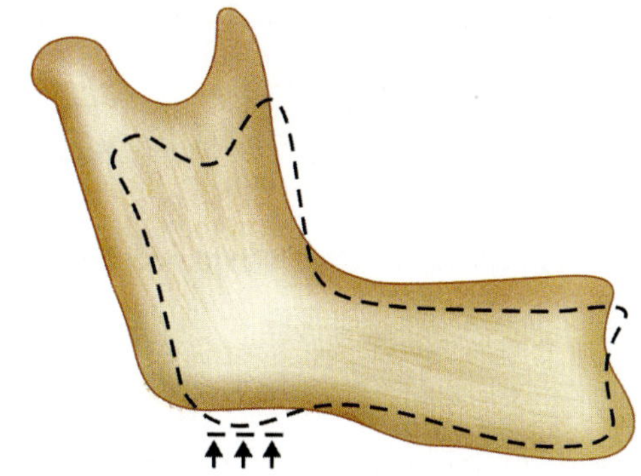

Fig. 5.51: Shape change in mandible with remodeling

2. The mental neurovascular bundle exits from mandible at right angles or even facing in a slightly forward direction at

birth. The regular remodeling and the forward shift of growing mandibular body changes the direction of the mental foramen during infancy and childhood. In adulthood, the mental foramen becomes to be directed backward. It occurs due to forward growth of body of the mandible and due to differential growth of bone and periosteum. The changed direction of mental foramen directs the administration of local anesthetic to the mental nerve. In infants and children, the syringe needle should be applied at right angles to mandibular body to enter the mental foramen, while obliquely from behind to achieve entry in mental foramen in the adults.

3. The position of mental foramen also changes in its vertical position with age. When teeth are present, it is located midway between the upper and lower borders of mandible. In the edentulous mandible, due to extreme bone resorption, it comes near the upper margin of the thinned mandible (Fig. 5.52).
4. Mandibular foramen lies at the level of OP in adults while at a level lower to OP in infants. So while giving the inferior alveolar nerve block, the needle is directed downward in the infants and is kept parallel to OP in adults.

Signs of Growth Completion

Physical signs are:

In males: Appearance of facial hair, body, pubic and axillary hair, hoarseness of voice, increased size or prominence of Adam's apple, increased size of penis, increase in height and weight.

In females: Appearance of pubic hair, increased size of breasts, onset of menstruation, increased weight, fat deposition on buttocks, etc.

Cephalometric signs: See CVMI

Skeletal indicators: Hand wrist signs, SMI, etc.

Dental indicators: Signs of canine calcification from OPG.

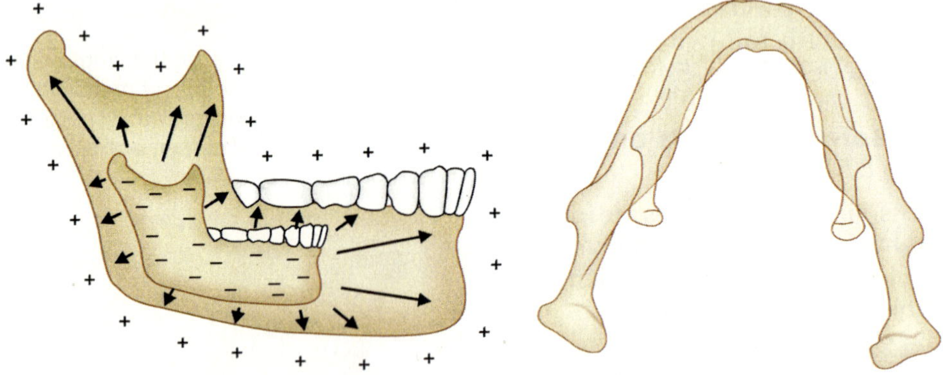

Fig. 5.52: Growth of mandible with remodeling when a child's mandible is superimposed on the adult mandible.

VIVA VOCE QUESTIONS

1. **What do you mean by growth?**
   It is an increase in size.

2. **What do you mean by development?**
   It is the progress toward maturity, i.e. growth + differentiation + translocation.

3. **What is the amount of the height increase?**
   Height increases by 5,000-fold in the prenatal period as opposed to only threefold increase during the entire postnatal period.

4. **What is the meaning of the term differentiation?**
   It is a change from generalized cell to a specialized kind, i.e. a change in quality.

5. **What is the meaning of maturation in context of the growth?**
   It expresses the qualitative changes which occur with age.

6. **What is the translocation of the bone?**
   It is **passive** growth of bone. It is a **change in the position** of whole bone. It depends on capsular matrix and is aka displacement of the bone.

7. **What are the components of the primary growth?**
   It is actual **translation** (passive growth) and remodeling of bones.

8. **What do you mean by secondary growth?**
   It is the **transformation** (periosteal) + sutural growth.

9. **What do you mean by transformation?**
   It is **active** growth. It is the apposition and resorption in a bone. It is a local change and occurs under the influence of periosteal matrix, and is aka the apposition and resorption in a bone.

10. **What do you mean by the intrinsic genetic factors and the epigenetic factors?**
    Intrinsic genetic factors mean those factors, which are inherent in the skull tissues themselves. The epigenetic factors mean that these factors are genetically determined, but manifest their influence in an indirect way by intermediary action on the associated structures (eye, brain, etc.). Modification of these soft tissues has a modifying effect on the primary craniofacial complex.

11. **What are the different mechanisms of bone growth?**
    a. Bone deposition and resorption = known as **bone remodeling.**
    b. Cortical drift = combination of bone deposition and resorption resulting in a growth movement toward the depository surface.
    c. Displacement = is the movement of whole bone as a unit. It is due to pull or push of different soft and bone tissues as they all continue to enlarge.
    d. Primary or active displacement = i.e. if bone gets displaced due to its own growth. For example, growth at maxillary tuberosity pushes maxilla anteriorly.
    e. Secondary or passive displacement = i.e. if the bone gets displaced due to growth and enlargement of an **adjacent bone**.
    f. Sutural growth.
    g. Enlow's expanding-V principle = many bones/parts of the bone have V-shape pattern of the growth, which occurs toward wider ends of the V due to selective apposition and resorption.
    h. Enlow's counterpart principle = states that the growth of any given facial or cranial part relates specifically to other structural and geometric counterparts in face and cranium.
    i. Neurotrophism = is a nonimpulse transmitting neural function which involves axoplasmic transport and provides for long term interaction b/w neurons and innervated tissues, which homeostatically regulates the morphological, compositional and functional integrity of these tissues.

12 **What are the different periods of prenatal growth and development?**
   It has been studied in three phases viz.

1. Period of ovum	0–2 weeks of IU age
2. Period of embryo	2–8 weeks of IU age
3. Period of fetus	after 8 weeks till birth.

13. How are the implants used as a method of studying the growth?

The implants are placed at particular sites in maxillary and mandibular bones. The subject is followed on a longitudinal basis by taking the lateral cephalograms at particular age of the subjects and studied. The position of implants does not change with growth and they are used for superimposing the serial cephalograms.

Various sites of implant placement in maxilla are:

1. Hard palate behind maxillary deciduous canines.
2. Below ANS
3. Zygomatic process of maxilla.
4. Border b/w hard palate and alveolar process medial to first molars.

14. Which are the various sites of implant placement in mandible?

1. In midline at the anterior aspect of symphysis.
2. Two pins on RHS of the body of mandible below first premolar, and below and b/w 2nd premolar and the 1st molars.
3. one pin on the RHS ramus at the level of occlusal plane (OP). This becomes free in the soft tissues as growth occurs due to resorption of anterior border of the ramus.

15. When does the midsagittal suture close?

It does not close until the middle of third decade of life.

16. What is the relation of age and the growth/ size of cranial base?

When related to the age, the size of the cranial base at

1. Birth is 55–60% of adult size,
2. 4–7 years is 94% of adult size, and
3. 8–13 years is 98% of adult size.

17. How does the ratio of the size of face vary with that of whole body with age?

When related to the age, the size of the face at Birth is 50% of the size of the body, at 4–7 years is 33% and at 8–13 years is 12%, i.e. 1:8 of the body size.

18. Which all bones are intramembranous in development?

1. Pure intramembranous: Frontal, zygomatic, parietal, palatal, maxilla, vomer, nasal, lacrimal.
2. Pure endochondral: Ethmoid, inferior nasal concha.
3. Mixed: Mandible, occipital, sphenoid, temporal.

19. What do you mean by the cephalocaudal gradient of growth?

Cephalocaudal gradient of growth means that the amount of growth of structures away from the head increases toward the caudal ends. For example, lower limbs grow more than the upper limbs; the mandible grows more and up to later age than maxilla.

It helps **decrease the overjet** which is especially marked during first 6 months of life. Mandible seems to erupt from below the cranium.

In newborn, the cranium is 8–9× larger than face, an example of the cephalocaudal gradient of growth. Later on, the facial growth catches up.

20. What is the general direction of growth of face with respect to skull and cranial base?

Downwards and forward.

21. From which pharyngeal arch, the maxilla and mandible are formed?

First arch, i.e. mandibular arch gives rise to maxilla and mandible, Meckel's cartilage, malleus, incus, muscles of mastication and the anterior digastric **m**.

22. How is the palate formed?

Palatal shelves arise from the maxillary processes. They first go vertically and then move horizontally with the lowered position of the tongue, then they fuse anteriorly with the primary palate (which arises from the median nasal process) and with one another. The fusion starts in the middle of the processes and proceeds anteriorly and posteriorly.

23. How does the growth in maxillary length occurs?

By apposition at maxillary tuberosity.

24. What do you mean by differential growth pattern?

Different tissues grow at different rates at different times. **Scammon's growth curves** show that lymphoid, nervous, somatic and genital tissues grow at different ages and rates. According to Scammon's growth studies, the lymphoid > neural > general > genital tissues growth.

Neural tissue is of adult size at = 6–7 years age.

Lymphoid tissue is 200% size at = late childhood phase, it starts involuting itself and becomes of normal size by 18 years age.

Genital tissues = grow at puberty, after it growth ceases. The start of menstruation in females and development of secondary sexual features in females is the sign of completion of growth in females. It starts increasing when the lymphoid tissues start decreasing at approx. 10–12 years of age.

25. How does the growth of general tissues relate with time?

Rapid growth occurs = up to 2–3 years age.
Slow growth = 3–10 years age
Rapid growth = after 10 years to 18–20 years age.

26. How does the development of face and neck region differ from other body parts?

Nearly all tissues of face and neck originate from ectoderm (including muscles and bone also, which elsewhere in the body originate from the mesoderm). Most of these tissues develop from NCC. Most of facial structures arise from NCC. Any interference with their movement leads to deformities, e.g. hemifacial microsomia, mandibulofacial dysostosis, i.e. Treacher Collins syndrome where both U/L jaws involved especially lateral face is involved due to excessive cell death in trigeminal ganglion which affects neural crest cells (NCCs).

27. Which is the most critical phase of the facial development?

Most of the problems, which result in craniofacial anomalies arise in 3rd stage of development, i.e. 19–28 days (4th week). It is the period in which the clefts develop, upto the 12 weeks IU age.

28. Which is the most common congenital defect of face?

CLP. Clefts arise during 4th developmental stage (first trimester).

29. Which is the most common congenital defect of the body?

Club foot.

30. Tell us a few points about the development of palate.

Formation of primary-palate is evident by 28–38 IU days, and of **secondary palate by 42–55 days IU.** The primary palate develops from the frontonasal process, while the secondary palate develops from the palatal shelves from the maxillary process. Fusion of the shelves progresses from A to P and reaches the soft palate.

31. What are the derivatives of primary palate?

It develops in the premaxilla and the alveolar process underlying it and part of the inside of the upper lip.

32. Which processes are involved in palatal development?

- Maxillary process
- Palatal process from maxillary process
- Frontonasal process = forms the premaxillary region
- It develops during 8–12 weeks of IU life.

Initial contact of palatal processes is in the central region of the palatal shelves.

- Ossification starts at 8th weeks of IU life.
- Midpalatal suture ossifies by 12–14 years of age.

33. How does the maturation of oral function progresses?

It follows **a gradient from anterior to posterior**, for example

Speech first sounds = bilabial	m, p, b
Tongue tip consonants	t, d
Sibilants	s, z
Posterior tongue positioning	r

34. When does the maxillary sinus develop?

It develops at around 3rd month of life.

35. When can you see the mandible developing in the embryo?

Mandible is recognizable in **shape at 8th week.**

36. What is the role of Meckle's cartilage during the mandibular development?

Although Meckle's C is a cartilaginous structure, still the development of mandible is mainly intramembranous, with only small part is endochondral. Meckle's C acts as a splint, around which the bone of mandible develops and the cartilage itself does not take any part in the bone formation.

37. Which areas develop by endochondral ossification in mandible?

Only three areas are endochondral in mandible, i.e. condyle, coronoid and mental areas.

38. What is the difference in the growth pattern of cranial base and cranial vault?

Cranial base (chondrocranium/neurocranium) grows endochondrally especially at synchondroses, bones of the cranial vault (desmocranium) develop by intramembranous growth and grow by sutural growth and remodeling. Cranial base is endochondral especially of midline structures. Desmocranium has neurocranial capsule and orofacial capsule.

39. What are the remnants of Meckle's cartilage?

These are malleus, incus, mental ossicles, spine of sphenoid bone, anterior ligament of malleus and sphenomandibular ligament.

40. Which is the first structure to develop in the primordium of lower jaw?

It is mandibular division of 5th N.

41. How does the growth of neurocranium and splanchnocranium differ?

Neurocranium = follows neural growth pattern, splanchnocranium (lower face) follows general/bodily growth pattern.

42. What is the difference between the growth of bone and the cartilage?

Cartilage grows both by interstitial and appositional growth. Bone grows by additive or apposition only (it can't grow by interstitial or expansile activity).

43. How does the condylar cartilage differ from the epiphyseal cartilage?

44. What is the difference of condylar cartilage with other hyaline cartilage of the body?

Epiphyseal C (if transplanted) can grow independently-so it is **a primary cartilage** with genetic potential. But, **condylar cartilage is secondary cartilage** and cannot grow after transplantation.

45. Where lies the biologic center of the growth of the face?

Stationary biologic center lies in the body of sphenoid bone. It is marked in the cephalogram by the position of **foramen rotundum**.

46. Mandible develops by how many ossification centres?

There is single ossification center for the development of each half of mandible. It appears in 6th week of IU life. It is present in the future premolar region, i.e. at the bifurcation of inferior alveolar n. in the mental and incisive branches. The ossification stops at the future mandibular lingula.

47. How does the growth of face and skull depend on functional matrices?

Up to 5th year, it is neurocranial dominance. After 5 year is the orofacial dominance of growth.

48. How are the epigenetic factors different from the genetic factors?

Epigenetic factors are genetically determined but influence in an indirect way by intermediary action on associated structures (eye, brain, etc.).

49. What is the influence of nasal septum on the growth of maxilla?

It is more important in anteroposterior growth than vertical growth of maxilla.

50. What are synchondroses? Which synchondrosis affects the growth of the cranial base?

Synchondroses are the sites of growth containing the intervening cartilage in between the two parts of the growing bone. So, the growth is cartilagineous here. There are four main synchondroses affecting the growth of cranial base specifically and the facial skeleton generally. These are:

- Sphenoethmoidal = close at 5–25 year (exactly unknown).
- Intersphenoidal = close at birth.
- Sphenooccipital = close at 20th year = main synchondroses and most important.
- Inter occipital = close at 3–5 years.

51. Which type of skeletal jaw malocclusion is seen in achondroplasia?

Skeletal class III relationship is present in this condition due to maxillary hypoplasia. It occurs due to absence of cartilagineous parts in the synchondroses of cranial base and hence the growth of cranial base is deficient. Since maxillary growth is affected by the growth of cranial base, so the maxillary AP deficiency is there.

52. What is the position of metopic suture?

It lies between the two halves of frontal bones before their fusion.

53. What is the direction of growth of the different craniofacial components?

a. Basal cranium = U/F
b. Maxilla = D/F
c. Mandible's condyle = U/B
d. Mandible = D/F.

54. What is the direction of mandibular rotation in horizontal and vertical growth patterns?

Mandible rotates in upward and forward direction in horizontal growth pattern leading to skeletal deep bite, while in downward and backward direction in vertical growth pattern leading to skeletal open bite.

55. What is the direction of condylar growth in horizontal and vertical growth patterns?

It is upward and forward in horizontal growth pattern, and upward and backward in vertical growth pattern.

56. What is the difference in growth sequence of cranium and the face?

Cranium growth occurs in **DW (H)**, i.e. growth in D is most rapid, with growth in W and H in that order. In **FACE, the pattern is HD (W), i.e.** H shows greatest incremental changes with age and W shows least incremental change with age. So **at birth, height of cranium and width of face are closest to adult size.**

In other words, the sequence of growth completion in cranium is HWD, while in face is WDH.

57. What is the difference in the velocity of growth of cranium and the face?

In cranium, the D > W > H; and in face there is H > D > W, i.e. at birth, the H of cranium and W of the face are the closest to the adult size.

58. How does the growth in female differ from the males?

Female pubertal spurt occurs 2–3 years ahead of that of male. Also, there are mostly only 2 spurts in females while males generally show 3 spurts. Females mature earlier than males.

59. Which is the basic maxillary skeletal unit?

Infraorbital neurovascular triad.

60. Which are the general features of maxillary growth?

a. Maxillary width is completed quite at early age (i.e. follows neural growth curve—as it is attached to cranial base.
b. Elongation of dental arches occurs at free (distal) ends only. Actual changes, which occur in maxilla, are controlled by EPIGENETIC FACTORS. Indirect genetic control is known as EPIGENETIC.
c. Growth completion sequence in dimensions with age is WDH (width earliest completed). It is important clinically, since orthodontic expansion works best during younger age.
d. The position of maxilla is dependent on the growth at the sphenooccipital and sphenoethmoidal synchondroses. It is because nasomaxillary complex is attached to cranial base.
e. While growth of cranial base is mostly endochondral, the growth of cranial vault and maxilla is intramembranous.
f. Early midface horizontal growth is tied to endochondrally induced anterior cranial base increase.
g. In late stages, vertical growth dominates the horizontal growth in maxilla.
h. Mainly sutural and remodeling leading to translation and transformation.
i. Midpalatal suture: does not start closing till 8–10 years of age.
j. Nasal septum shows endochondral growth.

61. How does the nasomaxillary complex grow in the face?

It is due to growth at sutures, surface remodeling, and displacement. Nasal cartilage also plays its role in its growth. A deficiency in nasal C for example, due to trauma, leads to a deficient maxilla.

62. What are the general features of growth of mandible?

a. It starts developing prenatally and is recognizable in shape by 8th week IU.
b. Lower jaw is the **first to develop** in the facial skeleton.
c. Its growth **follows general tissue growth curve**.
d. Ratio of alveolar plate length to the total mandibular length is relatively constant.
e. **At birth,** the size of mandibular arch is sufficient to accommodate all primary teeth if erupted.
f. Two halves of mandible fuse by 12–18 months age.

g. Main growth of mandible after birth occurs at condyle, ramus, alveolar bone.
h. D/F movement of mandible is primarily passive translation.
i. Mandibular growth is considered more of an **adaptive shift**.
j. **Active transformation** is seen as minor D/F changes but mainly U/B compensatory growth of ramus.
k. Mandibular growth is more sustained in boys than in girls, (i.e. up to 25 years age). Distance between mental foramina changes little after 6 years age, (i.e. width of mandible).
l. **Mental foramen** level changes with growth, from near mandibular border (infants) to middle of the body (in adults) to at alveolar crest (in edentulous patient).
m. Level of **mandibular foramen** lies below OP in children and at the level of OP in adults.

63. What do you mean by basal tubular part?

It protects mandibular nerve **(unloaded nerve concept)** and follows a logarithmic spiral in its D/F growth.

64. What is the most constant portion of mandible?

It is the ARC from F. ovale to mandibular foramen to mental foramen.

65. What structures are the functional matrices for the growth of alveolar bone?

Teeth are the main factors for the growth of alveolar bones. In a place where the tooth is congenitally missing, the bone is deficient. That is why, the enucleation of first premolar and 3rd molars tooth buds is not considered during the orthodontic treatment, till at least half of root development occurs.

66. Describe growth of chin?

Area of chin just above symphysis menti is resorptive, which gives the chin its prominence. The area at the pogonion is depository.

67. Describe the ramal growth

In infancy, the ramus is located at approx. primary first molar area.

Growth occurs along the **V-principle**. Anterior border is resorptive to provide space for eruption of permanent molars. Posterior surface is depository.

After **6 years of age**, the greatest increase in size of mandible occurs distal to first molars.

Ramal growth **provides space vertically** in which both U/L alveolar bones grow, the teeth being their functional matrices.

68. What is the concept of late mandibular growth?

It occurs in horizontal direction and is mainly responsible for lower anterior crowding, rather than mandibular third molars, which appears, develops or increases in the adult age/postpubertal age (20–30 years age).

Lower incisors tend to upright under the terminal horizontal growth increments, which occurs due to **U and F rotation of mandible**, leading to lingual movement of lower incisors and their crowding.

69. How does the growth of maxilla occur?

Maxilla is mainly **intramembranous** except
- Paranasal processes of nasal capsule
- Alveolar border of zygomatic process.

Two areas:
1. Neural and alveolar areas,
2. Frontal, zygomatic, palatal processes.

   A passive/**secondary displacement** of nasomaxillary complex is D and F due to cranial base growth.

   Primary displacement of nasomaxillary complex occurs by growth of maxillary tuberosity in posterior direction.

70. Where lie the ossification centers of the maxilla?

Three primary ossification centers of one above canine fossa for maxilla proper and two for premaxilla.

71. What is the prenatal growth of maxilla?

It arises from a single center of ossification into two areas based on the relation to the infraorbital nerve. These are neural and alveolar areas, and frontal, zygomatic and palatal processes.

Maxilla is an intramembranous bone except the paranasal processes of the nasal capsule and the cartilaginous areas at the alveolar border of the zygomatic process.

72. How do the craniomaxillary sutures affect the growth of maxilla?

Main sutures are frontonasal, frontomaxillary, zygomaticomaxillary, zygomaticotemporal, and pterygopalatine. All are oblique and parallel to each other, growth there moves the maxilla D/F or cranium U/B. But, sutural growth is secondary.

73. Describe condyle as the growth site of mandible?

Condyle is the major growth centre of mandible, it has **fibrocartilage,** which is a secondary cartilage, grows by proliferation of cartilage. **Condyle is the only bone in body** which shows **both interstitial and appositional growths.** Peak of condylar growth is at 12–14 years age and it ceases at around 20 years age.

Condyle grows in U and B direction-so mandible moves in D and F direction, along an arc, which runs from foramen ovale to mandibular foramen to mental foramen (**unloaded nerve concept**).

Condyles are not the primary site of mandibular growth, but are loci with secondary, compensatory growth potential.

74. Which are the various theories of growth?

1. Genetic
2. Sutural theory by Sicher
3. Cartilaginous theory by Scott
4. Functional matrix theory by Moss
5. von Limborgh's theory
6. Enlow's expanding V-principle
7. Enlow's counterpart principle.

75. Which is the most important theory of growth?

It is the **functional matrix theory by Moss.** It is based on the functional cranial component theory of van der Klaauw.

	FCC
Functional matrix	**Skeletal unit**
Periosteal matrix	1. Macroskeletal unit 2. Microskeletal unit
Capsular matrix	1. Neurocranial capsule 2. Orofacial capsule

76. Which are the two main functional matrices?

These are periosteal matrix and capsular matrix.

77. Which are the main theories of growth?

There are three main theories, i.e. Sicher's sutural theory, Scott's cartilagineous theory, Moss's functional matrix theory.

78. What is the idea behind functional matrix theory of growth?

It emphasizes that the osseous growth of the skull is entirely secondary. There is dominance of non-osseous structures of the craniofacial complex over the bony parts.

79. Which factors affect the growth as given by Von Limborgh?

1. Intrinsic genetic
2. Local epigenetic
3. General epigenetic
4. Local environmental
5. General environmental factors.

80. What is the major difference in various growth theories?

It is the location at which genetic control is expressed.

81. What is the difference between the growth site and the growth center?

Site is a location where growth occurs, **center** is a location **at which independent, genetically controlled growth occurs,** i.e. independent of environment.

82. Which are the two capsular matrices affecting the growth of face?

They are neurocranial and orofacial capsules.

83. What is a growth spurt?

The growth never occurs with uniformity. There are periods when there is an increase in growth. These are KA growth spurts.

	Female	*Male*
First peak (childhood)	3 years	3 years
2nd peak (Juvenile)	6–7 years	7–9 years
3rd peak (Prepubertal)	11–12 years	14–15 years

84. What are the main features of the growth spurts?

a. More boys to have 2–3 peaks.
b. Girls show only two peaks.
c. Very few girls show mixed dentition period growth spurt, but all show pubertal growth spurt.
d. So mixed dentition jaw changes (with functional appliances) is more successful in boys.

e. Females mature earlier (2–3 years) than males, so early treatment is more critical in girls than in boys.

f. During pubertal growth period, there is directional change from vertical to horizontal.

g. Growth modulation therapy is better and results are stable, if given during the spurts period.

85. What are Tweed's growth trends?

Based on the angles FMA, IMPA, FMIA, Tweed described growth trends in type A, B, C.

1. Type A = maxilla and mandible grow D and F in unison. It is seen by no changes in the ANB angle; 25% of patients are in this category.
2. Type B = here, entire growth D and F, but the maxilla grows more rapidly than the mandible, and so ANB angle increases, 15% patients belong to this category.
3. Type C = mandible grows rather D and F at a faster rate as compared to maxilla, it shows the decrease in ANB. 60% patients, i.e. largest amount of patients are in this category.

86. What are the periods of growth and dental development according to Hellman?

1. Stage I = Is the period of early infancy before the completion of the deciduous dentition.
2. Stage II = It is the period of late infancy at the completion of the deciduous dentition.
3. Stage III = Is the period of childhood when the permanent first molars are erupting or have taken their positions.
4. Sage IV = Is the period of pubescence when the second molars are erupting or have taken their positions.
5. Stage V = Is the period of adulthood when the third molars are erupting or have taken their place.
6. Stage VI = Is the period of old age when the occlusal surfaces of molars are worn off to the extent of obliterating the pattern of the grooves.
7. Stage VII = Designates the period of senility.

6

Clinical Significance of Growth and Development Concepts

INTRODUCTION

Knowledge of growth concepts, status and trends of an individual is very important to provide the best treatment to the patients. Craniofacial complex not only involves the bony components, but also the dental components. It is also important to have knowledge of natural events happening during growth and development, and during development of dentition. As we have discussed in previous sections, there are certain features which are called as self-correcting anomalies, which look like to be abnormal features to the parents. But, these natural events should not be disturbed mechanically, as they resolve themselves with further growth. An over-enthusiastic parent or clinician can do more harm than good by disturbing such natural events.

Most of the patients who come to consult an orthodontist are in various phases of active growth. It has been found that although Angle's class I malocclusion is the most common orthodontic condition, but the cases which come for orthodontic treatment are of Angle's class II variety. It is due to skeletal discrepancy in jaw relationship and poor esthetics. An early intervention of such a condition helps in achieving a normal skeletal relationship of the jaws, which gives an improved esthetics and a psychological boost to the patient.

Growth of the craniofacial complex is a dynamic phenomenon. It is not uniform throughout life and occurs in phases known as growth spurts, and differential growth. There are phases of rapid growth and slow growth. Any intervention done during the period of active growth helps in redirection of the growth to achieve a state of balance.

During the initial life of an individual, various changes in the dentition, dental relations, and skeletal relationships take place in all the three dimensions. Since the growth is a continuous, nonuniform process, it has major effects on these changes. The clinical significance of growth has been briefly discussed in the following section.

Timing of Growth

Active growth of craniofacial complex, although keeps on occurring during first 18 years of life, but there are phases when its speed is rapid. Those periods are called as growth spurts. Most important growth spurts occur during preadolescent and during adolescent years of age. These are the periods when maximum advantage of natural growth can be obtained through well-timed treatment procedures to stimulate or to redirect growth. Since, orthodontist mainly deals with the correction of middle and lower third of faces, thereby such timing of appropriate treatment has to be done according to the sequence of the growth completion in various parts of the facial complex.

Sequence of Growth Completion

As we have discussed in previous section, the facial skeleton follows the cephalocaudal gradient of growth. It means that the growth of parts of face which are near to cranium gets completed first. In view of this information, it is sure that the growth of maxilla will get completed before that of mandible. So, any treatment modality for growth-redirection of maxilla has to be used at an early age, as compared to mandible.

Also, the sequence of timing of growth completion is different in different planes of space. The growth in transverse dimension is first to be completed, and then in sagittal, and lastly in the vertical plane (WDH). In view of these facts, the transverse growth of maxilla gets completed first. So, any intervention to treat the maxillary constriction has to done as early as possible. Now, during preadolescent growth spurt, which is observed at around 8 years of age, it is the right time to achieve a skeletal expansion of maxilla. It is also helped by the patency of midpalatal suture, which can be easily activated and opened with normal physiological expansion forces. With age, the suture gets more inter-digitated and becomes difficult to open with normal forces. Then it will need heavy forces through RME. Also the skeletal effects diminish with age and dental effects start coming in more.

Treatment of sagittal dimension of maxilla also needs an early intervention. A maxillary deficiency needs protraction therapy, which is best done during the early age of 8–9 years, to obtain maximum advantage of ensuing active maxillary growth.

Also, if maxilla is protrusive, it has to be restricted with the help of head gear forces to prevent its further growth in sagittal direction. It is also best started during the early age esp the early or mid mixed dentition period, before the eruption of second molars. It should be started when second molars are well above the cervical part of first molars, but has crossed the apical third root of first molars. This headgear force will also help in distalisation of entire maxillary arch. A very early distalisation of upper first molars can lead to deflected path of eruption of second molars and their impaction. Treatment should be started at early age if there is more severe discrepancy, if the patient is cooperative in wearing such appliance.

Excessive vertical growth of maxilla leading to gummy smile and bite problems (deep bite if anterior region grows more, open bite if posterior region grows more), should also be addressed in early mixed dentition period to control the active maxillary growth. It can be done with the help of high-pull head gears.

Role of Growth Pattern on Treatment Decisions

Growth patterns have been divided in horizontal, average and vertical types. They influence the extraction decisions and anchorage planning. Horizontal growth pattern leads to development of skeletal deep bite, increased mandibular and ramal lengths, flat basal plane angles, short face, and strong masticatory musculature. These factors provide a strong anchorage and thus loss of anchorage in such cases is extremely difficult. It can be remembered as that the during anchorage loss, the molar has to walk along a straight path, under strong muscles, which is very difficult. Thus, such cases should be treated on nonextraction basis.

In vertical growth pattern, there is skeletal open bite, decreased mandibular and ramal lengths, steep basal plane angles, long face, and weaker masticatory musculature. These factors provide a weak anchorage and thus loss of anchorage in such cases is very fast. It can be remembered as that the during anchorage loss, the molar has to walk along a slope/inclined path, and muscular forces are weak, which do not prevent any movement of molar, thus leading to an easy mesial movement of molars. Thus such cases generally are treated on extraction basis depending on space requirements, and they need anchorage reinforcement by various methods.

Expansion

After the closure of mid-mandibular suture, there are least chances that the mandibular expansion can be achieved. The natural growth leads to attain an intercanine width at

9 years of age, after which there is no appreciable growth in this dimension. Once established, it cannot be increased without a 100% relapse potential, or otherwise a permanent retainer has to be placed. Lately, distraction osteogenesis has been used to expand the mandible in certain cases.

Expansion in Maxilla

The best time to expand maxilla is during preadolescent period, especially during 8–9 years of age. During that time, the spurt causes an increase in intercanine width, in consonance with an increasing intercanine width of mandible. Otherwise, if maxillary width does not increase at that time, it may lead to crossbite or premature contacts in this region. Also, the midpalatal suture is patent and not interdigitated at the younger age of the child, and can be easily opened / stimulated with lighter forces.

Mandibular Intercanine Width

Mandibular intercanine width gets completed by 9 years of age in both sexes. It is also supported by the erupting mandibular canines generally at that age. After that, any attempt to increase it leads to relapse or is subjected to permanent retention. Since there is no suture in mandible, a skeletal expansion cannot be achieved. Nowadays, the distraction osteogenesis procedure has given a hope to expand the constricted mandible skeletally, followed by a prolonged / permanent retainer to give time for soft tissue adaptation in new environment.

Maxillary Intercanine Width

Another phase of increase in basal maxillary intercanine width occurs during adolescent growth period, especially during 11–12 years age. It occurs by remodeling and increased functional demand, and is also aided by erupting maxillary canine, which generally erupts in a labial direction. This increased width also helps as a **safety-valve**, to prevent developing cross bite in this region. It is because during this phase of spurt, the mandible is growing in anterior direction thereby its wider posterior part comes in relation with narrower anterior part of maxilla. So, if maxillary width does not increase, it may lead to cross bite or premature contact.

If primary maxillary canines are prematurely extracted or lost, then the stimulus of increase in intercanine width is lost and maxillary width deficiency develops, leading to space deficiency. Also, the permanent canines either can get impacted or erupt in ectopic positions.

During **serial extractions**, the primary maxillary canines should be judiciously extracted at proper time, otherwise intercanine width gain will not be achieved, if premature extraction is done. Therefore, generally, in mandibular arch the sequence followed is CD4, while in maxillary arch, the sequence followed is D4C. It all depends on the sequence of eruption of teeth and the level of teeth in the jaw bones during eruption. To gain minor space, rather than extracting a primary tooth, its proximal sides can be sliced to accommodate the erupting tooth. Since, the teeth act as functional matrix for alveolar bone, a premature extraction of tooth leads to loss of this stimulus. Teeth should be extracted when their successors are near to alveolar crest area, and almost half root has completed.

Ugly-duckling Stage

It is a normal event during dentition development. It is seen during the age of 8–10 years. Maxillary canines develop very high near the nasal floor, and the last succedaneous teeth to erupt. It occurs when the maxillary canines start moving down during initial eruption. Since at this age, maxilla has not gained its proper width, and thus there is a physiological crowding in this area. When they move downward, they apply physiological pressures on roots of laterals which also gets transmitted to roots of central. It leads to root crowding and crown flaring and spacing of incisors. However, in late mixed dentition period, when the maxilla gains an intercanine width, and the canines reach near the alveolar crest level, this force gets transferred to crown region of incisors, and they start straightening. This is a natural phenomenon, and should not be disturbed orthodontically. If mechanical force is used to close the spaces, then there are chances of root resorption of upper lateral incisors because their roots will come in approximation to erupting canines during the root uprighting of lateral incisors.

Terminal Plane Relationship of Primary Molars and Effect on the Relation of Permanent Molars

Although the relation of permanent first molars depends a lot on the relation of primary second molars and sequence of their loss, but a great role is also played by the growth of mandible. It has been discussed in previous sections. A due consideration should be given to these factors during the development of dentition and space management. It has also been discoursed at page 102–104.

Space for Mandibular Incisors

During eruption of mandibular incisors, they generally erupt in a crowded position, seen during 6–8 years of age. A natural alignment of upto 2 mm gets achieved by natural growth of mandible, and under the influence of tongue pressure. More than 2 mm crowding does not resolve itself.

Myofunctional Treatment

In most of the cases, the myofunctional treatment is needed to correct the relation of mandibular retrognathism with the maxilla. It needs to bring mandible in a downward and forward direction. Since mandible follows cephalocaudal gradient of growth, it is the bone of face which grows till a later age. It follows a growth spurt in adolescent period of growth, at which time, if proper functional appliance is placed, can lead to enhanced growth of mandible. In boys, it is started in late mixed dentition or early permanent dentition stage. In girls, it should be started at an early age than boys, because they observe growth spurt 2 years earlier than boys. So, such a treatment can be postponed for boys till late MDP or early permanent dentition period, while in girls, the treatment should be started at an early age, at around 10 years of age.

Chin Cup Treatment

It is used to restrain the excessive forward growth of chin, which is leading to mandibular prognathism and skeletal class III. Clinically, the active mandibular growth occurs during preadolescent and adolescent growth spurts. So, chin with highpull headgen cup should be given at an early age, i.e. early mixed dentition period. Also, since mandible keeps on growing till late adult age, i.e. upto 18 years of age, the chin cup therapy has to be continued till that age to offset any forward growth effects.

In cases of any component of maxillary deficiency alongwith a mandibular prognathism, it should be treated at early preadolescent spurt age by maxillary protraction appliance to take advantage of active maxillary growth in anterior direction. The best appliance in such a situation is a combination of maxillary protraction with chin cup appliance.

Maxillary deficiency is almost often accompanied with **maxillary constriction**. Clinical experience has shown that before the start of maxillary protraction, a phase of RME should be given, which helps to loosen the circummaxillary sutures and hence the maxillary protraction is easy and faster. The maxillary expansion is best achieved during preadolescent growth phase, i.e. 8–9 years of age, which is also the best time to activate growth of deficient maxilla.

Effect of Growth Pattern and Direction

Growth patterns can be horizontal, normal and vertical directions. Horizontal growth leads to skeletal deep bite, while vertical growth leads to skeletal open bite. After orthodontic treatment of cases with horizontal growth, there are still chances of reappearance of deep bite due to upward and forward growth rotation of mandible. To prevent relapse of deep bite, the dynamic retention concept has been described by Nanda. He advised to use an anterior bite plane in upper Hawley's retainer during active growth period. It will prevent development of deep bite. In vertical growth cases, a high pull head gear applied at molars will not allow them to erupt and hence will prevent D and B rotation of mandible.

Vertical Growth of Ramus

Vertical growth of ramus occurs in consonance with the growth of condyle and downward growth of maxilla. It helps to growth of upper and lower alveolar bones also. During active periods of growth, with growth of ramus, the interocclusal gap is created, which is covered by eruption of teeth toward each other. This phenomenon helps to attain proper relation during orthodontic extrusion of buccal teeth, which gets balanced by ongoing vertical ramal growth. However, after the active growth period, any extrusion of buccal teeth is not balanced by equal ramal growth. It leads to premature contacts in molar regions, activation of masseter-medial pterygoid sling and hence relapse.

Late Mandibular Growth

During adult age, an increase of crowding in lower incisor region is observed. Initially, it was considered due to eruption forces of lower 3rd molars, but later on the research has shown that it is the late mandibular growth which leads to development of this crowding. During adult period till at least 45 years of age, the mandibular keeps on growing silently with most of the growth expressed in upward and forward direction. The mandible rotated anticlockwise and thrusts itself lingual to upper anteriors. It leads to transfer of forces on the lower incisors which then tilt lingually in a smaller arch, and leading to development of crowding. To avoid this, a permanent hard lingual retainer has to be placed in the patients. In some cases, it may also cause the flaring and spacing of upper incisors, which occurs due to mandible coming in close approximation of upper incisors and thus redirecting the forces on upper incisors leading them to move labially. It mostly happens when the upper lip is hypotonic and cannot counteract these physiological forces.

Soft Tissue Growth of Lips and Nose

Dynamic changes in dental, skeletal, and soft tissues of face occur over the entire period of active growth and even into the decades past the age of 20 years. Different facial types, i.e. long-face and short-face individuals have different growth and maturational patterns.

Growth changes in the soft tissue profile occur during active growth at a greater rate. Females show more growth as a percentage of their adult size (at age 18) than males. In males, the nose keeps on growing even after age 18. Upper lip length growth in both males and females is almost complete by age 15. The lip length in males increases more than the females. Even the increase in lip thickness is more in males than females and keeps on growing in males even at age 18. Growth at chin is also observed, which mainly occurs due to translation of mandible by growth in skeletal length of mandible.

Retention

It is a very important phase of orthodontics in which the post-treatment results are to be maintained with the help of appliances. The growth has a great deal of effect in retention. The late mandibular growth leads to appearance of crowding in lower incisors region. The horizontal growth pattern leads to development of deep bite, which needs to be controlled with the help of bite plane. In vertical growth, it may lead to open bite tendency, and thus high pull headgear is needed to retain. Mandible in class III cases keeps on growing till at least 18 years, and it needs night time wear of chin cup to control.

7

Stomatognathic System and Functions

INTRODUCTION

The orofacial region performs a number of functions, like respiration, deglutition, mastication, speech and vision, etc. Normal function helps in normal growth and development of craniofacial structures, as the function and the form are inter-related. According to Moss's concept of functional matrix of growth, the normal functions are required for normal growth and development. The tissues controlling that function are its functional matrices. More functional demands on jaws lead to more development of masticatory and other muscles, which in turn, leads to growth of jaws and craniofacial skeleton by remodelling, e.g. neanderthal man used to eat raw meat, which needed extreme force on jaws and thus more force generation by the muscles. It led to their robust jaws and other related bones. Raw food also led to more attrition of teeth on occlusal and functional surfaces. It helped to reduce the dental arch length and thus mesial shifting of the teeth, which helped to create the space for third molars, which were very rarely found to be impacted in them.

Any abnormal function or habit leads to deviation in the proper growth. Hence, understanding of the normalcy is important for diagnosis and treatment planning.

Mastication

It is a complex process which helps to assimilate the food in small pieces and mix it with saliva and enzymes to prepare it for swallowing. Infants who do not have teeth, there is no mastication. An infant resorts to mastication when his first molars erupt and come in occlusion. Before that, he just keeps on pushing the food between the gum pads. Murphy has described six phases of mastication as follows:

1. **Preparatory phase:** In this phase, the food is positioned by the tongue in the occlusion on the chewing side and the mandible moves to the same side.
2. **Food contact:** There is a momentary pause in chewing cycle during this period. Here, the sensory receptors evaluate the quality of food and the expected load on the masticatory apparatus.
3. **Crushing phase:** Food is broken in small pieces by equal activity on both the sides of dental arches. The food is shifted between sides with the help of tongue and cheeks. Crushing is fast during initial phase and gradually slows down.
4. **Tooth contact:** The teeth come in contact with each other and signify the end of crushing phase.
5. **Guiding phase:** The contact of teeth is unilateral and the mandibular molars transgress across the maxillary molars.
6. **Centric occlusion:** The teeth come to a definite and distinct stop.

Deglutition

It is an important function which helps to push the masticated food from the oral cavity to stomach via esophagus for further digestive processing. The swallowing pattern develops gradually, so it is different in infants than adults. It develops according to the changing needs of the child. There are mainly two patterns of swallowing, viz. infantile swallow and the mature swallow.

Infantile/visceral Swallowing

The infantile (visceral) swallow, is an essential function in neonates. It is closely associated with suckling, and both are well developed by about 32nd week of intrauterine life. Even in the intrauterine life, the fetus has been seen to suck the fingers. Process of suckling is different from sucking and should not be confused. During the process of suckling, the child brings his mandible forward and draws nipple into the mouth which is held between tongue and upper lip. The tongue comes between the gum pads in close apposition with the lips around the nipple to make a seal. The facial muscles help to stabilize the mandible. The mandibular elevators which play a prominent role in normal mature swallow, show minimal activity. The milk is directed to the pharynx by the peristaltic movements of tongue and mylohyoid muscle. During this process, the normal breathing is continued.

Characteristics of Infantile Swallow

Moyers described certain features of infantile swallow which are as follows: It is seen esp during suckling, when the child brings the tongue and the mandible forward. Tongue is placed between upper and lower gum pads, with the jaws apart. Mandible is stabilised by the muscles of seventh cranial nerve and the tongue. Swallowing is controlled by sensory interchange between lip and tongue. Extreme activity of mentalis muscle and other circumoral muscles is seen aiding in suckling.

Transitional Period of Swallowing

It marks the gradual change of infantile swallowing to mature swallowing pattern. During the early childhood, several maturational events occur that alter markedly the functioning of orofacial musculature. The eruption of incisors helps in more precise opening and closing movements of mandible; helps in a more retracted tongue posture, and initiates learning of mastication.

Initial occlusion is established when the primary first molars erupt and child shifts to solid food. At that time, the mandible does not protrude and tongue is contained within the dental arches. It initiates the development of mature swallow pattern.

Mature/Somatic Swallow

With the establishment of posterior occlusion when primary first molars erupt, the true chewing movements start, and the learning of mature swallow begins. The infantile swallowing gradually disappears with the establishment of buccal occlusion. Gradually, the fifth cranial nerve muscles take the role of mandibular stabilization during the swallow, while muscles of facial N learn the functions of facial expression. The transition from infantile to mature (somatic) swallow takes place over several month, aided by maturation of neuromuscular elements. Most children achieve most characteristics of a mature swallow at 12 to 15 months.

Characteristic Features of a Mature (Somatic) Swallow (Fig. 7.1)

Teeth come together in light occlusion. The mandible is stabilized by contraction of muscles of fifth cranial nerve. The tongue tip is held against the palate above and behind the incisors. Minimal contraction of the lips is seen during the swallow. Facial N muscles do not show any activity related with swallowing.

Phases of swallowing: The deglutitional cycle is divided into four coordinated phases.

1. Preparatory phase
2. Oral phase
3. Pharyngeal phase
4. Esophageal phase.

The preparatory phase: After assimilation, the food is gathered on the dorsum of the tongue. The teeth are brought in contact and a seal is created on buccal and labial side to avoid the escape of food toward the labial/ buccal vestibules.

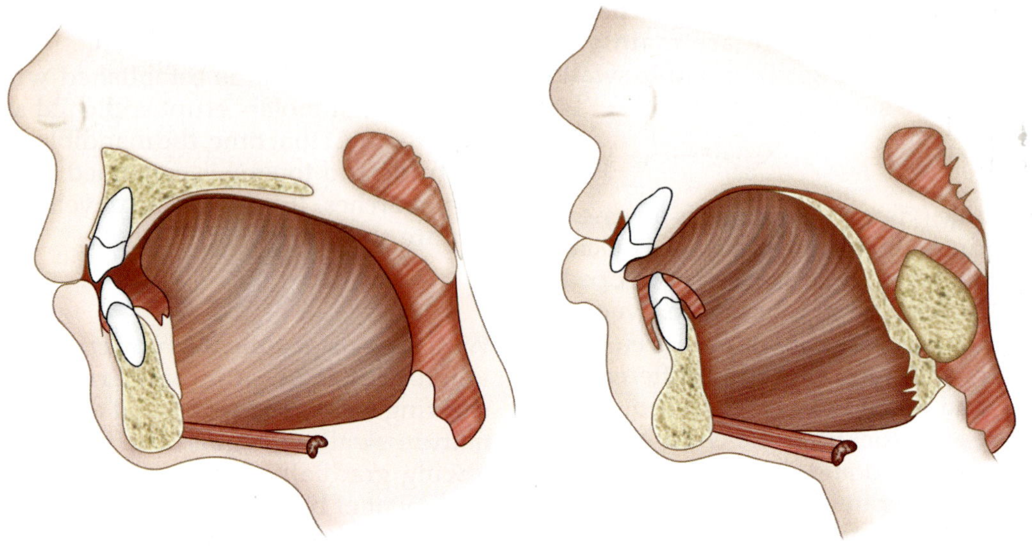

Fig. 7.1: Normal relation of teeth and tongue in the first figure, while second figure shows protrusion of tongue between incisors during tongue thrusting.

The oral phase: Soft palate rises to seal the nasopharynx so that the food does not go upwards. Posterior part of the tongue drops downward and backward to create the space for movement of food down the oro-pharyngeal part under the influence of movement of tongue. This is a voluntary phase. At the same time the larynx and the hyoid bone move upwards. The oral cavity is stabilized by the muscles of mastication, and maintains an anterior and lateral seal during this phase to avoid escape of food in labial buccal vestibules.

The pharyngeal phase: Once the food is pushed towards the pharyngeal part, further process becomes involuntary. This phase starts when food crosses the faucial pillars. The peristaltic movements push the food towards esophagus. The pharyngeal tube is raised upwards *en masse*, and the nasopharynx is sealed off by approximation of soft palate against the posterior pharyngeal wall (Pasavant's ridge). The hyoid bone and the base of the tongue move forward as both the pharynx and the tongue continue their peristaltic-like movement on the bolus of food.

The esophageal phase: When the food passes cricopharyngeal sphincter, the esophageal phase starts. It helps to push the food towards stomach. While the peristaltic movement carries the food through the esophagus, the hyoid bone, palate and tongue return to their original positions.

Abnormal Swallowing Patterns

Simple Tongue Thrust Swallow

It is seen in patients having an anterior open bite. There is a **teeth-together swallow**, but tongue-thrust is seen in the open bite region to create a seal. It typically displays contractions of mandibular elevators, the lips, and mentalis muscle to seal off the open bite during swallowing, and the teeth are in occlusion as the tongue protrudes into an open bite. The contraction of other facial muscles is minimal. This type of swallowing can also be seen as an adaptive mechanism to maintain an open bite created by factors like thumb-sucking.

The open bite in a simple tongue thrust is well-circumscribed, i.e. it has a definite boundaries of beginning and the end. Any history of prolonged digital or pacifier sucking is the most common etiologic factor for such open bite. The tongue thrust develops as an adaptation during swallowing to the open bite. Early control or removal of such causes can help in correction of open bite and abnormal swallowing pattern. It may also be found with hypertrophied tonsils which are not enlarged and/or inflamed sufficiently to prompt a tooth-apart swallow. The incidence of simple tongue thrust diminishes with increasing age, and its treatment is simpler and prognosis more certain than complex tongue thrust.

Complex Tongue-thrust Swallow

The complex tongue-thrust swallow is a more severe form of abnormal swallowing and is defined as a tongue-thrust with **teeth-apart swallow**. There is contraction of lips, facial and mentalis muscle (7th nerve ms), and lack of contraction of the mandibular elevators. Patient may present with strained—looks of the face. The open bite associated with a complex tongue-thrust usually does not have definite boundaries and is more diffuse than seen in simple tongue thrust. Examination of occlusion and the dental casts typically reveal a poor occlusal fit and instability of intercuspation. Patients with complex tongue-thrust usually demonstrate occlusal interferences in the retruded contact position. They are more likely to be mouth breathers and may have a history of chronic nasorespiratory disease or allergies. The incidence of complex tongue-thrusting does not diminish as much with age as does the simple tongue-thrust.

Retained Infantile Swallow

Retained infantile swallowing behavior is defined as a predominant persistence of the infantile swallowing reflex after the arrival of permanent teeth. The tongue thrusts strongly between the anterior and posterior teeth. Contractions of buccinator muscles are very strong. Such patients have inexpressive faces, since facial muscles are not being used for the delicate purposes of facial expression but rather for the massive effort of stabilizing the mandible during the swallow. Mastication is not proper since the occlusion is present on only one molar in each quadrant. The gag threshold is typically low. These patients generally take a soft diet as they are not able to masticate food properly due to no occlusal contacts. Food often is placed on the dorsum of the tongue and mastication occurs between the tongue tip and the palate.

Respiration

It is an inherent activity to survive. Normal orofacial development depends on the presence of normal breathing as per the functional matrix of growth concept. A proper nasal passage is needed for normal breathing. Breathing patterns can be nasal, oral or naso-oral. Nasal breathing is a normal and essential pattern. As the requirement and capacity of lungs increases, the more air inflow is required, and thus the size of nasal passage also increases. It helps in remodeling of nasal cavity, palate, maxilla and maxillary sinuses. Any partial or complete blockage in the nasal passage leads to abnormal form of respiration in the form of oral or oronasal breathing. It leads to a lowering of mandible and tongue, thus disturbing the muscular balance and hence abnormal development of dental arches and the jaws.

Speech

It is a learned activity. First speech sound of baby is **babbling** which appears at around 7–8 months of age. The speech develops by coordination of various parts of oral, pharyngeal and laryngeal cavities. The sound is produced in larynx by a process called **phonation**, which gets modified in the nasal, oral and throat passages by the process of **articulation**. The development of speech vowels and consonants starts anteriorly in the oral cavity and with time, it migrates posteriorly. The labial sounds are the first sounds to develop, followed by labiodental sounds and so on. Till the age of 3 years, the child learns to talk by making full sentences.

Listed below are the different manners, basic definitions, consonants and manner of production:

- **Plosives and stops:** A release of built up air pressure occurs with plosives; the pressure is not released for stops; e.g. p/b, t/d, k/g.
- **Fricatives:** A point of constriction causes friction in the breath stream that creates a sound; e.g. h, f/v, s/z, sh.
- **Nasals:** The breath stream goes mainly through the nose; e.g. m, n.
- **Semivowels:** Produced like vowels except there is greater constriction; e.g. w, y.
- **Liquids:** The tongue diverts the breath stream in the mouth; e.g. l, r.
- **Affricatives:** A stop is released with a fricative; e.g. ch, j.

Listed below are the different places, basic definitions and the consonants within each place of production:

- **Bilabial:** They are produced between the two lips; e.g. p, b, m, w.
- **Labiodental:** when the lower lip touches the incisal edges of upper teeth; e.g. f, v.
- **Linguodental:** They are produced by contact of tongue with the lingua surface of upper incisors; e.g. TH , th.
- **Alveolar:** They are produced by touching of tongue tip with the hard palate behind the upper teeth; e.g. t, d, s, z, n, l, r.
- **Palatal:** They are produced by escaping air between the dorsum of tongue and the roof of mouth/hard palate; sh, zh, y, ch, j.
- **Velar:** Back of soft palate; e.g. k, g, ng.
- **Glottal:** Back of mouth; e.g. h.

Normal speech development follows a normal functional and jaw development. Any abnormal dental and jaw development and abnormal functions can lead to development of faulty speech, although this is seen very rarely, especially in the absence of underlying disorder. Patients having abnormal habits and functions have speech problems. The /s/ sound is the most noticed speech error; while others errors are /z/, /sh/, /ch/, /j/, /d/, /t/, /n/, /l/ and /r/. When there is a combination of functional and abnormal habits, and related speech errors, it is often difficult to correct the speech problems through traditional speech therapy. The orthodontic intervention is needed to break the abnormal habits, which leads to development of normal morphology and thus the speech is improved. Cleft of lip/palate leads to defective speach and nasal away twane.

Functional Equilibrium of Muscles (Fig. 7.2)

The growth and development of bones depends on the functions, which are performed by surrounding soft tissues acting as functional matrices. Bone responds to functional demands by remodeling. Teeth and the supporting structures are surrounded by muscles, which are generally in a state of equilibrium. The shape of dental arches and the relation of teeth to each other are under the influence of such forces. During eruption, the teeth are guided in their proper position by these forces. The dental arches face two opposing forces, i.e. from labiobuccal aspect (lips and cheeks); and lingual aspect (tongue). The teeth lie in the **neutral zone** created by balance of these opposing forces.

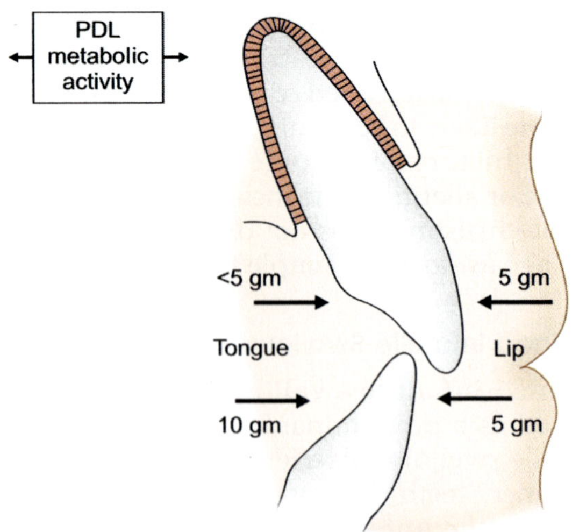

Fig. 7.2: Balance of circumoral forces with forces of tongue. However, note that there is another force component of less than 5 gm which is due to eruption forces of teeth *(Adapted from Proffit)*.

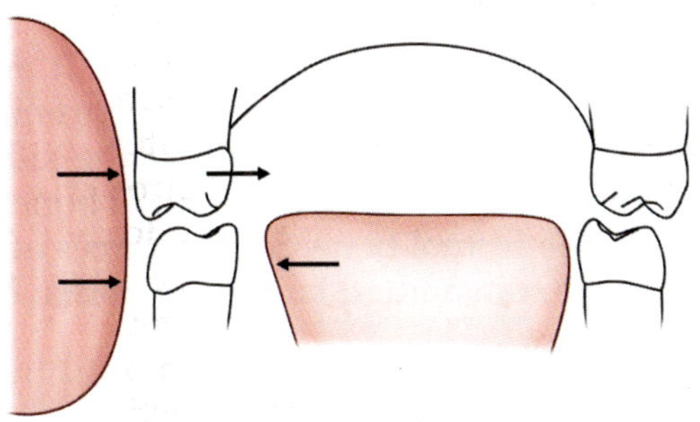

Fig. 7.3: Forces from the cheek and tongue are in equilibrium and keep the teeth in proper arch form.

Buccinators Mechanism (Fig. 7.3 to 7.7)

Fibers of superior constrictors, buccinators and circumoral muscles form a drape/sheath of muscles on labiobuccal aspect of the dental arches. Superior constrictors arise at pharyngeal tubercle, and then they intermingle with buccinators fibers and attach at pterygomadnibular raphe. The buccinator muscles intermingle with fibers of circumoral muscles at modiolus. This is called as buccinator mechanism. It is balanced by forces of tongue from inside. It helps in directing the erupting teeth and moulding the proper arch form. Any disturbance in the balance of these forces leads to maldevelopment of the dental arches and occlusion. Hyperactivity of muscles especially at modiolus leads to decrease in intercanine width and thus a narrow arch form.

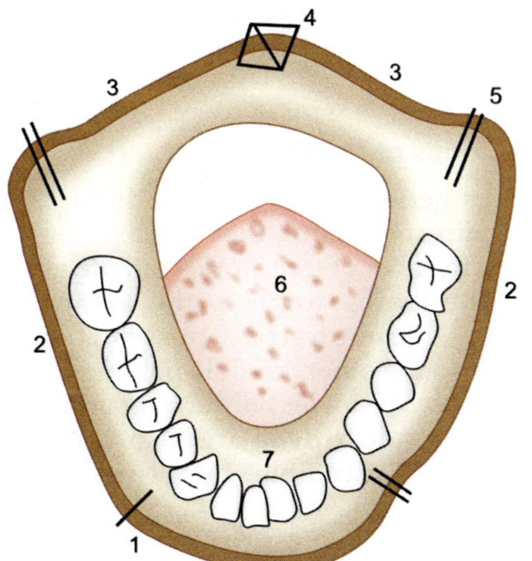

Fig. 7.4: Buccinator mechanism: 1. labial region; 2. buccal region; 3. superior constrictor muscle; 4. attachment of superior constrictor muscle. 5. pterygomandibular raphe; 6. tongue.

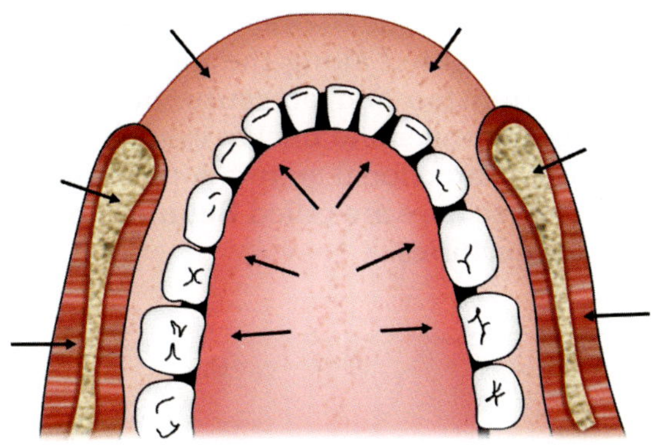

Fig. 7.5: Buccinators mechanism: a balance of circumoral forces with the tongue forces helps shaping the dental arch.

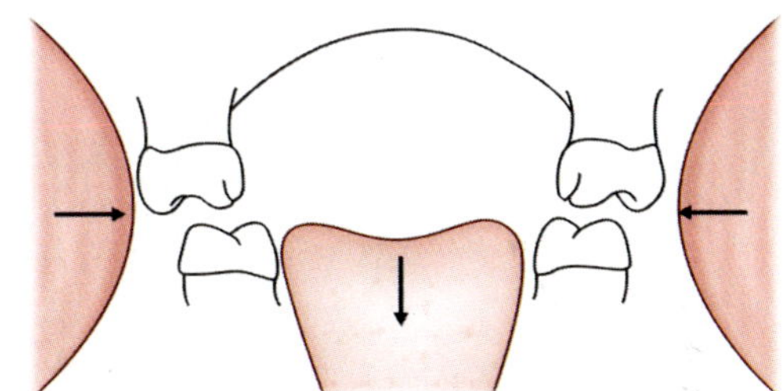

Fig. 7.6: Balance of buccal and tongue forces in shaping the buccal segments of the dental arch.

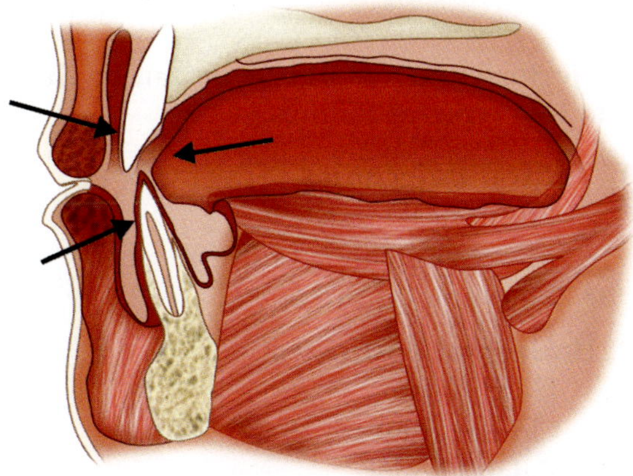

Fig. 7.7: Showing balance of labial and tongue forces in shaping the dental arch in anterior segments.

Trajectories of Forces (Fig. 7.8)

Stresses generated in the jaws during various functions pass along the long axes of teeth and get distributed to a wider area by getting transmitted along certain lines in the bones. These lines occur due to orientation of bony trabeculae, oriented along the pathways of maximum tension and pressure. Bone trabeculae get stronger and thicker in such areas as a result of functional adaptations to these stresses. These lines are called **Benninghoff's lines** or **trajectories.**

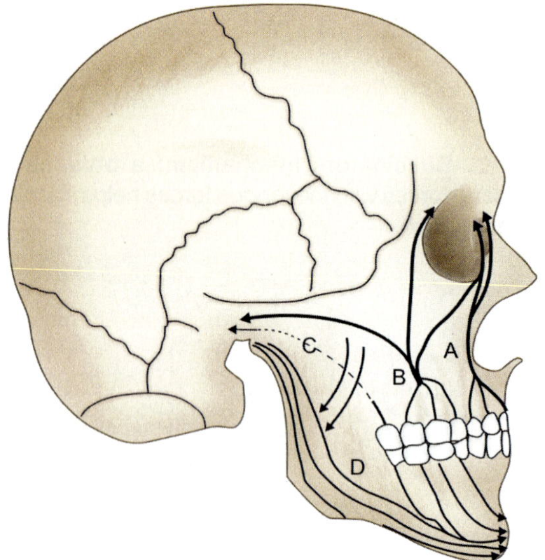

Fig. 7.8: Trajectories of forces in maxilla and mandible.

Trajectories in maxilla: They can be divided in two types as follows:

1. Vertical trajectories:
- Frontonasal buttress,
- Malar zygomatic buttress
- Pterygoid buttress

2. Horizontal buttresses:
- Hard palate
- Orbital ridges
- Palatal bones
- Zygomatic arches
- Lesser wing of sphenoid bone

Frontonasal Buttress

It is a vertically oriented trajectory. It arises from incisors, canines and first premolar region, and runs upward along the side of pirifrom aperture, the crest of nasal bone and ends in the frontal bone. So, the forces of this region are transmitted largely to frontal bone regions.

Malar Zygomatic Buttress

Crest of the zygomatic bone called as key ridge lies in relation to the mesiobuccal root of upper first molars in a normal dentoskeletal arrangemetn, and it is the area of thickened cortical bone. Almost 50% of total stresses generated during mastication are generated in the first molar regions only. MZ buttress helps to transmit the stresses from the posterior teeth especially second premolar and first molars, along the three paths:

1. Upward to the frontal bone through lateral wall of orbits.
2. Along the lower orbital margin/ridge which then joins the upper part of frontonasal buttress.
3. Through the zygomatic arch to the base of skull.

Pterygoid buttress: It helps to transmit forces from 2nd and 3rd molars to the base of skull.

Trajectories of Mandible (Fig. 7.9)

Stresses generated in the mandible pass in apical direction along the long axes of teeth. Thus, a number of trajectories radiate apically from the teeth, down to the mandibular border. A line of stress passes from one condyle to the other condyle passing through symphysis. The lower border of mandible and the mylohyoid ridges are also prominent buttresses of mandible, comprising of compact bones.

Wolff's Law of Bone Transformation (Fig. 7.10)

According to Wolff's law of bone transformation, the bone changes its external shape and internal trabecular architecture in

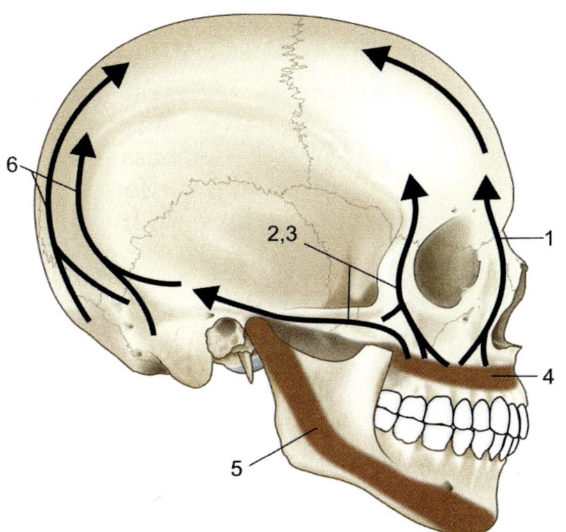

Fig. 7.9: Forces of mastication are transmitted from jaws to the skull along the trajectories of forces

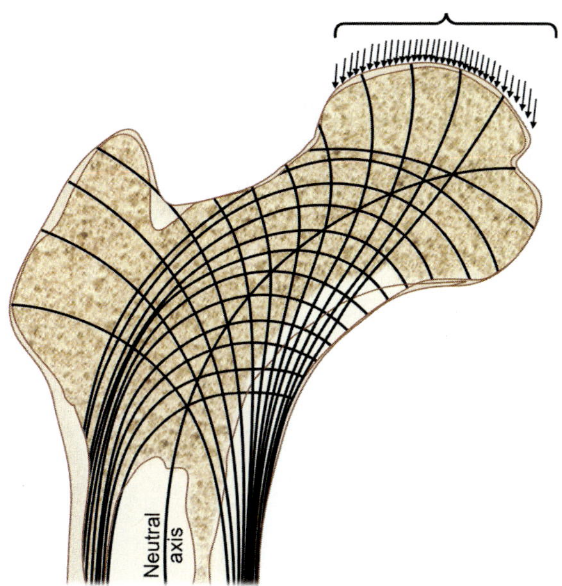

Fig. 7.10: Trajectories of force and trabecular orientation in long bone, according to Wolff's law.

response to the stresses acting on it. When stresses are applied on the bone, it responds by changing in form through remodeling. Areas of pressure and tension are created leading to bone resorption and apposition. The trabeculae are arranged perpendicular to the direction of forces to best resist them.

This phenomenon holds a wide significance for whole body generally, and in orthodontics particularly. During tooth movements, functional or orthopedic appliance usage, the forces are applied to the teeth which are transmitted to supporting bones. It leads to development of areas of pressure and tension around the teeth in PDL spaces. The bone resorption and deposition occurs respectively in these areas leading to remodeling of bone, the change in trabecular pattern of the bone, and thus tooth movement or/and change in external shape of the bone.

Koch described the concept of the **laws of bone architecture**. He described following laws of bone architecture (Figs 7.11a and b):

a. Inner structure and external form of human bones are closely adapted to mechanical conditions which exist at every point in the bone.
b. Inner architecture is determined by the definite and exact requirements of the mathematical and mechanical laws to produce maximum strength with minimal of material.
c. There is a close relationship between form and function of the bone. Any continued deviation from the normal function must be followed by a continuous structural adaptation to the altered functions.

In view of above facts, it can be decided that the external forms of maxilla and mandible are adapted to their functions. Abnormal form of bones develops due to pathological functions. This law can be applied to orthodontics very well. The bone deformity develops due to abnormal function and stresses. Then conversely, to treat the deformity, proper mechanical conditions can be created which can overcorrect the deformity and reverse the transformation process.

Conclusion

Knowledge of normal development and morphology is essential to differentiate from the abnormal morphology, so as to aid in the

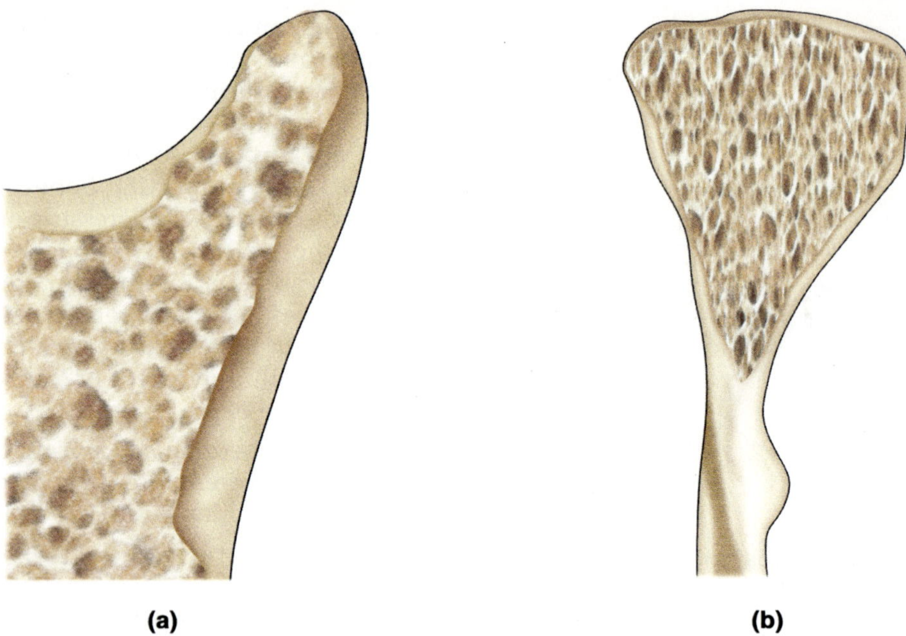

Figs 7.11a and b: Trabecular pattern in condyle and coronoid regions of mandible.

diagnosis and treatment planning. Growth and development depends on the function of associated tissues, and thus the normal function is very important for normal development. Any abnormal function needs correction so that the development may proceed in the normal direction. Therefore, all preventive, interceptive and corrective efforts should be done by the clinicians to achieve a harmonious relation of soft tissues and functions, so as to guide a proper growth and development of the facial tissues.

8

Development of Dentition

INTRODUCTION

Development of the dentition is a very important phase of life. The teeth start developing in the jaw bones in utero. They start erupting in the oral cavity at around 6 months of age. Eruption of first tooth of an infant is always eagerly awaited by the parents. From an orthodontist's point of view, the teeth act as "functional matrices" for the growth of alveolar processes of both the jaws. The absence of one or more teeth leads to deficient growth of the alveolar process in that area.

Development of the dentition can be broadly studied in four phases:

1. Gum pads
2. Primary dentition phase
3. Mixed dentition phase
4. Permanent dentition phase.

The Self-correcting Anomalies

Before discussing the various stages of dentition, we should know the normal features of the dentition. There are certain features observed during the development of dentition, which appear abnormal at that time. But these are the natural stages and are essential features of development at that time, and resolve automatically with the advancing development of dentition. These features should not be disturbed by any intervention, but a close and regular check-up must be done. Following are some of the features noted as self-correcting features.

Gum Pads Stage

Open bite; increased overjet; tongue in between gum pads; skeletal class II relationship.

Primary Dentition Period

Deep bite; primate spacing; small mandible; more upright incisors; primary spacing; FTP; skeletal class II relationship; whiter teeth.

Mixed Dentition Period

End-on molars; ugly-duckling stage; spacing between maxillary incisors; less than 2 mm of lower incisors crowding; lingual eruption of incisors.

Incipient Malocclusion

These are certain features which give an idea of expected space problems in future. Sometimes, if growth is favorable, they get resolved naturally. But if proper growth is not there, they contribute to crowding of teeth. These are, the lack of interdental spacing in primary dentition, crowding in permanent incisors in MDP and premature loss of primary canines especially mandibular due to erupting lateral incisors which cause root resorption of canines, if arch length is deficient in the mandibular arch.

GUM PADS (Fig. 8.1)

The alveolar processes/ridges from the time of birth till the eruption of first tooth are known as the gum pads. They are pink, firm and are covered by fibrous perriosteum. They are of somewhat horse shoe-shaped.

Grooves in Gum Pads

Dental Groove

Each gum pad is divided into two parts by a groove (called as dental groove), i.e. labio-buccal part and the lingual part. The former forms the major part of the gum pad, and has the deciduous teeth. The lingual portion is of relatively small size, and it loses its identity by merging with the tissue on the lingual aspect with eruption of the deciduous teeth. The dental groove is due to the invagination of oral epithelium into underlying connective tissue; and with eruption of the deciduous teeth, the dental groove disappears.

Lip Groove

Lip groove is on the external aspect of the arch and is not well defined.

Transverse Grooves

Each gum pad is divided into 10 small segments by grooves called as transverse grooves. These 10 parts correspond to the 10 developing primary teeth.

Lateral Sulcus

Transverse groove between canine and first molar region is called as lateral sulcus. They help in determining the interjaw relations at young age. Since the lower jaw is smaller than the upper jaw at birth, the lateral sulcus of lower arch lies distal to that of upper arch.

Gingival Groove

Gingival groove separates the gum pad from palate or the floor of mouth.

Most of the sulci and grooves present in gum pads at birth disappear with eruption of teeth.

Characteristics of Gum Pads

1. **Shape:** Both gum pads are almost similar to each other. The upper gum pad is U-shaped, while lower gum pad is horse shoe-shaped.
2. **Occlusal contact:** They touch in future primary first molar region only. It leads to the presence of anterior open bite (so it is a self-correcting malocclusion condition which does not require any treatment), which helps in anterior tongue positioning and making the lip seal during suckling (Fig. 8.2).
3. **Overjet:** Upper gum pad is wider and longer than the lower gum pad. When in occlusion, it covers the lower gum pad from all around, thus having a positive overjet in anterior and posterior regions.
4. **Skeletal class II effect:** Also, anterior overjet is more than normal, thus giving a skeletal class II effect, and thus a convex profile. It is due to smaller mandibular jaw as compared to upper jaw. The overjet diminishes markedly with age due to growth of lower jaw in accordance with

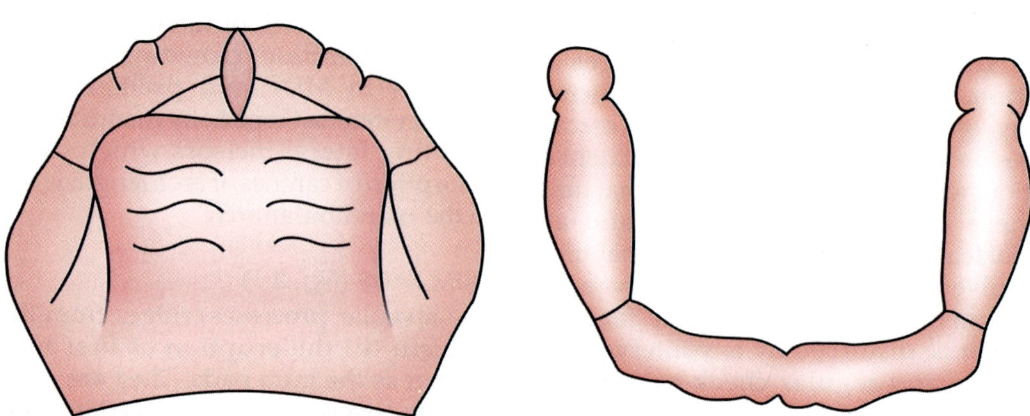

Fig. 8.1: Upper and lower gum pads

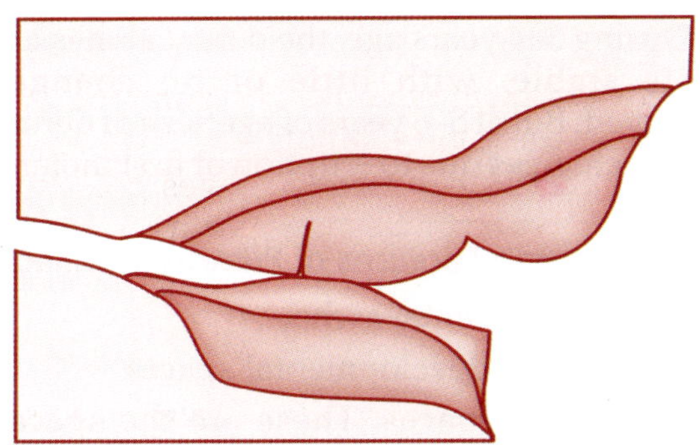

Fig. 8.2: Upper and lower gum pads occluding in future premolar region, with anterior open bite, and increased overjet.

the anteroposterior changes associated with cephalocaudal gradient of the skeletal growth.

5. **Neonatal jaw relationships:** Although the upper and lower gum pads touch in future primary first molar area, a precise bite or jaw relationship cannot be seen. Indeed at birth there is variability in the upper and lower gum pads, and so it can't be used as a diagnostic criterion for reliable predictions of subsequent occlusion in primary dentition.
6. **Anterior open bite:** The gum pads contact in the region of future primary first molar only, thus giving an anterior open bite. This helps in forward movement of tongue and making a tongue-lip seal during suckling. The mandible is controlled by the muscles of face, especially orbicularis oris, mentalis, etc. supplied by facial nerve. However, with the eruption of incisors, the child learns gradually to control the mandible with the masticatory muscles supplied by branches of mandibular nerve.

The space between the anterior segments of the gum pads has been classified as follows:

Class A: The maxillary and mandibular anterior segments lie in their respective planes.

Class B: In the maxillary, the incisor segments are higher than the canine segments, while in the mandibular, the anterior segments are in the same plane.

Class C: In the maxillary, the incisor segments are higher than the canine segments, while in the mandibular the canine segments are higher.

Class D: In the maxillary, the anterior segments are in the same plane, while in the mandibular, the canine segments are higher.

However, it has been found by studies that the anterior space between the gum pads at birth bears no relationship to future open-bite.

According to Leighton, the size of gum pads at birth may be affected by one of the following factors:

- The state of maturity of the infant at birth
- The size at birth as expressed by birth weight
- The size of the developing primary teeth
- Genetic factors.

Prematurely Erupted Primary Teeth

Natal teeth (i.e. present at birth), neonatal teeth (i.e. erupted during the first month), and pre-erupted (i.e. erupting during 2nd or 3rd months) may be present in some children. Teeth are generally the mandibular incisors. Familial tendency for these conditions also exists. They cause the problem during suckling. But, they should not be extracted without proper diagnosis, as they may be the normal primary teeth.

PRIMARY DENTITION PERIOD

It starts with the eruption of first primary tooth, usually the mandibular central incisors, at approx. 6 months of age; and extends upto 6 years of age till the eruption of first permanent tooth, usually mandibular first permanent molars (Fig. 8.3).

Sequence of Eruption

The sequence of eruption of primary teeth is ABDCE. Primary teeth start developing at 6th weeks of IU life. The first primary tooth erupts at approx. 6 months of age; and by 2½–3 years age, all primary teeth are present in the oral cavity. The lower teeth erupt before their upper counterparts, and females are ahead of males in eruption.

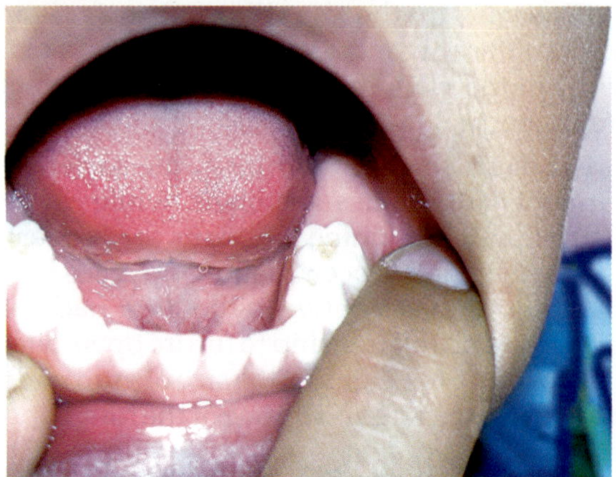

Fig. 8.3: Place for first permanent molar eruption.

Neuromuscular Consideration

The neuromuscular regulation of jaw relationship is important during the development of primary occlusion. During suckling before the eruption of incisors, the main jaw movement is forward and is supported by the facial muscles. After eruption of incisors, the mandibular movement is controlled mainly by masticatory muscles. As the new teeth erupt in oral cavity, the muscles learn to effect the necessary functional occlusal movements. First occlusal contact appears with eruption of D's. The teeth are guided into their occlusal position by the functions of muscles during active growth of facial skeleton. The low cusp height and occlusal wear also contribute to the adaptability of primary occlusion, with ensuing growth.

Before the incisors eruption, the mandible is moved in a forward direction for suckling. At this time, the articular eminence is flat, thereby allowing the forward movement of mandible. With growth, and with the eruption of incisors, the articular eminence also starts taking shape, and the incisal guidance is introduced by incisors. This IG is parallel to the height of articular eminence (which in turn provides the condylar guidance (CG). With further growth, and with eruption of permanent incisors, the articular eminence, CG and IG also increases, e.g. in class II division 2 cases, the IG and thus CG is longer due to deep bite.

During 3–4 years age, the dental arches are quite stable, with little or no changes observed. But at 5–6 years of age, size of dental arches changes due to eruption of first molars.

Characteristic Features of Primary Dentition

a. Shape of dental arches
b. Primary / developmental spaces
c. Primate spaces: These are the spaces found mesial to the maxillary cuspids and distal to the mandibular cuspids.
d. Deep bite due to upright incisors
e. Molar relationships.

Primary Dental Arch

Most primary arches are ovoid and show less variation in shape as compared to the permanent arches. In the early stages of development, the tongue plays an important role in the shaping of dental arches.

Occlusal Relation

At birth when the gum pads are in contact, the mandibular arch is posterior to the maxillary arch giving rise to **a skeletal class II relationship**. This difference reduces progressively with age, due to a cephalocaudal gradient of growth, leading to more growth of mandible than maxilla and thus reducing the skeletal class II effect. However, this skeletal class II relationship is a normal feature of dentition and no attempt should be performed to intervene with the nature at this stage.

First Occlusal Contact

The posterior occlusion / the intercuspation in primary dentition is first established by eruption and contact of primary first molars.

Molar Relation in Primary Dentition (Fig. 8.4)

According to Baume's classification of occlusion in primary dentition, there are 3 relations: according to the relation of distal surfaces of upper and lower primary second molars, as follows:

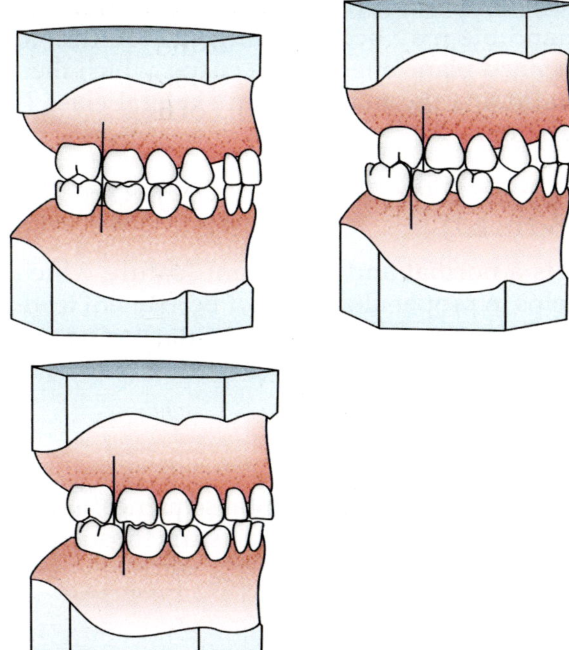

Fig. 8.4: Relation of upper and lower primary second molars: flush terminal plane; distal step; and mesial step relation.

1. Flush terminal plane — 76% (to be observed most critically)
2. Mesial step — 14%
3. Distal step — 10%

Flush terminal plane: When the distal surfaces of upper and lower primary second molars are in the same plane, it is the flush terminal plane (FTP). The mesiolingual cusp of maxillary molars occludes in the central fossa of mandibular molars. The mesiodistal width of the mandibular 2nd primary molar is more than the maxillary, giving rise to, *"flush terminal plane"*. Thus, the flush terminal plane relation is a normal relation of the developing dentition, and should not be disturbed with the treatment. The difference in the sizes of second primary molar and the second bicuspid is known as the **E-space**. This is greater in mandible than the maxilla, which is due to the fact that the size of mandibular second primary molar is large than the maxillary second primary molar.

When the terminal plane is straight, the first permanent molars are guided into an initial **"end-on" relationship** by the distal surfaces of primary second molars.

Mesial step: In mesial step, distal surface of lower second molar is mesial to that of upper second molar. It gives rise to skeletal class III tendency.

Distal step: In distal step, distal surface of lower second molar is distal to that of upper second molar. It gives rise to skeletal class II tendency.

Significance of the Primary Molar Relationships (Fig. 8.5)

They give an indication of future occlusion relation, and guide to achieve the permanent molar relationship in future.

Flush terminal plane:

- Change to end-on, if minimum growth differential is there.

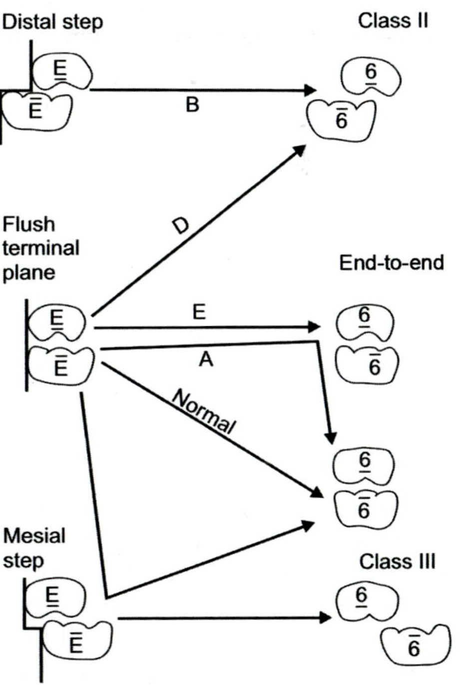

Fig. 8.5: Effect of deciduous molars relation on the relation of permanent first molars *(Redrawn from McDonald's)*.

- Change in class I due to loss of leeway space of mandibular E.
- Change in class II if maxillary E is lost before mandibular E.
- It can change to class I if lower second molar is lost before upper.
- Chances of change in class I are also achieved with the growth of mandible.

Distal step:

- It almost changes to Angle's class II molar relation. It is due to the already locked inclined plane relationship of primary molars in distal step fashion, that they guide the permanent molars in Angle's class II relation.
- Change to class II, if minimum growth differential is there.
- Change in end-on, by loss of leeway space and forward mandibular growth.
- Rarely, it can change to class I, if lower second molar is lost before upper.

Mesial step

- It almost changes to Angle's class III molar relation. It is due to the already locked inclined plane relationship of primary molars in mesial step fashion, that they guide the permanent molars in Angle's class III relation.
- It rarely changes to class I if upper second molar is lost before lower.
- It can also change to class I if minimum growth differential of jaws is there.
- Mostly, it changes to Angle's class III, due to loss of leeway space and forward mandibular growth.

Local Factors

Interproximal caries, sucking habits, or a skeletal pattern may produce a *"step"* rather than a flush terminal plane. In people with coarse diets, occlusal surfaces of primary teeth wear to a great extent. The removal of these cuspal interferences permits mandible to move forward as it is growing faster than the maxilla. It also helps in correction of skeletal class II relation. But if there is no natural occlusal wear, a functional retraction of the mandible may occur during closure due to inclined plane effect of the cusps, which then maintains the mandible in skeletal class II relation.

Spacing in Primary Dentition (Figs 8.6a and b; 8.7)

It is a normal and important feature which helps in proper alignment of permanent teeth in the arches. Following types of spacing can be observed.

Primary Spacing/Physiological/ Developmental Spacing

It is a normal developmental sequence, a self-correcting anomaly; and is an important

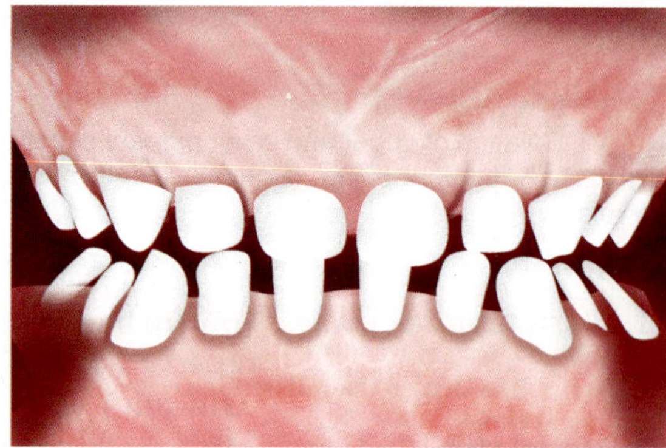

(a)

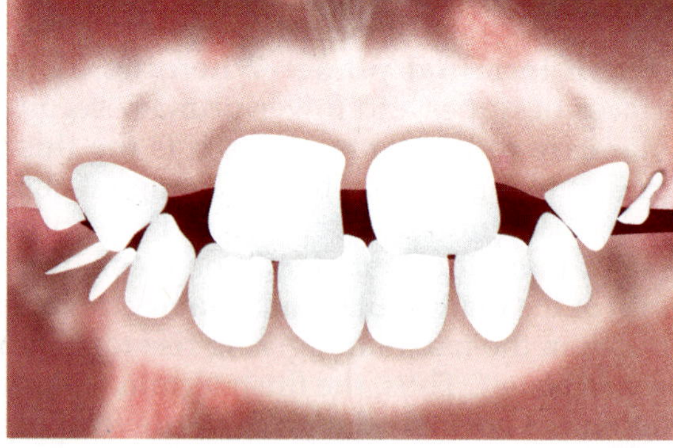

(b)

Figs 8.6a and b: Spacing in the primary dentition is important for alignment of permanent teeth in the dental arches because permanent teeth are bigger in MD size than primary teeth and need more space.

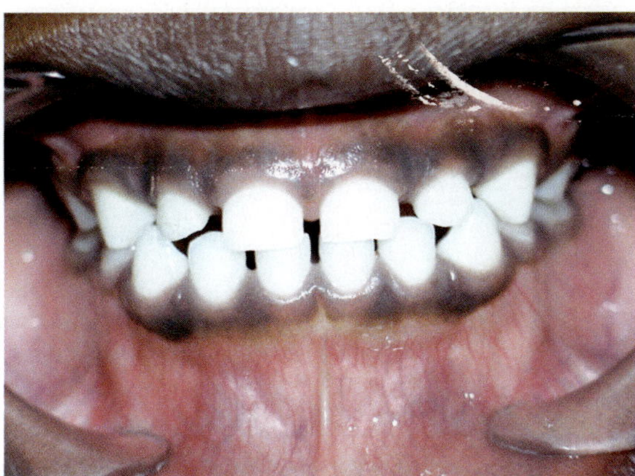

Fig. 8.7: An ideal condition of developmental spaces in primary dentition, which is important for alignment of the permanent teeth in arches.

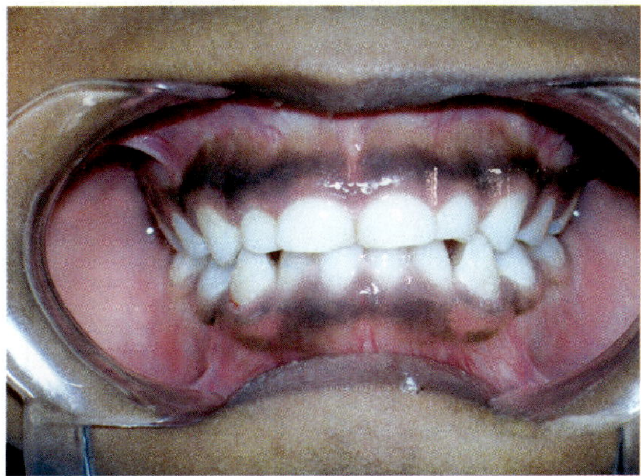

Fig. 8.9: Closed primary dentition, and mild crowding in lower incisal region. Crowding in primary teeth is a sure sign of future crowding in permanent dentition.

requirement for proper development of dentition. It appears due to active skeletal growth. It helps in proper alignment of permanent teeth which are wider than primary teeth. It occurs 70% of time in maxilla and 63% in mandible. Spaces are more in maxillary arch than the mandibular arch.

Open Dentition and a Closed Dentition (Figs 8.8 and 8.9)

If developmental spacing in deciduous dentition is present, it is known as open dentition. If there is no spacing, it is known as a closed dentition. Mean increase in the intercanine width is more in closed dentition as compared to open dentition, so that there is no excessive space for erupting incisors.

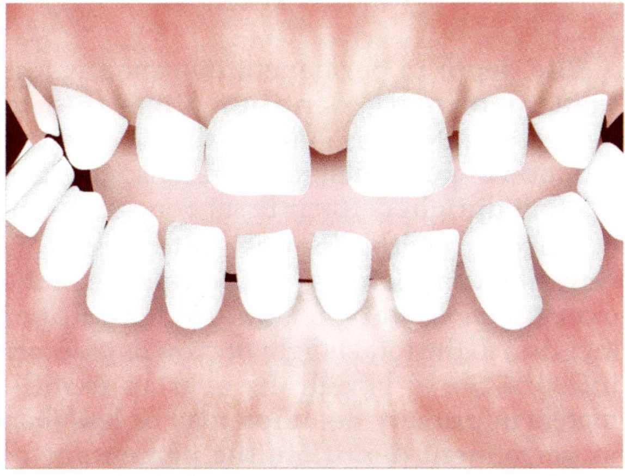

Fig. 8.8: Physiological spaces in both arches. It is known as open dentition.

Primate/Simian/Anthropoid Spaces (Figs 8.10 and 8.11)

These are found mesial to primary maxillary canines and distal to primary mandibular canines; named so as it is found in primates, i.e. between BC/CD. They help in proper interdigitation of canines, because of larger MD size of upper canine than lower, and presence of more I/D spaces in upper than the lower arch.

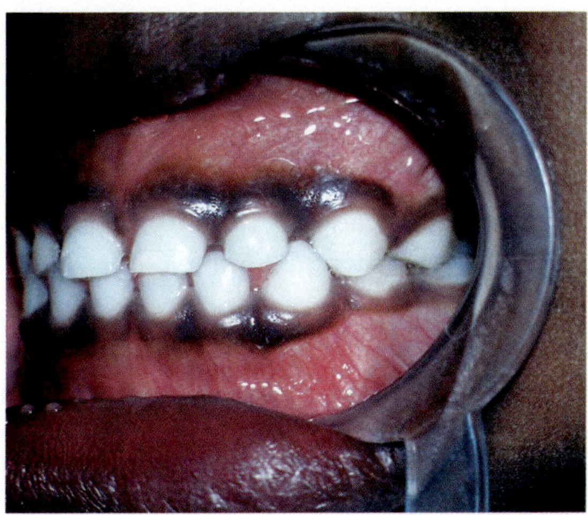

Fig. 8.10: Developmental and primate spacing in primary teeth which is a normal and necessary condition.

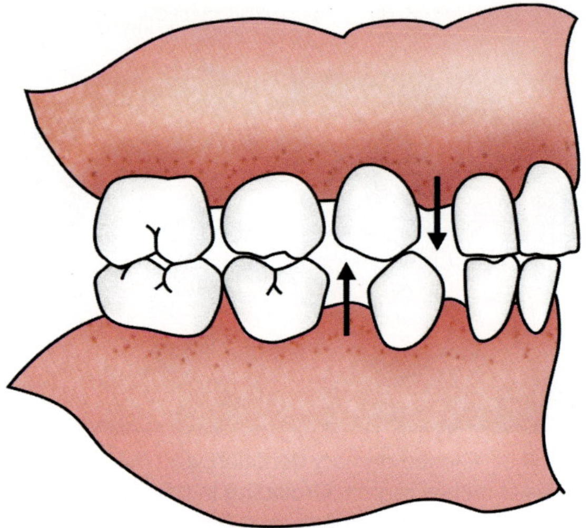

Fig. 8.11: Primate spaces in both arches, which are found mesial to canines in upper arch, and distal to canine in lower arch.

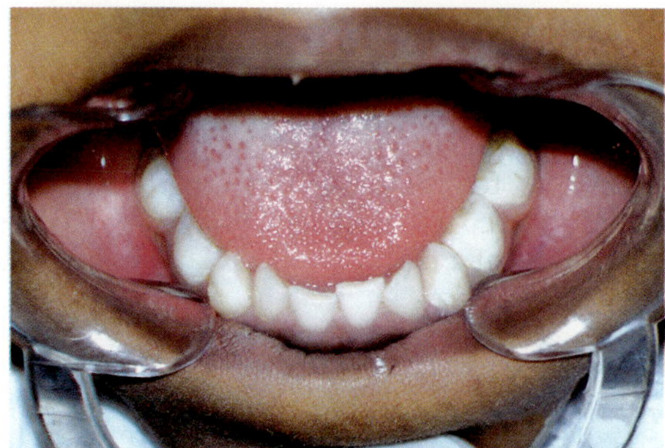

Fig. 8.12: Crowding in the primary dentition implies the space deficiency and a future crowding in the permanent dentition.

Importance of Spacing in the Primary Dentition (Fig. 8.12)

It helps in proper alignment of permanent teeth in the arches, since the size of permanent teeth are larger than the primary teeth. Given below in the table are the possibilities of crowding in permanent dentition depending on the amount of spacing present in the deciduous dentition.

Class	*In deciduous teeth*	*Crowding chances in permanent teeth*
I	Crowded	10 in 10
II	No spaces	7 in 10
III	< 3 mm spacing	5 in 10
IV	3–6 mm spacing	2 in 10
V	> 6 mm spacing	None

Deep Bite in the Primary Dentition

A relative deep bite exists in incisal region, which is due to more upright/vertical position of the incisors. It is due to a larger interincisal angle (170°) than in the permanent incisors (130°). It decreases due to attrition of primary incisors, eruption of primary molars and by forward mandibular growth (Fig. 8.13).

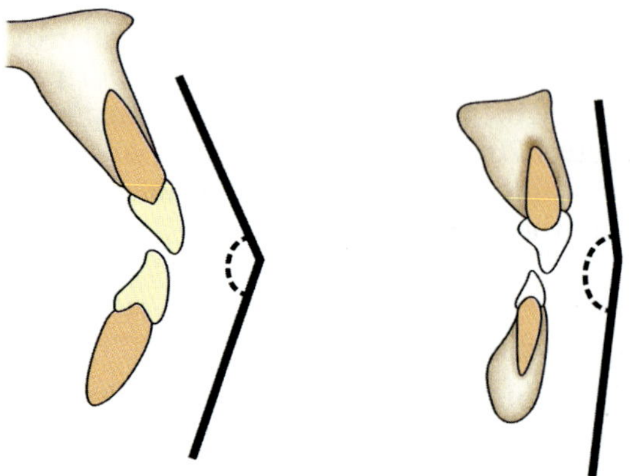

Fig. 8.13: Interincisal angle in permanent teeth is less than that in primary teeth, i.e. primary incisors are more upright in position.

Bite depth in permanent dentition is less than in primary dentition. It is due to decreased interincisal angle, due to forward eruption of permanent incisors. Also they are not that upright on their basal bone.

Since in orthodontics, bite depth is generally considered as the percentage of the overlap of lower incisors (by the upper incisors) to the total height of crowns of lower incisors. So, although the overlap in milimeters in primary dentition may be less than in permanent dentition, the percentage of overlap in primary dentition is more than the permanent dentition.

Self-correcting Anomalies

There are certain features of the dentition which are naturally present in developing dentition at various stages, they look abnormal features at that age, but are naturally-occurring and essential features of development of occlusion. They should be known to every dentist and should not be interfered with treatment procedures. The worried parents should also be comforted by proper explanation.

The following normal signs of primary dentition should be noted:

- Spaced anteriors
- Primate spaces
- Straight terminal plane
- Almost vertical inclination of anterior teeth
- Small mandible, convex profile.

Why a class III relationship is very rare in primary dentition period? Normally, in primary dentition, an equivalent of class III is never/very rarely seen, due to growth pattern of mandible, which lags behind the maxilla. Also C2D2 is not seen in primary dentition. However, abnormal growth can lead to such problems even in primary dentition (Figs 8.14 and 8.15).

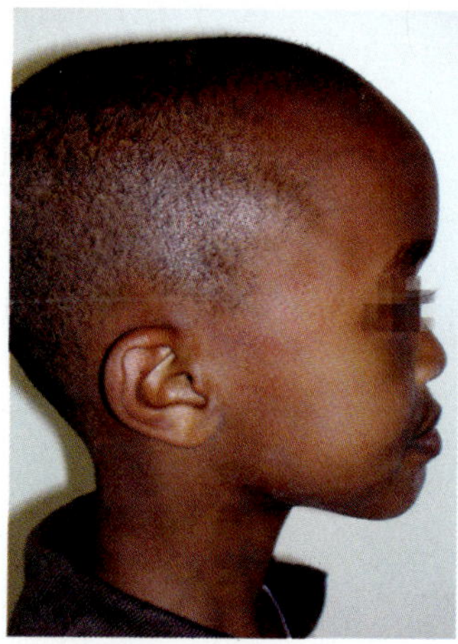

Fig. 8.14: Concave profile due to mandibular prognathism in a small child.

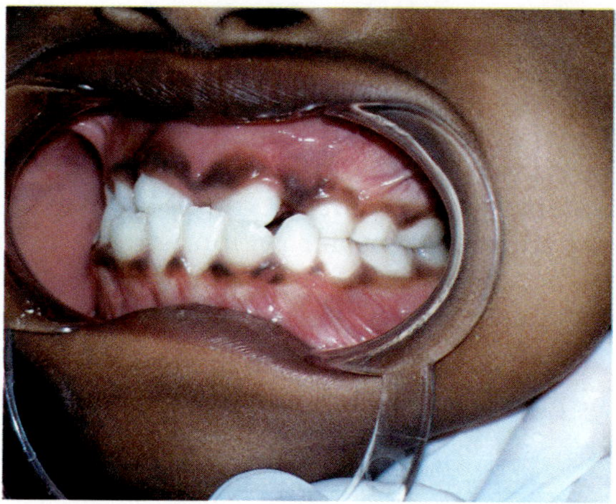

Fig. 8.15: Anterior crossbite and mesial step of primary E's.

THE MIXED DENTITION PERIOD

It is the period of dentition when a few primary and permanent teeth are present in the mouth. It begins with the eruption of first permanent molars at 6 years of age, generally in end-on relationship. It also marks the stage I of natural bite opening.

Natural Bite Opening (Fig. 8.16)

It is the decrease in the overbite due to eruption of the permanent molars in the oral cavity. It occurs three times in the life of an individual, i.e. at the time of eruption of first, second and third permanent molars. So, the permanent molars are called as natural bite openers.

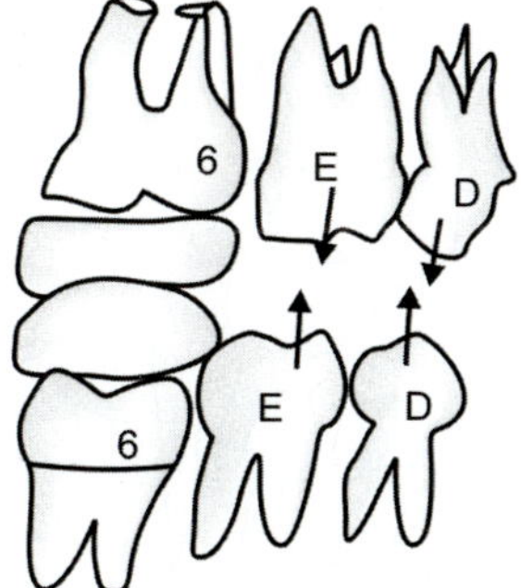

Fig. 8.16: Extrusion of primary teeth and thus correction of deep bite when the soft tissues on erupting permanent first molars lead to some occlusal gap in which primary teeth erupt.

Mechanism of Natural Bite Opening

When the molars erupt, the soft tissue overlying the molars is swollen and it comes in contact during mastication or swallowing and causes pain. So, the patients learn to keep the contact away from it. It causes a gap in the area anterior to molar region and leads to supraeruption of the teeth, and thus the bite opening.

Occlusal changes in the mixed dentition: The mixed dentition can be divided into three phases.

- First transitional period
- Intertransitional period/rest period
- Second transitional period.

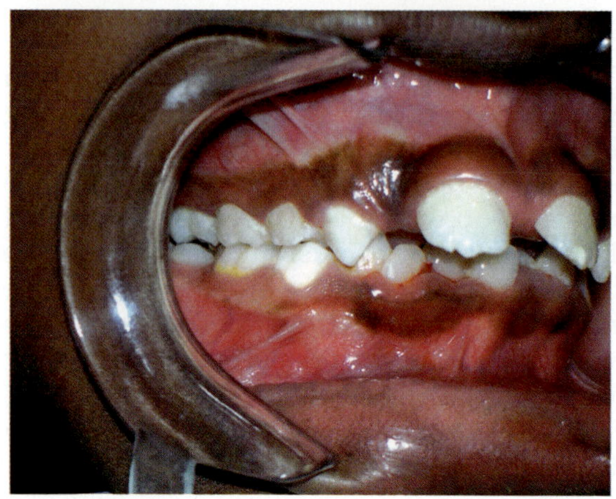

Fig. 8.17: Early mixed dentition stage showing lower incisal crowding.

First Transitional Period (Fig. 8.17)

It is also called as early mixed dentition period (MDP). It is characterized by emergence of first permanent molars and incisors teeth in lower and upper arches. Mostly, the lower teeth erupt before upper teeth. This phase is seen during 6–8 years of age. Here, we can see the three relations of permanent first molars, viz. end-on, class II, and class III, depending on the relation of primary second molars. Correction of end-on relation to class I occurs by utilization of physiologic space, leeway space and differential forward growth of the mandible (Figs 8.18 and 8.19).

Emergence of First Permanent Molars (Figs 8.20 and 8.21)

The mandibular first molar is generally the first permanent tooth to erupt at around 6 years. The first permanent molars are guided into the dental arch by the distal surfaces of the second deciduous molars. As discussed before, the mesiodistal relationship between the distal surfaces of the upper and lower second deciduous molars can be of three types:

1. **Flush terminal plane** (Fig. 8.22): The distal surfaces of the upper and lower deciduous molars is in one vertical plane

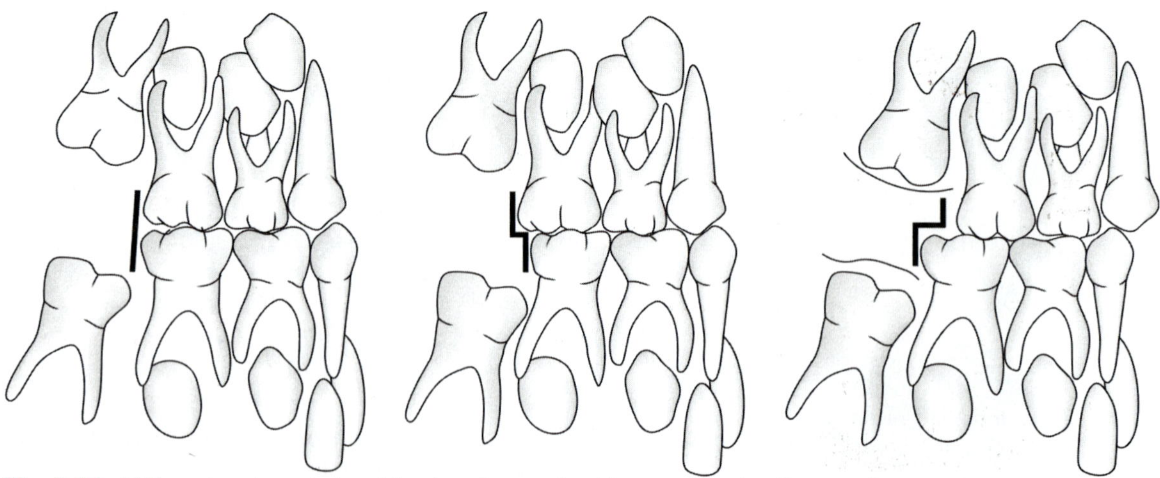

Fig. 8.18: Different molar relationships in primary dentition, and their effect on the eruption of permanent first molars relation *(Redrawn from Graber and Swain)*.

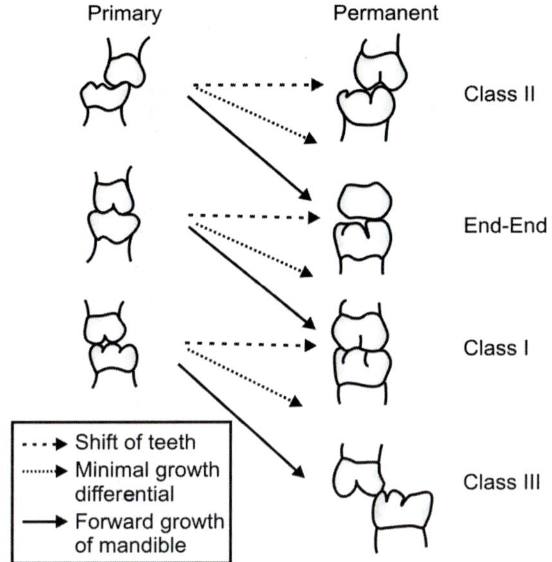

Fig. 8.19: Molar relation of primary teeth and the ensuing effect of growth on the final relation of permanent molars *(Redrawn from Proffit and Fields).*

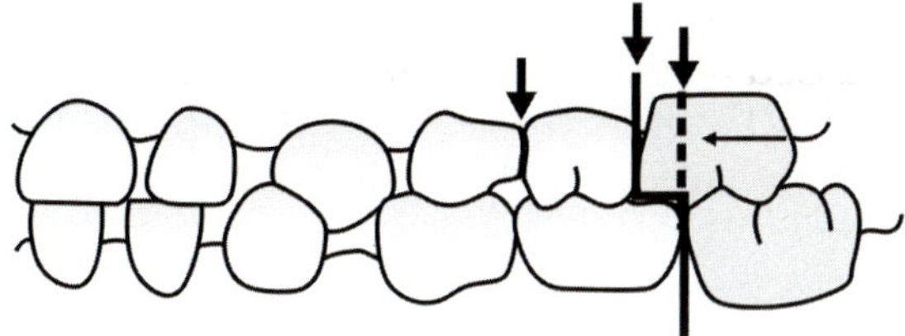

Fig. 8.20: How the distal caries on upper primary second molar leads to space loss with mesial migration of permanent first molar and thus a change in occlusal relation toward Angle's class II *(Redrawn from Graber and Swain).*

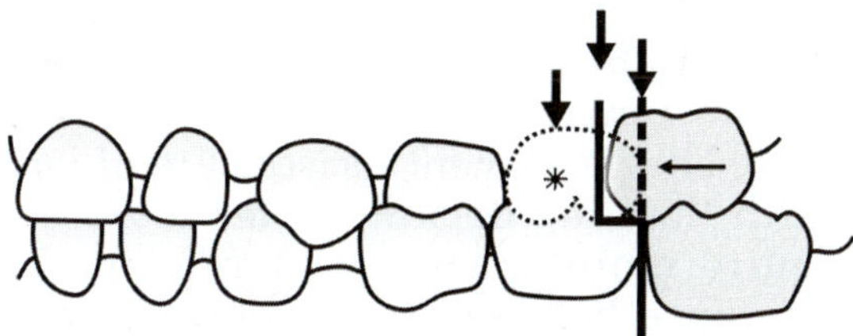

Fig. 8.21: How the early loss of upper primary second molar leads to space loss with mesial migration of permanent first molar and thus a change in occlusal relation toward Angle's class II *(Redrawn from Graber and Swain).*

called as flush or vertical terminal plane, thus the erupting permanent first molars are in end-on relationship. For them to end in class I molar relation, the lower molar has to move forward by 3–5 mm relative to upper molar. This occurs by utilization of physiological spaces and leeway spaces in lower arch and by differential forward growth of the mandible. The shift of lower molar from a flush terminal plane to class I relation, occurs by early and late shift.

Early mesial shift (Fig. 8.23): It is a phenomenon which is observed in open dentition at 6–7 years of age, and it occurs due to closure of primate spaces by pressure of erupting permanent molars. It leads to conversion of FTP relation into class I relationship. However, it is not a good feature as per the development of dentition, as it leads to a future space crunch in the arches, and generally leads to the development of crowding. An observant parent and an orthodontist can save this space loss by cementing proper appliance at a proper timing so as to avoid mesial movements of the permanent molars, e.g. lingual holding arch, Nance palatal arch, etc.

Late mesial shift: It occurs in closed dentitions at 10–11 years age (Fig. 8.24). First permanent molars shift mesially due to closure of leeway spaces after shedding of primary second molars. It also leads to loss of E-space, which may be utilised for alignment of teeth by the orthodontist. So, a close watch should be kept during this period and if possible and required, this space should be preserved by putting appropriate space managing appliances in the dental arches.

Since, the orthodontist has to be very vigilant regarding the maintenance of spaces during the mixed dentition period, this period can also be termed as space-age.

Many children lack the primate spaces. In these cases, the permanent

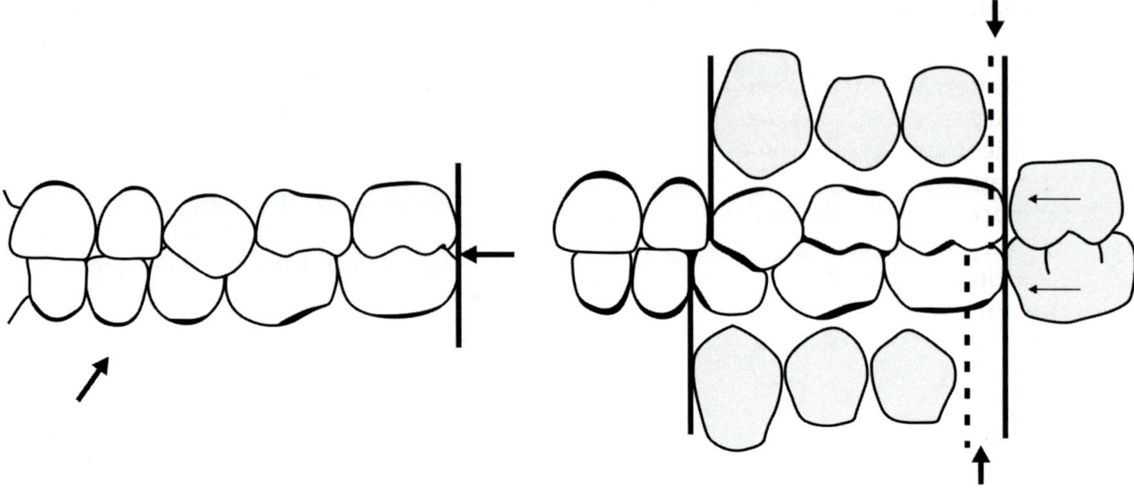

Fig. 8.22: Edge-on relation of permanent first molars when primary molars are in flush terminal plane relation. It gets converted in Angle's class I relation later on when leeway space is utilized *(Redrawn from Graber and Swain)*.

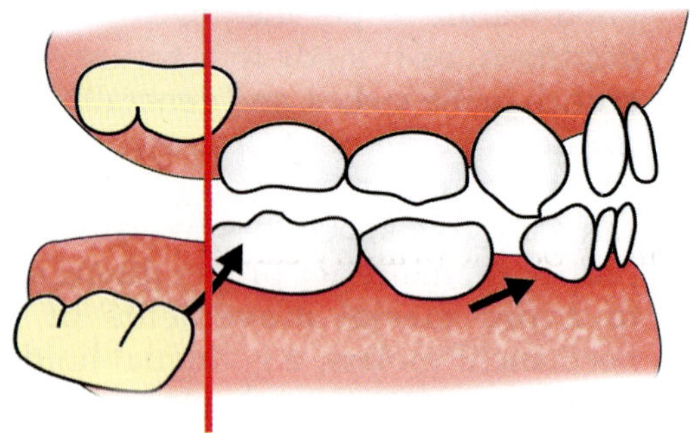

Fig. 8.23: Early mesial shift in the lower primate space.

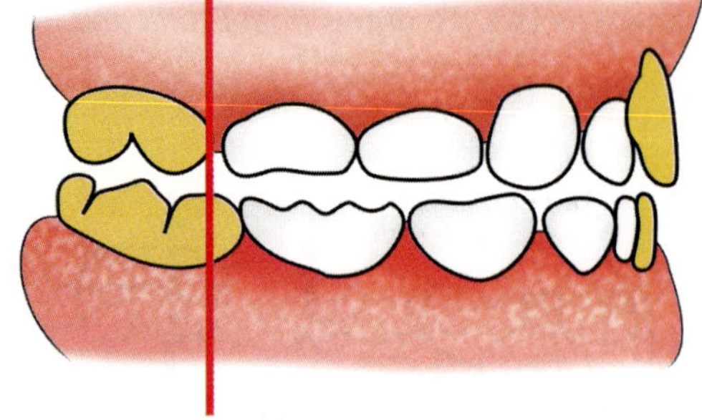

Fig. 8.24: Closed dentition, in which late mesial shift will take place when primary second molar will be lost

molars drift mesially utilizing the leeway space. This occurs in the late mixed dentition period.

2. **Mesial step terminal plane:** Here, the distal surface of lower primary 2nd molar is mesial to that of the upper. The permanent molars erupt directly into Angle's class I relation. It occurs due to early forward growth of mandible. If this differential growth of the mandible in a forward direction persists and is more, it can lead to skeletal and dental class III malocclusion.
3. **Distal step terminal plane:** It is characterized by the distal surface of the lower 2nd deciduous molar being distal to that of the upper. The erupting permanent molars generally are in class II relation.

The Exchange of Incisors

Incisal liability: The mandibular central incisors generally are first to erupt at 6–7 years. The permanent incisors are of larger width than the deciduous teeth. So, they require more space for alignment. This difference between the amount of space needed for the accommodation of permanent incisors and the amount of space available is called as incisal liability. It is 7.6 mm for the maxillary and 6.0 mm for the mandibular arch approximately.

The incisal liabilty exists in one of the three forms:

1. The favorable incisor liability is when primary spaces of the spaced dentition are sufficient to allow for the eruption of the permanent incisor without any crowding.
2. It is precarious when some amount of primary spacing is present in primary dentition. And then the individual must rely on secondary spacing to create sufficient space for the permanent incisors to erupt without crowding.
3. A difficult situation exists when the incisor liability is of such kinds that the growth and development will never be able to meet the space demands required by the permanent incisors, which leads to severe crowding and irregularities.

Naturally, the incisal liablity is overcome by following factors, known as **Warren Mayne's principles** (Table 8.1, Fig. 8.25).

1. Utilization of interdental spaces in the primary dentition.
2. Increase in the intercanine width
3. Change in incisor inclination.

Interdental spacings appear in both arches, especially in anterior region, with the ensuing growth. It occurs especially due to the transverse growth of jaw bases (remember, the sequence TSV). Sagittal growth mainly occurs distal to the molars, and does not contribute to any spacing in anterior region. It can also be seen that at this age, the transverse growth is more rapid, and also the growth in the transverse plane is first to be completed in the jaws.

Increase in intercanine width occurs more in males as compared to females, M > F, and more in upper arch as compared to lower arch, U > L. So, the girls have greater liability to incisor crowding.

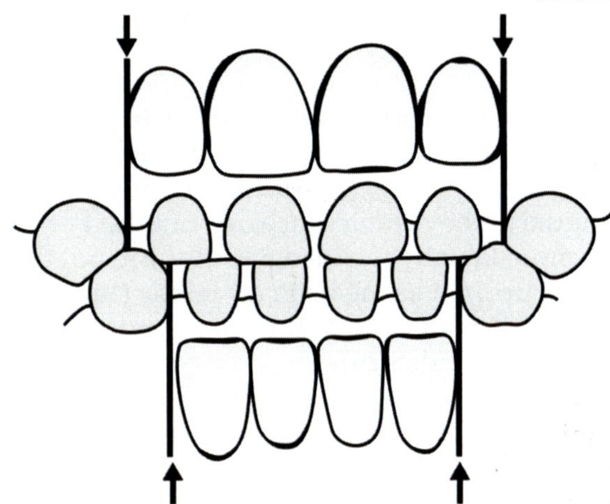

Fig. 8.25: Physiological spaces in incisal regions, and the compensation of incisal liability in both the arches. Note that how the presence of upper primate spaces helps in accommodation of bigger permanent incisors in the arch *(Redrawn from Graber and Swain)*.

By the age of eruption of lateral incisors, the intercanine width in each arch is gained by 3 mm. Also, an increase of 1.5 mm in upper arch is also attained with the eruption of upper canines. So, the primary canines should not be restricted by any clasps or space maintainer during this time.

Intercanine width in mandibular arch does not increase after 9 years of age in both the sexes. But in maxillary arch, it increases upto 16 years in males and upto 12 years in females. Thus, expansion of maxillary arch should be commenced in females at early age to take advantage of growth. In mandible, the arch expansion by natural development is possible till 9 years of age. It can be achieved by oral screen appliances or other passive/myofunctional appliances. Once the width of lower arch is established, it cannot be increased mechanically. Any attempt to increase the width needs

Table 8.1: Incisal liability

Method	*Maxilla*	*Mandible*
I/D spacing	0–10 mm, average 4 mm	0–6 mm, average 3 mm
Increase in intercanine width	4.5 mm	3.0 mm
Incisor position	2.2 mm	1.3 mm

a permanent retainer, otherwise it gets relapsed.

Forward position/eruption of incisors: It also contributes to some spaces in arches. The permanent incisors buds are positioned lingual to the primary incisors, but their erupt on more labially inclined, i.e. they are not that much upright as the primary teeth. Thus they acquire a wider arc of the circle and a larger perimeter (Fig. 8.26).

Repositioning of primary mandibular canines occurs distally, in the primate spaces when mandibular lateral incisors erupt and push the mandibular primary canine there, which also give approx. 1 mm space. But, this phenomenon does not occur in maxillary arch, as primate space is already between B and C there.

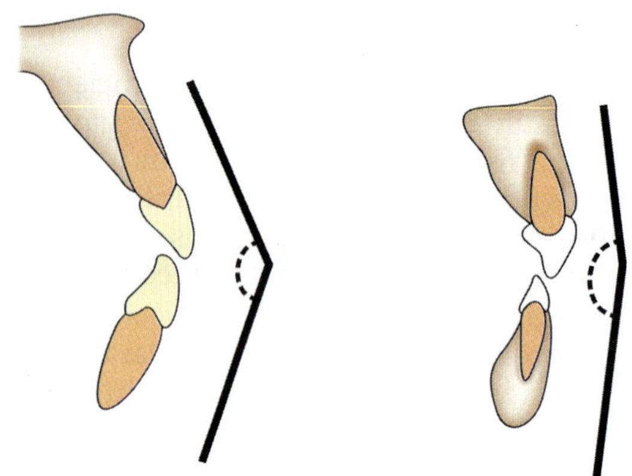

Fig. 8.26: Interincisal angle in permanent and primary dentition.

Secondary Spacing (Fig. 8.27)

It occurs in closed dentition with eruption of lower incisors, which pushes primary mandibular canine laterally. It creates space for proper eruption of maxillary lateral incisors. It helps to increase the intercanine width in both arches and increase in arch circumference in maxilla.

Normally, the lower incisors erupt in mild crowding stage. Crowding of upto 2 mm gets resolved by natural growth and alignment of teeth under tongue pressure. More crowding does not resolve by itself. Also, if any crowding does not resolve itself by the age of 8 years, it is highly unlikely to be resolved by any other natural process after this age, and will need some interceptive or corrective procedures later in life.

Also, the primary maxillary canines should not be extracted at an earlier age, esp during serial extractions. It is because erupting permanent canines help in increasing the intercanine width in maxilla. If primary maxillary canines are extracted at an earlier age, the stimulus of eruption of permanent canines is lost, which may lead to their impaction or deflection in their path of eruption. Also, the maxillary intercanine width increase is not proper. In some cases, if crowding is there, then it is better to slice the mesial surfaces of the primary canines, so as to provide some space for proper eruption/ alignment of the erupting incisors.

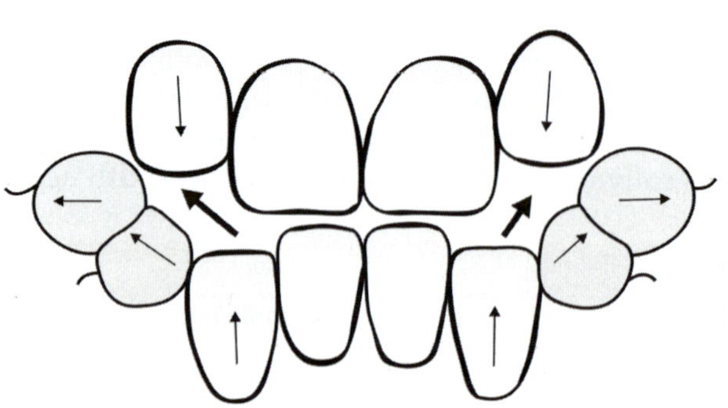

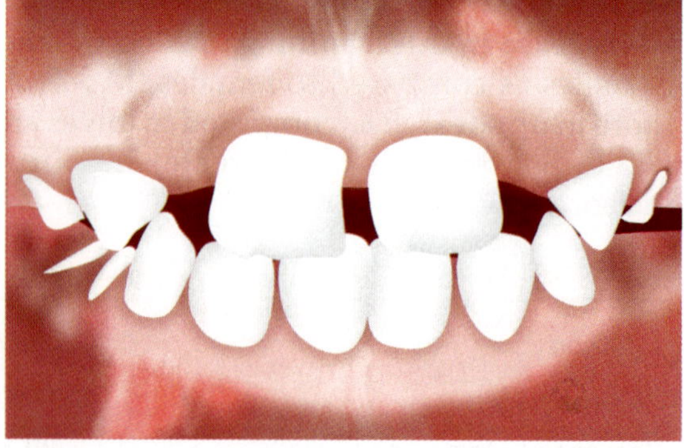

Fig. 8.27: Phenomenon of secondary spacing when erupting lower lateral incisors push the primary canines distally to gain space for alignment *(Redrawn from Graber and Swain)*.

Intertransitional Period

This is the phase when no change in status of dentition is observed, but only growth of the jaws is taking place. Thus, it can be considered as a stable phase or a **period of rest**. However, continuing skeletal growth helps in increasing the width and length of basal bones, which is to be subsequently used for the alignment of other succedaneous teeth. It generally extends in 8–9 years of age.

Second Transitional Period

It is also called as late mixed dentition period. It is characterized by replacement of deciduous molars and canines by their successors. It generally starts after 9 years of age with the eruption of mandibular permanent canines. This is an important phase of development, as the changes in dentition and jaw growth are rapid and going on simultaneously. It is the age of prepubertal growth spurt when basal jaw growth in length and width take place. According to Graber, the main growth spurts seen in children are as follows.

Spurt	*Females*	*Males*
Childhood	3 years	3 years
Juvenile	6–7 years	7–9 years
Prepubertal	11–12 years	13–15 years

The sequence of growth completion in face is WDH, i.e. width completes first, then the depth and then the height in the last. The jaws follow the same sequence as face, i.e. general growth curve. So, the treatment of expansion should be done at an early age to take advantage of the ensuing growth in width. The expansion should best be done in the age range of 8–10 years, followed by period of retention. In cranium, the sequence of growth completion is WHD, i.e. width completes first, then the height and then the depth in the last. The cranium follows the neural growth curve.

The following features are noted during this stage:

1. Ugly-duckling stage
2. Conversion of first molar relationship, by the use of leeway space of Nance.
3. Late mesial shift
4. Growth of jaws and reduction of bite depth, skeletal convexity, etc.

Leeway Space of Nance

The combined mesiodistal width of permanent canines and premolars is usually less than that of the deciduous canines and molars. The surplus space is called as leeway space of Nance. It is 1.8 mm in the maxillary (0.9 mm per side) and 3.4 mm (1.7 mm per side) in the mandibular arch. It is more in lower arch because the size of lower primary second molar is larger than upper. The difference in the size of primary second molar and the second premolar is called the **E-space**. It is bigger in lower than in upper arch. This space is utilized by the mesial drift of the permanent molars, more for mandibular molars, to establish an Angle's class I molar relation from flush terminal plane relation (Fig. 8.28).

Importance of this space: This space is generally gets used during eruption by mesial drift of permanent first molars after the loss of primary second molars. In certain cases, the conservation of this space becomes very important during the development of dentition, as an interceptive procedure. This preserved space can be used for alignment of teeth in the arches, when erupting 2nd premolars drift distally giving space for teeth anterior to them.

Indications of preservations: Certain conditions, e.g. closed dentition; cases of mild lower incisors crowding; loss of space due to premature loss of primary tooth especially in maxillary primary second molar region; cases requiring maxillary molar distalization to correct molar relationship, etc. The decision depends on the clinical accumenship of the orthodontist. But, conservation of this space can be very useful in future orthodontic treatment and can help convert an extraction case to a nonextraction case, and also helps in conservation of the anchorage.

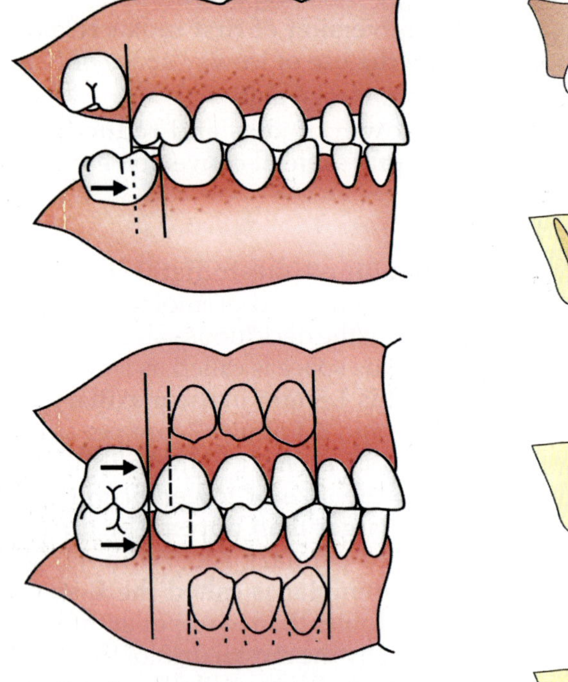

Fig. 8.28: Eruption of lower first molar in mesial position when there is mesial step. Second fig showing leeway space of Nance in upper and lower buccal regions. Note upper leeway space is less than lower.

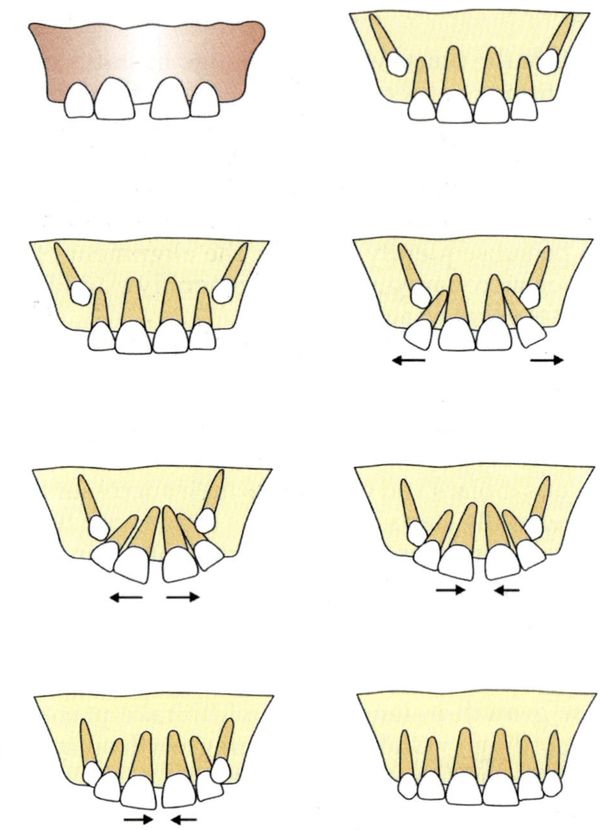

Fig. 8.29: Ugly-duckling stage: Note that the erupting permanent canines, while sliding along the roots of lateral incisors, lead to root crowding of incisors and flaring of crowns distally thus creating spaces. Later on, when canines slide along the crowns of lateral incisors, apply mesial forces thus closing the spaces and uprighting the crowns. Thus, it is a self-correcting anomaly.

Appliances needed: Certain appliances, e.g. transpalatal arch, Nance's palatal arch, lingual holding arch, etc. can be used to preserve this space. During fixed appliance therapy, this space can be preserved by making bent-in stop loops in the arch wires; by using open coil spring; by using arch sleeves; headgear, etc. which do not allow the molars to drift forward.

THE UGLY-DUCKLING STAGE (Fig. 8.29)

It is a transient or self correcting condition which starts in the maxillary incisor region between 8 and 9 years, when the permanent canines start their eruptive movements within the bone. Maxillary canines are generally the last succedaneous teeth to erupt in oral cavity as they have to traverse a very long path of eruption from their initial position near the floor of maxillary sinuses. As they erupt, they apply physiological forces and displace the roots of upper lateral incisors mesially. It results in transmitting the forces on roots of central incisors also, which also get displaced mesially, creating a **root-crowding**. In reciprocation, the crowns of incisors move distally, thus opening the spaces between them. This resultant divergence of crowns of incisors and spacing has been called by Broadbent as the ugly-duckling stage (Fig. 8.30).

Do not Disturb this Condition

This condition corrects itself when the canines erupt and the pressure of canines is transferred from the root to the coronal area of

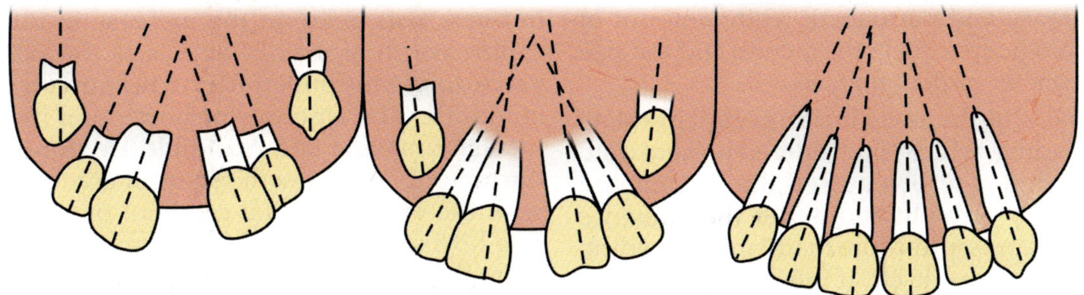

Fig. 8.30: Various phases of ugly-duckling stage.

incisors. It is very important to know here that this stage should not be disturbed by any orthodontic intervention, (unless the spaces present are more than normal, and inhibit the eruption of canines). If an attempt is done to close these spaces, it may cause root resorption of lateral incisors, which strike the canines during their orthodontic tipping movement. They may also cause deflection of path of eruption of canines leading to their impaction or malalignment.

A midline space between central incisors may also be present due to lower attachment of labial frenum. The frenum normally gets receeded due to growth of alveolar height with eruption of incisors. This space should not be attempted to close and we should wait till eruption of canines. Sometimes, it gets closed itself by the pressure of incisors causing pressure atrophy of frenum, thus removing the resistance / cause. But, if this space is larger due to some other factor, e.g. supernumerary tooth, or larger basal bone size, etc. and if it is expected to cause ectopic eruption of adjacent teeth, then it needs orthodontic intervention to close some part of the space.

Eruption of Permanent First Molars

It occurs at around 6 years of age, and the lower molar erupts before the upper molar. In majority of children, the first permanent molars erupt prior to the central incisor. The occlusal relationship that the first permanent molars initially obtain with each other is determined by the terminal plane relationship of the primary second molars which is generally end-on. During formation, the crowns of the maxillary molars face distally rather than occlusally. As the maxilla grows forward, space is created posteriorly, permitting the growth of maxillary tuberosity. It helps the first molar to rotate and by the time the crown pierces the gingiva, it is facing more occlusally.

Eruption of Incisors

Lower incisors generally erupt before upper incisors. In mandible, although the incisors erupt after permanent molars, they reach their clinical crown height earlier. The permanent incisors develop lingual to the roots of the primary incisors, causing their root resorption on lingual side, forcing them to get exfoliated. But, they erupt in a labially inclined direction in a larger perimeter as compared to the primary incisors. Also the interincisal angle of permanent incisors is less than the primary incisors. It helps in accommodating some incisal liability.

When the primary central incisors get exfoliated, their successors move labially under the influence of tongue pressure. The balance of forces of tongue and the buccolabial musculature help to attain a proper arch form. Sometimes, the primary incisors do not exfoliate but permanent incisors appear lingual to them, thus creating rotations and crowding. If this situation is allowed to progress, then it leads to development of crossbite of the tooth / teeth. The primary incisors should be extracted as soon as possible to pave way for permanent teeth to take their aligned position.

There are certain criteria which help to determine whether the permanent incisors will appear crowded or not are: size difference of primary and permanent teeth; amount of physiologic spacing in the arches; and the size of perimeter of dental arches.

Generally, the lower incisors erupt in a state of crowding, which is considered normal upto 2 mm. It gets resolved itself due to ongoing skeletal jaw growth and under the influence of tongue pressure. More than 2 mm crowding does not resolve itself. If this crowding is not resolved by the time the lateral incisors have completely erupted, i.e. 7–8 years of age, then it will need orthodontic intervention.

During eruption, the mandibular lateral incisors push the primary lateral incisors labially but also move the cuspids distally and laterally. It leads to closing the primate spaces, and helps to create some space (known as secondary spacing) for alignment of lower incisors.

When the mandibular primary cuspids are prematurely lost, the lower incisors may get tipped lingually under the influence of hyperactive mentalis, leading to increased overjet. It leads to a loss of space in dental arch from the anterior side, and is a strong indication of future crowding. It warrants a closer and regular follow-up of the case for a proper and timely guidance of eruption or serial extractions and may need LHA for prevention of lingual tipping. Lingual tipping of incisors also leads to labial eruption of permanent cuspid. A premature loss of primary canines occurs due to small arch or jaw size; and is an indication of future crowding.

The maxillary anterior dental segment is supported by the mandibular, providing functional stops against which the maxillary incisors erupt. The maxillary permanent incisors erupt with a more labial inclination than their predecessors and in a larger arch perimeter, thus reducing the incisal liability.

Safety Valve Mechanism

It is the nature's attempt to maintain a proper occlusion during growth. The intercanine width in mandible is completed at 9 years in females, and at 10 years in males. In maxilla, it is completed at 12 years in girls and at 18 years in boys. This delay in the increase in intercanine width of maxilla serves as the safety valve during the pubertal growth spurt for the mandible. The amounts of horizontal increments of maxilla and mandible are different during pubertal growth spurt, in accordance with the cephalocaudal gradient of growth. The horizontal increments of mandible are more than the maxilla. So when the mandible comes forward during growth spurt (mandible's forward growth being more than maxilla) and for long-time, its wider posterior part comes in approximation with a narrower anterior part of maxillary arch. If this relation gets maintained, it will lead to crossbite situation. Here, the maxillary intercanine width comes as a savior, and an increasing intercanine width helps in gaining a width of maxillary arch. This helps in adjusting the broader part of forwardly-moved mandibular arch to the maxillary arch, when mandible comes forward during growth.

Eruption of Canines and Premolars (Fig. 8.31)

Normal development of occlusion depends on factors like a favorable sequence of eruption; normal tooth size–arch size ratio without any discrepancy; a normal molar relationship with minimal loss of leeway space; and a favorable buccolingual relationship of the alveolar processes.

Mandibular Arch

The most favorable sequence of eruption in mandibular arch is 61234578. The cuspids erupt at 9 years of age and lead to a final gain in intercanine width. They help in maintaining the anterior arch perimeter and prevent the lingual tipping of incisors. On the contrary, if primary canines get lost prematurely, and there is time for eruption of permanent canines, the lower incisors tip lingually under the pressure of lower lips. It leads to the loss of their centric stops with maxillary incisors. Thus, they overerupt until they find the occlusal stops, either with upper teeth or the palatal mucosa, leading to deep bite. If first premolars erupt before the

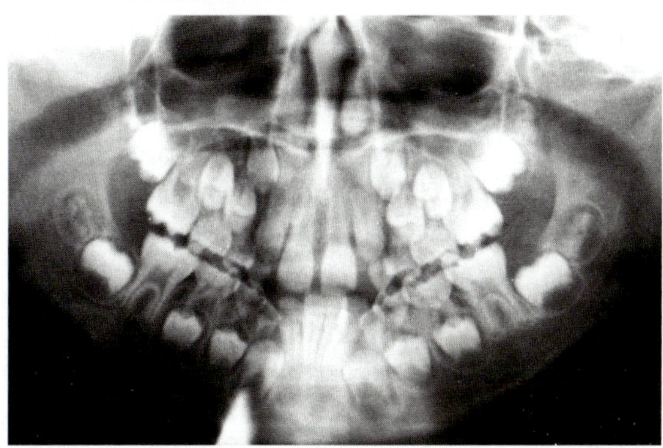

Fig. 8.31: OPG showing normal development of teeth.

canine / s, they take up some of the space meant for canines, and cause them to erupt into labioversion / labially blocked out situation.

Second bicuspid is the last tooth to erupt in lower arch. If space needed has been lost partially or completely (by gross caries or by premature extraction of primary 2nd molars without space maintainers, etc.), then there will be a shortening of the arch perimeter by mesial movement of permanent first molar. Then the said premolar gets either deflected buccally or lingually, or gets impacted. So it is necessary to maintain the arch space / perimeter by using space maintainer. All attempts should be done to maintain primary 2nd molars to avoid their extraction, or proper space maintainers should be given. It should be remembered that the primary teeth are the best space maintainers. In many cases, lower 2nd bicuspids are congenitally missing. There the primary 2nd molars may / may not be maintained depending on the crowding; need and consent of the patient / parents.

Maxillary Arch

The normal sequence of dental eruption in maxilla is either 61245378, or 61243578. Leeway space in upper arch is less than the lower arch due to difference in the size of primary 2nd molars. This leeway space is required for accommodation of the wider permanent teeth. Canines erupt generally at 11½–12 years age, and they help in increase in intercanine width during eruption. intercanine width is also gained by basal jaw growth during this age, as the adolescent growth spurt is active at this age. It helps in providing space for accommodation of canines. There should be no space loss during this phase; and also the permanent first molars must not be allowed to rotate and tip mesially. If space loss occurs, the cuspid is likely to be labially blocked out of the arch.

Maxillary anterior segment is easily displaced labially by thumb sucking, tongue thrusting, or a hyperactive mentalis muscle causing lower lip trap. And such displacement affects the eruptive pattern of the cuspid and bicuspid.

Eruption of Second Molars

The second permanent molars should erupt after eruption of canines. But, if permanent second molars erupt before second bicuspids but after the loss of primary second molar, they will force first molars to shift mesially. It leads to loss of leeway space and thus crowding / palatal eruption of second bicuspids. This condition should be recognised early and proper space maintainer should be given to prevent space loss.

The mandibular second molar appears before the maxillary and both of them generally appear after all teeth have erupted in the mouth. The eruption of maxillary second molar prior to the mandibular is symptomatic of developing Angle's class II malocclusion.

PERMANENT DENTITION PERIOD

When all the primary teeth have been lost, and the oral cavity has only the permanent teeth, this stage is called as permanent dentition period. Normally, it starts with the loss of either maxillary second primary molar or the canines, which are the last erupting permanent tooth. It generally starts at 11½–12 years of age.

Eruption of Second Molars

It starts erupting at around 12 years of age. The space distal to first permanent molars is created by continuing growth of maxillary tuberosity, and by resorption of anterior border of ramus. Generally, the lower molars erupt before the upper; and teeth in females erupt before males.

Dentition of Young Adults

Third molar eruption: They show great variability in calcification and eruption. Normally, they erupt in 18–25 years age. Their eruption has also been linked to crowding of mandibular incisors during late teen period, but has now been largely disapproved. Incisor crowding is more common in men than women. This late lower arch crowding has been found to be associated with the late mandibular growth phenomenon.

They get impacted also due to lack of space. It can be due to evolutionary trend of small size of mandible due to the use of soft food in modern civilisation, to use of softer foods and thus loss of functional stimulation for the growth of mandible. Also there is less proximal attrition and mesial shifting of teeth. Thus, space for third molar is not created.

Dimensional Changes

Maxillary and mandibular arch widths do not show appreciable changes. Once established, the mandibular intercanine width cannot be changed. The arch length also does not increase, but shows a continued shortening of arch perimeter due to attrition and mesial shifting of teeth from posterior side; and by lingual tipping of lower incisors under the influence of late mandibular growth.

Occlusal Changes

Both overjet and overbite decrease throughout the 2nd decade of life, probably due to forward growth of mandible. Natural bite opening effects are seen at the time of eruption of first, second and third permanent molars.

Conclusion

The development of dentition is a very important phase during the growth of individual. The teeth are directed in the arches under the influence of growth and muscular forces. The teeth act as functional matrices for the alveolar bone growth. The dentition passes through various phases which need to be monitored carefully to take the best advantages of growth of jaws, the spaces and eruption sequence of the teeth. With the help of proper appliances and monitoring, the developing malocclusions can be intercepted timely to reduce the severity or to completely eliminate the developing conditions. A proper knowledge of the normal features of developing dentition is very important, which should not be interfered. However, any mechanical interference in normal path of eruption should be removed timely for normal eruption of teeth and development of dental arches.

VIVA VOCE QUESTIONS

1. **How much mesial movement of the permanent first molar is required for attaining class I relation from the FTP?**
   Approx. 3.5 mm of movement of mandibular first molar forward with respect to maxillary first molar is required for smooth transition to class I relation in permanent dentition (i.e. a one-half cusp transition in molar relation).

2. **What is intertransitional period?**
   It is a quite period, at 8–10 years of age; here no change is seen in dentition. No teeth erupt during this time period.

3. **What is late mixed dentition/second transitional period?**
   It is the period of dentition in the age of 10–12 years when there is eruption of 3,4,5; Transition in chewing pattern develops in conjunction with eruption of permanent canines at age 12 years.

4. **What is leeway space of Nance?**
   It is the difference between MD sizes of CDE and 3,4,5; it is 1.8 mm in maxilla and 3.4 mm in mandible; it is mostly due to primary mandibular second molar size ka E-space (2–3 mm), helps in late mesial shift to achieve class I molars.

5. **What is E-space?**
   It is the space provided by the primary mandibular second molar when the second premolar erupts after its shedding. It is approx. 3 mm.

6. **What is space age?**
   It is the mixed dentition period (MDP). This is the most important phase of dentition development and should be very critically observed.

7. **Why the attrition is considered important in the primary dentition and mixed dentition period?**
   Pronounced attrition in MDP is observed to help in-decrease in deep bite, prevent interlocking of the cusps by flattening them and thus paving way for unhindered forward growth of mandible.

8. **How does the deep bite decreases during transition of dentition?**
   It occurs by eruption of permanent molars, attrition of incisors and forward movement of mandible due to growth.

9. **What is meant by secondary spacing?**
   It occurs in closed dentition with eruption of lower incisors, which pushes primary mandibular canine laterally. It creates space for proper eruption of maxillary lateral incisors. It helps to increase the intercanine width in both arches and increase in arch circumference in maxilla.

10. **What do you mean by tertiary spacing?**
    It is the spacing created due to extraction, etc.

11. **What is ugly-duckling stage of Broadbent?**
    In maxillary arch, at 8–9 years age, canines press the roots of laterals and so root crowding occurs, crowns move distally, spaces develop b/w crowns of incisors. It should not be disturbed till eruption of canines, as it is a self-correcting anomaly.

12. **How does the arch length change from mixed dentition period (MDP) to the permanent dentition period (PDP)?**
    It decreases by 2–3 mm when MDP changes to PDP, both from anterior and posterior sides. The anteriors erupt in upright situation and with growth of mandible. Also posterior teeth move mesially throughout life due to attrition, loss of leeway space and anterior component of force of occlusion. Also the arch width does not increase b/w 2½–6 years of age; and the arch perimeter does not increase b/w 2½–6 years of age.

13. **When is the largest arch length available in the dentition?**
    It is before eruption of first permanent molar.

14. **What are the signs of incipient malocclusion?**
    These are: the lack of interdental spacing in primary dentition, crowding in permanent incisors in MDP and premature loss of primary canines especially mandibular due to the eruption of lateral incisors which cause root resorption of canines if arch length is deficient in the mandibular arch.

15. Which are the self-correcting anomalies?

Gum pads stage	Primary DP	Mixed DP
Open bite	Deep bite	End-on molars
Increased overjet	FTP	Ugly-duckling stage
Tongue in between gum pads	Primary spacing	< 2 mm of lower
	incisors crowding	
	Primate spacing	
	Small mandible	
	More upright incisors	

16. How does the chewing pattern of child differ from that of an adult?

The adults open the mouth straight and then moves it laterally during chewing, while the child moves laterally.

17. What are various features of development of dentition?

18. What is natural bite opening phenomenon?

Natural bite opening occurs at 6, 12, 18 years of age, with eruption of permanent molars. There are 3 periods of natural bite opening according to Schwarz. At 6 years, when First molar erupts; at 12 years when 2nd molar erupts; at 18 years when 3rd molar erupts.

19. What are some other important features of dentition?

- U/L permanent incisors erupt lingual to primary teeth and move forward under the tongue pressure as they erupt.
- 7–8 years age = critical period
- Sudden change during the eruption of the CI and LI is shown by = 1.5 mm crowding in both M and F. Average female recovers slightly better than males.
- No great relief of crowding in incisor region is expected after full eruption of LI.
- Most crowding is generally seen in lower anterior segment.
- Occlusal contact is only 2–6% in 24 hours period.
- Primary incisors are more vertical and interincisal angle is greater causing deep bite.
- Mandibular CI, LI seem to erupt from lingual
- Maxillary LI = no labial gingival bulge. It is because the position of lateral incisor lingual to the central incisors.
- Maxillary second molar erupts D and F.
- Maxillary third molar erupts D and B and outward.

20. How does the apical inclinations of upper and lower teeth differ?

Axial inclination of maxillary teeth tend to converge apically especially at the end of the arch and mandibular axes tend to diverge following the curve of Spee. Crowns of maxillary posterior teeth and canines and of all mandibular teeth are lingually inclined, (labial root torque), whole of maxillary incisors are labially inclined (labial crown torque).

SELF-ASSESSMENT QUESTIONS

1. What are different types of crowdings?
2. What is the eruption sequence of primary and permanent teeth?
3. What is the eruption age of various permanent teeth?
4. Define chronologic age, dental age and skeletal age? Which is most reliable?
5. What do you mean by self-correcting anomalies?
6. What are the natal and neonatal teeth?
7. What do you mean by mixed dentition period (MDP)?
8. What is the natural bite opening?
9. What is mechanism of natural bite opening?
10. What is meant by first transitional period/ early mixed dentition period (MDP)?
11. What is meant by Early mesial shift?
12. What do you mean by late mesial shift?
13. What is incisal liability?

9

Occlusion

INTRODUCTION

Occlusion is one of the important areas of continuous discussion among dental professionals. All the treatment modalities consider occlusion as main source of guidance so that a comfortable and healthy relation of teeth can be maintained for longevity of the dental and supporting tissues. An understanding of the principles of occlusion and the relationship to oral health and disease is of paramount importance. There is a balance of forces of tongue, lips and cheeks at rest creating a neutral zone. This allows for the proper alignment of the teeth, development of dental arches, and normal facial development.

In the past, the occlusion was considered to be a morphologic entity rather than a biologic entity. It was considered as a static relation rather than dynamic relation. But with continued research and expanding knowledge, importance of the functional status of the patient's entire masticatory system including TMJ, supporting structures and neuromascular phenomenon has been acknowledged.

In dentistry, occlusion refers to the "relationship of maxillary and mandibular teeth when they are in functional contact during activity of mandible." The study of occlusion involves the entire stomatognathic system during the functional movements. The study of occlusion is essential for the proper understanding, and for achieving the objectives of orthodontic treatment. The establishment of a functional occlusion is one of the primary goals of the orthodontics.

Definitions

Occlusion: It can be simply defined as the relationship of the maxillary and mandibular teeth, as they are brought into functional contact.

According to glossary of prosthodontic terms, occlusion is defined as the static relationship between the incising or masticatory surfaces of the maxillary or mandibular teeth or tooth analogues.

McNeill defines occlusion as the functional relationship between the components of masticatory system, including the teeth, supporting tissues, neuromuscular system, temporomandibular joints and craniofacial skeleton. On the contrary, disocclusion as defined by Stallard is, "the separation of the teeth from occlusion, i.e. the opposite of occlusion".

Ideal Occlusion

It is a hypothetical concept, however, no ideal has been defined. It involves the theoretical concept of functional relationships which includes idealized principles and features that an occlusion should have. An occlusion should provide function, health and comfort. The important aspect of ideal occlusion now includes functional harmony, health and stability of stomatognathic system.

It is a hypothetical or theoretical concept based on the anatomy of the teeth and is rarely found in nature. As narrated by McDonald and Ireland, 1998, it involves a condition in which the skeletal bases of maxilla and mandible are of the correct size relative to each other and the teeth are in correct relationship in all three planes of space at rest. It can be used as a standard to which other occlusions can be compared and judged. Houston et al. (1992) suggested the following concepts of ideal occlusion in permanent dentition:

a. Each arch is regular; the teeth have ideal mesiodistal and buccolingual inclinations; and correct approximal relationship with each other.
b. The arch relationships are such that each lower tooth (except the central incisor) contacts the corresponding upper tooth and the tooth anterior to it. The upper arch overlaps the lower arch anteriorly and laterally.
c. In maximum intercuspation position of teeth, the mandible is in centric relation, i.e. both mandibular condyles are in symmetrical retruded unstrained positions in the glenoid fossae.
d. During mandibular movements, the functional relationships are correct. In particular, during lateral excursions there should be either group function or a canine protected/rise on the working side with no occlusal contact on the non-working side; while in protrusion, the occlusion should be on incisor teeth while buccal segment should disocclude.

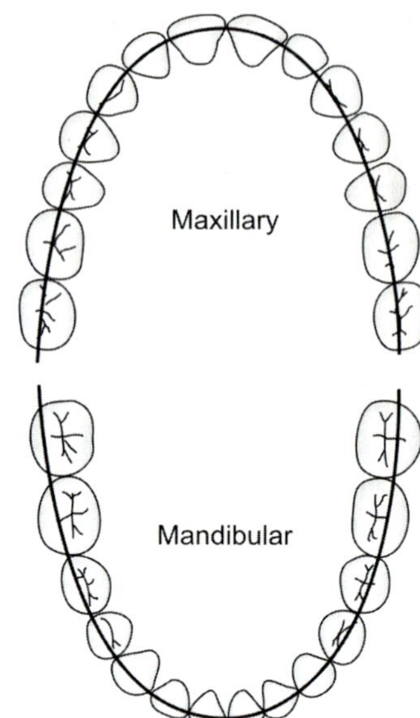

Fig. 9.1: Occlusion in upper and lower dental arches as described by Angle *(Redrawn from Proffit and Fields).*

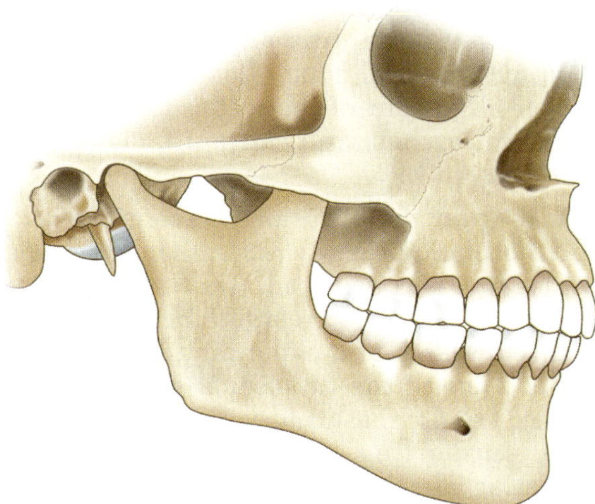

Fig. 9.2: Skull picture showing ideal arrangement of upper and lower teeth.

Normal Occlusion (Figs 9.1 and 9.3)

Angle (1899) had provided the first clear definition of normal occlusion. Angle defined occlusion as the relationship of the occlusal inclined planes of teeth upon jaw closure. Normal occlusion in orthodontics is an Angle's class I occlusion. The mesiobuccal cusp of maxillary first permanent molar should occlude in mesiobuccal groove of mandibular first permanent molar, and the teeth were arranged in a smoothly curving line of occlusion. An occlusion can be said to be normal, if the dental arches are well aligned, with a normal, nondamaging interrelation with the opposing arches, and is in a position of health and stability.

He defined upper first molars as the "key to occlusion". According to it, the position of permanent upper first molars is always constant and nonvariable. The position of mandibular first molars changes to attain either distoclusion or mesioclusion. He also introduced the concept of line of occlusion. It is the line along which the upper and lower

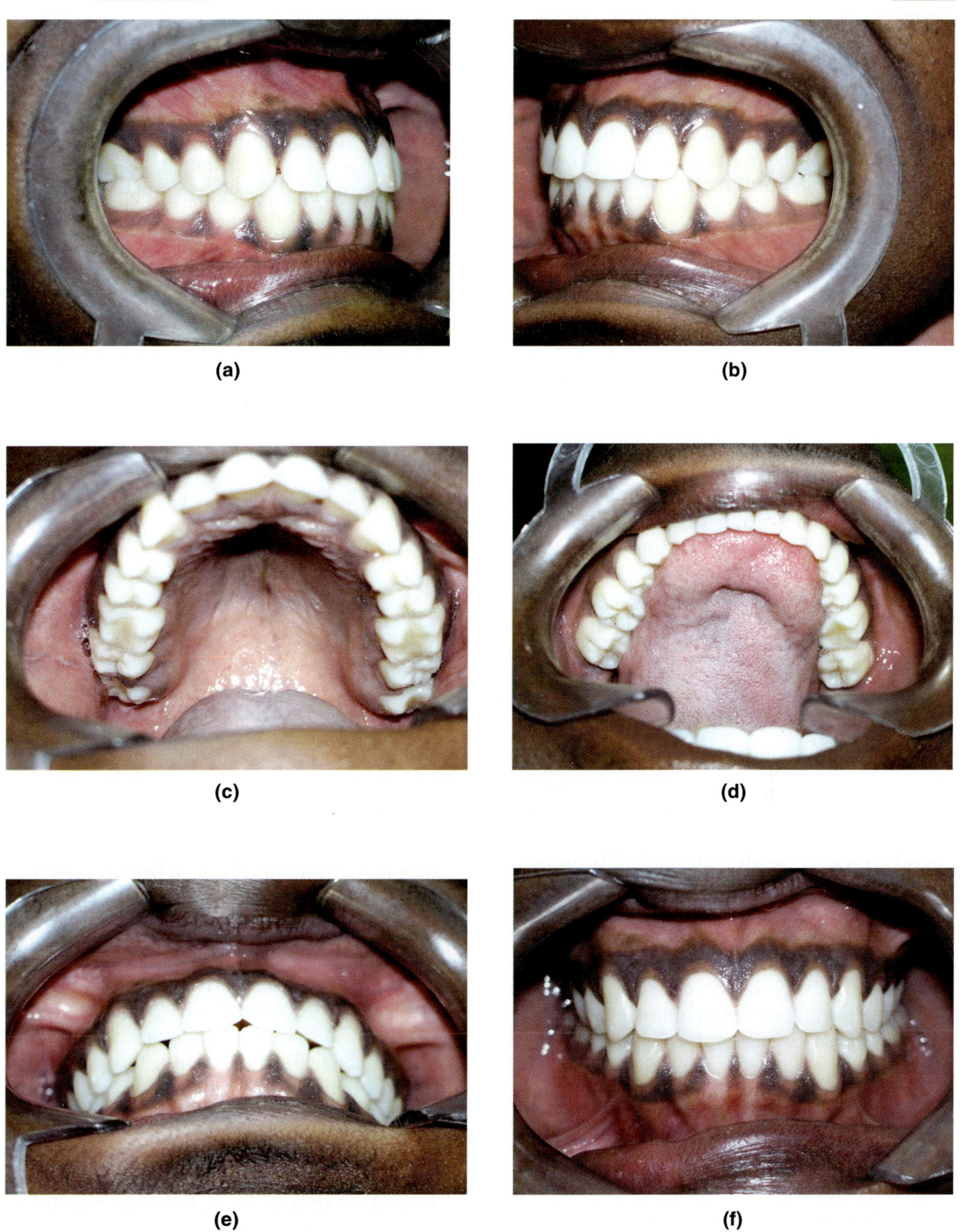

Figs 9.3a to f: Normal occlusion with well-aligned arches, normal overjet and overbite, and Angle's class I molars, with ideal teeth inclinations.

teeth occlude where "buccal cusps and incisal edges of the mandibular teeth should be concordant with the central fossae and cingulae of the maxillary teeth when the teeth are normally occluded", and according to him, it described the ideal arrangement of the teeth clearly and geometrically. It is a smooth, continuous, and symmetric curve.

From the hypothesis of constancy of upper first molars and the line of occlusion, he developed the philosophy that for a normal occlusion, all teeth should be present in the dental arches. So, his treatment philosophy revolved around nonextraction of the teeth.

Difference between Normal Occlusion and Class I Malocclusion

Normal occlusion and class I malocclusion shared the same molar relationship but differed in the arrangement of the teeth relative to the line of occlusion. Class I malocclusion does not have good alignment of teeth relative to the line of occlusion. According to Houston et al. (1992), a normal occlusion is an occlusion within the accepted deviation of the ideal and does not constitute aesthetic or functional problems.

Lischer and Simon tried to broaden the concept of occlusion by relating the teeth to the rest of the face and cranium. They related the teeth in occlusal contact to cranial and facial planes oriented outside the denture proper.

Andrew's Concept of Normal Occlusion

Andrews (1972) reported six significant occlusal characteristics in a study of 120 casts of nonorthodontics patients with normal occlusion. These are referred to as the "six keys to normal occlusion" as described below.

- Molar relationship
- Crown angulation
- Crown inclination
- Absence of rotations
- Absence of spaces
- The flat occlusal plane/curve of Spee.

Key I: Molar relationship: It has three features:

- Distal surface of distal marginal ridge of upper first permanent molar occludes with the mesial surface of mesial marginal ridge of the lower second molar.
- Mesiobuccal cusp of upper first permanent molar occludes within the groove between the mesial and middle cusps of the lower first permanent molar.
- The mesiolingual cusp of the upper first molar occludes in the central fossa of the lower first molar (Fig. 9.4).

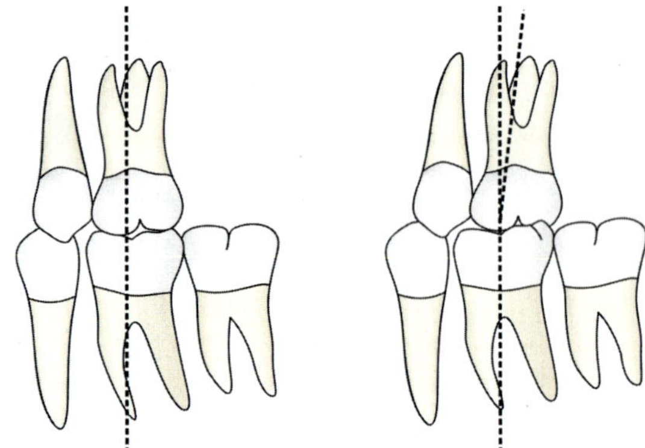

Fig. 9.4: First molars relationship according to Angle and Andrews, wherein later, the upper molar tips distally so that its distal marginal ridge occludes with mesial marginal ridge of mandibular second molar.

Key II: Crown angulation, the mesiodistal "tip": The gingival part of the long axis of crown is slightly distal to the occlusal part of that axis (Fig. 9.5).

Key III: Crown inclination, the labiolingual or buccolingual, "torque": The crowns of the maxillary incisors have incisal portion of the labial surface labial to the gingival portion of the clinical crown. In all other teeth, the gingival part is labial to incisal/occlusal part (Fig. 9.6).

Key IV: Absence of rotations: Teeth should be free of rotations. A rotated posterior tooth occupies more space in the dental arch, while a rotated anterior tooth occupies less space than normal (Fig. 9.7).

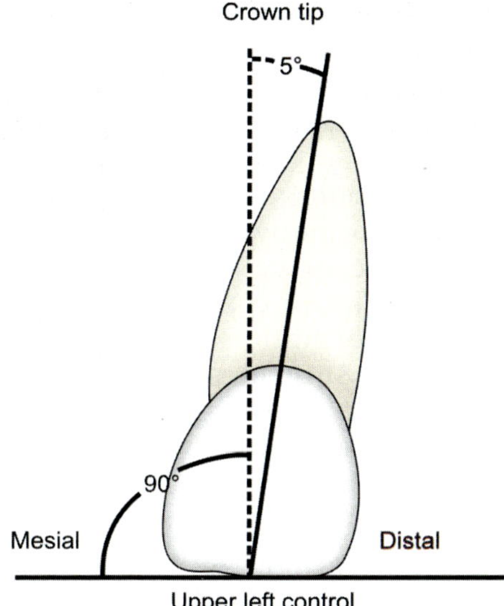

Fig. 9.5: Distal root tip of upper central incisor according to Andrews.

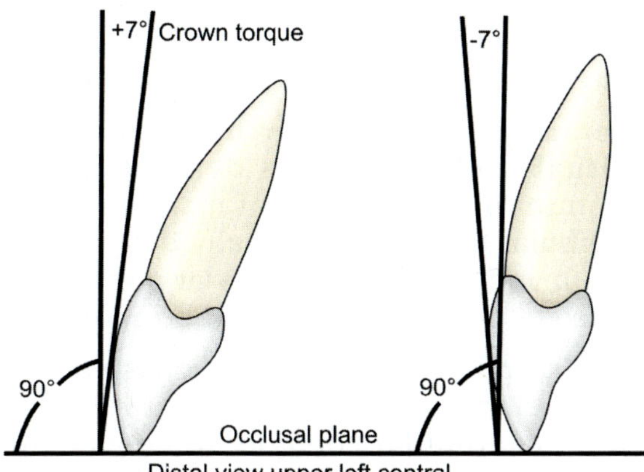

Fig. 9.6: Root angulation/torque of upper central incisor, according to Andrews.

Key V: Tight contacts: Contact points should be tight without any spacings.

Key VI: Flat curve of Spee: A flat occlusal plane is desirable for stability of occlusion.

Roth's Modifications

Roth (1981) added some functional keys to six keys to normal occlusion of Andrews concept. He described that:

a. Centric relationship and centric occlusion should be coincident.

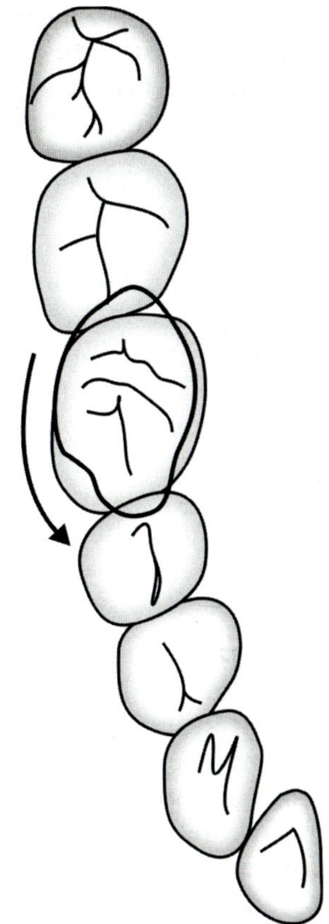

Fig. 9.7: A rotated posterior tooth in dental arch occupies more space.

b. In protrusive movements, the incisors should disclude the posterior teeth, with the guidance provided by the lower incisal edges passing along the palatal contour of the upper incisors.
c. In lateral excursive movements, the canine should guide the working side while all other teeth on that and the other side get discluded.
d. When the teeth are in centric occlusion, there should be even bilateral contacts in the buccal segments.

Physiologic/Pathologic Occlusion

Amsterdam defined two types of occlusion:

Functional occlusion: It is a static and dynamic relationship of teeth, which provides highest efficiency during all functional movements of the jaws. It provides minimum stress on TMJ, optimal function of the orofacial complex, stability and esthetics of the dentition and protection and health of the periodontium.

Physiologic occlusion is present when no signs of dysfunction or disease are present and no treatment is indicated. It is the one that adapts to the stress of function and can be maintained indefinitely. Characteristics of physiologic occlusion are: Physiologic occlusion has adapted well to its environment. It has no pathologic manifestations or dysfunctional problems. It is in a state of harmony and requires no therapy. It could be a malocclusion that is in a state of health.

Pathogenic Occlusion

It is defined as an occlusal relationship capable of producing pathologic changes in the stomatognathic system. In such occlusion, sufficient disharmony exists between the teeth and the TMJs to result in symptoms that require intervention. It is characterized by some of the following features:

Pulpal changes ranging from hyperemia to necrosis are found in the teeth.

Teeth may exhibit hypermobility, open contacts, or abnormal wear.

Periodontium: A widened periodontal ligament space may indicate premature occlusal contacts and is often associated with tooth mobility.

Musculature: Acute or chronic muscular pain on palpation can indicate habits associated with tension such as bruxism or clenching.

Temporomandibular joint: Pain, clicking or popping in the TMJ can indicate TM disorders, and the myofacial pain dysfunction syndrome (MPDS).

A therapeutic occlusion is the state achieved with specific therapeutic interventions to treat dysfunction or disease.

Traumatic occlusion: When occlusal forces exceed the adaptive capacity of the tissues, tissue injury results. The resultant injury is termed as trauma from occlusion. Thus, TFO, trauma from occlusion refers to the tissue injury, not the occlusal force. An occlusion that produces such injury is called traumatic occlusion.

It is the occlusion which provides abnormal stresses on the otherwise normal dentition, and is capable of causing injury to the periodontium if not corrected. It acts as a factor in the formation of traumatic disturbances in the structures of stomatognathic system. A nonphysiologic (or traumatic) occlusion is associated with dysfunction or disease due to tissue injury, and treatment may be indicated.

Balanced occlusion: This is the concept of complete denture prosthodontics. It helps in the stability of the dentures in the mouth during functional movements. It exists when there is a simultaneous contact of maxillary and mandibular teeth, on both the right and left sides, when the jaws are either in centric or eccentric occlusion.

Centric occlusion (intercuspal position, habitual occlusion): It is defined as the maximum intercuspation of maxillary and mandibular teeth. It is a dentally determined position, independent of condylar position. It can also be called as intercuspal position.

Centric relation: Centric relation is a bone-to-bone relationship of upper and lower jaws, i.e. the mandibular condyle in the glenoid fossa. Once centric relation is established, centric occlusion can be built to coincide with it. In many people, centric occlusion is ahead of centric relation by 1–2 mm which is considered a normal limit as it may not contribute to damage of periodontal structures.

It is a more dynamic maxillomandibular relationship in which the condyles are in there most superior, anterior and retruded position in the articular fossae, resting against the posterior slopes of the articular eminences with the articular discs properly interposed. The condyles articulate with the thinnest avascular portion of their respective discs.

Mandible rotates around a transverse axis passing through the condyles in the centric relation movement. The guidance of jaw by clinician in opening and closing movements, which has only rotational component without having any translation component, is referred to as a hinge axis movement. In this position, condyles are considered to be in the terminal hinge position.

Glickman et al concluded that there are 13 muscle attachments to mandible that provide a high degree of stability of position. These controlling muscles provide stability of postural resting position (PRP). Thus, the dentist must harmonize the abnormal vertical dimension at occlusion (VDO) with the normal VDR (postural vertical dimension at rest) in order to achieve success in orthodnotic therapy.

Importance of centric relation in orthodontics: Diagnosis and treatment planning depends on proper evaluation of occlusion in centric relation to determine exact maxillo-mandibular skeletal and dental relationship in all the three planes of space, e.g. a case of pseudo class III may be diagnosed a true class III if not evaluated in CR as it presents itself as anterior crossbite in maximum intercuspation relation, i.e. CO. So, the mandible should be manipulated backward to achieve a CR position for evaluation.

Eccentric occlusion: Any occlusion other than centric occlusion is the eccentric occlusion. It includes latero-occlusion, protrusive and retrusive occlusion. Lateral occlusion is the contact between opposing teeth when the mandible is moved either right or left side. Protrusive occlusion is the occlusion of the teeth when the mandible is protruded, i.e. mandible is anterior to centric relation. Retrusive occlusion is the occlusion of teeth when mandible is retruded, i.e. mandible is posterior to centric relation.

Schemes of the Occlusion Patterns

Bilaterally balanced occlusion: This requires having a maximum number of teeth in contact in maximum intercuspation in all excursive positions. It is a concept of complete dentures, to provide stability to the denture during function.

Unilaterally balanced articulation (group function): In a unilaterally balanced articulation, excursive contact occurs between all opposing posterior teeth on the laterotrusive (working) side only. On the mediotrusive (nonworking) side, no contact occurs until the mandible has reached centric relation. Thus, in this occlusal arrangement the load is distributed among the periodontal support of all posterior teeth on the working side.

Optimum occlusion: It is defined as an ideal relationship of maxillary and mandibular teeth combining a functional occlusion with the absence of malocclusion. Occlusal contact has been shown to influence muscle activity during mastication. With teeth in optimal occlusion, the load exerted on the dentition should be distributed optimally. Horizontal forces on the teeth should be avoided or at least minimized, and loading should be always be parallel to / along the long axes of the teeth for best distribution of forces in the larger basal areas of jaws. Loading of teeth occurs when cusps occlude in fossae of occlusal surfaces, rather than on the marginal ridges. This is facilitated when the tips of centric cusps are located centrally over the roots. Horizontal forces are also minimized if posterior tooth contact during excursive movements is avoided. Excessive horizontal forces lead to resorption of alveolar crestal bone (which is very weak and porous in nature), and thus the loss of support to teeth. To enhance masticatory efficiency, the cusps of the posterior teeth should have adequate height. The chewing and grinding action of teeth is enhanced if opposing cusps on the laterotrusive side interdigitate at the end of the chewing stroke. The mutually protected occlusal scheme probably meets this criterion better than the other occlusal arrangements.

Canine guidance (canine protected occlusion, canine rise): In this scheme, the labial surface of mandibular canine on working side comes in contact with the lingual surface of maxillary canine causing disarticulation of all other teeth. The contact is only in canine region on the working side.

Canines are best suited to accept the horizontal forces during eccentric movements. They have the longest and strongest roots and therefore the best crown/root ratio. They are also surrounded by dense compact bone, which tolerates the forces better than does the medullary bone found around posterior teeth. Another advantage of the canines is due to the sensory input provided by them and the resultant effect on the muscles of mastication. Fewer muscles are active when canines contact during eccentric movements than when posterior teeth contact.

Group function occlusion: In some patients, canines are not in proper position to accept the horizontal forces; so the other teeth must contact during eccentric movements. The most favorable alternative to canine rise is called group function. The Pankey-Mann concept, recently referred to more as the Pankey-Mann-Schuyler concept, is based on group function. The scientific rationale about this group function is that lateral stress generated on the posterior teeth during function might provide the necessary periodontal stimulus within a physiological tolerance, and also help in distribution of occlusal load to multiple teeth.

Mutually protected occlusion: It was advocated by Stuart and Stallard in 1960s. Here, centric relation coincides with the maximum intercuspation position. It is the occlusal scheme in which posterior teeth prevent excessive contact of the anterior teeth in maximum intercuspation. Also, the anterior teeth disengage the posterior teeth in all mandibular excursive movements. Posterior teeth act as stops for vertical closure when the mandible returns to its maximum intercuspal position. Posterior cusps should be sharp and should pass each other closely without contacting to maximize occlusal function.

The features of a mutually protected occlusion are as follows:

- There is uniform contact of all teeth in arches, when the condyles are in their most superior position.
- Stable posterior tooth contacts with vertically directed resultant forces.
- Centric relation is coincident with maximum intercuspation (intercuspal position) (CR = MI).
- There is no contact of posterior teeth in lateral or non-working side or during protrusive movements.
- Anterior tooth contacts harmonizing with functional jaw movements.

Rationale: The mandible is a lever of class III type which is least efficient of the lever systems. Effectiveness of forces exerted by muscles of mastication is notably less when the loading contact occurs farther anteriorly. The farther the anterior initial tooth to tooth contact occurs (that is the longer the lever arm), the less effective will be the forces exerted by the musculature and the smaller the load to which the teeth are subjected. Food is more easily chewed in posterior region than the anterior region due to more forces.

Characteristics

- There are stable and static contacts over the greatest possible number of teeth in centric relation.
- The long centric is defined as occlusal harmony with an anterior slide between centric relation and maximum intercuspation (1 mm) and a small amount of lateral freedom for accommodation of Bennett movement in the horizontal plane.
- During the working movements, there is harmonious contact on all the inclines involved for both anterior and posterior teeth.
- There should be no contact of teeth on the balancing side otherwise it may lead to injury of TMJs.
- An immediate disocclusion of the posterior teeth should occur during protrusive movements.

- Among all the factors of occlusion, i.e. CG, IG, CH, CC, CI; the most important factors of occlusion are condylar guidance/temporomandibular joints; incisal guidance; and Bennett movement. CG and IG are the anatomic factors which are not under the control of clinicians. So other factors, i.e. CH, CC, CI should be compensated for the best occlusal arrangement.
- In group function, several teeth on working side contact during the laterotrusive movement. It is a scheme of occlusion, in which during lateral excursion, the cusps of upper and lower posterior teeth glide in unison and disocclude the occusion on the opposite side.
- Any laterotrusive movement, contacts of more posterior than upto the mesial part of first molars are not desirable because increased amount of forces come into play as we reach near the fulcrum. Buccal cusp-to-buccal cusp contacts are more desirable during laterotrusive movements than are lingual cusp-to-lingual cusp contacts. The laterotrusive contacts (either canine rise or group function) provide adequate guidance to disclude the teeth on the opposite side of the arch (mediotrusive or nonworking side) immediately. Mediotrusive contacts are traumatic to masticatory system because the abnormal forces come into play. Hence, mediotrusive contacts should be avoided in developing an optimum functional occlusion. All these contacts should be in coordination with lateral compensating curves of occlusion so that proper disclusion occurs during mandibular movements.
- During protrusive movement of mandible, the mandible moves downward and forward guided by CG and IG. The IG should be set parallel to CG; and should be in coordination with COS and other curvatures of occlusion. It leads to disocclusion in posterior region. If there is contact in posterior region, then abnormal horizontal forces come into play leading to damage to the tissues. Therefore during protrusion, the anterior and not the posterior teeth should contact. The anteriors should provide adequate contact or guidance to disarticulate the posteriors. In class II division 2, cases, the incisors are extruded and deep bite is there, so the IG is not in consonance with CG. It leads to premature contacts and backward shifting of mandible during closure, and trauma to tissues and TMJ. So during treatment, the incisors are positioned such that they provide IG parallel to CG.

Types of Cusps (Fig. 9.8)

- **Supporting cusps:** These cusps fit in central fossae and marginal ridges of opposing teeth. They are also called as centric-holding cusps or stamp cusps, e.g. lower buccal and upper palatal cusps. They help in maintaining the vertical dimension of occlusion, and should not be reduced during occlusal equilibration.
- **Non-supporting cusps or shearing cusps:** They are also called guiding cusps. They contact and guide mandible during lateral movements, and help in shearing food, e.g. lower lingual and upper buccal cusps.

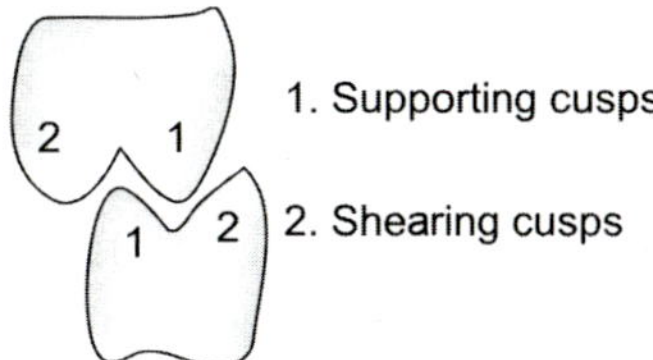

Fig. 9.8: Cusps on molars.

Occlusal Interdigitation

Occlusal interdigitation in humans is of two types:

a. Cusp-to-fossa relation
b. Cusp-to-embrasure relation.

- **Cusp to embrasure/marginal ridge occlusion:** Here, one stamp cusp occludes in the fossa of opposing tooth, and another cusp of the same tooth occludes into the embrasure area of two opposing teeth. This is a one tooth to two teeth relation occlusion.
- **Cusp-to-fossa relation:** It is a tooth-to-tooth arrangement. Here, the cusps of opposing teeth occluded in fossae of opposing teeth. This is a one tooth-to-one tooth relation. Advantages of cusp-fossa arrangement over cusp-embrasure arrangement are that the occlusal forces are directed towards the long axis of teeth in a better way. It leads to greater stability of the arch, and the chance of food impacting in the embrasures is less.

COMPENSATORY CURVATURES

The occlusal surfaces of dental arches and the teeth are not arranged as a flat plane, but they show mild amount of curvatures in antero-posterior and lateral planes. It is a natural phenomenon as it helps to avoid any abnormal forces falling on the supporting structures during mandibular functions, and they help to provide functional guidance during jaw movements.

Importance of Curvatures

The curvatures are natural adaptations of various functions and anatomical features of teeth, condyles, glenoid fossae, and articular eminences, e.g. D & F slope of articular eminence guides the mandible in D & F direction during protrusive movements. This is called as condylar guidance. This should be in consonance with incisal guidance provided by the lingual surfaces of upper incisors, on which incisal edges of lower anterior glide. If it is not, then abnormal forces may fall on TMJ and lower and upper incisors which lead to damage to PD tissues and TMJ tissues, e.g. (suppose in class II div 2 case), if a patient is having a deep bite, then his D & F slope articular eminence either should be parallel to the incisal guidance provided by the deep bite, otherwise the deep bite should be reduced to normal levels to avoid abnormal forces falling on lower incisors.

Similarly, the curvatures in lateral directions are also nature's gift to mankind. It is also in consonance with the lateral slopes of articular fossae of TMJ and the Bennett movement. They help to guide the mandible downward on the working lateral side, thus discluding it on the other side. This teeth arrangement should be replicated during occlusal treatment by proper torquing. During lateral movements, if the planes are flat, then the hanging palatal cusps of upper teeth will strike prematurely to cusps of lower teeth and make the mastication impossible.

As the mandible moves D & F during protrusion, and if there is no curve of Spee (i.e. if OP is flat and horizontal), then during protrusion, the molars will strike and get locked together and person will not be able to perform protrusive movements. Similarly, mandible moves D, F and medially during lateral movements esp on non-working side, and the curves help to avoid any premature contacts of teeth. There are certain curves defined by certain authors as follows.

Curve of Spee (Figs 9.9 and 9.10)

It is the anteroposterior/sagittal curve of the occlusal surfaces of lower teeth, which begins at the tip of lower canines and then follows cusp tips of premolars and molars, continuing as an arc through the anterior border of ramus and passing through the condyles. If it is extended, it forms a circle of 4 inches diameter. It has a concavity in lower arch and convexity in upper arch. In consonance with this curve of lower arch, the upper teeth show a reverse curve of spee.

It occurs due to mesial axial inclinations of the lower teeth, which gradually increase as we progress towards the molars from the canines. When the long axes of the lower teeth are extended apically, they seem to diverge. The upper teeth are adapted with the lower

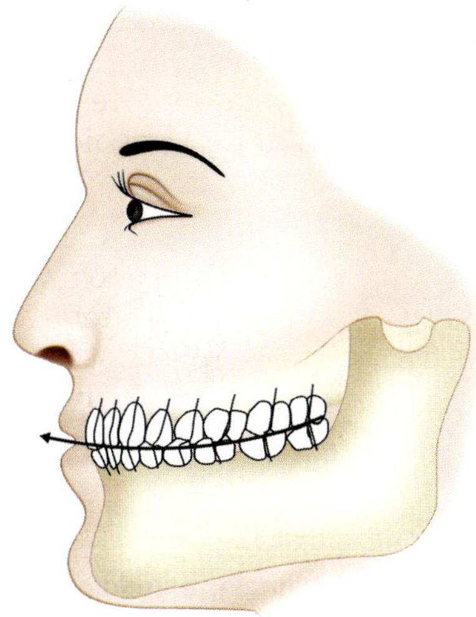

Fig. 9.9: Curve of Spee and the anterior component of forces.

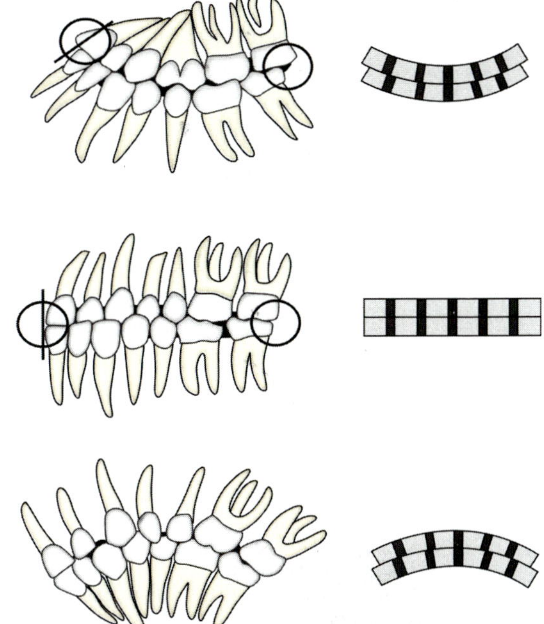

Fig. 9.10: Different types of curve of Spee: concave, flat, convex curves.

teeth for a proper relationship and the axes of these teeth converge when extended apically. Normal depth of COS is 1–2 mm in first premolar region measured in the region of marginal ridge. During orthodontic treatment, the occlusal plane is flattened, with zero curve of Spee, since with time, due to some relapse, it is expected to return and settle at 1–2 mm depth during retention period. COS, IG, and CG should complement each other during functional movements.

Curve of Wilson (Fig. 9.11)

It runs in a transverse/mediolateral direction of the arch, by contacting the buccal and lingual cusp tips of mandibular posterior teeth. It results from inward/lingual inclination of lower posterior teeth (the lingual crown torque), making the lingual cusps lower than the buccal cups on the mandibular arch. It is a U-shaped curve in coronal dimension. Due to lingual crown torque of mandibular teeth, when the long axes of the buccal teeth are extended apically, they seem to diverge.

A similar curve is present in upper arch also which is parallel to the lower curve. It is due to arrangement of the palatal cusps, especially

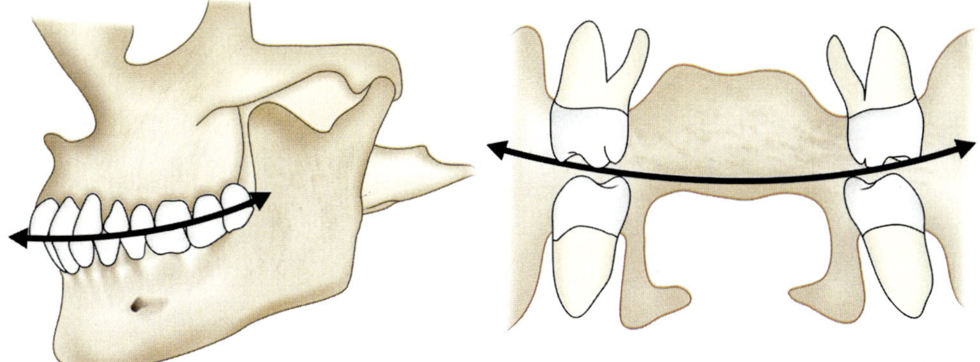

Fig. 9.11: Curve of Spee and curve of Wilson.

mesiopalatal cusps of upper molars which are slightly at a lower levels to that of buccal cusps irt the occlusal plane; the buccal cusps are higher than the lingual cusps in maxillary arch because of their size. Although maxillary posterior teeth also have a lingual crown torque, but it is of lesser degree as compared to the lower teeth. Curve of Wilson in the mandibular arch appears concave and in maxillary arch, it is convex. The lingual inclination of lower posterior teeth positions the lingual cusps lower than the buccal cusps. This design permits easy access to the occlusal table. As the tongue lays the food on the occlusal surfaces, it is stopped from going past the chewing position by the taller buccal cusps (Fig. 9.12).

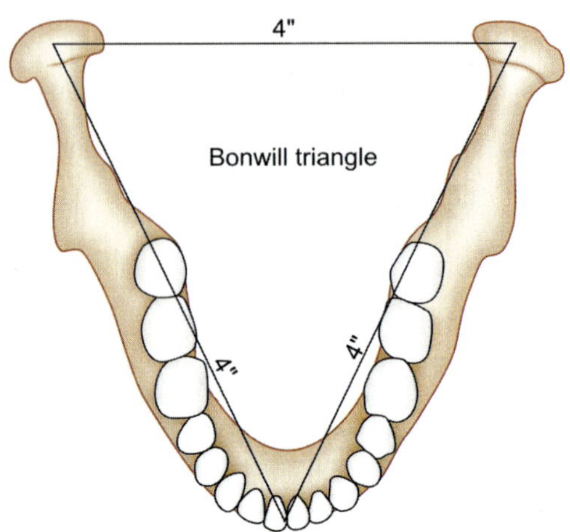

Fig. 9.12: Bonwill's triangle, extending from inter-incisal area to condylar region and intercondylar region as an equilateral triangle with 4 inches size each.

Curve of Monson

It is a 3D curve, where the curves of Spee, and Wilson have been combined in a segment of a sphere. It is obtained by extension of the curve of Spee and curve of Wilson to all cusps and incisal edges. He suggested that the mandibular arch adapts itself to a curved segment of a sphere of 8 inches in diameter with its centre in the region of glabella.

Conclusion

Different authors have described different features in a normal occlusion. Although a single system cannot completely describe the normal occlusion, different features from different systems can be incorporated to establish a scheme for a stable and healthy state of stomatognathic system. Occlusion should be considered as a dynamic issue, taking care of the teeth and supporting tissues to be in harmony with the functions for a stable and healthy tissue system. All the efforts should be done by clinicians to achieve a nonpathologic state of occlusion.

10

Classification of Malocclusion

INTRODUCTION

For the ease of referencing and communication, a wide variety of cases are grouped in different categories. This categorization is done based on some common clinical features pertinent to that category of cases. A classification system is a grouping of clinical cases of similar appearances for ease in handling and discussion. It is not a system of diagnosis, method for determining prognosis, or way of defining treatment. By using a classification system the clinicians can easily communicate among themselves, and think of a treatment objectives and the plan.

Advantages of Classification

- It helps in categorizing numerous different cases in smaller number of groups, based on common features.
- Every time, during describing the patient's nature of problems, all the signs need not be mentioned. A class of malocclusion mentioned itself gives most of the information to the clinicians about the nature of problems.
- It helps in easy communications and discussion among the colleagues.
- It helps in deciding the line and plan of treatment.
- It helps in simplifying the data storage.

Historical background: A number of classifications systems have found place in the literature. A brief review is as follows, however the details are irrelevant in the present scenario.

In 1850, Kingsley classified malocclusion according to etiology. He made a simple division into developmental or accidental.

Edward H Angle proposed his classification of malocclusion in 1889. Angle coined the term 'line of occlusion' which he defined as "the line with which in form and position according to the type, the teeth must be in harmony if in normal occlusion".

Calvin S Case in 1908 gave a classification from the stand point of treatment.

Italian Muzj in 1939 gave a classification based upon the facial types.

Lucin de Coster in 1939 included both the soft tissues and hard tissues in his classification.

Paul W Simon classified the teeth in relation to supporting bone framework.

Strang's classification defines the relation of teeth, arches and jaws to cranial anatomy.

Initially, the occlusion was studied as a static position, in a single dimension. But with increased knowledge, it has been considered as a dynamic entity with a three dimension view.

Occlusion: It is defined as the relationship of the maxillary and mandibular teeth as they are brought into functional contact, as defined in the glossary of orthodontic terms. Occlusion can be ideal, normal or malocclusion. Ideal occlusion is only a hypothetical idea, with no set criteria. However, the normal occlusion can be considered to be having certain features as given below.

The Characteristics of Normal Occlusion

- Correct axial position of the teeth
- Normal overbite and overjet
- Normal relationship of the individual teeth. There should be no abnormal rotation and axial inclination present, with minimal spaces or crowding.
- Normal relation of the dental arches with each other and the cranium and the face.
- The teeth should be in a harmonious balance with the soft tissues and associated structures, in a state of health, stability and pleasant esthetics.

MALOCCLUSION

It is the state of any deviation from the normal or ideal occlusion, as defined in the glossary of orthodontic terms.

Epidemiology of malocclusion: Many studies have been done around the world to find out the prevalence of malocclusion in different countries, races and ethnic group. There is wide variation of malocclusion prevalence found in different areas of world. Malocclusion has been found to be more in developed countries than the developing countries. It is mainly due to soft and sticky dietary habits of developed countries. In US, the prevalence of Angle's class I malocclusion is 60–70%; Angle's class II div 1 is 20–30%; and Angle's class III malocclusion is 5–10%. Although, class I malocclusion is more prevalent, but the in practice, the clinicians receive more cases of class II malocclusion for treatment, which is due to their affected esthetics and functions.

Angle has defined different classes of malocclusion based on the relation of upper and lower permanent first molars. Even, Andrew has also incorporated their interrelationship in his six keys to normal occlusion in a modified form. So, a brief knowledge of the anatomy of these teeth is mandatory for proper classification.

Anatomy of Maxillary First Permanent Molar (Figs 10.1a and b)

A maxillary first permanent molar has four major cusps and a supplemental cusp viz.

1. Mesiobuccal cusp
2. Distobuccal cusp
3. Mesiolingual cusp (largest)
4. Distolingual cusp
5. Supplemental cusp or tubercle of carabelli found on the lingual surface of mesiolingual cusp.

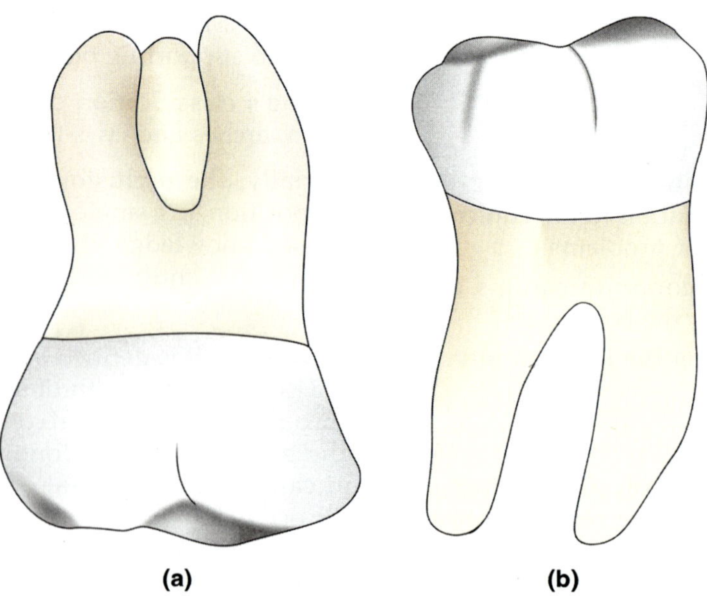

Figs 10.1a and b: Permanent upper and lower first molars

There is an oblique ridge running from ML to DB cusp. On the buccal surface, it has a groove separating MB from DB cusp.

Anatomy of Mandibular First Permanent Molar

A mandibular first permanent molar has five cusps, viz. mesio- and distobuccal, mesio, and distolingual and one distal cusp.

On the buccal aspect, there are two developmental grooves:

1. Mesiobuccal developmental groove
2. Distobuccal developmental groove.

Andrew's criteria of normal occlusion: With an extensive research spread of many years, Andrews proposed following six features of the normal occlusion. These are also referred as "six keys to normal occlusion" as postulated by him in 1970s. These are:

1. Molar relationship
2. Crown angulations
3. Crown inclination
4. Rotation
5. Tight contacts
6. Occlusal plane.

Molar relationship (Fig. 10.2): It has been described by three relations as compared to only one relation in Angle's system, as follows:

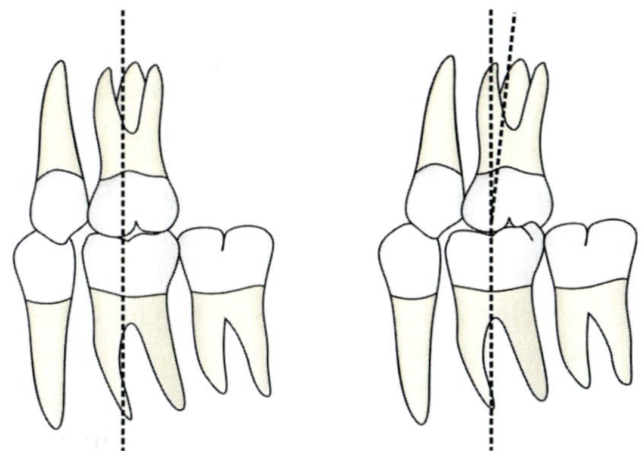

Fig. 10.2: Angle's first molar relation in first figure, while second figure shows Andrew's first molar relation, where upper first molar has tilted distally so that its distal marginal ridge can occlude the mesial marginal ridge of mandibular second molar.

1. The mesiobuccal cusp of the maxillary first permanent molar occludes with the mesiobuccal groove of the mandibular first permanent molar.
2. The mesiolingual cusp of the maxillary first permanent molar lies in the central fossa of the mandibular first permanent molar.
3. The crown of upper first molar is angulated in such a way that the distal marginal ridge of maxillary first permanent molar occludes with the mesial marginal ridge of mandibular second permanent molar.

Crown angulations: It depicts the TIP of the tooth, i.e. mesiodistal inclination or the second order relationship. It is measured in degrees as plus or minus. This degree is the measure of the angle formed between the long axis of the clinical crown and a line at 90° from the occlusal plane. If the gingival portion of the crown was more distal than the incisal portion, then a PLUS reading is given. And a MINUS reading is given when the gingival portion of the crown is mesial as compared to the incisal portion. So, all the teeth have positive readings, showing distal root tip. It shows that the roots of all the teeth are distally directed, i.e. they flare apically.

Crown inclination: It depicts the torque of the tooth, i.e. labiolingual position or the third order relationship. It represents the angle formed by the line which bears 90° to the occlusal plane and a line that is tangent to the most prominent part of the crown of the tooth, i.e. bracket site (Fig. 10.3).

A positive reading is given if the gingival portion of the tangent line is lingual to the incisal portion and negative reading is given if the gingival portion of the tangent is more labial to the incisal portion. So, all the teeth except maxillary incisors have negative readings, showing lingual crown torque.

Rotation (Fig. 10.4): There should be no rotations. A rotated anterior tooth takes lesser space in the arch thus leading to a space loss or in other words, it requires space for alignment during treatment. While, a

Andrews	*Central incisor*	*Lateral incisor*	*Canine*	*First pre-molar*	*Second pre-molar*	*First molar*	*Second molar*
Maxillary	5	9	11	2	2	5	5
Mandibular	2	2	5	2	2	2	2

Andrews	*Central incisor*	*Lateral incisor*	*Canine*	*First pre-molar*	*Second pre-molar*	*First molar*	*Second molar*
Maxillary	7	3	–7	–7	–7	–9	–9
	–1	–1	–11	–17	–22	–30	–33

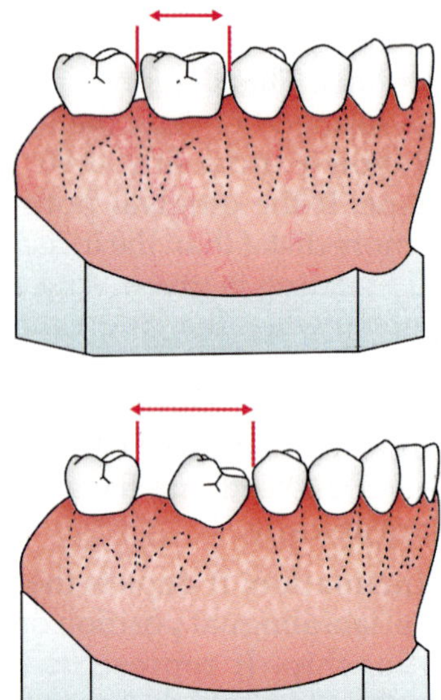

Fig. 10.3: Tilted posterior tooth takes more space in dental arch due to its shape, and thus helps to gain space in the arch when it is uprighted.

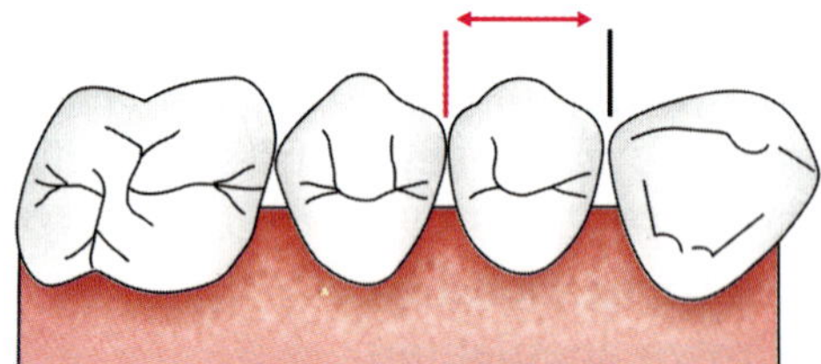

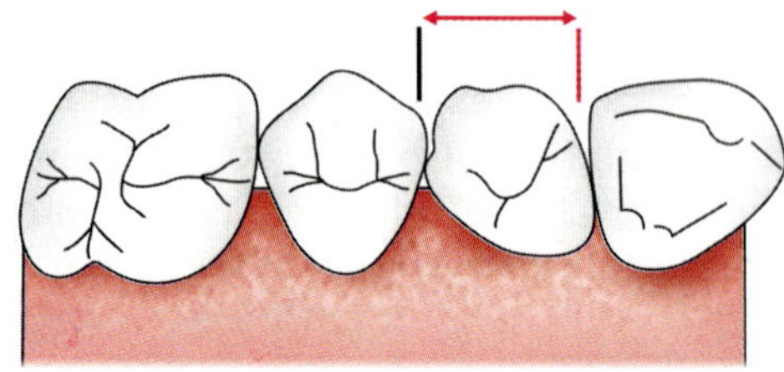

Fig. 10.4: A rotated posterior tooth takes more space in dental arch due to its shape, and thus helps to gain space in the arch when it is derotated.

posterior tooth covers more space in the arch or in other words, it provides space in the arch after correction (Fig. 11.5).

Tight contacts: The proximal contacts between the teeth should be tight with no spaces between them.

Occlusal plane: It should be flat or a slight curve of spee (Fig. 11.6).

Need of classification: A system of classification helps in following ways:

1. It helps in grouping of different malocclusion conditions which helps in referencing and sorting.
2. It helps in comparison of the features of different conditions.
3. It helps in discussion with the colleagues and the patients. Classification is an essential communication tool.
4. It helps in patient treatment planning. Treatment mechanics appropriate to that classification may be generally applied. It also helps in planning the orthopedic

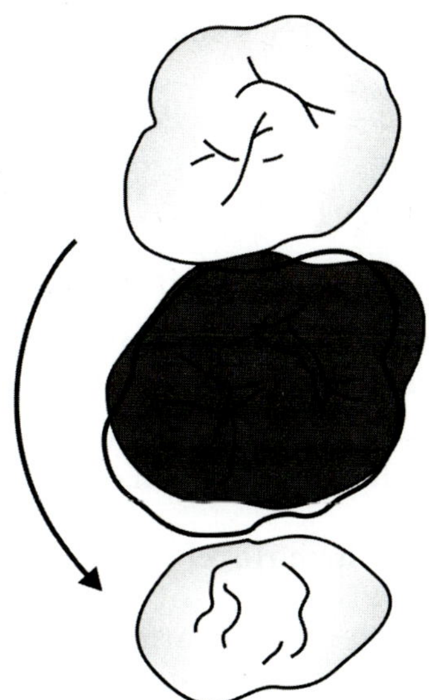

Fig. 10.5: Rotated molar occupies more space in the dental arch.

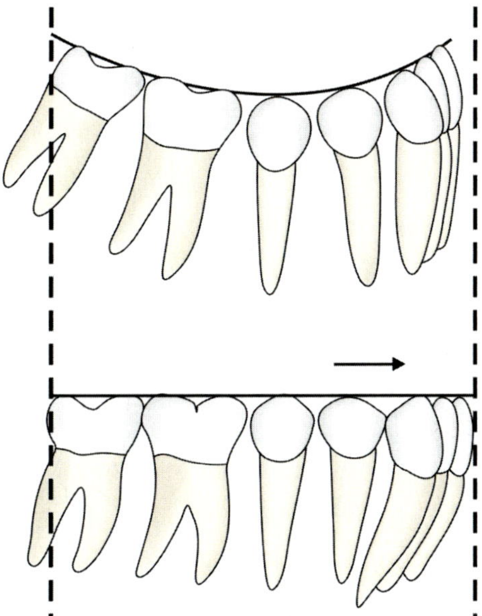

Fig. 10.6: Curve of Spee in the lower arch. To achieve a flat curve of Spee, it needs some space in the arch. Note that after flattening the curve, the lower incisors have moved forward.

appliances for achieving normal skeletal relations.

5. Generally, one of the goals in the treatment of a malocclusion is to achieve class I, which is considered as normal relation. However, there should be a consensus among orthodontists as to what constitutes ideal occlusion.

Requirements of a Good Classification System

- It should be easy to learn and remember, easy to discuss and easy to apply.
- It should not be confusing.
- It should consider malocclusion in all the three planes of space.
- It should consider the severity of the condition and the prognosis/results of treatment.
- It should consider etiology of the problem.
- It should be able to differentiate/compare between skeletal and dental contribution.
- It should help in planning the treatment.
- It should be easy to compare pretreatment and post-treatment condition of the problem.
- It should be easily transmissible.
- It should consider soft tissue relationships of the stomatognathic system.

Principles of orthodontic classification: For the establishment of classification, it is necessary to relate the face, the jaws and the teeth to the 3D of space, and with the growth status of the patient according to the following facts:

- Spatial relation of the teeth in all the three planes in the same arch and the opposing arches should be considered; and if possible, to the fourth dimension, viz. time.
- The growth of craniofaciodental tissues and the soft tissues and muscles of the face should be considered.
- The morphologic development and position of dental arches and their relation to one another and to the cranium and the face should be considered.
- Displacement of individual teeth or groups of teeth, and their inter-

relationship with teeth in the same arch and the opposing arch.

- Crowding accompanied by excessive mesial and distal displacement of the buccal and the labial segments of the teeth (Fig. 10.7).
- The dynamics of smile and relation to craniofacial and dental tissues should be considered.
- Growth of the jaws, soft tissues, etc. should be considered.

Systems of Classification and Terminology

Since last hundred years or more, a number of classification systems have been proposed. There are various systems of classification of malocclusion based upon the position of teeth in the arches, relationships of the arches, and skeletal discrepancies in all the three planes of space. Of all the classification methods as given below, two methods mostly referred are the Angle's system, and Ackermann-Proffit system. The various systems are:

- Angle's system, 1899
- Dewey's modification of Angle's system, 1915
- Simon system, 1930
- Lischer's classification, 1933
- Salzmann's skeletal classification, 1950
- Ackermann-Proffit classification, 1960
- Moyer's modification, 1973
- British society's incisors classification, 1983
- Katz classification, 1994
- Baume's classification of deciduous dentition, 1950.

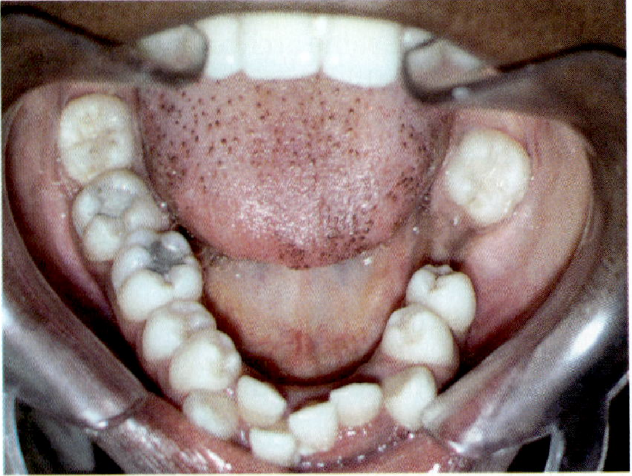

Fig. 10.7: Severe lower anterior crowding.

Types of Malocclusions (Figs 10.8 and 10.9)

A. In a simple way, the malocclusion can be classified as follows:

a. **Intra-arch malocclusion:** It includes individual malposition of tooth/teeth in its arch.

b. **Interarch malocclusion:** It is due to malrelationship of teeth with the opposing counterpart.

c. **Skeletal malocclusion:** It involves the abnormal positions of bony bases.

Individual teeth malpositions: The teeth in their dental arches may be in abnormal relation with the adjacent teeth, e.g.

- **Mesial inclination/tipping:** The crown/long axis of the tooth is inclined mesially.

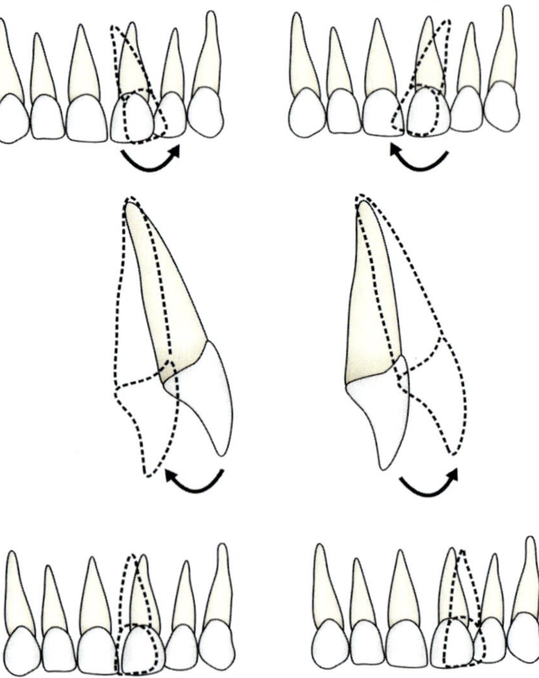

Fig. 10.8: Individual tooth malposition: distal inclination; mesial inclination; retroclination, proclination, mesial translation, distal translation of the tooth.

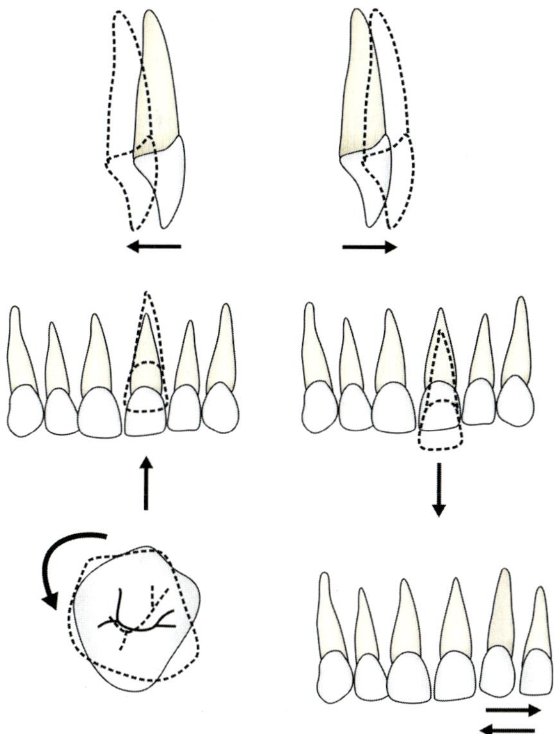

Fig. 10.9: Bodily lingual movement, bodily labial movement; intrusive position; extrusive position; rotation; transposition.

- **Distal inclination/tipping:** The crown/ long axis of the tooth is inclined distally.
- **Labial/buccal inclination/tipping:** The crown/long axis of the tooth is inclined labially/buccally. It is also called proclination (Figs 10.11 to 10.13).

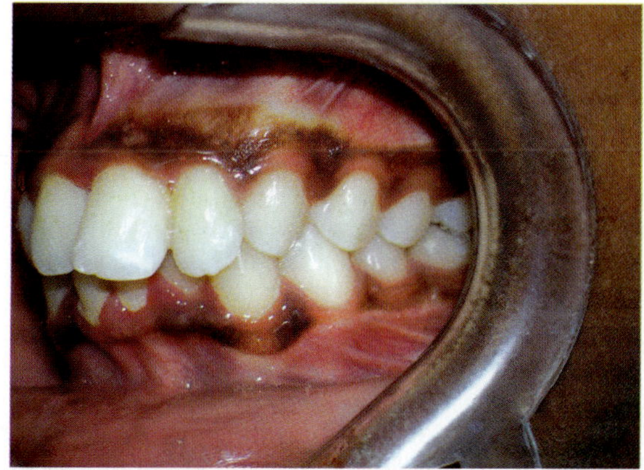

Fig. 10.10: Distal inclination of lateral incisor.

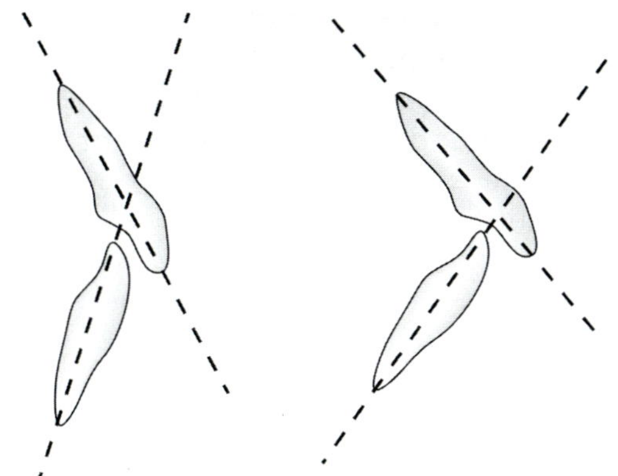

Fig. 10.11: Showing interincisal angles: normal in first fig, while second fig shows decreased angle due to proclination of upper and lower incisors.

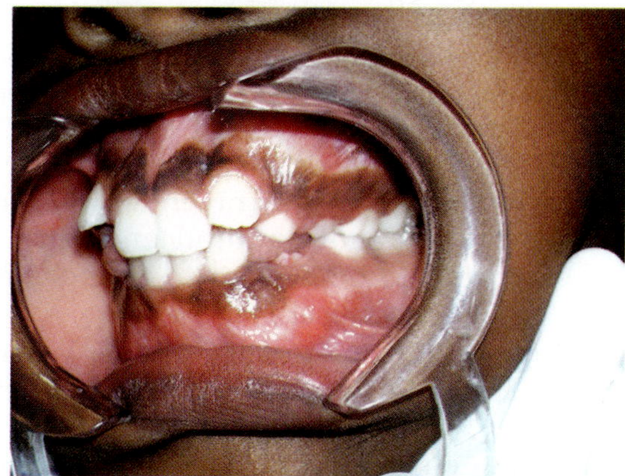

Fig. 10.12: Proclination of lateral incisors.

- **Lingual inclination/tipping:** The crown/long axis of the tooth is inclined lingually. It is also called retroclination.
- **Mesial displacement:** When a tooth is shifted bodily toward mesial side/ midline.
- **Distal displacement:** When a tooth is shifted bodily towards distal side/away from midline.
- **Labial or buccal displacement:** When a tooth is shifted bodily toward labial or buccal side.
- **Lingual/palatal displacement:** When a tooth is shifted bodily towards lingual or palatal side.

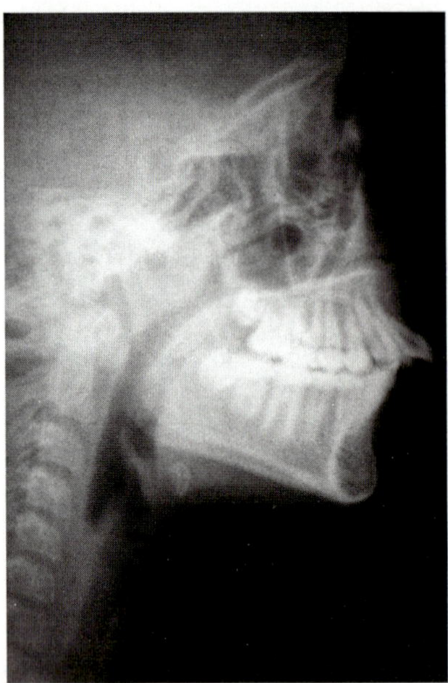

Fig. 10.13: Lateral cephalogram showing increased overjet due to proclination of upper incisors, and deep curve of Spee.

- **Infraocclusion or infraversion:** When the tooth is not erupted enough as compared to other teeth. The tooth is away from occlusal plane.
- **Supraocclusion or supraversion:** When the tooth is erupted more than the other teeth.
- **Rotation:** When a tooth has abnormal movement around its long axis. It may be of two types:
  - **Distolabial/mesiolingual rotation:** Distal aspect is more labially placed; or mesial aspect is more lingually placed.
  - **Distolingual/mesiolabial rotation:** Distal aspect is more lingually placed; or mesial aspect is more labially placed.
- **Transposition:** It is the term when two teeth exchange their places of normal eruption.

B. Another simple way to classify malocclusion is:

- **Dental:** Only teeth have malposition, on normally positioned bony bases.
- **Skeletal:** The bony bases have malrelation within themselves or with each other.
- **Skeletodental:** Both, the teeth and the bony bases are having abnormal relationship. Mostly, all the malocclusions are of this type, since any skeletal variation leads to compensatory adjustments of dental positions (Figs 10.14 and 10.15).

Skeletal malocclusion can be expressed in either one or all the three planes of spaces, (Figs 10.16 to 10.24).

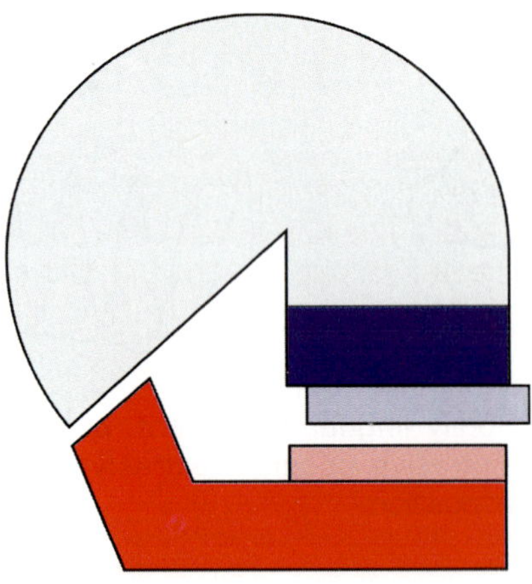

Fig. 10.14: Model diagram showing maxillary dentoalveolar proclination leading to dental class II relation and increased overjet.

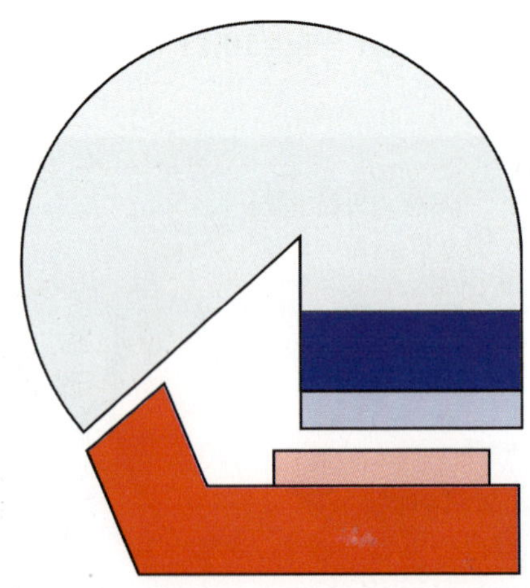

Fig. 10.15: Model diagram showing mandibular dentoalveolar retroclination leading to dental class II relation and increased overjet.

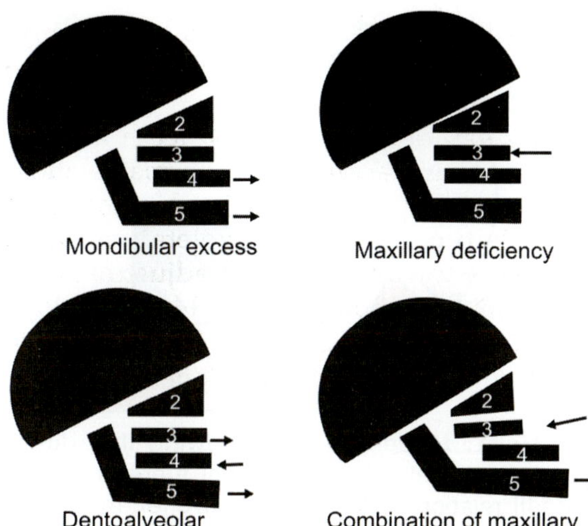

Fig. 10.16: Schematic representation of skeletal jaws disharmonies and dentoalveolar disharmonies which can be seen in different individuals, and thus influencing the treatment plans.

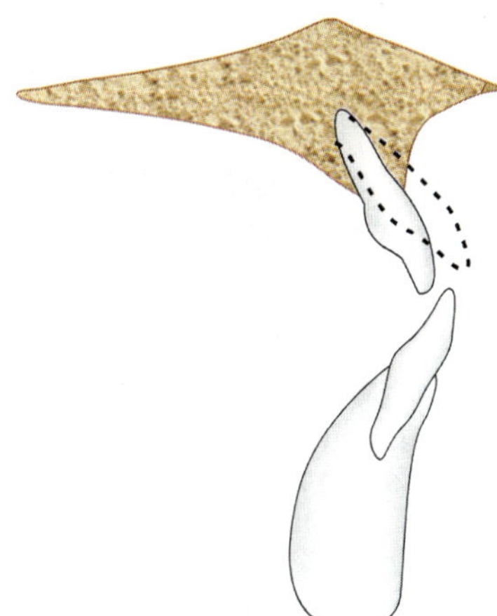

Fig. 10.17: Anterior crossbite due to lingual position of upper incisors. It happens when there is maxillary deficiency

- **In sagittal plane:** Prognathism and retrognathism of maxilla or mandible or both.
- **In transverse plane:** It is narrowing or widening of the jaw bases of maxilla or mandible or both.
- **In vertical plane:** It is expressed as increased or decreased facial height of maxilla or mandible or both. It can be expressed in anterior or posterior facial heights as well, e.g. SFS, LFS, etc.

C. The malocclusion can also be classified based on the deviations in different planes of space:

a. **Malposition in sagittal plane:** These are the conditions due to abnormal relation of teeth or jaws in AP plane of space. They are:
   - **Normal occlusion:** When upper and lower arches are normally related in centric occlusion.
   - **Prenormal occlusion:** When lower arch is forward to the normal position in centric occlusion.
   - **Post-normal occlusion:** When the lower arch is in a distal position to normal when in centric occlusion.

b. **Malpositions in vertical plane:** They include variations in bite depth; e.g. normal bite, deep bite and open bite (Fig. 10.18).

c. **Malpositions in transverse plane:** They include variations in arch width; e.g. normal, narrow, and wide. It contributes to development of cross bites which is

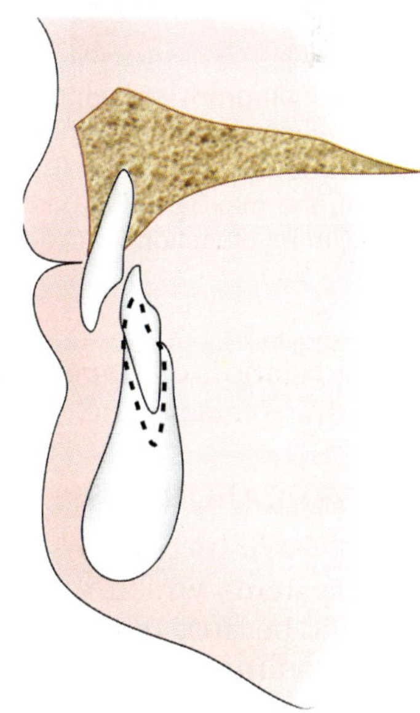

Fig. 10.18: Deep bite and decreased overjet in Angle's class II division 2 condition.

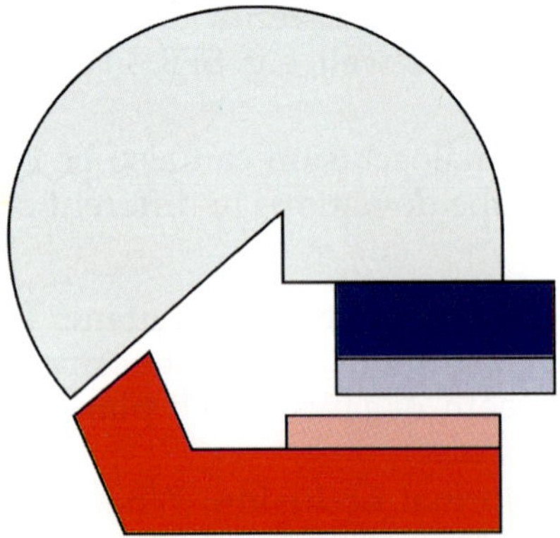

Fig. 10.19: Model diagram showing maxillary skeletal prognathism with dentoalveolar component leading to skeletal class II relation and increased overjet. It is treated with either headgear therapy to control the growth or by extraction of upper first premolars and then retraction of anterior segment.

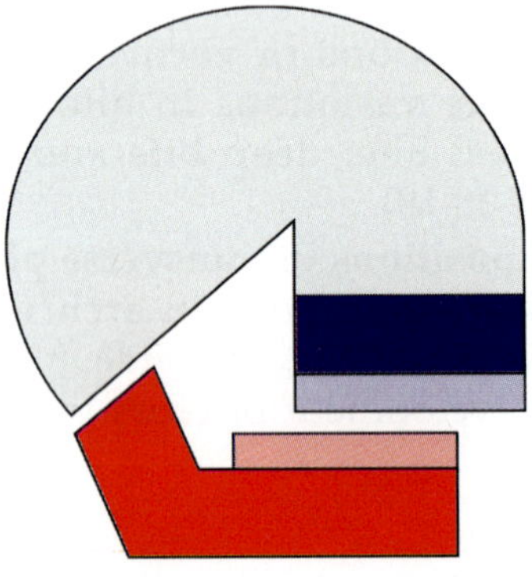

Fig. 10.20: Model diagram showing that due to mandibular skeletal retrognathism with dentoalveolar component, there is skeletal class II relation and increased overjet, the maxilla being normal. Such a case is treated with myofunctional appliances.

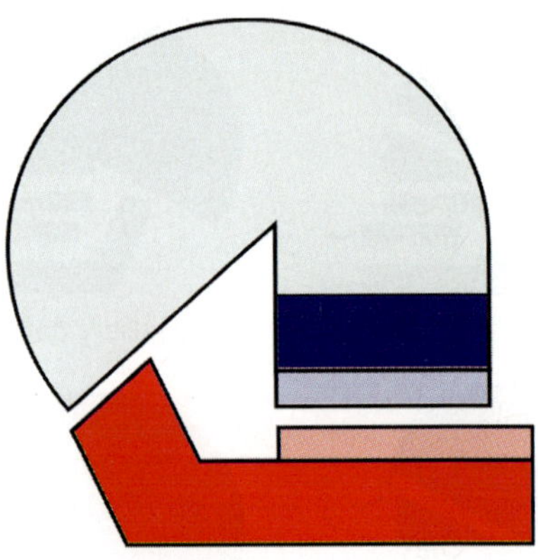

Fig. 10.21: Model diagram showing that due to mandibular skeletal prognathism, there is skeletal class III relation and a negative overjet, the maxilla being normal. Such a case is treated with chin cup appliances during growth stage, while mandibular set-back surgery is needed after growth completion.

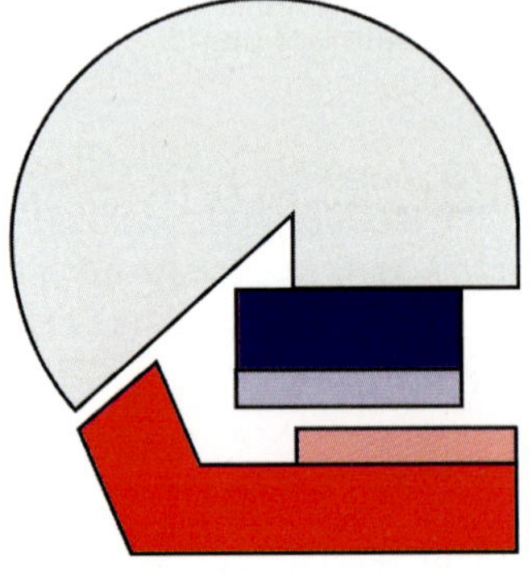

Fig. 10.22: Model diagram showing maxillary skeletal retrognathism leading to skeletal class III relation and negative overjet. It is treated with reverse headgear therapy to bring maxilla forward during active growth period or by surgical advancement of maxilla after growth completion.

abnormal relation of upper and lower arches in transverse plane.

ANGLE'S CLASSIFICATION (1899) (Fig. 10.25)

Before Angle, various authors proposed classification systems which were not universally accepted because of their complexity and difficulty in learning. The Angle's system was a revolutionary description as it was simple, easy to learn and apply. He divided all the malocclusion conditions in three broad categories based on the relationship of permanent first molars of upper and lower arches, which were easy to identify. It has following features:

Normal position of maxillary first molar: According to Angle, upper first permanent molar is fixed in its position in the jaw. Its normal position is that its MB root lies in line with the zygomatic buttress called as key ridge. Atkinson gave the term 'Key Ridge'. The key ridge is a ridge of bone descending

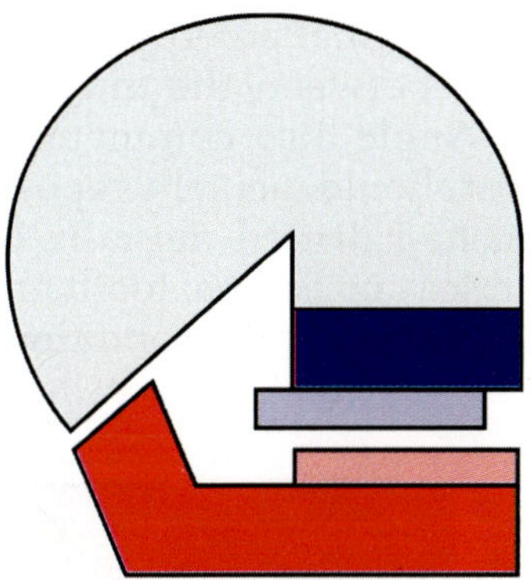

Fig. 10.23: Diagram showing normal skeletal jaw bases, but retropositioned maxillary dentition, leading to anterior crossbite and class III relation.

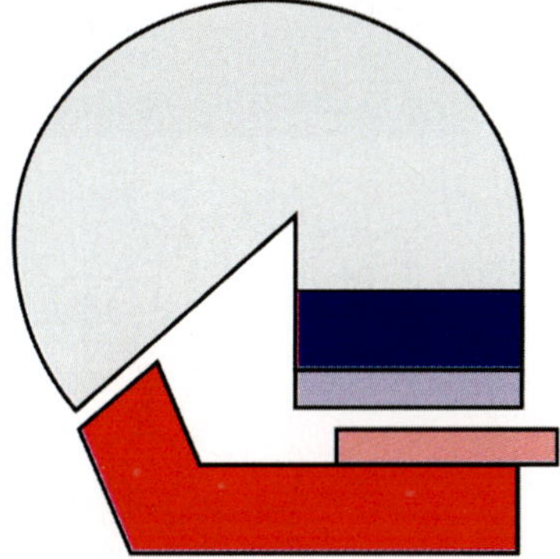

Fig. 10.24: Diagram showing normal skeletal jaw bases, but forward-positioned mandibular dentition, leading to anterior crossbite and class III relation.

downward and forward from the zygoma, which is the anterior edge of the jugal or molar buttress of the maxillary bone and which marks the union of the anterior and the posterior buccal walls of the antrum of Highmore. According to Angle, it is the mandibular first molar which contributes to development of class II or III relation, while the upper first molar is always fixed and normal in its position.

- Angle considered the maxillary first permanent molar as "fixed and in correct position" in the jaws, while only mandible was at fault, thus changing the position of mandibular first molar wrt maxillary first molars.
- The Angle system explains the malocclusion in the sagittal plane, i.e. the anteroposterior plane only.

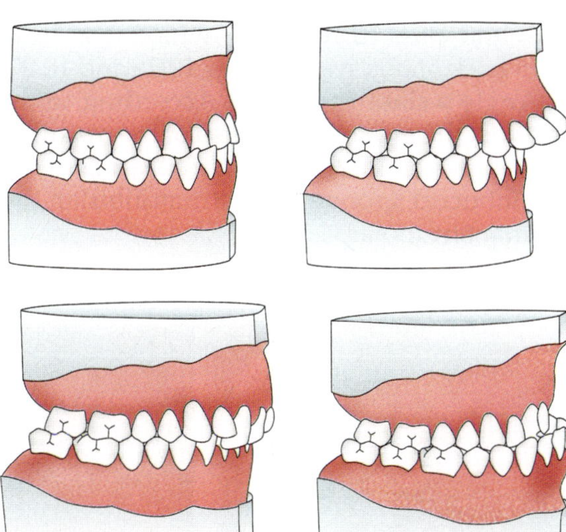

Fig. 10.25: Angle's class I, class II division 1, class II division 2, and class III malocclusions.

- He took the relationship of the mesiobuccal root of the maxillary first molar with the zygomatic buttress called as the key ridge, as the fixed reference. He considered that the mesiobuccal root always lies just below the crest of zygomatic buttress. The key ridge is a ridge of bone descending downward and forward from the zygoma, which is the anterior edge of the jugal or molar buttress of the maxillary bone and which marks the union of the anterior and the posterior buccal walls of the antrum of Highmore. Contemporary orthodontists, however, do not consider the anatomic interrelationship of the upper molar to the cranium as fixed and significant (Katz). He divided malocclusion in three broad categories, viz class I, class II and class III.
- All the classes have been proposed in reference to the relationship of mesiobuccal cusp of maxillary first molar to the mesiobuccal groove of mandibular first molars.
- He has described the change in molar relationship by full cuspal width or premolar width, rather than a partial shift, thus giving a wide range of approx. 9 mm (full cusp widths) between class II

and class III relations, which is a drawback of this system (Figs 10.26 and 10.27).

Angle's class I relation: According to this relation, the mesiobuccal cusp of the maxillary first permanent molar articulates in the mesiobuccal groove of the mandibular first permanent molar.

There is a normal anteroposterior skeletal relationship between the maxilla and the mandible. Angle also commented that the orthodontist should mentally reposition a first molar that had drifted mesially because of early tooth loss or ectopic tooth eruption for exact classification of the condition.

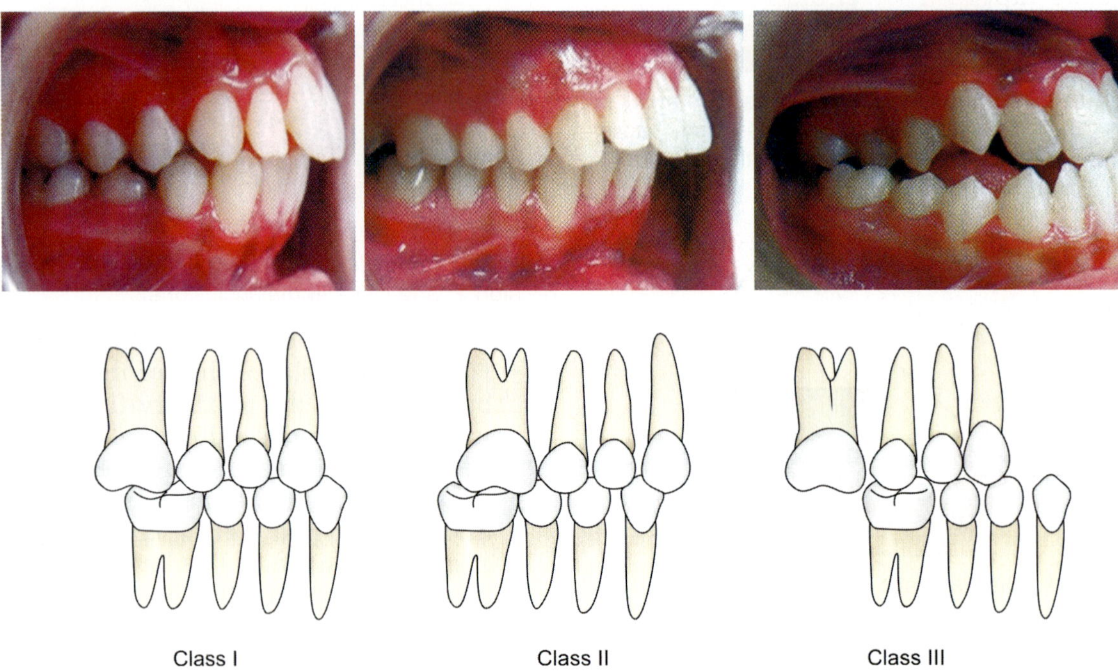

Fig. 10.26: Angle's class I, class II division 1, and class III malocclusions.

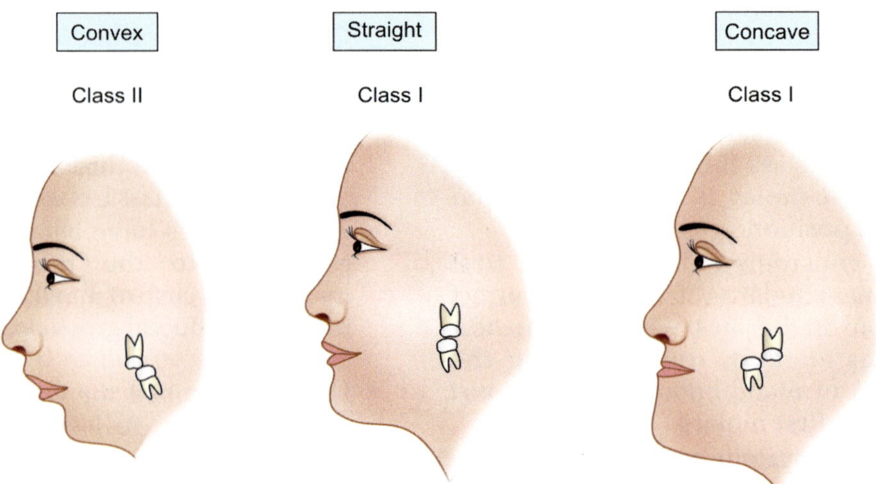

Fig. 10.27: Different Angle's molar relations/malocclusion and the profile of patients.

Angle's class II relation: The mesiobuccal cusp of maxillary first permanent molar articulates mesial to mesiobuccal groove of mandibular first molars, in interdental area between the mandibular second premolar and first permanent molar (Figs 10.28 to 10.31).

Here, Angle did not define the partial shift of the molar relationship, but this shift was of full cusp (approx. 4.5 mm). Those malocclusions in which there is a distal relationship of mandible to maxilla make up the class II.

Divisions of class II malocclusion: Angle further divided class II relation into divisions, based on certain common features of each division.

Division 1: A class II relation in which maxillary incisors are inclined labially, and increased overjet is present.

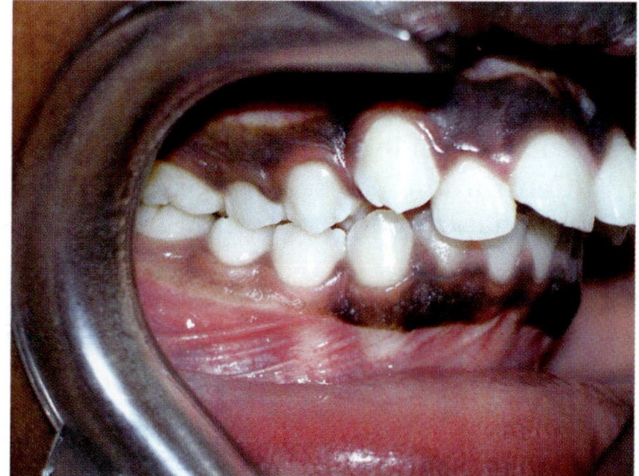

Fig. 10.28: Angle's class II molar and canine, and high level of upper canine, increased overjet, and crowding.

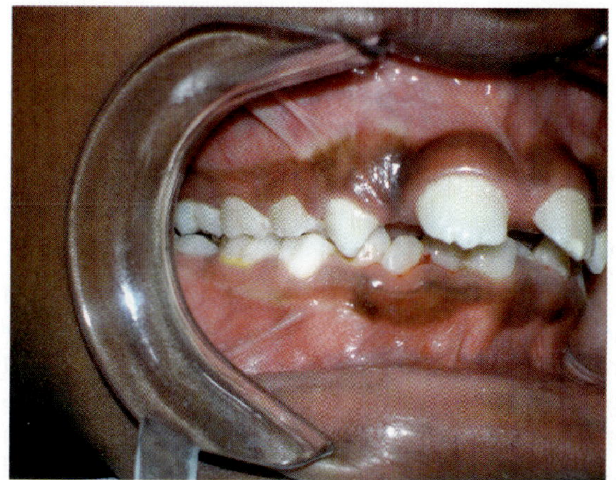

Fig. 10.29: Angle's class II molar and lower incisal crowding.

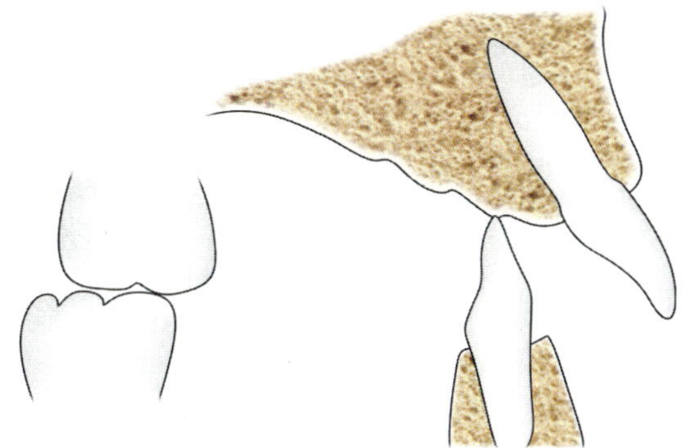

Fig. 10.30: Line diagram of Angle's class II division 1 malocclusion with complete, deep, traumatic bite.

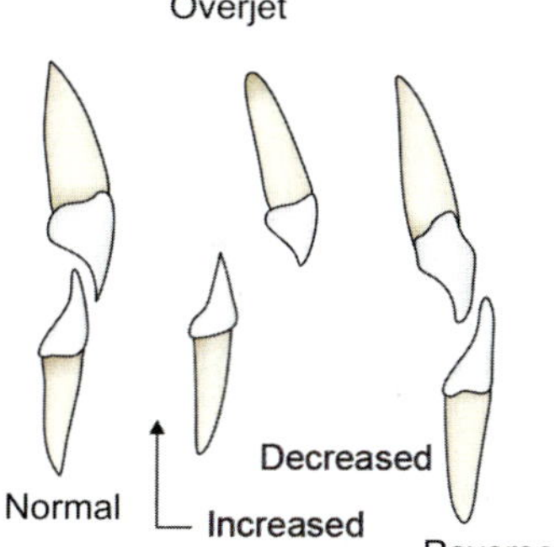

Fig. 10.31: Different overjets.

Division 2: A class II relation in which maxillary central incisors are inclined lingually, and maxillary lateral incisors have tipped labially and mesially, covering the distal of central incisors (types from RANI). The overjet is reduced, and there is deep bite of partial/complete/traumatic/more than 100% nature. There is a posterior shift of mandible during closure in centric occlusion which may be due to premature contacts or incisal guidance, thus retropositioning of the mandible occurs. It leads to development of skeletal class II relations.

Subdivision: Class II relation has been further subdivided based on unilateral presence of class II molar relation. When the distocclusion occurs only on one side, with a class I relation on the other side, it has been termed as subdivision.

Angle's class III relation: The mesiobuccal cusp of maxillary first permanent molar occludes distal to mesiobuccal groove of mandibular first molars, in distobuccal developmental groove of the mandibular first permanent molar. Those malocclusions in which there is a mesial relationship of mandible to maxilla form a skeletal class III. Here also, Angle did not define the partial shift of the molar relationship, but this shift was of full cusp (approx. 4.5 mm).

Subdivision: Class III relation has been further subdivided based on unilateral presence of class III molar relation. When the mesio-occlusion occurs only on one side, with a class I relation on the other side, it has been termed as subdivision.

Variations of Angle's classes: Although not described originally by Angle in his system, the continuous quest of knowledge and gain in experience has led to evolution of following terms which are important for diagnosis and treatment planning of the patients.

Super-class I: It was not described in Angle's system. This indicates a malocclusion in which there is tendency for class III relationship but the molar relationship cannot be described as class I either. However, according to some authors, it may be considered as shift of mandibular first molar mesially by less than half cusp width variation.

Pseudo-class I: Another modification was presented by Jan De Baets and Martin Chiarini in 1995 as "The Pseudo-class I: a newly defined type of malocclusion. It is an apparent class I molar and canine relationship with following features, that has developed too mesially because of a combination of factors like:

- Mesial rotation of the upper first permanent molar, which may be due to mesial shift of tooth during loss of leeway space.
- Lower incisors crowding.
- Lack of space for the lower canines to erupt.
- Mature pseudo-class I also have over-erupted lower second molar and anterior deep bite.
- The class I intercuspation in fact masks a mild dental class II.

Variations of Class II Division 2 Incisor Relations

Three types of incisal relations can be seen in class II division 2 as follows:

a. Central incisors in lingual inclination with lateral incisors in labial inclination.
b. Central and lateral incisors in lingual inclination with canines in labial inclination.
c. Centrals, laterals and canines in lingual inclination.

Deck biss: This is a condition in which there is bilateral class I molar relation, but the incisors are in a pattern resembling division 2 of class II category (Figs 10.32 and 10.33).

True class III: This is a skeletal class III malocclusion of genetic origin due to discrepancy in jaw positions. It may be due to

- Excessively large mandible or forwardly placed mandible.
- Smaller than normal maxilla or retropositioned maxilla.
- Combination of the above two.

The patient can present with normal over jet, edge or anterior crossbite.

Pseudo-class III: As the name suggests, it is a false position of occlusion in class III molar relation. It is produced by forward movement of mandible during centric occlusion due to a premature contact in incisal region, which leads the mandible to close in a forward position. It is also known as the habitual or the postural class III.

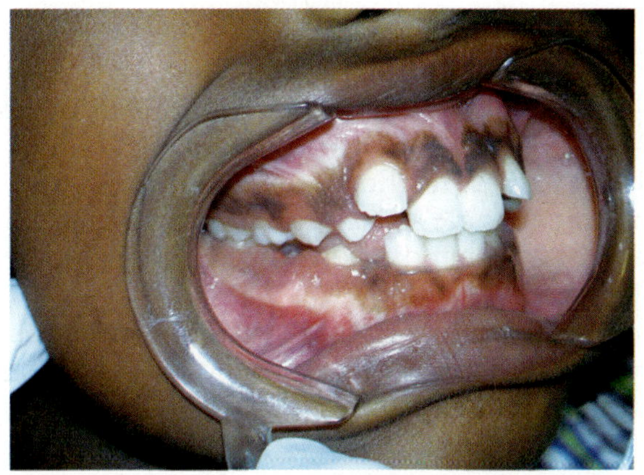

Fig. 10.32: Angle's class I molar relation, and upper incisors in division 2 pattern (Deck biss).

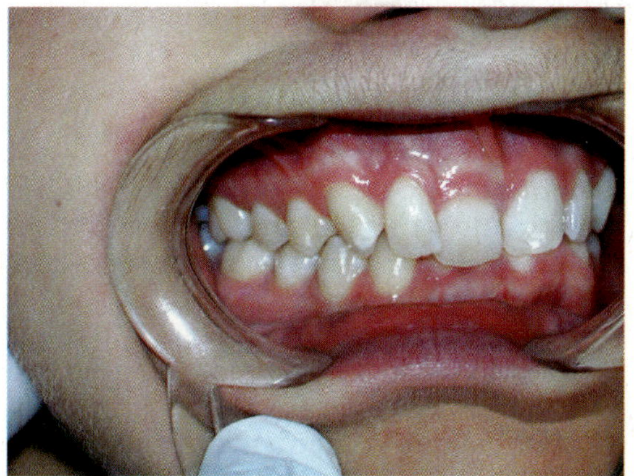

Fig. 10.33: Deep bite, Angle's class I molars, and incisors in division 2 pattern (Deck biss).

It occurs due to presence of prematurities forcing the mandible to slide forward during centric occlusion, e.g. anterior crossbites. It may also be seen in cases of premature loss of multiple deciduous posterior teeth or multiple missing buccal teeth; so the patient closes the mandible in a forward position to contact in the anterior teeth or a patient with enlarged adenoids, which forces the tongue forward and thus the mandible to close in a forward position.

Here, the skeletal relationship of jaws is generally normal toward class I. It is very important to treat this condition as early as possible, otherwise with ensuing mandibular growth and a countered maxillary growth (by anterior positioned mandible), it may convert in true skeletal class III, as the mandible does not face the restrictive effect of maxilla during this condition.

Class IV: It is seen when there is class III on one side and class II on the other side. This condition is very rare and seen in gross facial asymmetries. It was not described by Angle in his original classification, but finds mention in the literature.

Half-cusp relationship: Angle described the variation as full cusp change in the molar relation. However, in routine practice, many cases are seen which have less than full cusp or half cusp variation in molar relation. It may occur due to many factors, e.g. abnormal loss of leeway space; proximal caries; lack of growth; abnormal development due to habits, etc. Below are mentioned half cusp relations also.

Half-cusp class II: Here, the relation of lower first molar with upper first permanent molar is more than one-half cusp distal to that of normal relation. It may be due to either maxillary arch forward or mandibular arch backward or partial loss of leeway space.

Half-cusp class III: Here, the relation of lower first molar with upper first permanent molar is more than one-half cusp mesial to that of normal relation. It may be due to either maxillary arch backward or mandibular arch forward or loss of leeway space in lower arch.

Advantages of Angle's system:
- It is very simple to learn.
- Easy to use and reproduce.
- Easy for communication with fellow clinicians.
- Can be easily used during research to categorize the study subjects.
- It is not confusing, as it considers only molar relation in sagittal direction only. But this contributes to disadvantage in practice.

Drawbacks of Angle's classification: Although Angle's system is one of the simplest systems to remember and learn, it has a number of drawbacks. But despite of these drawbacks, it is still followed due to its simplicity. It has following drawbacks:

- Angle considered malocclusion only in anteroposterior plane, describing molar relation in sagittal plane only. He did not consider malocclusion in the transverse and vertical planes.
- Angle considered maxillary first permanent molars as fixed points in the skull which is not true.
- It gives only a dental relationship rather than skeletal relationship.
- It does not consider the soft tissues of the face.
- It does not consider the effect of growth, growth patterns and time factors.
- The classification cannot be properly applied if any of the first permanent molars are extracted or missing.
- The classification cannot be applied to the deciduous dentition.
- The classification does not highlight the etiology of the malocclusion.
- Individual teeth malpositions are not considered.
- Also it considers a large range of variation of approx. 9 mm by full cuspal width or half a molar width. It did not consider the partial cuspal variation.

According to Katz, another major concern regarding the Angle classification is the lack of a numerical quantification of the degree of class II or class III.

- Angle never intended his classification to depict class I as a treatment goal or "ideal," but as a range of abnormality between the extremes of full class II and class III.
- Friel, Arya et al have demonstrated the dynamic nature of permanent first molar position in the mixed dentition, which changes as the occlusion matures into the permanent dentition because of jaw growth and use of leeway space. Thus, the natural "adjustment" makes a molar-defined classification awkward in young patients.

DEWEY'S MODIFICATION OF ANGLE'S CLASSIFICATION

Since Angle's system did not consider the relation of incisors during categorization of class I and III relations, then in 1915, Dewey modified Angle's class I and Angle's class III categories depending on the relation/position of maxillary incisors.

Dewey's modification of class I: Class I has been divided in five types based on the position of maxillary incisors, as follows:

- **Type 1:** There is crowding of maxillary incisor teeth. The canines may be in axioversion, labioversion or infraversion. All the other individual tooth malposition may be present (Fig. 10.34).
- **Type 2:** Maxillary incisors are labially inclined and have spacing in between. There may be increased overjet (Fig. 10.35).
- **Type 3:** An anterior crossbite of individual or multiple teeth is present. The maxillary incisor teeth are in linguoversion to the mandibular incisor teeth (Figs 10.36 and 10.37).
- **Type 4:** A posterior crossbite is present of individual or multiple teeth, but the incisors and the canines are in normal alignment and the dental arches are in normal relationship.
- **Type 5:** The molars are in mesioversion due to mesial shifting after the loss of teeth in position anterior to the molars; the rest of the teeth are in normal relation.

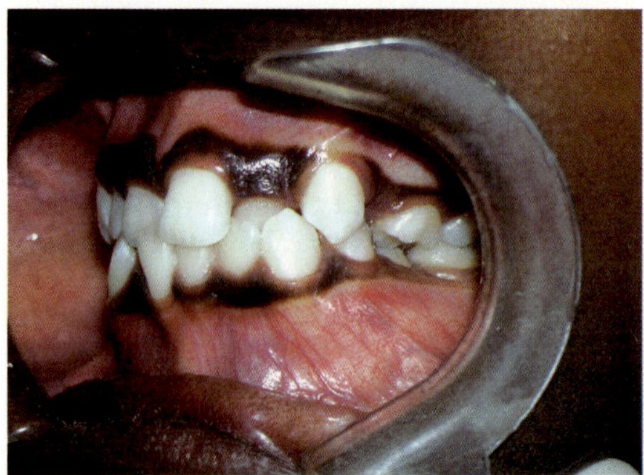

Fig. 10.34: Crowding and crossbite in anterior region.

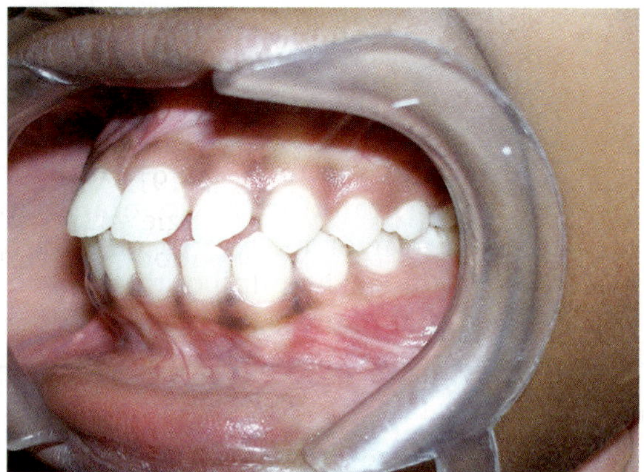

Fig. 10.35: Angle's class I molar relation, and spacing in anterior region (Dewey type 2).

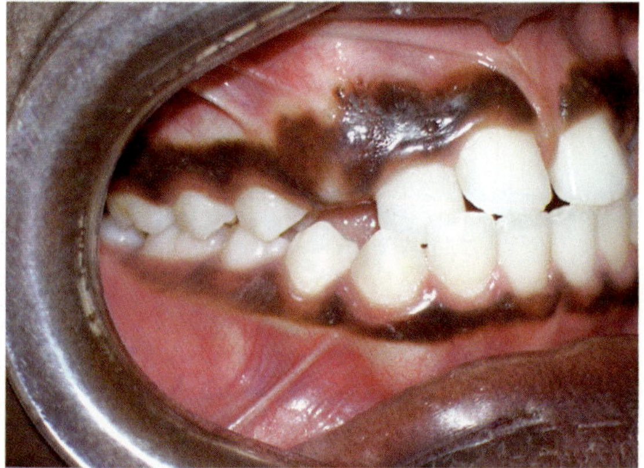

Fig. 10.36: Angle's class I molar relation, and single tooth crossbite of lateral incisor (Dewey type 3).

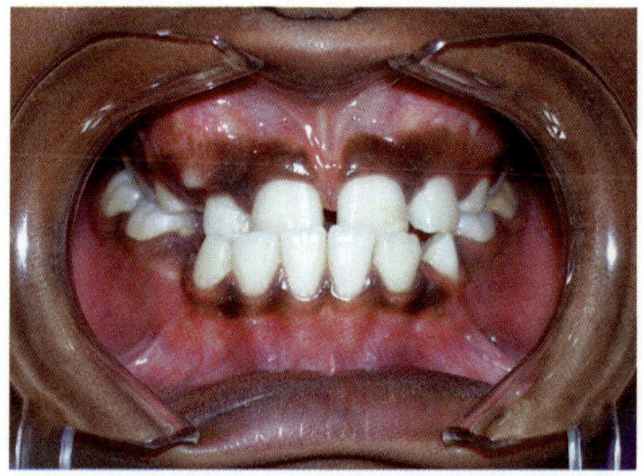

Fig. 10.37: Crossbite in anterior region involving multiple teeth.

If more than one of the above mentioned features are present in a patient, then in the diagnostic statement, all those types are mentioned, e.g. a patient having spacing in upper incisors, and a posterior crossbite in a class I malocclusion will be diagnosed as Angle's class I type 2, 4 malocclusion.

Dewey's modification of class III: Class III has been divided in three types based on the position of maxillary incisors as follows:

- **Type 1:** Appearance in these cases suggests that mandibular dental arch has been moved forward bodily. There is an edge to edge incisal relation in centric occlusion, with zero overjet.
- **Type 2:** The mandibular incisors are crowded and in lingual relation to the maxillary incisors. So, there is normal overjet relation.
- **Type 3:** The maxillary arch is underdeveloped. The maxillary incisors are crowded. The mandibular arch is well developed and the mandibular teeth are in normal alignment. There is an anterior cross bite and hence reverse overjet present.

LISCHER'S MODIFICATION OF ANGLE'S CLASSIFICATION

In 1933, Lischer proposed modified terms for the Angle's classes of malocclusion, as follows.

- **Neutroclusion:** It is equivalent to class I, i.e. there is normal relation of upper and lower arches.
- **Distoclusion:** It is equivalent to class II, i.e. there is a distal relation of lower arch to the upper arch.
- **Mesioclusion:** It is equivalent to class III, i.e. there is a mesial relation of lower arch to the upper arch.

Individual teeth malpositions: It was also described by Lischer. He added the word "version" to describe the deviation of the tooth in that direction. He described individual tooth malpositions as:

a. **Mesioversion:** Mesial to the normal position

b. **Distoversion:** Distal to the normal position
c. **Linguoversion:** Lingual to the normal position
d. **Labioversion or buccoversion:** Toward the lip or cheek
e. **Infraversion:** Away from the line of occlusion, i.e. infraerupted
f. **Supraversion:** Extended past the line of occlusion, i.e. supraerupted
g. **Axiversion:** Tipped, the wrong axial inclination
h. **Torsiversion:** Rotated on its long axis
i. **Transversion:** Wrong order in the arch, transposition.

SIMON SYSTEM (Figs 10.38 and 10.39)

Simon in 1930 proposed his system of classification. He was the first to relate the dental arches to the face and cranium in all the three planes of space. It is also famous as Simon's law of canines. The dental arches in Simon system are related to three anthropologic planes based on the cranial landmarks. The planes are the Frankfurt, the orbital, and the midsagittal planes, mutually perpendicular to each other.

- **Frankfort horizontal plane** is drawn as a straight line through lower margin of the bony orbit directly under the pupil of the eye, to the upper margin of the auditory meatus. FHP was among the first reference planes used in craniometry and agreed by consensus in 1889 at Frankfurt.
- **The orbital plane** is a perpendicular drawn to Frankfort horizontal plane from the lower margin of bony orbit directly under the pupil of the eye
- **Midsagittal plane** is the plane in antero-posterior direction passing through the median raphae of the palate; and is perpendicular to both the above mentioned planes.

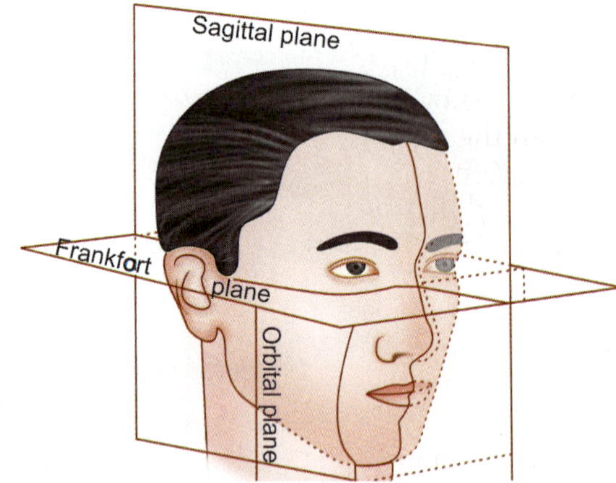

Fig. 10.39: Three reference planes used in Simon's classification of malocclusion to define the position of the teeth.

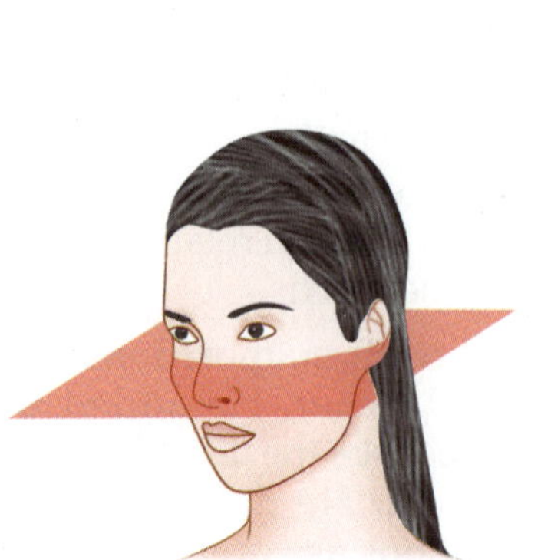
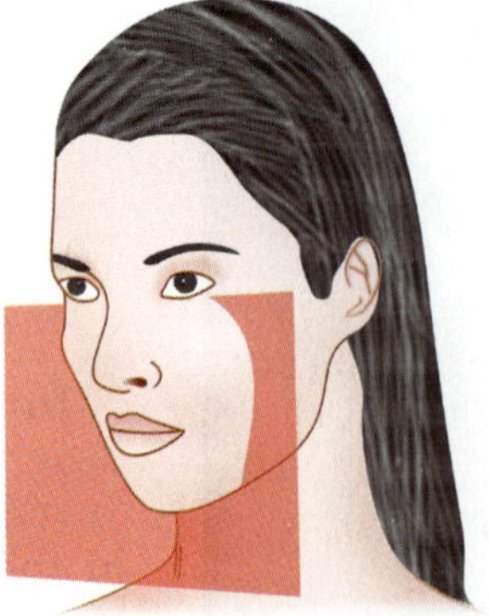
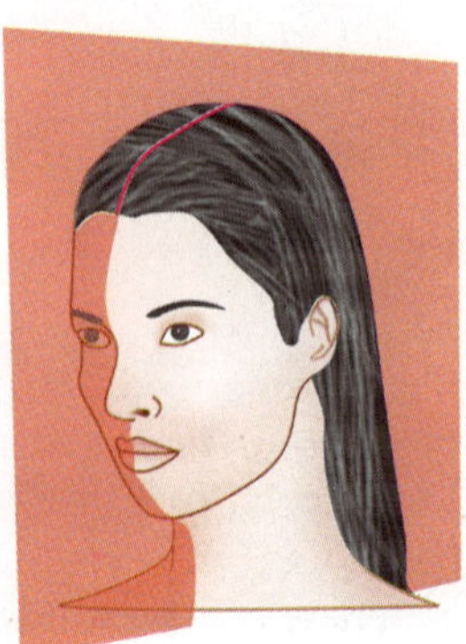

Fig. 10.38: Three planes of space used in Simon's classification: orbital, vertical and midsagittal planes.

Simon proposed a canine-based classification. His law of canine considered the orbital plane (a line drawn from orbitale perpendicular to Frankfort horizontal) as passing through the distal third of maxillary canine in an ideal occlusion. Maxillary canines have been used to evaluate ideal buccal occlusion. Maxillary canines are among the most stable dental units because they have the longest root and therefore very well anchored to the alveolar bone. The canine is the "keystone" tooth in the dental arch, and provides a buttressing support for the incisors, as well as the posterior teeth. Also, canines provide a vital protective function in lateral excursive movements, i.e. canine-protected occlusion.

According to Simon's law of canine, in an ideal occlusion, the orbital plane should pass through the distal third of upper canine, and when extended downward, it should pass through the buccal embreasure between mandibular canine and first premolars.

Relationships Described Based on Simon's System

1. **Anteroposterior relationships** (assessed with respect to the orbital plane, oriented left to right): The malocclusion is based on the distance of upper teeth or dental arch irt orbital plane.
   a. When the teeth or dental arch are placed anterior to the normal position with respect to the orbital plane, it is said to be in protraction.
   b. When the teeth or dental arch are placed posterior to the normal position with respect to the orbital plane, it is said to be in retraction.
2. **Transverse/mediolateral relationships** (assessed with respect to the midsagittal plane, oriented in AP direction): It is evaluated as the distance of teeth, or dental arch from this plane. It shows the deviations in transverse plane.
   a. When the dental arch or a part of it is nearer to midsagittal plane than the normal position, it is said to be in Contraction (e.g. narrowing of the arch).
   b. When the dental arch or a part of it is away from midsagittal plane or is wider than the normal, it is said to be in distraction (e.g. increased width of the dental arch).
3. **Vertical relationships** (assessed with respect to the Frankfurt plane, oriented flat parallel to OP)
   a. When the dental arch or a part of it is nearer to the Frankfort horizontal plane than the normal position, it is said to be in attraction, e.g. such a feature can be seen in short facial height; short face syndrome.
   b. When the dental arch or a part of it is farther apart from the Frankfort horizontal plane than the normal position, it is said to be in abstraction, e.g. such a feature is seen in long facial heights, long face syndrome.

CANINE CLASSIFICATION

It is based on the relationship of long axis of maxillary canine to the buccal embrasure between mandibular canine and first premolar. According to this relationship, following types can be classified.

Class I: when the long axis of maxillary canine lies exactly in the center of the buccal embrasure between mandibular canine and first premolar.

Class II: When the long axis of maxillary canine lies mesial to the center of the buccal embrasure between mandibular canine and first premolar. It may be due to maxillary prognathism; mandibular retrognathism or a combination of both.

Class III: When the long axis of maxillary canine lies distal to the center of the buccal embrasure between mandibular canine and first premolar. It may be due to maxillary retrognathism; mandibular prognathism or a combination of both.

Limitations: This canine system has a limitation as described by Katz, which is due to anatomy of maxillary canines. Due to asymmetric size and slopes of mesial and distal incisal ridges (mesial being smaller than distal slope), the central axis of maxillary canine does not bisect its cusp tip. So, tip comes to lie 1–1.5 mm mesial to the central axis. Hence its cusp tip does not directly fit into the embrasure between mandibular canine and the first premolar, but lies on the distal slope of mandibular canine.

Another objection to canine classification is due to its time of eruption. The upper canine is mostly the last succedaneous tooth to erupt. So, we have to wait until the patient is 12 years or more in slowly erupting patients. The deciduous canine cannot be used for classification as its mesiodistal width is less than its permanent successor, resulting in a central axis that is not coincident with the central axis of its future permanent replacement.

BENNETTE'S CLASSIFICATION OF MALOCCLUSION

He described malocclusion based on their etiology as follows:

Class I: Abnormal position of one or more teeth is due to local causes.

Class II: Abnormal development of a part or complete dental arch is due to developmental defects of the bone.

Class III: Any abnormal interrelation of upper and lower arches; and relation of either arch with the facial contour is due to development defects of the bones.

SALZMANN'S SKELETAL CLASSIFICATION

Salzmann in 1950 described a skeletal classification based on the relationship of jaws rather than the teeth, as follows:

Skeletal class I: The relation of skeletal bases of upper and lower jaws is normal in sagittal direction. The profile is orthognathic. The malocclusion is of purely dental nature. It has been divided as follows:

Division 1: It has local malposition of the teeth.

Division 2: The maxillary incisors are proclined.

Division 3: The maxillary incisors are retroclined.

Division 4: There is bimaxillary protrusion.

Skeletal class II: The mandibular jaw base is in a distal relationship with maxillary jaw base, i.e. mandible is retrognathic. It has been divided in following two types:

Division 1: Upper arch is narrow and crowding is present. There is retrognathic profile, and decreased vertical face height. Cross bite may also be present.

Division 2: Maxillary central incisors are retroclined, with lateral incisors in normal or labial inclination relation.

Skeletal class III: The mandibular jaw base is in a mesial relationship with maxillary jaw base. It is due to overgrowth of mandible, i.e. mandible and profile is prognathic.

INCISORS CLASSIFICATION (Fig. 10.40)

The British Standards Institute proposed in 1983 the incisor's classification (BS EN21942 part 1 (1992) glossary of dental terms), based on the relation of incisal edges of upper and lower incisors, as follows:

Class I: The lower incisal edges occlude with or lie immediately below the cingulum plateau (middle part of) the upper central incisors.

Class II: The lower incisor edges lie posterior to the cingulum plateau of the upper central incisors. Here, due to loss of functional opposition, the lower incisors usually supra-erupt leading to deep bite. There are two divisions:

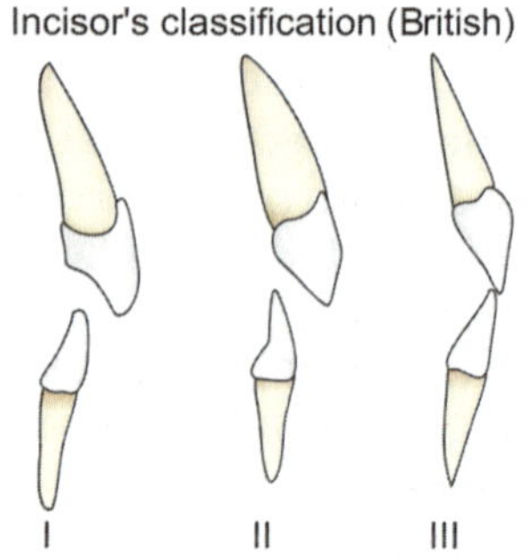

Incisor's classification (British)

I II III

Fig. 10.40: British incisor classification.

Division 1: There is an increase in the overjet and the upper central incisors are usually proclined.

Division 2: The upper central incisors are retroclined. The overjet is usually minimal but may be increased.

Class III: The lower incisor edges lie anterior to the cingulum plateau of the upper central incisors. The overjet is reduced or reversed.

KATZ'S CLASSIFICATION

It is a modified form of Angle's classification suggested in 1994 by Katz.

Class I: The most anterior upper premolar fits into the embrasure created by the distal contact of the most anterior lower premolar.

With this relationship, the canines also relate correctly in class I, as also the incisors. Here, molar relation is not considered. The occlusion functions and intermeshes properly and is considered class I, even though when one upper premolar correctly opposes two lower premolars, the molars are full Angle's class II position, and when two upper premolars oppose one lower premolar, the molars are full Angle's class III position.

Advantages of Katz Classification

1. It can be applied to the conditions whether all premolars are present or some premolar has been extracted for orthodontic treatment; whether one upper premolar opposes two lower premolars, whether two upper premolars oppose one lower premolar or whether only one premolar is present in each quadrant. So, it can be perfectly applied in normal, pretreatment, as well as treated cases.
2. Angle was in favor of nonextraction treatment to achieve class I relation with full complement of teeth as a goal. Since extractions are very common in orthodontics, there is a need to have an occlusion classification that works when teeth are extracted in only one arch also. In the rare instance where no premolar exists in a quadrant, then the central axis of the upper canine crown (not the cusp tip) should be used as a reference to the distal contact of the lower canine.
3. It can also be applied to deciduous and mixed dentition, which is an advantage over Angle classification. Here, the central axis of upper first primary molar should pass through the embrasure between both lower deciduous molars. The central axis of upper second primary molar is less accurate than first molars because of the leeway space. In cases, if upper first deciduous molar is prematurely lost, a line drawn through central axis of the edentulous space should bisect the embrasure between two lower deciduous molars.

Quantifying the Classification

Angle's classification lacks a numerical quantification of the degree of class II or class III. Katz's classification designates ideal cusp-embrasure occlusion (as described by Angle) as zero (0). A plus sign (+) is given to class II direction and a minus sign (–) to class III tendency. Also, the right side of occlusion is evaluated first, and then the left side. Thus, the ideal occlusion on both right and left sides is (0,0).

A study done by Sinh and Rinchuse in 1998 found Katz's classification having the highest reliability, The British Standard Incisor classification system was next highest, and Angle's classification system was the least reliable. The British, and particularly Angle, have poor definitions and descriptions of the classes, causing overlapping of categories where one class blends into another.

ETIOLOGIC CLASSIFICATION

Most of the systems described above do not consider the etiology of malocclusion for classifying them. Following is the classification based on the etiology of malocclusion.

- Osseous
- Muscular
- Dental.

Osseous: It includes problems in abnormal growth, size, shape, or proportion of any of the bones of the craniofacial complex, e.g. class III cases may be due to mandibular hypertrophy and class II may be due to mandibular deficiency.

Muscular: It includes problems due to malfunction of the dentofacial musculature. Any persistent alteration in normal function of the muscles may result in distorted growth of the facial bones or abnormal position of the teeth.

The muscular factors are:

- Functional slides into occlusion due to occlusal interferences
- Detrimental sucking habits
- Abnormal patterns of mandibular closure
- Incompetent normal reflexes, e.g. Lip posture
- Abnormal muscular contraction.

Dental: Dental problems involve primarily the teeth and their supporting structures.

This category includes:

- Malposition of teeth
- Abnormal number of teeth
- Abnormal size of teeth
- Abnormal shape or texture of teeth.

ACKERMANN–PROFFIT SYSTEM VENN DIAGRAM USED IN THE ACKERMANN-PROFFIT SYSTEM

Ackermann and Proffit in 1960s proposed a comprehensive system of classification, which considered the malocclusion in all the three planes of space, and considered the skeletal problems and the etiology of the malocclusion. It also gives an indication of the severity of malocclusion. The classification is described by using Venn diagram (Fig. 10.41). The classification considered five characteristics of malocclusion, and their interrelationships, divided in 9 groups. Those five characteristics are studied in that order as follows:

Characteristic 1: Alignment

Intra-arch alignment and symmetry are assessed from the occlusal view. Based on the findings, a dental arch can be classified as ideal / crowded / spaced.

Characteristic 2: Profile

It is assessed from the side of the face. It gives indications of skeletal relations and soft tissue morphology of the face. The profile can be convex / straight / concave. This also includes the assessment of facial divergence, i.e. anterior or posterior divergence.

Characteristic 3: Transverse Relationships

These include the transverse skeletal and dental relationships. Buccal and palatal cross bites, and midline deviations are noted in this plane. Asymmetries of facial complex are also noted. These are further divided as unilateral or bilateral conditions. Differentiation between skeletal and dental components is also made and noted.

Characteristic 4: Class

It is studied in the sagittal plane, where the AP relationship of teeth and jaws is noted. Here the relationship of teeth is assessed by Angle's classification as class I / class II / C1ass III. The skeletal and dental malocclusions are distinguished. The prognathism or retrognathism of the jaws is noted. Also the canine relation, and anterior cross bite, i.e. incisor relation are noted.

Characteristic 5: Overbite

The conditions are assessed in the vertical plane, i.e. bite depth, facial heights, etc. are noted. Variations in bite depth are described as normal bite / open bite / deep bite / collapsed bite. It may involve anterior and / or posterior regions. The skeletal nature of the vertical problem is also differentiated, e.g. deep bite may be skeletal due to decreased anterior facial height, or it may be purely of dental nature on a normal skeletal base or it may be a combination of both. Similarly, the open bite can be skeletal and/or dental nature. It also gives an idea of growth pattern of the face.

Details of AP system with nine groups: As mentioned above, AP system of classification helps to study the malocclusion in 9 groups which are briefly mentioned below. The malocclusion in three planes is studied in the order of TSV, i.e. transverse, sagittal and vertical planes (Fig. 10.41).

- First group represents the intra-arch alignment and symmetry.
- Second group represents the profile.
- Third group represents the transverse deviations.
- Fourth group represents the sagittal deviations.
- Fifth group represents the vertical deviations.
- Sixth group represents the malocclusions with transverse and sagittal deviations.
- Seventh group represents the malocclusions with sagittal and vertical deviations.
- Eight group represents the malocclusions with vertical and transverse deviation.
- Ninth group represents the malocclusions with deviations in all three planes of space, i.e. transverse, sagittal and vertical.

Nature of the severity of the malocclusion: As the deviations in the conditions increase,

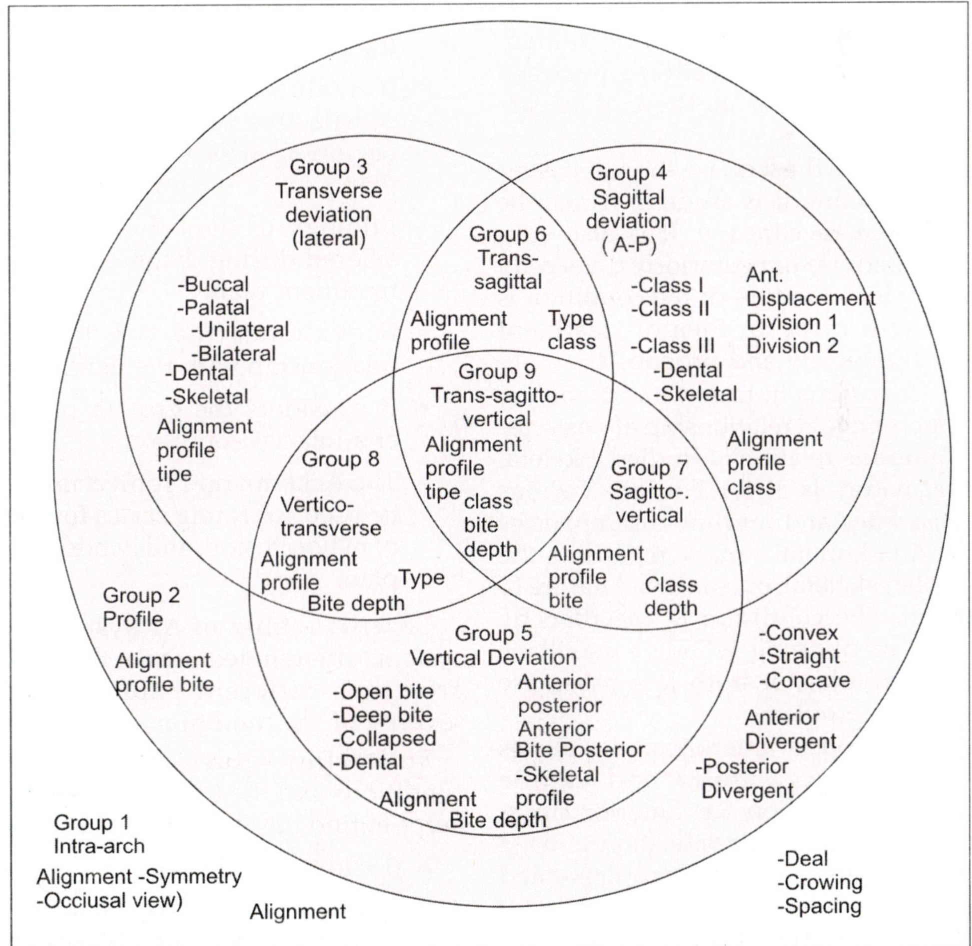

Fig. 10.41: Venn diagram showing the various components which should be studied to classify malocclusion in three dimensions, as suggested by Ackermann and Proffit.

it leads to the severe form of malocclusion and thus the nature of treatment and prognosis is affected, e.g. the condition lying only in 1–5 groups are not that complicated, as those lying in 6–8 groups. The problem lying in group 9 is the most complicated type. Also problems having skeletal component are more difficult to treat than only dental problems. Thus, AP system also helps to judge the prognosis and complexity of the treatment.

Procedure: Following five steps are followed for classifying any malocclusion using this system. During this system, the skeletal and dental nature of the problem and the etiology of the problem is also denoted side by side in each group.

Step 1: Alignment and symmetry of the teeth and dental arches is analysed. Alignment can be ideal; crowded; spaced; mutilated. Irregularities of individual teeth are described by using the Lischer's method of classification.

Step 2: Profile of the face, i.e. the soft tissues and factors affecting it is studied. It may be straight, convex or concave. It is also subdivided as anteriorly or posteriorly divergent. Skeletal and dental nature of the condition is studied. It also gives an idea of treatment objectives, complexity and prognosis.

Step 3: Deviations in transverse plane are studied. Buccolingual relationship of posterior teeth and midline relation is studied. Skeletal and dental nature is also recorded. Various buccal cross bites and midline discrepancies are noted. A judgment is made regarding the dentoalveolar, skeletal, or combined nature of the problem. The condition is specified by finding and mentioning whether maxillary and/or mandibular/or both jaw bases are involved in the problem.

Step 4: Deviations in anteroposterior planes are considered, e.g. molar and canine relations, incisor relation, i.e. anterior crossbite are noted. Angle's classification is used to note molar relation. It is also supplemented by noting the skeletal, dentoalveolar, or combined nature of the problem.

Step 5: Malocclusion in vertical dimensions are considered, e.g. bite depth (deep/open bite), growth patterns, facial heights, growth pattern, etc. are noted. The term bite depth is used to describe the vertical relationship. It can be normal bite; open bite, deep bite, and posterior collapsed bite. The nature of problem whether it is skeletal, dental or combined is also determined, along with the possible etiological factors.

Advantages of the Ackermann-Proffit System

AP system is the most comprehensive classification system till date. It has following advantages over other systems.

- It evaluates the malocclusion in three planes of the space.
- It evaluates the influence of dentition on the profile.
- It evaluates the skeletal and dental perspective of the problems from the beginning, which influence the treatment plan.
- Etiology of the condition is also considered during diagnosis and hence the treatment plan.
- It evaluates the soft tissue and its relationship with the dentition.
- It considers the growth pattern of the craniofacial complex.
- The Ackermann-Proffit classification can be used for rating scales for the severity of malocclusion, and hence the treatment plan.

Severity ratings of AP system: Under this system, different features of the malocclusion are given different values based on the severity of the condition as depicted below.

Following values are assigned to the conditions and the total score is taken, which helps to find out the severity of the condition.

- 0 = Ideal, no deviation
- 1 = Slight deviation from the normal, not enough to warrant treatment for this alone.
- 2 = Slight to moderate deviation

Characteristics	*Ideal*	*Slight*		*Moderate*	*Severe*	
Alignment	0	1	2	3	4	5
Profile esthetics	0	1	2	3	4	5
Crossbite	0	1	2	3	4	5
Angle class	0	1	2	3	4	5
Bite depth	0	1	2	3	4	5

- 3 = Moderate deviation from ideal, enough alone to justify treatment.
- 4 = Moderate to severe deviation from ideal, definitely needs treatment.
- 5 = Severe deviation to such an extent that the patient is handicapped.

Recent additions in the description of a malocclusion: In addition to the five characteristics of AP classification system, the smile characteristics are now being considered important from treatment viewpoint. Esthetic line of the dentition is the one seen when evaluating anterior tooth display. It follows the facial edges of the maxillary anterior and posterior teeth.

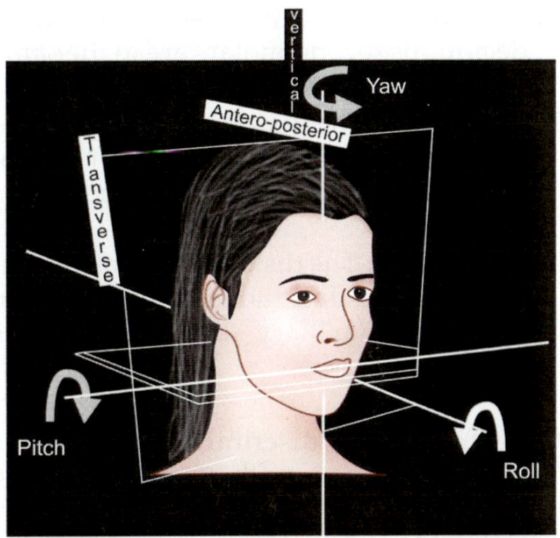

Fig. 10.42: Planes used in yaw, roll and pitch.

PITCH, ROLL AND YAW IN SYSTEMATIC DESCRIPTION (Fig. 10.42)

The terms pitch, roll and yaw are used in systematic description of the malocclusion. They help to describe the position of the teeth and jaw bases irt lips and cheeks.

Pitch: It is the characteristic showing an excessive upward/downward rotation of the dentition around the transverse plane, relative to the lips and cheeks. It shows incisal exposure, and the bite depth, i.e. normal bite/ open bite/deep bite. Pitch of the jaws and teeth relative to the soft tissue is evaluated by studying the relation with the intercommissure line. Pitch of the jaws and teeth relative to facial skeleton can be seen with cephalograms, where pitch is revealed as the orientation of the palatal, occlusal and mandibular planes relative to the true horizontal plane.

Roll: It is described as rotation of teeth or jaws around the sagittal plane on one or the other side. It depicts the asymmetric inclination/skewing of the incisal plane and the occlusal plane. It is evaluated in relation to the soft tissue using the intercommissure line, while in relation to facial skeleton, the interocular line is used.

Yaw: It is the rotation of the jaws or the dentition to one side or the other, around a vertical axis. It produces a skeletal or dental midline discrepancy which is defined as Yaw. It also produces different molar relations on both sides.

(These terms can be easily remembered as follows: the initials, i.e. PRY correspond to three planes in that order, i.e. TSV. TSV is also the order of planes used in AP system, and it is the sequence of planes, which depict the sequence of growth completion in different dimensions).

CLASSIFICATION OF MOLAR RELATIONSHIPS IN THE DECIDUOUS DENTITION

It was suggested by Baume in 1950s. The Angle's classification could not be applied to the deciduous dentition, as it was based on the relationship of permanent first molars only.

Reference point: The distal surfaces of upper and lower primary second molars are taken as the reference point. Following three relationships are determined based on this relation.

1. **Flush terminal plane:** When the distal surfaces of the maxillary and mandibular deciduous second molars are in the same line.
2. **Distal step:** The distal surface of mandibular second deciduous molar is distal to that of maxillary second deciduous molar.
3. **Mesial step:** The distal surface of mandibular second deciduous molar is mesial to that of maxillary second deciduous molar.

Classification for discriminating the class II by Moyer: Based on his cephalometric studies, Moyer in 1980s divided class II in six horizontal types and five vertical types as follows. However, they are not used much in the literature.

Horizontal Types

- **Type A:** Normal skeletal profile and normal anteroposterior position of the jaws. The dentition in the mandible is normally placed on its basal bone but the maxillary dentition is protracted.
- **Type B:** Displays midface prominence associated with mandible of normal length.
- **Type C:** The maxilla and the mandible are quite back in relation to the anterior cranial base. The lower incisors are tipped labially and the upper incisors are either upright or tipped labially.
- **Type D:** The mandible is smaller than normal. The midface is normal or diminished. The lower incisors are upright or tipped lingually and the upper incisors are tipped labially.
- **Type E:** There is a class II tendency even when the mid face is deficient and the mandible is normal. The dentition in both the arches are labially placed in comparison to their respective bases.
- **Type F:** It is a large heterogeneous group with mild skeletal class II tendencies.

Vertical Types

- **Type 1:** The anterior facial height is larger than the posterior facial height. The values of mandibular line, functional occlusal plane are somewhat more than normal and the palatal plane may be tipped downward while the anterior cranial base is upward. These cases are referred to as the long face type.
- **Type 2:** It is square face type. The mandibular line, functional occlusal plane and the palatal line are horizontal than normal. The gonial angle is less and the anterior cranial base is also horizontal. The incisors take a more vertical or upright position producing a skeletally imposed deep bite.
- **Type 3:** The palatal plane is tipped upwards anteriorly decreasing the anterior facial height predisposing to an open bite and if the mandibular line is steeper than normal then the open bite is worsened.
- **Type 4:** The mandibular line, functional occlusal plane and the palatal plane are tipped downwards and the gonial angle is obtuse. This malocclusion is associated with horizontal type B.
- **Type 5:** The mandibular line and the functional occlusal plane are placed normally but the palatal plane is tipped downward so there is a skeletal deep bite.

Conclusion

A classification helps in grouping of similar types of conditions in small groups. It helps in effective communication, discussion and treatment planning. A simple classification which is easy to understand and apply is the one which is most commonly followed by clinicians. However, a comprehensive system should be applied in routine practice so that it evaluates a condition in all the three planes of spaces, considering skeletal and dental nature and the growth pattern. It helps in determining the treatment plan and prognosis of the condition. Out of the many systems in literature, the Angle's system is the simplest one and is in use till today. The AP system is the most comprehensive system which evaluates the condition in all the three planes of the space and provides dynamic information of the condition.

Further Readings

1. Andrews. Six keys to normal Occlusion. Am J Orthod and Dento Orthop. 1972 p 296-309
2. Graber TM. Orthodontics Principle and Practice. WB Saunders. 1988. p 60-64
3. Moyer ME. Handbook of Orthodontics. St Louis. C V Mosby.1986.p 184-194
4. Proffit WR. Contemporary Orthodontics, St Louis.4ed. C V Mosby, 2007 p 215-230
5. Salzmann JA. Practice of Orthodontics, JB Lippincoat Company. 1966 p 416-423
6. Wheelers. Dental Anatomy, Physiology and Occlusion. 7ed. P 241-258, 274-280

11

Etiology of Malocclusion

INTRODUCTION

Etiology of malocclusion is the study of factors leading to creation of that condition. A malocclusion can occur due to a number of causes. Since the orthodontics deals with the treatment of malocclusion, it is very important to know the causes, so that "removal of causes" philosophy can be applied for the treatment. It can be helpful especially for the prevention and interception of the developing condition, by removing the cause and thus reducing the severity. Malocclusion is generally considered a developmental condition and has multifactorial etiology. Most of the time, it is not caused by a pathologic process but by moderate distortions in normal development. It may be caused by a single specific cause or by complex interactions among multiple factors influencing the growth and development which then result in malocclusion.

To simplify the study of the causes, various factors have been described and classified in various classification systems like:

- White and Gardiner's classification
- Salzmann's classification
- Moyer's classification
- Graber's classification.

Salzmann's Classification

He categorized the factors of etiology in following five categories which are interdependent (CDEFG):

1. Congenital
2. Developmental
3. Environmental
4. Functional
5. Genetics.

The etiology of malocclusion is infinitely complex. Dental and facial deformities may be the result of many etiological factors, such as hereditary factors, environmental factors, nutritional factors, endocrine dysfunction, premature loss or prolonged retention of deciduous teeth, malformed or supernumerary teeth, loss of permanent teeth, pathological entities, as well as abnormal pressure habits, all of which may function singly or be superimposed upon each other.

Although, many systems of classifications have been proposed, it is the Graber's classification which is simple to learn and apply in practice. Graber has broadly classified the causes under two categories: (1) general and (2) local factors.

General factors are those factors which affect the body as a whole, and whole or part of dentofacial complex.

Local factors are those factors which have a localized effect on the specific segment of developing dentition.

Heredity and environment are two very important active factors in the etiology of malocclusion. Heredity means that there are some patterns handed on by our ancestors which cannot he changed thereafter.

Galton's law of bisexual heredity quotes the mathematical proportion that can be inherited from our forefathers.

- One-half is derived from the parents
- One-fourth is derived from the grandparents
- One-eighth is derived from the great-grandparents

- One-sixteenth is derived from the great-great-grandparents, etc.

After heredity factors which cannot be changed, there are other environmental or acquired factors which influence the development to great extent.

General Factors

Various factors are:

1. Heredity
2. Congenital
3. Environmental:
   a. Prenatal: Trauma, maternal diet, German measles, maternal metabolism, smoking, alcohol intake, etc.
   b. Postnatal: Birth injury, cerebral palsy, TMJ injury, etc.
4. Predisposing metabolic, climate and infectious diseases, like endocrine imbalances; metabolic disturbances; infectious diseases.
5. Abnormal pressure habits and functional aberrations, like:
   - Abnormal sucking
   - Thumb and finger sucking
   - Tongue thrust and tongue sucking
   - Lip and nail biting
   - Abnormal swallowing habit, improper deglutition
   - Speech defects
   - Respiratory abnormalities: Mouth breathing, OSAS, etc.
   - Tonsils and adenoids
   - Psychogenetics and bruxism.
6. Dietary problems: Nutritional deficiency
7. Posture
8. Trauma and accidents.

Local Factors

1. Anomalies of tooth size: Macrodontia, microdontia
2. Anomalies of tooth shape: Malformed teeth, e.g. peg lateral, etc.
3. Anomalies in number of teeth: Supernumerary teeth, hypodontia/oligodontia, etc.
4. Abnormal labial frenum: Mucosal barrier during eruption
5. Premature loss of deciduous teeth
6. Prolonged retention of deciduous teeth
7. Delayed eruption of permanent teeth
8. Abnormal/deflected eruptive pathway
9. Impacted teeth
10. Ankylosis
11. Dental caries
12. Improper dental restorations.

General Factors

Heredity: It is one of the most important causes of malocclusions. Not only dentition, but all the tissues of body have a strong genetic influence, e.g. color of skin, hair, eyes, height, weight, facial features, intelligence, etc. These characteristics are controlled by multiple genes coming from both the parents. Conditions like clefts, diabetes, hypertension or hypotension, myopia, etc. have genetic links. Factors inherited can also get modified by various factors like prenatal and postnatal environment, hormones, abnormal habits, nutritional deficiencies, smoking and alcohol, etc. Racial and ethnic differences are all genetically-linked, e.g. Chinese and Japanese have different facial features than Africans and Caucasians, etc. Facial features, malocclusion types, growth pattern, tongue size, certain syndromes, etc. are genetically linked and are presented as either autosomal or sex-linked traits.

Heredity influence and specific dentofacial morphologic characteristics: Lundstorm in his study on twins concluded that heredity can determine the tooth size, shape and number, arch dimensions, like width and height of dental arch, height of palate, crowding and spacing of teeth, and the degree of overjet. There is probably a heredity influence on the position and conformation of perioral muscles to tongue size and shape, soft tissue peculiarities (characteristic and texture of mucosa, frenum size, shape and position).

Heredity racial influence: Dental characters, facial types, etc. show racial influences.

With the mixture of racial genes with genetic meltdown, the chances of occurrence of jaw size discrepancies and occlusal disharmonies are more. Studies also suggest a dominance of skeletal deficiency over the skeletal excess has been found due to racial mixtures, e.g. more of class II with mandibular deficiency, rather than class III with excessive mandibular growth is seen during the evolution of man. Thus, the jaw size seems to be reducing with evolution and so there is an increased frequency of third molar impaction, congenital absence of certain teeth and retrognathic tendency of mandible.

Hapsburg jaw: It was a characteristic trait of a European German royal family, where the generations had a large mandibular size leading to skeletal class III condition.

Hereditary facial types: Different ethnic groups have different shapes of the face and head. Hasund and Swersten has pointed out the sex-linked nature of facial width and dental arch shape. Mongoloids have a different facial pattern than Africans and Americans.

Achondroplasia: Here, there is early fusion of cranial synchondroses, epiphysis and metaphysic, and thus a lack of primary cartilageonous growth. Thus, the growth of cranial base and the limbs do not increase. There is maxillary growth deficiency leading to maxillary hypoplasia and a normal/big mandible. It leads to skeletal class III problem.

Congenital factors: These malformations are present at the time of birth, and they can be acquired or hereditary in nature. Hereditary conditions may not be present at the time of birth but may appear at any stage of life. Most common congenital condition of body is club foot, while that of face is cleft lip and palate. Congenital conditions can be due to a number of factors like genetic, endocrine, infections, chemicals and mechanical factors. They can be divided as general and local congenital abnormalities.

General factors causing congenital problems:

- Abnormal health of mother during pregnancy
- Malnutrition
- Endocrinal problems
- Infections, e.g. Rubella, Syphilis,
- Metabolic and nutritional disturbances
- Accidents during pregnancy and child birth
- Intrauterine pressures and posture
- Fetal trauma due to accidents
- Large size of cranium due to CSF collection, i.e. hydrocephalous.

Local factors leading to congenital conditions:

- Abnormal jaw development due to IU pressure
- Clefts
- Macro/microglossia
- Cleidocranial dystosis
- Maternal rubella infections.

Certain congenital conditions are:

Clefts of lip, palate and face: CLP are the most common congenital conditions of the face, with an incidence of 1: 700 live births on an average, with different incidence in different races. It generally occurs due to improper fusion of various embryonic processes of face in first trimester of the IU life. It may occur due to multiple factors like genetic influence, infections, smoking and alcohol, various drugs, etc.

Micrognathism (small jaw): Congenital variety is usually seen with congenital heart disease and Pierre-Robin anomalad. PR anomalad is a triad of mandibular micrognathia, cleft palate and glossoptosis. Micrognathia of maxilla is due to deficiency in the premaxilla.

Pierre Robin syndrome: Fetal malposition and interposition of tongue between the palatal shelves is probable etiology. Severe micrognathia and mandibular hypoplasia; U-shaped cleft palate and glossoptosis are important features.

Oligodontia: It is the lesser number of teeth than the normal complement due to congenital absence of certain teeth. It is also called as hypodontia or partial anodontia. The commonly missing teeth being the third molars, mandibular second premolar, maxillary lateral incisros, maxillary second premolars in that order. Butler's field theory has explained this pattern on the basis that human dentition has four fields: (1) molars, (2) premolar, (3) canine and (4) incisors. The teeth most distal in the field are most commonly missing. Canines are the least missing teeth. However, an exception is generally seen in mandibular incisor region where the central incisor is found missing more than the lateral incisor. Anodontia can be total or partial. Total anodontia is a very rare condition.

Maternal rubella infections: It is also known as German measles. It causes various congenital malformations. The crucial age is first trimester of IU life, during which the cell multiplication and differentiation is going on rapidly. It may lead to malformation of tissues and organs, and may cause dental hypoplasia, retarded eruption of teeth, and extensive caries.

Congenital syphilis: It leads to enamel hypoplasia especially of permanent first molars (mulberry molars).

Cerebral palsy: There is absence of muscular coordination and thus aberrant muscle activity resulting in malocclusion.

Pfeiffer syndrome: There is craniosynostosis, leading to maxillary hypoplasia and thus skeletal class III relation.

Other syndromes, e.g. Crouzon, Down syndrome, Pierre Robin anomalad, CLP, achondroplasia, hyperpituitarism, hormonal imbalance, etc. also lead to malformation of the dentoskeletal tissues.

Genetic Abnormalities

There are certain conditions which also have dental manifestations.

Cherubism: It occurs as an autosomal dominant disorder and with 100% penetrance in males and 50–75% penetrance in females, with 2:1 male predominance. There is a marked fullness of the jaws. Ectopic eruption, severe malocclusion is seen. Permanent teeth may be found missing or malformed as the developing tooth follicles are displaced.

Osteogenesis imperfecta: It occurs due to a quantitative defect in production of type I collagen which leads to fragility of bones. OI is the probably the most common inherited bone disease. It may/not be associated with dentinogenesis imperfecta. It is of following types:

- **OI type I:** Autosomal dominant, most common.
- **OI type II:** Autosomal recessive, most severe.
- **OI type III:** Both AD and AR.
- **OI type IV:** AD.

Clinical features: Classically, this condition includes fragile bones, blue sclerae, ligamentous laxity, hearing loss and dentinogenesis imperfecta. Primary teeth are more severely affected than permanent teeth. Crowns are described as shortened and bell shaped with cervical constriction.

Cleidocranial dysplasia: It is inherited as AD with high penetrance with wide variability in expression. A gene for this disorder has been mapped to chromosome 6p21. There is maxillary hypoplasia giving a relatively mandibular prognathic appearance. Midface deficiency and straight/concave profile is seen. Palate is narrow and high arched. There is increased incidence of submucosal clefts and complete or partial clefts of the palate involving the hard and soft tissues. Nonunion of symphysis of mandible and unerupted multiple supernumerary teeth are other features.

Crouzon's syndrome (craniofacial dysostosis): It is an AD disorder with complete penetrance and variable expressivity. Mutation in the fibroblast growth factor receptor 2 (FGFR2) gene which maps to chromosome 10q25-q26, causes this syndrome. Shallow orbits are the most common feature. Frog-like facies, midface hypoplasia and exopthalmos are striking features. Mandibular prognathism with nose resembling parrot's beak, maxillary hypoplasia, high arched palate, bilateral posterior lingual crossbites due to anrrow upper arch, and anterior open bite are the dental features.

Treacher Collins syndrome (mandibulofacial dysostosis): It is an AD disorder with high degree of penetrance but variable expressivity. Mutation in a gene of unknown function referred to as treacle which maps for 5q32–33.1 are responsible. Bird-like or fish-like facial appearance is characteristic. It includes various degrees of hypoplasia many bones, like mandible, maxilla, zygomatic process of temporal bone, external and middle ear. Oral findings include cleft palate, macrostomia, high-arched palate, dental malocclusion, apertognathia and widely separated and displaced teeth. The peculiar broad and concave nature of the inferior border of the mandible is characteristic.

Down syndrome (trisomy 21): It is found in 1 in 600–700 live births. Most cases of trisomy 21 are caused by nondysjunction, resulting in an extrachromosome. Skull is brachycephalic with flat occiput and prominent forehead. Frontal, sphenoid sinuses are absent and maxillary sinus is hypoplastic. Fissured tongue, macroglossia leading to open bite, excessive salivation, open mouth posture, decreased palatal width and length, bifid uvula, cleft lip and palate are main clinical features. There is delayed eruption of teeth, hypodontia, microdontia, crown root malformations are seen. Occlusal disharmonies, posterior crossbites, apertognathia, severe anterior teeth crowding are main malocclusion features.

Hemifacial atrophy: Progressive unilateral atrophy of the face, tongue, lips and salivary glands may show hemiatrophy. Developing teeth may show incomplete root development and delayed eruption.

Amelogenesis imperfecta: AI represents a group of hereditary defects of enamel unassociated with any other generalized defects.

Types:

- Hypoplastic—mainly AD.
- Hypocalcified—AD and AR.
- Hypomaturation—AD and AR.

Dentinogenesis imperfecta: The association between DI and OI is well recognized although each condition may occur independently

- **Type I:** AD generally. Both DI and OI present.
- **Type II:** Never occurs with OI. Autosomal dominant.
- **Type III:** Brandywine type. Same clinical appearance of teeth as types I and II but it may also show multiple pulp exposures in deciduous teeth.
- Growth of the jaws and the eruption pattern gets severely altered. However, the skeletal relation can be improved by distraction osteogenesis or orthognathic surgery after the growth is over. Based on careful diagnosis, the clinicians can plan the distraction device placement and the vectors of distraction.
- If there is disturbance in eruption, then guidance of eruption of teeth is planned to help the teeth to erupt in proper relationship and to reduce the future irregularity to a minimal. In case of developed malocclusion, the corrective orthodontic treatment is given. Abnormal tooth morphology is treated by using cast metal crowns on posterior teeth and jacket crowns on anterior teeth to prevent the fracturing of the enamel.

Environmental Causes

Prenatal Factors

- **Abnormal fetal posture:** It interferes with symmetric development of face. It is not directly associated with malocclusion but may be associated with abnormal pressure or imbalance. Most of the deformities are temporary and disappears with time with normal growth and development.

- **Maternal infections,** such as German measles and use of certain drugs during pregnancy, like phenytoin, thalidomide, excessive retinoic acid, etc., can cause congenital deformities, like cleft.
- **Smoking and alcohol intake** by expecting mother can lead to congenital deformities.
- **Environmental teratogens:** The term teratogen is referred to an environmental agent that causes congenital malformation. History of exposure to teratogenic drugs during the first trimester of intrauterine life of development could influence the incidence of cleft.

Ethyl alcohol: Fetal alcohol syndrome (FAS) is a pattern of mental and physical defects which develops in some babies when the mother drinks too much alcohol during pregnancy. Alcohol in a pregnant woman's bloodstream circulates to the fetus by crossing the placenta. There, the alcohol interferes with the ability of the fetus to receive sufficient oxygen and nourishment for normal cell development in the brain and other body organs.

Cigarette smoking: Maternal smoking increases the risk of orofacial cleft. Woman has approx a 30% increased risk of having a child with CLP and a 20% increased risk of having one with CP if she smokes during pregnancy. Cigarette smoking may act alone or synergistically with gene transforming growth factor (TGF).

Vitamin A: Severity of orofacial cleft is related to cell death in the first pharyngeal arch, induced by acute maternal exposure to 13-cis retinoic acid, a vitamin A analog during first trimester of human pregnancy (drug to treat cystic acne).

Folic acid deficiency: Folic acid deficiency is considered as the "universal teratogen" affecting virtually every organ and system in the body varying considerably. It causes neural tube defect. Shaw presented evidence that women above 35 years of age had a double risk of having a child with cleft lip and palate. Women above 39 years of age had a triple risk of having a child with cleft palate.

Postnatal Factors

Trauma: Forceps delivery can result in injury to the TMJ area of the infant, which can lead to ankylosis of TMJ. It leads to deficient mandibular growth and so a hypoplastic mandible. It is known as Vogel-Geischt, i.e. when during forceps delivery of a child, trauma occurs to his TMJ area, it may undergo ankylosis. Here, a severe class II skeletal relation is evident.

Predisposing Metabolic Climate and Disease

Endocrinal imbalance: Hormones have a very strong influence on the growth and development.

Hypopituitarism: It is due to a decrease in hormonal levels secreted by pituitary gland esp the growth hormone. The general growth of body is delayed, which also affects the craniofacial growth. The main features of malocclusion are delayed tooth eruption, incomplete root formation, smaller dental arch leading to malocclusion. There is retarded growth of supporting structures.

Hyperpituitarism: It is due to increased GH secretion, affecting whole body skeletal growth. Facial features include a long face, a large mandible because of excessive condylar growth leading to skeletal class III condition, strong and robust chin and gonial region, enlarged tongue, accelerated dental development; teeth tipped buccally/labially, etc.

Hypothyroidism: Growth retardation; delayed eruption of the teeth; maxillary protrusion; spacing; enlarged tongue.

Hyperthyroidism: Accelerated skeletal growth; irregular eruption of the teeth because of earlier shedding of deciduous and early eruption of permanent teeth, mild prognathism.

Hypoparathyroidism: Altered pattern of eruption; early exfoliation; enamel defects; sudden drifting; dentin dysplasia; partial anodontia.

Hyperparathyroidism: Demineralization; disappearance of lamina dura; mobility of teeth.

Metabolic Disturbances

Acute febrile diseases may also affect the dentition and its surrounding hard and soft tissue. If severity and duration is not prolonged the child is able to catch up and growth is possible.

Infectious diseases

- **Bacterial infection:**
  a. **Osteomyelitis:** Bone response to force is altered
  b. **Congenital syphilis:** It is vertically transmitted from the infected mother to the child. Main features are Hutchinson's molars, mulberry molars, enamel deficiency, extensive dental decay, small maxilla, anterior crossbite.

Viral infection:

- **Mumps:** Dental hypoplasia, retarded eruption, extensive caries, inflammation/congestion of gingiva
- **Measles:** Airway obstruction
- **Rubella:** Retarded eruption of teeth; congenital malformations, e.g. cleft lip and palate.

Nutritional deficiency: Nutritional deficiency during the periods of active growth may lead to deficient development, thus causing the malocclusion. Deficiency in protein and vitamin can lead to scurvy, beri beri, rickets, etc. leading to growth and dental development disturbances.

- **Protein deficiency:** Delayed eruption
- **Vitamin A deficiency:** Calcification of teeth is affected, retarded eruption
- **Vitamin B complex:** Cheilosis, retarded growth, pernicious anemia
- **Vitamin C deficiency:** Disturbed collagen fibers formation, bleeding gums, loosening of teeth
- **Vitamin D:** Disturbed calcification of teeth, poor quality of teeth, narrow maxillary arch, high palatal vault, under-developed mandible
- **Hypervitaminosis D:** Poorly calcified teeth, decalcification of bones, increased osteoclastic activity

Oral habits: Habit is defined as an "autonomic response to a situation acquired normally as the result of repetition and learning, strictly applicable only to motor responses" (Fig. 11.1). At each repetition, the act becomes less conscious and can lead to development of an unconscious habit. Abnormal habits lead to development of malocclusion as they apply abnormal pressures on the dentofacial tissues.

There are many abnormal pressure habits and functional aberrations affecting the development of dentofacial complex and dentition; e.g. thumb sucking, tongue thrust, lip and nail biting, abnormal swallowing habits, speech defects, respiratory abnormalities, tonsils and adenoids, pshychogenic habits and bruxism.

All these habits are functional aberrations and produce abnormal forces. These forces

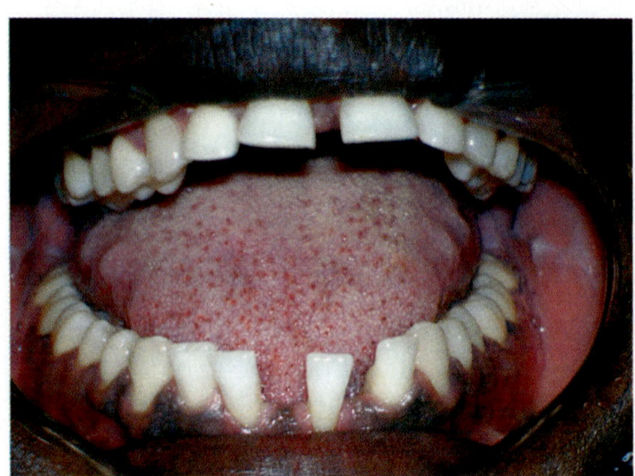

Fig. 11.1: Anterior spacing in arches due to anterior tongue thrust habit and large size of tongue.

can lead to development of deformity in the developing dentofacial unit. Severity of the deformity depends upon the trident of factors; i.e. intensity, duration and frequency of the habit. Habits have been dealt in details in separate section.

Posture: Poor posture may also lead to malocclusion. They lead to abnormal pressures on the tissues leading to abnormal development, e.g. children with abnormal sleep and sitting posture, children with scoliosis and kyphosis, patients on Milwaukee braces, have abnormal muscular pressures and imbalances.

Accidents and traumas: Injuries to dentoalveolar region may get unnoticed during the early years of life (Fig. 11.2). Trauma leads to nonvital teeth. The ankylosed teeth may lead to deflected path of eruption of other teeth. Injuries at condylar region may lead to ankylosis of TMJ and abnormal growth of the jaws.

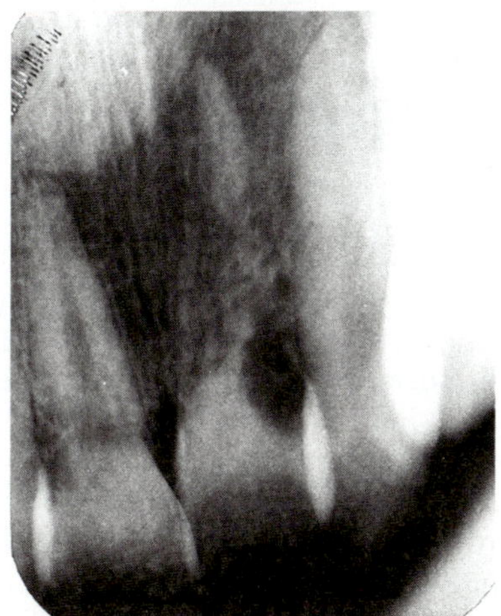

Fig. 11.2: Root resorption of incisor; has history of traumatic avulsion of tooth with reimplantation.

Local Factors

These are the factors which have their influence in localized area and lead to development of malposition of teeth. Various factors have been briefly described below.

1. **Anomalies of tooth size:** For a proper occlusal relationship of teeth, the sizes of upper and lower teeth should be proportional to each other. Bolton's analysis measures this proportion to find out the excessive tooth material which has to be adjusted by stripping or extraction to create a balance. Smaller or larger mesiodistal size of teeth leads to the development of malocclusion.
   a. **Microdontia** is the smaller size of the teeth. True generalized form of microdontia is rare. It is usually seen in pituitary dwarfism. Most common form of localized microdontia is maxillary lateral incisors called peg lateral. Smaller teeth lead to development of spaces in the arches.
   b. **Macrodontia** is larger size of the teeth. Also, there should be a balance in the total tooth material and the size of the jaw bases for proper alignment of the teeth. Larger sized teeth in normal dental arches lead to crowding.
2. **Anomalies of tooth shape** (Figs 11.3 to 11.8)**:** Abnormal shape of tooth or teeth leads to development of localized problems. It may be due to abnormal contours of teeth, e.g. peg laterals; or wider MD size of tooth at contact area and tapering towards the CEJ, leading to slippage of contacts. Abnormal size

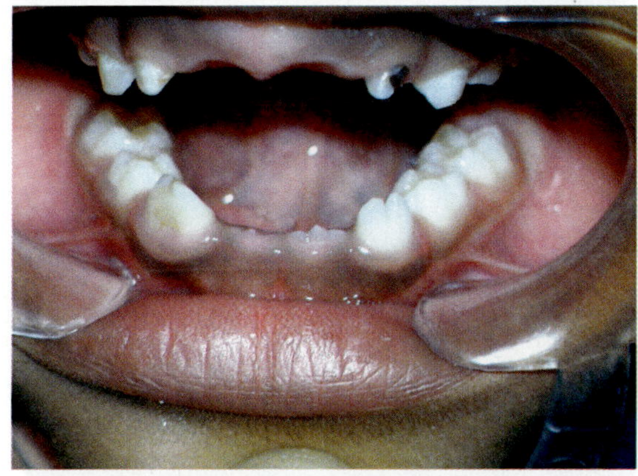

Fig. 11.3: Fused primary teeth on lower anterior segment. Absence of a primary tooth may also lead to absence of permanent tooth and deficient dentoalveolar growth.

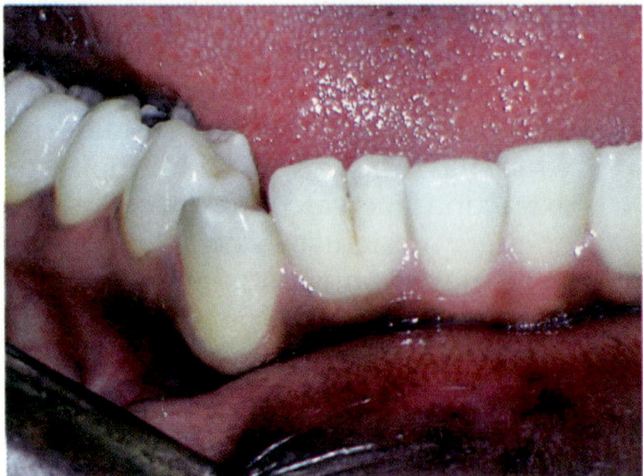

Fig. 11.4: A permanent lateral incisor which is oversized due to fusion of incisor with supernumerary tooth or oversized incisor with invagination, leading to bigger MD sized tooth, and thus creating space deficiency for erupting canine, which erupted labially out of the arch.

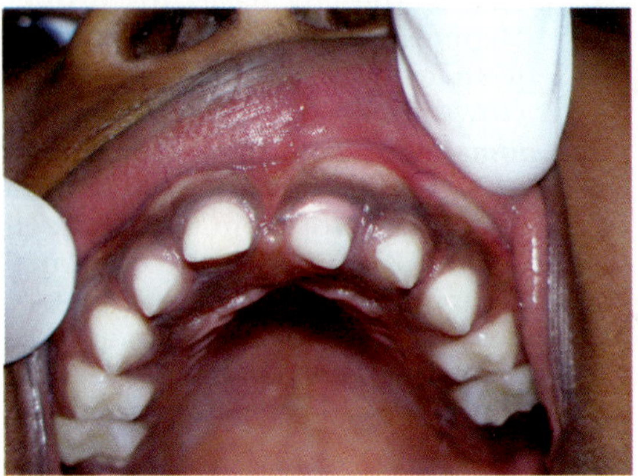

Fig. 11.5: Abnormal shape of primary upper central incisor.

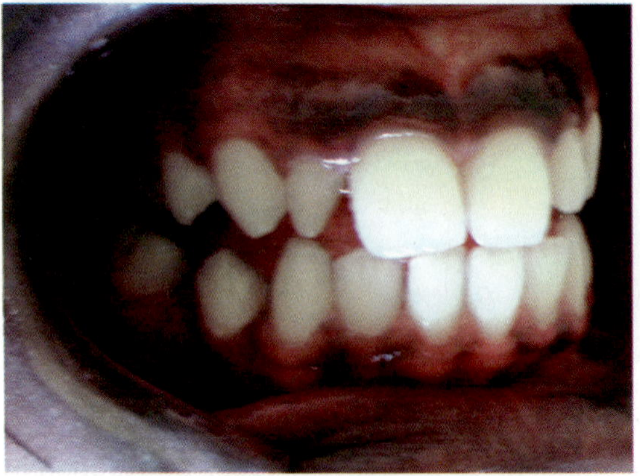

Fig. 11.6: Peg lateral incisor.

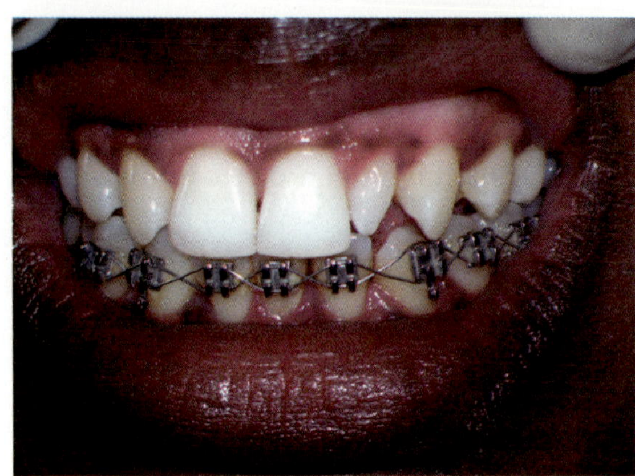

Fig. 11.7: Peg lateral on one side, and missing lateral incisor on other side.

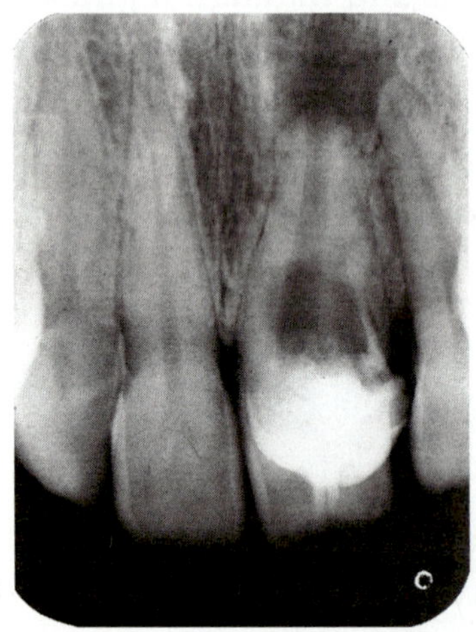

Fig. 11.8: Dental anomaly showing big MD width of central incisor, invagination, calcific mass / odontome on the tooth, root resorption, and associated periapical pathology.

may also develop due to fusion; gemination; twinning, etc. of the teeth. Fusion arises due to union of two normally separated tooth buds, it may lead to spacing, rotations, etc. Presence of Talon's cusps, extra-cusps on molars, etc. lead to improper relation of the teeth.

3. **Anomalies in number:** Increased or decreased number of teeth in the dental arches or jaws also leads to development of malocclusion:
   a. **Supernumerary teeth:** If teeth are more than normal complement of

teeth, they are called as supernumerary teeth. Most common supernumerary teeth are mesiodens, i.e. they are present in the midline between maxillary central incisors. They may be erupted or impacted; and may closely resemble the teeth of the group they belong to or may bear no resemblance. They generally lead to deflected path of eruption of teeth; non-eruption of adjacent teeth by blocking the path and space; delayed eruption of teeth; crowding; diastema, etc.

b. **Supplemental teeth** (Figs 11.9 to 11.18): Teeth that resemble closely to a particular group of teeth and erupt close to original site of these teeth.

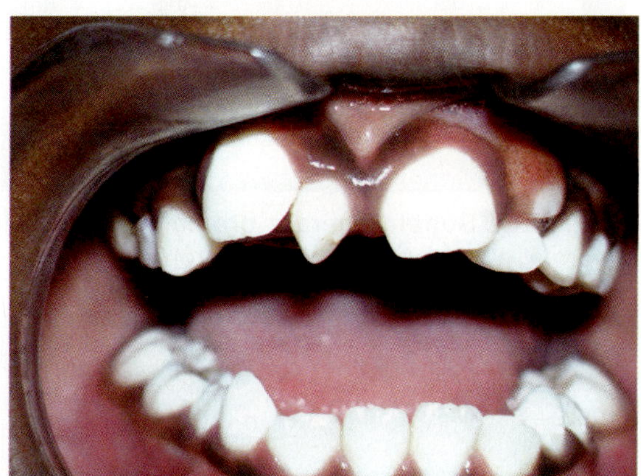

Fig. 11.9: Mesiodens leading to malocclusion in upper incisal region.

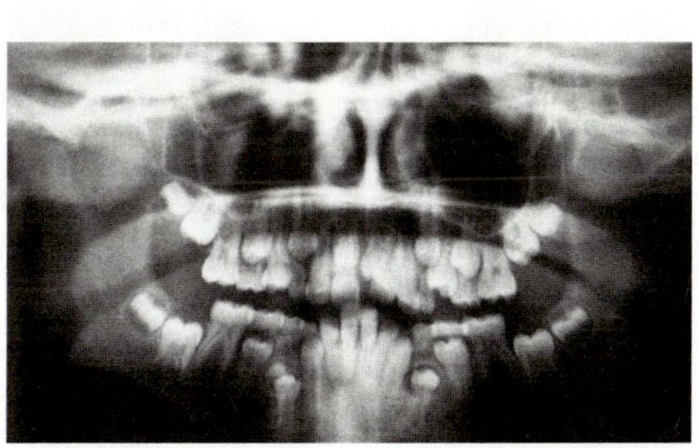

Fig. 11.10: OPG showing mesiodens leading to malocclusion in upper incisal region leading to deflection of central incisor.

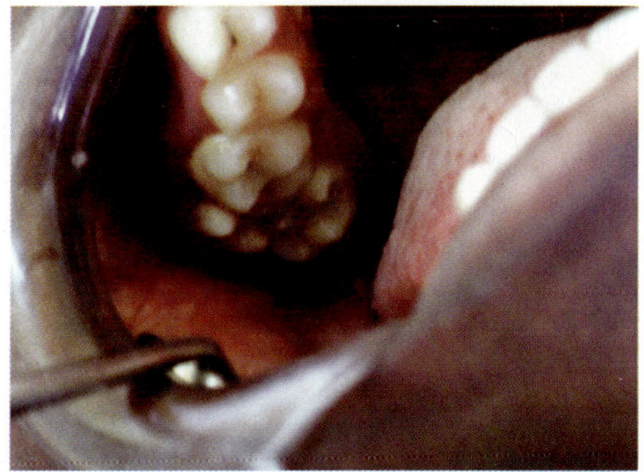

Fig. 11.11: A peg-shaped, small paramolar in second molar region leading to disturbed occlusion and gingival problems.

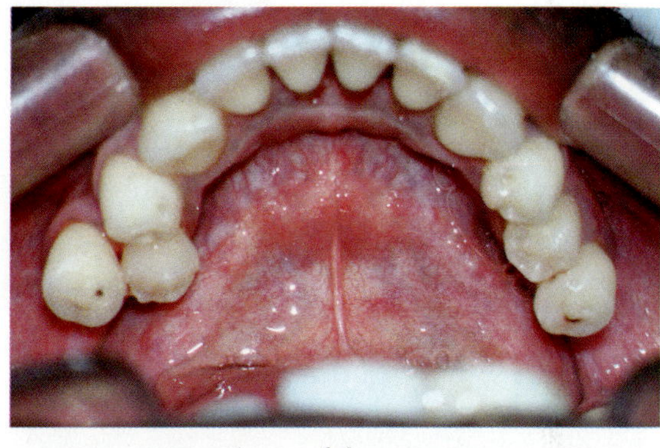

(a)

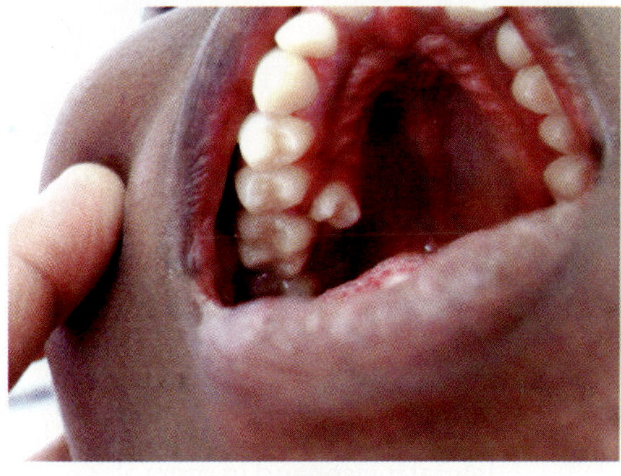

(b)

Figs 11.12a and b: Supernumerary premolar erupted lingually.

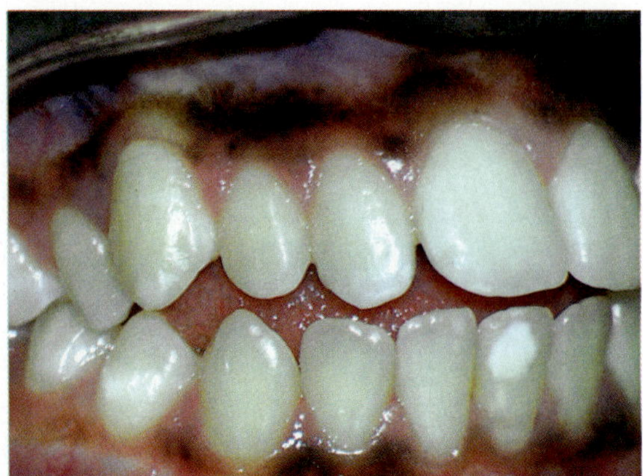

Fig. 11.13: Supernumerary lateral incisor in upper arch.

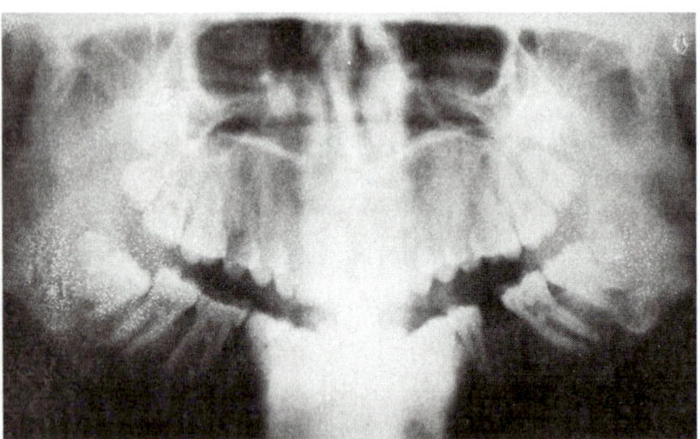

Fig. 11.14: Distomolar in each segment.

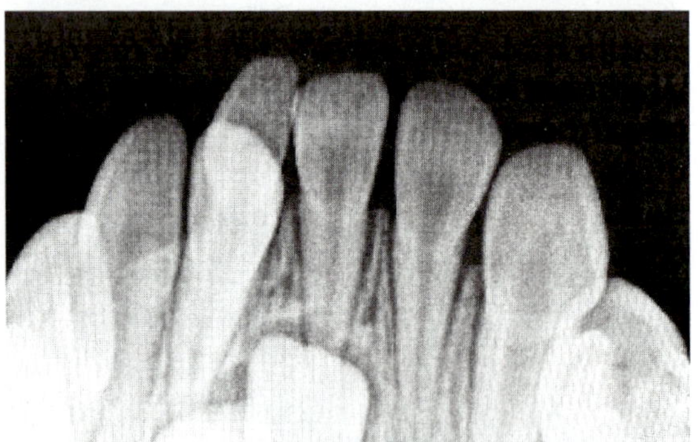

Fig. 11.15: Supernumerary primary incisor.

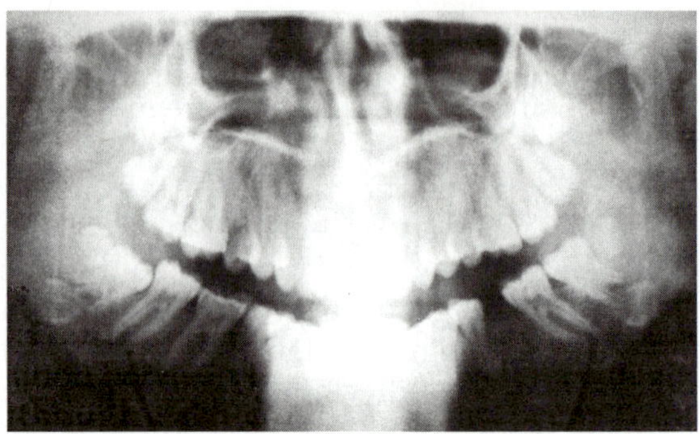

Fig. 11.16: OPG showing one distomolar in each quadrant of the jaws.

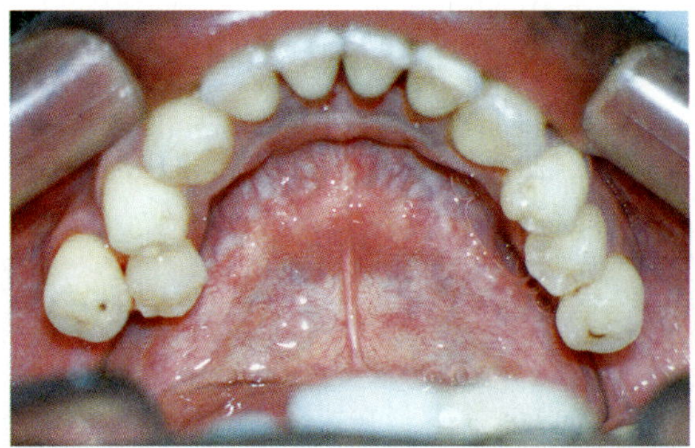

Fig. 11.17: Supernumerary premolar leading to abnormal alignment and gingival problems.

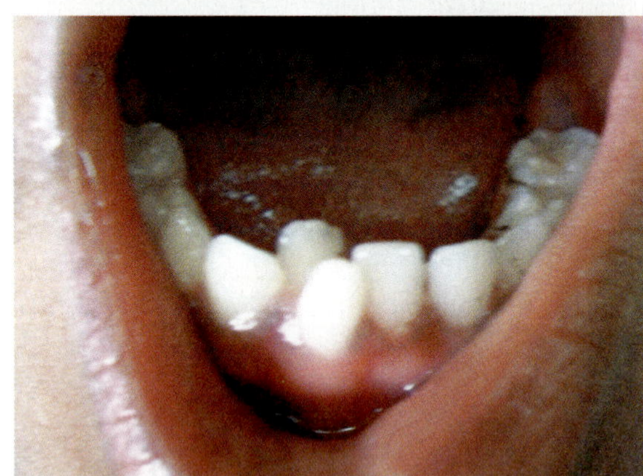

Fig. 11.18: Supernumerary primary incisor leading to crowding in deciduous dentition.

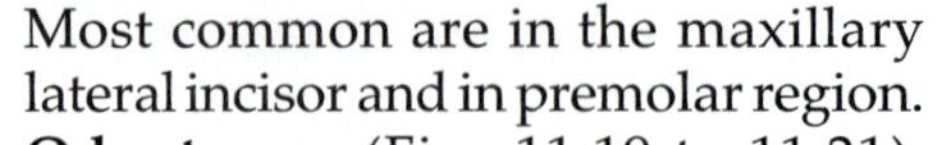

Most common are in the maxillary lateral incisor and in premolar region.

c. **Odontomes** (Figs 11.19 to 11.21): They are also the extra teeth or teeth-like structures in the jaws which do not bear a close resemblance to the normal anatomy of any type of teeth. They block the space or may lead to deflected eruption or impaction of adjacent teeth.

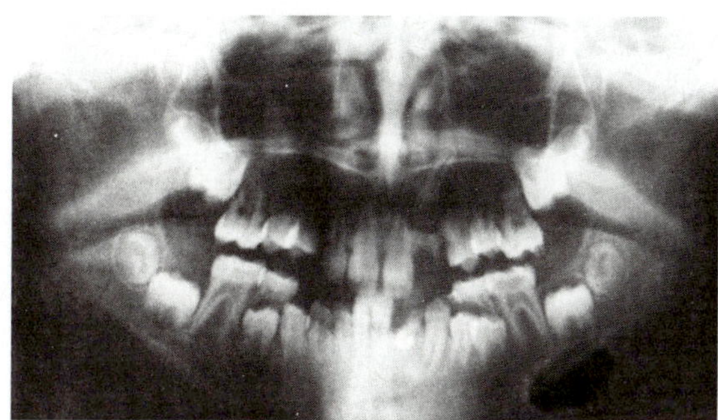

Fig. 11.19: Odontome-like structure on one side of lower jaw in anterior region leads to blocked eruption of teeth in that area.

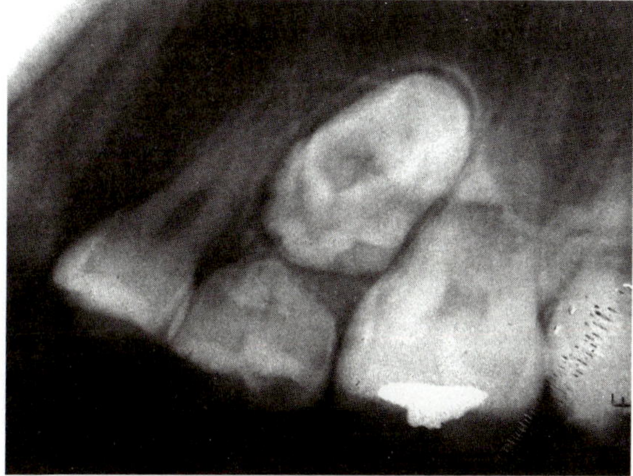

Fig. 11.20: Complex odontome-like structure in premolar region which has to be removed surgically.

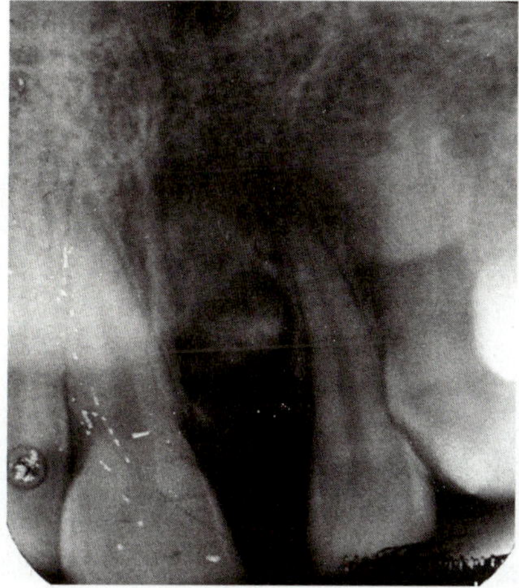

Fig. 11.21: An odontome-like structure in the midline in upper jaw and absence of corresponding central incisor.

d. **Missing teeth** (Figs 11.22 to 11.29a and b): It is a more common condition than supernumerary teeth. Absence of teeth may be classified as partial anodontia and complete/total anodontia. Partial anodontia/oligodontia/hypodontia is a condition of absence of some teeth (except 3rd molars). It is also seen in some syndromes, e.g. hypohydrotic ectodermal dysplasia. Complete/total anodontia is the absence of all teeth, which is a very rare condition. This condition leads to spacing between the teeth; masticatory and esthetic problems, aberrant speech and swallowing patterns. Adjacent teeth tend to shift in the space, which may lead to abnormal axial inclination of adjacent teeth. Unsightly appearance of the spaces generally leads the patient to come for treatment.

e. **Transposition of teeth** (Figs 11.30 to 11.33a and b): It is defined as the interchanged position of erupted tooth with another tooth in the same quadrant, leading to a change in natural sequence of permanent teeth. It can be complete and incomplete. Complete transposition means when the crown and root of transposed tooth completely shift in new location, i.e. tooth bodily shifts in its new

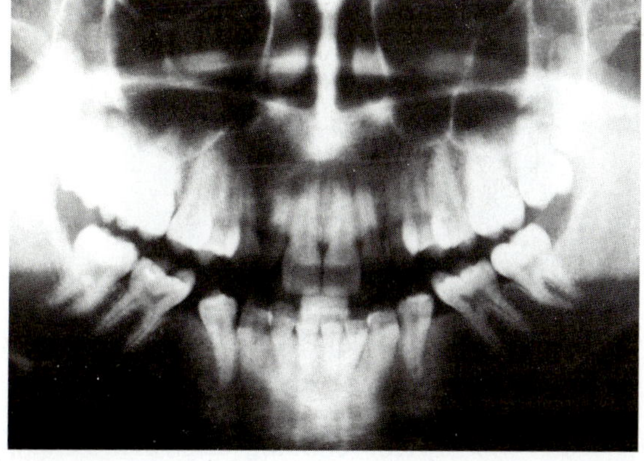

Fig. 11.22: Absence or extraction of lower second premolar leading to mesial tilting of lower molars.

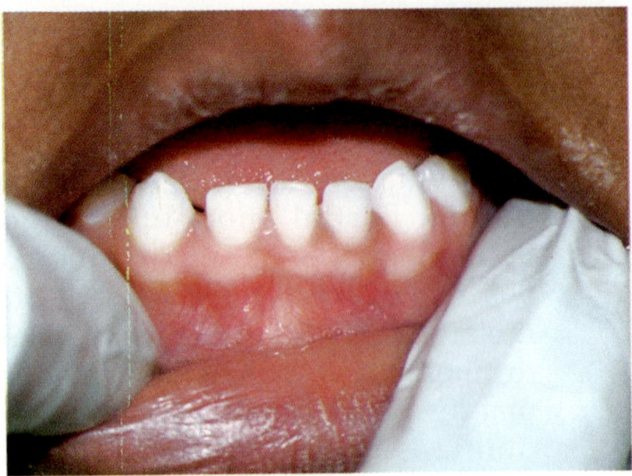

Fig. 11.23: Lower primary incisal region showing fused incisor, which may further lead to absence of permanent incisor and thus malocclusion in future.

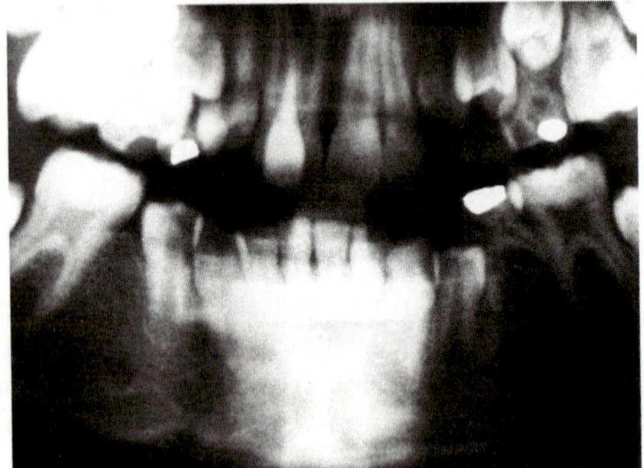

Fig. 11.24: Congenital absence of lower second premolars, with premature loss of primary second molar, and complete loss of space on one side.

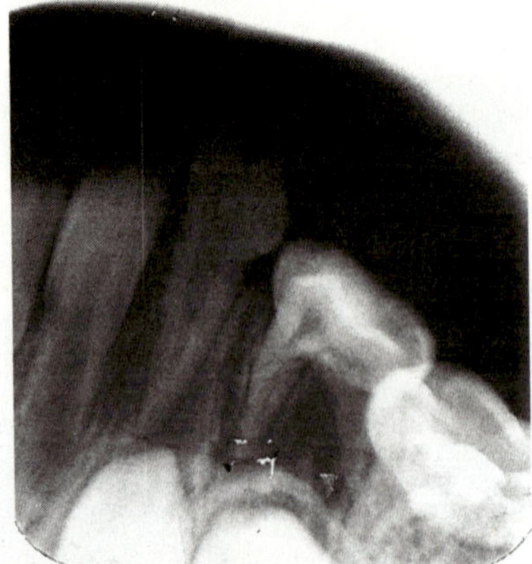

Fig. 11.25: Primary tooth showing fusion of two teeth, and thus absence of a primary and its permanent counterpart.

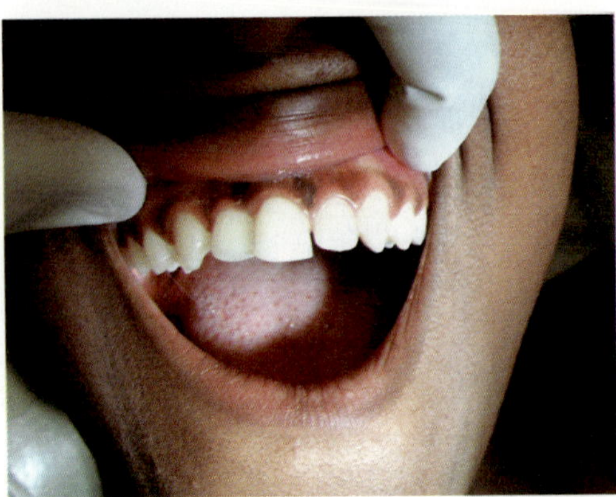

Fig. 11.26: Lateral incisor and canine migrated mesially after the loss of central incisor and non-maintenance of the space.

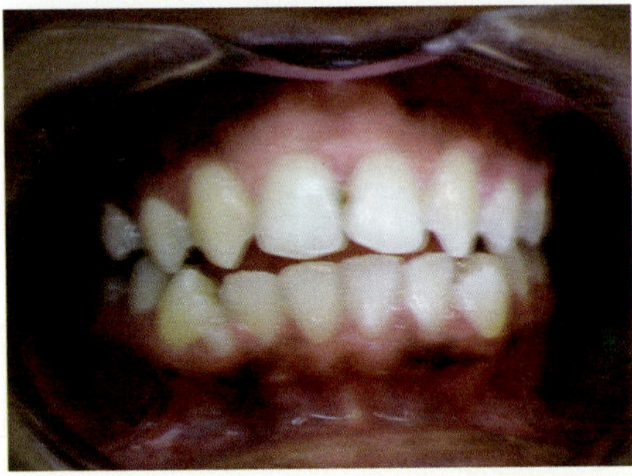

Fig. 11.27: Congenital absence of upper lateral incisors and mesial migration of both canines.

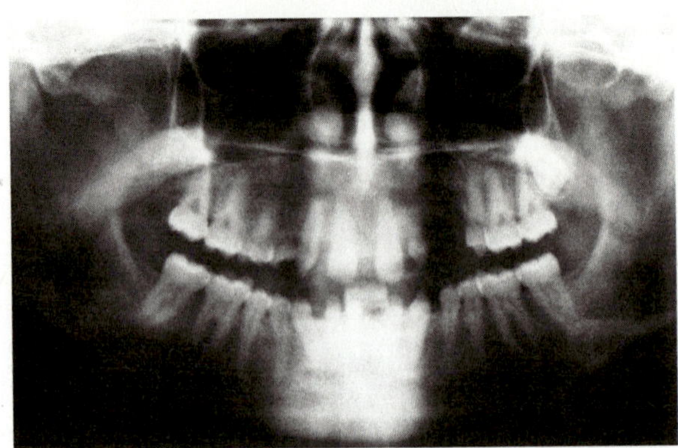

Fig. 11.28: OPG showing partial anodontia, leading to spacing and malocclusion. Generally, in partial anodontia, the MD width of teeth is also reduced.

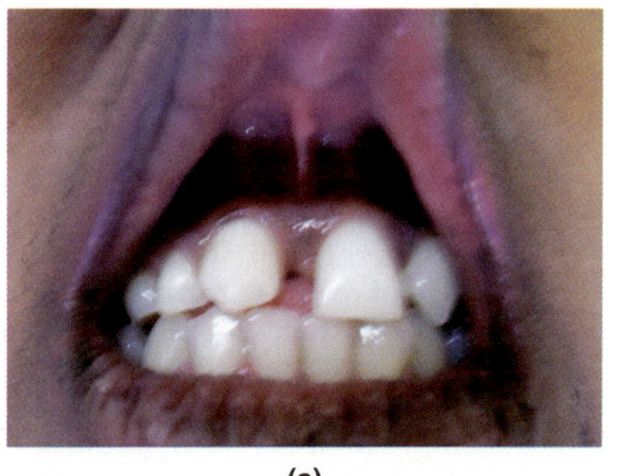

(a)

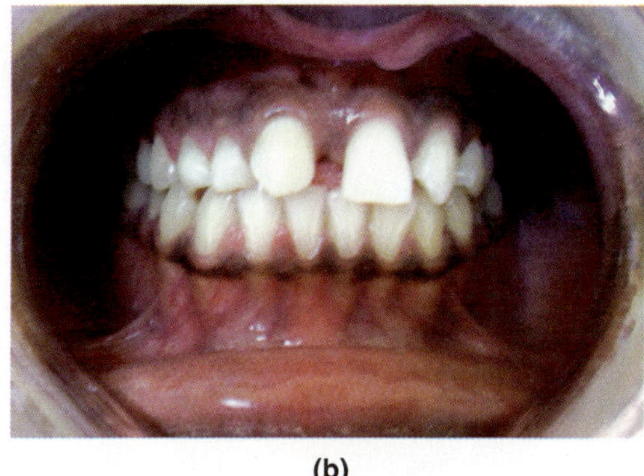

(b)

Figs 11.29a and b: Transposed upper canine due to absent central and lateral incisors on one side, and retained primary teeth.

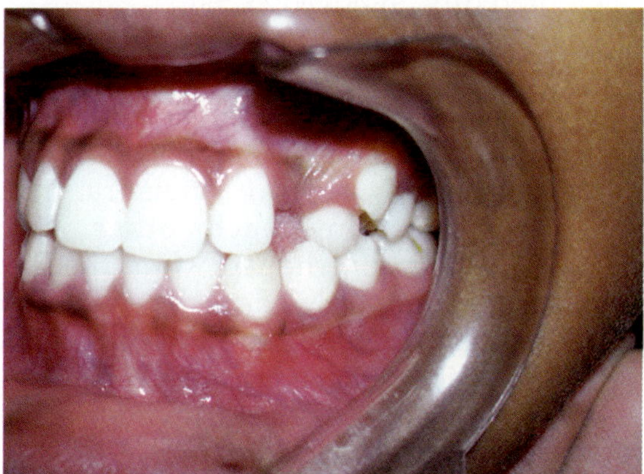

Fig. 11.30: Transposition of maxillary canine between two premolars and associated gingival problems.

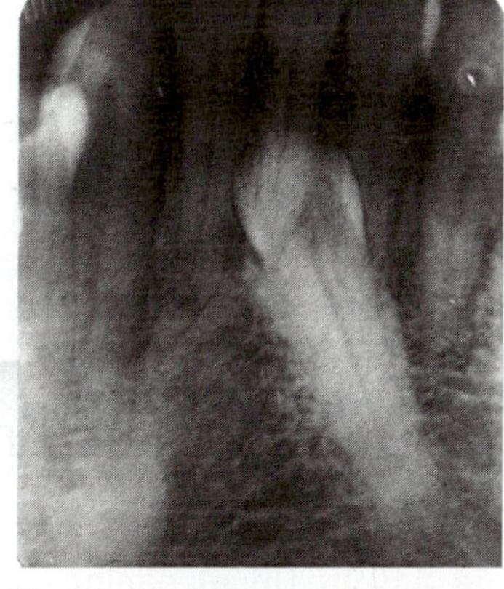

Fig. 11.31: Impacted and transposed mandibular canine as seen in IOPA view.

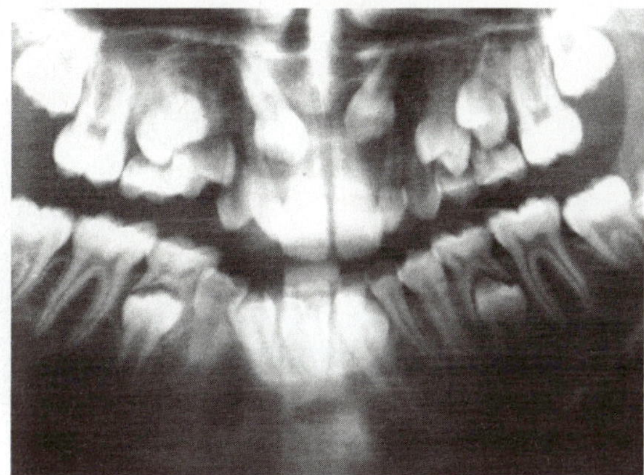

Fig. 11.32: Upper canines transposed between incisors

location. In incomplete transposition, the crown shifts while root remains in its original position. It may occur unilaterally or bilaterally. It is more common in maxilla than mandible. Left side is involved more than the right side, and is more common in females. Other dental anomalies like peg lateral, missing lateral incisors, retention of deciduous canines and/ or lateral incisors, malpositioned teeth, etc. are also seen with transposition. It can be divided into six main types, as related to their distribution as:

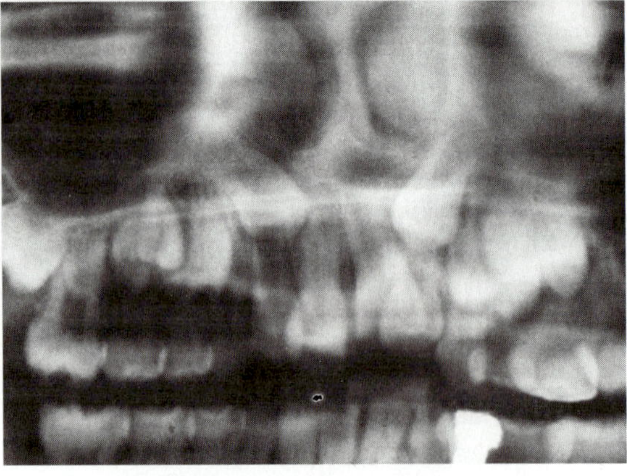

(a)

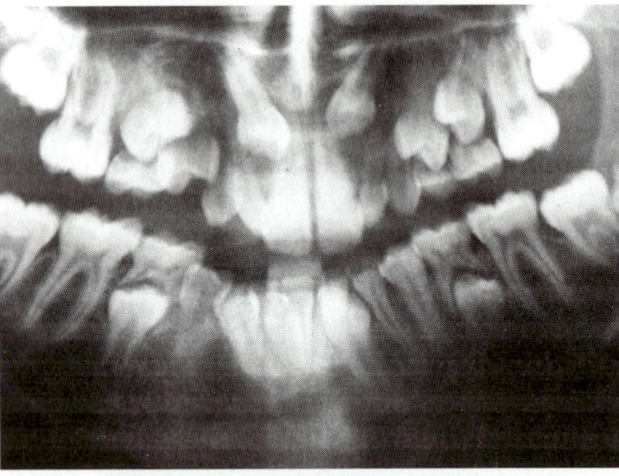

(b)

Figs 11.33a and b: Upper canines transposed between central and lateral incisors.

- Canine–first premolar (71%)
- Canine–lateral incisor (20%)
- Canine to first molar site (4%)
- Lateral incisor–central incisor (3%)
- Canine to central incisor site (2%).
- Mandibular lateral incisor to canine sites.

Causative factors include genetics; interchange in the position of tooth buds; trauma, mechanical interferences; and early loss of adjacent primary tooth. Mostly, the maxillary canine has been found to be associated with transposition. The guidance theory for canine eruption and long path of eruption of canine is also a possibility, since the canine develops high in the maxilla with a long path of eruption. Canines are also seen as transmigrated, i.e. they cross the midline partially or completely.

4. **Size of the jaw base** (Fig. 11.34): Imbalance between size of jaw bases and the tooth material also leads to development of malocclusion. If the MD size of teeth is normal, but the size of one or both jaw bases is smaller, it leads to development of crowding. If jaw bases are bigger, then it leads to spacing. However, with evolutionary trends, generally jaws are smaller in size leading to crowding. Bigger jaw size may be found to be associated with large tongue size, hormonal problem, heredity, syndromes, etc.
5. **Abnormal labial frenum** (Figs 11.35 to 11.37): A heavy fibrous frenum found attached to interdental papilla leads to midline diastema, as it prevents the two maxillary central incisors from approximating each other. It is generally fan-shaped when the lip is pulled outward. It does not contain any muscle fibers. Before the eruption of teeth, it is attached to the alveolar ridge with some fibres attached to the incisive papilla. Normally, it shifts sufficiently apically to the attached gingiva with the eruption of teeth and

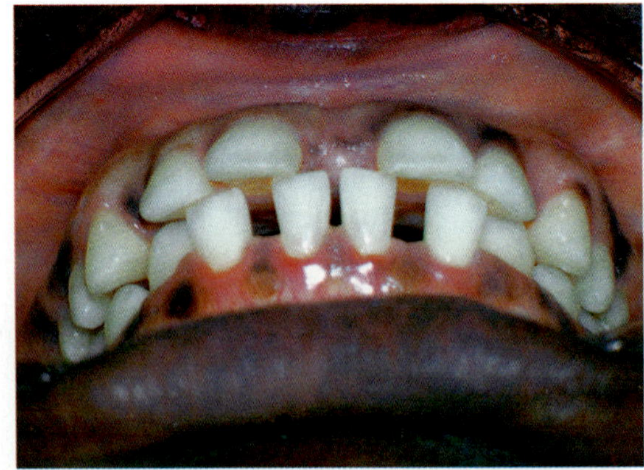

Fig. 11.34: Extreme spacing in anterior segments of arches. It occurs due to small MD size of teeth and/ or bigger skeletal bases of jaws, and in some cases, due to tongue-thrusting habits.

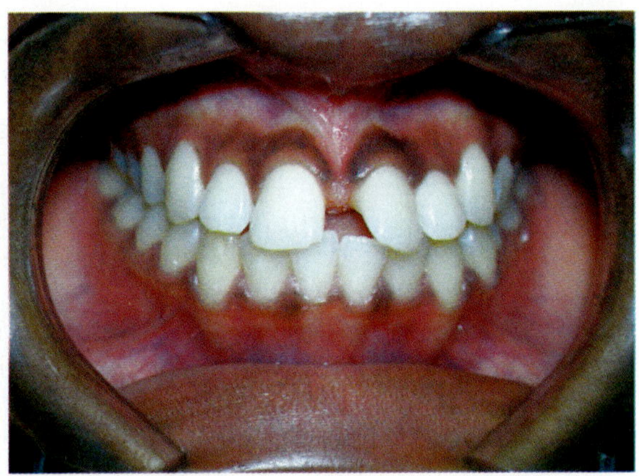

Fig. 11.35: Midline diastema and rotated incisor due to abnormal attachment of maxillary labial frenum.

alveolar growth. Normally, the frenum has migrated sufficiently superiorly by 10–12 years of age. If it does not move, it may cause midline diastema. It is diagnosed by blanch test.

The other causes of midline diastema are mesiodens, tongue thrust or thumb, sucking habits, small size of the teeth, e.g. peg laterals, midline cysts, periodontal disease, etc. and ugly-duckling stage.

Diagnosis: Blanch test is done to determine the attachment of frenum. The lip is pulled superiorly and anteriorly; any blanching in the incisive area of palate indicates fibers of frenum crossing the alveolar ridge. An IOPA X-ray film may show notching in the interdental alveolar ridge region.

Treatment: Closure of midline diastema should not be attempted till the eruption of maxillary canines, as sometimes it may automatically close. But if it does not close, then the space should be closed first orthodontically; and then surgical/Wanton's clipping of the frenum should be done. If surgery is done before space closure, the scar tissue may not allow space closure and leads to relapse. After space closure, the surgical removal of frenum leads to scar formation which helps in keeping the space closure by traction of scar firbres. However, if the midline diastema is more than 2–3 mm, it will not close spontaneously, and then the other causes of diastema should be explored and removed. Partial closure of midline diastema needs to be done if space is more. A permanent sturdy fixed retainer should be fixed for retention purpose after closure of diastema. It may also need supplementation by a labially fixed retainer at 1-1 in some cases.

6. **Premature loss of deciduous teeth** (Figs 11.38 to 11.49): It is an early loss of a primary tooth before the successor tooth has sufficiently advanced in its eruption status. If space is not maintained, then it can lead to decrease in total arch length due to space loss by migration of adjacent teeth in the space, leading to ectopic eruption; impaction of teeth; crowding; midline-shift. It is especially true for the posterior region, where space loss is faster, due to mesial direction of eruption of teeth, and anterior component of masticatory forces. It can also lead to delayed eruption of permanent teeth, because the alveolar bone and the overlying soft tissue becomes thickened, which takes more time to resorb during eruption of permanent teeth. Early loss of primary incisors does not lead to space loss due to natural presence of the physiological spaces, but it may delay eruption of permanent tooth. It occurs due to the thickening of bone and mucosal tissue in that area, and the eruption force may not be sufficient to pass that barrier at a normal pace. In such cases, we need to surgically incise the mucosa or bone to facilitate the eruption by removal of the barriers.
7. **Prolonged retention of deciduous teeth** (Figs 11.50 to 11.55): Primary teeth should get exfoliated just before the eruption of the successor tooth to provide space for them in the dental arch. However, sometimes some of the

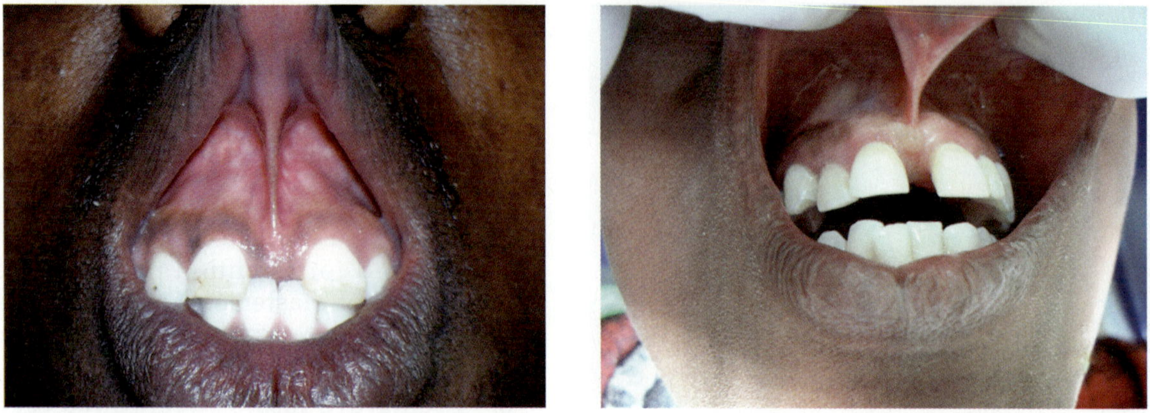

(a) (c)

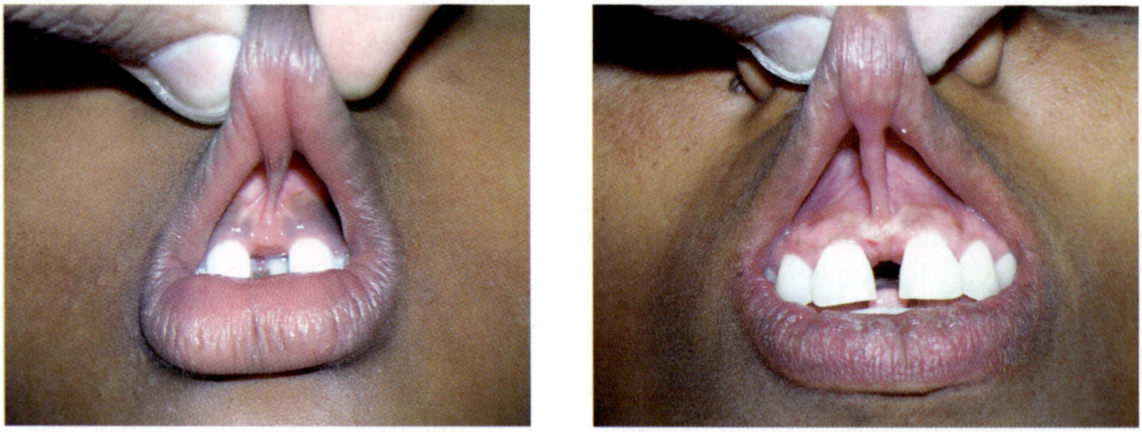

(b) (d)

Figs 11.36 a to d: Low attachment of maxillary frenum, and thick frenum lead to midline diastema. It is more common in African population.

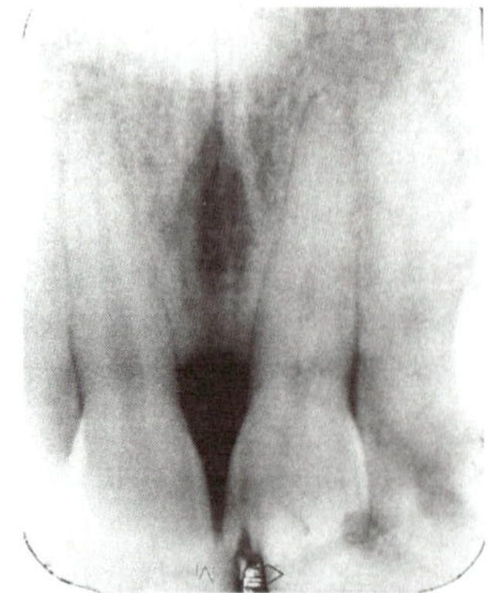

Fig. 11.37: IOPA view showing notching of the alveolar crest in upper central incisor region due to abnormal attachment of frenum.

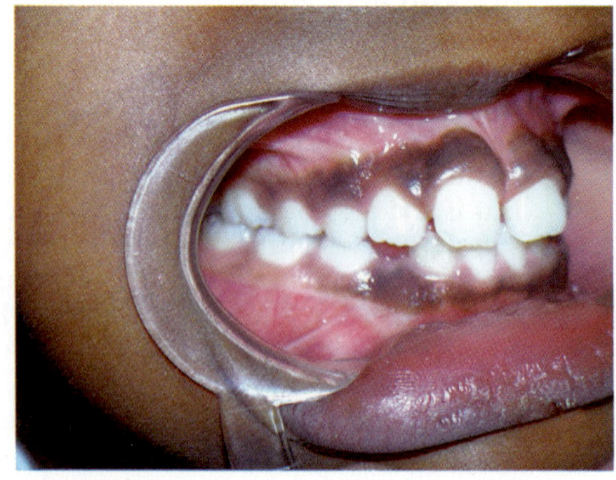

Fig. 11.38: Lower primary teeth have shifted mesially due to space loss

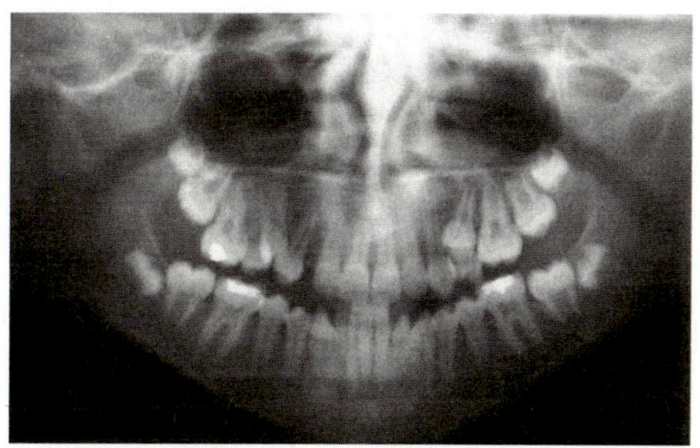

Fig. 11.39: Impacted upper second premolars due to space loss after premature extraction of primary second molars.

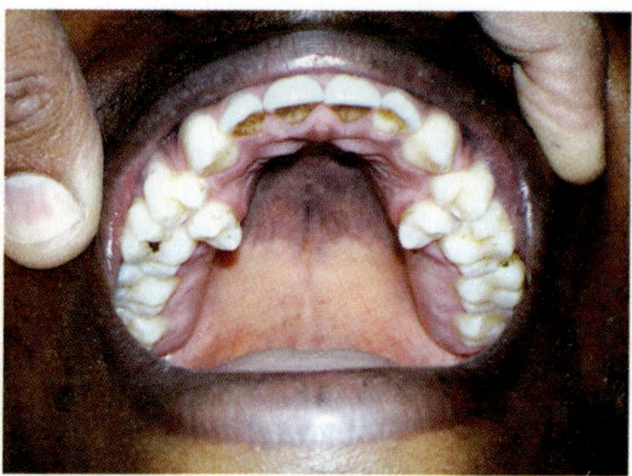

Fig. 11.42: Palatal eruption of upper second premolars due to space loss after premature extraction of primary counterparts.

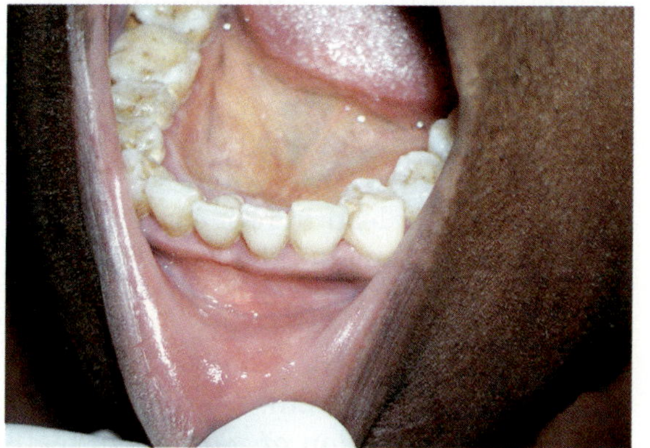

Fig. 11.40: Complete space loss after inadvertent removal of canine in childhood.

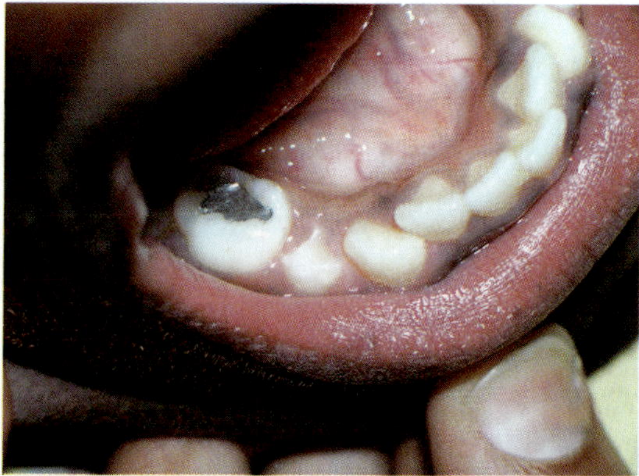

Fig. 11.43: Extreme space loss in premolar region leading to impaction of second premolars, and having less space for erupting first premolars.

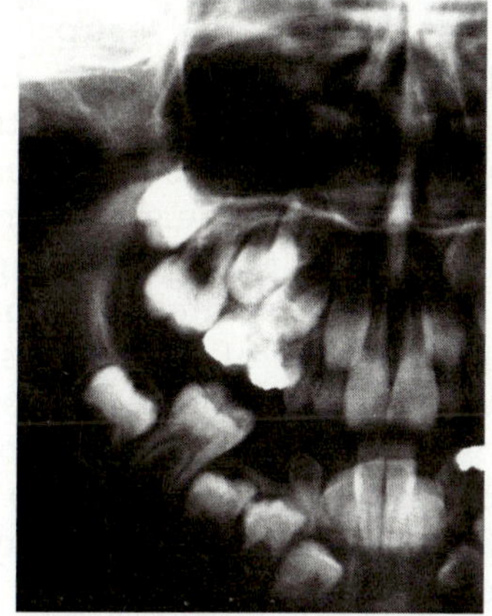

Fig. 11.41: Severe crowding developing in the jaws due to TSALD; space loss after premature extraction of primary teeth and not putting space maintainers; and may be some deficient growth, and hereditary reasons.

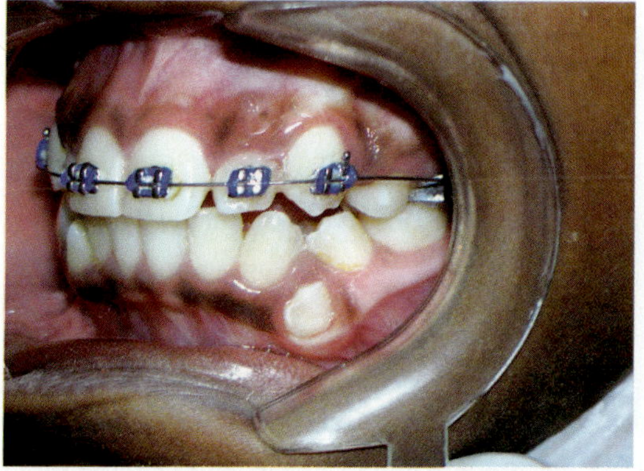

Fig. 11.44: First premolar erupted buccally due to full space loss in the region.

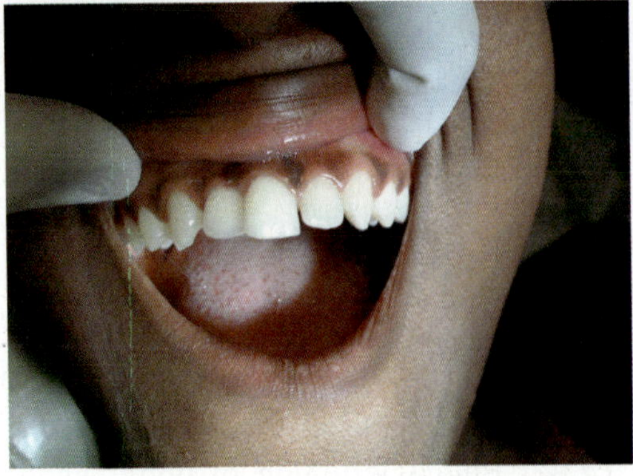

(a)

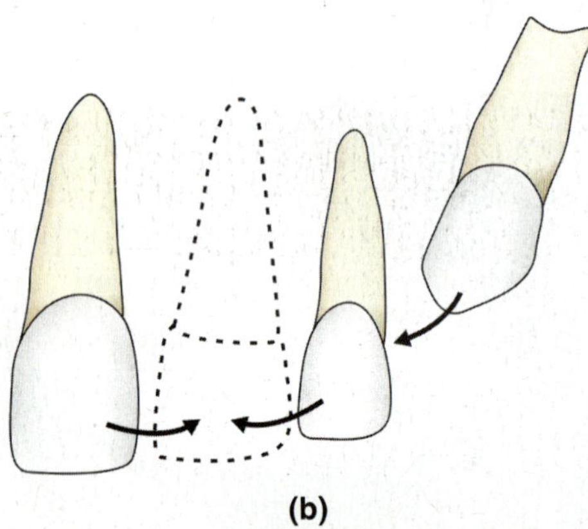

(b)

Figs 11.45a and b: Loss of permanent tooth and subsequent closure of space by shifting of adjacent teeth, e.g. central incisor leading to mesial shifting of lateral incisor and canine, leading to malocclusion and esthetic problems. The erupting canine pushes the lateral incisor mesially and leads to space loss if space maintainer is not inserted.

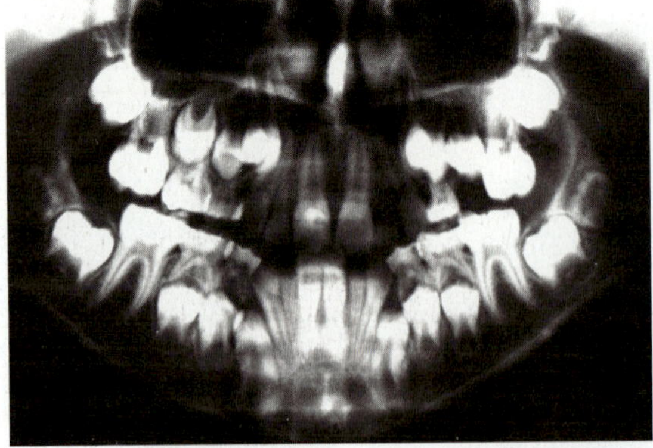

Fig. 11.46: Severe space loss in lower canine region which will lead to impaction of canine unless serial extraction procedure is done.

primary tooth is still present in the arch while the permanent tooth is seen erupting. Such overretained primary teeth lead to deflected path of eruption of the permanent tooth as they occupy the space meant for permanent tooth. Such a permanent tooth may erupt in cross bite and / or crowded state. It may also lead to impaction or transposition or transmigration of permanent teeth. This is mostly seen in lower incisors region and in premolar region also.

It may be due to many factors like space deficiency in the dental arch; absence of any underlying permanent teeth; endocrinal disturbances, e.g. hypothyroidism; hypopituitarism, etc. Congenital conditions, e.g. cleidocranial dysplasia, cherubism, etc. ankylosed deciduous teeth, etc.

If such teeth are not removed timely, then it may lead to root completion of the succedaneous teeth and later on they need orthodontic traction to be pulled in the arch, since a sufficient natural eruption potential does not remain in such teeth.

8. **Delayed eruption of permanent teeth** (Fig. 11.56): If the permanent teeth cannot erupt at a scheduled time despite the exfoliation of primary teeth. It results in ectopic eruption or impaction of permanent teeth. It may also lead to space loss due to shifting of adjacent teeth. There are many reasons for delayed eruption, e.g. presence of supernumerary teeth blocking the path, presence of heavy mucosal barrier; presence of deciduous root fragments; endocrinal disturbances; ankylosed teeth; premature loss of primary teeth; space loss due to early loss of primary teeth; any abnormal habit, etc.
9. **Abnormal eruptive path** (Figs 11.45; 11.49; and 11.57 to 11.59): It leads to eruption of teeth in abnormal location or ectopic eruption / transposition, etc. or impaction of teeth. It may be caused

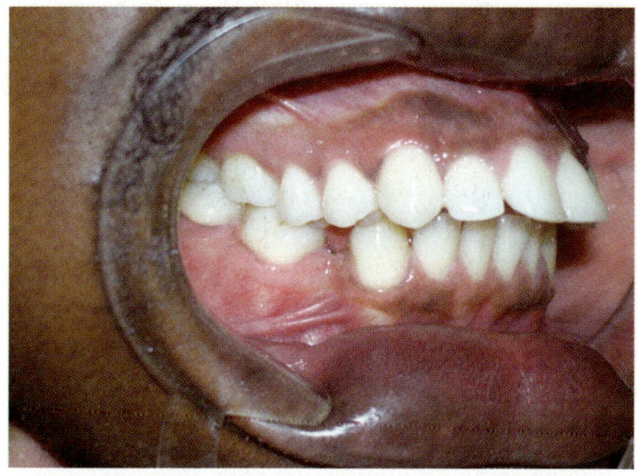

(a)

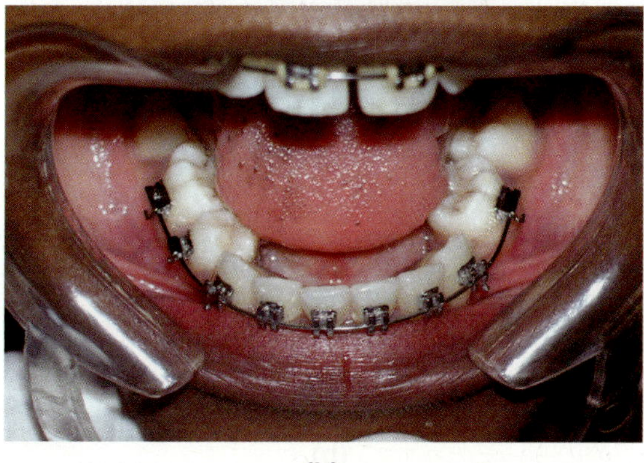

(b)

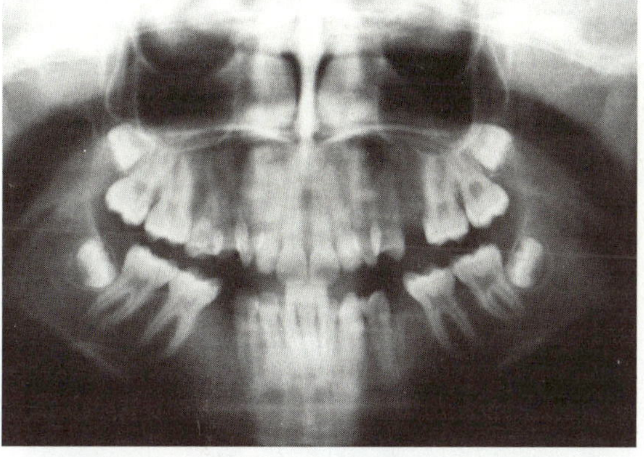

(c)

Figs 11.47 a to c: Extraction of two premolars on the same side of lower jaw by untrained dental professional and layman orthodontist, which also leads to malocclusion. See OPG also.

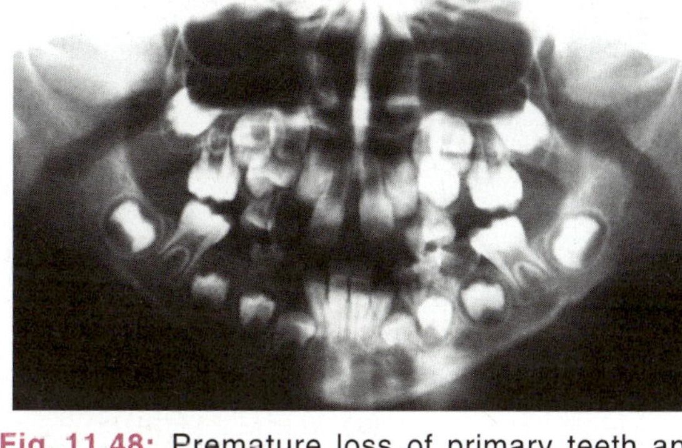

Fig. 11.48: Premature loss of primary teeth and space maintainer not being present will lead to space loss and thus ensuing future crowding and impaction of some teeth.

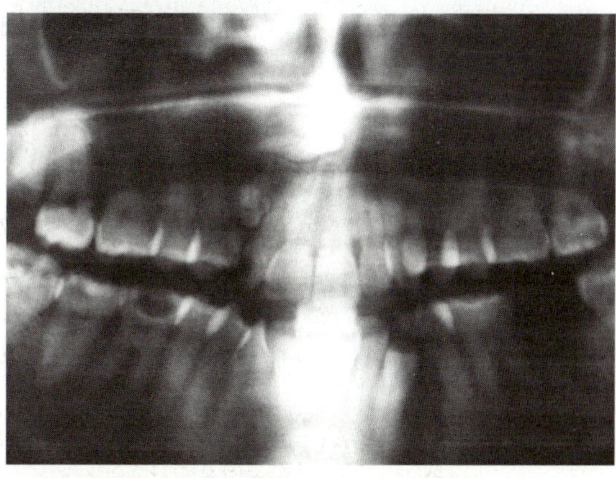

Fig. 11.49: Maxillary canine transmigrated in midline, and retained primary canine. These teeth cannot be aligned in arches orthodontically and need extraction.

due to arch length deficiency, presence of supernumerary teeth, odontomes, retained tooth/root, etc. which may divert a tooth from its eruptive path. Retained deciduous teeth might force a tooth to erupt along a path of least resistance rather than in place of deciduous teeth. Arch length deficiency or excess of tooth material may cause one or more teeth to deviate from their eruptive path.

It may also be caused if the tooth bud gets displaced from its ideal position due to trauma to primary teeth during childhood. Trauma to maxillary incisor region is common with their traumatic

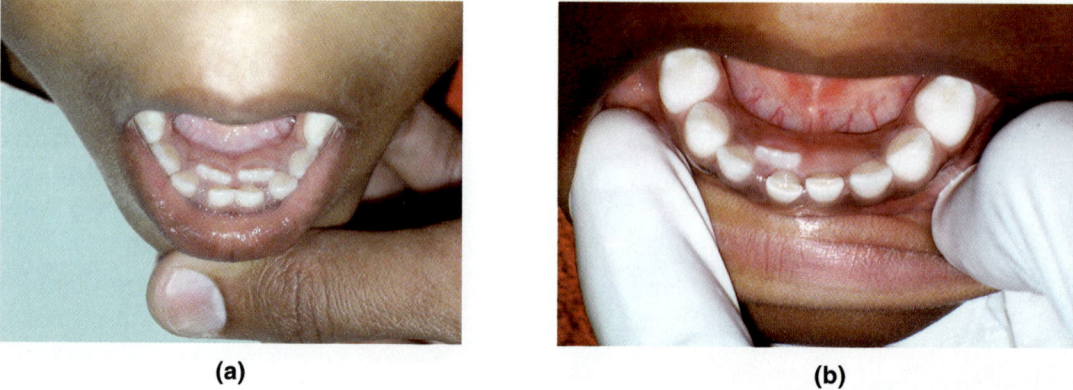

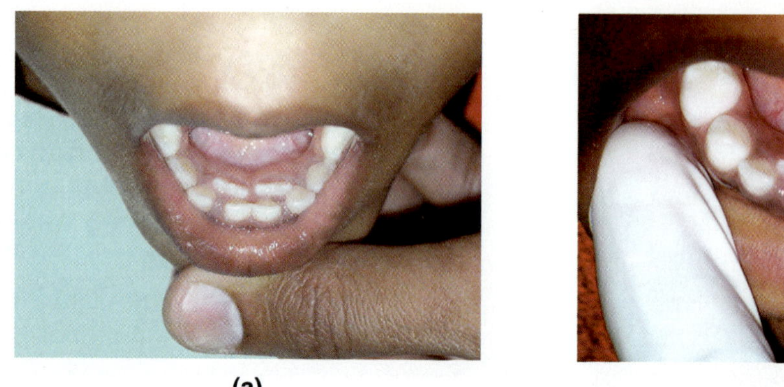

(a) (b)

Figs 11.50a and b: Permanent central incisors erupting lingual to retained primary incisors. Primary incisors should be removed so that permanent can take their place under the tongue pressure.

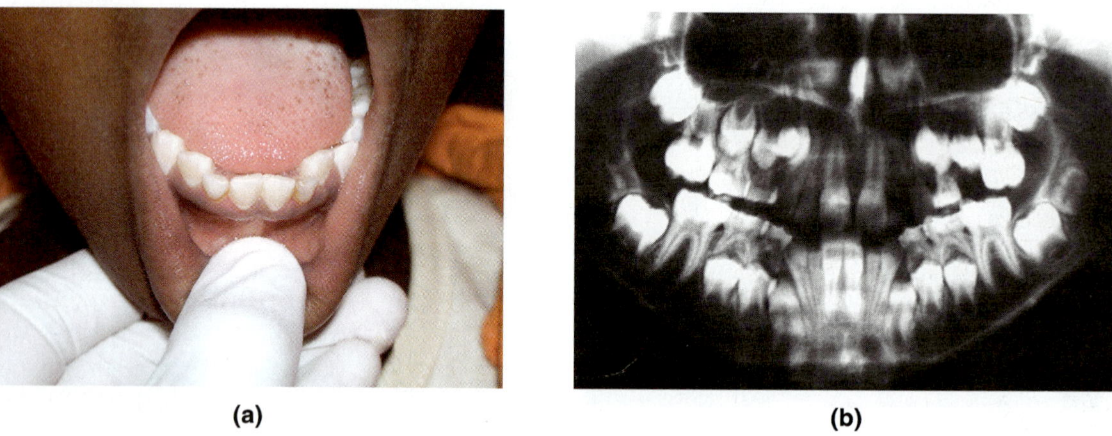

(a) (b)

Figs 11.51a and b: Retained primary incisors in lower incisal region lead to malalignment, and later on spacing when they are removed. OPG showing the retained primary incisors and their effect on the mandibular canines leading to their impaction.

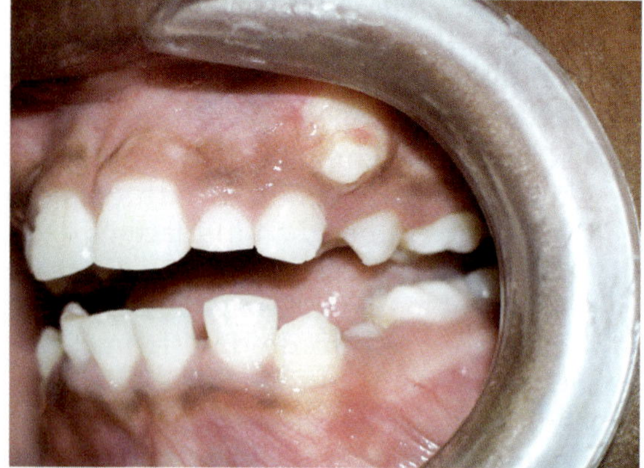

Fig. 11.52: Overretained upper primary lateral incisor leading to space discrepancy and thus labial eruption of canine.

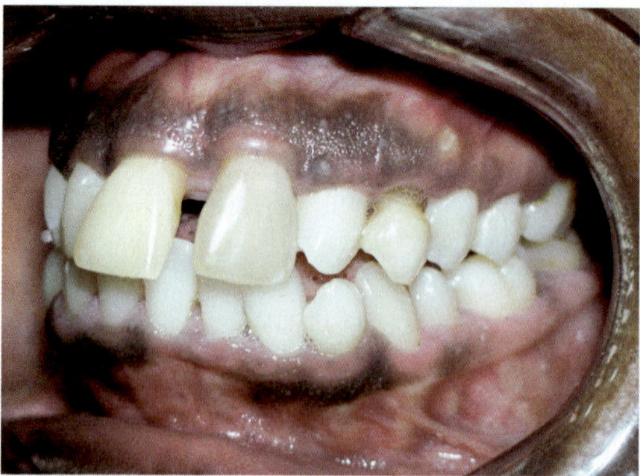

Fig. 11.53: Overretained upper primary canine, which may be due to impacted counterpart.

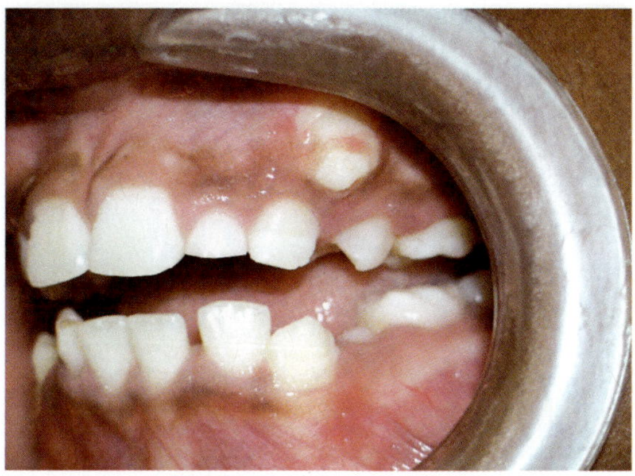

Fig. 11.54: Upper canine erupting out of arch because primary lateral incisor is retained and thus there is no space for canine.

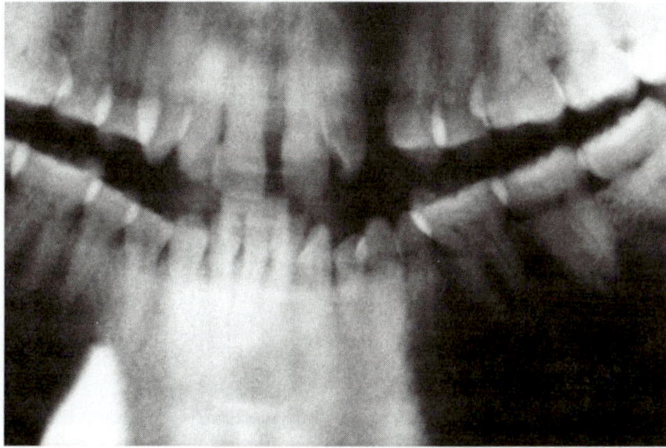

Fig. 11.55: Overretained mandibular canine and abnormally shaped premolar one side.

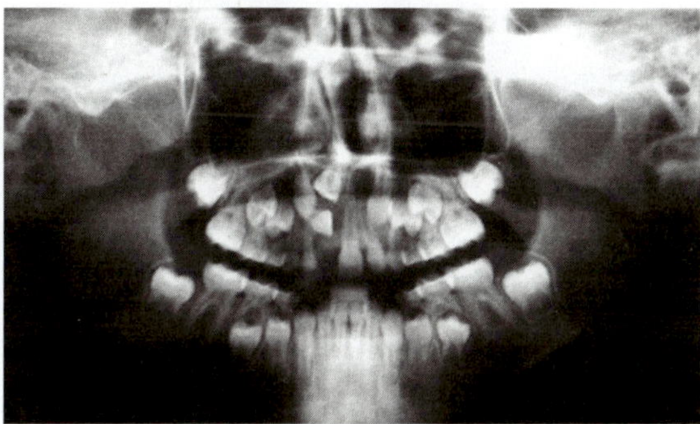

Fig. 11.56: High level impaction of incisors and canine on one side in upper jaw, leading to esthetic problem and malocclusion.

intrusion. It may lead to trauma to labial surface of permanent incisors (Turner's tooth) or displaced tooth bud or dilacerations of permanent tooth depending on the stage of tooth development.

Maxillary canine has been found to be the most common deflected tooth. It is because it has the longest path of eruption, as it develops near the floor of the orbit and is the last tooth to erupt in oral cavity. Any loss in arch length in this region occurs from both the anterior and posterior regions, so the adjacent teeth may impinge on its space. Abnormal position of its tooth bud is also the cause. It is generally deflected to the palatal side, leading to palatal eruption or impaction. It has also been found to transposed or transmigrate crossing the midline (Figs 11.60 to 11.62).

10. **Ankylosis** (Figs 11.63 to 11.65): It is the union of the root or part of a root directly to the bone without the intervening periodontal ligament. It is mostly caused by trauma to the tooth. It may be associated with certain infections, endocrine disorders, and congenital diseases, like cleidocranial dysostosis, etc. also. Chronic periapical infection of the tooth may also lead to ankylosis. If it occurs in primary tooth, that tooth does not get resorbed and exfoliate, thus leading to deflection or impaction of the successor tooth. It also leads to deficient alveolar bone height as the tooth acts as a functional matrix for the growth of the alveolar bone, thus the adjacent teeth keep on erupting leading to gain in alveolar bone. This tooth then has its occlusal level at a lower position than the adjacent teeth. This condition is known as submerged tooth. If not treated timely, the adjacent teeth may tilt in or supraerupt over the submerged tooth, further leading to occlusal problems. The same effects can occur, if permanent tooth gets ankylosed.

11. **Dental caries** (Figs 11.66 and 11.67): It is the most common oral disease of human and leads to irreversible loss of tooth structure. It is also an important cause of malocclusion. Caries can lead to early loss of tooth and thus shifting of adjacent teeth in the space, abnormal tipping or supraeruption (Figs 11.68 and 11.69). Unrestored proximal caries leads to a reduction of arch length by shifting of adjacent tooth. So, the proximal caries should be restored as early as possible to avoid space loss. It also leads to the loss of E-space, if caries affects proximal surface of primary second molars. E-space is very important for normal development of dentition and occlusion. It may be used

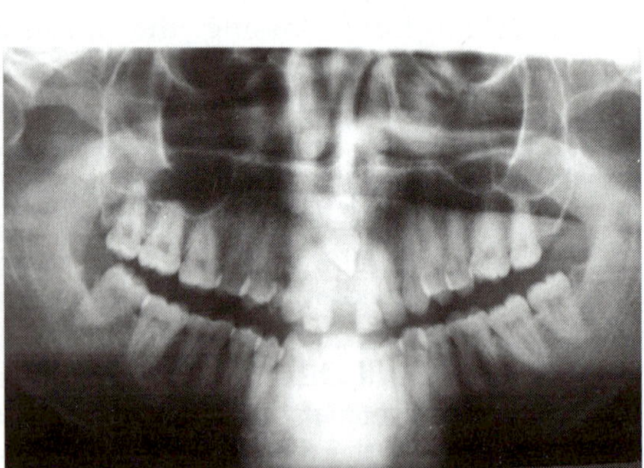

Fig. 11.57: Maxillary canine transmigrated between central incisors, associated midline diastema and malocclusion.

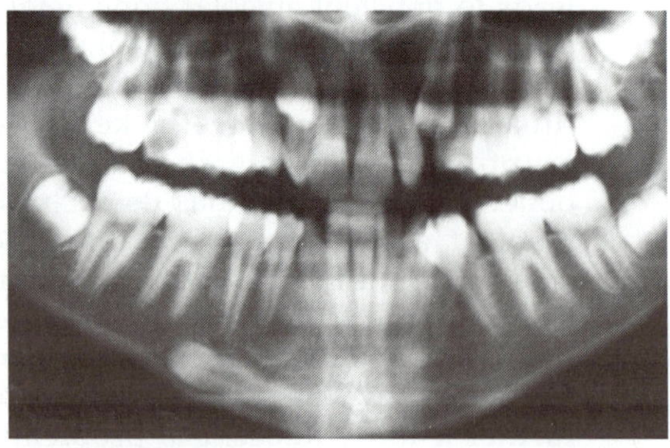

Fig. 11.58: Impacted lower canine, migrated apical to premolar and molar area.

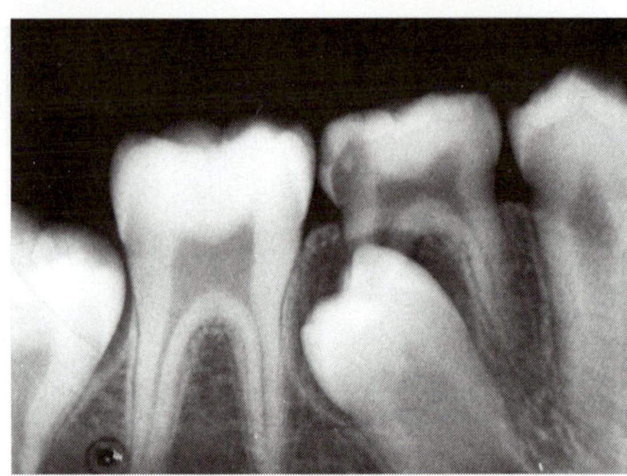

Fig. 11.59: Distally inclined premolar which may not erupt and may get impacted later on.

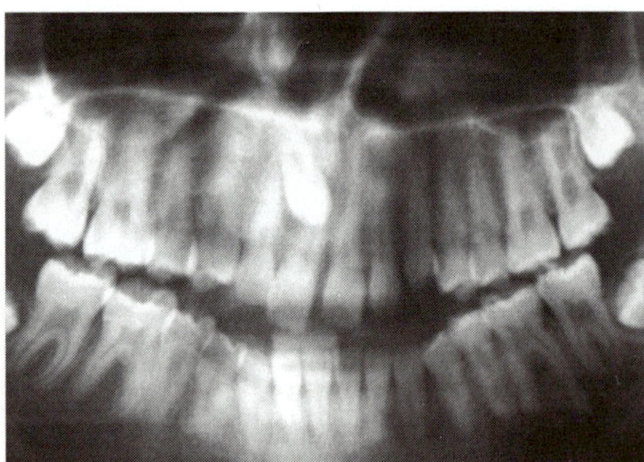

Fig. 11.60: Upper canine transmigrated in central incisor region, leading to extrusion, and may be root resorption of the central incisor.

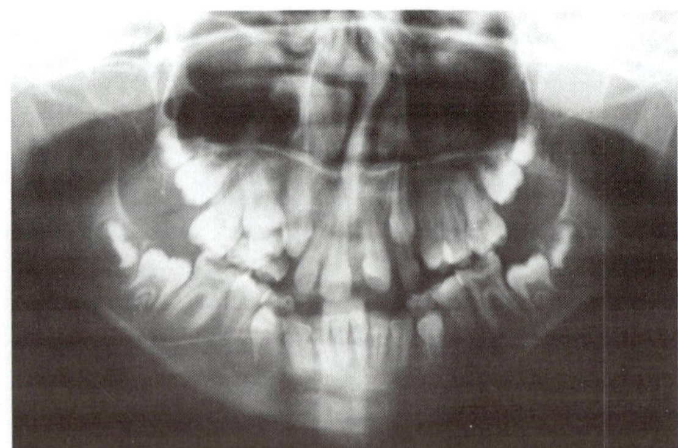

Fig. 11.61: Upper canine overlapping the lateral incisor on one side, due to lack of space for its eruption.

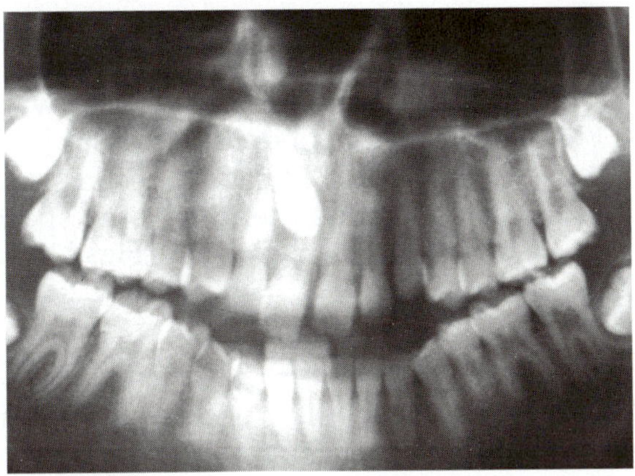

Fig. 11.62: Impacted upper canine leading to deflection of central incisor.

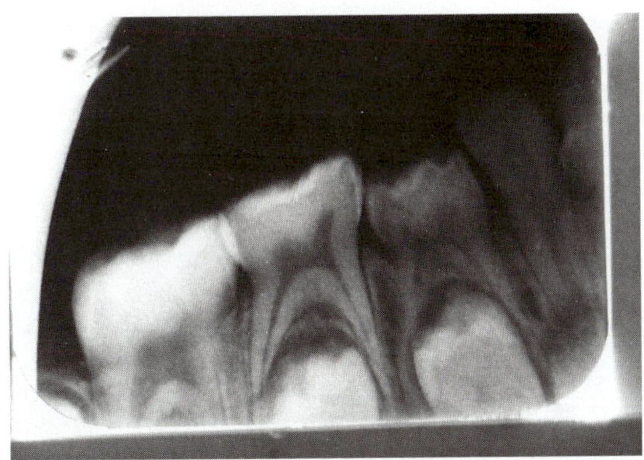

Fig. 11.64: Submerged primary first molar due to it being ankylosed, as there is no PDL space on both roots.

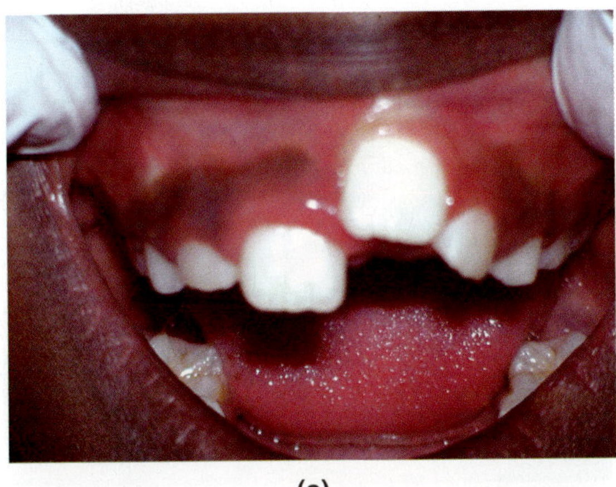

(a)

(b)

Figs 11.63a and b: High position of central incisor. It happens generally when there is trauma to this region and subsequent ankylosis of the tooth.

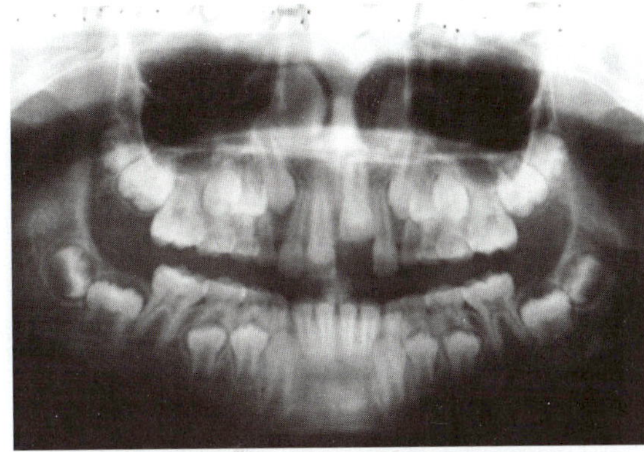

Fig. 11.65: Intruded / ankylosed central incisor after trauma.

during orthodontic treatment for alignment of irregular teeth. An early loss of primary second molars before the eruption of permanent first molar can lead to abnormal path of its eruption. So in such cases, a distal shoe space maintainer is inserted for eruption guidance. In adult patients, caries and periodontal disease lead to loss of teeth, leading to migration and supraeruption of teeth. Such patients require multidisciplinary treatment for occlusal restorations.

12. **Improper dental restoration:** Under-contoured proximal restoration leads to a decrease in arch length by mesial migration of adjacent teeth. Over-

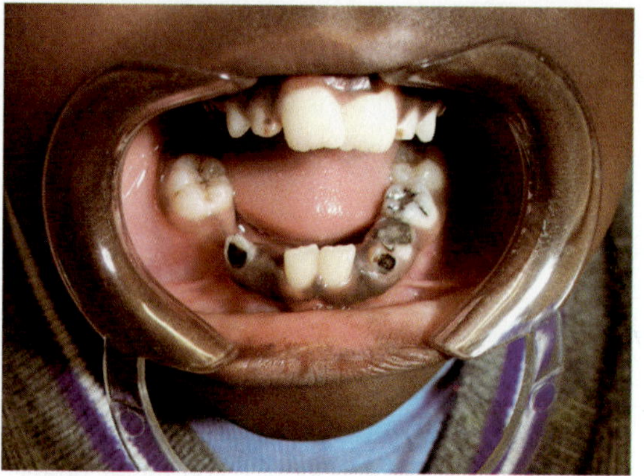

Fig. 11.66: High caries rate leading to loss of primary teeth, space loss and thus future malalignment of the teeth.

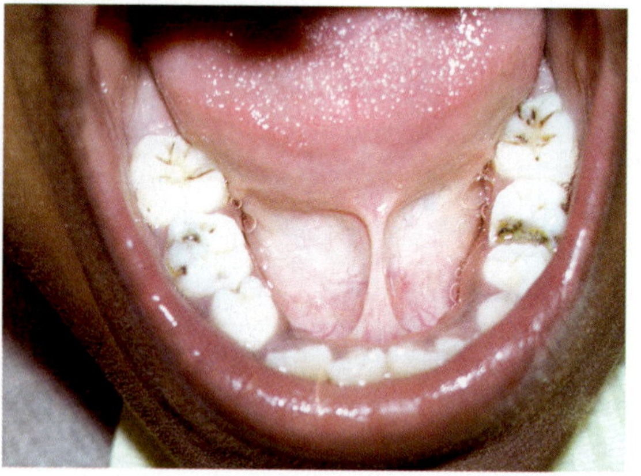

Fig. 11.67: Non-restoration of mesial surface caries on a posterior tooth leads to space loss by shifting of adjacent tooth in this cavity.

contoured restoration may cover the space to be occupied by the succedaneous tooth. It may also lead to functional shift of mandible during closure. Overhanging restorations or poor proximal contacts lead to periodontal breakdown due to food impaction. It may lead to abnormal mobility of teeth (Fig. 11.70).

13. **Periodontal disease:** It leads to weakening of periodontal support and thus pathological migration of teeth. It leads to malocclusion like proclination of teeth, increased overjet, overbite, change in incisal levels of adjacent teeth, rotation, spacing, premature contacts and mobility of teeth. Such conditions are commonly seen in adults with uncontrolled periodontal diseases.
14. **Truma to teeth:** It leads to the loss of a tooth, and thus the loss of the space leading to space deficiency (Figs 11.71a and b).

Other Causes (Fig. 11.70)

Molar bands interfering with eruption: In some cases, the margin of molar band may interfere the occlusal movement of the erupting tooth during the ongoing orthodontic treatment. In such cases, a regular IOPA X-ray

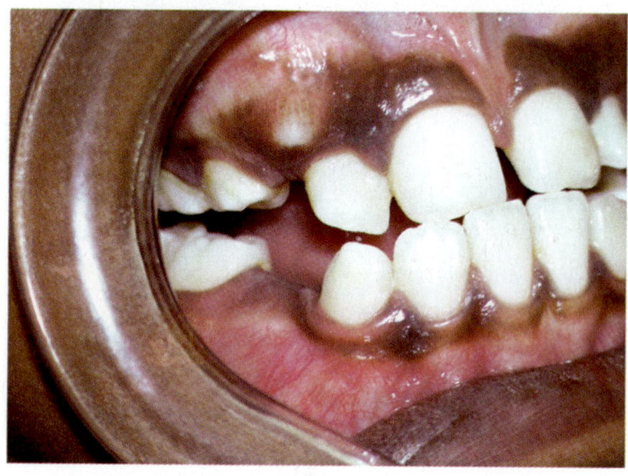

Fig. 11.68: Space deficiency for erupting upper canine, and rotation of adjacent lateral incisor.

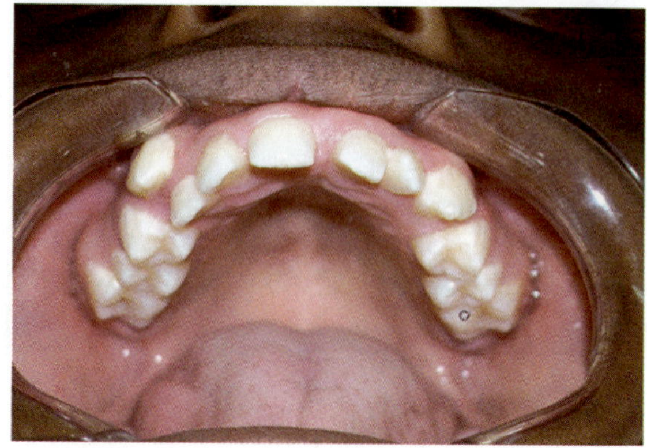

Fig. 11.69: Blocked out upper canine due to space deficiency.

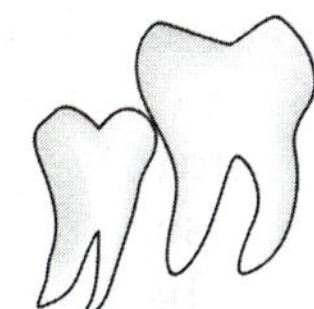

Second molar stuck below the HOC of first molar

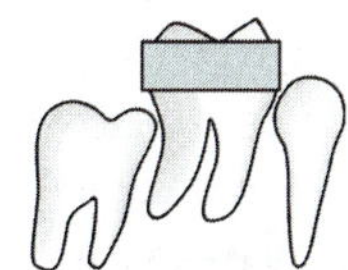

Eruption inhibited by abnormal edges on molar band

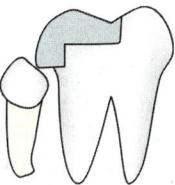

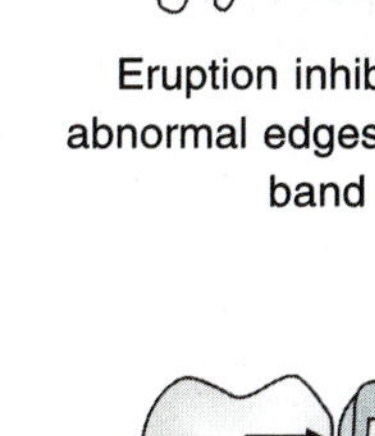

Large overhang of amalgam filling leading to interference of eruption of premolar

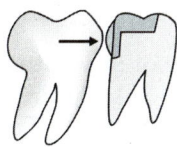

Proper contour of amalgam filling on the adjacent tooth helps in proper inclination and eruption of tooth

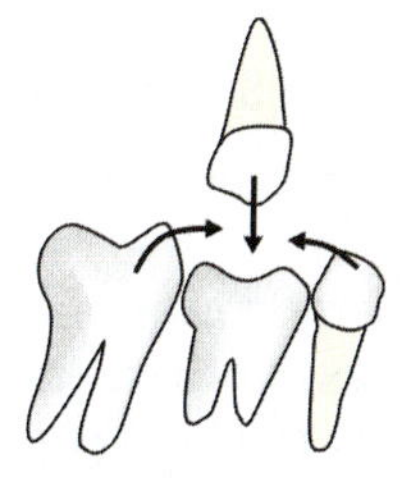

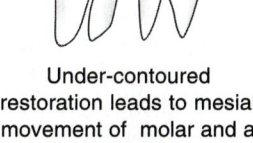

Under-contoured restoration leads to mesial movement of molar and a space loss

A submerged primary tooth and thus shifting of adjacent teeth in the space, leading to malocclusion and abnormal axial inclination of teeth.

Fig. 11.70: Figure showing different causes of malocclusion due to problem of dental eruption.

may be needed to assess their relation, and if needed corrective measure is taken by putting a disimpaction spring.

Similarly, the erupting tooth may get stuck below the HOC of the molar, due to space deficiency, and needs disimpaction spring to allow its eruption.

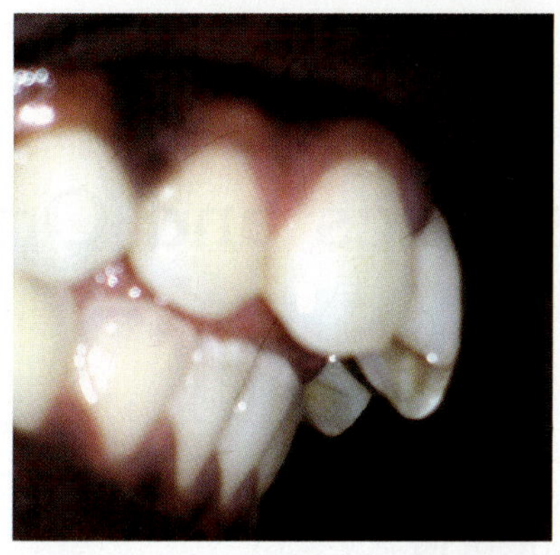

(a)

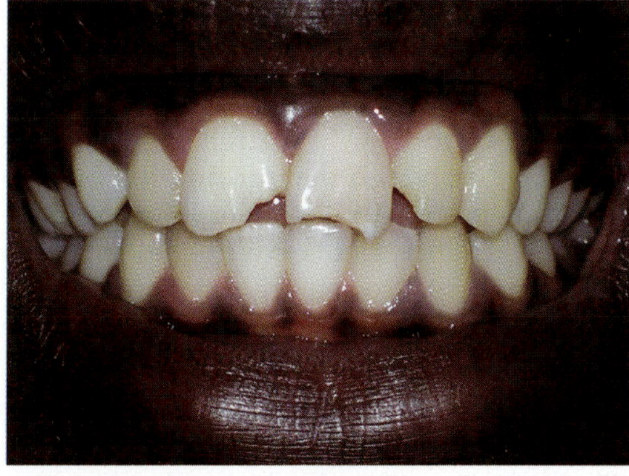

(b)

Figs 11.71a and b: Fracture of upper incisors due to trauma, which generally happens when the incisors are very proclined, making them prone to trauma and fracture.

Conclusion

Malocclusion has a multifactorial etiology. A proper diagnosis involves the examining the condition and its associated causes. Removal of the cause is important for treatment or reducing the severity of the condition and to prevent the treatment relapse.

12

Genetics and Orthodontics

INTRODUCTION

Genetics plays a great role in the growth and development of human body and any disturbance in the growth of craniofacial complex leads to malocclusion.

Types of studies: Main research studies which have provided the information on role of heredity on malocclusion are of two types: (1) Family studies and (2) twin studies. Twin studies have been done on the monozygotic twins and the dizygotic twins. Studies have been done to compare different races and ethnic groups also to determine the differences in the dentofacial patterns of different groups.

Twin studies: The classical twin approach for separating the effects of nature and nurture involves comparing identical (monozygous: MZ) and nonidentical (dizygous) twin pairs different. In MZ, twins reflect environmental factors whereas differences between dizygous (DZ) pairs are due to both genetic and environmental factors.

Etiology of the malocclusion: Genetic and environmental factors play important role in etiology of malocclusion. It has been shown by many family and twin studies. However, the characteristics are not controlled by a single gene, but they show a polygenic inheritance pattern.

Polygenic inheritance: The "normal" variation in dentition is a result of multiple rather than single genes. Normal variation means that the genetic defects or syndromes associated with the dentition are excluded, which may be caused by other associated factors like mutations also. Thus, the size or shape of the teeth, etc. is determined by many genes interacting with each other and the environment. Tooth size, tooth eruption, congenitally missing teeth, tooth morphology, etc. are affected by polygenic inheritance, as has been shown by various family and twin studies.

Genetic Studies on Growth

Growth and development of craniofacial complex is the result of interplay of genetic and environmental influences. Various twin studies confirm that the size and shape of body parts, the rate/progress of growth (fast maturing/slow maturing tendencies), fat deposition, growth patterns and the onset of growth events viz. menarche, dental calcification, dental eruption, ossification of bones and start of adolescent growth spurt, are controlled by genetic factors. The fast maturing and slow maturing tendencies run in the families and also in some racial and ethnic groups. Growth differences in males and females are also controlled by genetic factors, as Y chromosome in males is responsible to delay the growth and maturation in males to allow them to grow for a longer time. Individuals having XXY chromosomes (Klinefelter's syndrome) follow a growth pattern similar to males despite presence of two X chromosomes, whereas individuals having one X chromosome (Turner's syndrome) follow that similar to females in absence of Y chromosomes. Individuals having XYY chromosomes follow a growth pattern similar to males but result in increased height due to the presence of two Y chromosomes to allow them to grow for a longer period of time.

Genetic Studies on Malocclusion in Different Populations

Malocclusion in primitive human population was less prevalent than in modern population because of inbreeding leading to genetic isolation and uniformity. Certain morphological features are known to run in the family or in the races. Polynesian population had shown an unusual distinctive form of lower jaw with a smoothly curved gonial angle also termed as "Rocker Jaw". Short face with deep bite runs in White population whereas long face with open bite is prevalent in blacks. Such problem in facial height is due to inherited tendency of orientation of anterior cranial base. Increased inclination (saddle angle) leads to increased anterior facial height.

In modern civilization, outbreeding has led to an increase in malocclusion due to certain genetic differences between crossing populations. A study conducted on human population in Hawaii by Chung et al revealed increase in malocclusion as a result of outbreeding with European, Chinese, Japanese and other races.

Genetic Studies on Malocclusion in Family Members

About 40% of the dental and facial variations leading to malocclusion can be attributed to hereditary factors. Local occlusal variables are also under genetic control. Lundstrom 1984 emphasized that greater genetic influence is on skeletal pattern than the dental features. Also the soft tissues morphology and behavior show a genetic influence which in turn shapes the dentoalveolar structure, as described by van den Linden.

Best information on heredity can be obtained by twin studies involving monozygotic twins (MZ twins). Family studies using twins show that the difference between MZ twins are due to environment, while between dizygotic (DZ) twins are due to both genes and the environment. MZ twins show much resemblance due to similar types of growth pattern and biological ages indicating a dominating role of genetics in the growth and development.

Heritability of Skeletal Variables

Prognathic mandible in European Royal family has run in generations, which is termed as "Hapsburg Jaw". Mandibular prognathism was found to be transmitted as an autosomal dominant AD trait as confirmed by the pedigree analysis of Hapsburg family.

Skeletal class III: Mandibular prognathism has been shown to be strongly under genetic control while long face pattern with open bite being next in order. Even cranial base morphololgy, i.e. a more acute cranial base angle; short posterior cranial base and more anterior position of glenoid fossa, which contribute to mandibular prognathism is also controlled by multifactorial inheritance model, as suggested by Ellis and McNamara 1984, Singh et al 1997. A study on MZ and DZ twins has shown that certain areas, e.g. lateral surface of ramus, lingual symphysis and frontal curvature of mandible are predominantly under genetic control.

Skeletal characteristics in all the dimensions, i.e. anteroposterior, transverse and vertical have been found to be under considerable genetic control. Hughes and Moore in 1941 concluded that mandible and maxillary areas are under separate genetic control, and also certain parts of bones like ramus, body, symphysis of mandible are under different genetic and environmental influences.

Class II division 1: Harris in his study on class II div 1 cases found that mandible is significantly more retruded , body of mandible smaller and the overall length of mandible decreased as compared to class I, showing polygenic inheritance.

Syndromes: Most common congenital problem of face is *cleft lip and palate*. Craniofacial asymmetry can be caused by genetic factors or environmental factors including pathological change. Craniofacial asymmetry in certain conditions, e.g. neurofibromatosis and hemifacial microsomia is predominantly due to hereditary factors, which may occur on either side, i.e. right or left. Unilateral cleft lip cases usually are found to be on the left side roughly twice than that on right side. This preference, in absence of any environmental factors, leads to an assumption of it being associated to the genetic differences between the two halves of the body.

Heritability of Dental Variables
(Figs 12.1a to e)

Lundstrom 1948 in his study pointed out that dental arch width and length, overbite and crowding and spacing of teeth are influenced by heredity. Dental arch asymmetry also may be genetic or non-genetic in origin. Cranial type and facial type are genetically determined and are correlated with arch width, i.e. brachycephalic cranial type is associated with euryprosopic facial type and wide dental arch and dolichocephalic cranial type is associated with leptoprosopic facial type and narrow dental arch, so the arch width is found to be primarily under genetic control. Arch interrelationship assessed by maxillary and mandibular permanent first molar relationship likely to be reflection of anteroposterior skeletal relationship is also found to be under genetic influence.

Number and the size of the teeth: Osborne et al 1958 showed that tooth crown size is strongly determined by heredity. Variation in number of teeth ie hypodontia, supernumerary teeth, etc. and the size of teeth also shows a familial tendency, and polygenic inheritance. Abnormal shapes of teeth, e.g. maxillary lateral incisors and Carabelli cusps trait are strongly under genetic influence showing familial trends, showing a polygenic inheritance. Variation in eruption pattern of teeth eg impaction, ectopic maxillary canine; transposition of teeth and submerged primary molars all show familial tendency and strong genetic component having incomplete penetrance and variable expressivity.

Butler's Field Theory

There are certain specific teeth which show more variation than others. According to Butler's field theory 1939, the mammalian dentition can be divided into several developmental fields. There is a "key" tooth within each field, one that is more stable developmentally, and on either side of this key tooth, the remaining teeth within the field become progressively less stable. The three fields are those for molars / premolars, incisors and canines.

The molars / premolars field consists of the first molar as the key tooth, the second the third molars on the distal end of the field, and the first and second premolars on the mesial end. The theory predicts that the third molar and first premolar would be most variable in size and shape. It can be questioned that the third molar is agreed as the variable tooth but not the first premolar. Actually the earliest mammals had four premolars and some of the higher primates, including man, have lost the first two premolars. So the premolars that we refer to first and second should really be labeled third and fourth. The point is that as Butler's theory predicted, the premolars farthest from the first molar were the first to be lost in an evolutionary sense and therefore can be considered the least stable.

However, a modern modification of this concept considers the dental arch in four segments: (1) incisors, (2) canines, (3) premolars and (4) molars. It depicts that the distal tooth of each segment is most often missing congenitally.

In maxillary incisor region, the lateral incisor is found to be missing more often than the central incisor. However, an exception is noted in lower incisors region, where central incisor is found missing more often than the lateral incisor. Canines being the only teeth in their respective field, they are found missing least percentage of time. In premolar region, it is the second premolar which is found more often congenitally missing, and in molar region, the third molar is missing congenitally.

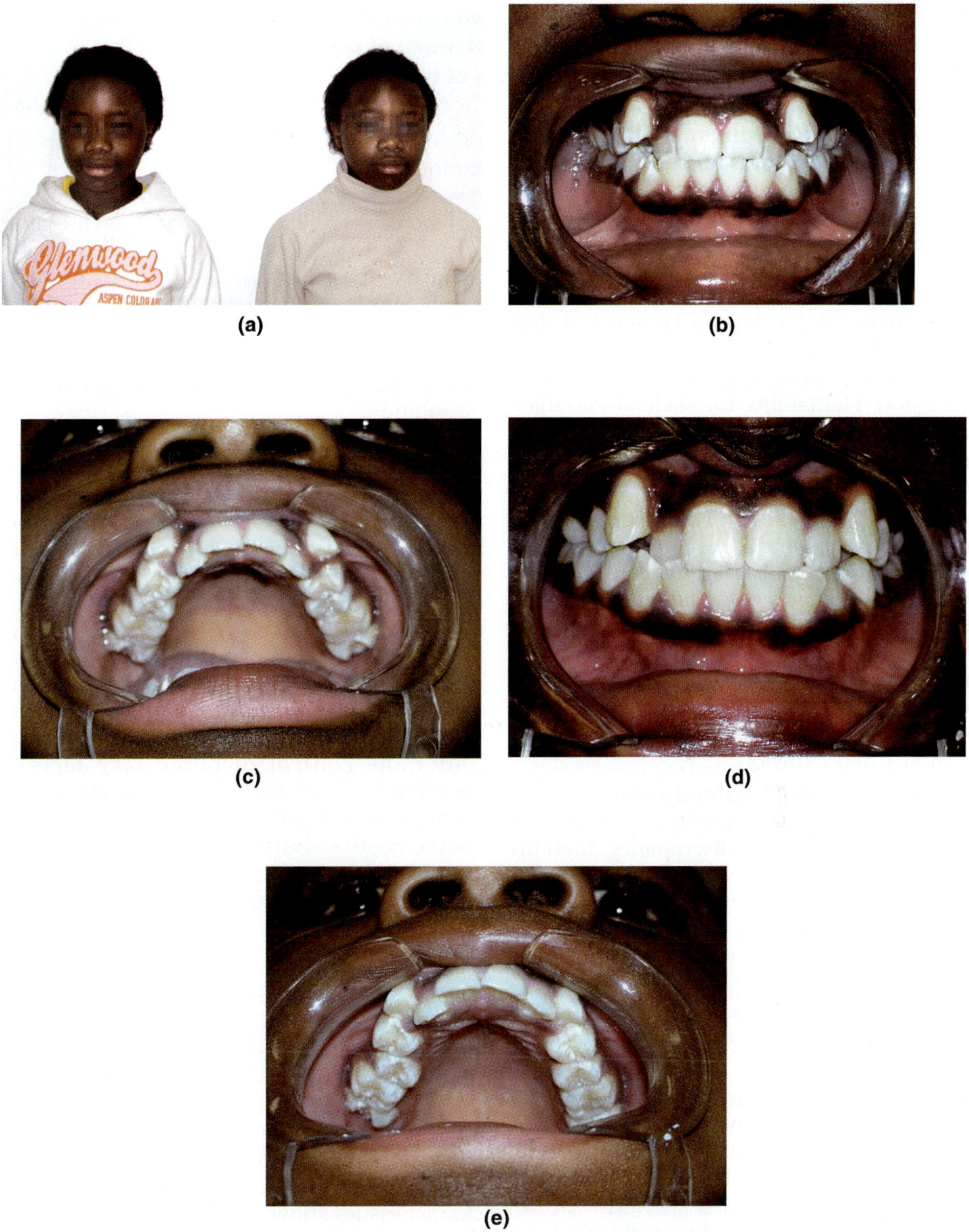

(a)

(b)

(c)

(d)

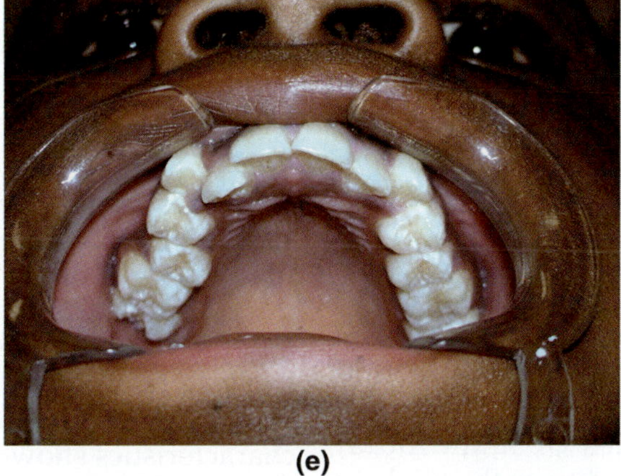

(e)

Figs 12.1a to e: Genetic link in development of malocclusion. These twin sisters have almost same type of dental alignment and malocclusion, although environmental factors also play a big role during dentition development.

Pattern of Inheritance from Parents to Offspring

Numerous differences exist in dentofacial characteristics of the individuals, even among family members. A multifactorial etiology, with genetics and environmental factors are main contributors to such variation. Skeletal dimension for parent-child pair have higher correlation coefficient than dental characteristics indicating skeletal dimension to be much under genetic influence than dental characteristics. It has been a known fact that craniofacial abnormalities are not monogenic but are multifactorial, i.e. gene – environmental interaction. Heritability for skeletal variables viz position of lower jaw, anterior and posterior face heights, and cranial base dimensions is stronger, while that of dental variables was low.

Class II division 1 malocclusion: Cephalometric studies have shown that mandible in class II is significantly more retruded than class I patients, with the body of mandible smaller and overall mandibular length reduced. These studies also show a higher correlation between the patients and his immediate family, thus supporting the concept of polygenic inheritance for class II division 1 malocclusion.

Class II division 2 malocclusion: Its main features are deep overbite, retroclined incisors, class II skeletal discrepancy, high lip line with strap like activity of the lower lip and active mentalis muscle. There is a tendency to a forwardly rotating mandibular movement, which contributes to deep bite, chin prominence, and reduced lower face height. Family and twin studies have shown the familial occurrence of class II division 2 malocclusion.

Class III malocclusion: Skeletal class III condition esp due to mandibular prognathism observes familial inheritance. It was seen as Hapsburg jaw in a German royal family. Various familial studies of mandibular prognathism suggest heredity as the etiology of this condition.

Cleft lip and palate: It is a very common congenital condition, and has a strong genetic link. The chances of CL/P increases in the children of parent/s having CL/P.

Contemporary View on Inheritance

Primitive population with low prevalence of malocclusion has drawn the attention of researchers. It was thought that the coarse diet put increased functional demands on the jaws which led to normal growth of jaws in primitive population. Changes in dietary habits to soft and processed food reduced the functional demands on the jaws, thereby causing lesser growth and less attrition of teeth, leading to malocclusion in the existing population.

Another aspect to explain the low prevalence of malocclusion in primitive population and high prevalence of malocclusion in the existing population came into view. The low prevalence of malocclusion in primitive population was explained on the basis of genetic isolation and uniformity since, all the individuals who were involved in mating, carried same genetic information. In modern times, genetic melting due to outbreeding led to increase in malocclusion. The skeletal characteristics are primarily under the control of hereditary factors showing less vulnerability of change under environmental influences, whereas dental characteristics showed low heritability and more vulnerability to change under environmental influences with advancing age.

Conclusion

Role of heredity in growth and development of dentoskeletal complex cannot be underemphasised. Genes from both the parent guide the formation of jaws, teeth, soft tissues and their inter-relationship. Malocclusion is not inherited in a simple Mendelian fashion, but shows a polygenic inheritance, accompanied by several environmental influences. Skeletal characteristics show much higher heritability than dental characteristics. Tooth size and shape, congenitally missing teeth, supernumerary teeth and median diastema are also under genetic control. Dental arch form and permanent first molar relationship, which are usually harmonious with certain skeletal pattern, are also under genetic influences. As during treatment, the genetically determined factors cannot be controlled, the main emphasis remains to control the environmental factors to treat or improve the malrelation. Knowledge of genetic pattern of an individual helps in determining his expected growth and facial pattern and hence the interceptive methods (e.g. functional appliance, dentofacial orthopedic Rx) can be preplanned and instituted timely to avoid development of a severity of the condition. Also, advanced consultation and advice can be provided to the future parents to plan their family in consultation with genetic experts to avoid any congenital conditions in their children.

Further Readings

1. Bishara SE. Textbook of orthodontics, WB Saunders, 2001.
2. Ellis E and McNamara JA Jr. Components of adult class III malocclusion. J Oral and Maxillofac Surg. 1984;42: 295–305.
3. Graber TM, Vanarsdall RL, Vig KWL (eds). Orthodontics: Current principles and techniques, 4th edition, St. Louis, Mosby, 2005.
4. Harris JE. Genetic factors in the growth of the head: Inheritance of the craniofacial complex and malocclusion. Dent. Clin. North Am 1975;19:151–60.
5. Lundstrom A. Tooth size and occlusion in twins. 2nd ed. S Karger AG, Basle, 1948.
6. Lundstrom A. Some asymmetries of the dental arches, jaws and skull, and their etiological significance. Am J Orthod 1961;47:81-106.
7. Moyers RE. Handbook of orthodontics. 4th edition. Year book medical publishers, Inc. 1988.
8. Proffit WR, Fields Jr HW, Sarver DM. Contemporary orthodontics. 4th edition, Mosby, 2007.
9. Proffit WR, Phillips C, Dann C IV. Who seeks surgical-orthodontic treatment? The characteristics of patients evaluated in the UNC Dentofacial Clinic. Int J Adult Orthod Orthognath Surg 1990;5:153-60.

13

Orthodontic Diagnosis

INTRODUCTION

Diagnosis is an important step to plan the treatment. In simple terms, it is the process of finding out the type of condition and its features, so that a patient-directed treatment can be planned. It helps us to determine the prognosis of case depending on its features. Diagnosis is defined as the statement of the condition of patient based on the information obtained from history, clinical examination, and other diagnostic aids, like radiological and lab examination. Prognosis is the expectation of the results to be achieved from the treatment in that particular patient. A treatment plan is defined as the blue print of the steps to be followed to treat the patient.

Orthodontic diagnosis deals with the identification of various characteristics and causes of the malocclusion. It helps in determining the course of treatment. Knowledge of the causes is important because the first step in treatment is "to remove the cause". So the diagnosis requires integration of scientific knowledge, with clinical experience and the common sense.

Diagnosis requires development of an adequate database. It is an orderly summarizing the obtained data base to a useful list of patient's problems, to which the treatment has to be directed. The data is derived from case history, clinical examination and diagnostic aids such as study casts, radiographs and photographs. The relevant information obtained from data base helps to develop a priority list/triage list, so that treatment objectives and plan can be defined. Triage list means the problems are sequenced such that the treatment is provided in that sequence to eliminate the problems.

Formulation of a problem list: It is separated in two parts: (1) pathologic problems and (2) development problems. Pathologic problems must be under control before the treatment of developmental problems is started. Problems should be arranged in order of priority, i.e. triage concept.

To determine treatment plan, four issues must be considered:

1. Timing of the treatment: Rx can be carried out at any time but should be done during active growth period for better and stable results. However, there are certain conditions which should be treated as soon as possible, so that the growth and development takes place normally.
2. The complexity of Rx required: Rx may be aimed at specific problem or may be comprehensive. Less complex cases can be dealt by general dentist. More complex cases should be dealt by specialists.
3. The predictability of success with a given Rx approach. On this basis, choice of Rx method is made if alternative methods are available.
4. The patients and parents goals and desires. Rx planning must be an interactive process. Patient must be involved in decision making process because patients' compliance is very important for success or failure of the Rx.

Diagnostic Aids

The information data for diagnosis is obtained from many clinical methods, known as the diagnostic aids. They have been divided in essential diagnostic aids and supplemental diagnostic aids.

Essential Diagnostic Aids

They are mandatorily required in all cases needing orthodontic treatment. They are simple and inexpensive. They are:

- Case history
- Clinical examination
- Study models
- Radiographs—IOPA, OPG; bitewing
- Facial photographs.

Supplemental Diagnostic Aids

They are required in only certain cases needing comprehensive intervention, for specific evaluation. Their need depends from case to case. They require specific equipments and thus are expensive. They are:

- Special radiographs:
  - Cephalograms—lateral and PA
  - Occlusal views
  - Skeletal lateral jaw views
- Functional records:
  - Incision—end to end bite
  - Phonation
  - Wide open mouth
  - Views with radiopaque media
- EMG
- Hand wrist X-rays to find out the bone age and growth status
- BMR and other endocrine tests
- CT scan and MRI
- 3D imaging
- Diagnostic setup
- Occlusograms
- Videofluoroscopy
- Model/cast surgery for surgical evaluations
- Photocephalometry
- Digigraphy
- 3D imaging.

Case History

It is the collection of the relevant information from parents and patient by interviewing them about the problem to aid in the overall diagnosis of the case.

Personal Details

Name: It is recorded for communication and identification of the patient. Addressing the patient by his name gives a positive psychological boost, and creates a friendly atmosphere. It helps in getting a better cooperation from the patient.

Date of birth and age: Date of birth and age of the patient should be recorded. Age factor is important in treatment planning (also refer to Chapter 6 on Clinical Significance of Growth). Briefly, we describe the importance of the age.

- It helps to get an idea of the growth status of the patient.
- It is also important to determine exact chronological age of the patient while doing research using his radiographs.
- **Self-correcting anomalies:** Certain malocclusion conditions are normal for that age and get corrected with growth. Age helps to determine the nature of malocclusion whether it is transient or established (e.g. ugly-duckling stage, etc.). Such conditions should not be disturbed with treatments.
- Certain Rx modalities are carried out during active growth period, e.g. growth modulation; while others may be carried out in post-growth period, e.g. surgery.
- There are certain conditions and such treatment modalities which if treated during active growth period give us the advantage of growth and neuromuscular adaptation leading to better and stable results, e.g. growth modifications, i.e.

treatment of growth problems like maxillary retrusion or mandible retrusion, expansions, etc. while other conditions should be treated in the post-growth period, e.g. orthognathic surgery.

Different Types of Ages

Biological age: It is determined from the skeletal, dental and morphological age and onset of puberty.

Skeletal age: It is determined from the radiographs, e.g. hand wrist; CVMI, etc. It is also called as biological clock. It is the best indicator to find the exact status of the growth and is the most important criteria to determine the course of treatment.

Chronological age: It is calculated from date of birth. It helps us to get an idea of the growth status of the patient. It helps to determine the nature of the malocclusion whether it is transient or established (e.g. ugly-ducking stage, etc.). The status of the child can be compared with the standards to determine whether the child is growing normally or not. However, this does not give us the exact status of growth.

Dental age: It is determined by the status of dental development and eruption. It can be determined by comparing the patient's dental status with the standard chronology tables of dental development. It can be determined by two methods: (1) stage of eruption of teeth and (2) stage of tooth mineralization on radiograph. A patient can have early dentition or delayed dentition. The stages of tooth development can be studied by Nolla's stage of dental development or by Demerijan's method.

The assessment of dental maturation from the panoramic radiographs can be done based on the method of Demirjian et al. They have described eight stages of calcification from A to H for each tooth.

Stage A: In both single-rooted and multi-rooted teeth, a beginning of calcification is seen at the superior level of the crypt. No fusion of these calcified points can be observed.

Stage B: Fusion of the calcified points forms one or more cusps which unite to give a regularly outlined occlusal surface.

Stage C: Enamel formation has been completed at the occlusal surface, and dentine formation has commenced. The pulp chamber is curved, and no pulp horns are visible.

Stage D: Crown formation has been completed to the level of the cementoenamel junction. Root formation has commenced. The pulp horns are beginning to differentiate, but the walls of the pulp chamber remain curved.

Stage E: The root length remains shorter than the crown height. The walls of the pulp chamber are straight, and the pulp horns have become more differentiated than in the previous stage. In molars, the radicular bifurcation has started to calcify.

Stage F: The walls of the pulp chamber now form an isosceles triangle, and the root length is equal to or greater than the crown height. In molars, the bifurcation has developed sufficiently to give roots a distinct form.

Stage G: The walls of the root canal are now parallel, but the apical end is still partially open.

Stage H: The apical end of the root canal is completely closed and the periodontal membrane is uniform around the root and the apex.

The Nolla's dental developmental stages are given below (Fig. 13.1).

Stage 0: Absence of crypt

Stage 1: Presence of crypt

Stage 2: Initial calcification

Stage 3: One-third of crown completed

Stage 4: Two-thirds of crown completed

Stage 5: Crown almost completed

Stage 6: Crown completed

Stage 7: One-third of root completed

Stage 8: Two-thirds of root completed

Stage 9: Root almost complete; open apex

Stage 10: Apical end of root completed.

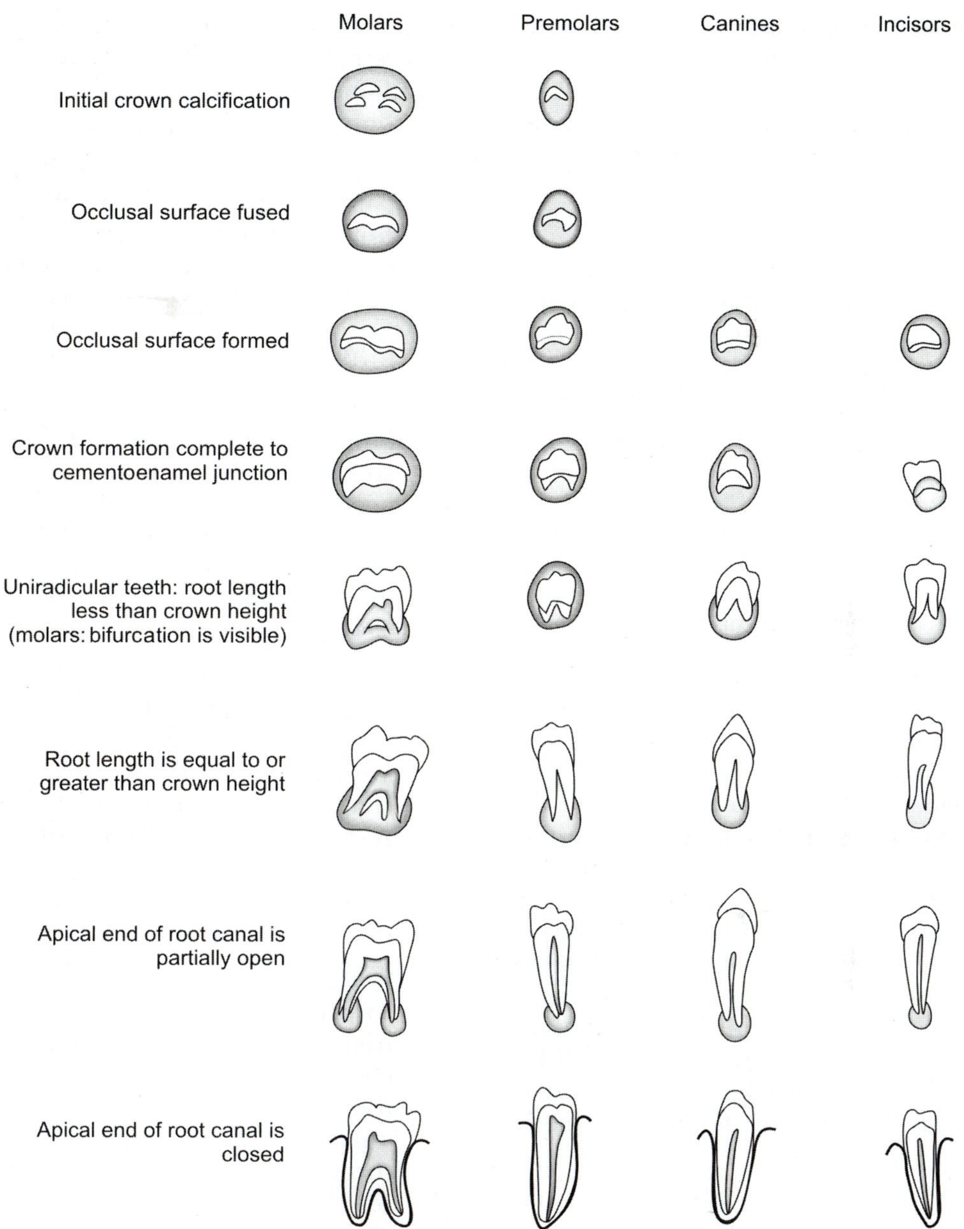

Fig. 13.1: Various stages of dental development as described by Nolla.

Sex: Growth spurts and events occur at different times in boys and girls. Growth in girls is 2–3 years ahead of boys, i.e. girls attain puberty and growth termination earlier than boys. Timing and number of growth spurts differ in males and females. Onset of growth spurts occurs at an early age in females than males. So, the growth modification (with, e.g. functional appliance) needs to be started earlier in females than the males, i.e. in late mixed dentition period in females, while in males it can be delayed till early permanent dentition period. Similarly, the expansion of maxillary arch in females has to be started before the males. If we think to start this treatment at the same age at early permanent dentition period for both sexes, then by the time we start the treatment, the active growth spurt in females may have passed while in boys, it is beginning to start.

Address, phone number and occupation of patient/ parents: Contact information of patient are important, as it helps to evaluate socioeconomic status (gives an idea of nutrition, prevalent diseases, awareness of the Rx, etc.). It also helps in selection of appliance and gives an idea of expected cooperation from the patient. Address and phone number is important for future correspondence, e.g. for reminding/resetting of the appointments; reminders for failed payments, etc.

Chief complaint: A patient who visits a doctor may have more than one problem but he tells the doctor the most bothersome problem first and then may be the other problems. Also, he may or may not be aware of the other problems. This chief complaint should be noted in patient's own words. It gives an idea about the priorities and desires of the patient. It should be discussed thoroughly and limitation of the Rx should be well informed. It also helps in discussing the treatment procedures and the results, as sometimes patients may say that they did not come with such a problem or they did not understand the scientific terms explained to them.

It is better if they write it themselves in the form provided to them. Alongwith, they should be informed about other problems also and their effect on the treatment planning, prognosis, cost and timing.

Medical history: A thorough medical history should be recorded. There are certain conditions in which orthodontic treatment may not be feasible to start or there may be inhibition of tooth movements. In certain conditions, there may be more chances of root resorption; while other warrant extra precautions to prevent cross-infections or bacteremia. However, there are few medical conditions which contraindicate the use of the orthodontic appliances, e.g.

- It is desirable to delay orthodontic Rx in patients suffering from epilepsy unless controlled. If the uncontrolled epileptic patient uses a removable appliance, it may get broken and the pieces may be aspirated by the patient leading to further complications.
- **Blood dyscrasias, e.g. hemophilia, leukemia, congenital heart conditions, sickle cell anemia, thalassemia, etc.** may need special management and antibiotic cover if extraction is required. There are abnormal bone and tissue response during orthodontics in such cases, e.g. sickle cell anemia, thalassemia, etc.
- **Mental and/or physical conditions** require special management. A violent, uncontrolled child will break the appliances and there will always be a chance of aspiration of broken elements. A depressed child will not cooperate with instructions and oral hygiene procedures, lending to failure of treatment. A proper cooperation will be a problem.
- **Trauma to jaws:** An insight into the history of facial and dental trauma should always be done. It may lead to disturbance to the jaw growth, TMJ ankylosis; facial asymmetry and disturbed occlusion. Trauma to teeth may lead to root fractures and resorption, mobility of teeth, nonvital teeth requiring RCT, calcified root canals, periapical pathoses, etc.
- Patients with uncontrolled diabetes have abnormal tissue response like gingival overgrowth, increased mobility of teeth, more bone resorption, infections, etc. A proper care is taken in such patients regarding force magnitude. A controlled diabetic can undergo orthodontic Rx like normal child but

should take proper care about oral hygiene, etc.

- **Osteoporosis and arthritis:** These patients are regularly on NSAIDs which slow the orthodontic response due to their prostaglandin inhibiting effects.
- **Rheumatic fever, artificial heart valves or cardiac anomaly** require antibiotic coverage during banding, extractions, oral prophylaxis, any minor or major surgical intervention, etc. to avoid SABE. Refer to section on antibiotic prophylaxis schedule.
- **Nasal conditions and related respiratory diseases** may affect normal growth of face and jaws by changing the head and jaw postures, while patient resorts to mouth breathing. It also leads to deficient development of nasal passage, nasal bone and bridge.
- Certain patients on cancer therapy with zoledronic acid given in certain conditions, like postmenopausal osteoporosis, etc. there is completely stopped tooth movement. This drug inhibits the osteoclasts and thus the bone resoprtion does not occur.
- In certain infections, like HIV, Hep B, Hep C, etc., special precautions should be taken to avoid needle stick or wire injuries, to avoid cross-infections.
- **Endocrine problems:** Patients on hormone replacement therapy should be dealt carefully. The details have been discussed in Chapter 63 on Drugs and Orthodontics.

Drug History

A complete drug history should be taken, as it may give idea of underlying diseases, which the patient is not able to express or never wanted to tell. Also certain drugs like aspirin, ibuprofen, steroids, etc. (inhibit prostaglandin synthesis may slow tooth movement); phenytoin sodium, immunosuppressants, etc. (may cause gingival enlargement).

Dental History

It should include the approximate time of eruption of primary and permanent teeth, history of extractions of teeth, restoration and trauma to dentition, etc. Knowledge of eruption schedule gives an idea of any delayed or fast eruption, which may be related with underlying endocrine problem.

History of any previous dental treatment and patient's experience gives an idea of patients and parents' attitude toward the treatment and their cooperation, e.g. a patient who had taken orthodontic treatment with removable appliance but did not cooperate and thus was not satisfied with the results, may put blame on the doctor and his treatment plan.

Prenatal History

It should include information on conditions of mother, status of nutrition, diseases, etc. during pregnancy and the type of delivery (forceps delivery may cause injury to TMJ and resulting growth abnormalities). Drugs taken during pregnancy should be noted, e.g. Tetracycline (staining of teeth); alcohol (fetal alcohol syndrome, CLP), thalidomide (defective limbs), etc. smoking by expecting mother; history of German measles to mother may lead to certain congenital problems in infant. Chemical and other agents capable of producing embryologic defects if given at the critical time are called teratogens. Some of the teratogens are given below. Aspirin, dilantin, cigarette smoke (hypoxia) cause cleft lip and palate; 6-mercaptopurine causes cleft palate; X-radiation can cause microcephaly; valium leads to CLP; while vitamin D excess can cause premature suture closure.

Postnatal History

This should include information on the type of feeding and nutrition, abnormal oral habits, milestones of normal developments and childhood diseases along with the drugs taken for the treatment, e.g. cystic fibrosis. Steroids taken for treatment of certain diseases affect bone growth. Milestones are certain physiological developmental stages which are achieved during the growth of an average child, e.g. social smiling; following the finger movements; sitting without support; standing; walking with support and without support, etc.

Family History

It gives an idea about the etiology of malocclusion, since there is always a genetic component to the condition, e.g. Hapsburg jaws, a skeletal class III condition of a German royal family; CLP; class II division 2, etc. Even the tooth size, shape, number, etc. are also genetically related. Monozygotic twins have more similar dental and skeletal conditions than the dizygotic twins.

Siblings: Number of siblings in a family and their dental health condition gives a good idea of the socioeconomic status of family and hereditary nature of malocclusion. More number of children per family means the nutrition may be deficient leading to growth problems, lack of cooperation from parents and patients, etc.

Social History

It helps to assess patient's affordability to bear the cost of the treatment and cooperation/ availability of patients for treatment during the entire treatment in follow-up. It also gives an idea of patient's attitude toward Rx and awareness.

General Examination

It is the assessment of general physical conditions of the patient, i.e. general health, stature, body type and posture, etc. Generally, the clinician starts to observe these features as soon as the patient enters the clinics.

- **Height and weight:** These findings provide a clue to assess physical growth and maturation; and future growth. It gives an idea of dentofacial growth and maturation. Some children are early maturers and gain height early in life, and also their growth is completed early; while some are late-maturers and they grow till later age.
- **Gait:** Gait is the way a person walks. It helps to assess any neuromuscular disorder. Certain disorders lead to skeletodentofacial problems, like crowding, narrow arches, mouth breathing, weaker muscles, abnormal facial growth, etc. and should be considered in treatment planning.
- **Posture:** It is the body position when a person stands. Abnormal postures affect craniocervical and maxillomandibular relationship, thus leading to malocclusion, e.g. scoliosis, kyphosis, etc. affect the alignment of spine and thus the cranium.
- **Body build/physique:** It also gives an idea of size and growth of facial bones. It has an association with the width of jaw bones and dental arches. The body has been classified in three types as follows:
  a. **Esthetic:** The person is thin (it is usually associated with narrow, V-shaped dental arches).
  b. **Plethoric:** The person is obese (it is usually associated with wide, square dental arches).
  c. **Athletic:** It is an average physique, (it is usually associated with average dental arches).

Sheldon has divided body types as:

- **Ectomorphic:** The person is tall and thin;
- **Mesomorphic:** The person is of average built.
- **Endomorphic:** The person is short and obese.

Extraoral Examination

It provides important information for diagnosis and treatment planning. A judgment of facial esthetics is very important which has to be balanced with the existing skeletal and soft tissue relationship. The face has to be evaluated in all the three planes, with the 4th dimension added as the "time", which indicates the active or completed growth period.

Extraoral components:
- Facial and growth pattern
- Asymmetry
- Profile
- Vertical imbalance
- Transverse imbalance

Transverse relationship:
- Facial asymmetry
- Cant of occlusal plane
- Posterior crossbites
- Skeletal midline
- Dental midline
- Horizontal fifths of the face
- Smile relationship

Sagittal relationships:
- Profile / nasolabial angle / nose size / chin position / mentolabial suclus / lip fullness and lip step.
- Skeletal facial pattern, face depth
- Facial divergence
- Angle's classification
- Canine relation
- Incisor relation, i.e. overjet
- Smile pattern

Vertical relationship:
- Deep or open bite or normal bite.
- Vertical facial height: small, average, large
- Vertical thirds of face
- Ratio of upper and lower face heights
- Lip competency
- Growth pattern.

Examination of face: It has to be evaluated in three planes of space, i.e. transverse, sagittal, and vertical. Ackermann and Proffit has defined their classification system in three planes in the sequence of transverse, sagittal, and vertical (TSV = WDH) planes, (it can be remembered that the sequence of growth completion of face is also in this sequence), thus the examination of face and intraoral examination should also be done in this sequence.

Transverse relationship:
- Facial asymmetry
- Cant of occlusal plane
- Posterior crossbites
- Skeletal midline
- Dental midline
- Horizontal fifths of the face.

Sagittal relationships:
- Profile / nasolabial angle / nose size / chin position / mentolabial suclus / lip fullness
- Skeletal facial pattern
- Angle's classification
- Canine relation
- Incisor relation—overjet
- Lip competency
- Smile pattern.

Vertical relationship:
- Deep or open bite
- Vertical facial height
- Vertical thirds of face
- Ratio of upper and lower face heights.

Morphologic analysis:

Shape of the head: It is observed from standing behind the patient, viewing at a right angle to the cranium. It provides an idea of growth pattern, and size and shape of dental arches. Shape of head is associated with the shape of face and dental arches shape.

Formula and value of cephalic index given by Martin and Saller 1957: Width of skull is measured between most prominent points on pariental bone, and the length of skull is measured from occipital to frontal bones between most prominent points.

$$\text{Cephalic index} = \frac{\text{Maximum skull width}}{\text{Maximum skull length}}$$

- Normal value = 76–80.9%
- Dolichocephalic: < 75.9
- Brachycephalic: > 81.

Based on the cephalic index, it can be divided in three types (Fig. 13.2):

1. **Brachycephalic:** The head is broad and short. The dental arch is wider. There may be spaces present in the arches.
2. **Dolichocephalic:** The head is long and narrow. The arches are narrow and V-shaped. Crowding may be present in these arches.

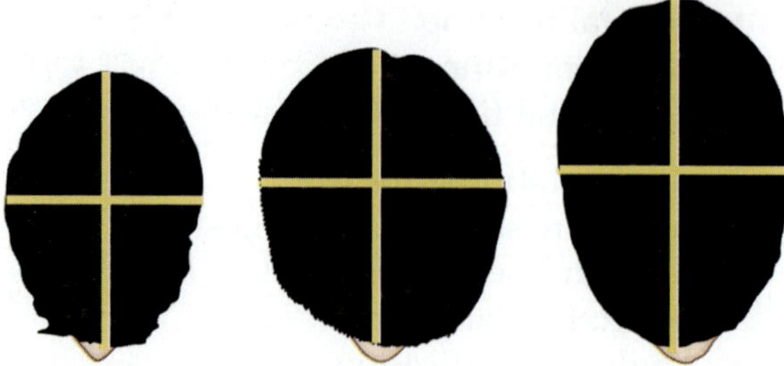

Fig. 13.2: Normo-, meso- and dolichocephalic shapes of head.

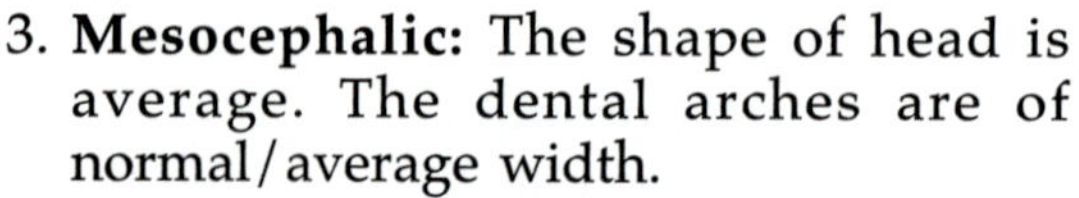

3. **Mesocephalic:** The shape of head is average. The dental arches are of normal/average width.

Facial type/form (Figs 13.3 and 13.4): It also provides clues about the growth pattern, shape and size of dental arches and presence of crowding or spacing. In simple terms, face can be classified as round, square or oval. However, based on facial index, the face is divided in following three types.

1. **Euryprosopic:** The face is short and broad. The dental arches are broad and wide. It corresponds to brachycephalic head form.
2. **Leptoprosopic:** The face is long and narrow. The dental arches are narrow. It corresponds to dolichocephalic head form.

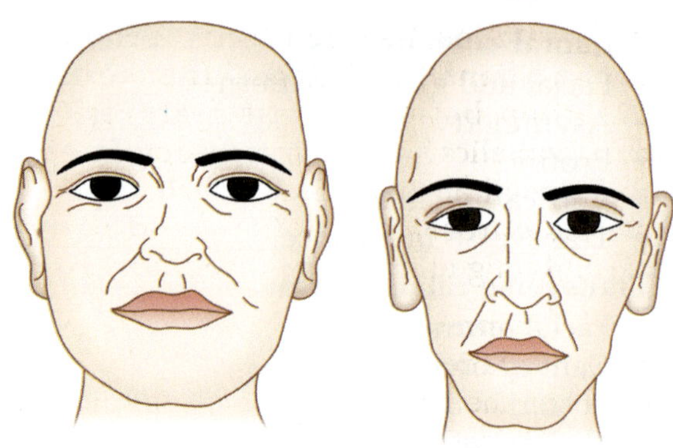

Fig. 13.3: Euryprosopic and leptoprosopic faces.

3. **Mesoprosopic:** The face and dental arches are of average size. It corresponds to mesocephalic head form.

Formula and value of Facial Index given by Martin and Saller 1957: Height of face is measured between points nasion–gnathion, and width of face is measured from point Zy-Zy.

$$\text{F. I} = \frac{\text{Morphologic facial height (Nasion—gnathion)} \times 100}{\text{Morphologic bizygomatic width}}$$

Normal value: 84–87.9%
Euryprosopic: < 84%
Mesoprosopic: 84–87.9%
Leptoprosopic: > 88%.

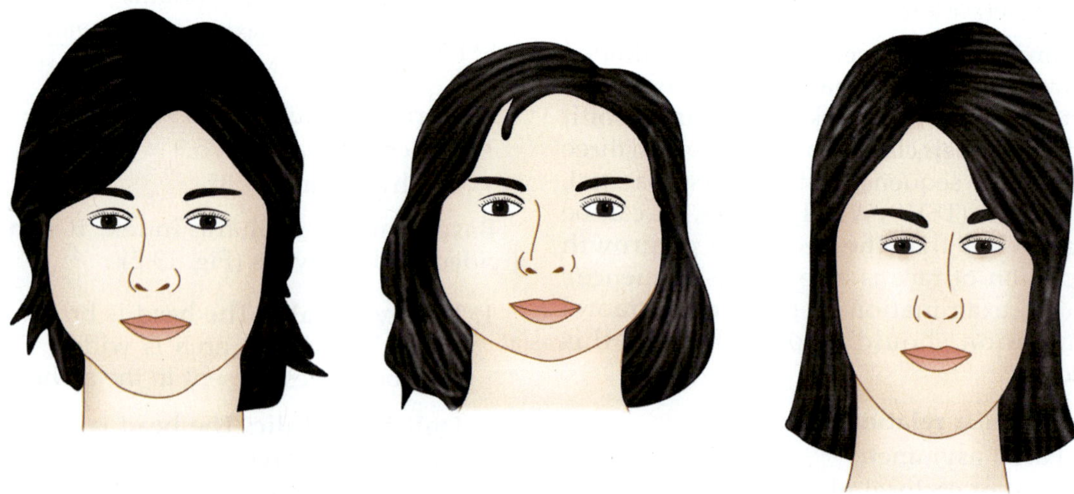

Fig. 13.4: Different facial types: mesoprosopic, euryprosopic and leptoprosopic.

Inter-relation between facial form, head form and dental arch form: There exists a correlation between these features. The brachycephalics have a euryprosopic face and broad dental arches; while dolichocephalics have leptoprosopic face (long and narrow face) and long and narrow dental arches.

Facial symmetry: To assess the symmetry of face, the patient's face is viewed either from the top of the cranium or from standing in front of the patient. It helps to determine the facial disharmony in transverse and vertical planes. There is always some degree of asymmetry present between the right and left sides of face, which is not much appreciable and is a normal feature. However, gross facial asymmetry may be due to many factors like trauma and impaired growth, certain congenital conditions, hemifacial atrophy or hypertrophy or unilateral condylar ankylosis and hyperplasia, etc. Gross asymmetry leads to a multitude of malocclusion conditions, malrelation of jaws and growth discrepancies.

Assessment of vertical skeletal relationships: The face is evaluated in vertical plane to determine the face height, growth pattern, the facial proportions and balance, etc. This information helps in treatment planning and prognosis.

Vertical thirds of the face (Figs 13.5a and b): Face can be divided in three parts in a vertical plane by passing lines through hair line; supraorbital ridge; base of the nose and inferior border of the chin. They are designated as upper, middle and lower third of face. In a well-proportioned face, these three parts are almost equal.

Lower third of face can be divided in two parts by passing line through the junction of lips. The upper lip occupies upper one-third part; while lower lip and chin occupy lower two-thirds part.

A markedly increased lower third face height is associated with vertical growth pattern and skeletal open bite. A decreased lower third face is due to horizontal growth pattern and skeletal deep bite.

The FMA angle, i.e. between FHP and MP can also be used for vertical estimation, a value of 25–30° is normal (Figs 13.6 and 13.7).

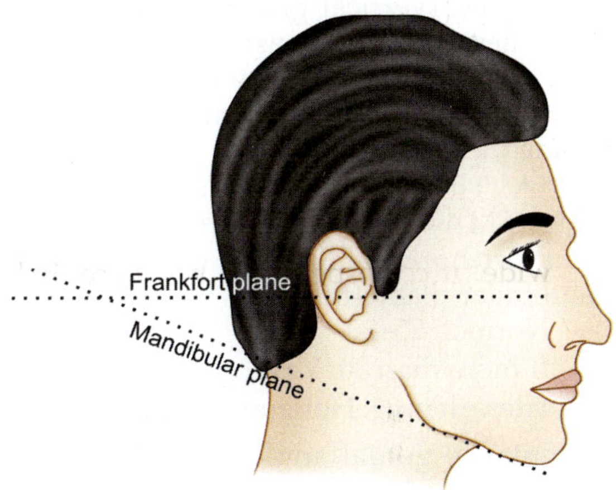

Fig. 13.6: Examining the Frankfort—mandibular plane angle clinically

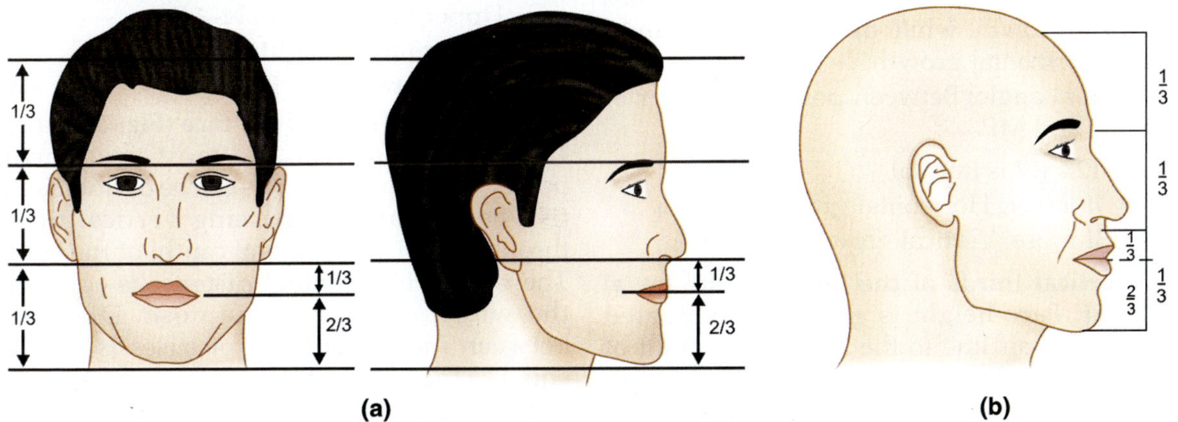

Figs 13.5a and b: Different vertical thirds of the face.

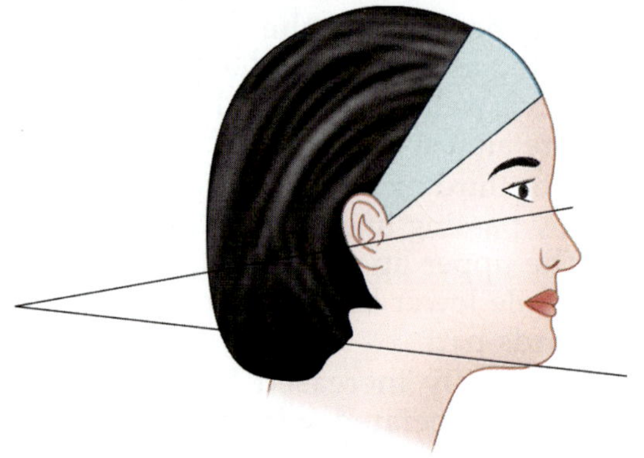

Fig. 13.7: Evaluation of Frankfort mandibular plane angle extraorally.

Location of the point of intersection of these two planes is estimated. Normally, these planes meet at the occipital region. In high angle cases, (vertical growth), these planes meet anteriorly in the mastoid region. In low angle cases (horizontal growth), these planes become more parallel and meet posteriorly outside the skull.

FMA: The Frankfort mandibular plane angle (FMA) which is made between the Frankfort horizontal plane (FHP) and the mandibular plane (MP).

- Normal: 25–30
- If more than 30: Vertical growth pattern
- If less than 25: Horizontal growth pattern

Similarly, gonial angle formed between posterior border of ramus and the lower border of mandible is also an indication for vertical estimation. A value of 128 $\pm$ 7 is considered normal. Increased value indicates vertical growth, while decreased value indicates horizontal growth.

Gonial angle: Between posterior border of ramus and MP:

- 128 $\pm$ 7 is normal
- If lesser: Horizontal growth pattern
- If more: Vertical growth pattern.

Vertical thirds of the face and the facial height: Face height is generally evaluated from the hair line to the lowermost point of chin. Vertically, the face can be divided in three equal parts: (1) upper, (2) middle and (3) lower third, in a balanced face, i.e. hairline to glabella; glabella to the base of the nose; and from the base of the nose to the lowermost point of chin.

Clinically, the vertical skeletal relations are assessed with face in profile and the teeth in occlusion, an estimate should be made of lower face height as a proportion of the total face height. From an orthodontist point of view, the face is divided in two equal halves vertically: distance from glabella (a point between eyebrows) to the base of the nose (junction of the nose with the upper lip) and distance from the base of the nose to the underside of the chin (Fig. 13.8).

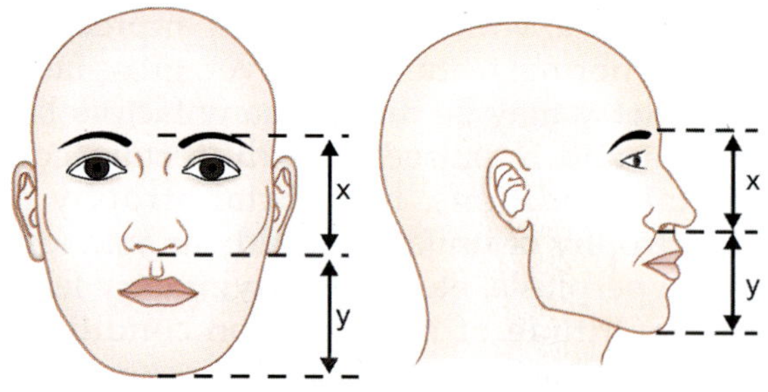

Fig. 13.8: Comparison of upper (x) and lower face heights (y): normally, ratio of x and y is 1 : 1.2.

Proportions of lips: Upper lip is one-third of lower third of face; and lower lip and chin are two-thirds of lower third of the face.

Cephalometrically, the total facial height is measure between N and Me points. It has two components, i.e. upper and lower facial height, i.e. between N-ANS and ANS-Me points.

- Total face height: N-Me
- Upper facial height: N-ANS
- Lower facial height: ANS-Me
- Normal ratio: UFH: LFH is 45:55 or 1: 1.2.

Horizontal fifths of the face (Figs 13.9 and 13.10): Face between the most prominent points on zygomatic bones can be divided into five equal parts by passing vertical lines through medial and lateral canthi of the eyes. The medial intercanthal distance is equal to the width of base of the nose. Distance between medial borders of irises is nearly equal to the width of mouth.

Facial profile analysis (Fig. 13.11): Facial profile is the outline of face as seen from the

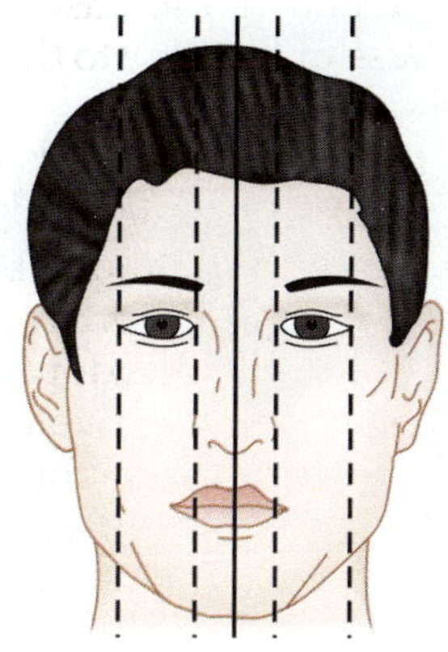

Fig. 13.9: Horizontal fifths of the face.

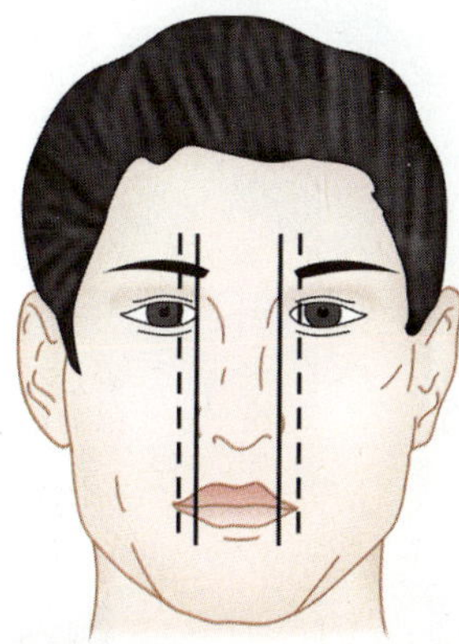

Fig. 13.10: Normal relation of nose width, width of mouth, and interpupillary width.

lateral view. It is also known as "poor man's cephalometric analysis". It helps in diagnosis of gross deviations in the relation of upper and lower jaws in sagittal and vertical dimensions. Profile also gives an idea of growth pattern and rotations. The profile is studied by relating the following three points:

1. Glabella, i.e. between eyebrows
2. At base of nose
3. Most anterior point of soft chin, i.e. soft tissue nasion, subnasale and pogonion.

It is assessed by studying the relation of two lines.

1. Line from forehead to soft tissue point A, the deepest point in curvature of upper lip (Gl′-A′).
2. Line from soft tissue point A to the soft tissue point Pog, the most prominent point on the chin outline (A′-Pog′).

Position of the patient: The patient is seated in the natural head position by either sitting upright or standing. Following 3 profiles can exist (Figs 13.11 to 13.16).

Straight profile: If these two lines form nearly a straight line ± 2 mm.

Convex profile: If these two lines form an inner angle much less than 180°, with the chin positioned behind. It may be due to maxillary prognathism or mandibular retrognathism or combination of both. It is generally seen in

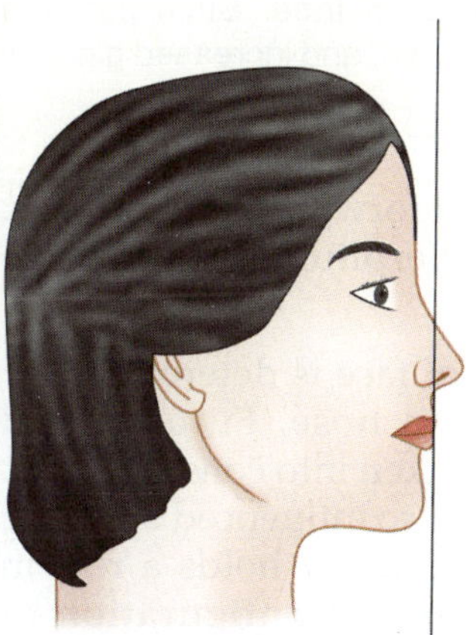

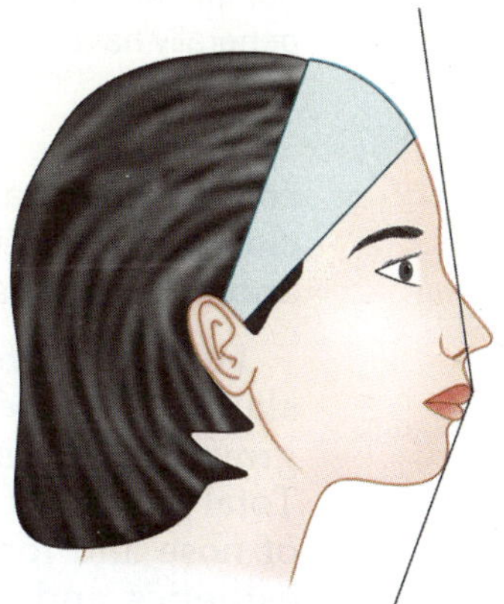

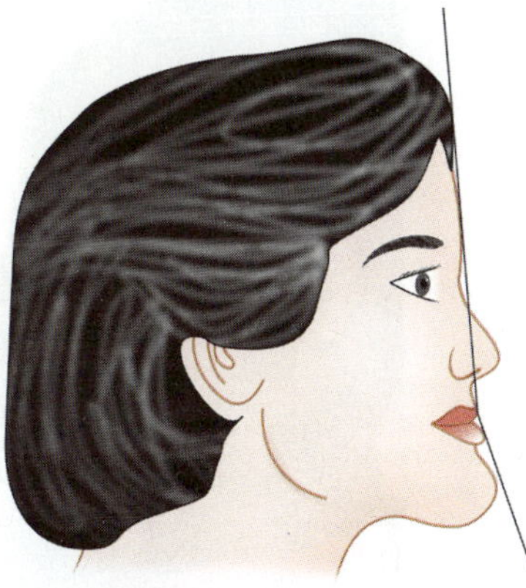

Fig. 13.11: Facial profile: straight; convex and concave.

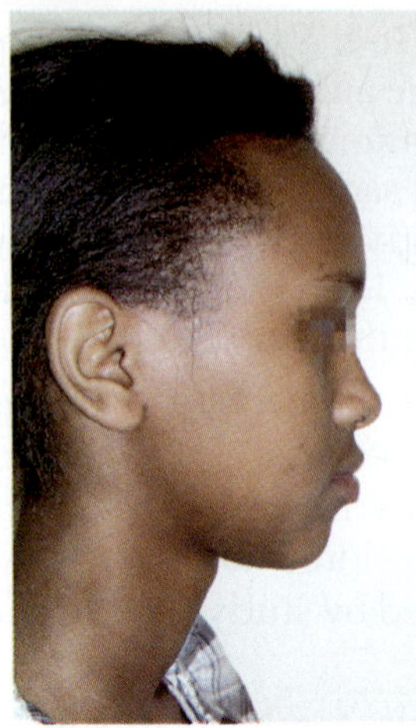

Fig. 13.12: Straight profile.

skeletal class II relations. It is more prominent in class II division 1 malocclusions and vertical growth patterns, where mandible gets rotated in downward and backward directions, i.e. anticlockwise.

Concave profiles: If these two lines form an inner angle much more than 180°, with the chin positioned forward. It may be due to maxillary retrognathism or mandibular prognathism or combination of both. It is seen in skeletal class III relation; forward closure of mandible due to premature contacts in incisor region, e.g. in pseudo-class III cases and the growth pattern where mandible gets rotated in upward and forward directions, i.e. clockwise, e.g. in hyperpituitarism, cleft lip and palate cases, etc.

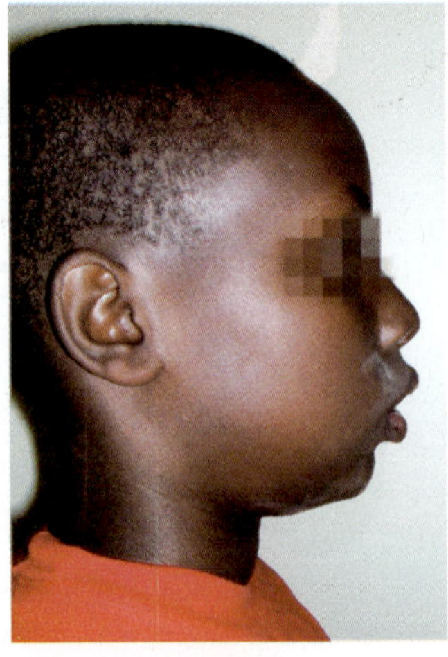

Fig. 13.13: Convex profile.

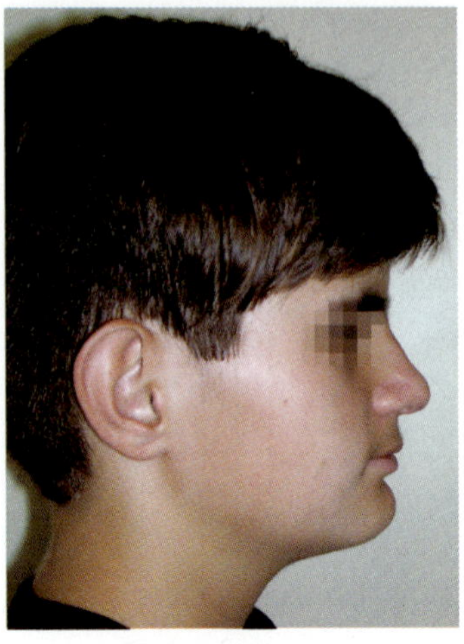

(a)

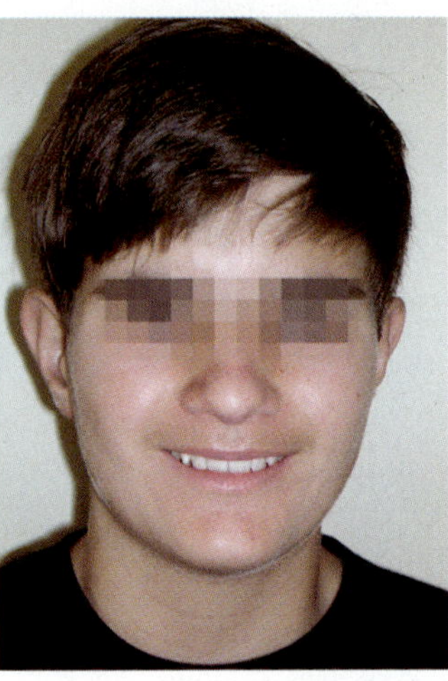

(b)

Figs 13.14a and b: Horizontal growth, prominent gonial region, and squarish face. Such patients generally have deep bite also, and increased gingival exposure.

Forehead: Profile of face is determined by slant of forehead and nose. Future nasal growth must also be taken into consideration. Total profile of face is also influenced by shape of nose and forehead; and it holds a role in esthetics and prognosis. Configuration of forehead is mainly racial and ethnic; it varies with age and gender. Lateral forehead contour

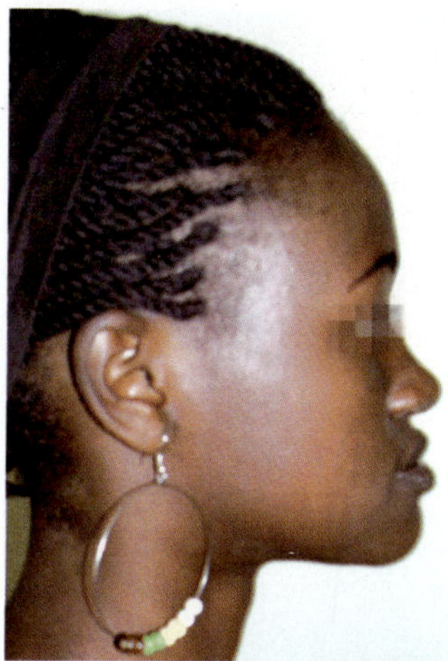

Fig. 13.15: Concave profile.

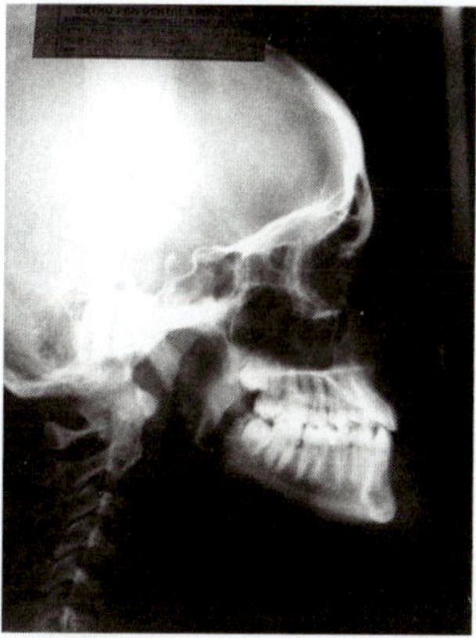

Fig. 13.16: Lateral cephalogram showing almost horizontal growth of face and skeletal deep bite.

can be flat; protruding or slanting steep/ oblique in different races. In steep forehead, the dental bases are more prognathic.

Facial divergence (Figs 13.17 and 13.18): Divergence is the anterior or posterior inclination of lower face in relation to forehead. It is studied in straight profile cases, and it may be of following types.

Straight/orthognathic: The line is straight and almost perpendicular to the floor.

Anterior divergent: The line is inclined anteriorly at the chin, i.e. slope of profile line is forward. Here, chin seems to be prominent.

Posterior divergent: The line is inclined posteriorly at the chin, i.e. slope of profile line is backward. Here, chin seems to be deficient.

Divergence is related to racial and ethnic background. It does not indicate a problem. But, concavity or convexity of profile may indicate an orthodontic problem.

Assessment of sagittal/AP jaw relationship: Skeletal patterns can be assessed clinically by seating the patient in an upright posture looking straight ahead, with the eyes directed at the horizon keeping, head in relaxed natural postural position (Fig. 13.19). Then, the relationship of soft tissue points A and B is assessed by using the index and middle fingers of the hand.

Maxillary base should lie about 2–3 mm anterior to the mandibular base when the teeth are in occlusion in skeletal class I. It is also called as orthognathic facial pattern. The position of hand is almost parallel to the ground.

In prognathic facial pattern or skeletal class II, the chin is behind, so the inclination of hand points upwards.

In retrognathic facial pattern or skeletal class III, the chin is forward, so the inclination of the hand points downwards.

Lips (Figs 13.19a and b): Lips are important components of face. They affect the smile and profile of face and hence esthetics. There are many factors affecting the morphology of lips like racial/ethnic; thickness of soft tissues; tonicity of orbicularis and mentalis ms; position of incisors: overjet/overbite; configuration of bony bases; and lip dysfunction, e.g. in mouth breathing; lip biting; sucking, etc.

During examination, you should look for the competence; size; position during rest; lip line; tone; position during smile, etc. Also, the lip length; width and curvature are studied. Normally, upper lip covers the entire labial surface of the upper incisors except incisal 2–3 mm at rest position. The lower lip covers the lower anteriors and the 2–3 mm of upper anteriors, i.e. incisal one-third of the upper anteriors at rest.

Length of upper lip is one-third (Sn-Sto) and the lower lip + chin (Sto-Me) is two-thirds of lower third of face height. In certain cases, e.g. with mouth breathing, thumb sucking, etc.

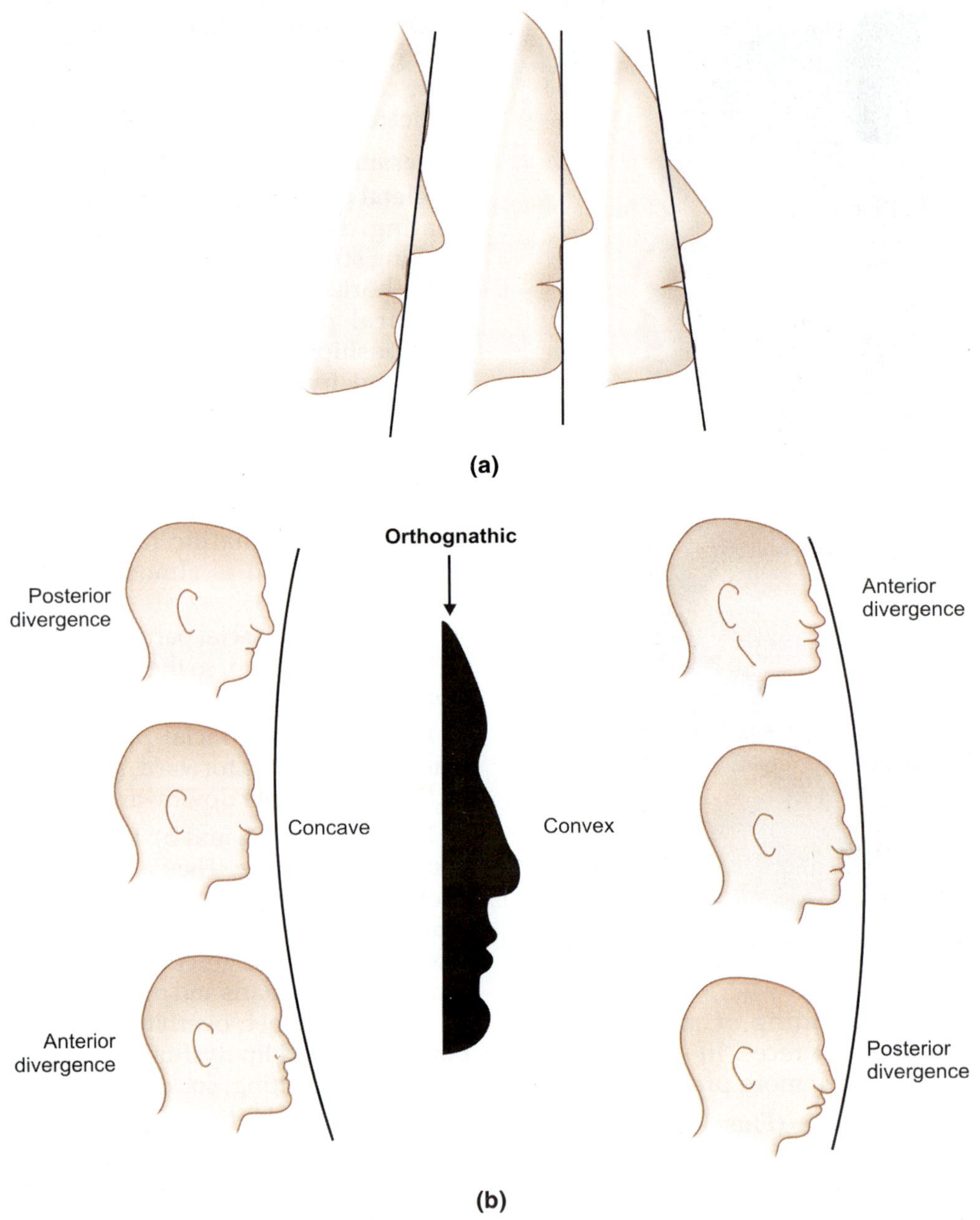

Figs 13.17a and b: Divergence pattern of a straight profile: posteriorly divergent, normodivergent, and anteriorly divergent

the upper lip is shorter and thus lips are incompetent.

Lip line: It is the crest of lower lip with respect to upper anteriors at rest.

In class II division 1, the lip line remains lower. In class II division 2, the lip line remains much higher occasionally covering the entire labial surface of the incisors, which is due to over-eruption of maxillary incisors.

Lips during smile (Figs 13.21 to 13.25):

- At rest, upper lip covers upto the junction of incisal and middle 3rd of

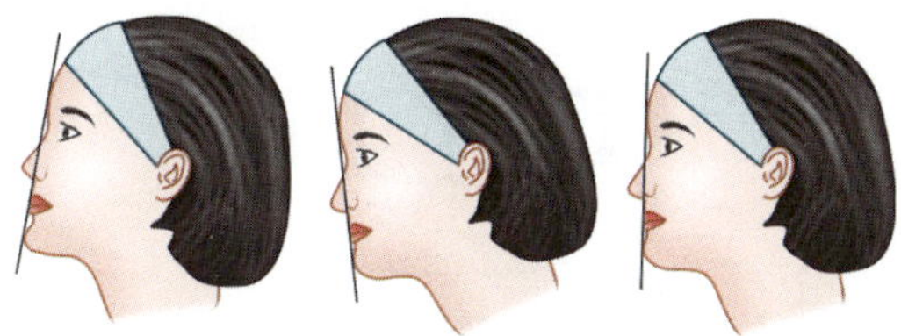

Fig. 13.18: Divergence of straight facial profiles: anteriorly divergent; posteriorly divergent, and normodivergent in that order.

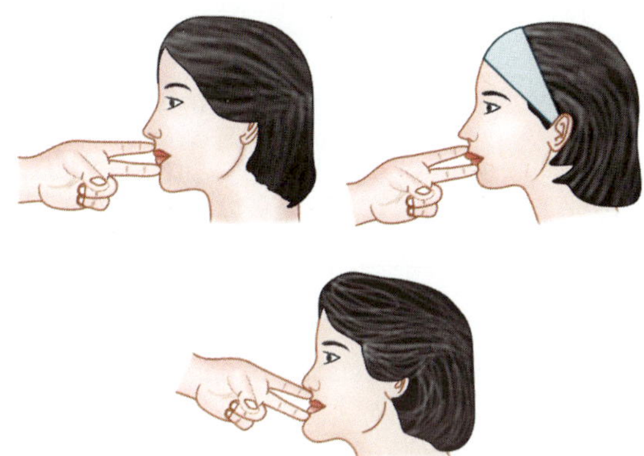

Fig. 13.19: Evaluation of the skeletal relation of the jaws during clinical examination of a patient, using index and middle fingers of the hand. In class I, the hand remains parallel to ground; in class II, the hand is bent towards the ground, while in class III, the hand is bent away from the ground.

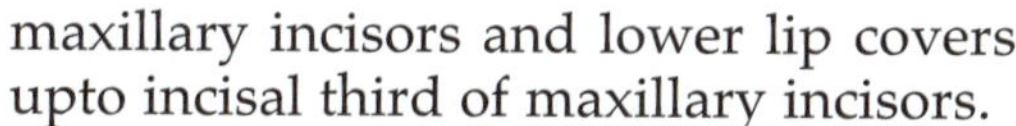

maxillary incisors and lower lip covers upto incisal third of maxillary incisors.

- At smile, the lower border of upper lip normally lies at $\pm$ 2 mm of the gingival margin of upper incisors. Smile arc, i.e. the upper margin of lower lip follows the incisal edges contour of upper anteriors, known as the consonant smile.
- Ideal exposure with smile is three quarters of upper incisor crown height to 2 mm of gingiva, it is more in females than in males. Lower lip lies parallel to the line joining the incisal edges of upper anteriors. It is then known as consonant smile.
- The smile may be toothy or gummy in case of abnormal morphology, e.g. deep bite, etc. Excess gingival exposure may

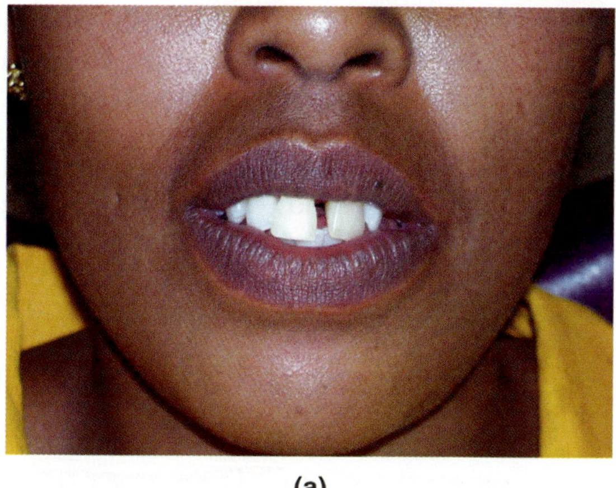

(a)

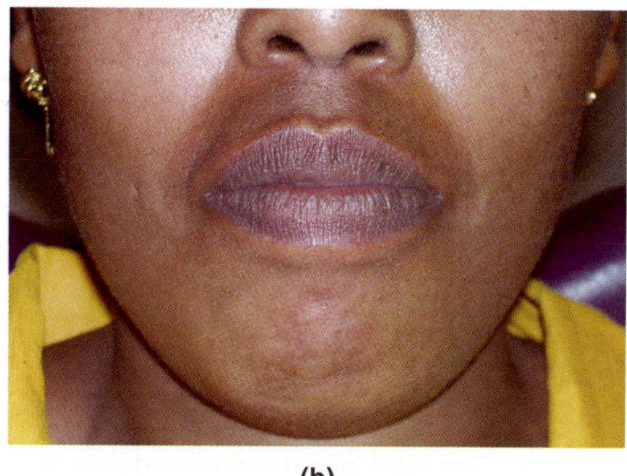

(b)

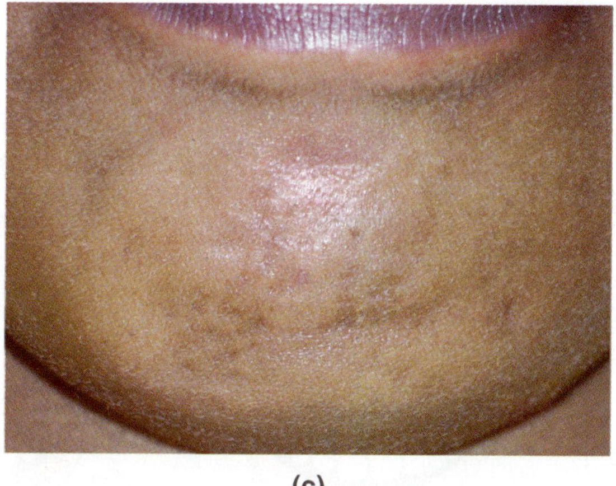

(c)

Figs 13.20a to c: There is puckering of chin tissues when incompetent lips are closed forcibly.

be caused by a short upper lip, vertical maxillary excess, long clinical crown, and/or large lip elevation with smiling. Deficient exposure etiologic factors include a long upper lip, vertical maxillary deficiency, and/or minimal smile lip elevation.

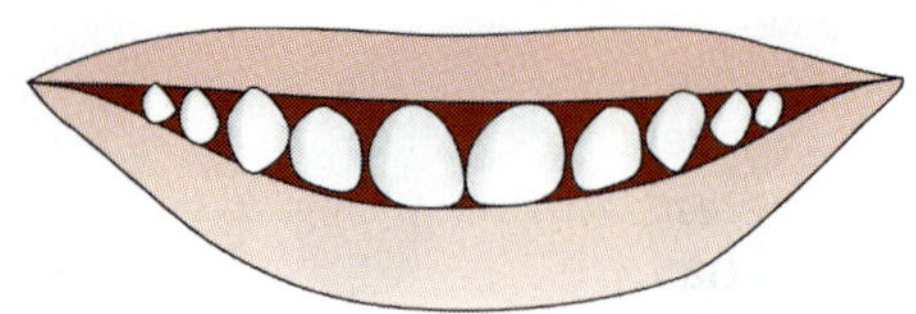

Fig. 13.21: An ideal consonant smile with border of upper lip is at the level of upper gingival margins, while the curve of lower lip follows the incisal curvature of upper anterior teeth.

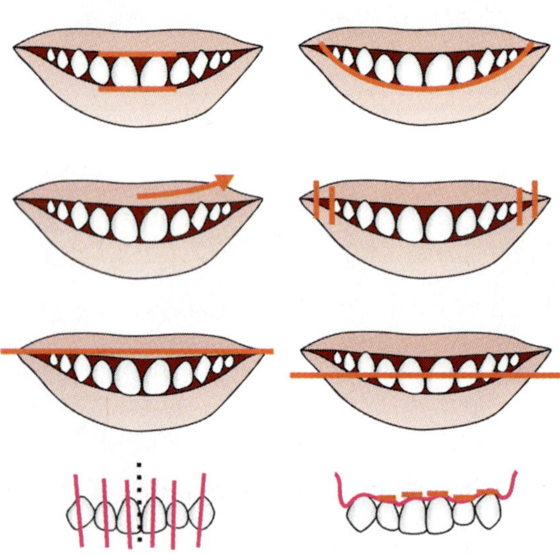

Fig. 13.22: The ideal incisal exposure during smile; lower lip relation to upper incisal edges; upper lip raise; buccal corridor; parallelism of OP; axial inclinations of upper anterior teeth; and level of gingival margins of upper anterior teeth.

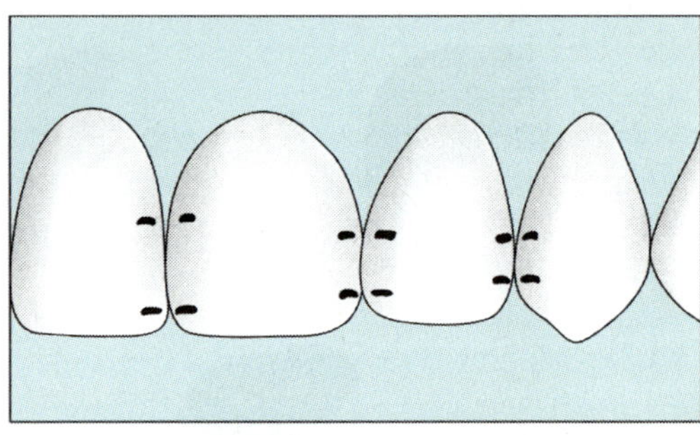

Fig. 13.23: The ideal relation of upper anterior teeth to each other.

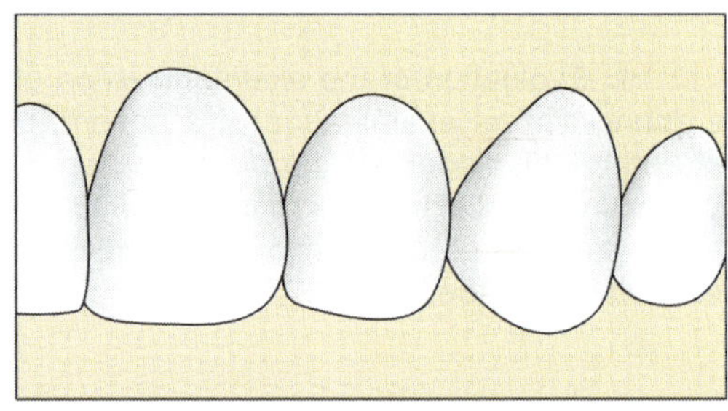

Fig. 13.24: The ideal relation of contact areas of upper anterior teeth to each other.

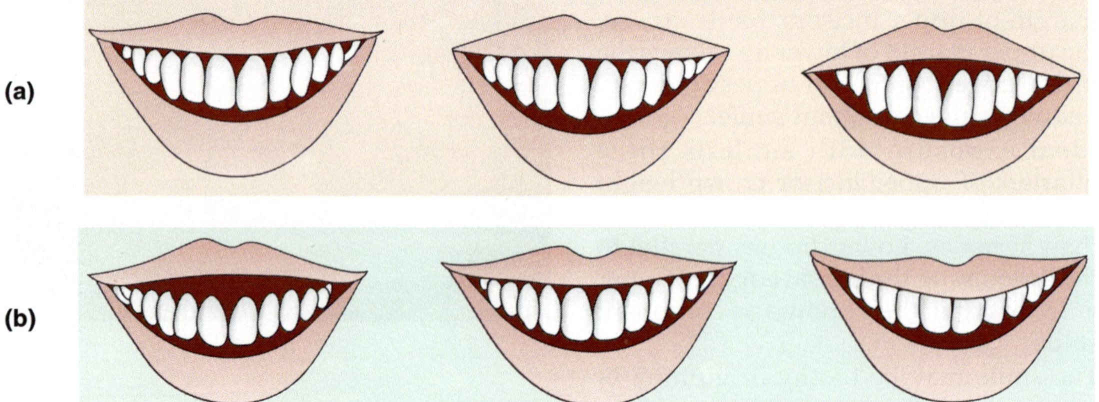

Figs 13.25a and b: The different types of smiles, e.g. ideal smile, gummy smile, etc.

Lip competency/seal: Three relationships are generally seen.

- **Competent lips:** Lips are in contact at rest or have 1–2 mm gap, without any effort.
- **Incompetent lips** (Figs 13.26a and b): Gap between lips at rest is more. It should be evaluated carefully because patient may close the lips deliberately which appears as puckering of chin soft tissue, i.e. orange peel appearance. Upper lip appears stretched and thinned with reduction of philtrum details. Flattening out of submental fold of lower lip and the dimpling over the anterior surface of chin are signs of contracted muscles. Incompetent lips can be due to various causes, e.g. short upper lip; increased dentoalveolar protrusion; mouth breathing; vertical growth pattern/long face, etc.
- **Potentially-competent lips:** The lips are of normal morphology and length, but due to extreme proclination of teeth, they remain incompetent.
- **Everted lips:** These are the hypertrophied lips with weak muscular tonicity, are associated with proclined teeth, e.g. in mouth breathing cases.

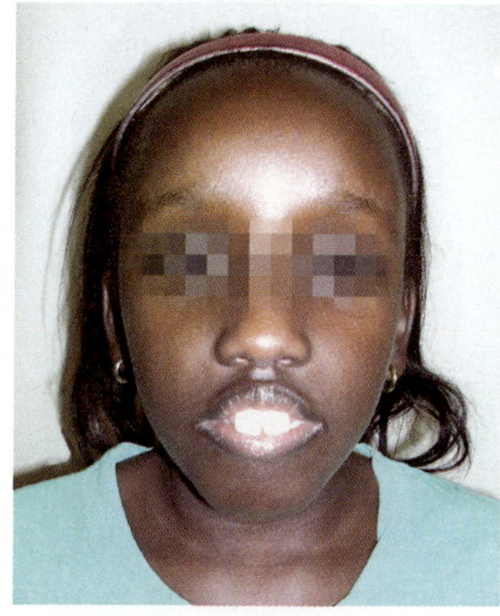

(a)

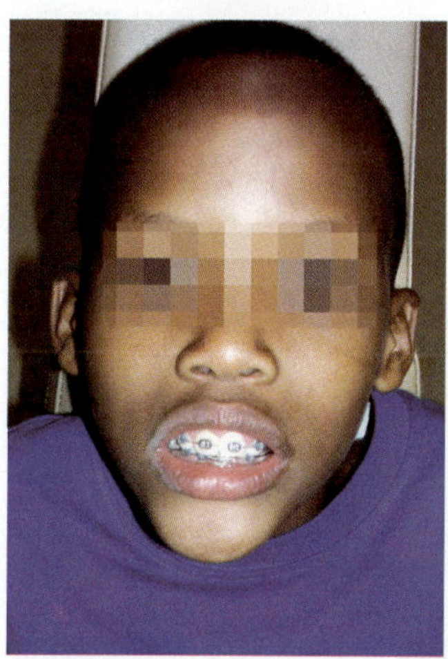

(b)

Figs 13.26a and b: Short upper lip, proclined upper incisors, and incompetent lips.

Lip steps (Korkhaus): Lip step is the relationship of upper and lower lips at rest position as seen from the lateral view. Normally, there is a slightly negative step, i.e. lower lip is slightly behind the upper lip. There is a positive lip step in skeletal class III; and an increased negative lip step in skeletal class II.

Tonicity of lips: It is the amount of strain in the lips. The lips may be normotonic/hypertonic/hypotonic.

Normotonic lips: These are the lips with no strain, and they are competent to each other. They are found in skeletal class I cases.

Hypertonic lips (Fig. 13.27): In cases of skeletal class II, in vertical growth, short upper lip, etc. the child is not able to approximate the lips without strain. It leads to increased strain in the lips. The increased strain in lower lip is seen as puckering of soft tissues of chin area and loss of mentolabial sulcus. Upper lip is seen as flattened with loss of philtrum details.

In skeletal class III cases with mandibular prognathism, the patient tries to approximate lips by straining the lower lip and chin tissues. In them, generally, the upper lip is found to be hypotonic.

Hypotonic lips: They are seen in patient having mouth breathing habit. The upper and lower lips become redundant and everted.

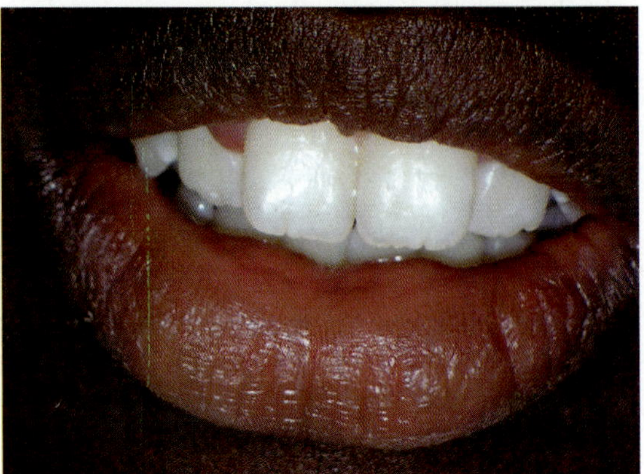

Fig. 13.27: Flaccid, incompetent lips, become dry with mouth breathing

Lip contour: Everted lips are the hypertrophied lips with weak muscular tonicity associated with proclined teeth, e.g. in mouth breathing cases.

Chin: It is an important part of face and has an effect on the profile and the esthetics of the face.

Chin prominence: Evaluation of chin is important because it affects the profile of face, and also gives us an idea of growth pattern of face. Usually Angle's class III and class II division 2 cases have prominent chin, while class II division 1 is associated with recessive chin.

Mentolabial suclus (Fig. 13.28): It is the concavity in soft tissues below the lower lip. Deep sulcus is common in class II division 1 cases due to everted lower lip or lip trap; and in class II division 2 cases associated with shorter face height. A shallow sulcus is seen in bimaxillary protrusions; and in skeletal class III with mandibular prognathism.

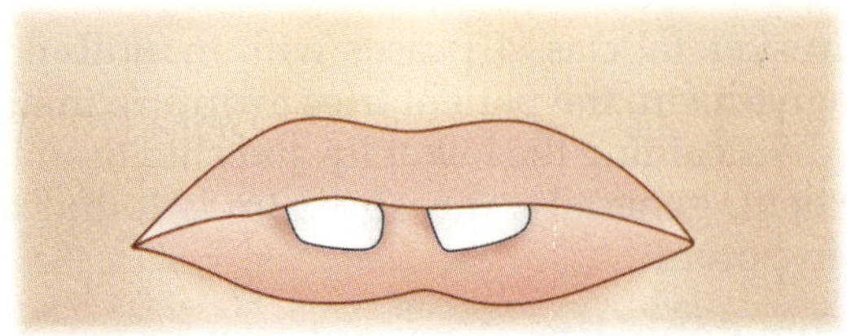

Fig. 13.28: Lower lip trap behind upper proclined incisors.

Mentalis activity (Fig. 13.29): Hyperactive mentalis muscle may be associated with incompetent lips especially in class II division 1. It causes puckering or dimpling of soft tissues of chin (orange peel appearance). In skeletal class III, lower lip hyperactivity may be present.

Nasolabial angle: It is the angle formed between lower border of nose and a line connecting base of nose and labrale superius (tip of upper lip) (Fig. 13.30). Normally, this angle is 102–110°. It affects the esthetics of face. It is reduced in the patients with proclined

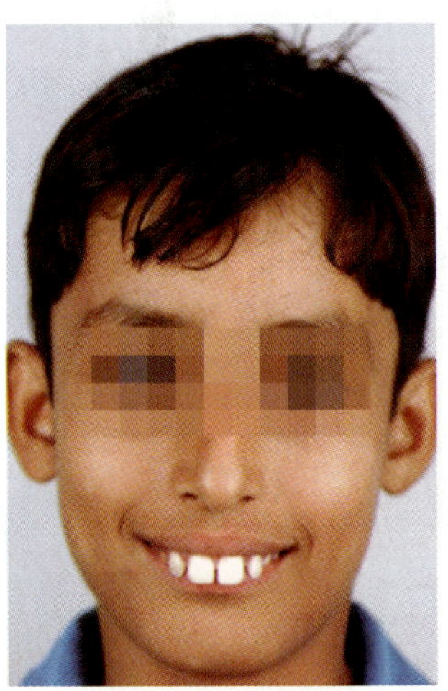

Fig. 13.29: Lower lip trap due to retrognathic mandible and increased overjet.

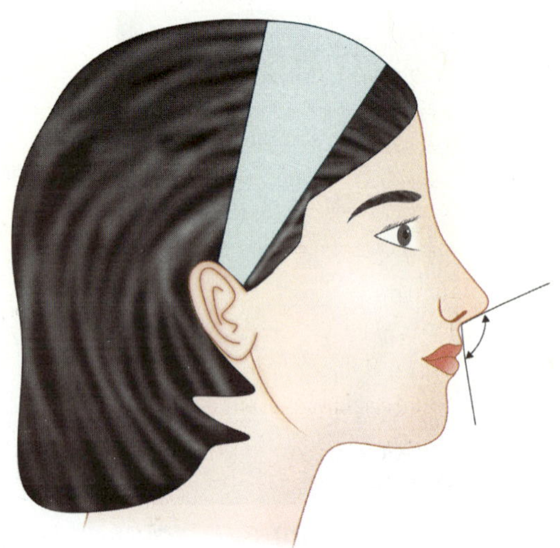

Fig. 13.30: Clinical judgement of nasolabial angle, normal range is 102–110°.

upper anteriors or prognathic maxilla and increased in retroclined maxillary incisors or retrognathic maxilla, e.g. class II division 2. It is also affected by the inclination of columella of nose.

Nose: It also affects the profile and esthetics of face and treatment considerations. Shape of nose varies in different races, and it is a hereditary feature. Different components of nose affect the total profile of nose and face. Length of nose is normally one-third of total facial height. Normally, there lies a relation of vertical length to the horizontal width of nose as 2:1. Width of nostrils are approx 70% of nose length (nasion to tip of nose).

Contour of nasal bridge can be straight, convex; crooked. Tip of nose can be pointed upward/elevated; downward/protruding; parrot-beak nose. Nostrils shape and size also differ in different races.

Nasal profile cannot be changed with orthodontic Rx, so rhinoplasty may be required for esthetic purposes in extreme cases. However, in some extraction cases, with the retraction of anterior teeth, the nose and the nasolabial angle may become prominent, giving a typical orthodontic-look to the face.

During examination, look for the signs of injury or any abnormality of nose.

Intraoral Examination

It can be divided in two steps, viz. soft tissue examination and the hard tissue examination.

1. **Soft tissue examination:** It involves the examination of:
   - Gingiva
   - Tongue
   - Lip and cheek frena
   - Palate
   - Tonsils and adenoids
   - Clefts
   - Oral hygiene status, etc.
2. **Hard tissue examination:** It involves the examination of:
   - Dentition
   - Caries index
   - Molar relationship
   - Canine relationship
   - Overjet (Fig. 13.31)
   - Overbite
   - Curve of Spee
   - Crossbites
   - Arch length discrepancy
   - Missing/supernumerary teeth
   - Anomalies.

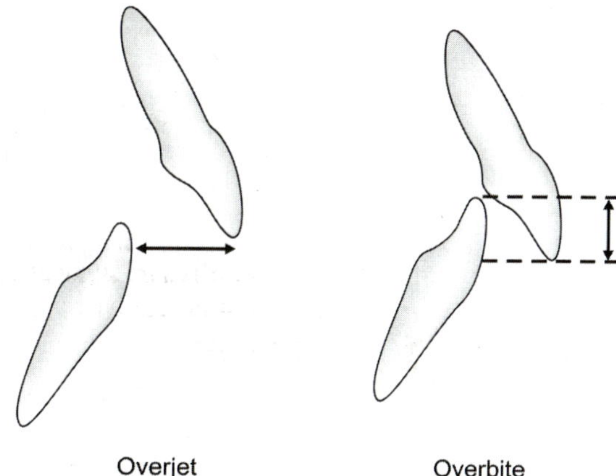

Fig. 13.31: Overjet and overbite measurement.

Soft Tissue Appraisal

Gingiva: Gingiva is examined for its features, like color, texture, plaque, bleeding; stippling, pocket depth, etc.

Gingivitis and poor oral hygiene should be noted and treated before starting the orthodontics treatment. If gingivitis is not treated, it may lead to more loss of bone, increased sensitivity of teeth, poor response to orthodontic forces and increased mobility of teeth.

- Attached gingiva level and any recession: gingival levels/clefts around each tooth should be noted. It is an indication of alveolar crest bone level around the tooth. A lower level of AG indicates loss of bone. So force levels are to be controlled there.
- Pockets around the teeth should be noted; it may be due to gingival hyperplasia also (e.g. a patient taking phenytoin, cyclosporine, etc.). A proper medical and drug history helps to

evaluate. The patient should be advised for meticulous oral hygiene maintenance, and the possibility of surgical/laser gingivectomy during the treatment.

Mouth breathing: Such children often present with everted and dry lips, and dry labial mucosa; anterior marginal gingivitis, etc. Anterior marginal gingivitis is usually associated with incompetent lips.

Trauma from occlusion (Fig. 13.32): Gingival clefts may be present around localized teeth due to TFO. Localized gingival recession due to traumatic occlusion may also be seen in crossbite, etc.

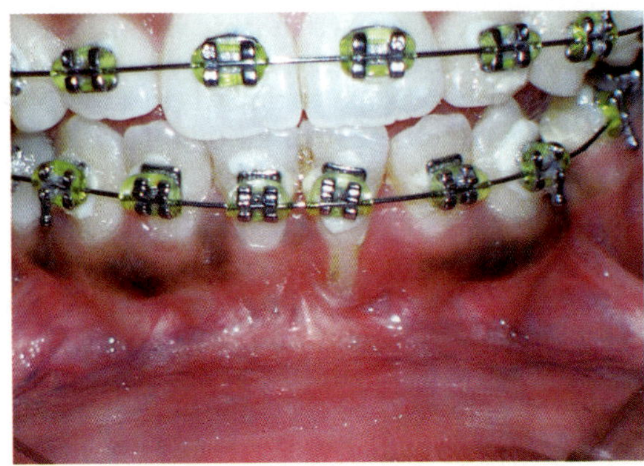

Fig. 13.32: Labial gingival recession in a lower tooth due to active lower frenum

Frenum: The position of freni is noted as abnormal attachment can lead to gingival recession; problem in soft tissue movements; spacing in teeth, etc.

- **Maxillary labial frenum**(Fig. 13.33): Normally at birth, it is attached at incisal papilla region which regresses in the vestibular musoca with dentoalveolar growth and eruption of maxillary incisors. But if does not regress, it remains attached as a band of heavy, fibrous structure and causes midline diastema. It does not contain muscle fibers. It affects the mobility of lips, and may affect the gingival levels leading to localized gingival recession.
- It is tested by Blanch test: Blanching of palatal tissues around incisive papilla occurs on stretching of upper lip. On IOPA X-ray, it shows a notching of the alveolar crest.
- **Lingual frenum** (Fig. 13.34): In many children, the lingual frenum can be seen attached at varied position between base of tongue and tip. Abnormal attachment can lead to reduced tongue mobility, affecting speech; and can also lead to flaring of lower incisors.

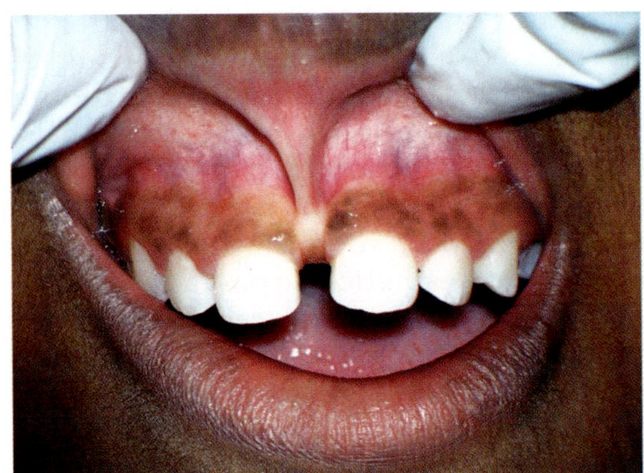

(a)

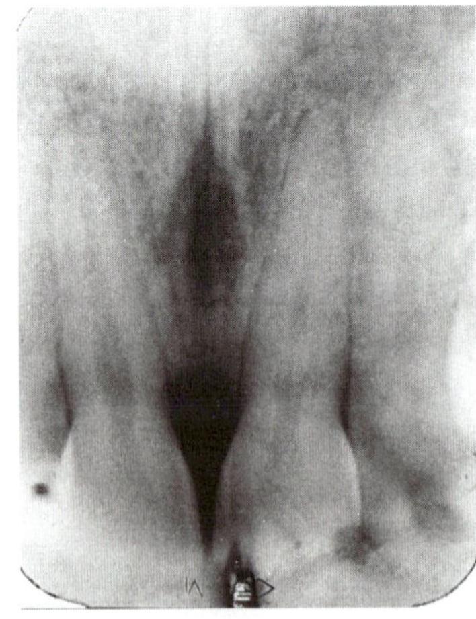

(b)

Figs 13.33a and b: Low lying heavy maxillary frenum and IOPA showing alveolar crest defect due to frenum and diastema also.

Tongue size, shape and posture: Tongue is a very important muscular tissue of oral cavity, and it also helps in facial growth as a part of functional matrix. It helps in establishment of occlusion and dental arch form by maintaining a balance of forces around the dentition. It is helpful for swallowing and speech. Shape, size, position, color and posture, habits, etc. should be noted while evaluating the tongue.

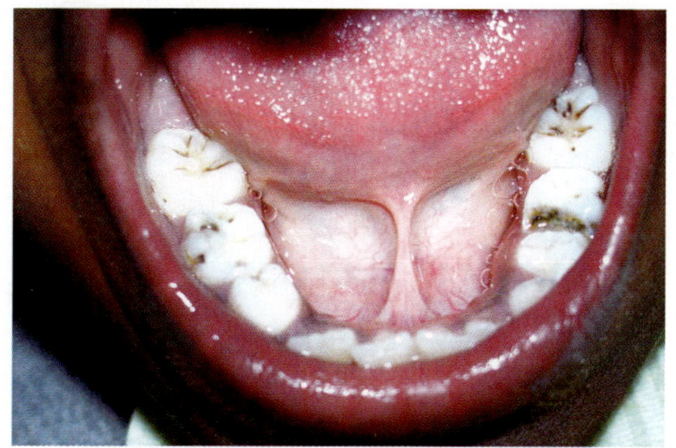

Fig. 13.34: Partial ankyloglossia due to abnormal attachment of lingual frenum on the tongue.

Size: Tongue can be normal, small, long or broad. Thus it affects the size, shape, etc. of dental arches. Large size tongue or macroglossia, although it being a rare condition and is seen in some diseases, e.g. amyloidosis, Down's syndrome, hypothyroidism, etc., leads to the development of wider arches, generalised spaces; proclined anterior teeth due to pressure from the tongue. It can be diagnosed by noting the scalloping of lateral borders; and covering occlusal surfaces of posteriors. Patient may be able to touch his nose and chin by protruding the tongue.

Position: Normally, the tongue rests with its tip in rugae area, with a mild gap between its dorsal surface and the vault of palate. Abnormal position of tongue often leads to development of malocclusion and abnormal facial growth due to affected functional matrix, e.g. if it lies in the floor of mouth, it may lead to wider lower arch and a narrow upper arch, due to disturbance of buccinators mechanism. Also, it leads to abnormal forward growth of mandible causing mandibular prognathism. Since there is no forward stimulus on maxilla, a maxillary deficiency can occur, thus leading to development of skeletal class III relations.

Habits: Tongue habits apply abnormal forces on dentoalveolar compelx, leading to abnormal development, e.g. tongue thrust habit leads to proclination of teeth and abnormal spacing. It may also lead to maxillary prognathism. It may be in anterior or lateral direction, and may cause the development of anterior or posterior open bite.

Palate

Hard and soft palate of the patients should be examined properly and the findings should be noted, as they influence the treatment planning.

- Palatal depth gives us an idea of the growth pattern and facial type of the patient. It is deep in dolicocephalic patients, while shallow in brachycepahlic patients. Maxillary arch is found to be narrow in dolichocepahlics, requiring expansion.
- Presence of swelling in palate may indicate an impacted / supernumerary tooth, odontome, cyst or bony pathology.
- Indentation or ulcerations in anterior area of palatal mucosa are due to deep traumatic bite, whereby the lower incisors bury themselves due to overruption. Some ulceration can be due to trauma or infections or cancer.
  - *Scar:* Scar may be due to cleft surgery; or due to healed ulcer or tumor surgery. These scars create a problem in proper maxillary arch development or treatment, as they apply resistance due to presence of fibrous tissue in them. Expansion done in a scarred palate is bound to relapse until a fixed study permanent retention is given.
  - *Clefts of palate:* CLP is one of the most common congenital anomaly affecting human kind. Cleft of palate lead to growth problems, speech defects and malocclusion.
  - *Rugae* (Figs 13.35a to c)*:* Relation of rugae to canines is a fare indicator of

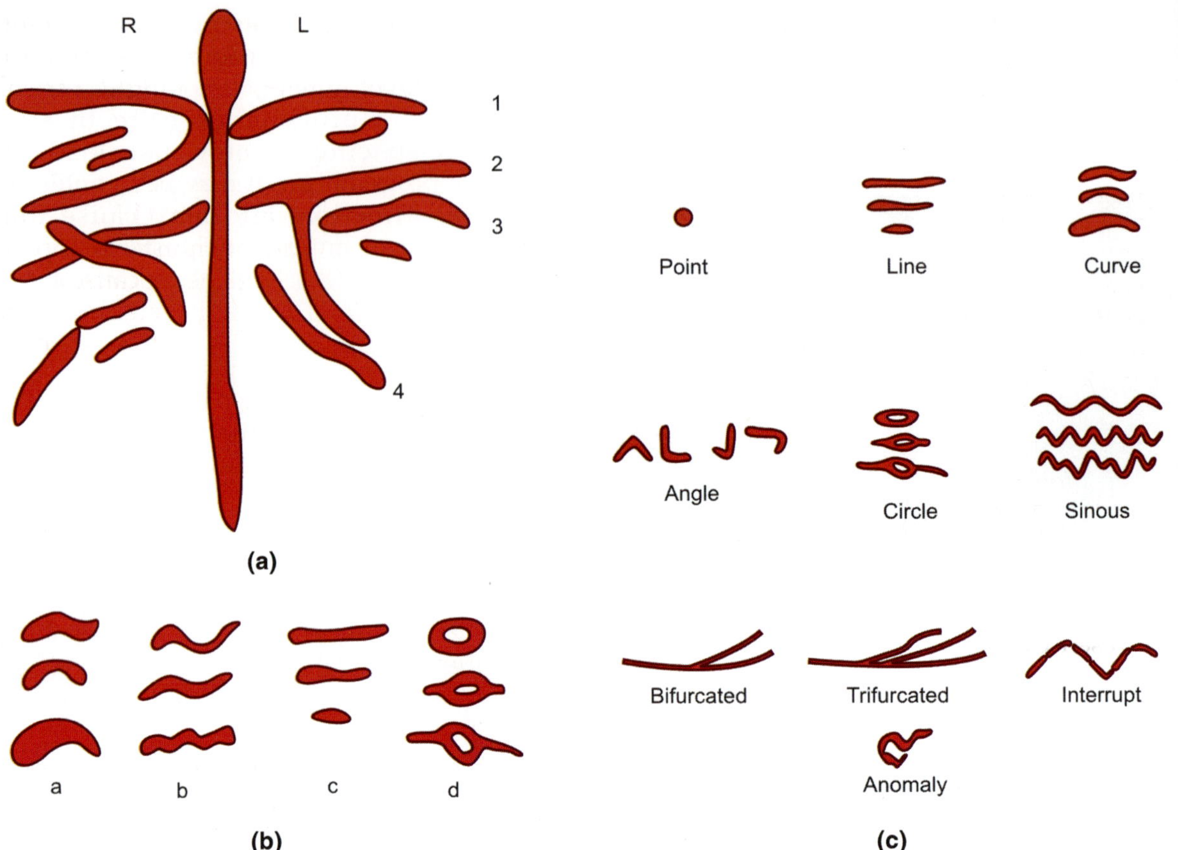

Figs 13.35a to c: Rugae pattern on the palate; and different types of rugae.

position of the dentition. Third rugae must be in line with maxillary canines. Thus, it helps to assess the maxillary anterior proclination.

Tonsil and Adenoids

Tonsils are the lymphoid tissues in the oral and pharyngeal spaces. Adenoids are present in the posterior pharyngeal wall and their inflammation and swelling leads to change in respiratory pattern from nasal to oral leading to mouth breathing. Inflamed tonsils may lead to alteration in tongue and jaw posture, thus upsetting the orofacial muscular balance leading to malocclusion and abnormal facial growth. Normally, the lymphoid tissues grow very rapidly to 200% till 10–12 years age, and then regress (see Scammon's growth curve).

DENTAL EXAMINATION

Certain features should be noted which are:

- Stage of dentition
- Number of teeth: Present/absent/supernumerary/impacted/unerupted
- Over-retained teeth; premature loss of teeth
- History of teeth extraction; trauma, etc.
- Shape, size and surface texture of teeth.
- Hypoplastic and malformed teeth
- Restorative status of teeth, filled or fractured teeth
- Caries, nonvital, RCT teeth; caries index
- Oral hygiene
- Wear facets on teeth
- Staining of teeth.

Stage of dentition: The present dental stage gives us the idea of age of the child, the teeth yet to erupt, and helps in treatment planning. There are certain features of dentition which appear abnormal and parents are concerned with them, but developmentally, they are normal for that stage. These are called as self-correcting anomalies or transient malocclusions. They should not be disturbed by any treatment, as it may disturb the normal development. Also, certain treatment procedures are to be initiated at an early stage, e.g. serial extraction, guidance of eruption, myofunctional treatment, etc. An idea of abnormal eruption can be judged if the present dentition stage does not correlate with the age of the patient, e.g. impacted tooth, missing tooth, etc.

Size of teeth: Small sized teeth lead to presence of spacing in the normal sized arches, while larger sized teeth lead to crowding and rotations, deflected path of eruption of teeth, impaction, etc.

Shape of teeth: Certain teeth may be of abnormal shape, e.g. peg lateral are the most common teeth. They have small MD size and conical shape, thus giving rise to spacing, unesthetic spaces and embrasures, affecting the smile. Certain supernumerary teeth may be having abnormal shape called as odontome, disturbing the occlusion and alignment.

Number of teeth: Increased or decreased number of teeth in the arches lead to development of malocclusion, e.g. crowding, spacing, midline deviation, disturbed molar relation, etc. Condition of decreased number of teeth is called as partial anodontia or oligodontia. Extra-teeth apart from the normal complement are called supernumerary teeth.

Any history of extraction of teeth should be noted. Loss of tooth leads to shifting of adjacent teeth leading to malocclusion.

Overretained teeth; premature loss of teeth: A note should be made regarding the overretained and/or premature loss of milk teeth. It leads to deviation of the path of eruption of teeth, loss of space and impaction, etc.

Dental caries: Before starting orthodontic treatment, all active caries lesions should be restored. Any white spot lesions WSLs, should be noted, and a remineralisation program should be chalked out by using topical fluorides, improving oral hygiene, CPP-ACP method, xylitol chewing gum, chlorhexidine mouth wash, etc. Patient should be advised to improve the oral hygiene, because braces act to harbor food causing increased caries risk. Long-standing caries lesion especially proximal caries lead to loss of space due to shifting of adjacent teeth in the spaces created by caries. Deep occlusal lesions can also cause cuspal-extrusion of opposing teeth.

Nonvital teeth and RCT teeth: Such teeth should be noted. Nonvital tooth may be due to trauma to teeth, it may be having periapical pathology and should be treated before orthodontic treatment. Due to trauma, teeth may be ankylosed and do not move with orthodontic forces. RCT tooth should be noted as they have weaker structure due to biomechanical preparation (BMP) and loss of water. However, RCT tooth is not a contraindication for orthodontic movement, because a only vital PDL is required for OTM.

Restorative status of teeth, filled or fractured teeth: Presence of fillings, jacket crown or bridge, etc. should be noted. Some teeth may be having deep fillings esp tooth colored fillings, which may become symptomatic during the course of orthodontic treatment. Fractured teeth restored with composites may cause problems with bonding. PFM best view for records/OPG is the metallic crowns may require banding rather than bonding. Otherwise, they may need special materials to bond the orthodontic attachments. Such teeth are generally seen in adult patients. It also gives idea of caries status and oral hygiene of the patient. Abnormally contoured fillings, overhangs, etc. should be noted and removed.

Wear facets on teeth: Wear facets and attrition status of the patient should be noted as they may be due to parafunctional habits or abnormal dental relations. In adult patients with normal attrtional loss of enamel, the contact areas and marginal ridges become flattened and pose problems during banding. Habits may apply abnormal forces on supporting tissues and may traumatize them, which may need certain precautions during orthodontics. Occasionally, separators cannot be passed through them due to the marginal ridges being flattened, the rubber separators break. Such teeth generally need brass wire separators or Kesling's separators, but due to heavy masticatory contacts, such wire separators also get lost or break.

Surface texture: Enamel surfaces of teeth should be evaluated, e.g. hypoplastic, hypomineralised teeth, etc. fluorosis, enamel hypoplasia due to trauma, i.e. Turner's tooth, white spot lesions due to initial caries, etc. can lead to change in treatment options.

Stained teeth: Intrinsic stains may be due to fluorides, tetracyclines, trauma, etc. which may lead to enamel hypoplasia and discolorations, and sometimes pose problems with bonding. Also they look unesthetic. Since, during course of orthodontic treatment, there are chances of development of white spot lesions, a record of already present staining is important, so as to educate the patient for hygiene and treatment, etc.

Dental and Orthodontic Findings

A thorough examination is done in all the three planes, viz. transverse, sagittal, vertical (TSV) planes. Noting the features helps in treatment planning and further evaluation during the treatment phase:

- Molar relation
- Canine relation
- Incisor relation
- Overjet and overbite (Fig. 13.36)
- Midline: Skeletal/dental; upper/lower
- Arch size, shape and symmetry and individual arch form
- Individual tooth alignment
- Crossbites
- Crowding/spacing/rotations

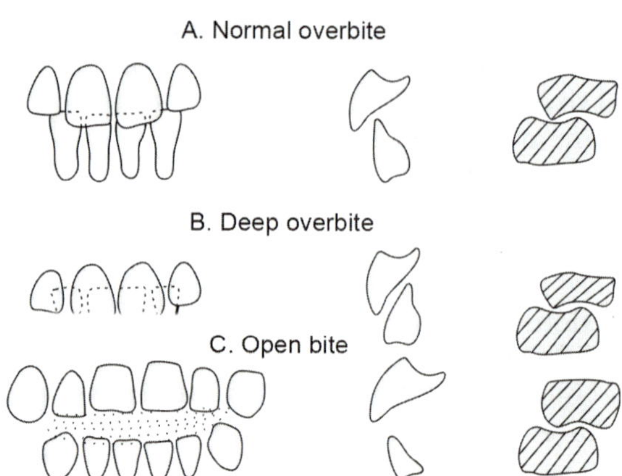

Fig. 13.36: Normal bite, deep bite and open bite.

- Tooth size-arch length discrepancy
- Curve of Spee: flat/1–1.5 mm.

Functional Analysis

The growth of cranio-orofacial complex is related with the normal functions of stomatognathic system. The diagnostic procedure should be a culmination of dynamic evaluation of skeletodental complex and the associated functional units, rather than a static examination of teeth and bones. The maxillofacial complex is involved with functions, like mastication, swallowing, speech, breathing, vision and smelling. Various components to be evaluated for functional analysis are as follows.

- Assessment of the postural rest position and freeway space
- Evaluation of path of closure: CR-CO discrepancy
- Prematurities during closure: point of first contact during closure and presence of mandibular slide/shift
- Assessment of respiration, swallowing and speech
- Examination of TMJ
- Excessive mobility of individual teeth
- Position of upper and lower lips wrt maxillary and mandibular incisors and tongue position during functional movements

- Tongue position and pressures exerted during functional movements.

Assessment of the postural rest position and freeway space:

Postural rest position is defined as the position of mandible at which the opening and closing muscles of the jaw are in a state of minimal contraction. It is the position at which everybody remains for most of the time throughout the day and night.

At this position, there exists a space between upper and lower teeth/jaws which is called as freeway space or interocclusal gap (IOG). Normally, IOG is 2–3 mm in canine-first premolar region. IOG has a strong influence on the treatment planning. It should not be encroached by extrusion of teeth, as then the dentition comes in premature contact, applying abnormal forces leading to relapse and abrasion of teeth and trauma to TMJ. Also, the muscles get activated and apply a continuous traumatizing force on the periodontium.

Excessive IOG is present in deep bite and horizontal growth cases. Patients who are in growth period, the extrusion of posterior teeth can be done to open the bite, because this extrusion is balanced by the vertical growth of ramus. This phenomenon is used while treating a case with myofunctional appliance.

There are various methods to evaluate the postural rest position and the IOG. During examination, the patient is asked to sit upright with unsupported back, and to look straight ahead, preferable in his own eyes in a distant mirror.

- **Phonetic method:** The patient is asked to say some consonants like C or M or to repeat words like Missisippi, Ram, etc. The mandible returns to the rest position after few seconds. At this point, the patient is advised not to change this relation. The dentist can separate his lips to note the IOG.
- **Command method:** Patient is asked to swallow and relax. The mandible comes to a rest position after this exercise.
- **Non-command method:** Some patients may not cooperate with the command as they become nervous. So, he is observed as he speaks or swallows while talking to him about some unrelated topics. Also, the patient can be left unattended for few minutes and is observed from a distance to evaluate the rest position.

Few methods to measure the free way space are:

- **Direct extraoral method:** It is one of the most common methods used. Two points are marked on nose and chin in the area unaffected by the movement of jaws, in the midline. The distance between these two points is measured at rest position VDR, and at occlusal position, VDO. The difference between them is the IOG, i.e. VDR-VDO = freeway space.
- **Direct intraoral method:** The distance between upper and lower teeth in the canine-first premolar region is directly measured in the mouth of patient with the help of vernier calipers.
- **Indirect extraoral method:** In patients who are apprehensive or nervous, this method can be used. Two cephalograms are taken, one at CR and other at CO position, and the difference is calculated. The disadvantage is that the patient is unnecessarily subjected to radiation doses. Kinesiography is another method to evaluate IOG.

Path of closure: Path of closure of mandible from maximum opening to rest position and then to centric occlusion should be noted. The patient is asked to close the mouth slowly from maximum opening and any deviation is noted. It may be an indication of TMJ problem.

The patient is first asked to stop at the first dental contact (point of first contact and the position of midlines and other dental relations are noted. Then, he is asked to close in CO and any deflected path of final closure, midline, etc. are noted. This process helps us to find out any prematurities, displacement or tooth guidance. It is important to note in cases of unilateral posterior cross bite and in some cases of anterior cross bite.

Lateral path of closure: Generally, posterior cross bites are bilateral due to narrow maxillary arch, but during closure, the mandible gets deflected to close in most comfortable position of CO, giving a clinical impression of a unilateral condition. Treatment of such a condition is bilateral expansion of maxillary arch. If there is no deflection, the defect may be unilateral asymmetry of either arch and may require different treatment approach.

Similarly, anterior path of closure/deflection during closure due to premature contacts in incisor region leads to anterior cross bite and pseudo-class III condition. If this is not treated, it may turn in true skeletal class III condition during ensuing growth.

A backward path of closure is seen in class II division 2 due to lingually inclined maxillary incisors and may cause abnormal pressure on TMJ tissues, and attrition of incisors at approyimating system.

Range of mandibular motion: ROM during various protrusive/retrusive/lateral excursions is noted. Any deviation from normal should be evaluated further regarding TMJ health, trauma or ankylosis, etc.

Excessive mobility of individual teeth: It should be noted by using mirror handle in one hand and by finger tips of other hand. It may be due to abnormal forces and TFO, which may have caused damage to periodontium.

Position of upper and lower lips with respect to maxillary and mandibular incisors during various functional movements is noted. Various smile features are also noted.

Tongue position, habits and pressures exerted during functional movements, like swallowing and speech, are noted. Any lisping, etc. is noted.

Assessment of respiration: Respiration is a fundamental function having a strong influence on the growth of craniofacial complex. Mainly, three types of breathing patterns have been noted viz. nasal; oral; and oronasal. Abnormal breathing pattern leads to abnormal growth of tissues. So, it is very important to diagnose and treat the abnormal breathing. Any DNS and other nasal pathology should be examined to find out the causes.

There are some tests which can help to find out the mode of respiration.

- **Water test:** Patient is asked to hold the water in mouth with lips closed for a long time. If he is able to keep it in mouth without difficulty, it means he can breathe through nose. The mouth breather finds it difficult to keep water in mouth.
- **Mirror test:** A double-sided mirror is held below the nostrils, between nose and mouth. Fogging on nasal side shows nasal breathing, while on mouth side shows oral breathing.
- **Cotton test:** It can also be called as butterfly test. A small wisp of cotton is placed below the nostrils. If it moves down, it shows nasal breathing. It can also be used to find out the unilateral nasal blockage.
- **Observation of nares:** External nares show dilation during breathing in nasal breathing, while there is no change in mouth breathing.

Examination of TMJ

Examination involving palpation and auscultation of TMJ and muscles involved with mandibular movements should be done to ascertain the health of TMJ. TMJ plays an important role in growth also.

Examination should note features, e.g.

- Normal range of mandibular movements: maximum protrusion; maximum opening; lateral excursions.
- Any deviation in the path during closing and opening movements. Deviation while opening/closing: When mandible moves from rest to CO position. Deviated path of closure due to occlussal prematurities have adverse effect on TMJ health.

- Symptoms like clicking; crepitus; pain of muscles or in TMJ.
- Limitation of jaw movements; hypermobility and morphologic abnormality.

Evaluation of Swallowing

In a new born child, the size of tongue is relatively large than the oral cavity, and it protrudes between the gum pads. It helps to make lip seal during suckling. It is called as infantile swallow and it is seen till 1½–2 years of age. The infantile swallowing starts changing to mature swallow when the buccal teeth start erupting. If infantile swallow persist, it may lead to abnormal development and malocclusion. It can be indicated by following features:

1. Protrusion of tongue tip to make seal with upper lip.
2. Contraction of perioral muscles during swallowing.
3. Absence of molar contacts during swallowing.
4. Escape of saliva from between the teeth during swallowing.
5. Spaces between the teeth.

Speech

Speech is affected in certain malocclusion. It may be due to improper movement of tongue, improper relation of lips, teeth and tongue, and improper escape of air during speech, e.g. patient having cleft palate have a nasal twang. In tongue thrust habit, there is lisping during speech. In anterior open bite, there is improper contact of tongue, lips and teeth.

Orthodontic Study Models

Models are the positive replica of teeth and surrounding tissues. They are one of the essential diagnostic aids and help us to study the position of teeth in all the three planes of space; and also from the lingual side. A lot of information can be gathered from them; however, they themselves are not the complete diagnostic records. They act as pretreatment record, and are used for comparison of the progress of treatment; for educational purpose; for treatment planning, etc. These are obtained at various stages of treatment to records and progress of treatment.

Information obtained from study models:

- Number of teeth present
- Shape, size and position of teeth
- Intra-arch and interarch relation of teeth
- Classification of malocclusion
- Overjet, overbite, crossbite
- Upper to lower midline
- Palatal contour: Sagittal/transverse
- Teeth measurements
- Arch form and symmetry
- Arch width
- Incisors midline to jaw midline
- Curve of Spee
- Vertical tooth malpositions
- Horizontal tooth malpositions/rotations
- Crowding/spacing
- Abnormal tooth morphology
- Arch length determinations
- Axial inclination of teeth: Incisors/canines/molars
- Factes of wear
- Muscle attachments/frenum, etc.
- Gingival recession
- Useful for Kesling's diagnostic setup
- To determine TSALD
- Lingual occlusion.

Squash Bite Record

- Squash bite record should be taken before start of treatment. This helps to articulate the casts, and to find out exact occlusal relationship. It is especially a helpful record in open bite cases to articulate the models in proper relationship, TMD cases, facial asymmetry, premature functional shifting cases, etc. At the end stages of treatment, it helps in articulating the casts and helps on planning of occlusal equilibration to achieve maximum intercuspation and to avoid any premature contacts in the post-treatment occlusion.

- A bite record is valuable to help the orthodontist to relate the upper and lower cast correctly in proper occlusion. It can be taken with wax sheet but they get distorted with time. So, the polyether- or silicon-based elastomeric impression materials must be used to make this record. Proper articulation of casts is necessary for proper surgical planning also.
- Two layers of soft base plate wax are roughly shaped to arch form and warmed in water, placed on lower arch and patient is guided and asked to close in centric occlusion. Care must be taken as children are prone to give a protrusive relationship or may not close completely.
- A wax bite should always be taken in patients with open bite as there are no proper anterior stops of occlusion; where multiple posterior teeth are missing; or where there is any doubt about proper articulation of the casts.

Advantage of Study Models

- They are the permanent records of patient's pretreatment and other stages of occlusion.
- They are 3D representation of a patient's dentition.
- Occlusion can be studied from every aspect especially lingual aspect.
- Accurate measurements TSALD can be made of the teeth and arch lengths and width for treatment planning.
- They help in the assessment of the treatment progress.
- They can also be used for discussion of the case with patients/parents and the fellow colleagues.
- They are helpful in explaining the Rx plan and progress to patients.
- They are useful for transfer of the cases to other doctors to depict the pretreatment stage and the present stage if the patient requires that.
- They can also be used to discuss with the patients to alleviate their anxiety before start of the treatment. It can be done by showing them the progress of treatment of some other cases.
- They are helpful in motivation of patient and to explain treatment plan as well as progress to patient and parents.
- Study models are useful to transfer records in case the patient is to be treated by another clinician
- They are also used for research purposes, e.g. for evaluating pretreatment and post-treatment changes in dentition; changes during retention period; changes in arch widths; to determine and compare Bolton's ratio in various races, etc. to name a few.
- They are also used for study and teaching purpose.
- The working models can also be used for fabricating the appliances in the lab.
- They are also used for diagnostic setup or orthognathic surgery planning/mock surgery, e.g. Kesling's diagnostic setup.

Requirements of Ideal Study Models

They should accurately reproduce all the details of erupted teeth; surrounding soft tissues and the full depth of the sulci, without any distortion.

They should be trimmed symmetrically and should be pleasing to the eyes. It helps to immediately assess any asymmetry in the arch forms.

The bases should be trimmed parallel to the OP.

The back of the base is trimmed perpendicular to the OP.

When placed on the back, they should represent the accurate occlusion, and should not disocclude.

Gnathostatic Models

They are the models where the base of maxillary model is trimmed parallel to the FHP.

Parts of study model: They are divided in two parts:

1. Anatomic portion
2. Artistic portion.

Anatomic portion: It is that part of study models which is comprised of teeth and its surrounding structures recorded by the impression. It is usually made of type II stone plaster, green in color or orthokal stone, white in color, which is the latest requirement for fabricating study models.

Artistic portion: Artistic portion is the base of the model made of white POP, and built in a standardized manner. It supports the anatomic portion. It helps in orienting the models and depicting the occlusion of patient. It also gives a pleasing appearance to the models. In a well made model, the ratio of anatomic to artistic parts is 3:1. Now, plastic and rubber base formers are available for forming the artistic part. Depending upon the stage at which the study models are made, they can be called as pretreatment models, stage models and post-treatment models.

The steps involved in making study models are:

- Impression making
- Disinfection of impressions
- Pouring of the impression
- Basing and trimming of the casts
- Finishing and polishing
- Identification marking and storage.

The Impression Technique

- An accurate impression recording dental and surrounding tissues with full depth of labial and lingual sulci and freni trimmed in function, is an important requirement for making ideal study models. The maxillary impression should cover hard palate and should not extend on soft palate. The impressions should be free of any air bubbles.
- Irreversible hydrocolloid/alginate impression materials are widely used for this purpose. Quick/medium setting type is recommended.
- **Selection of trays:** Comfortably fitting sterilized trays are selected, covering last erupted molars and having a 3 mm clearance all around. High flange plastic orthodontic trays which extend deep in vestibules must be used. Rim lock trays which prevent overflow of the impression material are also good choice. Smaller or larger trays distort the surrounding tissues and thus provide inaccurate impression.
- Strip of soft utility wax can be adapted to the tray periphery to hold the alginate and to assist in reproducing the details of vestibular fornix. It also reduces the pressure and irritation due to tray metal rim on the tissues during impression making procedure.
- Ask the patient to rinse the mouth to remove any food particles. Wipe the teeth with a cotton roll to reduce the salivary bubbles before impression making.
- Due to greater chance of gagging, the posterior periphery of upper tray should be adequately dawned with a roll of utility wax to avoid flow of alginate down the throat. In patients having gagging problem, local anesthesia should be applied to the soft palate area.
- The impression material should be mixed as per manufacturer's instructions to obtain a good mix, and is loaded in the tray.
- Generally, lower impression should be taken so that the patient gets adapted to the procedure and taste and feel of the material. It helps to prevent anxiety and gagging in upper impression.
- A blob of impression material may be placed in the palatal vault of the patient just behind the incisors before inserting the tray if the operator desires, to ensure the elimination of trapped air and to ensure a faithful reproduction of palatal tissues.
- The tray should be inserted so that the anterior periphery of the tray fits under the lip. The tray is then pressed to force the alginate out into the mucobuccal fold to record muscle attachments.

- At the same time, the tray is gradually rotated to fit on the arch. The impression should be stabilized at this point. The muscle molding is done to record the details.
- A good maxillary and mandibular impression will show a "peripheral roll" and will record muscle attachments. Both, the retromolar pad in the lower jaw and the tuberosity in the upper should be included if possible.
- Child patient should be explained the procedures, materials and trays before making an impression, using Tell-Show-Do technique. A pre-impression "mouth wash cocktail of a colored pleasant tasting alginate commercial mouth wash can be used in children. It is a pleasant experience for the apprehensive child. It removes debris and reduces the surface tension of the teeth and tissues, thus reducing bubble formation during the impression making.

Disinfection of Impression

This is done to avoid transfer of infection, etc. from impression to the models, which are to be handled very routinely during treatment.

The impressions should be washed under the running water for few minutes till they are clear of blood, saliva and the food particles.

Then they should be placed in 2% glutraldehyde solution for 10 minutes before pouring.

After disinfection, they should be again washed under water.

Pouring the Impression

A good quality white orthodontic stone is used to pour the impressions. It should be strong to avoid breakage of important tooth portions as they are permanent records, and yet allows easy trimming of the base. The impression is rinsed to remove saliva, mucin, blood and debris, etc. that might reduce the quality of surface reproduction. A diluted solution of detergent or commercial debubblizers is also available for this purpose.

A mechanical vibrator should be used to eliminate bubbles during casting the impression, and it also permits the use of heavier mix. A "heavier mix" is much easier to handle and produces a strong cast with less inherent air-entrapment.

Put the plaster at one end of the impression carefully and slowly vibrate it around to the opposite side, adding small amounts of material at the initial point of insertion.

Basing and Trimming of the Cast (Fig. 13.37)

The stone cast is carefully separated from the impression without breakages and its margins are trimmed to clearly define the vestibules with 2–3 mm margin all around. Care should be taken not to damage or trim the anatomic part of the casts. The dental plaster for base making is mixed according to manufacturer's instructions and spread on a clean glass or a ceramic slab. Otherwise, preformed plastic or rubber base formers can be used. The maxillary cast is placed in this mix of plaster, and is manipulated with the help of a glass slab to align its occlusal plane parallel to the floor. Allow the plaster to set. Start trimming the base of the upper cast as follows:

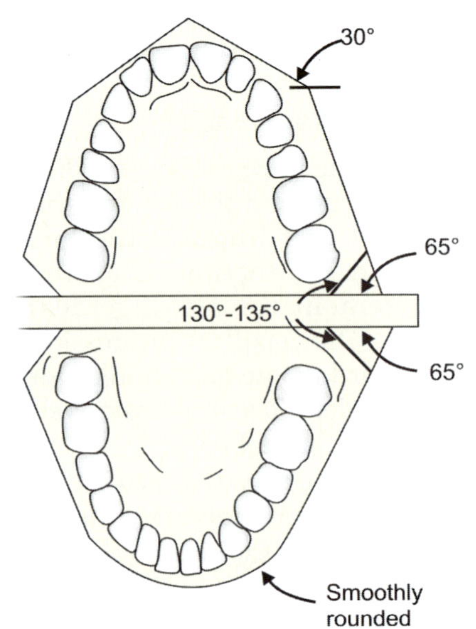

Fig. 13.37: Base fabrication of orthodontic casts.

Step 1: Record the height of cast at maximum depth of the sulcus; usually it is in the canine region. This height represents the height of the anatomic portion. Approx. one half of this height should be the artistic portion. Make a mark on the plaster base for the height of the artistic portion and then trim the excess base in such a way that the occlusal plane is parallel to the floor, and the back of the model.

Step 2: The anterior portion of base is trimmed in the form of a Gothic arch with the apex at the midline and the sides extending up to the canine region, at 5–6 mm from labial surfaces of anterior teeth.

Step 3: Posterior end of the base is trimmed perpendicular to midline of the palate, leaving at least 5 mm of plaster posterior to the last erupted tooth. Trim the sides of the cast parallel to the buccal surface of posterior teeth, 5–6 mm from the buccal surfaces of teeth.

Step 4: The angle between the posterior end of the base and the smaller sides is trimmed at an angle of about 120° and is 13–15 mm long. The longer buccal sides are again cut at approx 120° to the smaller cuts and should be 5–6 mm from the buccal surface of teeth. So, the base of upper model has seven sides.

Step 5: Check for the symmetry of both the sides and correct it, if necessary. Block the air bubbles with a fresh mix of dental plaster. Remove any excess plaster present on the surface of the anatomic portion and roughly finish the base of the model using a coarse stone.

Step 6: The lower cast is placed on upper cast in occlusion and then is placed in the mixed plaster on glass slab or base former. The cast assembly is manipulated so that the base of maxillary cast is parallel to the floor, thus automatically paralleling bases of both casts parallel to each other, floor and OP. While positioning the cast in the dental plaster, the wax bite recorded from the patient is used to seat the casts in occlusion.

Step 7: Trim the height of lower base like the upper. Later, trim the posterior end and the sides corresponding to that of the upper cast. But, the anterior portion of the lower cast is gently rounded off instead of forming a gothic arch as shown in diagram. So, the base of upper model has six sides.

Step 8: Put both the casts in occlusion and trim the posterior ends together in such way that they stay in occlusion when placed together on posteriors ends. Repeat this procedure on all sides except in the anterior region. This is the conventional method of constructing the study models.

Now, many commercials gadgets have made the job of preparing study models easier and are less time-consuming. They are:

Rubber base formers: Rubber base formers are available commercially and many study models can be prepared very quickly by casting the impression in stone plaster and forming the bases using these base formers. They not only help in saving the time, but they also help in conserving the material. They are available in different sizes.

Plastic model bases: These are made up of impact resistant plastic. The stone cast of upper and lower arch is occluded using a wax bite and placed into these plastic model bases using dental plaster. Upper and lower bases are held together by plastic hinges. This plastic models base eliminates the job of finishing the models, as they are left permanently.

Orthodontic base unit: It is an optional unit. By using this unit all the models can be prepared uniformly to the same height of about 6 cm.

Finishing the models: This is a very important step to make models pleasant to look and handle. After properly drying of models under natural sun light or in an oven under low heat for few hours, the bases are trimmed with the help of sand papers of different grits, starting from coarse to finer grits. The bases and corners are finished till they feel smooth and devoid of any visible scratches and air voids.

Soap flakes are melted in water and boiled in a broad flat bottomed vessel. After cooling this solution, immerse the models in it for few hours. Once the soap solution is cold and gels, the models are removed from the gel and dried. Now, the surface of the cast is polished with a piece of silk cloth or chamois which gives glossy appearance of the models. Model gloss is commercially available for finishing the models instead of the soap flakes.

Identification of Study Model

Name, age, sex, date of impression/starting of case and orthodontic case no. are marked on both the casts. It can be marked on the base of the cast or sides in front or at the back. But, a uniform method of identification should be followed.

Method of Identifying Models

1. Writing directly on the sides of the models using a permanent marking pen.
2. Typing the details on paper slips and sticking them to the model. But with time, they get lost and thus create problems in identification.
3. Punched tapes made from the tape making machine can also be stuck on the model.
4. Shallow cavity of 1 × 5 cm to a depth of 1 mm can be cut on the posterior aspect of the cast. The typed details can be placed in the cavity and sealed with clear autopolymerising acrylic resin.

Diagnostic Setup (Figs 13.38a to f)

This method to help in treatment planning was proposed by Kesling, so it is also known as Kesling's diagnostic set up. It is done to determine the proper intra-arch and interarch relations of teeth, in various combinations of extractions and non-extraction in one or both arches. Thus, it helps in deciding the teeth to be extracted or not, and thus in treatment planning, and simulating the tooth movements. An extra-set of models is made in POP to do this.

Uses

1. It is used to visualize and determine the effect of stripping or extractions and the orthodontic tooth movements on final outcome of occlusion.
2. It helps to determine which teeth should be extracted in the arches, and the anchorage planning.
3. It can help in discussing various corrective procedures and thus motivating the patients.
4. It can help in determining and visualizing TSALD.

Procedure

The upper and lower casts are fixed in occlusion with the help of wax bite record, and scoring should be done on the sides of the casts to determine the occlusion. The last erupted molars should not be removed from the casts as they act as index of the pretreatment occlusion. Numbers are marked on all the teeth for identification before they are cut away from the casts. The cuts are placed 3 mm apical to gingival margins and vertical cuts are placed to separate the individual teeth. Then they are placed in the casts with the help of wax in desired positions to simulate the orthodontic treatment and desired removal of teeth. Various combinations of dental extractions can be tried before reaching the final plan. Thus, patient can be motivated by showing the final outcome.

If a diagnostic setup is planned when the patient is examined, then the models can be prepared in a modified way so as to reduce the efforts of cutting. After taking the impressions, small pieces of radiographic films can be placed in the interdental areas extending till half of the roots, in the impression itself before pouring. Later on, only horizontal cuts need to be placed for removal of teeth from the casts.

Model surgeries for the orthognathic surgery planning: Models are also and must be used for OGS planning and for making the surgical splints. They also help to determine the type of orthognathic surgery; areas of surgical incision and the amount of the bone to be removed, and the direction of bone movements during surgery.

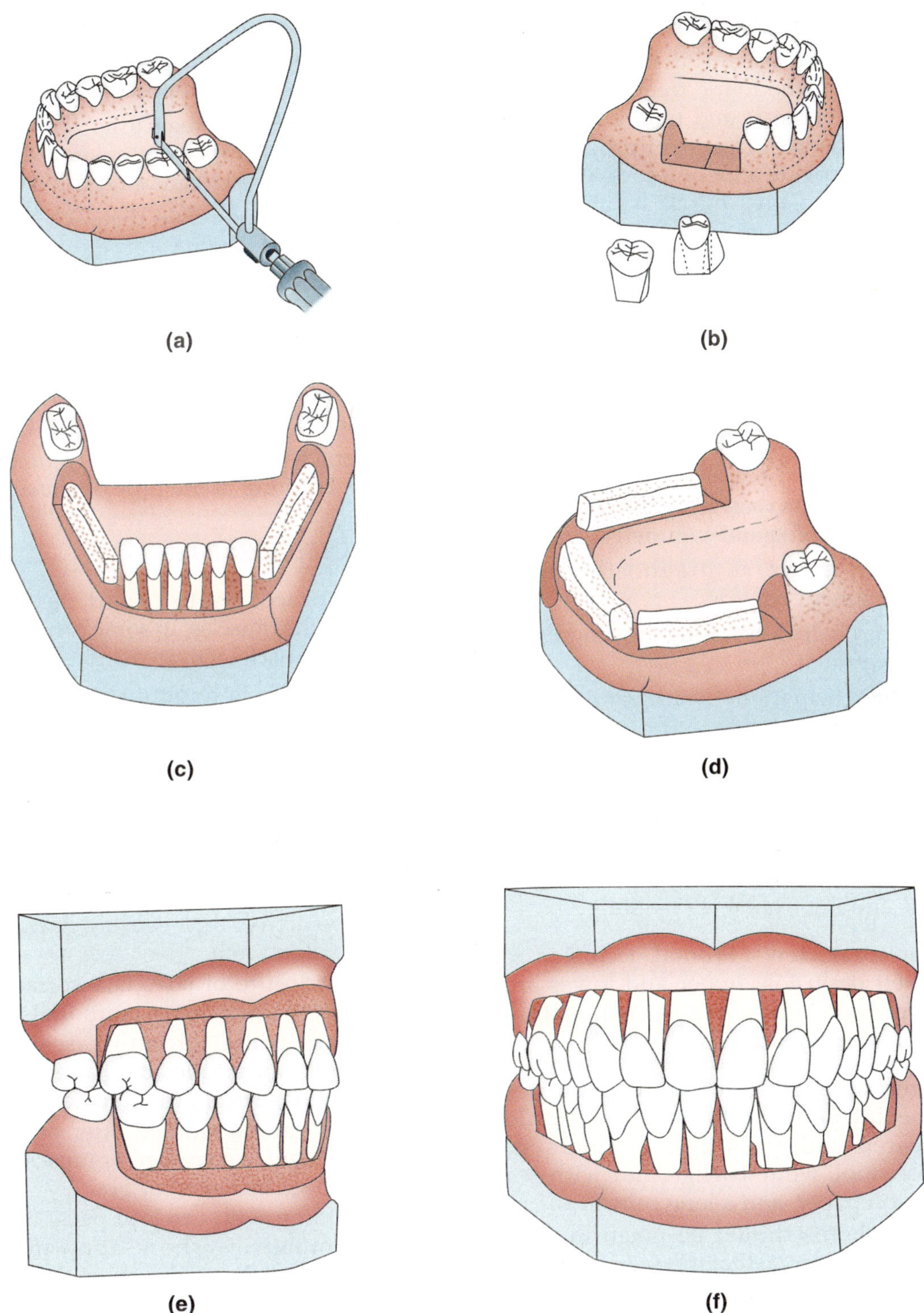

Figs 13.38a to f: Different steps of Kesling's diagnostic setup. The teeth are separated individually from the upper and lower casts except last molars; they are marked; and reset in wax in different combinations of extractions to determine the best possible extraction pattern.

PHOTOGRAPHS (Figs 13.39 and 13.40)

They are also essential records in comprehensive orthodontic treatment. They are taken for diagnosis and treatment planning; for comparison of treatment progress stages, etc. They provide a lot of information on soft tissue morphology, muscle habits and facial expression.

Pre-Rx assessment of lips, chin, nose, facial symmetry and smile can be made. Apart from these, any soft tissue abnormality; pressure spots on tongue; discolored and broken teeth, nasal and cranial asymmetry, etc. should also be recorded.

Uses

- They help in assessing the facial balance, type, profile and symmetry.
- They serve as diagnostic and pretreatment records.
- They help in assessing the progress of the treatment.
- They help in motivating and discussing with the patient.

Views needed: Extraoral and intraoral photos are taken. At least following views are taken.

Extraoral views: Frontal, profile, oblique facial, smiling frontal, 45° smiling.

Intraoral views: Frontal occlusion, right and left occlusion, upper and lower arches, overjet from side, any abnormal features of teeth and soft tissues.

Procedure: For orthodontic photography, a special photographic room should be prepared with flash lights, camera stand, stable stool, white background with scaling or graph paper, and a long mirror.

The photos should be taken in a standardized manner so that they can be compared with other set of photos taken at a later stage.

For taking extraoral photos: The patient should be relaxed, and should be sitting on a stable stool without back rest.

The FHP and interpupillary line is kept parallel to the ground.

Lips should be in repose, i.e. unstrained.

Camera settings regarding aperture, distance from the subject, etc. should be kept constant so that they can be repeated in future.

A fixed reproducible distance should be used for taking photos.

A small piece of known length of metric scale or any other object can be placed on the backside of wall of patient, which should also be included in photos. It will help to calculate the amount of magnification and to apply correction if required.

Patient should look directly in the lens without blinking at the time of clicking.

ELECTROMYOGRAPHY

It is the procedure to record the electrical activity of the muscles. In some conditions, the abnormal muscle-activity is noted, e.g.

1. Upper lip is hypofunctional in severe forms of class II division 1. During swallowing, the lower lip becomes hyperactivated due to increased mentalis activity and pushes the upper incisors from lingual side, thus increasing the overjet.
2. In certain forms of habits and class II division 1, the buccinators muscle is hyperactive, thus causing narrowing of maxillary arch.
3. Overclosure of jaws is associated with increased activity of temporalis m.
4. In horizontal growth cases, most of muscles of mastication have more force than in vertical growth cases.
5. EMG can be studied after orthodontic treatment to see whether muscle balance has been achieved or not.
6. Children with cerebral palsy and other asymmetries show abnormal EMG patterns.

CT scan and **CBCT:** It is one of the latest diagnostic modality. It can be used to study detailed features of hard tissues, e.g. TMJ morphology, sinuses, etc. Recently, CT scans

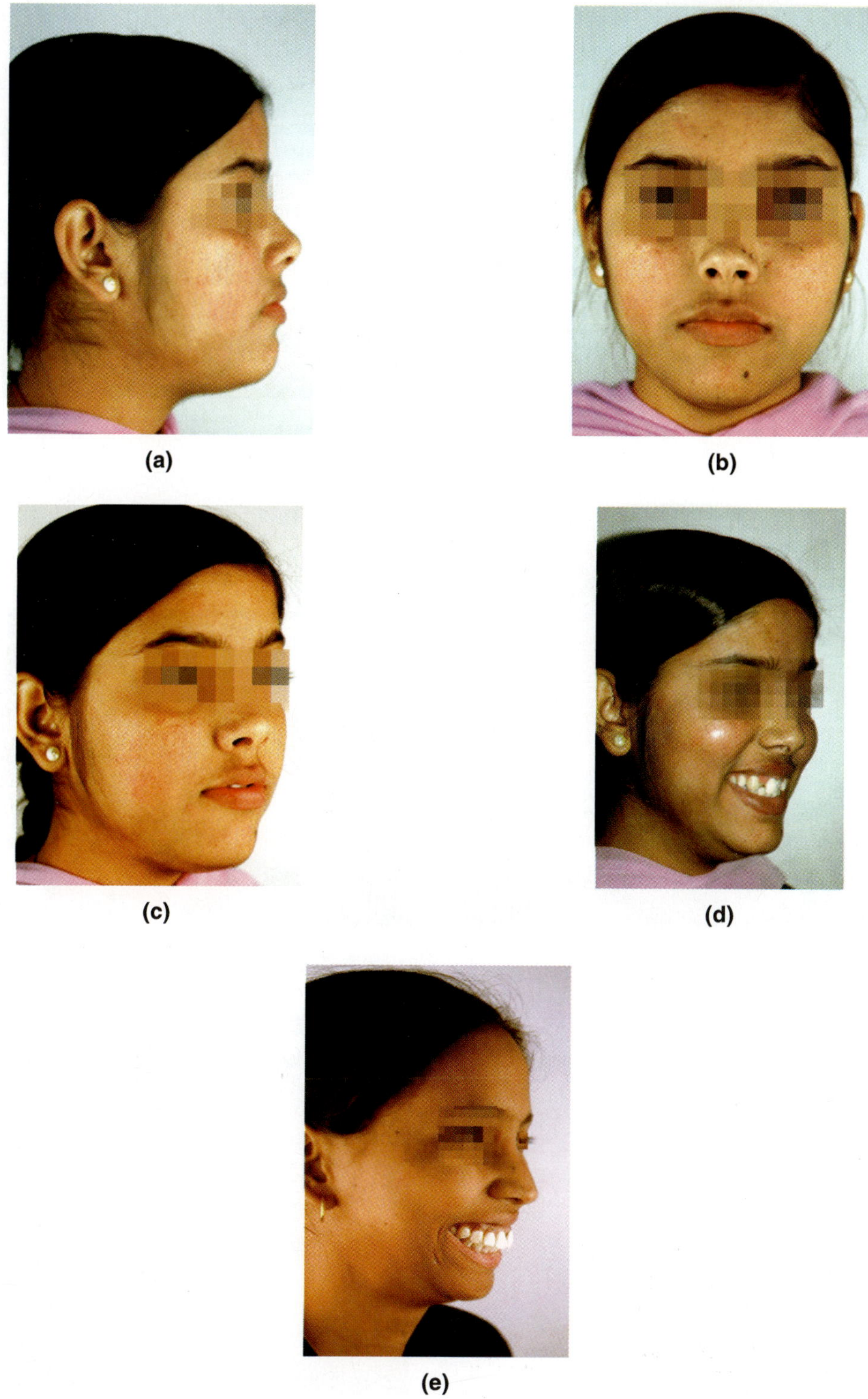

Figs 13.39a to e: Extraoral photos for records: Lateral view, frontal view, oblique lateral view, and oblique lateral smiling view.

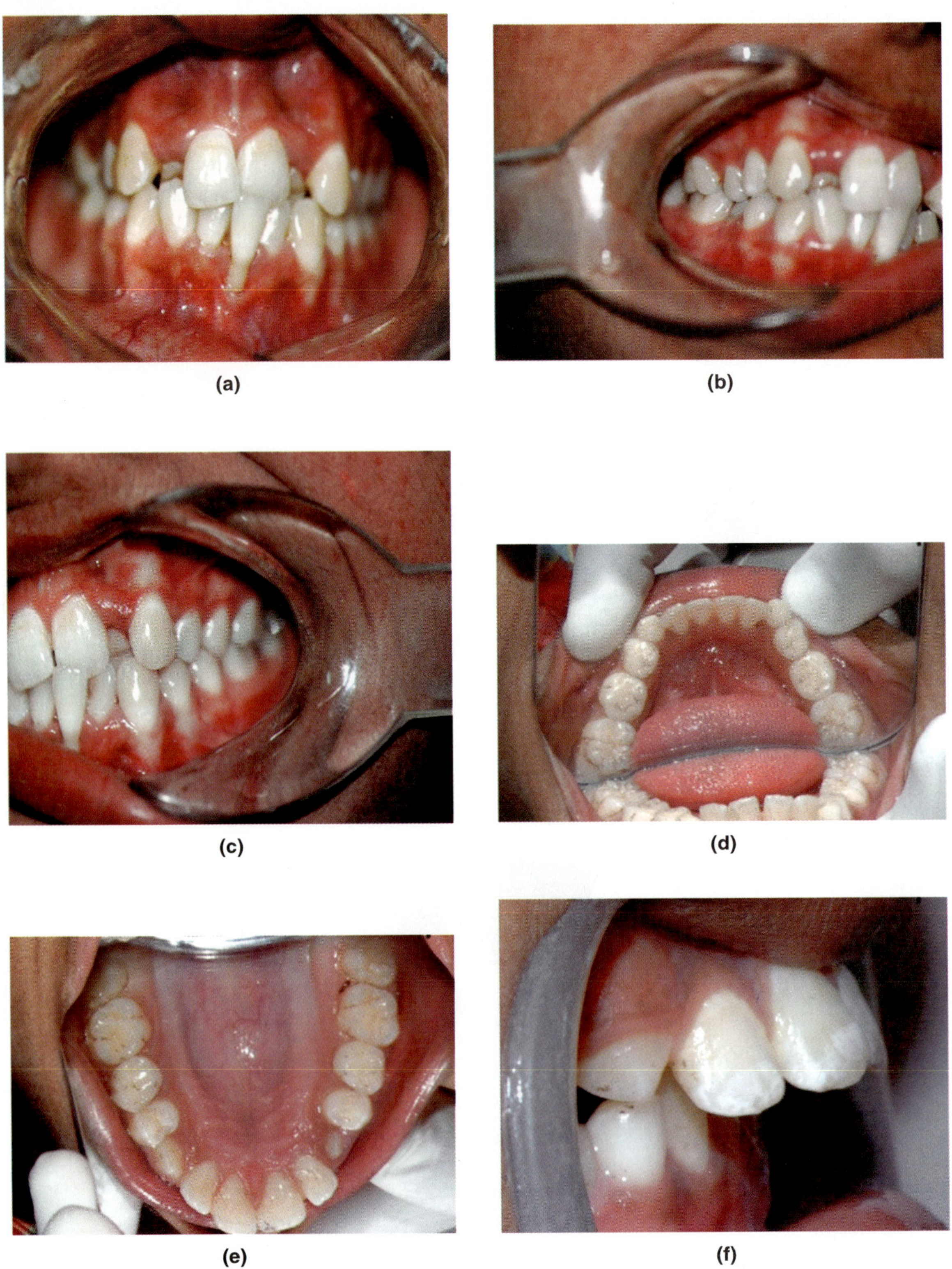

(a) (b) (c) (d) (e) (f)

Figs 13.40a to f: Intraoral views: Frontal, right buccal, left buccal, lower arch, upper arch and overjet.

are being used to study bone morphology before microimplants placement.

MRI: It is used to study soft tissue structures, e.g. TMJ disk.

Radiographs

Radiographs are important tools for diagnosis and required during diagnosis and treatment planning phase. However, they are not complete diagnostic records; but help in confirming and augmenting the information from examination.

Some of the views which may be required are IOPA, bitewing, occlusal views of maxilla and mandible, OPG, lateral and PA cephlograms, and hand wrist X-rays.

Uses from radiographs: Radiographs are one of the easiest and cheapest diagnostic tools available in medical field. They provide a lot of information to the clinician, as follows.

- General development of dentition, size, shape, position and state of development of teeth
- Pattern and amount of root resorption of primary teeth
- Status of eruption of permanent teeth
- Presence or absence of teeth/supernumerary tooth/impacted teeth
- Character of alveolar bone and lamina dura and periapical areas
- Morphology and axial inclination of the roots of teeth
- Pathologic conditions, e.g. caries, root fractures, apical infections, cysts, etc.
- To assess craniofaciodental morphology of the patient.
- For study and research purposes.
- For studying the progress of the case with treatment.

There are two types of radiographs used for diagnosis:

1. Intraoral views
2. Extraoral views.

Intraoral views: Generally, IOPA, bitewings and occlusal X-rays are used.

IOPA views: They are used to study the teeth and the supporting structures, e.g. periapical lesions; caries; morphology of root canals, etc. They provide the best views of teeth esp incisors and their roots without much distortion, since they are positioned closest to the tissues. They are also used for assessing the bone quantity and bone levels before microimplants placement.

They are taken by two techniques: (1) paralleling technique and (2) bisecting angle technique.

Paralleling technique: This is the best technique because the central rays of X-ray beam are at right angle to long axis of teeth and the film. It leads to least distortion. Here, the film is placed parallel to the long axis of teeth, supported by cotton role.

To take the best views, the film holders (e.g. XCP-DS from Dentsply, also called extended cone projection) are used and they hold the cone of X-ray tube at right position, e.g. Endoray, which helps in precise angulation and alignment of film to the X-ray cone. They prevent cone cutting and help in precise positioning of the films and cone.

Bisecting angle technique: Here, the central ray of X-ray beam is at right angle to the line which bisects the angle between long axis of teeth and axis of film. It incorporates some distortion in image.

Uses of IOPA films: Full mouth IOPA radiographs are generally taken before orthodontic treatment. They are used to:

1. To study the quality, quantity, height and contour of alveolar bone and supporting structures.
2. To assess the presence or absence of teeth; impacted tooth or odontome, etc.
3. To assess periapical pathologies, root fracture, root ragments, caries exposure, etc.
4. To assess ankylosis and root resorption, if any.
5. To assess size of unerupted teeth for space analysis purpose.
6. To study stages of root development, calcification, etc.

7. To assess root parallelism during treatment.
8. To see any supernumerary tooth and their morphology.
9. To assess the axial inclination of roots
10. To determine size and shape of unerupted teeth especially for calculating TSALD.

Disadvantages of IOPA

1. Many radiographs are required to assess the whole dentition, which needs patient cooperation, proper technique and proper storage.
2. It may be problematic in children, as they may not allow too many radiographs.
3. If patient has high gagging reflex, trismus or limited mouth opening, it may not be possible.
4. Storage is also problematic.

Advantages

1. They give us clear picture of tissues as they involve less distortion, as the film is closer to the tissues.
2. Low radiation dose to patient even for full mouth set of radiographs.
3. Can give us localized views of areas of the interest.
4. Less equipment cost, can be taken on chair-side.
5. No sophisticated equipment required.

Radio-visio-graphy (RVG): It is the latest technique of taking IOPA views. The X-rays strike a sensor placed in the mouth, the signal is fed in the computer, where it is manipulated by a specific software. The picture comes instantly on the screen. The image quality can be manipulated to see the proper findings. There is no need of physical films, no need of developing and fixing cycle; and no hassels of storage. The images are stored in the computer hard drive and can be easily retrieved. They can be sent through e-mails or in CD/flash drive to other doctor or to the patient. Only disadvantage is that the equipment is very costly, e.g. Heliodent from Sirona, etc.

Bitewing radiographs: They record mainly crowns of upper and lower teeth in one film, without much of roots and supporting structures. The uses are:

1. To detect proximal caries lesions mainly.
2. To study alveolar bone and crest level.
3. To assess height and contour or the shape and inclination of alveolar crest.
4. They also depict interdental calculi, restorations overhangs, secondary caries, etc.

Procedure: Special bite wing tabs are available in which the IOPA film can be secured and patient is asked to bite on the tab to stabilize the film. The central ray of X-ray beam is directed through the interdental area perpendicular to the film. A good quality picture without much distortion can be obtained.

Occlusal views: They are intraoral views taken for upper and lower arches separately. They help us to assess a larger part of dental arches, including palate and lingual areas of mandible and floor of mouth. Whole of the arch can be included in one film.

Uses

1. To locate impacted teeth, supernumerary teeth, pathologies, etc.
2. To assess mid-palatal suture for expansion planning and during expansion treatment procedures.
3. To assess location of incisive foramen.
4. To assess any buccolingual expansion of bones due to pathologies.
5. Help to assess stone in salivary ducts,
6. Help in diagnosis of fractures of basal bones.

Disadvantages

1. Cannot give exact location and inclination of impacted teeth especially maxillary canines.
2. May be uncomfortable in small oral cavity due to larger size of films.
3. Roots morphologies of teeth cannot be assessed.

4. Periapical areas are not properly assessed, as the rays pass almost parallel to the roots. So, IOPAs will be required.

Extraoral Radiographs

They are used to assess larger areas of craniofacial region in one film.

Main views required are:

- OPG,
- Lateral cephalograms
- PA cephalograms.

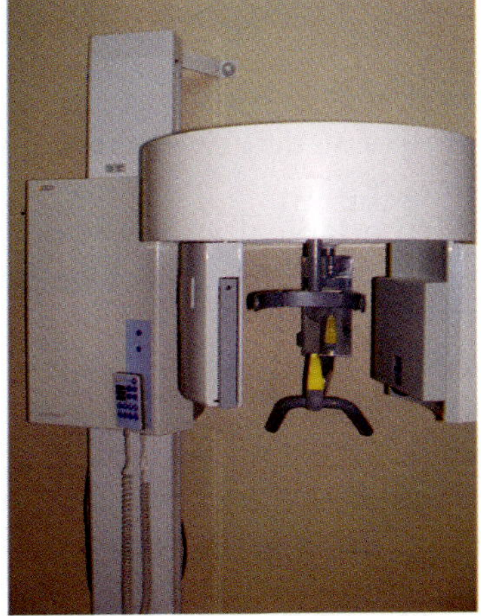

Fig. 13.41: OPG machine.

PANORAMIC VIEW (Figs 13.42 and 13.43)

OPGs are important pictures as they show both the jaws with the teeth and supporting structures and TMJs in one film.

Uses of OPG:

1. They become permanent record of the patient
2. All the erupted, unerupted teeth, their supporting tissues, can be seen on a single picture.
3. The stage of root development, dental eruption stage, and their relation with adjacent teeth can be seen, it helps in guidance of eruption.
4. TMJ morphology especially condyle and articular eminence can be visualized.
5. Any impacted teeth, supernumerary teeth, odontome, pathology, etc. can be seen.
6. Morphology of lower border of mandible, condylar neck and ramal morphology can be seen. Axial inclination of teeth can be evaluated
7. It can be used for research purpose.
8. It can be used for assessing the growth stage of the patient by examining the developmental stage of the roots of mandibular second molars, canines, and premolars.

Disadvantages of OPG are:

1. Costly, sophisticated and special equipment is required.
2. Radiation dose is high.

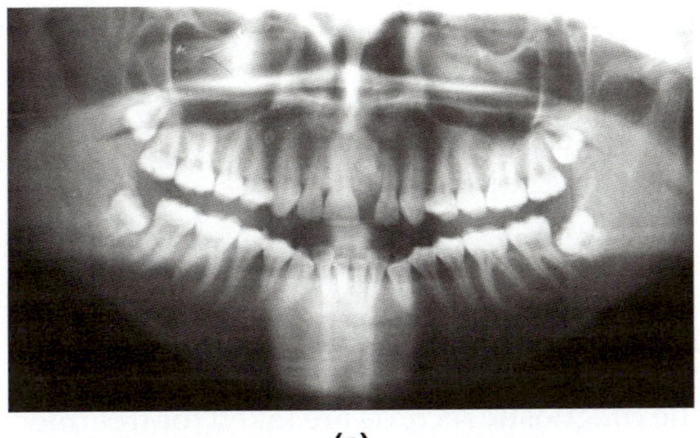

(a)

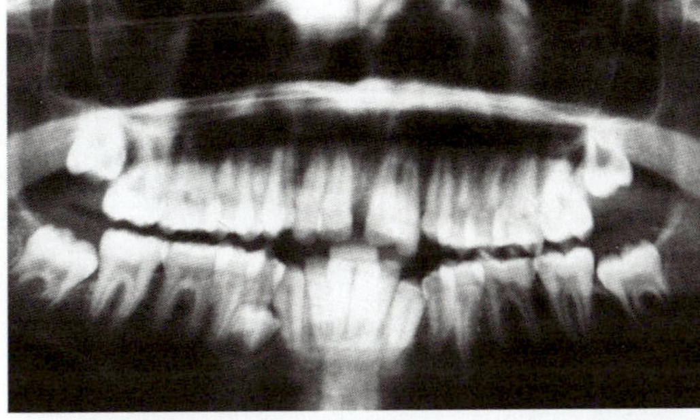

(b)

Figs 13.42a and b: OPG can be used to assess bone quality, pathologies, dentition stages, absent/ impacted/ supernumerary teeth, etc.

3. It takes approx. 12 seconds to take a full picture.
4. Distortion, magnification and overlapping of structures occur especially in incisal regions.
5. Proper periapical and interdental areas in incisal regions cannot be studied. It needs IOPA view.
6. Proper inclination of incisors cannot be studied.
7. Teeth and their supporting structures are not as clear as IOPA and contain magnifications approx. 15–30% depending on the machine, so the information in the area of interest esp incisal areas, is to be supplemented with other views.

CEPHALOGRAMS (Fig. 13.43)

They are specialized, standardized views taken from a special equipment called cephalostat. They are must for orthodontic diagnosis and treatment planning for a comprehensive treatment case. They are also used for research purpose and help in assessing growth status of the patient by studying cervical vertebrae. Details have been discussed in another chapter.

Other Radiographs

Hand-wrist radiographs (Fig. 13.44): They are taken to assess growth markers in hand and areas wrist of an individual. They may be taken as flat-hand views and glass-holding views for clarity of bones in question.

They help in assessing skeletal age of the child to help in treatment planning for growth modulation. The details will be given in Chapter 16 on Skeletal Maturity Indicators.

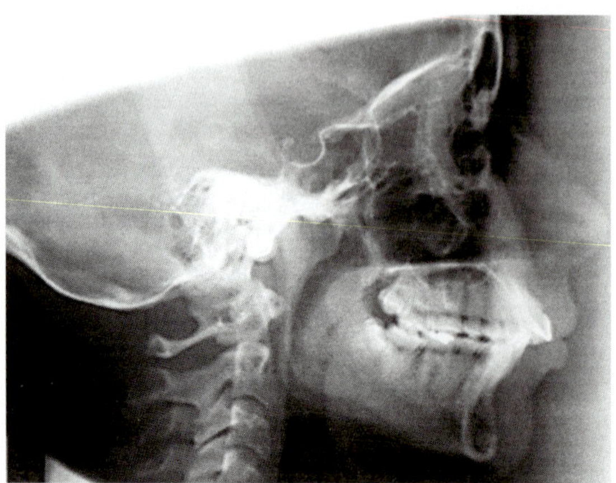

Fig. 13.43: Lateral cepahlogram.

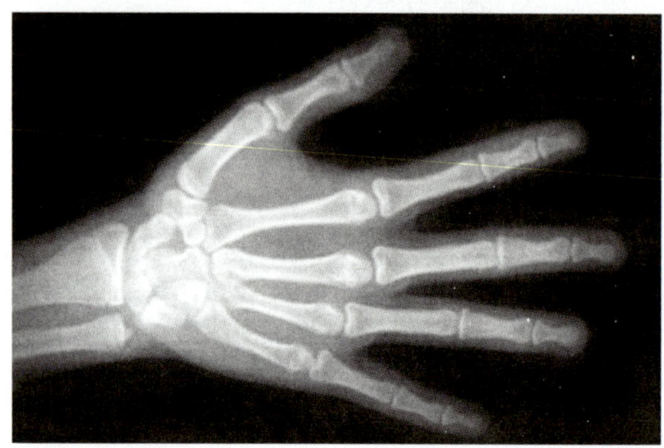

Fig. 13.44: Hand-wrist morphology of a mature child. Note that all the epiphyses and diaphyses of phalanges and radius bone are fused, confirming completion of growth.

Recent Advances in Diagnosis

Many other diagnostic instruments have been incorporated and used for orthodontic treatment planning. Some are:

- MRI (Fig. 13.45)
- CT scan/tomography/CBCT
- Xeroradiography
- Photocephalometry
- Digigraph
- Occlusograms
- Digital subtraction radiography
- Finite element methods
- Laser holography
- Cineradiography
- Fluoroscopy.

Their discussion is out of scope of this book.

Conclusion

The diagnostic records are taken for treatment planning, discussion with patients and parents, and for future reference. They are also used for comparing the progress of treatment

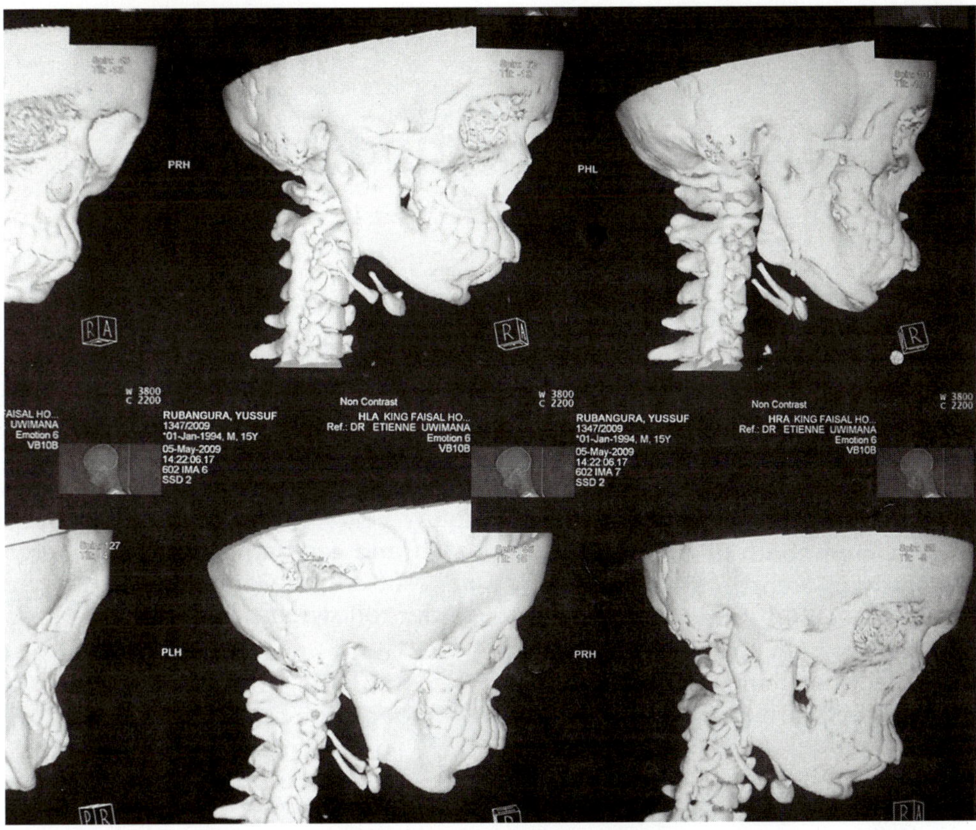

Fig. 13.45: MRI of face and TMJ showing ankylosis.

and can be used for retrospective cross-sectional and longitudinal studies. They should be obtained at every stage of treatment and thus they help in guiding and planning further course of treatment. Their value cannot be undermined and thus they should be stored safely. In the age of digitization, the storage of records has become quite easy through occlusography, digigraphy and holography. But, computers are also prone to viruses and corruption, thus back-up copies should always be kept.

14

Model Analysis in Orthodontics

INTRODUCTION

Study models are the essential diagnostic aids in the orthodontics. They are obtained at the pretreatment stage to study the relationship of teeth to the basal bones and to each other. They provide a 3D view of both dental arches and help in the study of occlusion in all the three planes of the space and especially from the lingual side. They help the orthodontist to evaluate the space deficiency or excess for the diagnosis and the treatment planning. Ideal requirements of models and their advantages have been mentioned in the chapter of diagnosis. In this chapter, we will discuss various methods for analyzing the space requirements during treatment.

PURPOSE OF MODEL ANALYSIS

1. To find out the TSALD, the space discrepancy or excess for treatment planning.
2. To assess the ratio of upper and lower teeth sizes for best extraction and stripping decisions (of course, aided by other diagnostic and structural factors) for the best-fitting occlusion.
3. To assess the width of dental arches to find out the requirement for expansion of dental arches.
4. To determine whether skeletal or dental expansion is needed.
5. To find out the proclination of teeth especially upper, and the need for their retraction. It also helps to determine the need for extraction of teeth.
6. To determine amount of stripping needed for creation of space, and which teeth need stripping.

Various methods have been proposed since many years, a few of them has been mostly used and are being discussed here. For the sake of convenience, we can divide them under following heads (Fig. 14.1):

1. To **determine TSALD,** e.g. Carey's analysis, Bolton's, Moyer's mixed dentition analysis, Hukaba's analysis.
2. To **determine arch widths,** e.g. Ashley Howe's, Pont's, Linder Harth index, Korkhaus'.
3. To **determine requirement of stripping:** Peck and Peck ratio; Bolton's ratio.

PRINCIPLES OF SPACE ANALYSIS

Space analysis is a comparison of the amount of space available in dental arches for alignment of the teeth and the amount of space required to align them properly. It may also be termed as tooth size-arch length discrepancy, TSALD. These methods of analysis may be broadly divided into following 2 types.

- Mixed dentition space analysis
- Permanent dentition space analysis

There are three basic approaches for space analysis:

1. Measurement of teeth on radiograph, e.g. Nance analysis
2. Estimation from proportionality tables, e.g. Moyer's analysis
3. Combination of radiographic and prediction table:

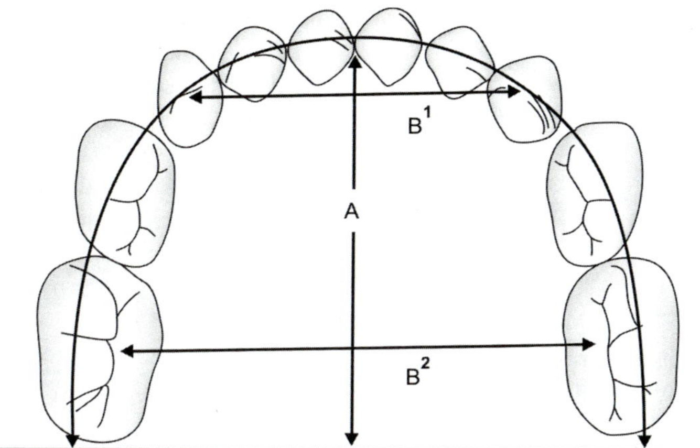

Fig. 14.1: Diagram showing intercanine width (between cusp tips) and intermolar (between central fossa) width measurements. Curve along the arch shows how to measure the arch circumference, while line A shows anteroposterior arch length.

- Tanaka Johnston analysis
- Staley and Kerber analysis.

Mixed Dentition Analysis

Measurement of Teeth on Radiographs (Huckaba's Analysis)

The structures on the radiograph appear magnified as compared to the original structures. This method is applied to determine the exact MD size of unerupted tooth by elimination of the magnification factor. It is done by comparing the size of unerupted and erupted teeth on the cast and radiograph. It requires undistorted IOPA radiographic image of that area, and the study model. It helps to nullify the radiographic enlargement (magnification factor) of the image of the teeth. With the help of a divider and scale, following three readings are taken from cast and the radiograph. The tooth which is present both on the cast and the radiograph is chosen:

a. MD width of erupted PM on the cast (true width), i.e. X1
b. MD width of erupted PM on the radiograph (apparent width), e.g. Y1
c. MD width of unerupted PM (true width), i.e. X2
d. MD width of unerupted PM on the radiograph (apparent width), i.e. Y2

The following formula is used for estimation.

$$\frac{\text{True width of Erupted PM (X1)}}{\text{Apparent width Erupted PM (Y1)}} = \frac{\text{True width of unerupted PM (X2)}}{\text{Apparent width of unerupted PM (Y2)}}$$

So $\mathbf{X2 = X1.Y2/\ Y1}$

Nance Analysis (Fig. 14.2)

It was proposed by Nance, 1940. It helps to determine the amount of space present in the arch and the amount of the space required when the permanent teeth will erupt. It helps to determine the MD widths of permanent teeth from cast and radiographs, by comparing the size of primary teeth and nullifying the radiographic enlargement, like in Hukaba's analysis.

Nance's Radiographic Measurement

Estimated width of unerutped permanent/ RG width of unerupted permanent tooth = Clinical width of primary/RG width of primary. Thereby:

- Estimated width of unerutped permanent = clinical width of primary × RG width of unerupted permanent tooth/ RG width of primary.

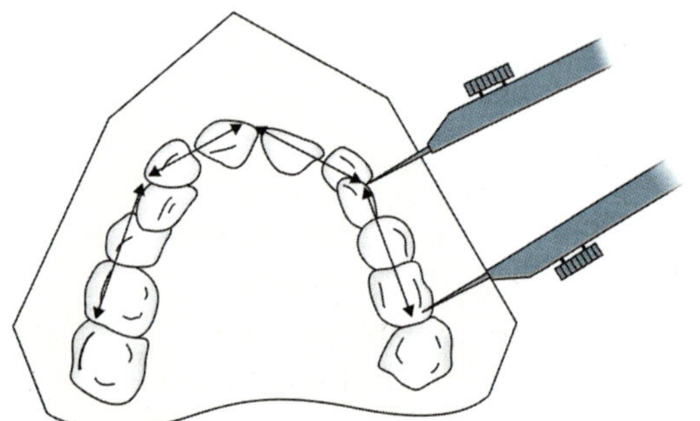

Fig. 14.2: Measurement of arch length in incisal and buccal regions, mesial to permanent first molars (Nance's analysis).

It helps to determine the exact width of the unerupted permanent tooth, as the radiographic correction gets applied through the ratio stated above. Thus, the widths of all the unerupted teeth are estimated and recorded.

1. The estimated widths of the unerupted teeth are calculated and recorded on a grid.
2. The MD widths of all the permanent teeth are summed and recorded for each arch. This gives the space required. (total tooth material).
3. The brass wire is adapted from mesial of first permanent molar from one side to that of other side and the length is recorded for each arch.
4. The leeway space is subtracted from the space available for each particular arch, e.g. 3.4 mm for the lower and 1.8 mm for the upper arch. This gives the space available.
5. The difference of steps 3 and 4 gives us the discrepancy, whether crowding or spacing. Based on this finding, the treatment plan, e.g. guidance of eruption, serial extraction, etc. can be planned. And a future estimation of crowding can be done which helps in future treatment planning.

Estimation from Proportionality Tables (Moyer's Analysis)

It was suggested by Moyer (1969). It helps to determine amount of space needed for alignment of canines and premolars, after the incisors have erupted. The combined mesiodistal width of the lower four incisors is used to predict the size of both the lower and upper unerupted canines and premolars.

Why only lower incisors are used? Because they are the first erupted teeth in the arches. And they have least variation in anatomy and eruption.

Procedure:

1. Visualize the aligned upper and lower incisors along the dental arch, if they are crowded.
2. Measure the space left behind between distal of lateral incisors and mesial of permanent first molars, for 345 in all the four quadrants.
3. Measure the mesiodistal width of lower four incisors with boley gauge and add.
4. By using Moyer's probability chart and incisal width value, find out the MD width of upper and lower 345 at 75% confidence level. However, this confidence level is different for different ethnic groups the charts for them are available in literature and should be referred for the particular race. However, recent studies have proved that it cannot be applied reliably to all types of population at 75% level, since this study has been done on the Caucasians only.
5. Compare the space available and space required in all the four quadrants by comparing findings of steps 2 and 4. This will give us an estimation of crowding/spacing for treatment planning. Consideration of loss or maintenance of leeway space should also be kept in mind.

Advantages:

- It is an easy and reproducible method.
- It has minimal error.
- It can be done with equal reliability by beginner and the expert.
- It is not time consuming.

- It does not require special instruments.
- It can be used for both the arches.
- No radiographs were required.

Tanaka Johnston Method

It was developed in 1974, another way to use the width of lower four incisors to predict the size of unerupted canines and premolars.

Steps: The MD widths of lower four incisors and summed up. Then following formula is used to find the combined width of 345 for upper and lower arches.

Half of the MD widths of lower 4 incisors + 10.5 mm	Estimated width of lower 345 for one quadrant
Half of the MD widths of lower 4 incisors + 11 mm	Estimated width of upper 345 for one quadrant

Advantage: It is a simple, quick and easy method. It does not need radiographs, and tables for estimation of the sizes.

Disadvantage: It tends to overestimate the size of canine and premolars.

It shows more amount of error for estimation of the sizes. It cannot be used for every race and gender. It gives a generalized idea of the size of the teeth.

Hixon-Oldfather Conversion Table

It uses the sum of mesiodistal width of one permanent mandibular central incisor and lateral incisor with the diameter of unerupted first and second bicuspid measured on an IOPA of same side to predict the actual space required for the eruption of cuspids and bicuspids. Corresponding values are assessed from the comparison table proposed by them. But, this method is not generally used.

Combination of Radiographic and Prediction Table (Staley and Kerber Method)

It is a modification of Hixon-Oldfather method. This method is used only for mandibular arch. It requires periapical radiograph. It is quite an accurate method.

Steps:

- **From the cast:** Mesiodistal widths of lower central and lateral incisors is noted for each lower quadrant.
- **From the periapical X-rays:** Mesiodistal widths of first and second premolars are noted for each lower quadrant.
- The sum of these widths is used on the prediction chart to determine the combined widths of lower canine and premolars in particular quadrant.

Interpretation of Mixed Dentition Analysis

1. When crowding is 1–4 mm, arch length is maintained and periodic examination of patient is done.
2. When crowding is predicted more than 4mm, patient is likely to develop crowding of permanent teeth that will require orthodontic treatment.
3. If crowding is more than 6 mm, serial extraction can be recommended.

Permanent Dentition Analysis

Some methods for cast analysis used in permanent dentition are used for different purposes. But, the information obtained from them is correlated and assimilated to reach the treatment planning. Some methods are as described under following headings:

1. To assess the need for expansion: Pont's index; Ashley Howe's analysis
2. To assess inclination of teeth: Korkhaus anterior arch length index
3. To assess palatal depth: Palatal index by Korkhaus
4. To assess arch perimeter tooth material discerpancy: Ashley Howes, Carey's analysis
5. To assess tooth material arch perimeter discerpancy:

- Bolton's ratios
- Peck and Peck ratio
- Little's irregularity index.

Pont's Analysis

It was introduced in 1909 and is proposed for French population. It is done for the upper arch only. It helps in determining the width of the dental arch, i.e. whether the dental arch is narrow or normal. And is there any need for arch expansion.

Reference teeth: Maxillary incisors are used for reference.

Sum of the mesiodistal (MD) size of 4 maxillary incisors is used to determine the ideal arch width in PM and molar areas. Steps involved in this analysis are:

- Determination of sum of incisors (SI)
- Determination of measured PM value (MPV) in mm, i.e. from distal pit of first premolar of one side to distal pit of first premolar of other side
- Determination of measured molar value (MMV) in mm, i.e. from mesial pit of permanent first molar of one side to mesial pit of permanent first molar of other side (Fig. 14.3).
- Determination of calculated PM value (CPV) mm
  $$\frac{SI \times 100}{80}$$
- Determination of calculated molar value (CMV) mm
  $$\frac{SI \times 100}{64}$$
- The measured and calculated values are compared in premolar and molar regions, respectively.

Inference:

1. If calculated value is greater than measured, i.e. measured value is less than the calculated value, it shows the need for expansion of upper arch in the required region to gain space (i.e. MPV < CPV or MMV < CPV).
2. Difference also quantifies how much expansion is required in the required region (i.e. CPV-MPV; CMV-MMV in mm).
3. But if it is greater than calculated value, then no scope of expansion.

Disadvantages:

- It does not include an assessment of mandibular arch. It is considered that the mandibular arch has to adjust according to maxillary arch.
- It is done for French population only. Reliability of index should be tested in other populations. Population specific data is needed for exact estimation.
- It also overestimates the desired arch width by an average of 2.5–4.7 mm, which leads to overexpansion, and then later on relapse.

Korkhaus Analysis

It is also done for upper arch only. It is used to determine ideal arch widths in molar and premolar areas, like Pont's index, but it uses Linder-Harth's index for this purpose. He proposed two indices, viz.

1. Anterior arch length index
2. Palatal height index.

1. **Anterior arch length index:** Formula for calculating the standard value of upper anterior arch length is:

Sum of upper incisors × 100/160

- **Actual distance** between the midpoint of a line joining the mesial pit of upper first premolar of one side to the other side, and the labial surface of most anteriorly positioned central incisor in cases of irregular teeth or the 'incision' point, i.e. a point between two upper central incisors in well-aligned teeth.

Inference:

- This analysis tells about both arch width and ideal positioning of anterior teeth.

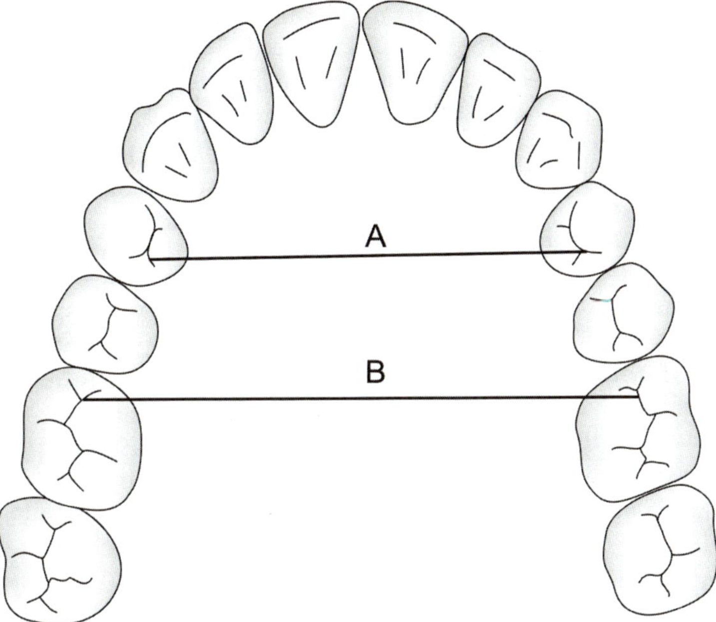

Fig. 14.3: Diagram showing interpremolar (between distal pits) and intermolar (between mesial pits) width measurements.

According to this analysis, for a given width of incisors, there exists a specific value of the distance between the midpoint of a line joining the mesial pit of upper first premolar of one side to the other side, and "incision" point, i.e. a point between two upper central incisors.

- The lower anterior arch length is 2 mm shorter than upper anterior arch length.
- If the perpendicular distance from inter premolar line is more than ideal, then the teeth are proclined. If it is less, then they are retroclined.

2. Palatal height index: This index was introduced in 1939. Purpose of this index was to evaluate the palatal height and shape. Palatal height is the perpendicular distance from the midline raphe to the level of OP in permanent first molar region.

Posterior arch width is measured between the mesial pits on occlusal surface of upper permanent first molars. Palatal height is the perpendicular distance from the line connecting the mesial pits of upper first molars.

Formula for PHI = Palatal height × 100/ posterior arch width.

Average value for palatal index is 42%. PHI increases with increased palatal height or decreased arch width. Such cases need expansion to normalize the PHI. It decreases with decreased palatal height or increased arch width. There, further expansion of maxillary arch is contraindicated.

- **Increased value** shows that the palatal vault is high relative to transverse arch development. It occurs in dolichocephalic, dolichofacial patients, where the arch is narrow and the palate is deep, e.g. in thumb sucking habit, mouth breathing habit, rickets, etc.
- **Decreased value** shows that palatal vault is shallow. It occurs in brachycephalic, brachyfacial patients, where the arch is wide and the palate is shallow.

Ashley Howe's Analysis (1954)

Ahsley Howe considered that the dental crowding is due to deficient arch width rather that the arch length. He found that a relationship exists between the total MD widths of upper 12 teeth (6–6 teeth) and the dental arch width in the first premolar area. This analysis is done for upper arch only. It helps to find out the tooth material-arch width discrepancy for determining the need for expansion and/or extraction and the treatment planning.

Steps:

Determination of total tooth material (TTM): Is the sum of MD widths of 12 upper permanent teeth between first molars.

Determination of premolar diameter (PMD): Is the distance between buccal cusp tips of first premolars.

Determination of premolar basal arch width (PMBAW): The canine fossa is present distal to canine eminence of upper canine. Width of the apical base, viz the junction of basal bone and alveolar process, of dental arch is measured between the canine fossae. If canine fossa is not clear, the measurements are made 8 mm below the crest of the interdental papilla distal to the canine.

Inference: The PMBAW and PMD are compared.

If PMBAW is more than PMD, the arch expansion is possible. In such a case, the teeth can be flared buccally by dentoalveolar expansion thus correlating dental alveolar and basal arch widths, which is a stable position.

If PMBAW is less than PMD, the arch expansion is not possible. If expansion is attempted in such a case, the premolar and other teeth will flare buccally, i.e. tipping occurs, which is an unstable condition, and may also lead to gingival recession on buccal aspects due to lost torque.

He also predicted that to achieve the normal occlusion with full complement of the teeth, the basal arch width in first premolar area should be 44% of the TTM.

PMBAW ratio: The ratio between the apical base width at the first premolar region and the total tooth material is called the PMBAW percentage.

PMBAW % = PMBAW × 100 / TTM.

a. If PMBAW % is 37% or less: There is a basal arch deficiency, and it indicates the need of extraction for treatment.
b. If PMBAW % is 44% or more: Then, the case can be treated without extraction, and some other methods of gaining the space can be used.
c. If PMBAW % is 37–44%: It is a borderline case, which may/may not need the extraction of teeth. It needs a more subjective treatment planning considering other parameters, like growth pattern, nasolabial angle, age, dental status, etc.

Carey's Analysis (1946)

It is one of the most widely used and simple analysis. Since most of the malocclusion is due to the discrepancy between arch length and the tooth size, this analysis helps to determine extent of this discrepancy. It is performed on the lower cast. Same analysis on upper cast is called arch perimeter analysis.

Determination of arch length available (ALA) (Fig. 14.4): The arch length anterior to first permanent molars is measured by using a soft brass wire. The wire is placed from the mesial surface of the first permanent molar of one side and is passed over the buccal cusps of

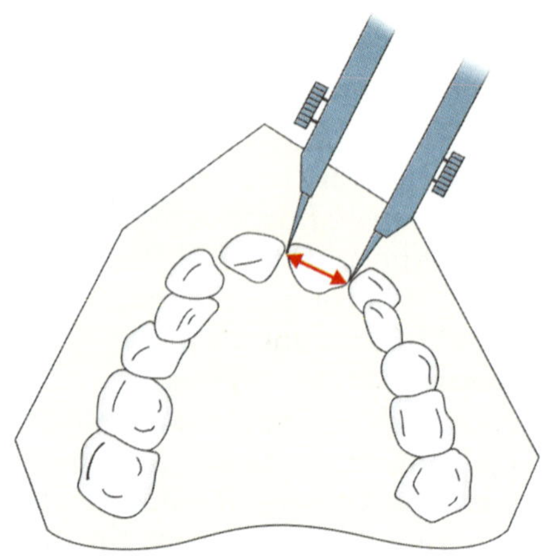

Fig. 14.4: Measurement of MD width of a tooth.

premolars/primary molars and along the anterior on the cingulum areas and is continued on the opposite side to mesial of first permanent molar. Thereby, it also helps us to determine the space available in the dental arch for the accommodation of the permanent teeth in a mixed dentition.

Determination of total tooth material (TTM): Mesiodistal widths of teeth anterior to first molars (5–5) is measured and summed up.

Inference: A difference of ALA and TTM is taken.

If ALA more thanTTM, it implies that there is spacing and thus no need of extraction.

If ALA less than TTM, discrepancy is negative depicting crowding. If it is:

- 0–2.5 mm, it implies that there is minimal tooth material excess. Such cases can be treated with space gaining and/or proximal reduction can be carried out.
- If 2.5–5 mm, it indicates the need to extract second PM
- If it is more than 5 mm, it shows the need to extract the first PM
- In cases of mixed dentition, the leeway space should also be considered for calculating the ALA. The 3.4 mm of space is subtracted from the ALA before calculating the actual discrepancy.

Profitt's Analysis

Profitt has given the following values of TSALD for determining the requirement of extraction. According to him.

1. **If TSALD is less than 5 mm:** It is a nonextraction case. So, different methods of space gaining can be applied to treat the case.
2. **If TSALD is more than 5 mm but less than 9 mm:** It is a borderline case. Other factors like growth pattern, nasolabial angle, growth completion, etc. should be considered for extraction planning.
3. **If TSALD is more than 9 mm:** Definite case of extraction.

However, latest trend in orthodontic treatment is nonextraction method, rather than extractions. A self-ligating bracket technique named as Damon system claims to treat the malocclusion by expansion of the dental arches. Still proper diagnosis and consideration of factors like age, growth, peak height, etc. is done to decide the extraction or nonextraction treatment plan.

Bolton's Analysis

It was introduced by Bolton (1958). According to him, the tooth size is an important factor to be considered for the case analysis and treatment planning. Most of the malocclusions occur due to the abnormalities in the tooth size, e.g. large or small MD widths of teeth leading to spacing, crowding, etc. According to Bolton, there exists a proportional relationship between the MD widths of upper and lower teeth. If the proportion is balanced, then there will be a proper alignment of teeth and proper interarch relation in anterior and posterior segments.

This analysis helps us to find out the disproportion between the upper and lower teeth. These days, it has gained such an important significance, that it is called as the "sixth key of normal occlusion".

Steps: MD widths of all the 12 teeth in upper and lower arches are measured and noted in a tabular form. Then, the following measurements are made.

1. Sum of mandibular 12
2. Sum of maxillary 12
3. Sum of mandibular 6
4. Sum of maxillary 6

Ratios: Two ratios are obtained from the above data, i.e.

1. Overall ratio
2. Anterior ratio

Overall ratio: It is the percentage relationship of mandibular 12 to maxillary 12 teeth.

$$\text{Overall ratio} = \frac{\text{Sum of mandibular 12} \times 100}{\text{Sum of maxillary 12}}$$

Normal value of overall ratio is 91.3% and standard deviation 1.91.

a. If overall ratio is less than 91.3, it shows the excess maxillary tooth material (since maxillary tooth material is the denominator in formula). So for the treatment and a balanced relation of upper and lower teeth, we have to reduce the tooth material in maxillary arch. It can be done either by extractions or by stripping, depending on the amount of TSALD. The amount of excess maxillary tooth material is calculated by the following formula:

Discrepancy in maxillary teeth = maxillary 12 – (mandibular 12 × 100/91.3)

How to calculate the discrepancy?

Since Overall ratio, i.e. 91.3 =

$$\frac{\text{Sum of mandibular 12} \times 100}{\text{Sum of maxillary 12}}$$

So, sum of maxillary 12 (expected) = sum of mandibular 12 × 100/91.3.

Difference (excess) = maxillary 12 of patient– maxillary 12 expected.

This excess has to be relieved by stripping of the teeth or if difference is large, combined with other factors, extraction may need to be done.

b. If overall ratio is more than 91.3, it shows the excess mandibular tooth material (since mandibular tooth material is the numerator in formula). The amount of excess mandibular tooth material is calculated by the following formula:

Discrepancy in mandibular 12 = mandibular 12–(maxillary 12 × 91.3/100).

Two anterior ratio: It is the percentage relationship of MD width of mandibular anteriors to maxillary anteriors.

$$\text{Anterior ratio} = \frac{\text{Sum of mandibular 6} \times 100}{\text{Sum of maxillary 6}}$$

Anterior ratio is 77.2% and standard deviation 1.65.

Inference:

a. If in a patient, the anterior ratio is less than 77.2, it indicates a maxillary tooth material excess. The amount of excess maxillary tooth material which needs to be reduced, is calculated by the following formula:
   = Maxillary 6 – (mandibular 6 × 100/77.2)

b. If value is less than 77.2, then the excess lies in mandibular tooth material. The amount of excess mandibular tooth material is calculated by the following formula:
   = mandibular 6 – (maxillary 6 × 77.2/100)

Drawbacks: Significant differences exist between different ethnic population, the same values cannot be applied to every population. So different ratios should be calculated.

Peck and Peck Analysis

This analysis was proposed by Harvey Peck and Sheldon Peck (1972). It is done in lower arch only.

Rationale: According to them, most common malocclusion seen is crowding of lower incisors. So, there should exist a relation between the mesiodistal and the faciolingual dimensions of the lower incisors. Purpose of this article was to evaluate tooth shape deviations of the mandibular incisors. This index helps us to find out the requirement of stripping in an incisor.

The findings of this study are based on two groups of young females (45 subjects with perfect mandibular incisor alignment, and 70 subjects with malocclusion).

$$\text{Index} = \frac{\text{Mesiodistal crown diameter in mm} \times 100}{\text{Faciolingual crown diameter in mm}}$$

Desirable MD/FL index values are:

- Mandibular central incisor: 88–92
- Mandibular lateral incisor: 90–95.

Higher values of the mesiodistal/facio-lingual index show that the MD width of the particular incisor is more, leading to the crowding in lower incisor region. So, a treatment planning can be done as which tooth will need the stripping to normalize the ratio.

Lower values will show that the teeth are narrower in width, and thus spacing can be expected in the incisor region, which needs to be built-up by composites or PFM restorations.

Tweed's Arch Perimeter Analysis

According to Tweed, if the teeth are not in a stable relationship with their basal bones after the treatment, this may lead to relapse. The lower incisors should be at right angle to their basal bone for stability. So, a dental oriented analysis alone is not adequate. A facial oriented analysis has to be done to evaluate the teeth with their basal bone. It is done for mandibular arch only. The mandibular arch is planned first, around which the upper arch is correlated. It is calculated by following components:

1. Arch length discrepancy
2. Tweed's head plate correction
3. Depth of curve of Spee.

Note: 1. for correction of 1°, space required is 0.4 mm in each quadrant.
2. For 1 mm, correction of curve of Spee, space required is 1 mm

Step 1: Calculating arch length discrepancy (ALD):

a. Arch perimeter: A soft brass wire is adapted from mesial surface of first permanent molar of one side to that of the other side, passing through the incisal edges. It is the arch perimeter.
b. Total tooth material: A sum of MD widths of 10 teeth mesial to permanent first molars is calculated.
c. Difference of values obtained in steps a and b above, is the arch length discrepancy.

Step 2: Tweed head plate correction, (HPC):

- It is measured on a lateral cephalogram. The amount of dental protrusion or retrusion is assessed and the correction is incorporated into the analysis. The incisors should be upright on their basal bone. The proclined incisors are retracted during treatment, which need the space and thus add to the total discrepancy. Retroclined incisors are flared during treatment, wcich give the space and thus reduce the total discrepancy. The values of Tweed's analysis are used for this purpose. It depends on the following values of FMA and FMIA.
- When FMA is 21–29, the FMIA should be 68°.
- When FMA is 30° or greater, FMIA should be 65°.
- When FMA is 20° or less, the IMPA should not exceed 92°
- As proposed by Tweed, if for a specific FMA, the FMIA did not correspond, then an objective line is traced on cephalogram to form the required FMIA. Then the distance between this objective line and line that passes through the actual long axis of mandibular incisors was measured on the occlusal plane. This figure is multiplied by two for right and left sides. The total was the cephalometric correction, HPC.
- It can also be calculated by the difference in the values of present FMIA and corrected FMIA, which is then multiplied by 0.8 mm. It is considered that for correction of each degree of FMIA, a space of 0.4 mm/degree/side of the dental arch is required.

Step 3: Depth of curve of Spee (COS): COS should be flat after the treatment, which then settles to 2 mm with time. Treatment of deep bite due to deep COS needs flattening of COS. Correction of curve of Spee also requires space. For correction of each mm of COS, a space of 0.5 mm/mm/side is required. So, e.g. for correction of 4 mm COS, an extraspace of 4 mm will be required.

Total discrepancy: It is calculated by summing the values of steps 1, 2, and 3, viz. ALD + HPC + COS.

Based on the total discrepancy, the decision of extraction or non-extraction is taken during the treatment of a case.

The Irregularity Index

It gives us a quantitative score of mandibular anterior alignment. It was proposed by Robert M Little in 1975. It is done on mandibular casts only. It determines the total of millimeters distances from the contact point on each incisor tooth to the contact point that it should touch.

- Measurements are obtained directly from the mandibular cast, with the help of a caliper held parallel to the occlusal plane.
- Each of the five measurements represents a horizontal linear distance between the anatomic contact points of the adjacent teeth.

All the measurements were added and the readings were compared to as follows:

- 0 perfect alignment
- 1–3 minimal irregularity
- 4–6 moderate irregularity
- 7–9 severe irregularity
- 10 very severe irregularity.

Total Space Analysis

It was suggested by Levern Merrifield. It helps to find out the discrepancy in different segments of the dental arch. It is considered mainly in mandibular arch. It involves teeth, jaw and soft tissues.

Since the facial esthetics has been of paramount importance in orthodontics, therefore, to achieve the harmony in facial profile and the stability of dentition, the soft tissue parameter is also considered in this analysis and the Tweed's method of head plate correction is included to find out the exact amount of discrepancy. It also considers the growth of mandible and the possibility of future crowding/impaction of third molars. The total discrepancy and the segmental discrepancy help to plan the extraction of teeth required especially also the third molars. The steps are as follows.

A. **Anterior area:** It is canine to canine segment. The space needed and space required are calculated as usual and discrepancy is calculated. It helps to decide the stripping, or incisal extraction. Arch length discrepancy is measured by conventional method, i.e.
   - **Space required:** Total tooth material can be calculated by adding the MD sizes of permanent incisors and canines. In mixed dentition, Hukaba's mixed dentition analysis is used to calculate TTM. The values obtained for mandibular incisors on the cast and those for the canines on the radiograph were added to space required.
   - **Space available:** The space available is measured by a soft brass wire from mesial surface of first primary molar or premolar on one side to another, passing through buccal cusp and incisal edges of remaining teeth.
   - **Discrepancy:** The difference obtained for space required and space available was the discrepancy.
   - **Tweed's cephalometric correction:** It is calculated by calculating the difference with patient's and proposed FMIA and multiplying by 0.8 mm. This is added to total discrepancy.
   - **Soft tissue modification:**
     1. It is derived by measuring Z-angle of Merrifield and adding the Tweed's cephalometric correction (in degrees). It measures the soft tissue protrusion of lower lip. A line is drawn from Pog′ to most prominent lip and extended to FHP. The lower internal angle is the Z-angle. It is affected by the proclination of incisors.

     If corrected Z angle is more than 80°, the mandibular incisor inclination is modified as necessary (up to an IMPA of 92°).

If corrected Z angle more than 75°, then the additional uprighting of incisors is required along with cephalometric correction.

2. If lip thickness is less than chin thickness, then the difference is calculated, which is multiplied by 2 and is added to space required.

   If lip thickness is less than or equal to chin thickness, no soft tissue modification is required.

B. **Middle area:** It is the segment involving premolars and first molars. The discrepancy is calculated as usual, to which COS is added. It helps to decide about premolar extraction. Curve of Spee is calculated as follows.

$$\frac{\text{Right side depth} + \text{left side depth} + 0.5 \text{ mm}}{2}$$

The COS should be flat. To correct the COS, the space is needed equal to the depth of COS. This is added to the space required.

C. **Posterior area:** Space required is calculated by adding the MD widths of 2nd and third molars. If they are unerupted, then radiographic enlargements are adjusted.

The estimated value of permanent third molar = actual size of permanent first molar × apparent width of third molars/apparent width of first molars.

- **Predicted space:** It is the space estimated to increase with growth of mandible in ramal area. It is considered to be 3 mm per year (1.5 mm on each side) till 14 years in girls and 16 years in boys. So, age of patient is subtracted from 14 or 16 years and the difference is multiplied by 3 to get the space increase estimated.
- Space available is measured by measuring the distance along the occlusal plane between a tangent to distal surface of first permanent molar to the anterior border of ramus of mandible.
- Space deficit = (space available + space predicted) – space required.

Miscellaneous findings

Relation of incisive papilla: A line passing through the posterior margin of incisive papilla which is drawn perpendicular to the midpalatal raphe, passes through the canines.

Relation of rugae and canines: First primary rugae should be in line with maxillary canine.

According to Rickets, the line connecting DB and ML cusps of first permanent maxillary molars should pass through the maxillary canine in a normal dentition. If it does not pass, then there is rotation of the molar present.

Stages of Dental Eruption

1. DS 1: Incisors erupting, early MDP
2. DS2: Incisors erupted, intermediate mixed dentition
3. DS3: Canines or premolars erupting, late mixed dentition
4. DS4: Canines and PMs fully erupted, adolescent dentition
5. DS5
6. DS 6

Conclusion

Model analysis is a very important part of orthodontic diagnosis and treatment planning. It helps in estimating the degree and severity of malocclusion in three planes of space. They help us to find the need of extraction, expansion, stripping, etc. and help us to decide the methods of gaining the space for alignment of the teeth. Mixed dentition analyses give us a picture of the developing condition which can be timely intercepted by utilizing the child's innate potential of growth. This timely intervention helps to reduce the severity of the condition in future. Hence, the value of model analysis cannot be overlooked during diagnosis and treatment planning.

MODEL ANALYSIS CHART

CAST ANALYSIS

A. MESIODISTAL DIMENSIONS:

	RIGHT SIDE						LEFT SIDE					
UPPER TEETH												
TOOTH NO.	6	5	4	3	2	1	1	2	3	4	5	6
LOWERTEETH												

B. SUM OF MD WIDTHS:

TEETH NO.	UPPER	LOWER
2–2		
3–3		
5–5		
6–6		

C. LABIOLINGUAL DIMENSIONS OF LOWER INCISORS:

SIDE	RIGHT		LEFT	
TOOTH NO.	2	1	1	2
LABIOLINGUAL WIDTH				
PECK AND PECK RATIO				
NORMAL VALUE	90–95	88–92		

D. CAREY'S ANALYSIS:

	UPPER	LOWER
ARCH LENGTH AVAILABLE – ALA		
TOTAL TOOTH MATERIAL – TTM, 5–5		
DISCREPANCY		

E. BOLTON'S RATIO:

	NORMAL VALUE	PATIENT VALUE	DIFFERENCE
MD 6–6			
MX 6–6			
MD 3–3			
MX 3–3			
ANTERIOR RATIO = MD 6 X 100/MX 6	77.2		
OVERALL RATIO = MD 12 X 100/MX 12	91.3		

F. TRANSVERSE DIMENSIONS:

	UPPER	LOWER
PMD-BUCCAL CUSPS		
FIRST PREMOLAR WIDTH		
(DISTAL PITS) MPV		
FIRST MOLAR WIDTH		
(MESIAL PITS) MMV		
PMBAW-CANINE FOSSAE		
INTERCANINE WIDTH		
KORKHAUS-DISTANCE B/W PM		
1 LINE TO CENTRE OF MX 1.		

	PATIENT VALUES		DIFFERENCE
PONT'S INDEX UPPER		LINDER HARTH'S	
ARCH ONLY		INDEX	
MPV DISTAL PIT			
MMV MESIAL PIT			
CPV = SI X 100/80		CPV = SI X 100/85	
CMV = SI X 100/64		CMV = SI X 100/64	

ASHLEY-HOWE'S INDEX: FOR UPPER ARCH ONLY

TTM 6–6
PMD-BUCCAL CUSP
PMBAW – CANINE FOSSA
PMBAW% = PMBAW X 100/TTM < 37% 37–44 > 44%

Further Readings

1. Ash M. Wheeler's Dental Anatomy, Physiology & Occlusion. 7th ed. Singapore : harcourt brace & company asia pte ltd;1940.
2. Bolton WA. Disharmony in tooth sizes & its relation to the analysis & treatment of malocclusion. Angle Orthod 1958; 28: 113-30.
3. Dirthoft BI. Dental holography – Earlier Investigations & prospective possibilites. Adv Dent Rest 1987 Oct; 1(1): 8-13.
4. Graber T.M.Orthodontics Principles and Practice:3rd ed;2001,AITBS publishers,New Delhi.
5. Graber T M, Vanarsdall R L, Vig K W L: Orthodontics: Current principles and techniques; 4th ed, 2005, Mosby.
6. Hajeer MY, Millett DT, Ayoub AF, Siebert JP. Applications of 3D imaging in orthodontics: part II.J Orthod. 2004 Mar; 31 (1): 62–70.
7. Hixon EH, Oldfather RE. Estimation of the size of unerupted cuspid & bicuspid teeth. malocclusion. Angle Orthod 1958.
8. Mcdonald Ralph E, Avery David R., Dean Jeffery A. Dentistry For child & adoloscent.8th ed. St louis: Mosby; 2004.
9. Peck s, Peck H.Crown dimensions & mandibular incisor allignment. Angle Orthod 1972.
10. Proffit W R: Contemporary Orthodontics; 4th ed, 2007, Mosby.

15

Cephalometrics

INTRODUCTION

Orthodontic diagnosis involves the assessment of the craniofacial structures, the interrelationship of teeth, jaw bases, soft tissues and the surrounding skeletal structures. These information help in appropriate treatment and anchorage planning, and give an insight into expected results. Cephalometrics is an important diagnostic method used in orthodontics. It helps in assessment of relationship of various craniodentofacial structures on a radiographic film.

As the name suggests, cephalometrics is made of two words, viz cephalo means head, and metrics means study. Cephalometrics is the study of head. Before the advent of cephalometry, the assessment of facial proportions was based on the artistic standards of harmony, beauty and symmetry.

Historical Perspective

Measurement of body parts and especially skull and face has been the area of interest from time immemorial. Ancient artists used to measure the dimensions of body parts, face and smile features, and replicate them in their paintings. The sizes of hands, etc. were used as the units of measurement of sizes of walls, houses, etc. and were also used to assess the time.

Clinical use of the body dimensions was also prevalent in ancient times. Measurement of body parts was known as **anthropometry**. Initially, it was used to measure the size of bones found during excavations. But later on, it was adapted to living persons. Antrhropometry had been used in orthodontic diagnosis, where the measurements were done directly on the face of the patient by marking certain points. But, it was not able to reveal exact skeletal relationship because of the thickness of soft-tissues. However, this method can be used for longitudinal studies.

Craniometry is the direct measurements made on skulls of dead persons. It is more reliable than anthropometric values since there is no soft tissue intervening. But it cannot be used on living person, and it cannot be used for longitudinal studies. Also, the soft tissue envelop makes direct measurements unreliable and less accurate. Also, the intraoriental and skeletal midline structures cannot be assessed and measured correctly. Only, external surface measurements can be correctly made.

Cephalometry: With the discovery of X-rays in 1895 by Roentgen, a new era started in medical science. In 1922, Pacini standardized the radiographic head views by fixing the distance of X-ray source to film. In 1931, a new world opened in the science of orthodontic, when Broadbent from USA and Hoffrath from Germany simultaneously presented a standardized cephalometric technique, and the machine was termed as cephalostat. Cephalometrics is defined as the study or measurement of the structures of head on a cephalometric radiograph, which is known as cephalograms or head plate.

Advantages

- Measurements can be done on living persons.

- The longitudinal studies can be done.
- Midline structures are also seen clearly on the films, which can be measured properly.
- Technique is reproducible.
- The X-ray films act as long-time records, which can be used for comparison and research purpose.
- The films can be overlapped on certain stable anatomical structures to evaluate the progress of treatment.
- Digital forms of pictures can be stored in hard drives of computers, and can be electronically transmitted for further discussions with fellow colleagues.

Disadvantages

- It represents 2D view of 3D structures.
- Machine is costly.
- Radiographic magnification tends to give over-estimation of values especially linear measurements. However, it needs correction during assessment.
- Patient has to be exposed to X-rays.

Equipment (Figs 15.1 and 15.2)

Cephalograms are standardized X-ray films which are taken with a specialized machine called as cephalostat. It consists of following parts:

- X-ray source.
- Head holder to hold the head in particular position and it can be adjusted for height.
- Forehead clamp is used to stabilize the head in vertical plane.
- Ear rods are placed in external auditory canal of patient to make him stable so that he does not move or rotate his head side to side.
- Orbital pointer is used to adjust the inclination of face so that FHP is parallel to the floor.
- Nasal pointer to augment the face position and to depict the point "nasale".
- Film cassette with intensifying screens and film cassette holder.

Specifications: The distance between the X-ray source and the mid-sagittal plane of the patient is fixed at 5 feet. Thus a standardized film can be obtained every time. The machine generally operates at 70 kvp, 7 mA, and for 0.7 seconds as the exposure time. However, improvements have been incorporated in machines to reduce the radiation exposure and to change settings according to size and age of the patient. Now, with the digital models, the image is directly seen on the computer screen where it can be seen for any discrepancy. If required, the exposure can be repeated immediately. The films can be

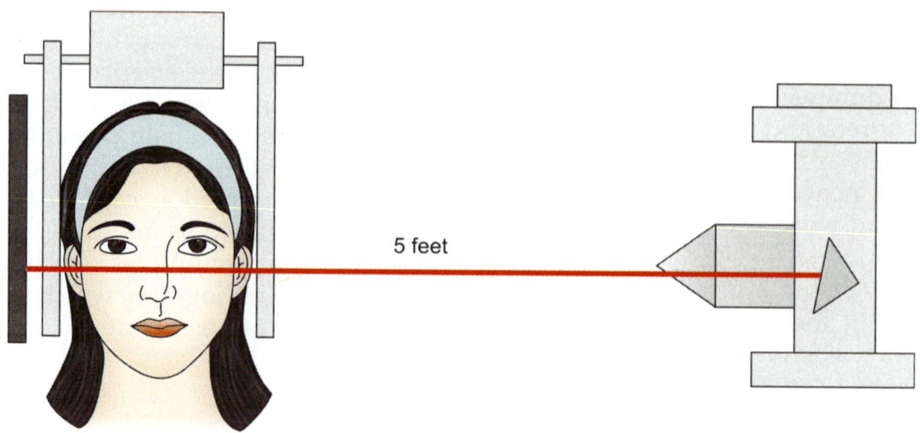

Fig. 15.1: Line diagram of cephalostat and position of the patient.

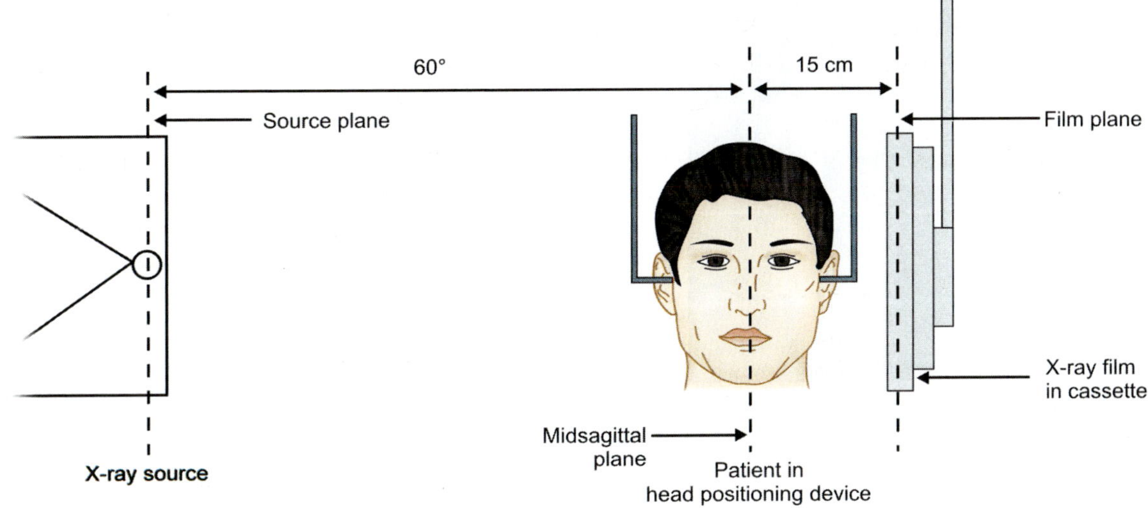

Fig. 15.2: Line diagram showing the cephalostat and position of the patient related to X-ray source and film holder.

directly printed by printers, and there is no need of settings like dark room, water tank and developing and fixing chemicals. Analysis of cephalometry has also gone digital with the help of certain software.

Technique: For obtaining the cephalograms, the patient can be made either to sit or stand upright without any strain in the body as per the machine's design. Patient's head is stabilized in the head holder, supported by the nasal support, and the ear rods are gently placed in the external auditory meatus. The orbital pointer is adjusted to make his FHP parallel to the floor. But, latest recommendation advises that the NHP should be kept parallel to the floor instead of FHP. The patient is asked to keep his teeth in centric occlusion, with the facial tissues, lips, etc. in relaxed position, and swallow and relax. The film cassette is kept on the left side of the face of patient. Natural head position (NHP) is attained by placing a long mirror at least 6 feet in front of the patient and he is asked to see directly in his eyes.

Types of Cephalograms (Figs 15.3 and 15.4)

Cephalograms are of two types:

1. **Lateral cephalogram:** It is the main view and is required in all the orthodontic patients. It gives us the lateral view of craniofacial structures, in vertical and sagittal dimensions. Since it is a 2D image of 3D structures, so the face cannot be evaluated in transverse dimension with it. It is used to measure various angles, dimensions and proportions of face, growth pattern, anchorage requirements and soft tissue balance of facial structures.
2. **Frontal/PA cephalogram:** It is obtained by placing the film near the face of patient and X-ray source is at the back of head at

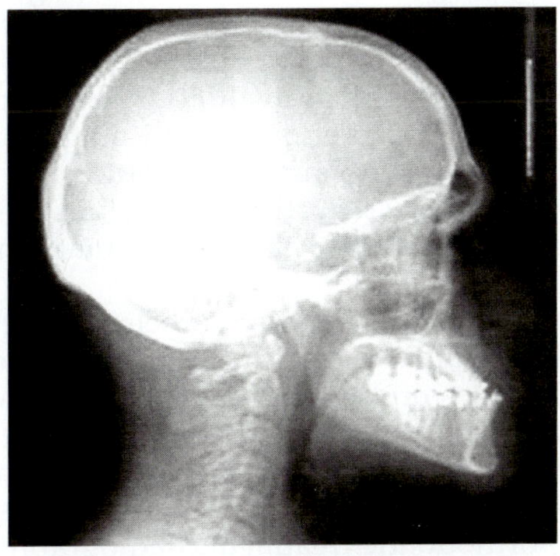

Fig. 15.3: Lateral cephalogram

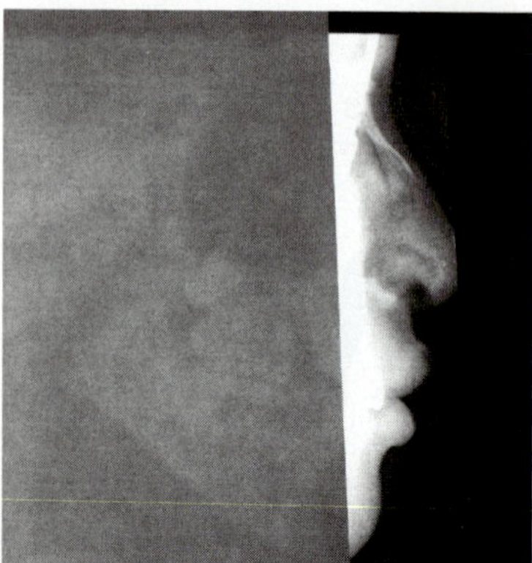

Fig. 15.4: Partially obscured lateral cephalogram showing the soft tissue facial profile of the patient.

a fixed distance. Rest of the technique remains the same as described above. It is used to assess the vertical and transverse dimensions of face. It is mainly needed in facial asymmetry cases.

Uses of Cephalograms

Cephalometrics is one of the most essential diagnostic aids in orthodontics. It has multitude of uses as follows.

- **Diagnosis:** It helps in orthodontic diagnosis by studying the relation of skeletal, dental and soft tissue structures.
- **Treatment planning:** The information obtained is used for treatment planning.
- **Growth assessment:** It is useful in predicting the growth-related changes. It helps in assessment of growth direction and pattern.
- It also helps in evaluation of skeletal maturity level or growth maturation level by studying CVMI status.
- **Facial classification:** It helps in classification of the skeletal and dental abnormalities.
- **Anchorage planning:** It helps in anchorage planning, by integration of various values of growth pattern, status, facial pattern, soft tissue relations, etc.
- **Treatment progress evaluation:** It is also used in evaluation of the progress of orthodontic treatment. Radiographs of different stages are superimposed and compared to evaluate the changes in facial and dental structures. They help us to modify the treatment plan and modalities, if required.
- **Surgical planning and evaluation:** It is also used to plan orthognathic surgical treatment and changes associated with surgical treatment.
- **VTO:** It is used in assessing the visual treatment objectives for myofunctional therapy, orthodontic changes and surgical treatments. Tracings of cephalogram are made, and cut, the pieces are then refixed by tapes in different positions to evaluate the best combination of surgical procedures. This information guides the surgeon for appropriate treatment plan and also can be used to discuss the expected changes with the patients.
- **Research:** It is a valuable tool in research work. Serial radiographs can be taken to assess the growth. It can be used to obtain serial radiographs for comparison and future researches.
- **Computerized assessment:** The digital pictures of cephlogram can be directly fed into the computers. With the help of various treatment planning softwares, the desired changes in skeletal an soft tissues can be seen on-screen, which help in motivating the patients and obtaining their consent.
- **Digigraphy:** The cephalograms can be digitized with the help of digitisers, the details are recorded in computer and are assimilated by a software. That soft ware gives the results of various cephalometrics analysis and their interpretation within seconds, and thus a lot of human effort and time is saved. These details can be printed to be kept in files of patients or for transferring the case to the other doctor.

Evaluation of Cephalograms

To assess a cephalogram, the student should be aware of the basic anatomical features of the head. It involves the knowledge of certain anatomical landmarks which are used to draw certain planes and angles. Outlines and landmarks are traced on the acetate paper using a view box in a darkened room, and a pointed 2H black lead pencil. The film is traced on an acetate sheet, various points are located, planes are drawn and angle and dimensions are measured. The bilateral structures which show double image, are bisected and that outline is used for measurements. As discussed above, the softwares are available which help in making complex measurements in no time. These measurements are even corrected for the race, age and different analyses. They also help in treatment planning, by simulating tooth movements and surgical repositioning, and thus can be used to discuss the plan with patients and to motivate them.

CEPHALOMETRIC LANDMARKS

Landmarks are the points representing certain anatomical structures in the craniofacial region and are marked on the tracing of cephalograms. They are used to draw planes, angle and lines for angular, linear and proportional measurements. These measurement help to analyse the size, position and balance of the structures, and help in diagnosis, treatment planning and prognosis.

Types

A. Landmarks are of two types: (1) anatomic landmarks and (2) derived landmarks.

1. **Anatomic landmarks:** They can be directly located in the bony structures. They represent the actual anatomic structures.
2. **Derived landmarks:** They are located or drawn with the help of other anatomic landmarks, and are projected on the skeletal structures.

B. They can also be classified as hard tissue landmarks which are present on hard structures, and soft tissue landmarks which are identified on soft tissue structures.

C. Hard tissue landmarks can be bony landmarks and dental landmarks.

D. Some landmarks are midline landmarks and others are surface landmarks.

E. Some landmarks are intracranial landmarks (e.g. sella, Ptm, Bo, Ba, etc.); while others are extracranial landmarks (e.g. Co, N, etc).

Requirements of Landmarks

- They should be easily identifiable and definable.
- They should be easily locatable.
- They should be reproducible with minimal location error.
- They should represent proper anatomical structure and location.
- They should be reliable for measurements and superimposition of serial cephalograms.

Common landmarks used in cephalometrics (Figs 15.5 to 15.8): There are numerous landmarks defined by various authors for general and specific purpose, but all cannot be used and remembered for general purpose orthodontic planning. Some of the important landmarks used in cephalometrics are as follows. Some of these points also have their soft tissue counterparts, which are marked on the soft tissue outline in immediate vicinity of

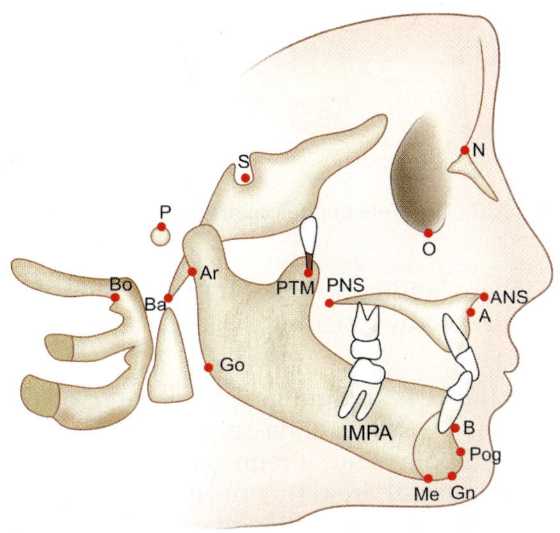

Fig. 15.5: Various hard tissue landmarks in a cephalogram.

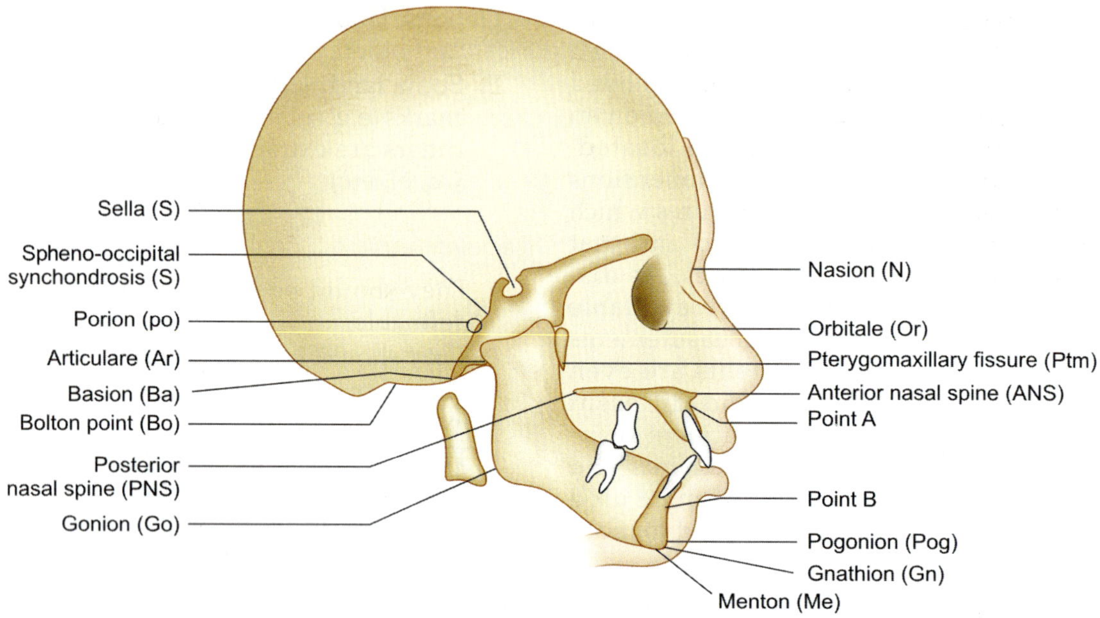

Fig. 15.6: Various hard tissue cephalometric landmarks.

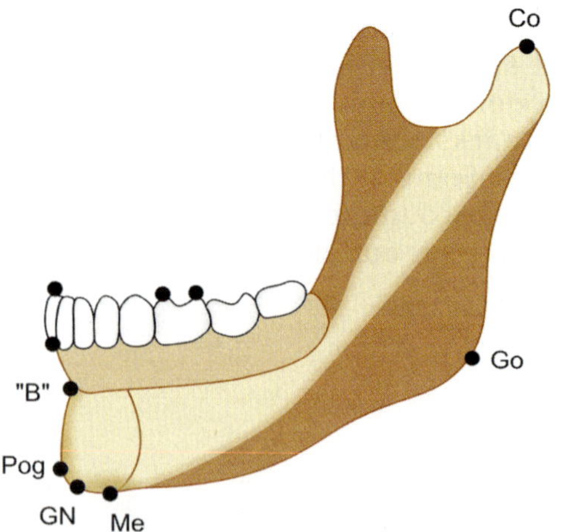

Fig. 15.7: Different cephalometrics landmarks on the mandible.

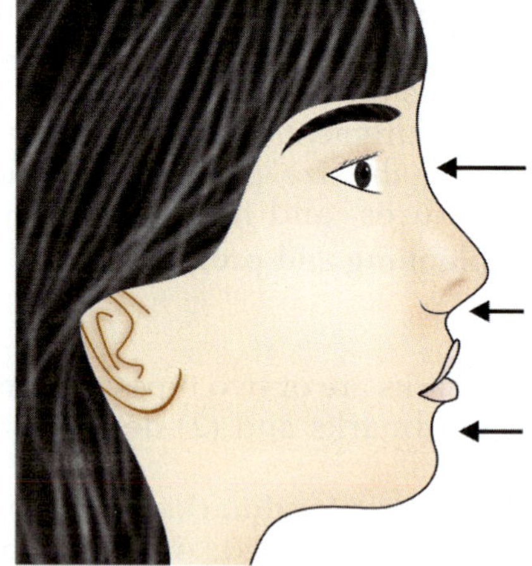

Fig. 15.8: Tissue nasion, point A, point B.

that hard landmark. The soft tissue landmarks are marked by an (′), e.g. N′, A′, B′, Pog′, Me′, Gn′, etc.

Sella: It is the geographic center of the pituitary fossa or sella turcica. It is a constructed point since it represents the centre of an anatomical area. It is used as a reference point for superimposition of cephalograms. It is considered as cranial-center. It is a midline, intracranial landmark.

Nasion (N): It is the anterior-most point on frontonasal suture in the midsagittal plane. It is an anatomical, midline, extracranial landmark.

Anterior nasal spine (ANS): It is the anterior-most tip of the sharp bony process of maxilla at the lower margin of the anterior nasal opening. It represents the anterior limit of hard palate. It is an anatomical, midline, surface landmark.

Point A (subspinale): It is the deepest point in the maxillary anterior alveolar process. It is the most posterior midline point in the concavity between the anterior nasal spine and the prosthion. It was considered as a skeletal point not affected by orthodontic forces. But, research showed that it is a malleable point and is affected by orthodontic movement of teeth, since the alveolar process gets remodeled with OTM.

Point B (supramentale): It is the counterpart of point A (of maxilla) on the mandibular. It is the deepest point in the anterior/labial outline of mandibular alveolar process. It is the most posterior midline point in the concavity of the mandible between the most superior point on the alveolar bone between lower incisors and pogonion.

Pogonion (Pog): It is the most anterior point on the bony chin.

Menton (Me): It is the inferior most point on the symphyseal outline of the bony chin.

Gnathion (Gn): It is the point located by bisecting the line joining Me and Pog and projecting it on the chin outline. So, it is a constructed point.

Condylion: It is the most superioposterior point on the outline of condyle.

Articulare (Ar): It is the point seen as the intersection of posterior border of ramus and the inferior outline of occipital bone.

Basion (Ba): It is the lowest point on anterior rim of the foramen magnum.

Bolton (Bo): It is the intersection of the outline of occipital condyle and the foramen magnum at the highest point on the notch posterior to the occipital condyle.

Gonion (Go) (Fig. 15.9): It is the point projected on the curvature of the angle of mandible, which is located by bisecting the angle formed by lines tangent to the posterior border of ramus and the inferior border of the mandible. It is a constructed point.

Orbitale (Or): It is the inferior-most point on the inferior rim of the bony orbit.

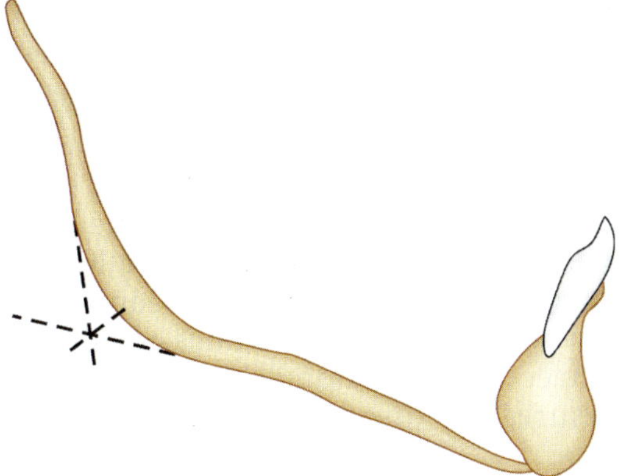

Fig. 15.9: How to construct the Go/gonial point.

Posterior nasal spine (PNS): It is the posterior-most point of the spine of palatine bone constituting the hard palate. It is the posterior limit of hard palate. It is obtained by extending the outline of pterygomaxillary fissure inferiorly and intersecting the palatal bone.

Porion (Po): It is the most superior point on the outline of metal ring of ear rods, representing the external auditory meatus. It is of two types: (1) machine porion and (2) anatomical porion (Ricketts). Machine porion is easily locatable, and is a nonanatomical/constructed point; while anatomical porion is difficult to locate.

Pterygomaxillary (Ptm) fissure: It is teardrop-shaped radiolucent figure behind the maxilla, the contour of which is formed anteriorly by maxillary tuberosity and posteriorly by anterior curve of the pterygoid process of the sphenoid bone. Its superior-posterior point is called Ptm point. It is the area where foramen rotundum opens and is considered as the geometric centre of cranium. It is a stable area of cranium according to Ricketts, and is used for superimposition of serial cephalograms for growth studies and other research in orthodontics.

Key ridge: It is the extension of zygomatic buttress which corresponds to the mesiobuccal root of permanent maxillary first molars in normal occlusion. It is also called zygomaxillary, and is the lowest point of the zygomaticomaxillary ridge.

Glabella: It is the most prominent point on forehead in midsagittal plane in between eyebrows, just above the bridge of nose.

Various Planes used in Cephalometrics

The landmarks are joined to make certain planes which are used to measure angles to depict the relationship between various components of the head. Planes are also used to project certain landmarks on them and to measure the distances between various points.

Types: They can be divided as horizontal planes and vertical planes.

Reference planes: These are those planes which are considered stable during the growth period. These are used for superimposition of serial cephalograms and also as the common plane for measurement of different parameters during particular cephalometric analysis, e.g. Downs analysis uses FHP as the reference plane, while Steiner's analysis uses SN plane as reference plane.

Horizontal planes: Commonly used horizontal planes are (Fig. 15.10):

SN plane: It is formed by joining points S & N, and represents the anterior cranial base. It is one of the most common reference plane used in orthodontics. It is considered stable after 5–6 years of age, since by that time most of the growth of cranial base is considered to be achieved. However, researches have shown that with time, the position of points S and N changes in vertical dimension, and thus the inclination of SN plane can also change.

FHP: Frankfort horizontal plane is constructed by joining points Po and Or. It was decided to be one of the first reference planes for orienting the skulls in craniometry and anthropometric studies, and a consensus was reached in 1889 in Frankfurt, Germany to use it as a reference plane. For taking cephalograms,

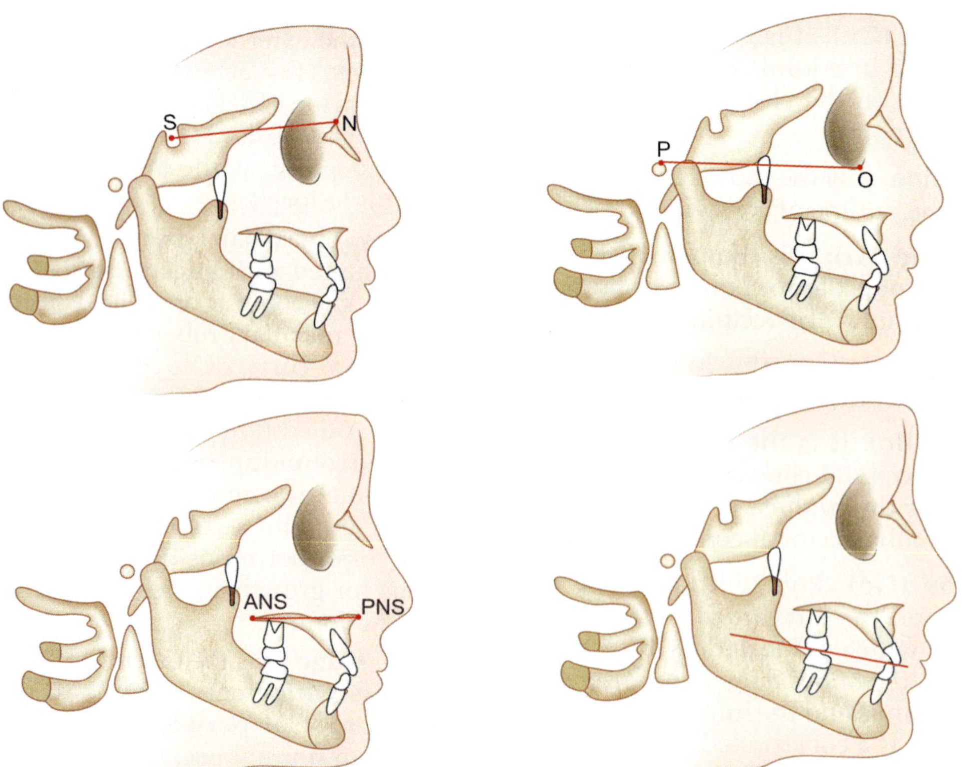

Fig. 15.10: Various horizontal planes: SN, FHP, PP, OP

it is oriented parallel to the ground. It is used in Tweed's and Downs analyzes. Ricketts also adapted it in his cephlometric analysis, but he used anatomic porion instead of machine porion.

Palatal plane: It is formed by joining ANS and PNS. It represents the base of maxilla, or roof of oral cavity.

Occlusal plane (Fig. 15.11): It denotes the orientation of dentition of the patient. It can be constructed in two ways: (1) bisecting occlusal plane and (2) functional occlusal plane.

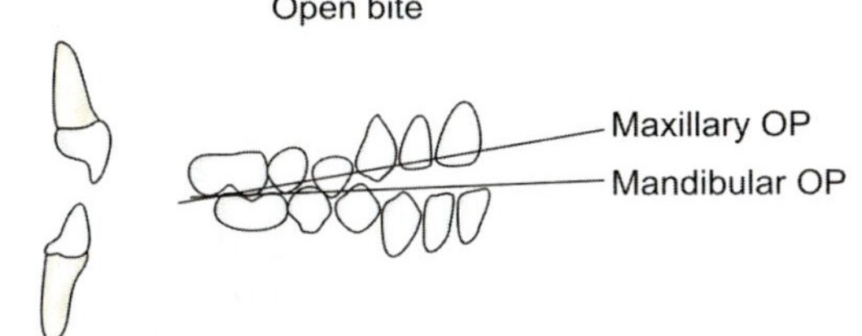

Fig. 15.11: Occlusal plane in an open bite case: Maxillary OP, mandibular OP.

BOP: It is constructed by joining the two points bisecting the molar occlusion in posterior region and the overbite anteriorly.

FOP: It is constructed by bisecting the buccal occlusion and extending it anteriorly. It is used in Wits analysis.

In anterior open bite case, there are two occlusal planes, i.e. maxillary occlusal plane and madibular OP. They extend from posterior occlusal point to the incisal edges of respective incisors.

Mandibular plane: It denotes the base of the mandible. It can be constructed by joining points Go–Me (Downs), Go–Gn (Steiner's), or a tangent to the lower border of mandible (Tweed), depending on the analysis being done.

NHP: Natural head position is the recent addition. It is used in orienting the face of patient while taking cephalograms and photos.

Broca defined the natural posture of the head as the posture of the subject when standing with his visual axis horizontal. It can be obtained by asking the patient to see in his eyes in a mirror placed at some distance from him while taking the X-ray. It has been shown to be correlated to craniofacial morphology, future growth trends, and to respiratory needs. It helps to orient the individual according to their most common posture.

Basion–sella plane: It is formed by joining points Ba to S. It represents the cephalometric posterior cranial base, however, anatomically, it being the middle cranial fossa.

Basion–nasion plane: It is formed by joining points Ba to N. It represents the total cranial base.

Bolton plane: It joins Bo to N points.

VERTICAL PLANES (Figs 15.12 and 15.13)

Various common vertical planes used in cephalometrics are:

Facial plane: It extends from nasion to Pog and represents the anterior limit of face.

A-Pog line: From point A to Pog. It represent anterior limit of denture.

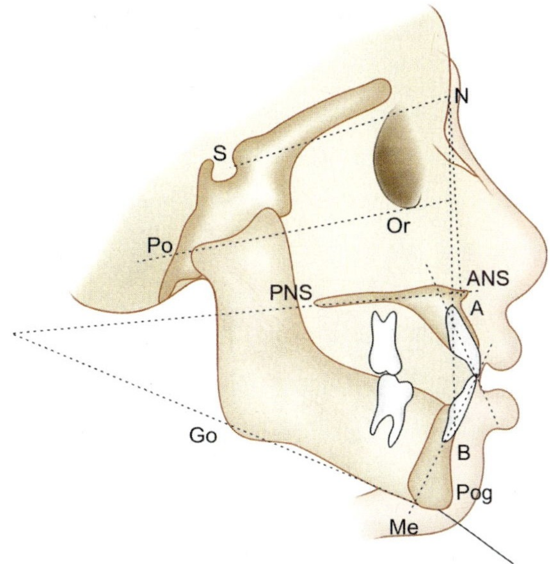

Fig. 15.12: Various vertical and horizontal planes: SN plane; Po–Or / FHP plane; ANS–PNS is palatal plane; Go–Pog is mandibular plane; N–Pog is facial plane; NA and NB lines for anterior limit of upper and lower alveolar processes.

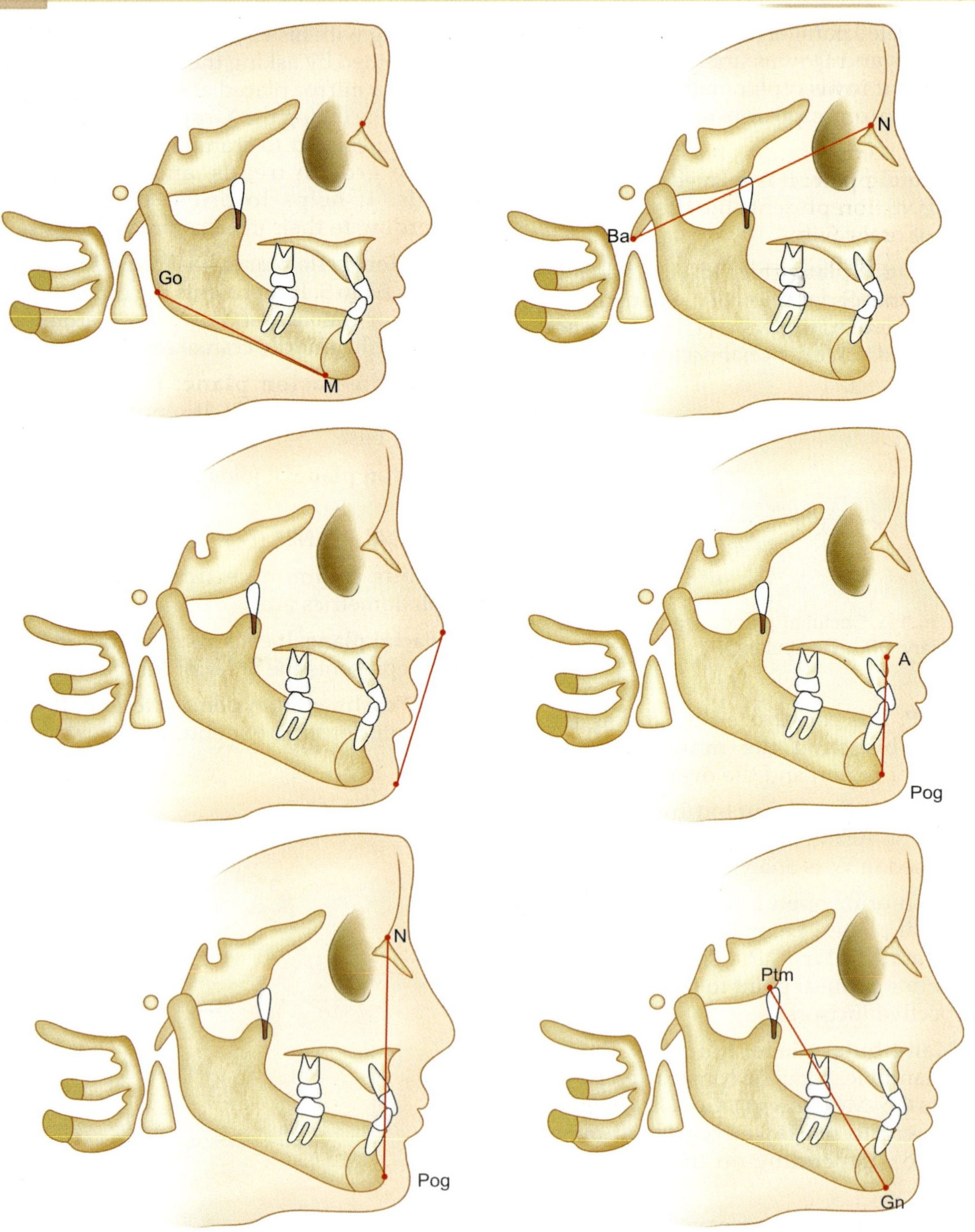

Fig. 15.13: Various planes: GoM—mandibular plane; BaN—basion-nasion plane; Rickett's E-line; A-Pog plane; N-Pog plane; facial growth axis—Ptm-Gn plane.

NA and NB lines: From point N to points A and B. They represent the sagittal position of upper and lower dentition irt anterior limit of cranial base.

Facial axis or growth axis: It is made by joining the points Ptm and Gn. It represents the direction of growth of face as a whole. Steiner uses S-Gn plane for measuring the growth direction/pattern.

E-plane: Esthetic plane, a soft tissue plane from anterior point on nose to soft tissue chin, Pog′.

Various analyses have been proposed by researchers for diagnosis and treatment planning depending on the requirements with their advantages and disadvantages, and most of them are the beyond the scope of this book. However, most common analyzes used in cephalometry are Downs analysis, Steiner's analysis, Wits analysis, soft tissue analysis and Tweed's analysis.

Downs Analysis (Figs 15.14 and 15.15)

It is one of the most commonly used cephalometric analyses. It was proposed by WB Downs in 1948. His findings are based on 20 Caucasian subjects in the age range of 12–17 years. It has 10 parameters, of which five are skeletal and five are dental. He also presented a graphic interpretation of his findings, which is called as "wigglegram", which represents the normal dentoskeletal features. The values lying outside of Wiggle immediately tell us about the deviations and the problems of patient.

Reference plane used: FHP (Po-Or) has been used as the reference plane to obtain all the values of analysis.

Skeletal Parameters

There are five skeletal parameters which are the facial angle; angle of convexity; A-B plane

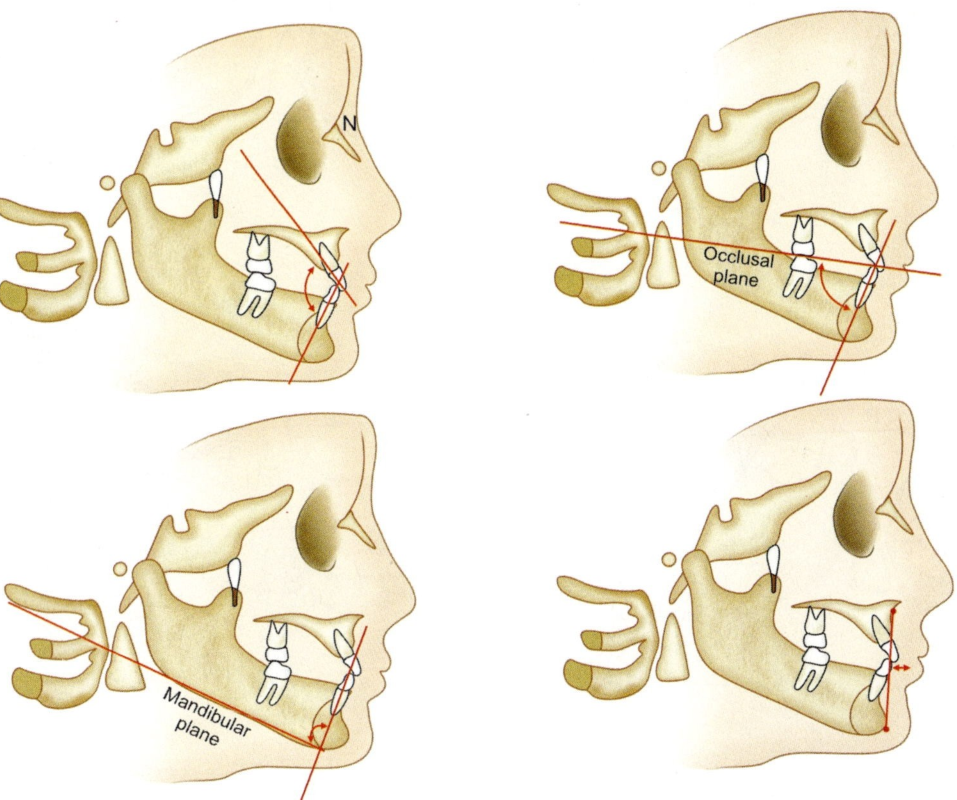

Fig. 15.14: Downs' analysis parameters.

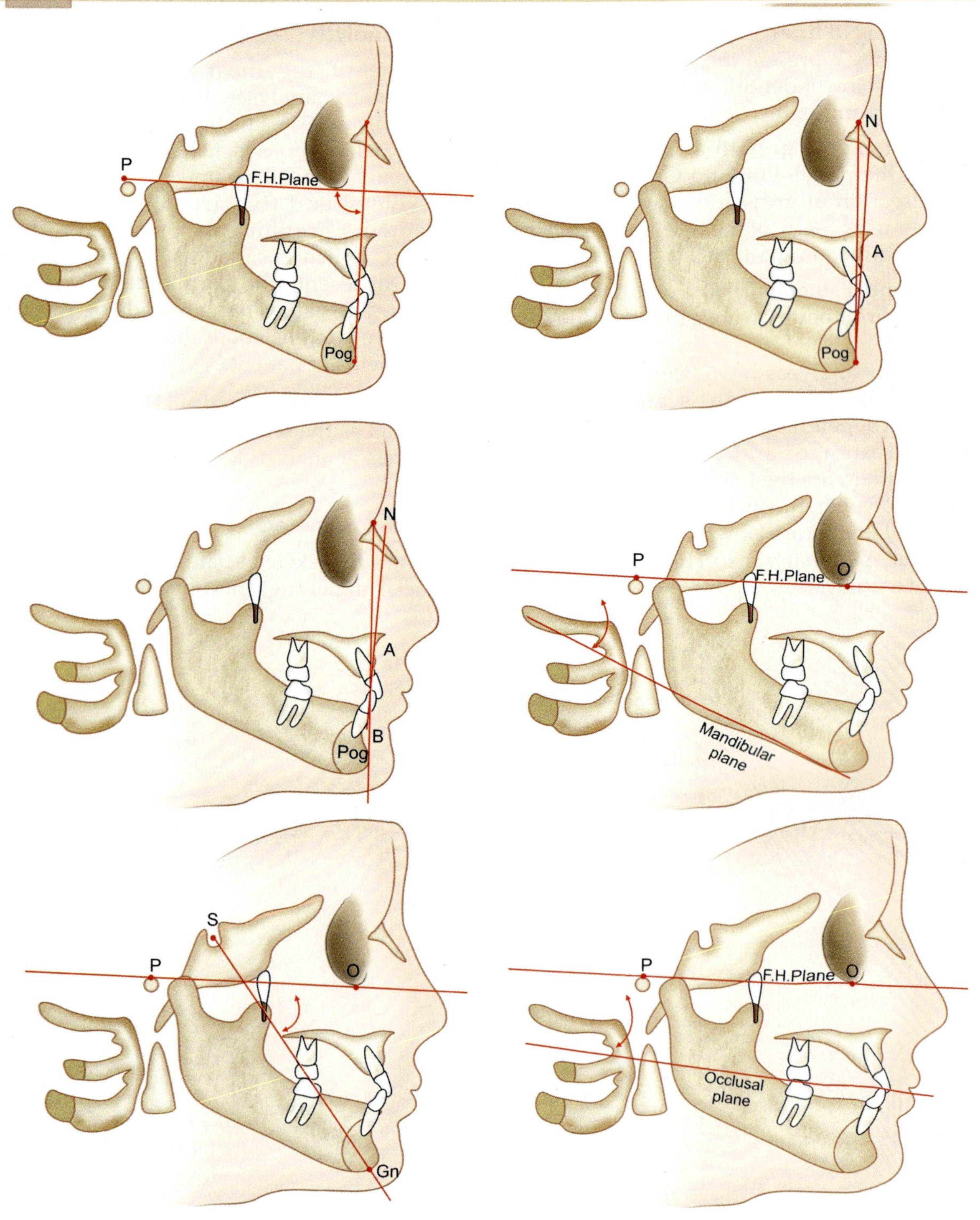

Fig. 15.15: Downs' analysis parameters: FHP is the reference plane.

angle; mandibular plane angle, and Y-axis angle.

1. **Facial angle:** It is the inside inferior angle formed by the intersection of nasion-pogonion (facial plane) plane and the FH plane. Its average value is 87.8°, with a Range of 82–95°.

   Inference: This angle gives us an indication of the antero-posterior positioning of the mandible in relation to the upper face.

   Lesser angle indicates posterior position of mandible / small mandible (skeletal class II, convex profile); while greater angle indicates anterior position of mandible / larger mandible (skeletal class III, concave profile).

2. **Angle of convexity:** This is the superior angle formed by the intersection of a line from nasion to point A and a line from point A to pogonion. It helps to depict the convexity or concavity of face. It also gives an idea of the facial profile. Its average value is 0°, with a range of –8.5° to +10°.

   Inference: A positive angle or an increased angle suggests a prominent maxillary denture base relative to a normal mandible or a retrognathic mandible relative to normal maxilla or a combination of both. It contributes to a convex profile and a skeletal class II pattern.

   A negative angle or a decreased angle suggests a prominent mandible relative to a normal maxilla or a retrognathic maxilla relative to normal mandible or a combination of both. It contributes to a concave profile and a skeletal class III pattern.

   However, the normal / abnormal position of individual maxilla or mandible can be found by other parameters (e.g. SNA, SNB, etc.).

   It can also be calculated by measuring the inside angle N-A-Pog and subtracting the value from 180. For example,

   Angle of convexity = 180 – angle N-A-Pog.
   \+ ve value = convexity
   \- ve value = concavity.

3. **A-B plane angle:** This angle is formed between a line connecting point A and point B and a line joining nasion to pogonion. Its mean value is –4.6°, with a range of –9°–0°. This angle indicates position of maxillomandibular dentition in sagittal plane in relation to the facial plane. Its value is generally negative since point B is posterior to point A. But, a higher negative value indicates prominent maxilla or retropositioned mandible, depicting skeletal class II relation.

   However, a +ve value indicates a prominent B point or a retrognathic A point, thus contributing to skeletal class III relation.

4. **Mandibular plane angle:** Downs used MP as a tangent to the gonial angle and the lowest point of the symphysis. MP angle is formed by the intersection of mandibular plane to FH plane. Its mean value is 21.9°, with a range of 17°–28°. It indicates the growth pattern of the patient, and helps in anchorage planning and extraction decisions.

   Inference: An increased mandibular plane angle suggests a vertical growth pattern, and a hyperdivergent facial pattern. A decreased mandibular plane angle suggests a horizontal growth pattern, and a hypodivergent facial pattern. It also helps us to classify skeletal nature of the bite depth. Increased angle indicates skeletal open bite, while decreased angle indicates skeletal deep bite.

5. **Y (growth) axis:** This anterior-inferior angle is formed by intersection of growth axis, i.e. the sella-gnathion line with the F-H plane. Its mean value is 59°, with a range of 53°–66°. It denotes the direction and pattern of growth of patient.

Inference: An increased value suggests a vertical growth pattern, and a hyperdivergent facial pattern. It also indicates a downward and backward rotation of mandible, e.g. seen in skeletal class II patterns.

A decreased angle suggests a horizontal growth pattern, and a hypodivergent facial pattern. It also indicates an upward and forward rotation of mandible, e.g. seen in skeletal class III patterns.

Dental Parameters

Five dental parameters are cant of occlusal plane; interincisal angle; incisor-occlusal plane angle; incisor-mandibular plane angle; and upper incisor to A-Pog line distance.

1. **Cant of occlusal plane:** This angle is formed between the occlusal plane and the F-H plane. Downs used the bisecting occlusal plane through the region of the overlapping cusps 1st molar and bisecting overbite. The mean value is 9.3°, with a range of 1.5°–14°.

   Inference: It indicates the slope of dentition in the face in relation to the FHP. It helps us to correlate the growth pattern with the slope of dentition, thus helping in anchorage planning, treatment mechanics and extraction decisions. It also gives insight into the bite depth and nature of bite, i.e. skeletal or dental deep bite, of the patient.

   A decreased angle is generally is seen in horizontal growth pattern, where skeletal deep bite is more common. It is generally associated with dental deep bite, due to decreased posterior alveolar heights.

   An increased angle is generally is seen in vertical growth pattern, where skeletal open bite is more common. It may be associated with dental open bite, due to increased posterior alveolar heights.

2. **Interincisal angle:** This is the posterior inside angle formed by the intersection of long axes of upper and lower central incisors. Its mean value is 135.4°, with a range of 130°–150.5°.

   Inference: It represents the inclination of incisors to each other, i.e. their interrelationship. A smaller value denotes proclined teeth, while increased value denotes upright or retroclined teeth. But, it does not specify whether the proclination or retroclination is due to upper or lower teeth or both. The angle may decrease if only upper teeth are proclined, with lower teeth at normal axial inclination, and vice versa. So, other parameters from other analyzes have to be studied to find out which teeth are at fault.

   The decreased angle is found in class I bimax proclination and class II division 1 malocclusion cases; and increased in class II division 2 , and some class III cases.

3. **Incisor occlusal plane angle:** It is the inside-inferior angle formed by the intersection of long axis of lower incisor with occlusal plane, and it is read as a deviation from 90° as plus or minus value. Average value is 14.5 with a range of 3.5°–20°.

   Inference: It helps to find the inclination of lower incisors on their basal bone. An increased value indicates proclination of lower teeth, while decreased value indicates retroclination or more uprighting of lower teeth on the basal bone. This angle should be used with interincisal angle for proper interpretation.

4. **Incisor mandibular plane angle:** It is an inside superior angle, formed by the long axis of lower incisor with mandibular plane, and then it is evaluated as a deviation from 90° as plus or minus value. Average value is 1.4 with a range of –8.5° to + 7°.

   Inference: It also helps to find the axial inclination of lower incisors, and helpful in treatment planning. An increased / positive value indicates proclination of lower teeth, while decreased / negative value indicates retroclination or more uprighting of lower teeth on the basal bone. This angle should be used with interincisal angle for proper interpretation.

5. **Upper incisor to A-pog line:** It is a linear distance measured between the incisal edge of the maxillary central incisor and the A-Pog line, which represents the anterior limit of upper and lower jaw bases. Its mean value is –2.7 mm, with a range of –1 mm to +5 mm.

   Inference: It helps to find out the position of upper incisors in a sagittal plane. Negative value means the tooth is behind the line representing retroclination, while an increased value indicates proclination of upper teeth.

   Wigglegram: The values obtained by Downs analysis are plotted on the graph with mean values on a vertical straight line, and the upper and lower limits on the right and left side of it. It represents the normal skeletal and dental pattern of the patient. Values lying outside that wiggle represent the deviations from the normal.

Steiner Analysis (Figs 15.16 and 15.17)

It was presented by Cecil C Steiner in 1950s with the idea of providing information of skeletal, dental and soft tissue relationship. It also helps in visualized treatment objectives, VTO, based on cephalometrics parameters, arch length discrepancy and soft tissue factors. It can be evaluated by his graphic representation called as "Steiner's sticks". He divided it into three parts, viz.

1. Skeletal analysis
2. Dental analysis
3. Soft tissue analysis.

He has used SN plane as the reference plane, since SN plane represents anterior cranial base and is considered one of the most stable area after 5–6 years of age.

A. Skeletal Parameters

1. **SNA angle:** It is the inside inferior angle formed by the intersection of SN plane and a line joining nasion and point A. This angle indicates the anteroposterior position of the maxilla in relation to the cranial base. Its mean value is 82°. An increased value indicates forward positioned/prognathic maxilla with respect to cranial base, while a decreased value indicates posterior positioning/retrognathic maxilla.
2. **SNB angle:** It is the inferior inside angle between the SN plane and a line joining nasion to point B. This angle indicates the anteroposterior positioning of the mandible in relation to the cranial base. Its mean value is 80°. An increased value indicates forward positioned/prognathic mandible with respect to cranial base, while a decreased value indicates posterior positioning/retrognathic mandible.

   Correction factor: However, in many patients, values of SNA and SNB can be decreased or increased, but still they may be having normal balance of the face. It is due to variation in the inclination of SN plane within the cranium. To eliminate this discrepancy, the correction should be included in the values. This correction is obtained by measuring the angle between FHP and SN planes. Since FHP is oriented parallel to ground, so any variation in angle is due to changed orientation of SN plane. A normal value is 7–8°. Any deviation from this value is the correction factor which is either added (if FHP-SN angle is increased) or subtracted (if FHP-SN angle is decreased) in values involving SN plane.
3. **ANB angle:** It is formed by the intersection of lines joining nasion to point A and nasion to point B. It can also be calculated as the difference between angles SNA and SNB.

   It indicates the relative skeletal sagittal position of the maxilla and mandible to each other. Its mean value is 2°. A range of 0–4 is considered normal. An increased value indicates a skeletal class

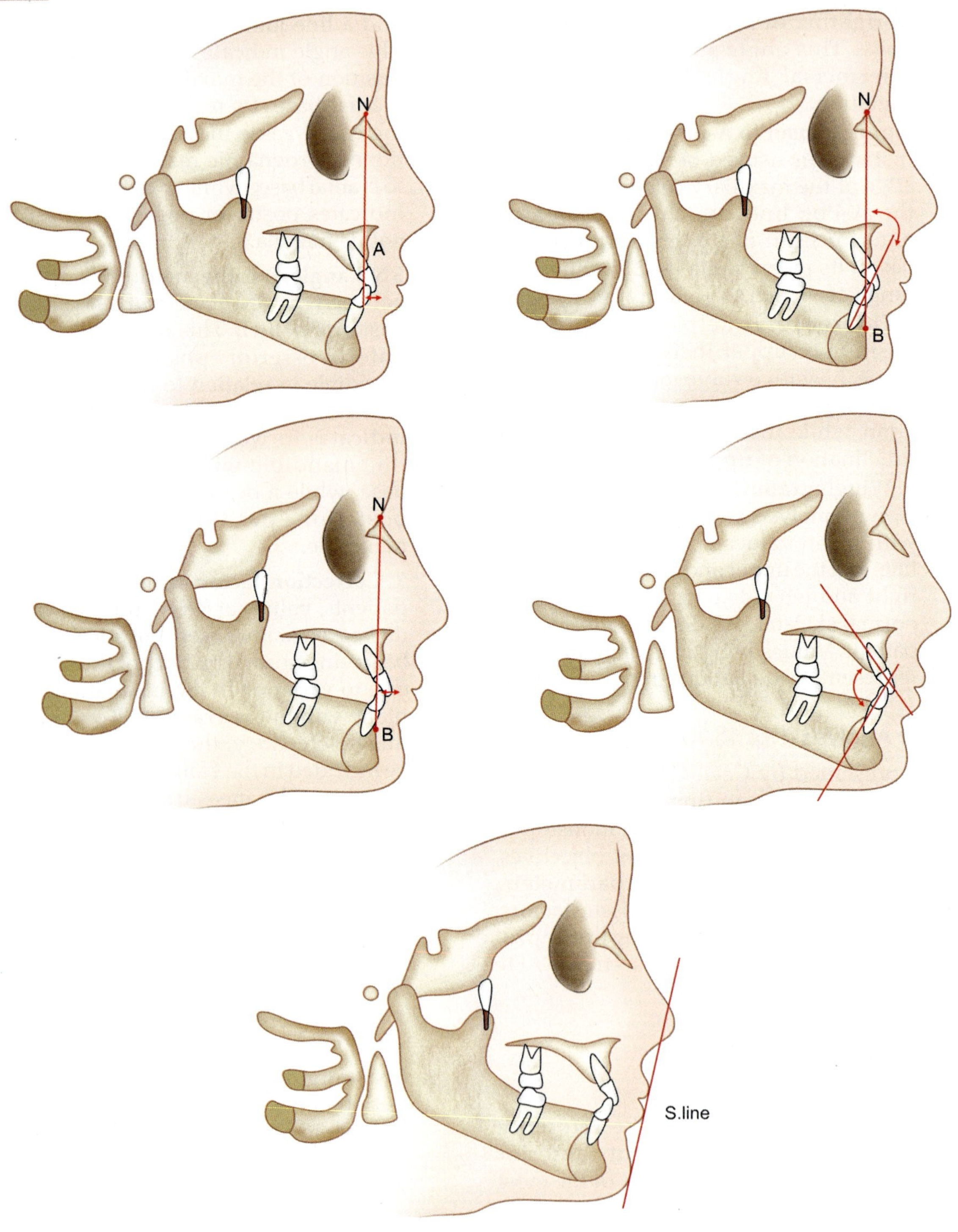

Fig. 15.16: Steiner's analysis parameters.

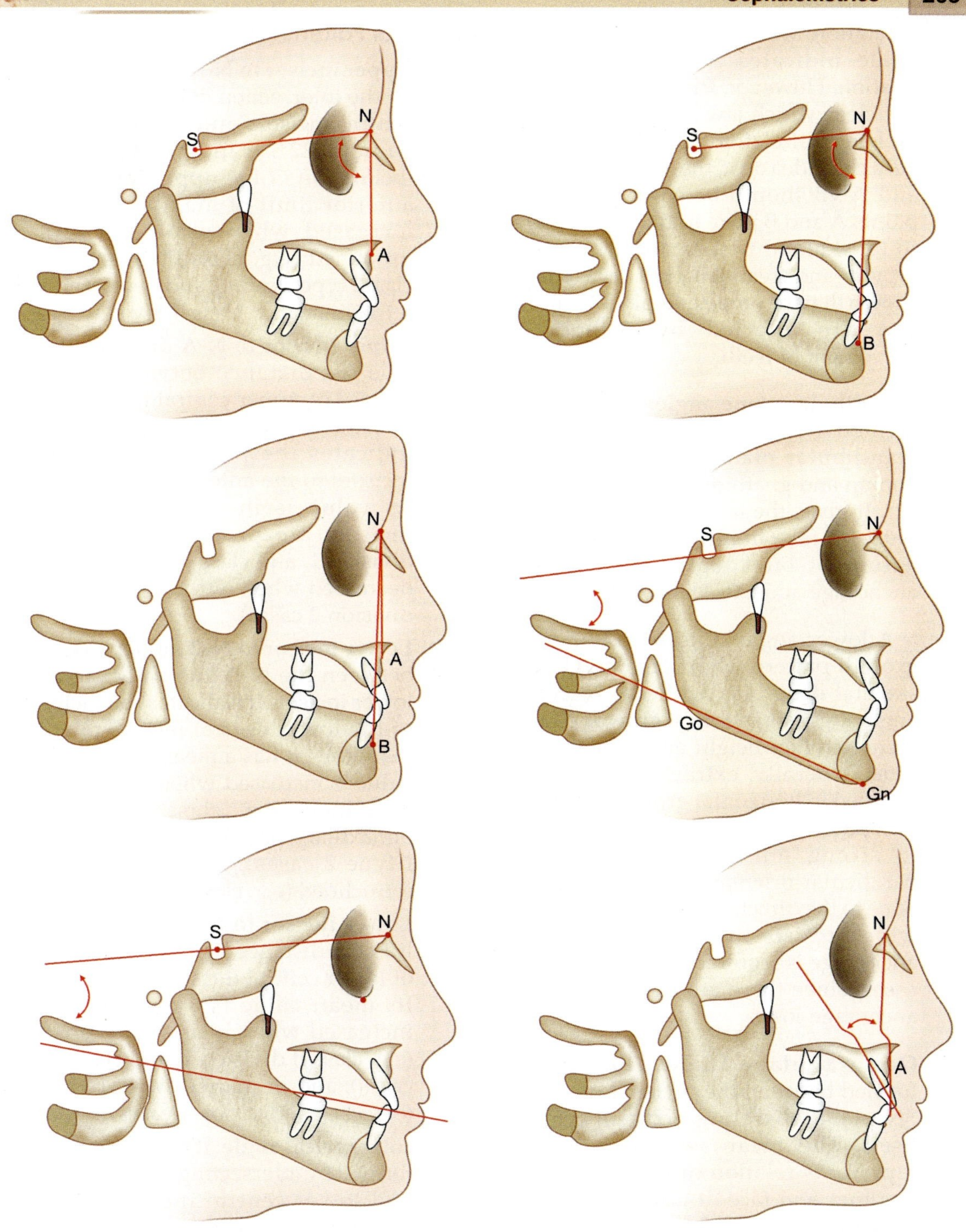

Fig. 15.17: Steiner's analysis parameters: SN plane is the reference plane.

II relation, while a decreased/negative value indicates a skeletal class III relation. However, from ANB itself, it is not clear which jaw has contributed to skeletal malrelation and how much. To get a clear idea on it, the angles SNA, SNB and ANB should be correlated. Also, points A and B were initially considered to be skeletal points not affected by growth and treatment, but research has shown that they are dentoalveolar points and are affected by orthodontic movement of teeth.

4. **Mandibular plane angle:** It is the angle formed between SN plane and the mandibular plane (a line connecting gonion and gnathion). Its mean value is 32°. It gives the information for growth pattern, face height and the skeletal nature of bite depth, and helps in anchorage and extraction planning.

   A lower angle indicates a horizontal growth pattern, short face height and skeletal deep bite, while an increased angle suggests a vertical growth pattern, increased face height and skeletal open bite. Generally, extractions should be avoided in horizontal growth pattern, as the space closure is difficult in them due to strong musculature and a perpendicular orientation of trabeculae of bone to the direction of tooth movement, which resists the forces. Maximum anchorage is required in vertical growth cases, since there are more chances of anchorage loss.

5. **Occlusal plane angle:** This angle is formed between the occlusal plane and SN plane. Bisecting occlusal plane is used. The mean value is 14.5°. It represents relation of dentition to the cranium and face. It also indicates the growth pattern of the face. Its value is increased in vertical growth cases and decreased in horizontal growth pattern. That way, it also indicates the skeletal bite depth, viz open bite or deep bite.

B. Dental Parameters

1. **Upper incisor to N-A angle:** It is formed by the intersection of long axis of upper central incisors and NA line. its mean value is 22°. It indicates the relative inclination of the upper incisors to the anterior limit of maxilla. Its value is increased when upper incisors are proclined (e.g. class II division 1, and class I type 2 cases); and decreased when retroclined (e.g. class II division 2 cases).
2. **Upper incisor to N-A distance (linear):** It is the distance between the labial surface of upper central incisor and the NA line. Its mean value is 4 mm. It also indicates the position of the upper incisors to the anterior limit of maxilla. Its value is increased when upper incisors are proclined (e.g. class II division 1, and class I type 2 cases); and decreased when retroclined (e.g. class II division 2 cases).
3. **Lower incisor to N-B angle:** It is formed between the N-B line and long axis of lower incisor. It indicates the inclination of the lower central incisor relative to mandible. It has a mean value of 25°. Its value is increased when the incisors are proclined (e.g. class II division 1, bimaxillary proclination cases and class I type 2 cases); and decreased when retroclined (e.g. class II division 2 cases).
4. **Lower incisor to N-B distance (linear):** It is the distance between labial surface of lower central incisor and the NB line. Its mean value is 4 mm. Its value is increased when incisors are proclined (e.g. class II division 1, and class I type 2 cases); and decreased when retroclined (e.g. class II division 2 cases).
5. **Inter incisal angle:** It is the internal angle formed by intersecting long axis of upper and lower central incisors. Its mean value is 131°. It indicates the relative proclination or retroclination of upper and lower incisors. Its value is decreased when incisors are proclined (e.g. class II division 1, and class I type 2 cases); and

increased when retroclined (e.g. class II division 2 cases). However, this angle does not specify which incisor viz upper or lower is at fault and to what extent. This finding is to be corroborated with all the four dental parameters discussed above.

C. Soft tissue Parameter (Fig. 15.18)

S-line: This is the line extending from soft tissue contour of the chin to the middle of an S formed by the lower border of the nose. The lips in a well-balanced face should touch this line at relaxed position.

If the lips are located beyond this line, then they are protrusive. If the lips are behind this line, they are retrusive.

THE WITS APPRAISAL (Figs 15.19a and b)

This method of evaluation of sagittal relationship of the skeletal bases of maxilla and mandible was suggested by Alex Jacobson in 1975 at Witswatersand university. That is why it has been named as Wits appraisal. It is a measure of the extent to which the maxilla and the mandible are related to each other in the antero-posterior or sagittal plane. The wits appraisal is used to corroborate the findings of ANB angle, and in cases where the ANB angle is considered not so reliable due to factors such as position of nasion and rotation of the jaws. Also, its values can help to correlate other measures for sagittal relation of the jaws.

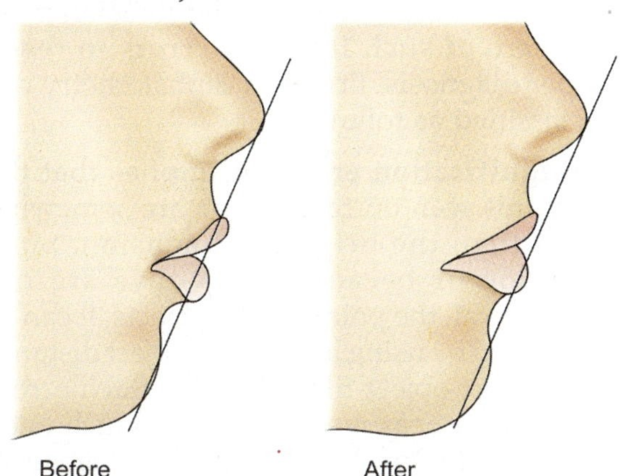

Fig. 15.18: Improvement in soft tissues/lips balance with E-plane.

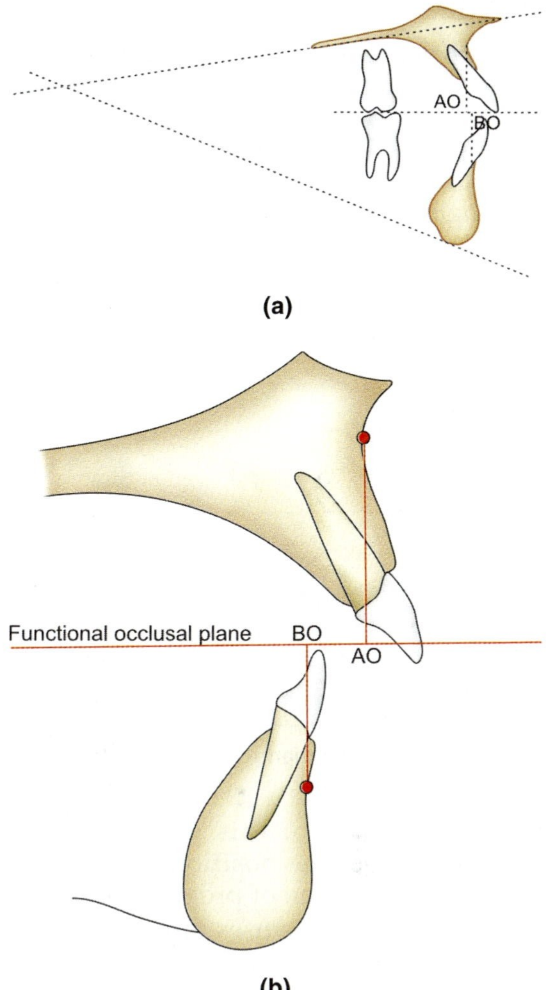

Fig. 15.19a and b: Wits' analysis.

Method: A functional occlusal plane FOP is drawn through the overlapping cusps of first premolars and first molars. Perpendiculars are drawn to the occlusal plane from points A and B. The points of contact of these perpendiculars on occlusal plane are termed AO and BO. The distance between points AO and BO gives the anteroposterior relation between the two jaws. In males, BO is ahead of AO by 1 mm (i.e. Wits = –1.0 mm), while in females, the points AO and BO coincide (i.e. wits = 0.0 mm). In case of skeletal class II, BO is usually behind AO (a positive value) while in skeletal class III pattern, the point BO is located ahead of AO (a negative value).

TWEED'S ANALYSIS (Fig. 15.20)

This cephalometric analysis was proposed by Charles Tweed in 1954 with his continued research for stability of post-treatment results of his patients. With continuous evaluation of cephalograms of those patients, he found three angles in succession which could help to determine the treatment plan and prognosis of the case, anchorage requirements and extraction decisions.

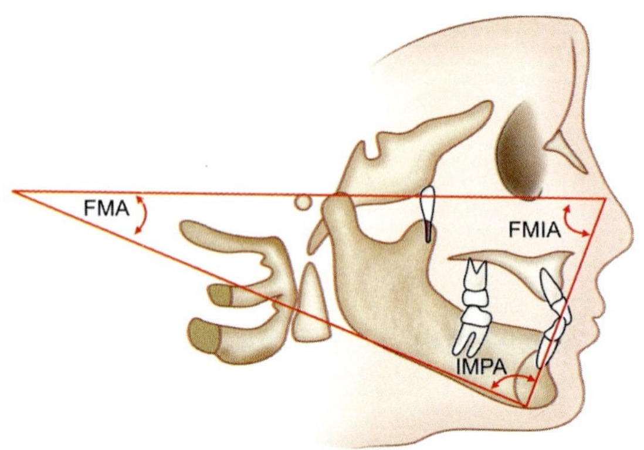

Fig. 15.20: Tweed's triangle and related angles.

Main objective of this analysis is the determination of the position of the lower incisor and evaluation of prognosis of a case.

The Tweed analysis uses three planes that form a diagnostic triangle. That is why it is also called as Tweed's triangle. These planes are:

a. Frankfort horizontal plane, Po-Or
b. Mandibular plane, Go-Me
c. Long axis of lower incisor.

Thus, the three angles formed in the triangle are FMA, IMPA, and FMIA angles.

Frankfort mandibular plane angle (FMA): It is formed by intersection of FHP and mandibular plane (Go-Me). Its mean value is 25°, with a range of 22°–30°. It indicates the growth pattern of face. Increased value suggest vertical growth pattern, while decreased values indicate horizontal growth pattern. It also helps in planning the anchorage.

Incisor mandibular plane angle (IMPA): It is the inside-upper angle formed by intersection of long axis of lower incisor with the mandibular plane. It indicates the inclination of lower incisors in relation to mandibular base. Its mean value is 90°, with a range of 85–95.

Value is increased in class II division 1, and bimaxillary proclination cases, while decreased in class II division 2 cases, in lip trap cases, lip sucking habit cases, thumb sucking habit cases, etc.

Increased IMPA during treatment indicates loss of anchorage; instability of results post-treatment; may indicate permanent retention of lower incisors, etc.

Frankfort mandibular incisor angle (FMIA): This angle is the inside angle, formed by the intersection of the long axis of the lower incisor with the FH plane. It was the main angle proposed by Tweed and he considered it a very important parameter to define the esthetic of the face. Its mean value is 65°. It should be compensated depending on the growth pattern of the patient. It also helps in calculating the arch length discrepancy by including head plate correction.

Errors in Cephalometry

Cephalometry has always been an important tool for the diagnosis and treatment planning of orthodontic cases. However, it is not immune to errors. Since any radiograph is a 2D image of 3D anatomical structures, the inherent errors come in play. Also, the errors related with the equipment are there. To interpret the cephalograph, the clinician must be aware of such inherent errors to reach proper diagnosis. Errors in cephalometry can be classified as follows:

Magnification errors: It implies that the structures seen on radiograph are somewhat larger than the original dimension. Such errors occur because the X-rays are not parallel to all the points of the objects. It can be minimized by using long focus-object distance and a short object-film distance. Such errors only affect linear measurements which need correction factor, but the angular measurements are not affected which can be used during analysis without correction.

Magnification correction factor: It can be calculated and applied during the measurement. A known length (say 5 cm) of metallic strip/wire/scale can be placed on the film-cassette during taking the X-rays. Its shadow will come on the film. The magnification factor can then be calculated by taking the ratio of original length to the length of shadow. It can then be incorporated for correction during analysis.

Distortions: Since anatomical structures are 3D, so different magnifications can occur at different depths of field. Certain structures and landmarks are not midsagittal but are usually bilateral, which cause the formation of dual images on the film. Also the rotation of patients head in any plane of space can lead to distortion. These errors can be minimized by using the midpoint of the bilateral structures. Stabilizing the head by using ear rods, orbital pointer and forehead/nasal rest also minimizes the distortion.

Measurement errors: These errors occur during the measurements of various linear and angular parameters due to human error during tracing and locating the landmarks. Digitizers and computerized plotters and analysis softwares have been found to decrease such errors. They also decrease the time for analysis and avoid human fatigue.

Errors in landmarks identification: These errors occur due to following factors:

Quality of radiograph: Poor radiographs do not show clear outlines of anatomical structures and thus lead to location errors. Poor contrast of films can be due to improper settings of kV and mA, thus causing differentiation of adjacent structures difficult. Good contrast can be obtained by using proper films and kV levels.

Movement of tube, film or object can lead to blurring. These should be stabilized during exposure. Long time taken during radiography can lead to shifting of head by the patient. Exposure time can be reduced by increasing the current (mA) settings.

Improper development of films can be the cause of poor quality films. It can be avoided by using proper method of development, proper concentration of solutions used, etc. Nowadays, the digital imaging with dry printing of the image has improved the clarity of images.

Landmark location: Errors in analysis can occur due to problem in the landmarks location. Certain landmarks are also difficult to identify due to overlapping by anatomical structures, e.g. porion, bolton, etc. If such landmarks are to be used during analysis, then good quality films and using average values from multiple identification of same landmark can be helpful.

Operator bias: Variations can occur during landmark location between different operators. So during serial cephalometric evaluation, same person should identify and trace the landmarks, and also the films should be obtained by using same machine and same settings.

Conclusion

Cephalometrics is a tool of great value in orthodontic diagnosis and treatment planning. Various methods have been developed by researchers to identify the skeletal, dental and soft tissue deviations in the position of various components. Normal values in different races have been established, which are referred for comparing the patient's values, which in turn help in defining the diagnosis, and planning the treatment.

Various soft tissue parameter help to determine the esthetics of face and to determine the changes needed to improve the smile and esthetics. Cephalometrics has proved itself as a valuable research tool beyond doubt. Latest modification of digital imaging, various softwares for analysis and orthognathic surgical planning have helped to better understand the nature of deviation, and discussion with the patients to show them the expected changes. It has helped to obtain a better cooperation of patient during the treatment.

16

Skeletal Maturity Indicators

INTRODUCTION

Malocclusion is a complex interaction of genetic and environmental factors, and it affects growth of the craniofacial complex, leading to malrelationship of skeletal components. Since the growth is a very important aspect in orthodontics, an understanding of the growth events is of prime importance to plan the treatment for the patients. Certain features of skeletal development can be assessed by various methods to know the present status of growth of the patient. They involve study of certain skeletal markers, stages of development of teeth and dentition, age of the patient, etc.

The status of growth can be studied as skeletal age, dental age and the physiological age. But, there exist variation in the information obtained from them. The method based on dental development is not considered as a reliable method because of variation in dentition development pattern. Similarly, age of the patient also does not correlate reliably with the growth status. Skeletal age has been considered as the most reliable method to find out the growth status of the patient.

Biological age, skeletal age, bone age and skeletal maturation are the synonymous terms used to describe the maturation status of the patient. There exist individual patterns in timings, duration and velocity of growth, the assessment of skeletal age is important for the treatment planning, along with sexual dimorphism. Growth status has an important influence on the treatment goals and outcome of treatment. Certain treatment modalities, e.g. myofunctional treatment, head gear treatment, dentofacial orthopedics, orthognathic surgery, expansion, serial extraction, etc. are largely influenced by the growth status of the patient.

Knowledge of growth and development of craniofacial complex is very important for treatment planning. Growth status of the patient at the time of treatment guides the orthodontist to decide the treatment modality. As we have studied, the growth is not a continuous process but has periods of acceleration and deceleration. So, it is very important to know the extent of remaining growth of the patient for treatment planning. Assessment of skeletal age helps to determine the extent of any remaining or active growth in individual and what percentage of growth can be expected.

Phases of Child's Development

In simple terms, the child's age can be divided in following phases, i.e. newborn (ages 0–1 month); infant (ages 1 month –1 year); toddler (ages 1–3 years); preschooler (ages 4–6 years); school-aged child / preadolescent (ages 6–13 years); adolescent (ages 13–20). From orthodontic point of view, the stages of preadolescent and adolescent are very important, as during these years, the active growth of maxilla and mandible occurs, which can be guided and redirected to achieve proper skeletal relationship and occlusion.

Proffit has defined the phase of adolescence as "the transitional period between juvenile stage and adulthood during which the adolescent growth spurt takes place, the secondary sexual characteristics appear, fertility is attained, and profound physiologic changes occur".

Clinically, the developmental status of a child can be judged by some changes in the body of the child, e.g. sudden increase in height and weight, i.e. peak height velocity; onset of menstruation in girls; voice change in boys; skeletal ossification, etc.

"Right appliance at the right time" is the key to successful growth modulation. It is the skeletal growth status of the person which matters for the growth modulation, rather than the actual age. The age can be expressed through number of methods, e.g.

Assessment of Age

Age of a person can be classified as follows.

- Neurological
- Chronological
- Morphological
- Skeletal
- Mental
- Secondary sex character age
- Dental age.

Neurological age: It is defined as the development of simple reflexes, the increasing complexity and development of nervous system and its dependent functions. Examples are smiling, sitting up, walking with support (developmental milestones).

Morphological age: It involves the assessment of somatic growth and development. Its basic indicators include height and weight.

Mental age: It is the indicator of intellectual development of the child.

Growth charts: Growth charts are plotted by using the data of height and weight in relation to chronologic age of the child. It is used to understand growth pattern in terms of deviations from the usual pattern and to express variability quantitatively.

It is used by pediatricians to follow the growth of the child over a period of time. It helps to evaluate the growth pattern, variability, and predictability. The growth is studied in percentiles and various percentiles ranges have been determined in the graph. The data of a child can be plotted on the growth charts. The main information gained from them is that the child's data after plotting lie in a particular percentile range, e.g. if the child's data lies on 40th percentile range, it means that 40% children are growing parallel to him, but rest 60% children are growing more than him. However, during growth, if the child remains in his percentile range, his growth is considered occurring normally. But if there is drastic deviation from his original growth percentile range, then the cause has to be looked into.

Chronological Age

It is defined as age since date of birth. It is a poor indicator of maturity. It is a poor indicator of the growth status of the child since there are variations in the growth rates of different children. It gives a rough idea to predict the rate and magnitude of facial growth. But that information is reliable for growth modulation. The children may be early maturing, late maturing and average maturing. This rate of growth is governed by the genetic pool of child.

Sexual/Pubertal Age

It is expressed by the physical changes coming in the body of children, e.g. in girls: If the onset of menstruation has occurred, it indicates that the peak height velocity (PHV) has been attained and the growth rate is decelerating. Girls' menarche occurs approx 1.1 years after PHV. Menarche occurs at a bone age of 13.1 years and it is considered as a highly reliable indicator of PHV. The growth is almost complete with the onset of menstruation. Therefore when planning for orthodontic treatment if menarche has occurred then PHV has passed, and only little growth will be remaining.

Secondary sex character age: Appearance of SSC is an indication that the growth of the body is towards completion, and little or no growth is remaining, e.g. in boys: If a boy has a childish/prepubertal voice, it indicates that the peak height velocity has not been reached. Beginning of the voice change indicates that the boy is in the pubertal spurt. If boy has attained a male voice, the growth rate has begun to decelerate.

The boys attain a "pubertal voice" 0.2 years before PHV; "Male voice" (pitch of adult voice) occurs approx 0.9 years after PHV. However, the SSCA is of little value in boys.

There are other physical changes also as has been mentioned before, which indicate that the pubertal growth spurt is progressing or near completion.

Dental Age

It is indicated by level of crown and root development, and level of dental eruption. Dental age correlates well with chronological but less with skeletal age. It is not a good indicator of growth status of the person. There are racial variations also, e.g. early eruption in Asians; and late eruption in Eastern and South European groups is seen. It is not a reliable method because the eruption time and sequence gets altered due to general and local factors.

Methods to determine dental age: Dental age of the child is determined by the status of the calcification, root development and the teeth erupted, which is compared to average chronological data. The chronology of dental eruption gives an estimate of the age of the child. Radiological development of root of lower canine has been found to be an accurate method to correlate dental age to skeletal age and second molars.

Skeletal Age

Skeletal/anatomical age is considered to be the most reliable method of growth and age assessment for orthodontic purposes. It is the measure of level of skeletal development of the individual and it helps to find out the extent of any remaining growth. The growth status can be accurately determined through the skeletal maturation indicators, SMIs. These are the different and sequential natural ossification and bone-development stages. This information is used by orthodontist to decide the timings and the type of treatment and the prognosis. It helps to predict adolescent growth spurt for timing of orthodontic treatment.

Difference between males and females growth status:

- Females mature faster than males. Generally, there is a difference of 2–3 years.
- Females generally show only two growth spurts while males show three growth spurts.
- Females tend to achieve a higher percentage of their total statural growth than males during early adolescence
- Female showed greater growth velocities and earlier maturation in stature.
- Growth velocities diminished more rapidly in females than in males.
- Their dental eruption is also ahead of that of males.
- They achieve early growth completion of facial complex as compared to males.

These findings hold an important clinical significance. The growth modulation treatment should be started in females at an early age as compared to males. This decision should not be based on the dental age, e.g. if a myofunctional appliance needed is given at an early permanent dentition stage, then it may be a delayed treatment device in girls, that the growth spurt may have already passed, while it may be at an appropriate time in males.

Methods to determine skeletal maturity indicators: Different methods have been proposed to know different SMIs which help to determine the growth status of an individual. Some of the most common methods used are as follows.

- Hand and wrist radiographs
- IOPAs for assessment of phalanges
- Cervical vertebrae on lateral cephalogram

- Tooth mineralization on OPG
- Maturation of frontal sinus
- Maturation of midpalatal suture
- Maturation of patella

Requirements of an ideal maturity indicator method: A maturity indicator should have following features:

- It should be safe and non-invasive.
- It should use minimum radiation dose.
- It should be able to determine growth status accurately.
- It should be reproducible.
- It should be cost-effective.
- It should be able to be used for all age-groups.

Clinical Importance

Main aim of interceptive orthodontic treatment is to harmonize the skeletal relation of upper and lower jaws. To achieve this goal, growth modulation is done during the period of active growth by the orthodontist and thus the knowledge of growth status and pattern is of utmost importance. It helps to determine the treatment plan and the appliance, and the best age to initiate the growth modulation treatment. The maturity indictors are the periodical sequence of events of ossification and the skeletal maturation of different bones occurring at specific timings in the body. Hence, the knowledge of maturity indicators is important. They help the clinician to determine the growth pattern and direction, growth rate, and the amount of growth expected. This way, they are used to decide the timing to start the treatment; and to decide the method of treatment.

Since there are individual variations in timing, duration and velocity of growth, the determination of skeletal age of the patient helps in determine a patient-specific treatment plan.

The skeletal age determination with the help of radiographs is based on the fact that different ossification centres appear and mature at different age of the individual, which follows a particular sequence.

Due to different rates of growth in different children, they can be divided as:

1. Early maturers
2. Normal maturers
3. Late maturers.

Advantages of Radiographs

These X-ray views are used for diagnosing the growth status of the patient before growth modification treatment, expansion treatment, functional appliance treatment and to help to guide for planning the orthognathic surgery. They are also used as pretreatment records, and can be used for longitudinal or cross-sectional research studies.

A. Hand and wrist radiographs: It is one of the oldest and most used methods for skeletal age determination by studying stages of various bones in the wrist area. It is considered as the biological clock. Rowland in 1896 took first H and W radiograph. Rotch and Crampton in 1,900 tabulated indicators of hand and wrist. Greulich and Pyle compiled different stages of growth by their longitudinal study and established the standard values. Grave and Brown 1976 determined six ossification centers for skeletal age assessment. Fishman in 1982 proposed 11 indicators for skeletal growth.

Anatomy of skeleton of the hand-wrist region (Figs 16.1 and 16.2): The hand-wrist region is made up of 29 bones, i.e. ends of radius and ulnar bones, eight carpal bones, five metacarpal bones, and 14 phalanges. Initial workers studied the level of development of mainly three bones for the purpose of growth assessment. These were hook of hamate, pissfrom and sessamoid (HPS) bones. Further researchers added other bones and development sequences to determine the bone age.

The carpal bones (Fig. 16.3): There are eight carpal bones. They are arranged in two rows of four bones each, i.e. proximal row and the distal row. Proximal row is near the distal/terminal ends of radius and ulna. Carpal bones in this row arranged from distal to medial side (thumb to little finger side) are

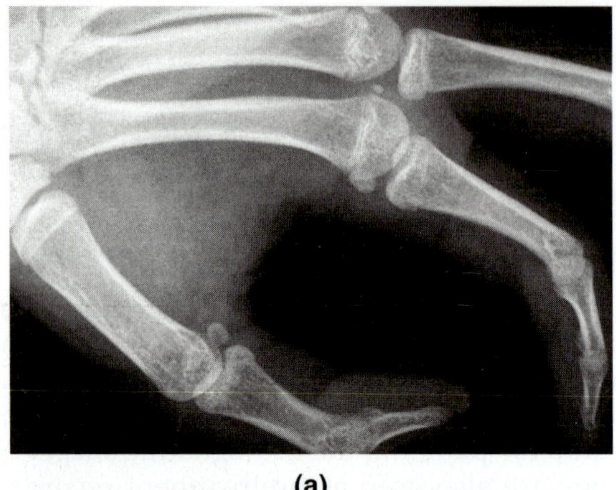

(a)

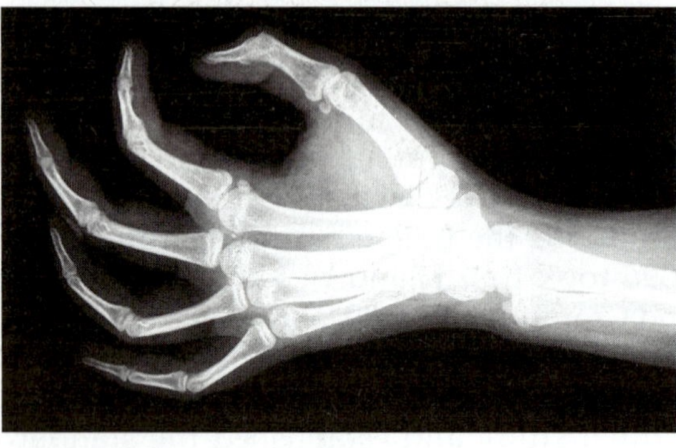

(b)

Figs 16.1a and b: Glass-holding view of hand. This view helps in better image of adductor-sesamoid bone which lies near the thumb. You can also see two other bony nodules at the base of index and middle fingers, which is considered normal findings in some individuals.

scaphoid, lunate, triquetral and pissiform. The bones in the distal row from distal to medial side are trapezium, trapezoid, capitates and hamate (they can be remembered as *Sneh Lata Tamatar Paka, Tere Tamatar Kachchey Hain*).

Metacarpals: They are five bones of the palm. The proximal ends are near carpals, while the distal ends are near phalanges.

Phalanges: They are 14 in number. Each finger is having three phalanges, with thumb having only two. They are referred as proximal, middle, and distal phalanges, the proximal being near the metacarpals. Phalanges ossify in three stages, which are:

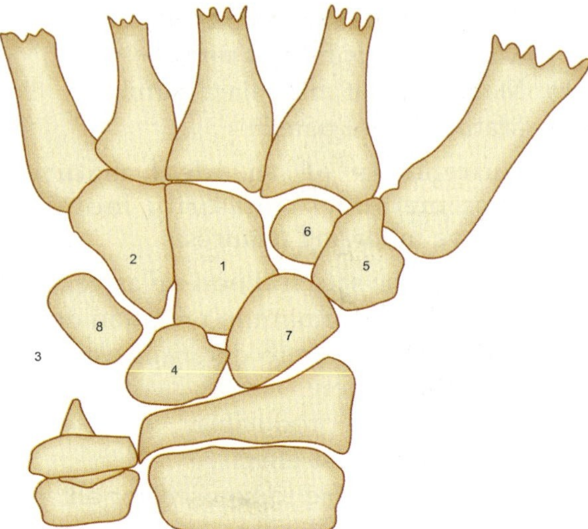

Fig. 16.2: Hand-wrist anatomy. The wrist has 8 carpel bones in a grown up child.

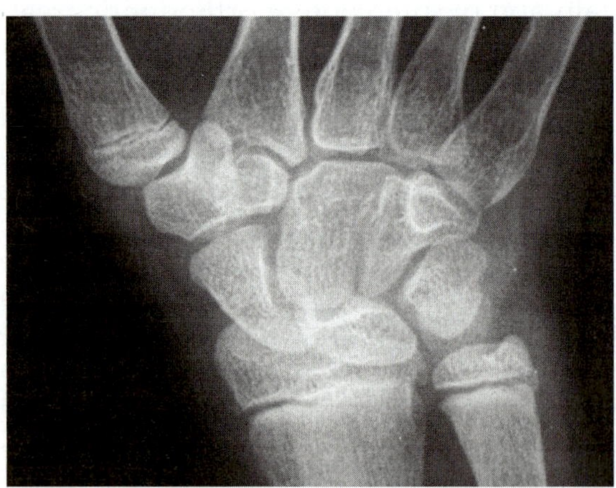

Fig. 16.3: Anatomy and bones in wrist region, wrist has 8 carpal bones.

1. Epiphysis and diaphysis are equal in width.
2. Epiphysis caps the diaphysis
3. Epiphysis fuses with diaphysis.

Hand-wrist radiograph: Early method included the study of three bones of wrist, i.e. hook of HPS. The sequence of events and hence the growth status can be briefly described as follows (Table 16.1):

a. **Prepubertal stage:** Appearance and initial ossification of hook of hamate is seen in prepubertal growth spurt period.

Also, the initial ossification of pissiform is seen before pubertal spurt. It is evident after the ossification of hook of hamate.

b. **Onset of pubertal growth:** Beginning of the calcification of sesamoid bone in thumb indicates the beginning of the pubertal growth spurt. Increased ossification of hook of hamate also occurs.

c. **Pubertal growth acceleration:** Progress of calcified sesamoid occurs. It also sees the onset of peak height velocity, PHV.

d. **Pubertal growth deceleration:** It is characterized by fully calcified sesamoid bone. It may later on fuse with the metacarpal bone. Thus, a fully calcified sesamoid indicates that there is no active growth left. Its appearance indicates the finishing of growth spurts.

e. Appearance of adductor sesamoid of thumb generally corresponds to the beginning of pubertal growth spurt, i.e. onset of PHV, equivalent to stage 2 of CVMI. MP3 cap stage heralds the peak of pubertal growth spurt, which is equivalent to stage 3 of CVMI; or Fishman's SMI 6.

B. Singer's method of assessment: Singer in 1980 proposed his method and determined 6 stages of development. These are described in Table 16.2.

Table 16.1: HW Assessment

Growth phase	*Ossification stage*
Prepubertal	• Initial ossification of hook of hamate • Initial ossification of pissiform
Onset of pubertal growth	• Beginning of the calcification of sesamoid • Increased ossification of hook of hamate
Pubertal growth acceleration	• Progress of calcified sesamoid • Onset of peak height velocity, PHV
Pubertal growth deceleration	• Fully calcified sesamoid bone

C. Hagg and Taranger's method: They described a method in 1982 for skeletal assessment using MP3 of left hand finger. Following stages were determined relative to the PHV.

- **S = Sesamoid** is usually attained during the acceleration of pubertal growth spurt, i.e. onset of PHV.
- **Stage F:** The epiphysis is as wide as the metaphysis. About 40% of the individuals are before PHV. Very few are at PHV.

Table 16.2: Singer's method

Stages	*Features*
I. Early	• Absence of hook of hamate • Absence of pissifrom • Epiphysis of proximal phalanx of second finger is narrower than diaphysis
2. Prepubertal	• Initial ossification of hook of hamate and pissiform • Epiphysis of proximal phalanx of second finger is equal to diaphysis • It is the stage prior to adolescent growth spurt. Significant amount of mandibular growth is possible.
3. Onset of pubertal growth	• Beginning of calcification of sesamoid bone • Increased calcification of hook of hamate and pissiform • Epiphysis of proximal phalanx of second finger is wider than diaphysis
4. Puberal	• Calcified sesamoid bone • Capping of diaphysis of middle phalanx of third finger by the epiphysis
5. Pubertal deceleration	• Fully calcified sesamoid bone • Fusion of epiphysis of distal phalanx of third finger with its diaphysis
6. Growth completion	• No active growth sites seen

- **Stage FG:** The epiphysis is as wide as the metaphysis, and there is a distinct medial or lateral (or both) border of the epiphysis forming a line of demarcation at right angles to the border. About 90% of the individuals are one year before or at PHV.
- **Stage G:** The sides of the epiphysis are thickened, and there is capping of the metaphysis, forming a sharp edge distally at one or both sides. About 90% of the individuals are at or one year after PHV.
- **Spurt H:** Fusion of the epiphysis and metaphysis has begun. About 90% of the girls and all the boys are after PHV but before the end of the pubertal growth spurt.
- **Spurt I:** Fusion of the epiphysis and metaphysis is completed. All individuals except a few girls have ended the pubertal growth spurt.

D. Bjork, Grave and Brown method: They divided the skeletal maturation in 9 stages as given in Table 16.3.

E. Fishman's skeletal maturity indicators: Fishman proposed a system for evaluation for skeletal maturation in 1982, Fishman made use of four anatomical sites located on the thumb, third finger, fifth finger and the radius. He proposed 11 adolescent skeletal maturity indicators (SMI's) covering the entire period of adolescent development. The Fishman's system uses four stages of bone maturation (Figs 16.4 and 16.5), i.e.

- Epiphysis as wide as diaphysis.
- Appearance of adductor sesamoid of thumb
- Capping of epiphysis
- Fusion of epiphysis DP3

These 11 SMIs can be broadly divided into 4 stages as follows:

Stage no. 1 width of epiphysis as wide as diaphysis:

1. Third finger proximal phalanx (PP3 width).
2. Third finger middle phalanx (MP3 width).
3. Fifth finger middle phalanx (MP5 width).

Table 16.3: Bjork et al method

Stage	*Features*	*Significance*
1PP2	Epiphysis and diaphysis of proximal phalanx of index finger are equal.	It occurs approx. 3 years before the peak of pubertal growth spurt slow rate of growth
2MP3	Epiphysis and diaphysis of middle phalanx of middle finger are equal.	maximum long bone growth imminent
3	Epiphysis and diaphysis of radius are equal. Initial ossification of hook of hamate and pissiform.	
4S	Initial ossification of sesamoid bone seen. Increased ossification of hook of hamate and pissiform.	Beginning of pubertal growth spurt
5MP3 cap	Capping of diaphysis by epiphysis of middle phalanx of 3rd and proximal phalanx of thumb and radius is seen	Peak of pubertal growth spurt
6DP3u	Fusion of epiphysis and diaphysis of distal phalanx of middle finger	End of pubertal growth spurt; long growth over
7PP3u	Fusion of epiphysis and diaphysis of proximal phalanx of little finger	
8MP3u	Fusion of epiphysis and diaphysis of middle phalanx of middle finger	Past maximum growth
9RC	Fusion of epiphysis and diaphysis of radius	End of growth

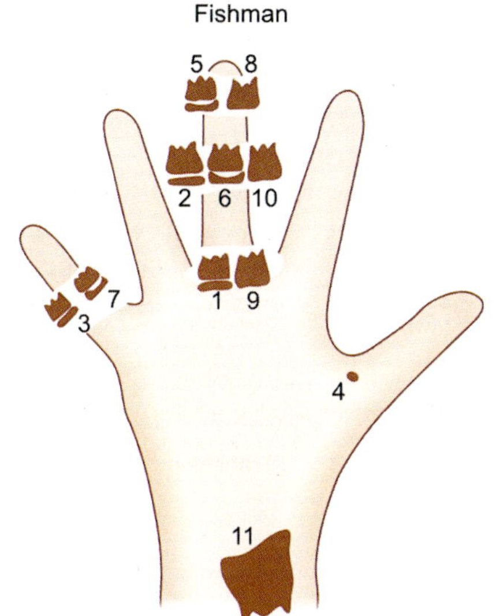

Fig. 16.4: Eleven growth stages of Fishman's skeletal maturation index *(Adapted from Fishman)*.

Stage no. 2 ossification of:

1. Adductor sesamoid of thumb (S).

Stage no. 3 capping of epiphysis:

1. Third finger distal phalanx (DP3 cap).
2. Third finger middle phalanx (MP3 cap).
3. Fifth finger middle phalanx (MP5 cap).

Stage no. 4 union of epiphysis and diaphysis:

1. Third finger distal phalanx (DP3u).
2. Third finger proximal phalanx (PP3u).
3. Third finger middle phalanx (MP3u).
4. Radius (Ru).

He described eleven adolescent SMIs found on these six sites and covering the entire period of adolescent development. The SMI can be arbitrarily divided into periods of accelerating velocity (SMI 1–3), high velocity (SMI 4–7), and decelerating velocity (SMI 8–11).

SMI 1–3: Initiation of pubertal growth spurt

SMI 4: PHV

SMI 5–7: Acceleration of pubertal growth spurt

SMI 8–10: Deceleration of pubertal growth spurt

SMI 11: Finishing of pubertal growth spurt.

F. Skeletal maturation evaluation using cervical vertebrae or cervical vertebrae maturity indicators (CVMI) (Figs 16.6–16.9 and Table 16.4): The continued quest for a

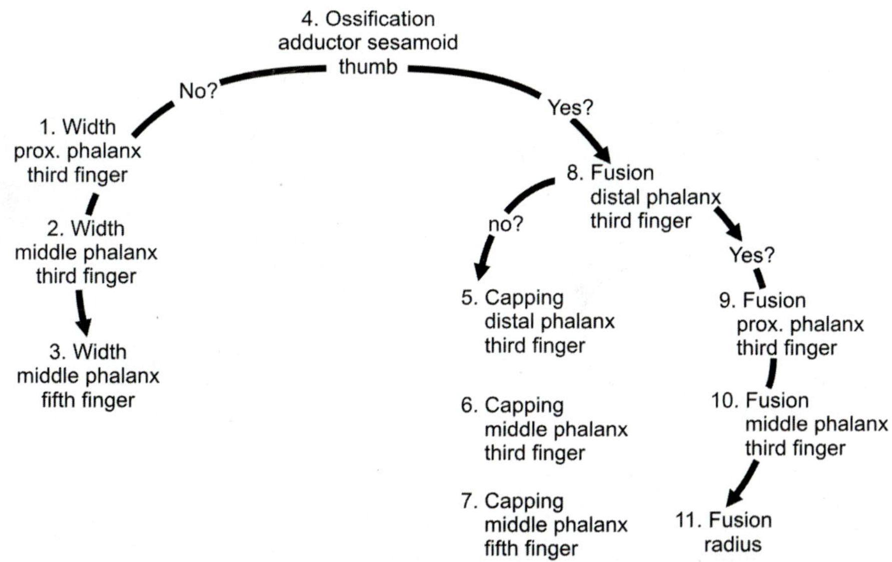

Fig. 16.5: Eleven growth stages of Fishman's skeletal maturation index. There are 2 main stages to note during reading the hand-wrist X-ray, viz stage 4, i.e. appearance of adductor sesamoid; and then stage 8, i.e. fusion of DP3. Appearance of the stage 4 or 8 indicates that now you have to look for stages beyond that stage *(Adapted from Fishman)*.

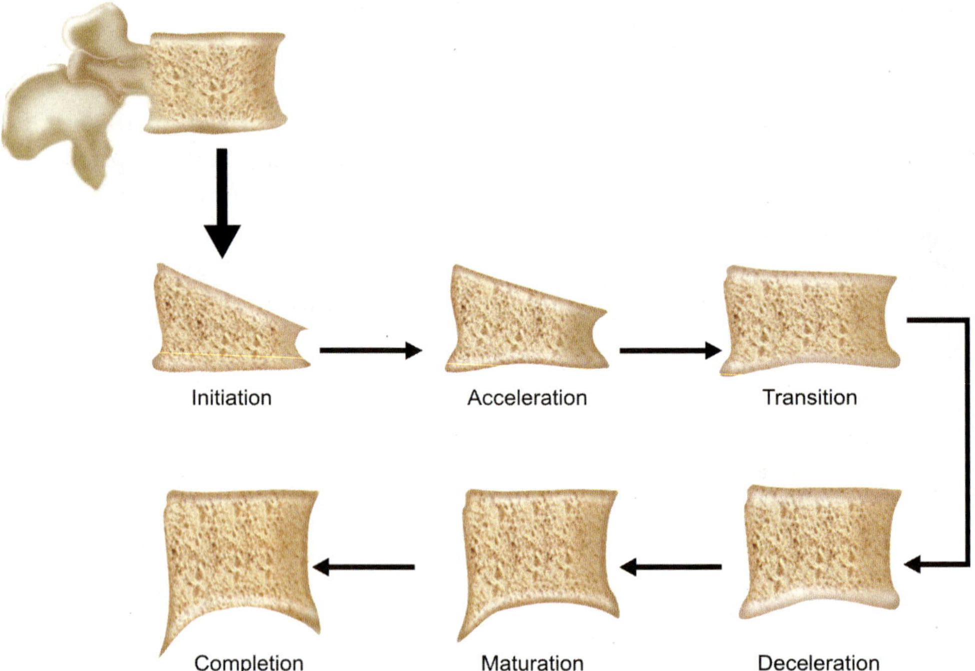

Fig. 16.6: Six stages of cervical vertebrae maturation, CVMI.

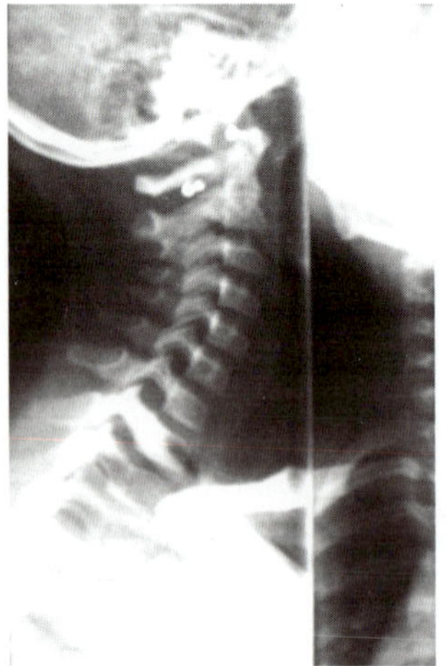

Fig. 16.7: Stage 1 of CVMI.

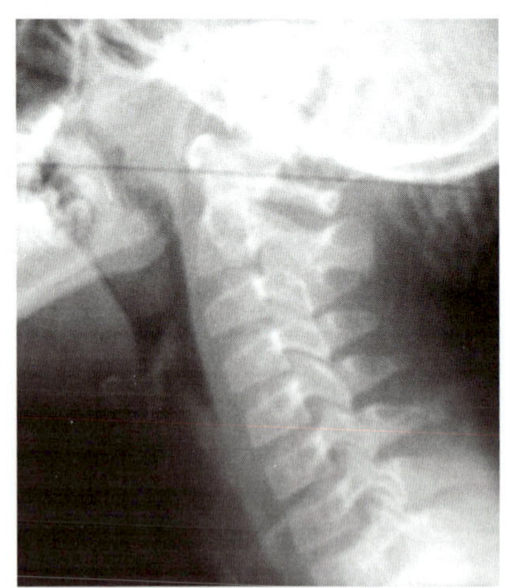

Fig. 16.8: Stage 2 of CVMI.

better SMI method has always been a driving force to find out new methods. A new method of skeletal maturation determination using cervical vertebrae has been proposed by Hassel and Farman in 1995. The shapes of bodies of cervical vertebrae are different at different levels of skeletal maturity. It changes from a relatively wedge-shape to square and then to a vertically rectangular shape, i.e. it changes with the increase in vertical height of the vertebral bodies, which is in consonance with the increasing height and skeletal

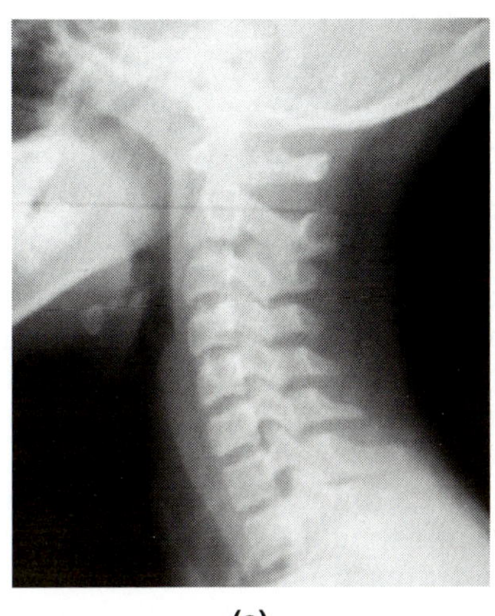

(a)

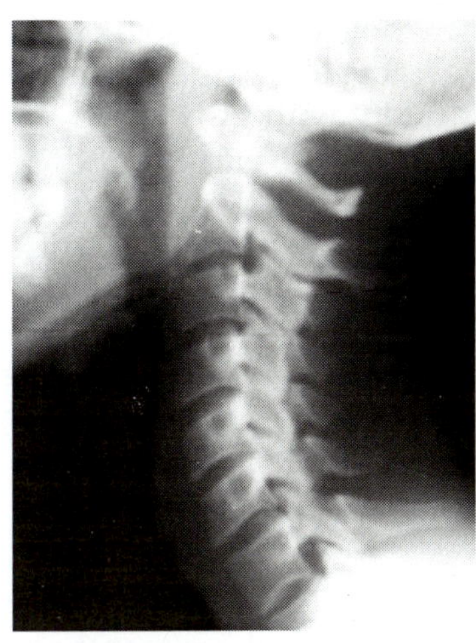

(b)

Figs 16.9a and b: Stage 6 of CVMI.

Table 16.4: CVMI

Stages	*Growth status*	*Growth expected*	*Inferior borders*	*Shape*
Initiation	Indicates the beginning of adolescent growth spurt	80–100%	Of C2, C3 , C4 are flat	Wedge, superior vertebral borders, body tapers from posterior to anterior
Acceleration	Growth acceleration begins	65–85%	Concavities developing in C2, C3, but C4 has flat border	Bodies of C3, C4 nearly rectangular
Transition	Growth acceleration towards peak height velocity, PHV	25–65%	Distinct concavities at C2, C3 Concavity developing at C4	C3, C4 rectangular
Deceleration	Deceleration of adolescent growth spurt	10–25%	Distinct concavities at C2, 3, 4	C3, 4 more nearly square in shape
Maturation	Final maturation of vertebrae	5–10%	More accentuated concavities	C3, 4 square in shape
Completion	Completion of adolescent growth	Little or no growth remaining	Deep concavities	Vertical height more than horizontal dimension

maturity of the whole body. Also, the inferior borders of vertebrae change from flat to increasing concavity with growth.

Fishman's correlated various SMI index stages and the shape, size and curvature of the lower border of cervical vertebrae at different levels of skeletal development to reach the results. Nowadays, it has become one of the most used methods to determine the stage of the skeletal maturity and any remaining growth of the person.

Advantages

1. The main advantage of this method is that it does not need a separate radiograph. The CVMI can be studied in the routine lateral cephalometrics view taken as a preliminary record for pretreatment diagnosis.
2. The total radiation dose is lesser.
3. It is easy to learn and reproduce.
4. This method can be used to correlate with other methods and is being widely used for research purpose.

The shapes of the vertebral bodies, and curvature of their lower borders were studied at different ages. They proposed following 6 stages of vertebral development.

Correlation of CVMI with Fishman's stages:

- Initiation: SMI 1, and 2
- Acceleration: SMI 3, and 4
- Transition: SMI 5, and 6
- Deceleration: SMI 7, and 8
- Maturation: SMI 9, and 10
- Completion: SMI 11.

CVMI: Bacetti 2005 correlated that

- Prepubertal growth stage: at CS1–CS2
- Pubertal stage: CS3, CS4
- Post-pubertal stage: CS5, CS6
- Pubertal peak: Between CS3 and CS4.

Raja Gopal and Kansal (2002) found a high correlation between six MP3 stages and six stages of CV maturation.

Level of GCF during growth stages:

Different stages of CVMI have been classified by Perinetti, et al 2011 as:

- Prepubertal stages: CS1 and CS2
- Pubertal stages: CS3 and CS4
- Postpubertal stages: CS5 and CS6

According to their study, there is a correlation between skeletal maturity as judged by CVMI and the level of gingival crevicular fluid, GCF-alkaline phosphatase enzyme levels.

It has been found that the activity of GCF-alkaline phosphatase enzyme was increased by two times during pubertal stages as compared to prepubertal and postpubertal stages.

Clinical application of CVMI knowledge in orthodontics and dentofacial orthopedics:

1. It helps to detect the growth status and hence the optimal time to start treatment.
2. If stages of CS1 and CS2 are present, then wait for at least 1 year to start the functional treatment, as there is no active growth.
3. If concavity is present on C2, it indicates that the growth spurt is approaching, and it will peak 1 year after this stage.
4. CS3 is the ideal time to start functional appliance, as the peak is expected within this year.
5. Timing for class III can be decided, e.g. a deficient maxilla can be protracted orthopedically during prepubertal phase by at least 2 mm. If the treatment is given at puberty, it helps to restrict mandibular growth by around 4.5 mm.
6. Rapid maxillary expansion should be done before peak.
7. The treatment directed to enhance or restrict mandible should be started during circumpubertal growth period.

G. Maturational evaluation by using stages of ossification of midpalatal suture: It mainly helps to determine the appropriate time for expansion of maxilla to achieve skeletal effects. The midpalatal sutural interdigitation increases with age, and thus expansion effects are seen as lesser skeletal and more dental changes. Also, the maxilla completes its growth first in the transverse dimension. As the age increases, the chances of skeletal changes in width of maxilla diminish. It has been found that it is best to accomplish the maxillary expansion before SMI 9. The deal time to commence the maxillary expansion is during SMI 1–4 stages or during 8–10 years of age. That time, the suture is soft and not interdigitated, so less orthopedic forces are needed to separate 2 halves of maxilla.

H. Tooth mineralization as an indicator of the pubertal growth spurt: Dental development can be used as a potential predictor of skeletal maturity. It can be assessed either by the stage of dental eruption or the stage of tooth calcification, the latter being more reliable. Using OPG to assess skeletal maturity by studying developmental stage of teeth has several advantages. It is easy to use and remember as the dental professionals are more familiar with the stages of dental development than the skeletal maturity indicators in hand-wrist region. Also, no additional X-ray exposure is needed since OPG are routinely taken before the orthodontic treatment.

Demirjian et al method to assess dental maturation: Eight stages of calcification from A to H are described for each tooth as studied on OPG.

Stage A: In both single rooted and multi rooted teeth, a beginning of calcification is seen at the superior level of the crypt. No fusion of these calcified points can be observed.

Stage B: Fusion of the calcified points forms one or several cusps which unite to give a regularly outlined occlusal surface.

Stage C: Enamel formation has been completed at the occlusal surface, and dentine formation has commenced. The pulp chamber is curved, and no pulp horns are visible.

Stage D: Crown formation has been completed to the level of the cementoenamel junction. Root formation has commenced. The pulp horns are beginning to differentiate, but the walls of the pulp chamber remain curved.

Stage E: The root length remains shorter than the crown height. The walls of the pulp chamber are straight, and the pulp horns have become more differentiated than in the previous stage. In molars, the radicular bifurcation has started to calcify.

Stage F: The walls of the pulp chamber now form an isosceles triangle, and the root length is equal to or greater than the crown height. In molars, the bifurcation has developed sufficiently to give roots a distinct form.

Stage G: The walls of the root canal are now parallel, but the apical end is still partially open.

Stage H: The apical end of the root canal is completely closed and the periodontal membrane is uniform around the root and the apex.

Chertkow in 1980 proposed a method based on the observation of pattern of calcification and stage of mineralization of teeth having a close relationship with the skeletal maturation of the individual. He used the mineralization pattern of mandibular canine to determine the skeletal maturity. Mandibular canines were used due to their uniformity of development. He showed that the mandibular canine **Stage G coincided with the appearance of adductor sesamoid bone (stage 2 of CVMI), which corresponds to PHV**.

Females mature faster than males as various studies show that the appearance of each skeletal stage is earlier in females than in males. In other study, Stage F of tooth calcification has been found to be corresponding to onset of PHV (stage 2 of CVMI) and Stage G of tooth calcification in canine; first premolar and second molar may correspond to peak of pubertal growth spurt (stage 3 of CVMI). Root formation of the canine as well as the first premolar gets completed in majority of subjects at stage 5 of CVMI. For all the teeth except third molar root formation was completed at stage 6 of CVMI. In a nut-shell, it can be agreed that tooth mineralisation stages mandibular canines and second molars can be used for skeletal maturation assessment.

Hagg and Bjork found appearance of adductor sesamoid of thumb marks the beginning of pubertal growth spurt, i.e. the onset of PHV, which corresponds to stage 2 of CVMI (Fishman's SMI 4). Stage F of tooth calcification corresponds to onset of PHV. Bjork found that MP3 cap stage was very closely related to the age of pubertal maximum growth velocity which corresponds to stage 3 of CVMI (Fishman's SMI 6). Stage G of tooth calcification in canine; first premolar and second molar may correspond to peak of pubertal growth spurt.

Summarily,

- Stage 2 of CVMI = Fishman's SMI 4 = Stage F of tooth calcification = onset of PHV.
- MP3cap stage = Stage 3 of CVMI = Fishman's SMI 6 = Stage G of tooth calcification in canine; first premolar and second molar = peak of pubertal growth spurt.

Some studies also show a significant association between the stages of calcification of mandibular second molar and the skeletal maturity stages of middle phalanx of third finger (MP3).

- Calcification stages D and E of mandibular second molar indicated a pre-peak of pubertal growth spurt.
- Stages F and G indicated the peak of pubertal growth.
- Stage H marked the end of pubertal growth spurt.

Mittal, et al in 2011 found a correlation of CVMI and Demirijan stage of second molar development irt to the stage of pubertal growth spurt as shown in Table 16.5.

Table 16.5: CVMI and Demirijan stage of second molar development

Demirijan index Second molar	CVMI	Stage of pubertal growth spurt
E	2	Prepeak of pubertal growth spurt; onset of PHV
F, G	3,4	Peak of pubertal growth spurt
H	5,6	End of growth spurt

Conclusion

An active growth period is the important phase of the growth during which growth modulation can be positively achieved. It helps to attain a normal skeletal jaw relationship. It can be best be known by skeletal age determination by using various maturity indicators. Rather than using various complex methods, now, the CVMI and the mineralization stages of teeth can be used reliably for assessing the growth status by using lateral cephalograms and OPG. These are having an additional advantage since OPG and cephalograms are the routine records for orthodontic patients, and thus an additional radiation exposure can be avoided, and they can be remembered and applied easily.

17

Electromyography in Orthodontics

INTRODUCTION

All the muscles of body are in a state of continuous remodelling to match their functional requirements. Overuse of muscles leads to its hypertrophy, with an increase in its total mass. Atrophy occurs when the muscle is not used causing a decrease in muscle mass. Electromyography (EMG) is a record of the action current showing muscular activity under diverse functional conditions.

Electromyographic Technique

EMG is defined as the recording and study of the intrinsic electrical properties of skeletal muscle to determine whether the muscle is contracting or not. An electrode is introduced into the muscle and the action potential is noted in the cathode-ray oscilloscope. Electromyograph is the instrument used in EMG. Electromyogram is the record obtained by electromyography. The several skeletal muscle fibers contract at almost the same moment, and a minute electrical potential is generated, which is dissipated into the surrounding tissue. This is referred to as an action current or an action potential which is recorded in the oscilloscope. The current generated is so small that it must be amplified many thousand times to be recorded. Two main types of electrodes are used, viz. surface (or "skin") electrodes, and inserted electrodes (usually wire or needle). Needle electrodes are superior to surface electrodes, as the quality of the electromyogram is better. There is a risk of infection associated with the use of needle electrodes. They may also be painful. Surface electrodes are non-invasive and have lesser risk of infection. But, some loosening of the electrodes may occur during nerve stimulation giving rise to errors.

Electromyography in Orthodontics

EMG in dentistry was introduced by Robert E. Moyers. He observed that the normal relations of teeth to each other in the same and opposite jaws were influenced by muscular balance. Main important muscles in orthodontics are muscles of mastication (masseter, temporalis, and medial and lateral pterygoids); buccinators, mentalis, orbicularis oris, and superior constrtictor of phayrnx. Genioglossus muscle which is responsible for the protraction of the tongue is also important. These muscles help in proper growth and development of craniofacial skeleton, and the dental arches/dentition.

Role of muscles: According to Moss's growth concept, the soft tissues guide the growth of hard tissues. Proper muscles coordination and function leads to normal growth. A balance of extraoral and intraoral muscular forces leads to development of normal arch forms. Any disturbance in the muscles activity, e.g. due to abnormal habits; due to syndromic abnormalities of muscular development and coordination, etc. the jaw growth is affected. Such effects have been discussed in relevant chapters of growth, etiology and habits. Abnormal contraction of muscles leads to deficient growth, e.g. hyperactivity of mentalis muscle leads to deficient chin growth; hyperactivity of buccinators leads to constricted maxilla, etc.

Lip and Cheek Activity in Sucking Habits

Ahlgren found that profound lip and mentalis (perioral) activity was developed during thumb and dummy sucking, while the cheek (buccinator) activity was less evident, showing light to moderate activity as compared to control normal children. Activity at rest in perioral muscles was pronounced among thumb and dummy suckers, while buccinator activity was negligible.

Electromyographic activity during swallowing: EMG activity of facial muscles is different during normal and abnormal swallowing. In the normal mature swallow, the mandible rises, the teeth come together during the swallow, and the lips touch lightly. There is no facial muscles contraction. The temporal muscle contracts as the mandible is elevated.

But, during the teeth-apart swallow, there is no contraction of the temporal muscle. Here mentalis muscle and lip contractions are needed to stabilize the mandible. Winders found that the buccal and labial muscles do not contract during swallowing, except in anterior open bite.

In tongue thrust swallowing, the tongue comes more forward than normal to make an oral seal to help the swallowing procedure. So the tongue muscle, especially the genioglossus muscle, responsible for protrusion of tongue, hypertrophies. A hypertrophic muscle has increased electromyographic activity because of increased motor units. The electromyographic activity after habit correction returns to normal levels.

Effect of Pain from Orthodontic Treatment on EMG Activity

Pain affects the muscle activity even when it does not originate in the muscle itself or in the related joint. Orthodontic pain on teeth tends to reduce muscle activity during function.

EMG activity in class II malocclusion patients: In contrast to class I malocclusion in which the muscle-function is usually normal (except in open bite cases), most class II division 1 malocclusions involve abnormal muscle activity. In class II division 2 malocclusions, there is dominance of posterior fibres of both the temporalis and masseter muscles. Pancherz found less electromyographic activity in the masseter and temporal muscles than the controls in patients with class II division 1 malocclusion during maximal biting in centric occlusion. During chewing, the class II subjects showed less electromyographic activity in the masseter muscle than in the normals. No differences were found between the two groups for temporalis. The impaired muscle activity in class II cases may be attributed to diverging dentofacial morphology and unstable occlusal contacts.

In many class II division 1 conditions, the mentalis muscle is hyperactive and the upper lip is hypofunctional. The lower lip contracts in upwards and forward direction during swallowing leading to labial movement of maxillary incisors. The buccinator muscle also may contract excessively. EMG studies verify this clinical observation. In class II division 1 malocclusion, posterior fibres of the temporalis muscle seem to exert greater influence than with a normal occlusion. Overclosure with concomitant retrusive posterior temporalis and deep masseter activity can create antero-posterior discrepancies.

Electromyographic findings in functional appliance treatment: The "pterygoid response" is seen in patients using FA which begins during the first few months of appliance placement. It is the newly acquired position of superior head of lateral pterygoid muscle under the influence of FA treatment for class II condition. After few months of treatment, when the clinician tries to push the mandible backward, the mandible does not go to its pre-treatment position. Hence, it is a good sign of treatment and also shows that patient is using the FA properly. It is due to the increased tonic activity of superior head of the lateral pterygoid muscle, seen during maintenance of the postural position of the mandible as well as during functional movements. A distinct change in muscle activity occurs after the first few days or weeks of appliance wear. It is characterized by a decrease in the EMG activity of posterior temporalis muscle, an increase in the activity of masseter muscle, and most significantly an increase in the function of superior head of lateral pterygoid muscle. This increased activity in the superior head of lateral pterygoid muscle then acts to stimulate condylar growth in a favorable direction. EMG activity of masseter, digastric, superior and inferior lateral pterygoid muscles decrease with functional appliance treatment.

EMG studies on class III subjects: The integrated EMG activity of masseter and temporal muscles in class III cases is less than in normal occlusion subjects. It is believed that correction of anterior crossbite in class III patients increases EMG activities of masseter and anterior temporal muscles, or improves coordination of bilateral masseter and anterior temporal muscles.

EMG activity in cleft lip and palate patients: Studies have evaluated EMG characteristics of masticatory muscle in operated unilateral CLP patients with anterior crossbite compared with normal individuals. Patients with unilateral CLP had a higher activation level of masseter and temporalis muscles in rest position.

Conclusion

The role of musculature in development of normal skeletal morphology, the dentition and the dental arch form is very important. Buccinator mechanism is one of the main systems needed for proper development of dental arches and dentition. Functional matrix concept of growth by Moss has described the importance of the soft tissues on growth and development. Any disturbed muscular function leads to development of malocclusion, as the compensatory changes in the dental and skeletal relationship occur. The masticatory and the facial muscles are intimately associated.

Premature occlusal contacts and compensatory muscle activity tends to change bony morphology, accentuating the malocclusion and it leads to an adaptive activity of muscles. It leads to a vicious circle of abnormal activity and development/sustenance of abnormal occlusion.

EMG is an important diagnostic tool to determine the abnormal functioning muscles. With improved equipments of EMG and its easy accessibility, more definitive studies can be done to determine the exact malfunctioning muscles, and this information can be used to plan proper treatment to solve many growth and malocclusion problems.

Further Readings

1. Brodie, A. G., Angle Orthod., 1953, **23**, 71–77.
2. Graber, T. M., Am. J. Orthod., 1963, **49**, 418.
3. Pancherz, H., Am. J. Orthod. Dentofac. Orthop., 1980, **77**, 679–688.
4. Meenakshi Iyer and Ashima Valiathan: Electromyography and its application in orthodontics. Current Science, Vol. 80, no. 4, 25 February 2001 503
5. Moyers, R. E., Am. J. Orthod., 1949, **35**, 837.

18

Biology of Tooth Movement

INTRODUCTION

To treat a malocclusion, the teeth are to be moved in the jaw bones to the desired positions. It can only be achieved by application of forces on the teeth, which get distributed to the bone and periodontal tissues, to initiate biochemical process in the bone and supporting tissues. Proffit described the orthodontic tooth movement occurring as a result of a biological response to an externally applied force. OTM occurs when prolonged forces are applied on the tooth, which get transferred to the supporting tissues, the bone remodeling occurs around the tooth, resulting in the movement. So, the bone under pressure due to compression of periodontal ligament (PDL) gets resorbed, while the bone gets deposited under tension due to stretch of PDL fibers. Accurate and precise control of tooth movement can be optimized with the proper use of mechanics and knowledge of the subsequent tissue response.

Tooth Supporting Tissues (Fig. 18.1)

Orthodontic treatment involves the use and control of forces acting on teeth and associated structures. During tooth movement, changes in the periodontium occur, depending on the magnitude, direction and duration of the force applied. The periodontium (peri = around, odontos = tooth) comprises four tissues, viz. the gingiva, the PDL, the root cementum, and the alveolar bone.

Gingiva

The gingiva is further differentiated into the free and attached gingiva. Free gingiva is in close contact with enamel surface, and its margin is located 0.5–2 mm coronal to cementoenamel junction. The attached gingiva is firmly attached to underlying alveolar bone by connective tissue fibers and is therefore comparatively immobile. The predominant tissue component of the gingiva is the connective tissue, which consists of collagen fibers (66%), fibroblasts (5%) and vessels, nerves and matrix (35%).

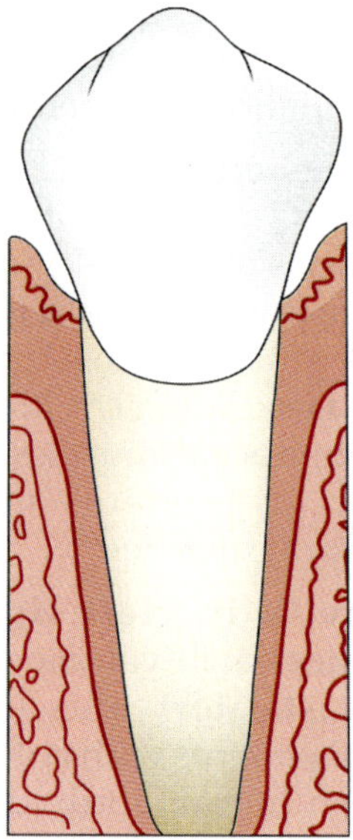

Fig. 18.1: Normal periodontal anatomy.

Periodontal Ligament

PDL is approximately 0.25 mm wide, vascular and cellular connective tissue surrounding the roots of teeth and joins the root cementum with the lamina dura or alveolar bone proper. This type of joint is called as gomphosis. It is hour-glass-shaped, and a vital PDL is a very important component for OTM. If there is deficiency of PDL, e.g. in ankylosis, the tooth movement is impossible. The PDL acts as a channel to distribute the forces applied on the teeth into the alveolar bone.

The true periodontal fibers, the principal fibers, develop in conjunction with the eruption of tooth, and are described in the following groups: alveolar crest fibers (ACF), horizontal fibers (HF), oblique fibers (OF) and apical fibers (AF). The fibrils of PDL are embedded in a ground substance which contains connective tissue polysaccharides (glycosaminoglycans), salts and water.

Root Cementum

It is a specialized mineralized tissue covering the root surface. It does not contain any blood vessels, has no innervations, and is characterized by continuing deposition throughout life, which may lead to hypercementosis in some cases. The PDL fibers at attached to cementum on one side and to the alveolar bone on other side, acting a cushion in between. Properties on are cementum in relation to orthodontics have been widely studied by Darendililer et al but the details are out of scope of this book.

Alveolar Bone

Alveolar bone surrounds the tooth to a level approximately 1 mm apical to the CEJ, in the area where transseptal fibers are attached on the neck of the tooth. The alveolar bone further consists of two components, the alveolar bone proper and the alveolar process. The part of the alveolar bone that covers the alveolus and helps in attachment of fibers of PDL is referred to as lamina dura, which is a cortical bone. The alveolar bone is constantly renewed in response to functional demands with the help of osteoblasts and osteoclasts. The osteoblasts produce osteoid, consisting of collagen fibers and a matrix that contain mainly proteoglycans and glycoproteins. The bone is covered with the periosteum, which functions as an osteogenic zone throughout life.

Bone tissue: Bone is a specialized mineralized connective tissue made up of an organic matrix of collagen fibrils embedded in an amorphous substance with mineral crystals precipitated within the matrix. Bone is of two types, i.e. compact/cortical bone and cancellous/trabecular bone.

Tooth Movement

The relationship of teeth and the supporting structure is a dynamic phenomenon, i.e. it keeps on adapting and remodeling throughout life depending on the function. Following types of tooth movements can be seen in the dentition in the life of an individual.

Physiologic Tooth Movement

It is a natural phenomenon occurring in the dentition throughout life. It includes tooth eruption, migration/drifting of teeth, and changes in tooth position during mastication. It means, primarily, the slight tipping of the functioning tooth in its socket cushioned by PDL when masticatory forces are applied on the teeth, and, secondarily, the changes in the tooth position that occur in young person during and after tooth eruption. The teeth and their supporting tissues have a life-long ability to adapt to functional demands and hence drift through the alveolar process, a phenomenon called physiologic tooth migration. This physiologic drift is essential to maintain stomatognathic form and function. With age, the enamel attrition especially on proximal surfaces also leads to physiological migration of teeth. Even after the extraction of tooth, the adjacent and opposing teeth start migrating in the space, if that space is not preserved.

Pathologic Tooth Movement

Carranza defined it as "displacement that results when the balance among the factors that maintain physiological tooth position is disturbed by periodontal disease," e.g. due to bone loss around the teeth, even the normal forces become pathologic and lead to shifting of teeth. It occurs most frequently in the anterior region, but posterior teeth may also be affected.

Orthodontic Tooth Movement (Fig. 18.2)

Since the teeth are moved more rapidly under the influence of orthodontic forces during treatment, the tissue changes elicited are consequently more marked and extensive. Orthodontic treatment is based on the principle that if prolonged pressure is applied to a tooth, movement of the tooth will take place due to bone remodeling.

Bone Modeling and Remodeling

According to Wolff's law (1892): "Every change in the form and function of bone or of their function alone is followed by certain definite changes in their internal architecture, i.e. orientation of trabecular pattern, and equally definite alteration in their external conformation, in accordance with mathematical laws". Bone's turnover occurs through remodeling via cell-mediated resorption and deposition which leads to change in the size and shape of bone.

Remodeling means in certain areas of bone, the resorption occurs, while in other areas, the deposition occurs. It helps in changes in size and shape of the bone. It occurs with the help of osteoblasts and the osteoclasts. Bone deposition and resorption occurs along periosteal and endosteal surfaces. It also helps in maintain the thickness of alveolarbone.

When the force is applied on a tooth, the areas of pressure and tension are created in the PDL. Bone on pressure side is resorbed on the PDL side, while it is formed in the marrow spaces, thus maintaining the alveolar thickness. On tension side, bone is deposited in the PDL side but gets resorbed in marrow area. Thus the tooth moves in the bone, maintaining the thickness of bone.

Histology of Tooth Movement

When forces are applied on the tooth, areas of pressure and tension are created in the PDL. Area of pressure is formed in the direction of tooth movement and the area of tension in the opposite direction. Bone resorption occurs on the pressure side and bone deposition on the tension side. Histological changes depend on the amount and duration of the applied forces and can be studied under two broad headings:

A. Changes occurring due to lighter forces
B. Changes occurring due to heavy forces.

A. Changes Occurring due to Lighter Forces

When forces are applied on the tooth, areas of pressure and tension are created in the PDL.

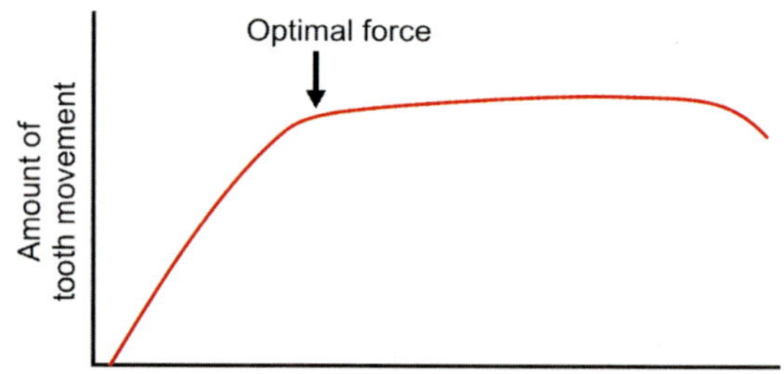

Fig. 18.2: A continuous tooth movement is achieved when forces are kept within optimal limit.

Changes on pressure side (Fig. 18.3): Under lighter forces, the PDL gets compressed to approximately one-third of its width. Its vascularity increases due to increased capillary blood supply, and thus number of fibroblasts, osteoclasts, etc. increases. Osteoclasts are the multinucleated giant cells formed by coalescence of local macrophages from the

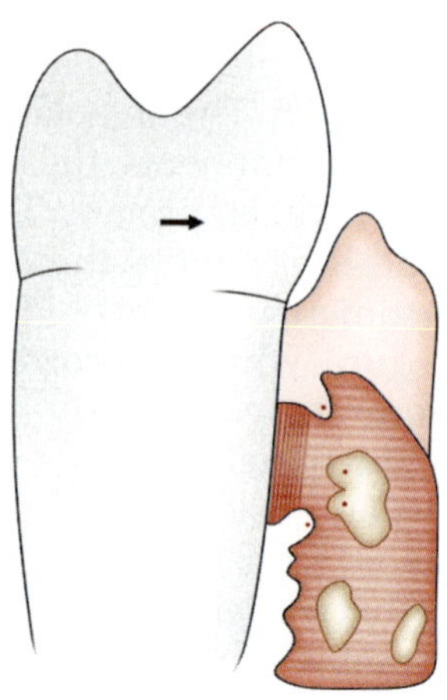

Fig. 18.3: Bone resroption area on the side of tooth movement being depicted by arrow.

PDL and also from the monocytes. They have ruffelled border, and house in Howship's lacunae in the bone. They resorb the bone in the alveolar plate just adjacent to the PDL. Thus the bone resorption occurs directly adjacent to the area of pressure. This type of bone resorption is the frontal/direct resroption.

When bone resroption is occurring near PDL side, simultaneous bone deposition also occurs in subjacent marrow area to maintain the width of the alveolar bone. A change in the orientation of bony trabeculae also occurs under the influence of forces. In normal unstressed bone, they are parallel to the long axis of the teeth, i.e. almost parallel to the forces of mastication so that these forces are distributed along them in the bone. When orthodontic forces are applied, the trabeculae become horizontally oriented, i.e. become parallel to the direction of orthodontic forces. This trabecular pattern comes back after the forces are removed, i.e. during the retention period.

Changes on the tension side: As the tooth shifts in the socket, PDL fibers get stretched as they get splayed in their intermediate zone. Thus the PDL width increases on the tension side. Increase in vascularity leads to migration of fibroblasts and osteoblasts which cause deposition of osteoid, the uncalcified precursor of bone, in the PDL immediately adjacent to the lamina dura. Osetoid is the tissue which is resistant to resorption. Osteoid becomes calcified in due course of time. Simultaneously, the bone resorption occurs in the alveolar bone on marrow side to maintain the width of bone and socket.

Secondary remodeling changes: Osteoblastic and osteoclastic changes occur in the areas of tension and pressure in the PDL side of the alveolar bone, respectively. However, to maintain the width of alveolar bone around the tooth, the resorption and deposition of bone also occur in the bone marrow side of the alveolar bone just below the areas of tension and pressure. These are called secondary remodeling changes.

B. Changes with Heavy Forces (Fig. 18.4)

Crushing of PDL occurs on the pressure side as the tooth shifts completely in the socket under the heavy forces. As the root approximates the alveolar bone on the pressure side, it compresses the PDL and leads to the occlusion of blood vessels. It causes necrosis and hyalinization of PDL in that area. As the PDL gets necrosed, it does not help in bone resorption in that area. Thus, the bone does not resorb by frontal resorption. However, the undermining resorption of bone occurs just beneath the hyalinized area on the subjacent marrow side and alveolar bone around the hyalinized zone. It leads to shifting of the tooth in the direction of applied force, thus relieving the pressure area. After that, the hyalinized tissues get removed.

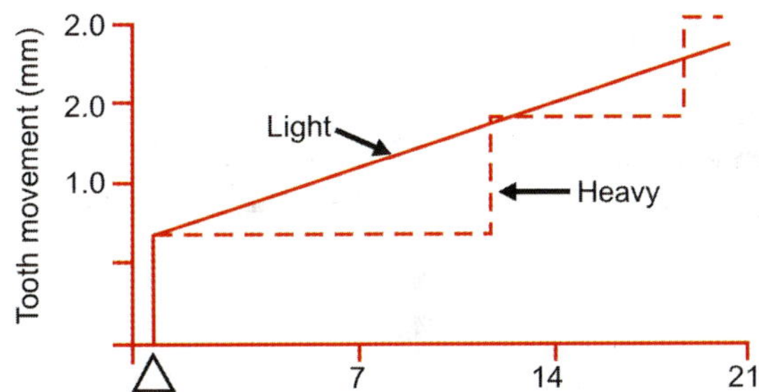

Fig. 18.4: Spurts of tooth movement with heavy forces (in dotted line), while continuous movement due to lighter forces (shown by solid line).

On the tension side, the overstretching of PDL causes the tearing of blood vessels and ischemia. So, under the influence of heavy forces, there is more osteoclastic activity on both the sides due to hyalinization and then its removal through undermining resorption, thus leading to widening of PDL and loosening of tooth in the socket. It also leads to pain and hyperemia of gingiva, and may also lead to discoloration and devitalization of the tooth.

Concept of Optimum Forces (Fig. 18.2)

The tooth moves in the bone when a force is applied on the tooth, thus causing pressure (force per unit area) on the PDL. Oppenheim and Schwarz in 1920s defined optimum force as "the amount of force which moves the teeth most rapidly through the bone in the desired direction, with the least possible damage to tissues and with minimum patient discomfort". It is generally considered in the range of capillary blood pressure. Its value is 20–26 gm/cm^2 root surface area (RSA). RSA also correspond to the anchorage value of the tooth. RSA of different teeth vary due to size and number of the roots, e.g. lower incisors have least RSA and molars having maximum RSA. Proffit has described the values of RSA of different teeth as shown in Table 18.1.

Table 18.1: Showing RSA of different teeth (from Proffit and Fields)

Tooth	*Maxillary*	*Mandibular*
Central incisor	230	170
Lateral incisor	194	200
Canines	282	270
Premolar	254	240
First molar	533	475
Second molar	450	450

Since the applied force gets distributed over the RSA. So, the amount of force required also varies with the teeth to be moved. The bigger teeth require more force to create adequate pressure (force per unit area) to initiate the OTM.

Advantages of Optimum Force

- Vitality of PDL and tooth is maintained.
- There is no marked mobility of the teeth.
- It helps to initiate the cellular response in PDL.
- It helps to produce frontal/direct bone resorption, thus reducing the treatment time.
- It does not lead to root resorption.
- It causes no pain.

Types of the bone resorption: Two main types of bone resorption patterns are seen during the OTM. It depends on the type/amount of the forces being used for OTM.

Frontal/direct resorption: The light forces lead to the frontal/direct resorption. Frontal resorption is preferred phenomenon during orthodontic treatment rather than the rear resorption.

Undermining/rear resorption: Heavy forces lead to undermining/rear resorption.

Differences Between Frontal and Rear Resorption

Frontal resorption: It occurs when light forces are used. This type of bone resorption occurs just below the area of pressure on alveolar bone on the PDL side, occurring in the lamina dura. Lighter force does not lead to crushing of PDL and capillary occlusion, thus the bone resorbing are supplied from the capillaries on the PDL side.

Less time is needed to initiate and continue the OTM, since the time is not wasted to remove the hyalinized area (as will be discussed in rear resoption). It causes minimum damage to and thus maintains the health of supporting tissues. So, the forces used are within the physiological limits. OTM is fast and continuous, i.e. it does not stop in between. There occurs little or no root resorption. Also, the patient does not feel pain. Vitality of pulp and the PDL is maintained.

Rear resorption: With the application of heavy force, there occurs crushing of PDL, and occlusion of capillaries. Excessive pressure leads to necrosis of PDL in that area which becomes devoid of cells, thus leading to hyalinization of tissues in that area. Due to occlusion of capillaries, the bone-resorbing cells cannot be supplied from the PDL side. Since the hyalinized areas are devoid of cells, the bone resorbing cells are derived from the bone marrow rather than the PDL. Thus, the bone resorption occurs on the marrow side below the hyalinized area of PDL, i.e. it occurs from the rear/the bone marrow side in areas of pressure, rather than in the area of bone in direct contact with the area of pressure. As the bone resorbs, the hyalinized are is removed, the pressure is relieved, and the tooth moves.

Heavy forces applied during the treatment lead to more damage to the tooth and supporting tissues. In such cases, the initial tooth movement occurs after a gap of few days (equal to the time taken to remove the hyalinized tissues), and thus more time is taken to initiate OTM. OTM stops until hyalinized tissue is removed. It also leads to more root resorption.

Hyalinization: Hyalinization is a tissue-degeneration characterized by formation of a clear, homogenous substance in the tissues. A hyalinized zone is formed as the localized cell-free area of over-compressed periodontal tissue in the areas of pressure, when heavy forces are applied, e.g. during OTM or during application of orthopedic forces for controlling the maxillary growth, during RME, etc.

Hyalinization is more frequently seen in adult patients even with lighter forces. In them, the bone is less pliable. Also they may have periodontal disease leading to decreased bone support to the teeth with lesser effective PDL and RSA, thus increasing the effective pressure (P = F/A) on the PDL.

The following changes are observed during formation of hyalinized zones.

1. There is a gradual compression of the periodontal fibers leading to their shrinkage.
2. Some nuclei disappear, while some become pyknotic.
3. The compressed collagen fibers gradually become cell-free, and some changes occur in the ground substance also. The vascular walls breakdown causing a loss of their contents in the surrounding tissues.
4. Osteoclasts are formed in marrow spaces and areas adjacent to the hyalinized area of PDL after 20 to 30 hours. There is a gradual increase in the number of young connective tissue cells around the osteoclasts.
5. In the hyalinized areas, the pressure in PDL is relieved by undermining bone resorption which occurs in the marrow area subjacent to the hyalinized PDL areas.

The appearance of hyalinized zone indicates that the PDL is not vital/functional in this area and so the bone resorption cannot occur. Since this part of PDL is necrotic, it is not able to supply the required cells for bone resorption. A vital PDL is very important for supplying the bone-resorption/deposition cells. So unless this necrotic tissue is removed, the bone resorption will not start.

The removal of hyalinized tissues occurs by 2 mechanisms:

1. Osteolclasts differentiate from the intact peripheral periodontal membrane and the adjacent bone marrow spaces, which lead to resorption of alveolar bone.
2. Necrotic tissue is removed by the cells which come through the invading blood vessels from the periphery of compressed zone. The cells penetrate the hyalinized tissue and remove the dead tissue by phagocytosis and enzymatic action.

Thus to relieve the necrotic and pressure area, the bone resorption starts from the bone-marrow side, which relieves the pressure in PDL side and also provides cells for the removal of necrotic tissues. Once this necrotic tissue and hylanized zone is removed, the tooth starts moving as the direct bone resorption process starts.

Width of the zone of hyalinized tissue depends on the amount of the force. Greater the force, wider the area and vice versa. Location of hyalinized zone depends on the type of the tooth movement, e.g. in tipping, this zone is formed near alveolar crest, while during bodily movement, it is near middle 3rd of the root.

Tissue Response in Periodontium during Hyalinization

PDL is one of the most important tissues during orthodontic tooth movement. Biochemical changes start in the tissues with the application of forces, leading to tooth movement within the alveolus. It is seen initially by narrowing of the periodontal membrane and shifting of the tooth, particularly in the marginal area. The tissue reveals a glass-like appearance in light microscopy, termed hyalinization. It represents a sterile necrotic area, generally limited to 1 or 2 mm in diameter. The process displays three main stages:

- Degeneration
- Elimination of destroyed tissues
- Establishment of a new tooth attachment.

In the secondary period of tooth movement, width of the PDL increases considerably. The osteoclasts attack the bone surface over a much wider area and, if the force is kept within lighter limits, the direct bone resorption occurs. The fibrous attachment gets reorganized by production of new periodontal fibrils, which get attached to the parts of newly deposited bone.

The deposition of new bone osteoid is seen after 30–40 hours on the tension side. Bone resorption also occurs on the marrow side of the alveolar bone to maintain the dimension of supporting bone. The original periodontal fibers become embedded in the new layers of osteoid.

PHASES OF ORTHODONTIC TOOTH MOVEMENT (Fig. 18.5)

Storey described three phases of OTM, i.e. the first, where rapid movement takes place through the periodontal ligament space; the second, where movement occurs relatively slowly, or not at all; and finally, a stage where teeth begin to move rapidly." Burstone has described three phases of OTM.

1. Initial phase
2 Lag phase
3. Post-lag phase

The Initial Phase

A rapid movement is seen during this phase as the tooth gets displaced within PDL space and it also includes the mechanical displacement due to deformation of supporting bone. This tooth movement does not involve any bone resorption, is mechanical in nature, and is only under the influence of applied force. Both light and heavy forces cause it. It is in the range of 0.4–0.9 mm and usually occurs within first week.

The Lag Phase

During this phase, no tooth movement is seen. The biochemical process starts on the pressure side which prepares for the bone resorption in this area before any further tooth movement

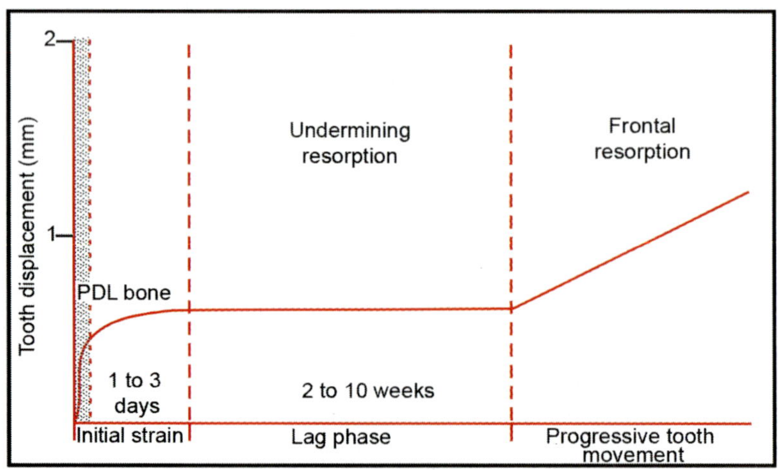

Fig. 18.5: Different phases of orthodontic tooth movements *(Adapted from Graber's for illustration purpose only).*

can commence. Also the hyalinized tissues, if any, have to be removed. This stage usually lasts from 2 to 3 weeks. It depends on the factors like amount of the force, density of alveolar bone, age of the patient, etc. Lighter force cause small hyalinized area, thus needing lesser time to be removed and vice versa.

The Post-Lag Phase

After the hyalinized tissues get removed, the tooth movement commences, associated with cellular activity of resorption and deposition of alveolar bone. This movement is biological type as it occurs after the bone resorption has occurred. This may be rapid or slow. It occurs spontaneously after lag phase has finished in the area of removed bone. It does not need any additional force. Direct bone resorption takes place.

Interrupted Lag Phase

According to Reitan, little or no movement occurs during the hyalinization period or lag phase. But, it has been observed that movement can occur after reactivation of the force before undermining resorption has eliminated the hyalinized areas. This might be termed an interrupted lag phase.

THEORIES OF ORTHODONTIC TOOTH MOVEMENT

Following theories have been proposed to explain the process of OTM.

- Blood flow/fluid dynamic theory (Bien, 1966)
- Pressure-tension theory (Schwarz, 1932)
- Bone bending/piezoelectric theory (Farrar, 1876)

Fluid Dynamic Theory

This theory was proposed by Bien in 1966, and is also called as blood flow theory. PDL is a hydrodynamic system, fluid-filled tissue. PDL fluid system is made of interstitial fluid, cells, ground substance, blood vessels and PDL fibers. According to this concept, when pressure is applied, the OTM occurs due to changes in the fluid dynamics of PDL. PDL is confined between two hard surfaces, i.e. bone and cementum, which is not pliable under pressure. So, there is limited movement of fluid. Under pressure, PDL behaves like a hydraulic mechanism, i.e. a **shock absorber**. When pressure is applied, the fluid moves out of the PDL-interstitial spaces toward apex and cervical margins, and the tooth movement occurs. This is called "squeeze-film effect" by Bien. When force is removed, the fluid is replenished by diffusion through the capillary walls. Orthodontic forces cause compression of PDL. Blood vessels of PDL get trapped between the principal fibers and their stenosis occurs. The vessels above the stenosis then balloon out thus forming aneurysms. According to Bien, there is changed chemical environment at the site of stenosis due to decreased oxygen levels in the areas of pressure. These aneurysms help in escape of blood gases in the interstitial fluid, which creates favorable environment for bone resroption. However, this theory does not hold good support and has been largely rejected.

The two main theories which have been accepted and are considered complementary to each other to describe the biological changes taking place during OTM are the pressure–tension theory and the bioelectric theories.

Pressure Tension Theory

This theory is based on the work of Oppenheim (1911), Sandstedt (1905) and Schwarz (1932). It states that areas of "pressure" and "tension" are created in PDL when forces are applied on the tooth. Compression of fibers and vascular channels occurs on pressure side, and stretch of fibers on tension side. Bone resorption occurs on pressure side (osteoclasts) and the deposition occurs on tension side (osteoblasts). Depending on the type of tooth movement and force direction, different areas of pressure and tension are created in PDL.

According to this theory, the chemical signals are generated in the tissues which act as stimuli which lead to cellular differentiation and ultimately the tooth movement. Under pressure, PDL gets compressed and the blood flow is decreased there, while in the areas of tension, it is usually maintained or increased. This alteration in blood flow leads to changes in the chemical environment. These chemical changes lead to release of other biologically active agents, stimulating other cellular activity. These chemical messengers stimulate remodeling of alveolar bone and tooth movement.

A minimum threshold of force duration of 4–8 hours is needed to initiate the chemical changes in the tissues. Any force of lesser duration is not effective, while prolonged duration helps in increasing the amount of tooth movement. With applied pressure, the increased levels of cyclic adenosine monophosphate (cAMP), also called as the "second messenger", appear after about 4–6 hours of continued pressure. Also, other chemicals like prostaglandin E and interleukin-1 beta levels increase within the PDL. Prostaglandin E (PGE2) is an important mediator of the cellular response during OTM. Certain drugs, e.g. NSAIDs inhibit its production, and thus negatively affect the OTM. PGE has an unique property of stimulating both osteoclastic and osteoblastic activity, thus it is an important mediator of tooth movement. If its production is decreased, the OTM slows down considerably. Parathyroid hormone injections induce the production of osteoclasts in only a few hours. But with external pressure is the stimulus, the response is much slower and it may take upto 48 hours before the osteoclasts appear in the compressed PDL.

Thus this theory can be summarized in three stages: (1) alterations in blood flow in PDL due to the applied pressure, (2) formation and release of chemical messengers and (3) activation of cells leading to bone resorption.

Bone-bending and piezoelectric theory or the bioelectric theory: This theory is based on the generation of electrical signals in the bone upon application of pressure. Farrar in 1876 described the idea that due to pressure, there is bending or deformation of the alveolar walls. He suggested that this bone bending may be a possible mechanism for causing tooth movement (Fig. 18.6).

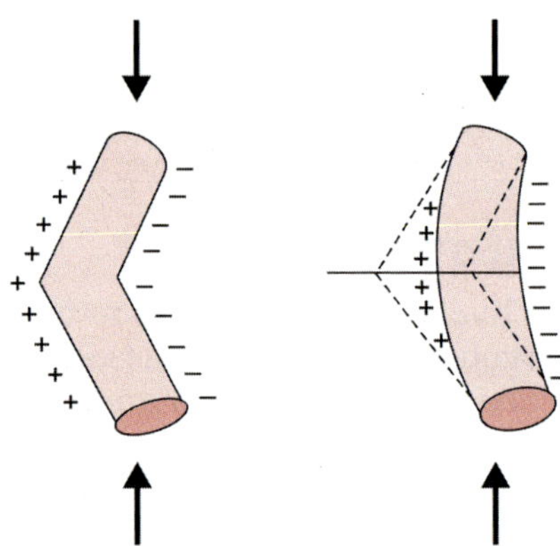

Fig. 18.6: Piezoelectric effect due to bone bending when force is applied on the bone.

This concept is based on the fact that a crystalline structure leads to generation of electric potential when it gets deformed under the applied force. It is due to distortion in crystal lattices leading to the movement of the electrons along the slip-planes. Bone is a crystalline structure due to its components, i.e. collagen, hydroxyapatite, collagen-hydroxyapatite interface, mucopolysaccharides, etc. It leads to generation of peizoelectric current in bone. Further, ions in the fluids surrounding the living bone interact with these electrical fields. These currents of small voltages are called streaming potentials.

Electric signals initiating the tooth movement are piezoelectric. Piezoelectricity phenomenon is seen in many crystalline materials where the deformation of the crystal structure produces a flow of electric current as electrons are displaced from one crystal lattice to another. This phenomenon is called piezoelectricity.

Piezoelectric signals have two characteristics (Fig. 18.7):

1. A quick decay rate: It means that when a force is applied, a piezoelectric signal is generated. But, it quickly comes to zero even though the force is maintained, since the new crystal structure becomes stable.

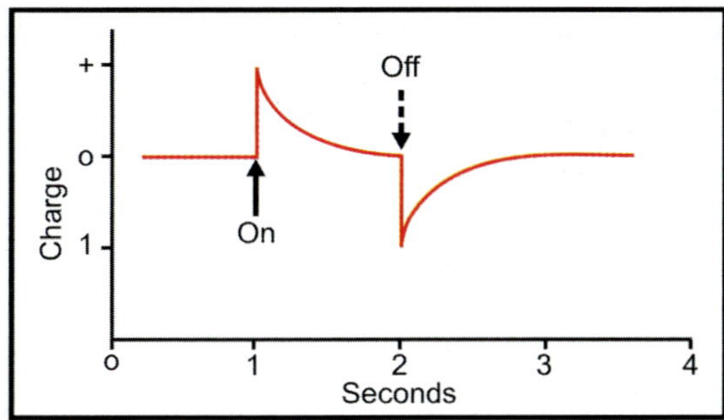

Fig. 18.7: Generation and an early decay of the piezoelectric current on application of forces *(Adapted from Profit and Fields for illustration purpose).*

2. When the pressure is released, the crystals return to their original shape, i.e. again a change in crystal structure occurs. It leads to a reverse movement of electrons toward the original sites, which again generates a current, again a momentary current due to quick decay rate. This rhythmic activity produces constant development of electrical signals. These electric stimuli help in bone remodeling changes. With pressure, the alveolar bone bends, thus creating areas of concavity and convexity. Areas of concavity are negatively charged and lead to the bone deposition. The areas of convexity are positively charged and lead to bone resorption.

Orthodontic Forces

Force is defined as a push or pull applied on the object, and has both magnitude and direction. In orthodontics, the forces play a major role by inducing certain chemical and electrical changes in the tissues leading to tooth movement. In orthodontics, forces can be classified variously.

1. Orthodontic and orthopedic forces, according to the induced changes.
2. Light and heavy forces, according to magnitude of forces
3. Continuous, intermittent, and interrupted forces, according to the force decay rate.
4. Degree/levels of forces according to Schwarz.

Orthodontic forces are the forces which lead to tooth movements, they are lighter in magnitude, and they get distributed to the PDL and alveolar process (Fig. 18.8).

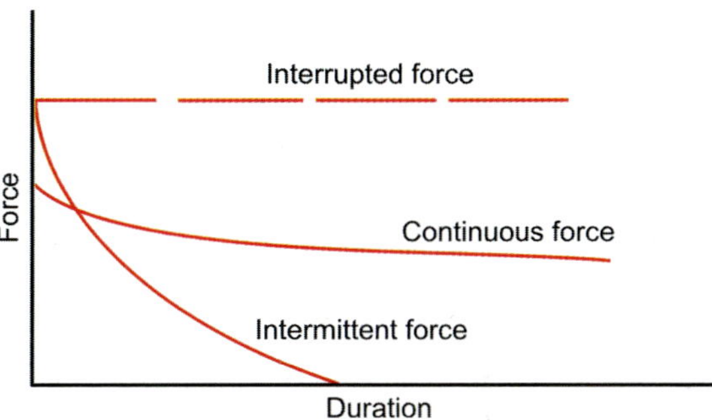

Fig. 18.8: Different types of forces used in orthodontic treatment.

Orthopedic forces are heavy forces which act on the basal parts of the jaws. They are not used for tooth movement, but are used for achieving changes in the jaw bones. The effects of these forces depend on many factors which are magnitude, duration, and direction of force.

Light forces: They are lighter in nature, and are generally within the physiologic limits. They do not crush the PDL, and lead to direct bone resorption. The orthodontic forces should be lighter in nature.

Heavy forces: They are of higher magnitude. They lead to crushing and hyalinization of PDL. They lead to undermining resorption during OTM. But if used for orthopedic changes, they are best suitably distributed to the basal bones and sutural system of craniofacial complex.

Continuous forces (Fig. 18.9): These are the forces which are maintained at some appreciable level (as a fraction of originally applied force) between the two consecutive visits. Fixed orthodontic appliances use light continuous forces.

Interrupted forces: These are forces whose force level declines to zero between activations.

Intermittent forces: These forces abruptly fall to zero intermittently when an appliance

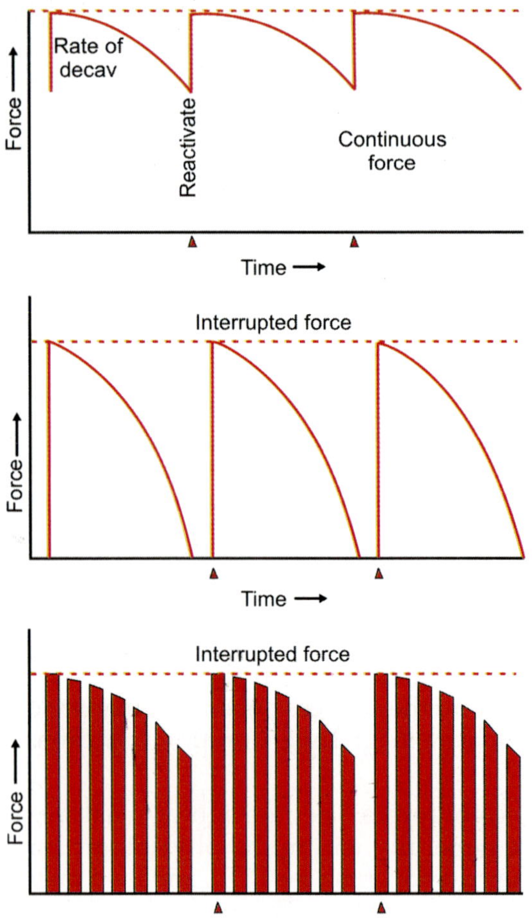

Fig. 18.9: Diagram showing the different types of forces used in orthodontic treatment. Note their decay pattern in relation to time *(Adapted from Proffit).*

is removed by the patient. These forces are produced by those appliance which need patient-cooperation, e.g. removable appliances, headgear, removable myofunctional appliances, chin cup, etc. The orthopedic appliances are generally used for few hours per day rather than using them continuously. Thus when the patient removes the appliance, the force immediately comes to zero.

In clinical practice, light continuous forces are the best, but heavy, intermittent forces can be clinically acceptable. But, the heavy continuous forces should be avoided. In clinical orthodontics an interrupted tooth movement may have certain advantages. A rest period helps in repair of the trauma/damage and reorganisation of newly formed tissues during the tooth movement. Also, the interval between two visits should be at least 3–4 weeks, as it gives ample time for the repair of the tissues. Some clinicians have proposed that reactivation should be done at 6–8 weeks intervals.

Four degrees/levels of the forces according to Schwarz are:

First degree: Force which is too gentle or of too short duration to produce any tooth movement.

Second degree: It is the ideal force; it produces the OTM without the tissue damage.

Third degree: The force which exceeds capillary blood pressure and could produce damage; but it is reversible, if pressure is removed.

Fourth degree: The force which produces irreversible damage in the investing tissues. It is followed by strangulation of apical vessels and death of the pulp.

Types of tooth movements: For correction of malocclusion, the teeth need to be moved in all the three planes of the space. The three basic tooth movements are tipping, translation, and rotation. Different types of tooth movements achieved during orthodontic treatment are:

- Tipping
- Translation/bodily movement
- Rotation
- Extrusion
- Intrusion
- Torquing/controlled root movement/controlled crown movement.

Types of Tooth Movement and Tissue Reactions in Supporting Tissues

When the forces are applied for tooth movement, the areas of pressure and tension appear in the PDL, depending on the pattern of the applied forces. In such areas, biochemical reactions occur leading to socket remodeling, and thus the tooth movement.

A. Tipping: This is the simplest form of orthodontic tooth movement, produced when a single force is applied against the crown of a tooth. Tooth rotates around its center of Resistance, a point located about halfway down the root. It is uncontrolled type of tipping movement. During this movement, the crown moves in one direction, while the root moves in the opposite direction. The amount of displacement of crown and root from their initial position takes in place in the ratio of their distances from the Cres (Figs 18.10a and b).

Areas of pressure and tension: Areas of pressure appear at two sites ie near the root apex on one side and at the crest of the alveolar bone on the opposite side. Areas of tension also appear at two sites opposite to the areas of pressure (Figs 18.11 to 18.15).

B. Torque: It is a controlled type of tipping movement, which can be of two types: (1) controlled crown movement and (2) controlled root movement.

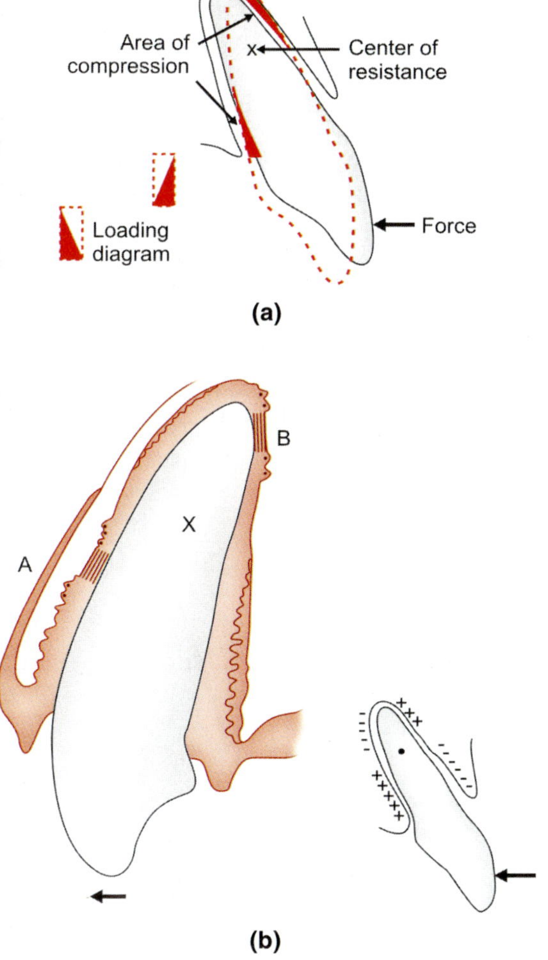

Figs 18.10a and b: During tipping movement, there are 2 areas each of pressure and tension on opposing sides in PDL.

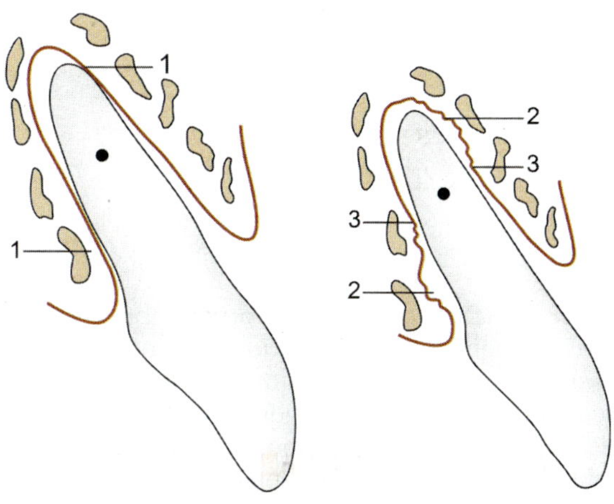

Fig. 18.11: When tipping forces are applied, the tooth rotates around Cres and opposing pressure areas (1,1) are generated in PDL; where later on bone resorption takes place (2,3).

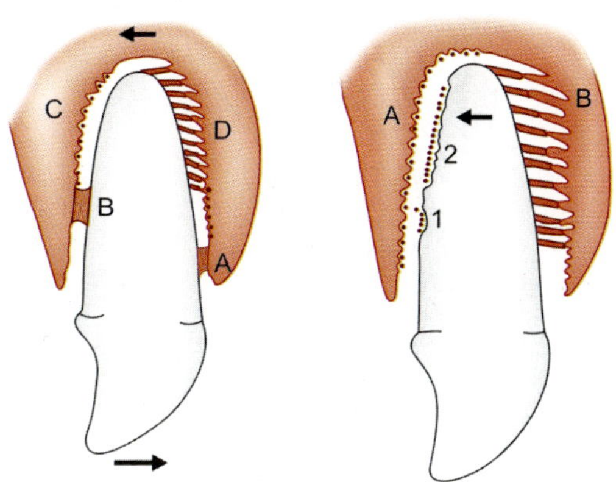

Fig. 18.12: Areas of bone and root resorption (1,2,A,C) during tipping movement, and 1,2,A during translatory movement; while areas of bone deposition as B and D. Note that there is stretching of PDL fibers on tension side in PDL which then helps in bone apposition *(Adapted from Graber and Vanardsdall for illustration purpose)*.

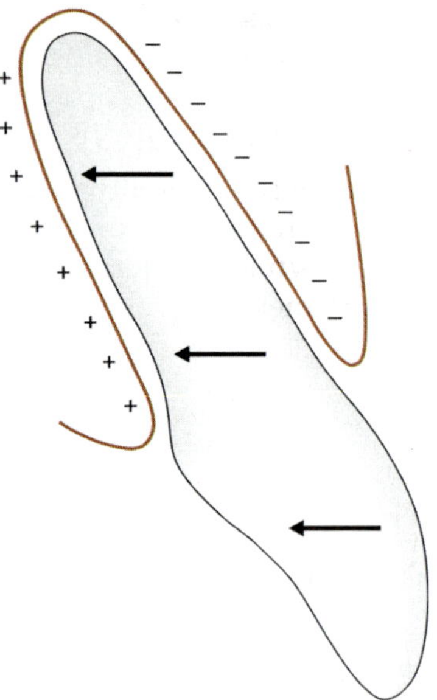

Fig. 18.13: During bodily movement, the pressure areas are generated through the whole length of PDL towards the direction of movement where bone resorption occurs on PDL side, but to maintain the thickness of alveolar wall, the bone deposition also occurs on the bone marrow side (Note that +++ signs in palatal region are due to bone deposition on marrow side), while in tension areas, opposite action takes place ie bone is deposited on PDL side, while removed from marrow side.

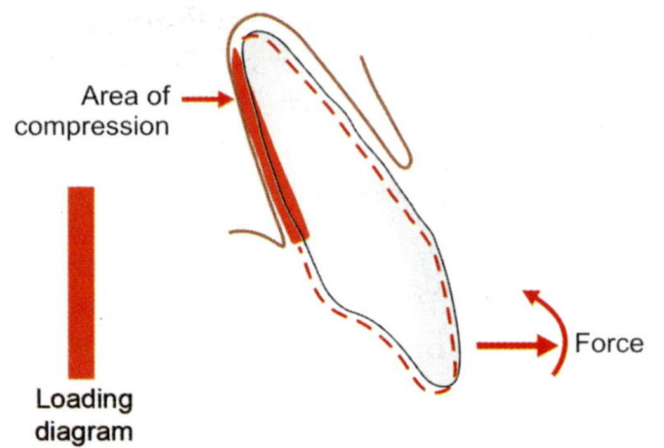

Fig. 18.14: Full PDL is loaded during bodily movement of tooth as seen by bold red strip.

In controlled crown movement, the crot gets shifted to the apex of the root, while only crown moves either in labial or lingual direction, depending on the type of force applied. It can be called as crown torquing. The pressure area is located in an area between the alveolar crest and the middle region of the root.

In controlled root movement, the Crot gets shifted to the incisal edge, while only the root moves either in labial or lingual direction, depending on the type of force applied. It is called as root torquing. The pressure area is located in an area between the apex of root and the middle region of the root.

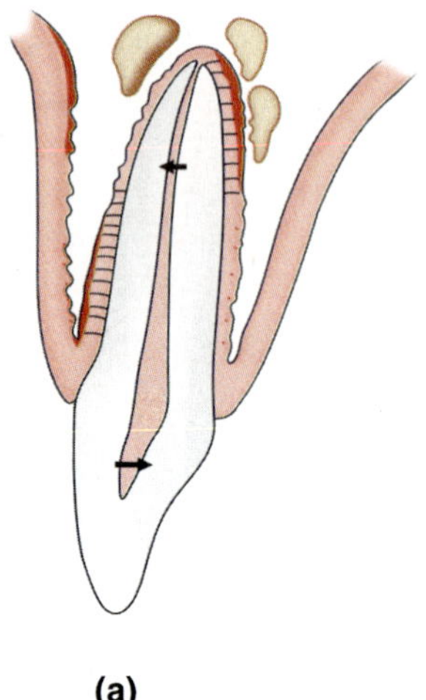

(a)

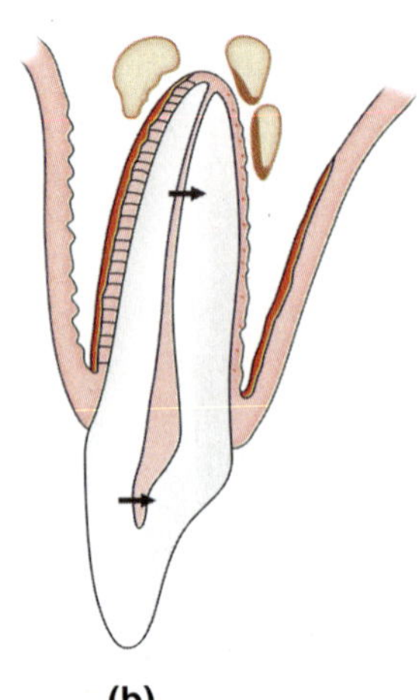

(b)

Figs 18.15a and b: Areas of bone resorption and deposition during OTM: Tipping movement has 2 areas of bone resorption and depositions one on each side of root; while bodily movement has one area of bone resorption and deposition. Arrows show the direction of tooth movement.

During torquing, lighter forces should be applied, otherwise root resroption can occur, because the applied forces are concentrated at small areas only, thus increasing the pressure. Reitan and Kvam (1971) showed that 50 gm of force was sufficient to cause root movement without any undermining resorption.

C. Bodily movement/translation: Bodily movement is the most desirable type of movement. It is also called translation. For achieving a bodily movement, the force should pass through the Cres. of the object. Since the tooth is having its Cres within the alveolar bone, and the translation force cannot be applied directly on it, so it is achieved by applying a system of forces, ie a force and a couple, the mean of which passes through the Cres to cause bodily movement (Figs 18.12 to 18.14).

The force is distributed over the whole alveolar bone surface creating the area of pressure in PDL in the direction of movement, and area of tension on the opposite side PDL. The applied forces are distributed along a larger PDL area thus creating lesser pressure (P = F/A). So force of a greater amount is required than that for tipping movement. In the bodily movement, the hyalinization periods are shorter than in tipping movements. The PDL on the pressure side is considerably widened by the resorption process. There is gradually increased stretching of the fiber bundles on the tension side. New bone layers are formed on the tension side along these fiber bundles.

D. Rotation (Fig. 18.15): Pure Rotation of a tooth occurs around its long axis, and requires a set of forces which are equal in amount, acting in opposite direction parallel to each other and separating by a distance. This is called as couple. Since there is no net force acting on the Cres, only rotation movement occurs, without any tipping or translation. Clinically this movement is viewed from the occlusal view. During rotation, the force is distributed over the entire PDL, rather than over a narrow vertical strip, so larger forces can be applied than in other tooth movements.

Most teeth to be rotated create two pressure sides and two tension sides. Bone resorption takes place in the pressure side, which may be a combination of direct and undermining resorptions. On the tension side, new bone spicules are formed along stretched fiber bundles arranged more or less obliquely. Furthermore, the periodontal space is considerably widened by bone resorption after rotation.

During rotation, the transseptal fibers get stretched and activated. These free gingival fibers mainly contain elastic fibers, thus leading to relapse. Transseptal fibers are the gingival fibers which are attached near the cervical areas of two adjacent teeth, and traversing the intervening alveolar septum between two teeth. Since they do not have an attachment to the bone tissues at either ends, but to the cementum, they do not reorganize so easily, but remain stretched. The periodontal fiber bundles and the new bone layers of the middle and apical thirds of PDL rearrange themselves after a fairly short retention period (Reitan 1959) (Fig. 18.16).

Generally, the time required for the readaptation of tissues after orthodontic treatment is 3–4 months for the readaptation of periodontal fibers; 6–9 months for bone and

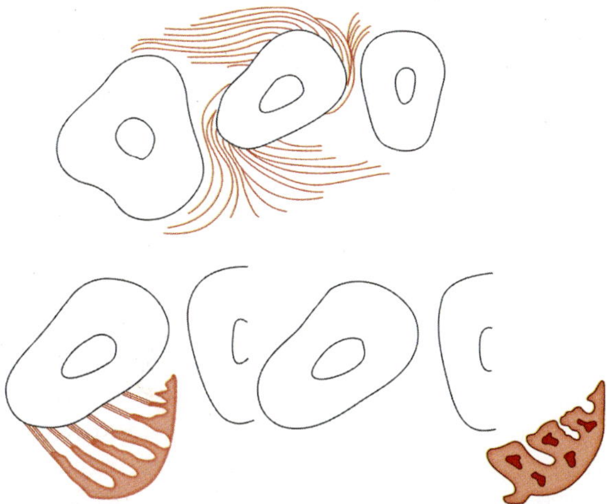

Fig. 18.16: During correction of rotations, the supracrestal alveolar fibers get stretched, which lead to relapse unless retained for a long period *(Adapted from Graber for illustration purpose).*

trabecular adaptation; 9–12 months for gingival fibers arrangement. So the main cause of relapse is the gingival fibers.

To retain a derotated tooth, at least 232 days of retention period is needed, and still there are chances of relapse. Therefore, over-rotation has been recommended. A permanent fixed retainer is the best choice in such cases, as part of patient cooperation is eliminated. Also CSF (circumferential supracrestal fibrotomy) is recommended after derotation of the tooth. This procedure was suggested by Edwards, where the stretched elastic and other fibers are cut with the help of BP knife through an incision given till the alveolar crest. New fibers formation occurs at the new position of the tooth.

E. Extrusion: It is the bodily displacement of a tooth along its long axis in an occlusal direction. Extrusive movement does not produce any areas of compression within the PDL, but only areas of tension are created due to stretch of the fibers of PDL esp in areas of alveolar crest and the periapical region. A more prolonged stretch of the supra-alveolar fiber bundles occurs than the principal fibers of the middle and apical third regions. The periodontal fiber bundles elongate and new bone is deposited in these areas of tension exerted by these stretched fiber bundles. They get rearranged after a fairly short retention period. However, in adult patients, the fiber bundles take more time for rearrangement. This movement requires low force levels since the forces are to be distributed to a smaller area of the PDL. The forces should be in the range of 25–30 gm (Fig. 18.17).

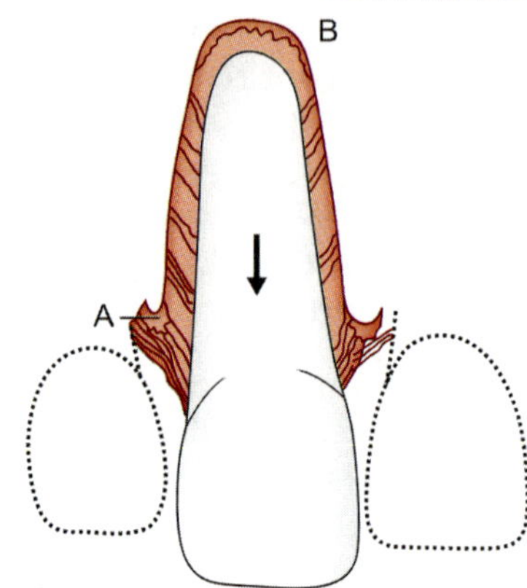

Fig. 18.17: During extrusion, the bone is deposited on alveolar crest and apical areas.

F. Intrusion: This is the bodily displacement of a tooth along its long axis in an apical direction. The area of pressure is created in the apical area. No areas of tension are created during intrusion. Relaxation of free gingival fibers occurs during intrusion (Free gingival fibers alveolar crest fibers run from alveolar crest to the cementum in an occlusal direction). Lighter force is required because the force is concentrated in a small area at the tooth apex. If a heavy force is used during intrusion, then heavy pressure is created in the apical area, thus leading to root resorption and devitalization of tooth. Most of the times, during orthodontic treatment, the anterior teeth need to be intruded. But in some cases, the posterior teeth also need intrusion to treat the anterior open bite cases, but this is very difficult. Recently, this movement has been achieved with the help of micro-implants, bone plates, etc. (Fig. 18.18 and 18.19).

An intruding movement may therefore cause resorption of bone in the apical and marginal alveolar crest regions. Rearrangement of the principal fibers occurs after a retention period of 2–3 months. Intrusion of

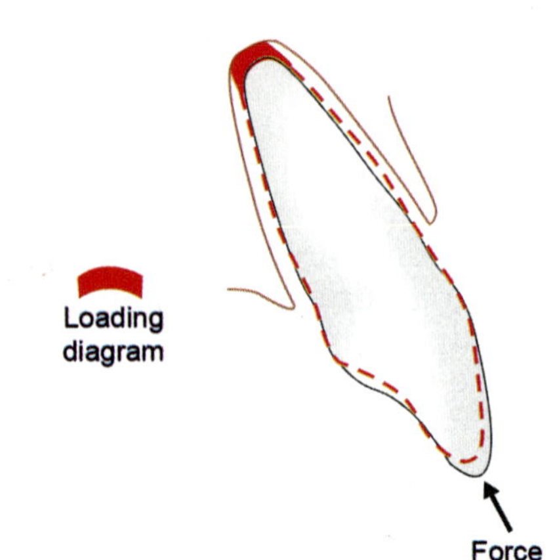

Fig. 18.18: During intrusion, the bone is resorbed on alveolar crest and apical areas.

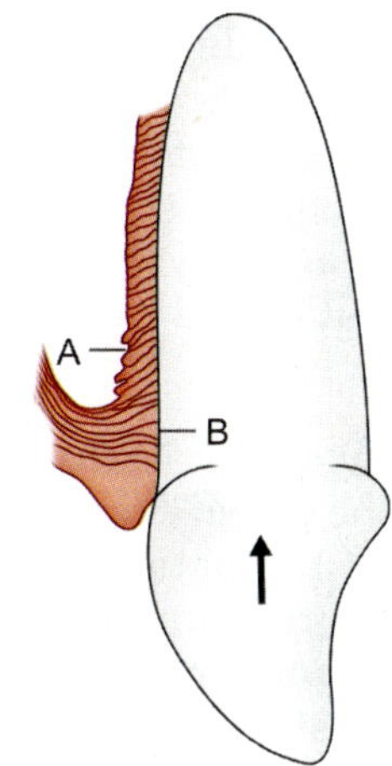

Fig. 18.19: Intrusive forces lead to stretching and activation of PDL fibers which lead to relapse.

teeth is a difficult movement and only small amount of movement can be achieved.

Forces required for different types of tooth movements: Table 18.2 gives the approximate values of forces needed for different tooth movements. The values are inclusive of some force loss for overcoming the friction and resistance provided by the base archwires.

Table 18.2: Forces required for OTM

• Tipping	-	50–75 gm
• Bodily movement	-	100–150 gm
• Intrusion	-	15–25 gm
• Extrusion	-	50–75 gm
• Torquing	-	50–75 gm
• Uprighting	-	75–125 gm
• Rotation	-	50–75 gm

Tooth Movement by Extraoral Forces

Extraoral forces can be divided into two categories. Heavy extraoral forces are used to redirect abnormal facial bone growth. They are also known as orthopedic forces. They influence the direction of bone growth and associated tooth position during treatment. Orthopedic forces lead to hyalinisation in the PDL areas and thus no tooth movement takes places, hence all the forces get distributed to the basal bones. Such forces are intermittent in nature. The second type of extraoral force is lighter in nature and is used for the movement of teeth. This is known as orthodontic force. These are applied through head gear to move the teeth, in cases requiring maximum anchorage, e.g. canine retraction and incisor retraction can be achieved through J-hook headgear. Intrusion of upper incisors can also be achieved by using HPHG with J-hook.

Factors Influencing Tooth Movement

Many factors play important role during the tooth movement. They have been described below.

Analgesics: Pain is one of the most common effects of orthodontic forces. So, some pain killers may be needed during orthodontic treatment. Many drugs have been used to alleviate pain; e.g. asprin, NSAIDs—ibuprofen, acetaminophen, diclofenac sodium and diclofenac potassium, etc.

During the biochemical changes after force application, the prostaglandins are produced which help in bone resorption. NSAIDs, e.g. ibuprofen, used as anti-inflammatory agents during OTM as pain killers lead to suppression of synthesis of prostaglandins which reduces pain. But, this also leads to slowing of the tooth movement due to suppression of PGs and hence more time is required.

Acetaminophen is another drug used as pain killer. It is the preferred medication for during orthodontic treatment because it does not interfere with localized inflammatory processes. However, studies have shown that NSAIDs are superior to acetaminophen and aspirin for relief of orthodontic pain. NSAIDs are effective orthodontic analgesics, but they may reduce the rate of tooth movement, and they should not be administered for long periods of time. However, if the initial dose is given before the force application and for a short duration (3 days), then NSAID is very effective analgesic, and it does not increase the treatment time.

Inflammatory agents: Such chemicals are produced in the tissues during OTM, e.g. prostaglandins, IL-1β and leukotrines. In experimental studies, inflammatory cytokines have been administered to enhance orthodontically induced bone remodeling, e.g. prostaglandin E2 (PGE2) administration to primates, which help in increased rate of OTM. But, they also have an increased risk of root resorption which is proportional to the increase in the rate of tooth movement.

Oral misoprostol, a PGE1 analog, used in rats at a dose of 10 μg/day for 14 days, increased the amount of orthodontic tooth movement, showed lesser risk of increased root resorption than PGE2.

PGE2 with simultaneous administration of calcium gluconate was tested in rats (2003), and an acceleration in tooth movement without root resorption was noted. It was concluded that Ca ions stabilize teeth against root resorption when the rate of tooth movement is enhanced by PGE2.

The effects of local administrations of PGE2 and 1,25-dihydroxycholecalciferol (1,25-DHCC) on orthodontic tooth movement was compared in a study (2004), and 1,25-DHCC was found to be more effective in modulating bone turnover during orthodontic tooth movement.

Distraction osteogenesis: Distraction osteogenesis is a method for generating new bone by progressively distracting the two segments of bone after complete osteotomy of a bone. Essentially, it is a bone modelling procedure that produces perivascular woven bone, which then condenses and remodels to mature lamellar bone. The method is currently being adapted for many orthodontic applications such as canine retraction, molar intrusion, segmental translation, recovery of ankylosed teeth, and interdental expansion. RME is R from of DO.

Nitric oxide (NO): Localized NO production is a known biochemical mediator of osteoclastic induction in an inflammatory environment, that is, in the presence of cytokines such as IL-1β, IL-6, and TNFα. Recent studies have suggested that NO is an important mediator in the response of periodontal tissue to orthodontic force (2002). Inducible nitric oxide synthetase (iNOS), a receptor that controls NO production, also mediates bone loss systemically in estrogen-deficient mice (2003). Estrogen exhibits anti-inflammatory activity by preventing the induction of iNOS and other inflammatory components.

Systemic diseases: Many systemic conditions affect the OTM. A proper medical and drug history of the patient should be taken before starting orthodontic treatment. Some diseases of relevance are rheumatoid arthritis, cystic fibrosis; osteomalacia; diabetes; osteoporosis; hyperparathyroidism; leukemia, sickle cell anemia; thalassemia, osteopenia, osteogenesis imperfecta, etc.

Iatrogenic response of supporting tissues in orthodontics: Application of forces for orthodontic treatment may also lead to certain iatrogenic effects on the teeth and the investing tissues. Various clinical, radiological and histological investigations have been conducted to assess the damage to root substance and supporting tissues.

Gingival inflammation: The most important factor causing gingival inflammation is bacterial plaque. Patients with fixed appliances have increased retention sites for plaque. Banding causes more plaque than bonding.

Alveolar bone loss: Some amount of loss of alveolar crest bone is generally seen during orthodontic treatment. Patients having periodontal diseases are more prone to this loss. Orthodontic treatment may also aggravate a pre-existing plaque-induced gingival lesion and cause loss of alveolar bone and periodontal attachment. It is very important to keep the gingival tissues healthy before and during orthodontic treatment. Also, the orthodontic tipping leads to shift supragingival plaque into a subgingival position, resulting in the formation of infrabony pockets. Compressed gingiva in the extraction site between teeth that have been moved together can produce a long-lasting epithelial fold.

Marginal bone recession: It is the displacement of soft tissue margin apical to the CEJ, with subsequent exposure of the root surface. It is generally due to localized plaque-induced inflammation, and sometimes in combination with orthodontic therapy.

Changes in the gingival dimensions and marginal tissue position during orthodontic treatment are related to the direction of tooth movement. Labial and buccal movements result in recession due to reduced facial gingival dimensions. It is due to thin labial cortical plates. The alveolar bone dehiscence leads to marginal recession. To avoid these problems, the tooth should be moved exclusively within the alveolar process.

Pulpal reaction: Modest transient inflammatory response is seen in the pulp at at the beginning of the treatment. This may cause some discomfort for few days after activation of the appliances, but the mild pulpitis has no long term significance. Devitalization of pulp and discoloration of the tooth may occur when heavy forces are applied. A vital PDL (non-ankylosed) is of paramount importance for OTM, rather than the pulp, so the endodontically treated teeth can be normally moved during orthodontic treatment. But, it should be kept in mind that the endodontically treated teeth are more prone to root resorption during orthodontics than the vital teeth.

Root resorption: Ketcham (1929) was the first to highlight the root resorption during OTM. Two types of root resorption may occur in connection with orthodontic treatment: Superficial surface resorption that undergoes repair, and apical resorption which may lead to permanent root shortening. It occurs due to heavy forces applied continuously for a long period. It is frequently preceded by hyalinization of the PDL. The necrotic hyalinized tissue and alveolar bone are removed by phagocytic cells, e.g. macrophages, foreign body giant cells, and osteoclasts, which may also lead to root resorption in certain unprotected surfaces on the root. Root resorption then occurs around this cell free tissue, starting at the border of the hyalinized zone.

Post-treatment stability: Relapse is inevitable in orthodontics, as almost 30–40% relapse is bound to happen. Retention appliances are used to maintain the corrected positions of teeth and the occlusion during reorganization and remodeling of the periodontal tissues and transitional changes during growth, dentoalveolar development and muscular adaptation. Retention is thus a continuation of orthodontic treatment. During retention, new bone fills in the spaces between bone spicules, resulting in a dense bone tissue, which prevents relapse. Therefore, to avoid relapse, a tooth should be retained until total rearrangement of the structures involved has occurred.

An orthodontic movement in the direction opposite to that of the functional tooth migration (i.e. mesial) is more liable to relapse than one in which the directions correspond. So, the distalized tooth is more likely to relapse.

The main remodeling of PDL occurs near the alveolar bone. Unlike the PDL, the supra-alveolar fibers are not attached in bone, but are attached in cementum of adjoining teeth, and hence have less chance of being reorganized. Also the remodeling of gingival connective tissue is not as rapid as PDL fibers.

The transseptal fibers stabilize the teeth against separating forces and help to maintain the contacts of adjacent teeth. But during closure of spaces, they get bunched up and thus activated, which may lead to opening of spaces. Transseptal fibers get stretched on one side and get compressed on other side when the teeth are moved proximatly and thus get activated. It leads to relapse unless maintained for a longer time. It happens esp inextraction cases. The fibrils connecting heavy maxillary frenum attachments to the alveolar process need a very long period of remodeling. The extraction sites retain a tendency to reopen. The compressed gingival tissue in the extraction sites may produce a long lastingepithelial fold or invagination.

Also, the fibrils connecting heavy maxillary frenum attachments to the alveolar process need a very long period of remodeling. The extraction sites retain a tendency to reopen. The compressed gingival tissue in the extraction sites may produce a long lasting epithelial fold or invagination. Also, an increased amount of glycosaminoglycans may be responsible for possible relapse after orthodontic treatment, i.e. reopening of the extraction sites.

Conclusion

Forces are needed to move the teeth for correction of malalignment. Lighter forces should be used so that they do not lead to trauma to the tissues. Movement of teeth can be accomplished in three planes of space with the help of orthodontic appliances. Initial application of force may lead to pain for first 2–3 days, which can be controlled by certain analgesics. But, analgesics should not be given as a routine since they can delay the biochemical response and hence OTM. Heavy forces are traumatic to the teeth and investing tissue in that they can lead to root resorption, pain, alveolar bone loss, devitalization of pulp, etc. But, heavy forces are helpful for orthodpedic correction and skeletal anomalies of jaws if used judiciously and at the time of active growth period.

19

Mechanics of the Tooth Movement

INTRODUCTION

When forces are applied to the teeth, these forces are distributed to the alveolar bone through the PDL. As we have studied in previous chapter, the areas of pressure and tension are created in the PDL and bone, causing biochemical changes effecting the tooth movement. However, the forces have the different effects depending on the way they act on the teeth and adjacent tissues. Since, tooth is solid object, as per the laws of physics, it has a centre of resistance Cres, where its mass is concentrated. But, it is not a free body, and is bound by the bone, so the force applied on the tooth does not behave as it has effect on a free body. The Cres of tooth lies in the approximate center of root which is buried inside the bone. So, the forces cannot be directly applied on the Cres of tooth to cause a bodily movement, rather a combination of force and moment has to be applied. That is why, laws of physics have to be understood and applied precisely on the tooth or teeth to achieve the desired tooth movement within the confines of the bone.

Mechanics can be defined as that branch of engineering science, which describes the effect of force on the body.

Definition of terms: Before beginning to discuss control of root position, it is necessary to understand some basic physical terms that must be used in the discussion:

- **Force:** It can be defined as a push or pull applied on the body, which changes or tends to change the position of rest or motion of the body. It is a vector quantity, so it has both, the magnitude, the direction and a point of application. It is measured in the units of grams. Force is defined in units of Newtons (mass X acceleration), is usually measured in weight units of grams or ounces.
- **Center of resistance:** A free body has the center of resistance as the center of mass. Center of resistance of a tooth is approximately at the midpoint of the embedded portion of root (i.e., about halfway between the root apex and the crest of the alveolar bone). It is a fixed point in the tooth, but its position varies if level of alveolar bone changes, e.g. in periodontal disease.
- **Moment:** When a force acts at a distance from the Cres, then a moment is generated. If the line of action of an applied force does not pass through the center of resistance, a moment is created. A moment is defined as the product of the force with the perpendicular distance from the point of force application to the center of resistance. It is measured in units of gm-mm (or equivalent). Thus, a combination of a force and the moment

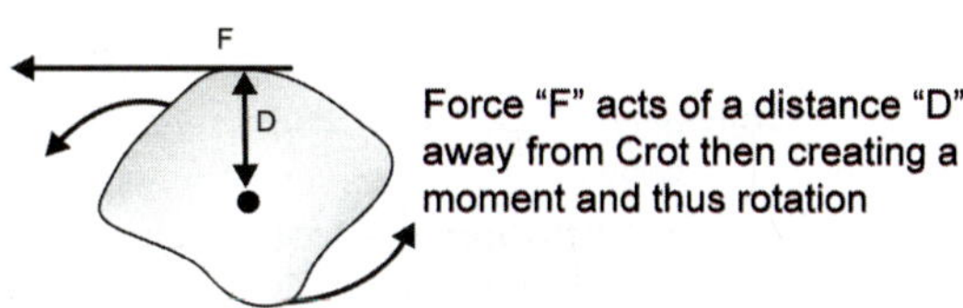

F
D
Force "F" acts of a distance "D" away from Crot then creating a moment and thus rotation

Fig. 19.1: When force is applied at a distance from the center of rotation Crot of the tooth, it generates a moment.

is simultaneously acting on the tooth, which helps to move the tooth and also tends to rotate the object around the center of resistance. A well-controlled combination helps to move the tooth bodily or torquing, etc. (Fig. 19.1).

- **Couple:** It is a combination of two forces equal in magnitude and opposite in direction, separated by a distance. They lead to generation of a pure moment, since the translatory effect of the forces cancels out. It is used for pure rotation around its center of resistance.
- **Center of rotation:** It is a point around which rotation actually occurs when a tooth is being moved. It can be controlled when a force and a couple are applied to any desired location for the desired tooth movement. It is variable according to applied forces; it can move on the tooth or out of the tooth within a measurable distance; and can also reach upto infinity. Its position thus affects the tooth movement (Figs 19.2 and 19.4).
- **Pressure:** When a force is applied on the tooth, it is perceived as pressure on the surrounding tissues. Pressure is defined as force per unit area. It is measured in units of gram per square mm. It is the pressure which is responsible for creating the areas of pressure and tension in the periodontium.

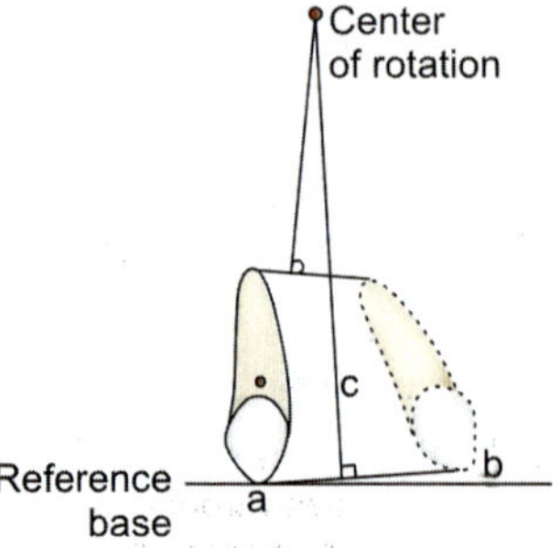

Fig. 19.2: How to find the center of rotation for a tooth which is being moved orthodontically. Join the pre-Rx and post-Rx apices, and the incisal edges. Then draw perpendicular lines on these lines. The point of intersection of these perpendicular lines is the Crot.

- **Stress:** It is defined as the force applied per unit area, and it corresponds to the pressure. It can be tensile, compressive and shear types.
- **Strain:** It is the change in dimension per unit dimension which occurs in the body when force is applied. It can be tensile compressive and shear types.

Stress and strain are interrelated phenomenon. Stress is an external force applied on the body, while strain is the result of stress generated in that body. Changes in the stress/strain distribution in peridontium after application of orthodontic forces triggers remodeling processes that makes tooth movement possible (Fig. 19.3).

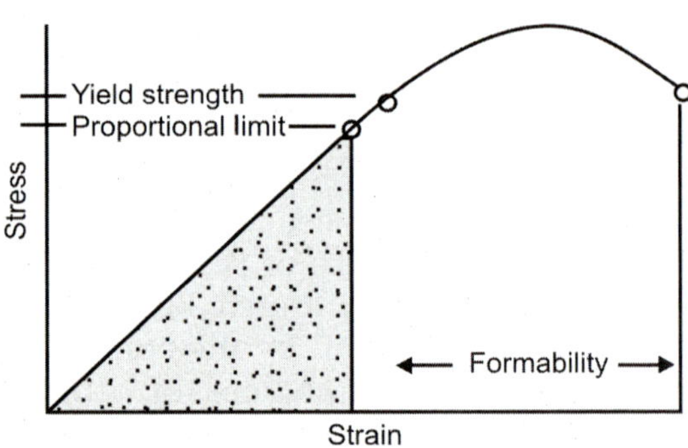

Fig. 19.3: Stress-strain curve of the elastic materials

Center of mass: All objects (finite) behave as if the entire mass is concentrated onto a single point.

CENTER OF RESISTANCE

Every free body has its mass concentrated at a single point, which is called as center of gravity, at which it is perfectly balanced. When a force is passed through this point, it leads to the bodily movement/translation of the body. But a tooth is not a free body, as it is constrained in the alveolar bone. So, a single force cannot be applied directly passing through its centre of resistance. In a single rooted tooth, it lies on the long axis of tooth between one-third to half of the root, apical to alveolar crest. In a multi rooted tooth, it lies 1–2 mm apical to furcation, between the roots

Cres has also been found for a group of teeth, for the entire upper and lower arches, and for the jaws. To achieve bodily movement of these entities, knowledge of Cres is important to plan the appropriate mechanics. It is analogous to the Cmass for restrained bodies.

Different locations of Cres (Figs 19.5 and 19.6)

- Cres of a single rooted tooth: Between one-third to half of the root, between apex and crest of alveolar bone.
- Cres in multirooted teeth: Near the bifurcation/trifurcation of the roots at midroot level, as explained by Nanda.
- Cres of maxillary incisors (especially for intrusion): Distal to lateral incisors (Nanda).
- When canines are also included, the Cres shifts distally

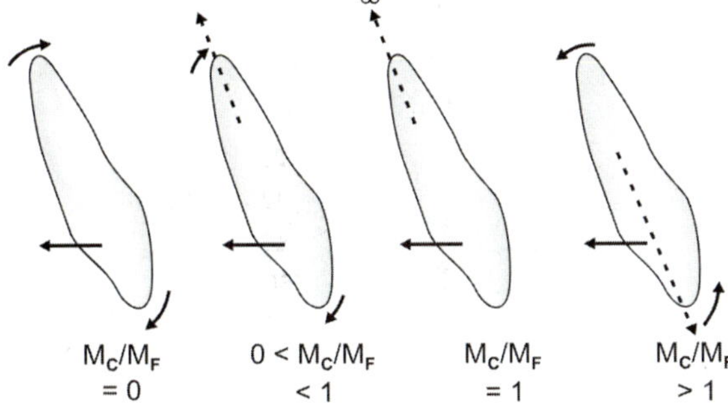

Fig. 19.4: Ratio of moments and the location of Crot in different tooth movements, e.g. Crot is at infinity for bodily movement of tooth.

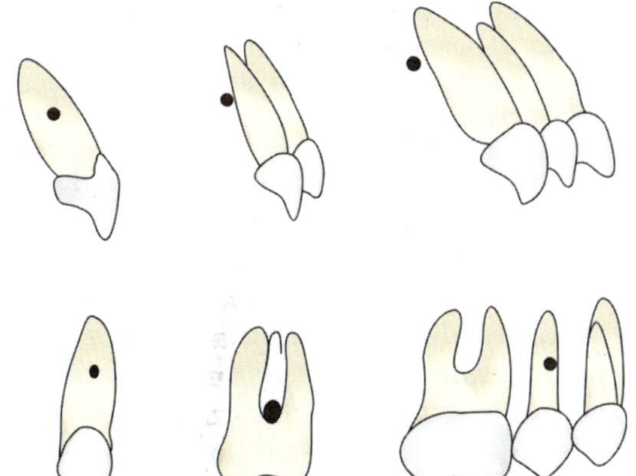

Fig. 19.5: Location of Cres of various teeth or group of teeth.

- Cres of maxilla lies slightly inferior to orbitale as described by Nanda; in the zygomaticomaxillary suture (Fig. 19.7).
- Cres of maxillary and mandibular dentitions lies in the apical region between first and second premolars, (Proffit) (Figs 19.7 and 19.8).

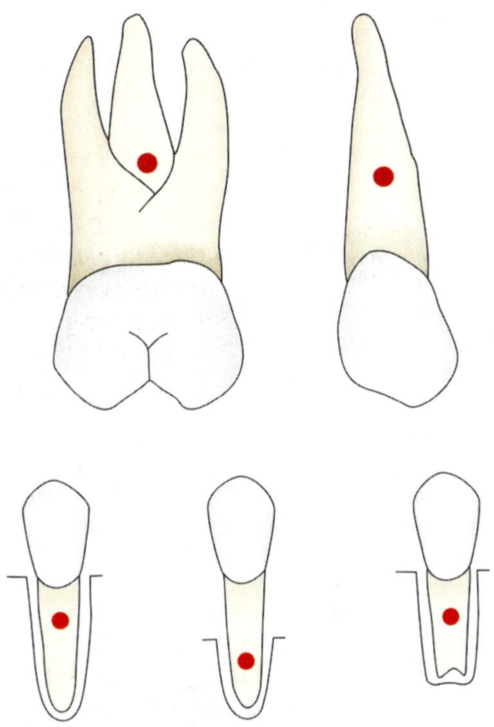

Fig. 19.6: Center of resistance by red dots in different teeth. Note that with loss of alveolar support to the root, the Cres moves apically.

Importance of Cres: A force passing through the Cres of a free body leads to its bodily movement. Since a direct single force passing through Cres cannot be applied on the tooth, so a combination of forces is required on the crown of the tooth/teeth to achieve a bodily movement. The resultant of these forces should pass through Cres to achieve bodily movement (Fig. 19.10).

Location of Cres is affected by length of the root, number and morphology of roots, and the level of the alveolar bone (Fig. 19.6). In long-rooted tooth, the Cres gets shifted towards apical side. Also if the alveolar bone level is high, the Cres is toward cervical side,

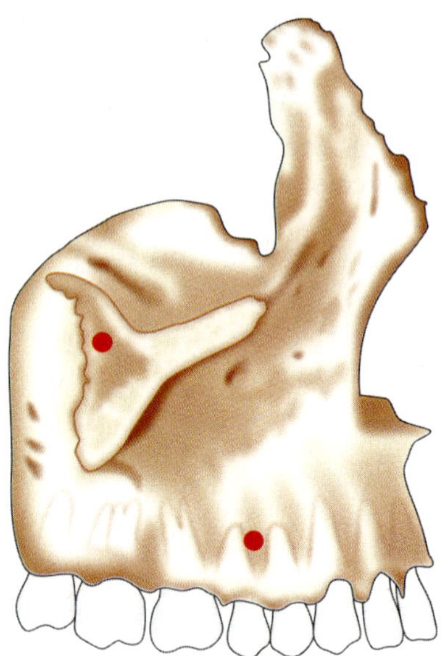

Fig. 19.7: Center of resistance by red dots for maxilla in the zygomaticomaxillary suture area, while for maxillary dentition in between upper premolars midroot region.

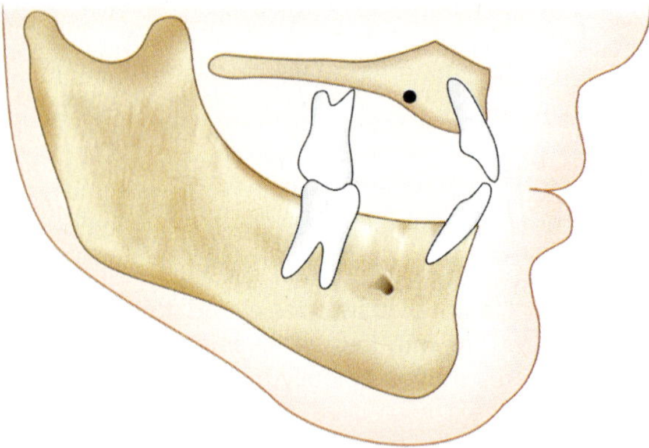

Fig. 19.8: Black dot showing the Cres of upper anterior segment of the teeth (3-3). So for bodily movement of this segment en-masse, the force should pass through this Cres.

while if alveolar bone level is low, e.g. in periodontitis cases, the Cres shifts toward the apical side.

Moment: It is the measure of the potential of rotation of the applied force on the body. Forces cannot be applied directly through Cres of the tooth, but to the crown of the tooth. The point of application thus lies at a distance from the Cres. Due to this, a component of rotation comes into play by the applied force, along with a linear component of displacement. This tendency to rotate the tooth is called moment. It is calculated by multiplying the magnitude of the applied force by its perpendicular distance from the Cres. It is measured as gm/mm (Fig. 19.9).

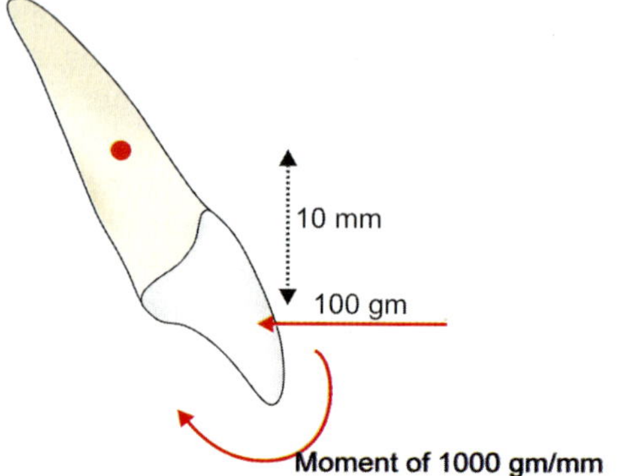

Fig. 19.9: Moment is generated when the force is applied at a distance from the Cres.

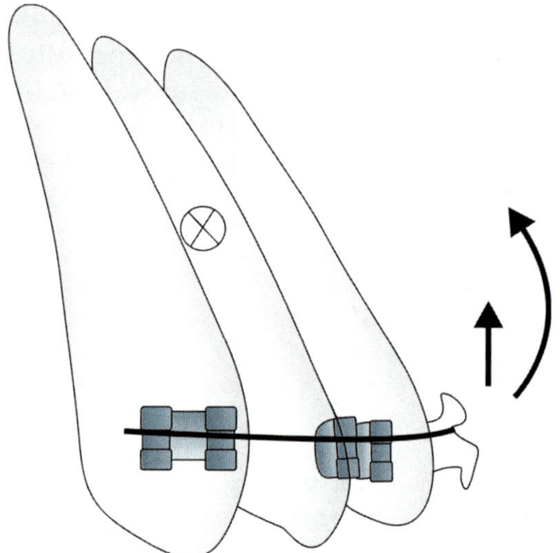

Fig.19.10: Cross-mark showing the Cres of upper incisors segment of the teeth (2-2). Intrusive forces lie anterior to this Cres and thus introduce a moment which leads to flaring of incisors. It should be counteracted by applying retractive forces on incisors either by headgear or by using class I or II elastics as the case may be.

Thus, $M = F \times d$.

d = perpendicular distance from Cres to the line of action of the force.

More is the force, more is the moment, and thus more tendency of rotation of the body under the given force. Similarly, greater distance leads to greater moment for a given force. The side effect of this generated moment is that it leads to the rotation of the apex of tooth in the direction opposite to that of the crown, i.e. tipping. More force leads to more moment and hence more tipping. If bodily movement is desired during orthodontic treatment, the moment has to be controlled by reducing the force applied. Also, a counter-moment has to be applied on the tooth so that the apex and crown move in the same direction to achieve bodily movement.

So, there are two factors which can be adjusted to achieve a desired moment, i.e. force and the distance. Generally, the distance (between Cres and the point of application/ bracket of the force) is fixed for a given tooth, thus the force is varied to achieve desired moment.

CENTER OF ROTATION (Fig. 19.11)

It is the point about which a body rotates when a force is applied. It is different from the Cres. It is not a fixed point, because it can be changed by varying the force and the moment, according to the type of tooth movement desired. Its location can be on the tooth or outside the tooth and even at infinity.

Different locations of Crot are depending on the movement desired:

- For pure translation movement, Crot is at infinity.
- In controlled crown tipping, i.e. crown torquing, it is at root apex.
- In controlled root tipping, i.e. root torquing, it is at the incisal edge.
- In uncontrolled tipping, it is between apex and Cres.
- During pure rotation, it lies on the long axis of the tooth.

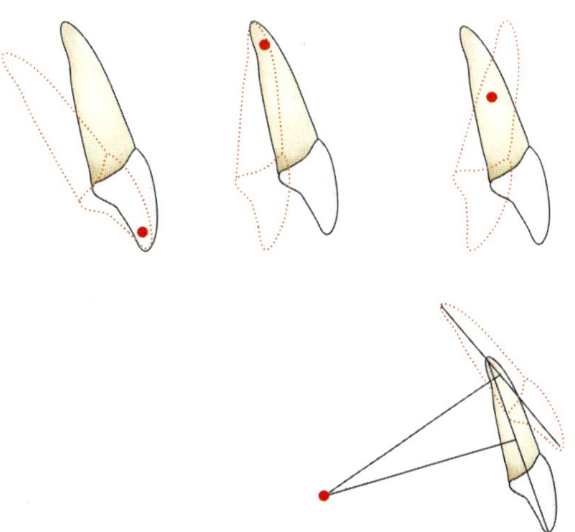

Fig. 19.11: Different locations of Crot for different types of tooth movement during orthodontic treatment, viz root torquing, crown torquing, tipping and extrusion, respectively.

TYPES OF THE TOOTH MOVEMENTS (Fig. 19.12)

To correct the positions of the tooth, the tooth moves in all the three planes of space under the influence of orthodontic forces and mechanics. Generally, following types of tooth movement can be achieved.

- Tipping or uncontrolled tipping
- Pure translation or bodily
- Pure rotational
- Extrusion
- Intrusion
- Torquing, i.e. controlled crown or root tipping.

Tooth movement	*Location of Crot*
Tipping, uncontrolled movement	At the junction of apical and middle third of root
Bodily/translation	At infinity
Rotation	Center of crown on occlusal or incisal aspect on the long axis
Torquing, controlled root movement	At the incisal edg
Controlled crown movement	At the root ape
Extrusion/intrusion	Along the long axis

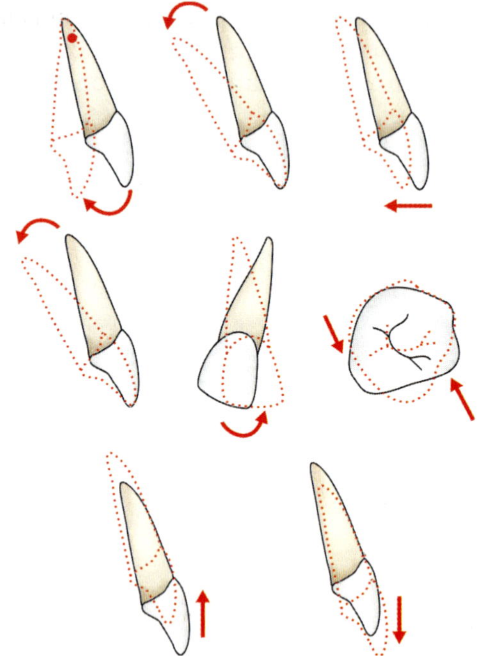

Fig. 19.12: Different types of tooth movements: controlled crown movement, controlled root movement (variation of torquing); bodily or translation movement; axial correction, rotation correction, intrusion and extrusion, respectively.

Each type of tooth movement is due to judicious control of the amount of applied moment and force. The ratio of the applied counter moment and the applied force experienced at the Cres is called the moment-to-force ratio. The M/F ratio of the applied force and moment determines the type of movement at the center of rotation.

Tipping: It is the simplest type of tooth movement. When a force is applied to the crown of the tooth, it leads to the movement of both crown and root of the tooth in opposite directions. However, this displacement is not necessarily equal and opposite, since it depends on the location of Crot. Tipping is the movement when there is a greater movement of the crown than the root. Center of rotation lies apical to the Cres. During uncontrolled tipping, the Crot lies between Cres and root apex. In case of controlled tipping, it lies at the root apex (Fig. 19.13).

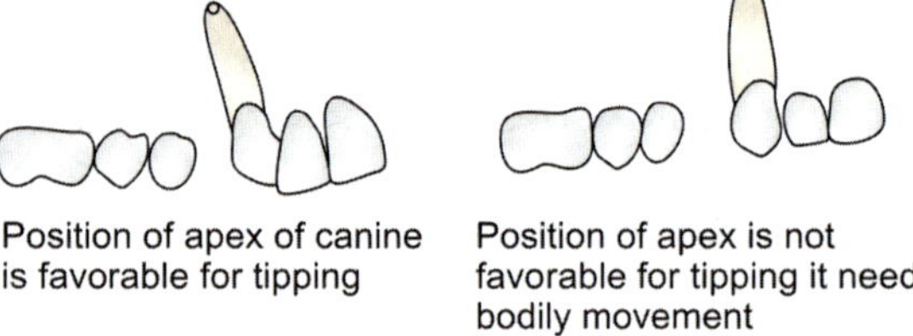

Position of apex of canine is favorable for tipping
Position of apex is not favorable for tipping it need bodily movement

Fig. 19.13: Favorable position of canine apex for tipping in first fig, while in second fig, the apex position dictates a bodily movement of the tooth.

Suppose the distance of the point of application of force is at a distance of X from Crot and the apex of the tooth is at distance Y, then the displacement of crown and root of the tooth will be in the ratio of X:Y.

Tipping can be of two types:

Uncontrolled tipping: Here, a tooth rotates around the Crot which lies between Cres and apex of the tooth. In this movement, the crown moves in one direction while root moves in opposite direction.

Controlled tipping: This is the type of OTM where only the crown or the root moves in the desired direction. It can be controlled crown tipping or the controlled root tipping. These movements are also called as torquing. Torquing is a difficult movement. It requires a combination of force and moments to achieve.

In controlled crown tipping, there is minimal movement of the root. The Crot lies

Type of OTM	*M/F ratio*	*Location of Crot*
Tipping		Apical to Cres
Uncontrolled tipping	0:1–5:1	Between Cres and root apex
controlled tipping	7:1	At the root apex
Translation	10:1	Infinity
Root movement/torquing	12: 1	Incisal or bracket

at the apex of the tooth root. Here, the root is fixed in its position, but the crown is made to move either in labial or lingual direction. The Crot lies at the apex of the tooth. It can be labial crown torquing or lingual crown torquing.

In controlled root tipping, there is minimal movement of the crown. The Crot lies at the incisal edge of the tooth. Here, the crown is fixed, but the root is made to move either in labial or lingual direction. The Crot lies at the incisal edge of the tooth. It can be labial root torquing or lingual root torquing.

Translation or the bodily movement: Crown and root of the tooth move in the same direction to an equal distance. Here, the Crot lies at the infinity. The line of action of the resultant of the forces passes through the Cres of the tooth (Fig. 19.14).

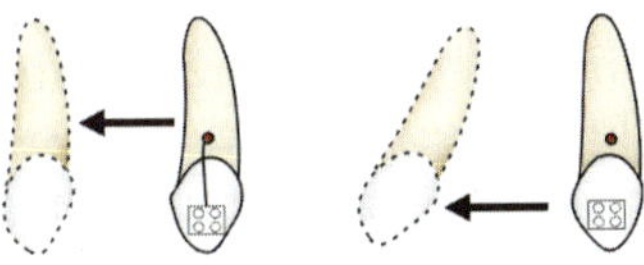

Fig. 19.14: When force is applied through Cres then it leads to bodily movement; while if force is away from Cres, then it leads to tipping.

Intrusion: This is the type of bodily movement of tooth when it is moved inside the alveolar bone, i.e. in the apical direction, along its long axis. However, sometimes it is accompanied with some tipping also.

Extrusion: It is also a type of bodily movement of the tooth. This is opposite of the intrusion, i.e. tooth moves along the long axis in the occlusal direction, i.e. away from the apical area.

Rotation: It is the movement of a tooth around its long axis, under the influence of couple, i.e. two equal forces acting in opposite direction separated by a distance. Here, The Crot lies on the long axis of the tooth, on the centre of the occulsal surface.

Uprighting: Many times, the teeth have abnormal mesiodistal inclination of the roots, with the crown in opposite direction. It may be in the malocclusion itself or it may occur during closure of extraction spaces especially with the Beggs technique. Thus, the correction of root position in the MD direction is the called as the uprighting of the roots.

IDEAL PROPERTIES OF AN ARCHWIRE MATERIAL

For orthodontic purposes, the archwires are used which help in applying the forces for initial alignment of teeth, for levelling of curve of Spee; for expansion of arch, etc. They also help as a channel along which the teeth slide while moving. Different types of archwires are needed depending on the situation and treatment stage and plan. Generally, the wire should possess some of the following qualities.

- Flexibility and range during initial alignment,
- Low stiffness (in most situation),
- High range,
- High strength, especially when it is needed for expansion, and for sliding mechanics.
- High formability: to make loops, etc. for applying required forces.
- Weldable or solderable, so that hooks or stops can be attached to the wire.
- It should also be reasonable in cost.
- Biocompatible, non-corrosive, non-allergic.

In contemporary practice, no one archwire material meets all these requirements, and the best results are obtained by using specific arch wire materials for specific purposes.

Properties of the wire: The archwires are made of different types of materials, e.g. SS, NiTI, TMA, Co-Cr, etc. which have different properties. However, the basic properties of the material are defined below.

Strength: It is the maximum stress required to fracture a material. The maximum load the wire can sustain is the ultimate tensile strength.

Stiffness: It is the resistance to elastic deformation; it is determined by modulus of elasticity (MOE).

Toughness: It is the energy required to fracture a material.

Resilience: It is the capacity to absorb mechanical energy without plastic deformation/amount of energy absorbed by a structure when it is stressed not to exceed its proportional limit (PL). It should be small for metalceramic restorations.

Modulus of resilience: It is the energy required to stress a structure to its proportional limit. Gold alloys have the lowest.

Proportional limit is the point at which any permanent deformation is first observed. Elastic limit and proportional limit may be used interchangeably. A point at which a deformation of 0.1% is measured is defined as the yield strength.

Three main properties of orthodontic wires are strength, stiffness and range. These depend on the diameter and the length of the wire; and the material of the wire used. Mathematically, for a cantilever spring, these can be described as below.

Strength is = D^3/L, i.e. strength increases in cubic proportion to increased diameter, and decreases in proportion to increased length.

Stiffness is = D^4/L^3 it increases if the diameter is increased or the length is decreased and vice versa.

Range is = L^2/D, i.e. range increases by square of increased length and decreases by increased diameter of the wire.

They are interrelated by the formula:

Strength = stiffness × range, i.e.

$D^3/L = D^4/L^3 \times L^2/D$

Stiffness and springiness are inversely related, i.e. stiffer wires are less springy. As the stiffness increases, the range decreases.

Effect of diameter: When the diameter of a round wire is doubled, it increases the strength by 8X. Doubling the diameter, however, decreases springiness by a factor of 16 and decreases range by a factor of two.

Effects of length: Springiness increases as the cubic function of the change in the length and its range increases as the square of the change of length. On doubling the length of a cantilever beam, its springiness increases by eight times and its range by four times, and the strength decreases proportionately.

Longer/thinner wires can be deflected over a larger distance under lighter forces, their load-deflection rate is less and they provide a more gentle force system. Also, force decay is less, e.g. if a spring made of lighter wire can be deflected to 5 mm under 50 gm of force, its LDR is 10. As the tooth movement occurs, the force loss is 10 gm/mm, so almost a constant force is applied on the tooth. On the other hand, a heavy-wire spring needs 50 gm force for 2 mm deflection, its LDR is 25. So, the force immediately falls to half value when tooth moves by 1 mm. So, force decay rate is very high.

Thus it can be concluded that thinner wire have more range and springiness but less strength. Similarly, the longer wire has more range but less strength and stiffness.

In orthodontics, lighter forces are needed, so the active component, i.e. springs, etc. should be made with thinner and longer wires. Wire length can be increased by incorporating loops/helices in the springs.

On the other hand, the retentive components should be made of thicker wires, so that they are strong and resist deformation due to masticatory and other forces.

Stiffness and springiness are proportional to the slope of the elastic portion of the force-deflection curve. The more horizontal is the slope, the springier is the wire; the more vertical is the slope, the stiffer is the wire.

Range is defined as the distance to which the wire can be bent elastically before a permanent deformation occurs. If the wire is deflected beyond its yield strength, it will not return to its original shape.

Resilience is the area under the stress-strain curve out to the proportional limit. It represents the energy storage capacity of the wire.

Formability is the amount of permanent deformation that a wire can withstand before failing. It represents the amount of permanent bending the wire will tolerate (while being formed into a clinically useful spring, for instance) before it breaks.

Load-deflection rate of the wires: It is the property according to which, how much distance a wire can be deflected on application of load without permanent deformation. If same force causes more deflection in one wire than the other wire, the former wire will apply less force for a unit deflection and also the force decay will be slower in it.

Heat treatment of the wire/recovery heat treatment: The stresses are generated in the SS wires due to cold working, when the wire is bent, the slippage of matrix planes occurs. The stresses get concentrated at the points of bending, making them weak and vulnerable to fracture. The heat treatment is done to release those stresses, and to regain the stiffness of wires. Stress relief heat Rx done at 370–480° C for 11 minute removes residual stresses. In SS wires, the heat treatment leads to increased MOE; increased YS; decreased ductility; increased modulus of resilience. As a chair side procedure, it can be done by heating the wire on the flame till it becomes straw-colored. It should not be heated red hot, otherwise the wire becomes dead.

Conclusion

Orthodontic treatment needs movement of teeth in the bone. The forces are applied on the teeth which generate biochemical response in the tissues. The forces should be kept in lighter range for physiological, pain free response. Direction and magnitude of applied forces influence the direction of tooth movement. Knowledge of Cres and Crot of the teeth is necessary to plan the line of action of forces. Also, the different arch wire materials possess different properties which are judiciously exploited in different situations. Flexible wires are used during initial alignment phase, while heavy, stronger wires are used during sliding and retraction of teeth. The clinician should also be aware of the side effects associated with reciprocal forces generated during tooth movement so that they can be controlled and / or used for the required tooth movements. However, detailed discussion of elaborate mechanics is beyond the scope of this book.

20

Anchorage in Orthodontics

INTRODUCTION

The word anchorage has been derived from the word anchor of a ship, which act as a resistance/brake to the movement of ship in the waters. To cause the orthodontic tooth movements, a force has to be applied, which gets distributed as pressure in periodontal tissues (force per unit area). Every force has two points of attachments.

According to the Newton's third law of motion, "to every action, there is an equal and opposite reaction". So when force is applied to move a tooth or a group of teeth, one point of attachment provides the resistance and the other point moves towards or away from the other point. In the oral cavity, the point providing the resistance to movement serves as anchorage. In orthodontics the goal is to maximize desired tooth movement and minimize undesirable effects. Orthodontic anchorage is defined as a resistance to unwanted tooth movement. Generally, in most of cases, the anterior teeth need to be moved back. So, the posterior teeth are used as anchorage unit. But, in some cases, the anterior teeth have to be used as anchorage unit for mesial movement of posterior teeth.

Anchorage is an important consideration in orthodontics, for the following reasons:

- It indicates the resistance required to prevent undesired tooth movement while permitting the desirable movement.
- It is indicative of the type of the resistance teeth offer.
- It also indicates the type of movement that may be expected.
- It also helps in determining the type of appliance which should be used to produce the desired tooth movement, and the anchorage.

Methods to Improve Resistance

Resistance of the teeth can be increased by some methods:

Bodily Resistance of the Anchor Teeth

The force-producing mechanism may be stationary in type, so that the tooth, if it moves at all, supposedly will move in a bodily manner rather than by tipping.

Modifications in the Archwires

The archwire may be modified such that it produces a bodily movement of the tooth rather than tipping.

Using more Teeth in Anchor Unit

Anchorage can also be increased by incorporating more teeth into the portion of the dental arch where movement is not desired, than in that portion of the dental arch, where movement is desired. Anchorage depends on the total root surface area, RSA of the involved teeth. Here, more teeth are engaged in anchorage unit than the teeth to be moved in the same dental arch, so that the applied force is distributed over a larger area. The total RSA of anchor unit should be more than the active unit. More the teeth in anchor are, better is the anchorage.

Performing Tooth Movements in Parts

Anchorage can also be taken care of by breaking the tooth movements, e.g. rather than doing en-masse retraction of anterior, it may be done in two steps: (1) canine retraction and (2) incisors retraction separately. After canine retraction, the canine can be incorporated inanchorage unit.

Definitions

Graber has defined anchorage as "the nature and degree of resistance to displacement offered by an anatomic unit when used for the purpose of effecting tooth movement".

Proffit has defined anchorage as "resistance to unwanted tooth movement". Moyers has described it as "resistance to displacement." According to him, during tooth movement, there exist active elements and resistance elements.

Classification

Many classifications have been proposed for anchorage.

Moyers: According to Moyers:

Depending on the position of anchorage units: it can be:

- Intraoral / extraoral / muscular
- Intramaxillary / intermaxillary
- Cervical / occipital / cranial / facial

Depending on the movement achieved:

- Simple / stationary / reciprocal

Depending on the number of teeth involved in anchorage units:

- Single / compound / reinforced

Ricketts introduced

- The cortical anchorage.

Nanda: According to him, there are three types of anchorage situations depending on the amount of space closure required by movement of active and reactive units.

1. **A-anchorage:** Critical / severe; here, 75% or more of the extraction space is needed for anterior retraction.
2. **B-anchorage:** Moderate; here, relatively symmetric extraction space closure (50%) is done by movement of active and reactive units.
3. **C-anchorage:** Mild / noncritical; here, 75% or more of space closure by mesial movement of posterior teeth, or by anchorage loss.

According to Burstone, following three groups of anchorage have been defined based on the anchorage loss.

- **Group A:** Posterior teeth contribute less than one-fourth to total space closure.
- **Group B:** Posterior teeth contribute from one-fourth to one-half to total space closure.
- **Group C:** Posterior teeth contribute more than one-half to total space closure.

Another classification is according to the anchorage requirement as: minimum, moderate or maximum anchorage (Fig. 20.1).

Minimum : More than one-half extraction space can be lost by mesial movement of the anchor teeth. Anchorage requirement is very low.

Moderate : one-fourth to one-half of the extraction space can be lost by mesial movement of the anchor teeth. Anchorage requirement is medium (Fig. 20.2).

Maximum : Less than one-fourth extraction space can be lost by mesial movement of the anchor teeth. Anchorage requirement is very high (Fig. 20.3).

Absolute anchorage: It means that there is no space loss of the extraction space by mesial movement of anchorage unit. So, whole of the space can be used for retraction of anterior teeth. It is provided by using microimplants and bone plates. Since there are no dental units used as anchorage, there is no anchorage loss, thus it has been called absolute anchorage. It has been discussed later on.

Skeletal anchorage system (SAS): SAS, the anchorage provided by using bone plates fixed in the bone near the dental units. Thus,

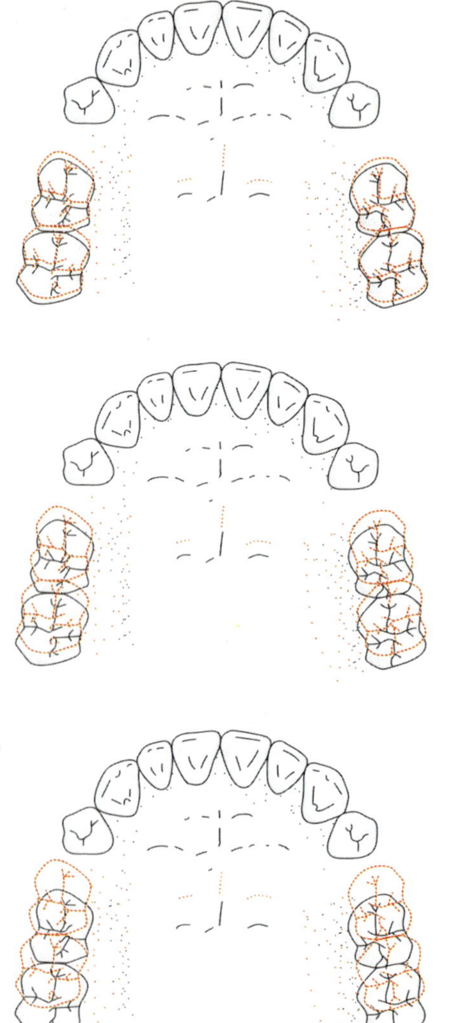

Fig. 20.1: Types of anchorage: maximum, moderate and minimum anchorage *(Adapted from Graber and Vanarsdall).*

the anchorage is provided by the bones, so it is called skeletal anchorage.

Cortical anchorage: This concept was introduced by Ricketts, especially in lower arch. By torquing, the roots of molars were brought closure to the cortices of mandible. The cortical bone is very difficult to resorb, and thus the anchorage is increased, as there occurs no tooth movement.

Muscular anchorage: It is provided by the muscles, e.g. lip bumper transmits the forces of lower lip to the first molars and prevents its

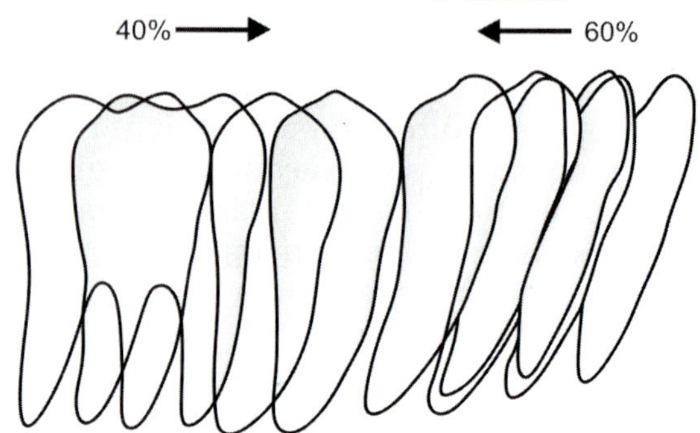

Fig. 20.2: Moderate anchorage condition where the 40% extraction space is lost by mesial movement of buccal teeth, while 60% space is closed by retraction of anterior teeth *(Adapted from Graber and Vanarsdall).*

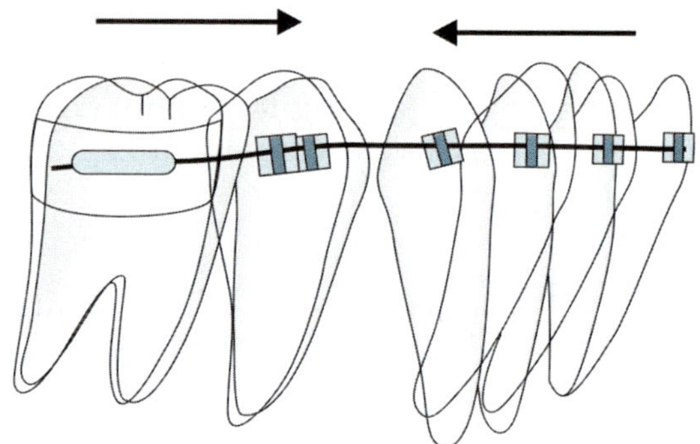

Fig. 20.3: Maximum anchorage with minimum mesial movement of buccal teeth *(Adapted from Graber and Vanarsdall).*

mesial movement. Also, the forces of upper and lower lips can be used to move back the spaced and proclined upper incisors with oral screen (Fig. 20.4).

Definitions

Simple anchorage: It is the resistance in which the anchor units move, by tipping. It is the type of dental anchorage in which the force tends to displace or change the axial inclination of anchor teeth. Here, the resistance of anchor unit to tipping is used to move other teeth. It is used mainly in removable appliances.

Stationary anchorage: Here, anchorage unit provides resistance by bodily movement of anchor teeth, i.e. if they move at all, they move bodily only. It is the type of anchorage

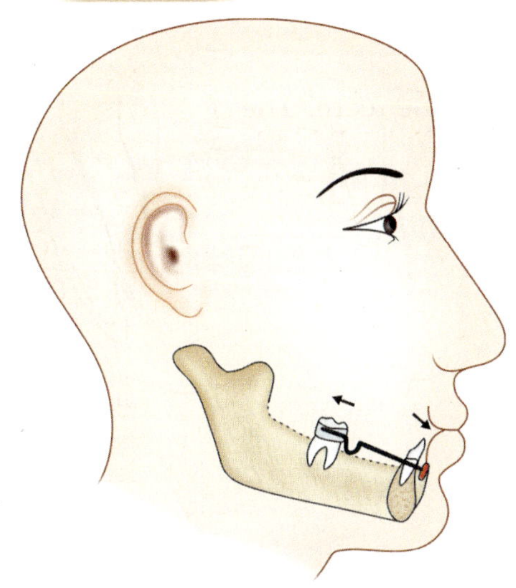

Fig. 20.4: Cross-section diagram showing position and action of lip bumper. Arrows show that molars achieve an uprighting effect under the forces from lower lip, while lower incisor move labially under tongue forces.

in which the applied force tends to displace the anchorage unit bodily. It is considerably stronger than the simple anchorage units. It refers to the advantage that can be obtained by pitting bodily movement of one group of teeth against tipping of another, e.g. retraction of mandibular incisors using first molars as anchorage.

Reciprocal anchorage: Anchorage in which the resistance of one or more dental units is utilized to move one or more opposing dental units in equal and opposite direction, e.g. diastema closure; correction of posterior cross-bite through cross-elastics; bilateral expansion, etc. (Figs 20.5 to 20.8).

Extraoral anchorage: This is the anchorage obtained by the sources outside the oral cavity. It can be obtained from occipital, cervical, frontal, chin, nasal or parietal bony areas or a combination, e.g. by using head gears, reverse face masks, chin cap, etc.

Intraoral anchorage: This is the anchorage obtained by the sources in the oral cavity only, e.g. from teeth, palate, lingual tissues or upper and/or lower arches, e.g. by using elastics, TPA, LHA, NPA, VHA, involving the more number of teeth, etc. and using the removable appliances.

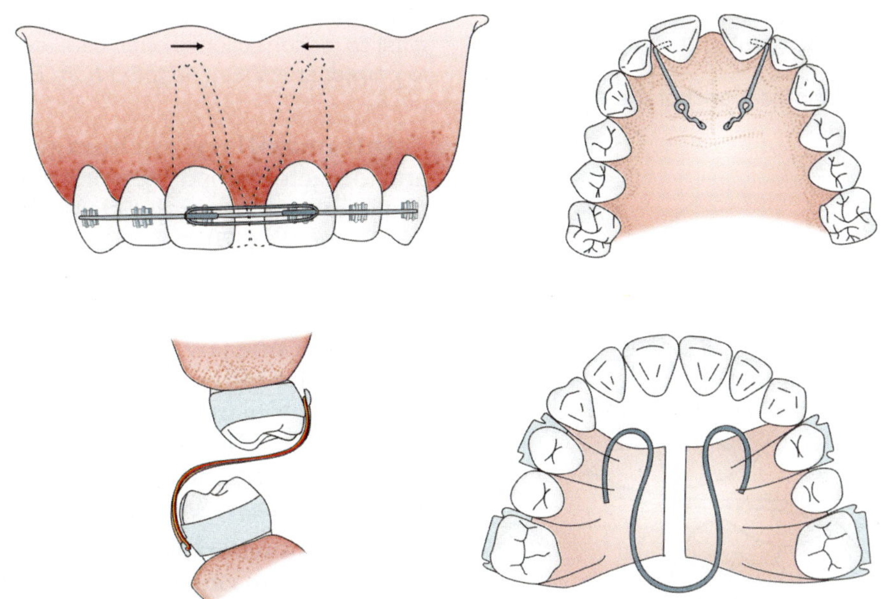

Fig. 20.5: Examples of reciprocal anchorage: Closure of midline diastema with elastics/elastic thread; closure of midline diastema with finger springs; cross-elastic to treat crossbite; Coffin's spring for transverse expansion of upper arch.

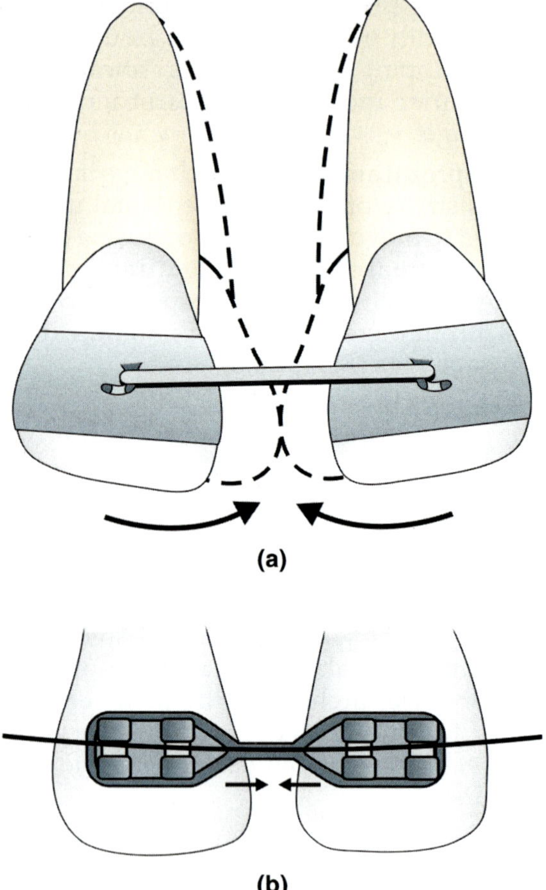

Figs 20.6a, b: Reciprocal anchorage for treatment of midline diastema.

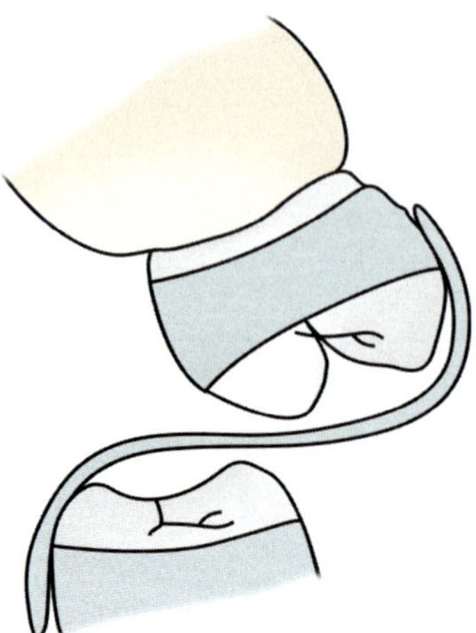

Fig. 20.7: Reciprocal anchorage for treatment of crossbite.

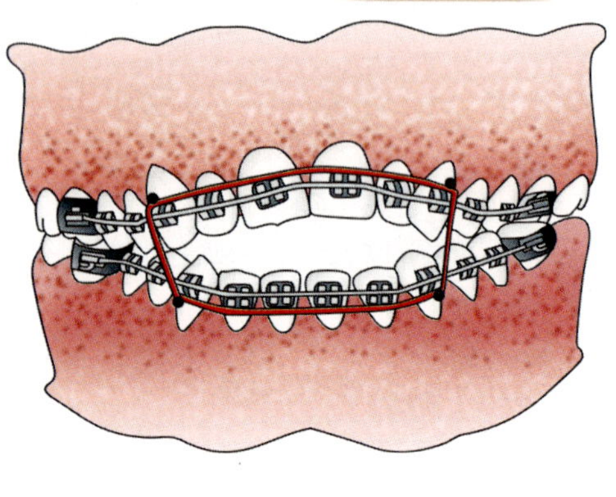

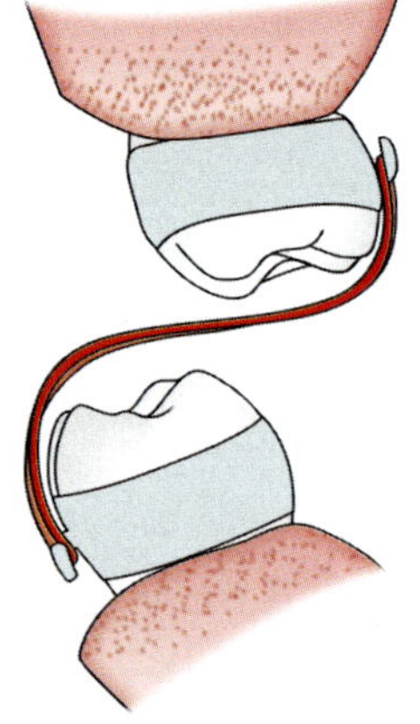

Fig. 20.8: Reciprocal anchorage: Anterior box elastics for correction of open bite; and cross-elastics to correct crossbite *(Adapted from Bhalaji)*.

Intramaxillary anchorage: This is the anchorage obtained by using the units in the same jaw/arch, e.g. by class I elastics, TPA, LHA, etc. (Fig. 20.9).

Intermaxillary anchorage: This is the anchorage obtained by the resistance units situated in one jaw to cause the tooth movement in the other jaw, i.e. the anchorage is obtained by using the units in the opposing arch, e.g. class II and III elastics, cross-elastics, vertical elastics, check elastics, triangular/box elastics; settling elastics, etc. (Fig. 20.7 and 20.8).

Baker's anchorage: When anchorage of one arch is used to cause tooth movements in the opposite arch, it is called the Baker's anchorage, e.g. class II, and III intermaxillary elastics. This pattern was suggested by Baker (Fig. 20.9).

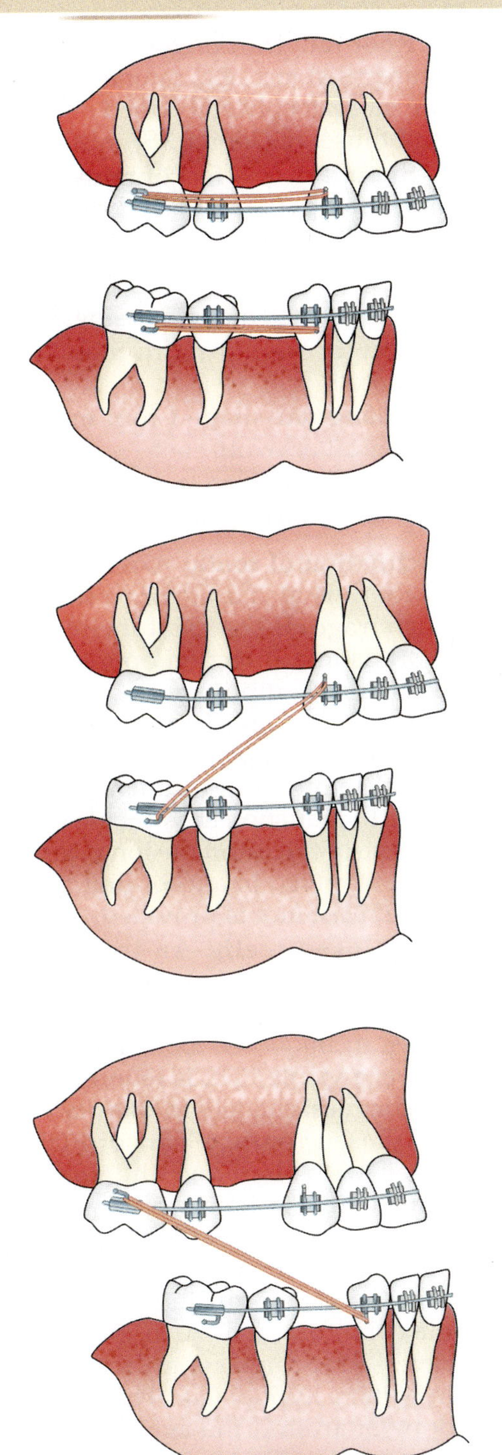

Fig. 20.9: Intermaxillary and intramaxillary anchorage through class I, class II, and class III orthodontic elastics.

Single/primary anchorage: It is the simplest form of anchorage in which only one tooth acts as anchorage. The tooth with larger alveolar support or root surface area, RSA acts as anchorage, while smaller tooth is moved.

Compound anchorage: It is the form of anchorage where more than one tooth is used in the anchorage unit.

Complex anchorage: It is the form of anchorage where different types of anchorage methods are used.

Reinforced/multiple anchorage: It is the anchorage where more than one type of resistance units are used, e.g. using TPA, more teeth, palatal tissues, and extraoral appliances, etc. It helps to wider distribution pressure and thus reduces pressure on the anchor units moving them down the slope of the pressure-response curve.

Hammock anchorage is provided by PDL.

Muscular anchorage: It is provided by the circumoral muscles. The forces generated by the muscles can be used for tooth movement, e.g. by lower lip using the lip bumper can be used to direct the forces on first molars. It may help in movement of the teeth, mostly by tipping. But most of the time, it helps in augmenting the anchorage by applying a distal force in the molars, thus controlling their mesial movement.

Cortical anchorage: According to Ricketts, when the roots of lower molars are torqued in the buccal cortical plate of mandible under heavy forces, there occurs the hyalinization of PDL, which does not allow the mesial movement or the loss of anchorage due to heavy cortical bone. It acts as the cortical anchorage. The anchorage is provided by the mandibular cortex.

Tooth-borne anchorage: It is the type of resistance which is provided by the dental units alone.

Tissue-borne anchorage: It is the type of resistance which is provided by the soft tissues in the oral cavity, e.g. in removable appliances without clasps.

Tooth-tissue-borne anchorage: It is the type of resistance which is provided by both teeth and tissues in the oral cavity, e.g. removable appliance with clasps as retentive elements.

FACTORS AFFECTING ANCHORAGE

Anchorage is affected by various factors, e.g. tooth shape, root shape, number of roots, bone quality, periodontal support; age of the patient; movements required, etc.

1. **The teeth:** Whenever some teeth move in the bone, the other teeth act as anchorage unit. Generally, the posterior teeth act as anchorage unit, since most of the malocclusions require retraction of anterior teeth for correction. The anchorage potential of teeth depends on a number of factors, e.g. root form, root length, number of roots, root surface area, root size and root inclination.
2. **Root form:** It is a very important factor in anchorage. Roots can be of three types according to the cross-section, i.e. round, flat and triangular.

   Round roots are in found in mandibular bicuspids, maxillary second bicuspid, MB root of maxillary molars, etc. They can resist horizontal forces in any direction, but they have least anchorage potential.

   Flat roots: They are present in mandibular incisors, and mandibular molars. They best resist movement in mesiodistal direction, but not in labiolingual direction due to their sharp edges.

   Triangular roots: They are found in maxillary incisors and canine roots. They offer maximum anchorage potential.

   Size and number of roots: Multirooted teeth and teeth with larger roots offer more anchorage. It all depends on root surface area. More RSA, the more is anchorage resistance.

   Root length: Longer roots provide more resistance, e.g. canine roots. They are more deeply embedded in the bone and thus have larger RSA also.

   Summary of effect of roots and root morphology: The roots of teeth have a major influence on the anchorage provided. It is summarized below.

   - Multirooted more than single-rooted
   - Longer rooted more than shorter rooted
   - Triangular-shaped root more than conical or ovoid root
   - Larger surface area more than smaller surface area.

3. **Inclination of tooth:** Axial inclination of tooth is also a factor to determine anchorage. If the axial inclination of tooth is in a direction opposite to the direction of applied force, it provides more anchorage. Tweed's method of anchorage preparation involved the distal inclination of anchor units. It leads to reduction in the angle between the line of force and the long axis of the teeth involved in anchor unit and thus more resistance is provided.
4. **Ankylosed teeth:** An intentionally ankylosed tooth can also be used for absolute anchorage. It is not possible to move an ankylosed tooth. For a tooth to move, a viable PDL is required for the biochemical changes to take place. In an ankylosed tooth, a part of PDL gets fused with the bone and so a tooth cannot move. Clinical success has been obtained by intentional ankylosing the maxillary primary canines, which are then used for pulling the deficient maxilla forward with the help of reverse face masks, to treat cases of maxillary hypoplasia. This process is done at around the age of 8 years, to take full advantage of maxillary growth. Intentionally ankylosed teeth, however, have limited longevity since the roots ultimately resorb and the teeth exfoliate. Also, their location may

not help in optimal correction of the skeletal deformity. Also, the intentional ankylosis of tooth affects the future eruption of the successor tooth.

5. **Age of the patient:** Younger patients have softer bones as compared to adults. Thus, tooth movement is easier in younger patients. More anchorage is needed in adult patients for OTM due to lesser cancellous bone. Also lighter forces are needed in adults.
6. **Periodontal support:** Anchor tooth having lesser PD support provides lesser anchorage, and thus amenable to anchor loss. So, multiple teeth may be needed in anchorage unit to provide adequate support.
7. **Periodontal disease:** A tooth associated with PD disease looses a part of alveolar bone support, and thus its anchorage potential is decreased. An active gingival or PD disease gets aggravated during application of forces, and leads to rapid loss of supporting tissues / bone, etc. It also leads to decreased potential of anchor units. Thus, before the start and during the orthodontic treatment, all the active gingival and PD diseases should be controlled.

Forces required for various orthodontic movements: Different tooth movements need different amount of forces, as described in the literature and depicted in Table 20.1.

Table 20.1: Forces required for various orthodontic movements

Type of tooth movement	*Forces needed*
Tipping	50–75 gm
Body/translation	100–150 gm
Intrusion	50–75 gm
Extrusion	50–75 gm
Rotation	50–75 gm
Uprighting	75–125 gm

8. **Type of tooth movement:** Tooth which is free to tip has a less anchorage value than a tooth (which is moving bodily), i.e. which is restricted in tipping by the application of a force couple.
9. **Quality of bone:** Cortical bone provides better anchorage than cancellous bone. Anchorage loss is more in maxilla than mandible, due to more cancellous bone in maxilla. Mandibular teeth provide better anchorage than maxillary teeth due to dense bone and direction of trabeculae. Trabeculae in mandible are oriented perpendicular to the roots of teeth, thus providing maximum resistance.
10. **Growth pattern of the face/jaws:** Anchorage requirements are maximum in vertical growing cases, but their anchorage resistance is less and thus chances of anchorage loss are more. It is due to the poor quality of supporting bones, weaker muscles, and position of posterior teeth on a more sloped basal bone. On the other hand, in horizontal growth cases, the anchorage resistance is maximum, while anchorage requirements are less. In such cases, anchorage loss is difficult. It is due to strong muscles, denser and thicker bones, with trabeculae aligned perpendicular to the direction of tooth movements. Also, the molars sit on an almost horizontal plane, and thus their mesial movement is difficult. Such cases, e.g. Angle's class II division 2 cases, should be avoided to be treated by extractions, as the closure of spaces by mesial movement of molars is a nightmare. Nowadays, the use of TAD, BAD, etc. have simplified the space closure mechanics.
11. **Muscular pattern/forces:** As discussed above, patients of horizontal growth pattern have stronger muscles than the vertical growth cases. Anchorage resistance is more in former than in later cases.
12. **Musculature:** Circumoral muscles can also be used for anchorage, e.g. lips can be used to augment anchorage of molars by using the lip bumper appliance in upper and / or lower arches.

13. **Alveolar bone and basal bones:** Certain areas of basal bones can be used to augment the anchorage potential of teeth, e.g. hard palate, and the lingual area of mandible. Appliances can be made to cover as large area of palate as possible so that the reactionary forces can be distributed to larger areas. In mandible, the flanges of removable or functional appliances can be extended deep in the vestibules to involve the larger area.

INTRAORAL SOURCES OF ANCHORAGE

Anchorage can be obtained from intraoral tissues, e.g. teeth, palate, alveolar bone, basal jaw bone, and the muscles.

EXTRAORAL SOURCES OF ANCHORAGE

These include cranium, back of the neck, frontal bone, zygomatic bones, mandibular symphysis and even chest has been used for anchorage. Using them, the burden on the teeth can be minimized, and the anchorage loss is reduced to minimal. But, they need absolute patient cooperation (Fig. 20.10).

Headgears use occipital, frontal, cervical areas and the parietal bones for anchorage. They are used for distal movement of dentition or to control the forward growth of maxilla. Reverse face mask and chin cup use frontal bone and mandibular symphysis for anchorage. Some authors have used chest for extraoral source of anchorage.

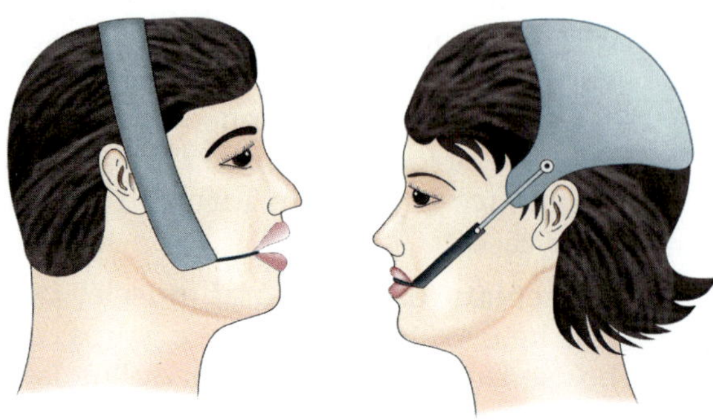

Fig. 20.10: Extraoral anchorage with the headgears.

TEMPORARY ANCHORAGE DEVICES

TAD / bone anchorage devices (BAD): as there is always a loss of the extraction space by undesired mesial movement of anchor units, there was a need of absolute anchorage. Authors have used certain microimplants, bone plates, etc. to obtain the anchorage. These devices are called TADs as they are to be removed after treatment.

SKELETAL ANCHORAGE SYSTEM

SAS implants serve as the anchorage source, as they do not have any PDL, but get engaged with the bone through osseointegration, similar to an ankylosed tooth. They cannot move even under heavy force, so the implants provide absolute anchorage. Osseointegration has been defined by Brånemark and co-workers as the direct contact between vital bone and the implant surface.

OSSEOINTEGRATED DENTAL IMPLANT SUPPORTED TOOTH

It can also be used as an absolute anchorage method, since the implant is joined to the bone and it does not move under orthodontic forces.

SIGNS OF ANCHORAGE LOSS

Anchorage loss is the unwanted movement of anchor teeth during the orthodontic treatment. It leads to insufficient space left for anterior teeth retraction, and thus the desired treatment may not be obtained. Certain signs are observed which indicate anchorage loss, which are change in pretreatment molar relationship, mesial tilting / rotation of the molars, labial movement of the incisors, reduction of extraction space without appreciable movement of active unit, etc. Anchorage loss should be minimised to achieve desired results.

Anchorage reinforcement and anchorage savers: These are the modalities used during treatment to avoid the anchorage loss. The anchorage can be reinforced with different methods, like incorporating more teeth in anchor unit, dividing the tooth movements;

using additional appliance, e.g. transpalatal arch (TPA), lingual holding arch (LHA), vertical holding appliance (VHA), lip bumper, removable appliances, head gear, nance palatal arch, microimplants, etc.

Anchorage value: Depending on the size of teeth and number of roots and other factors, various teeth have been assigned some anchorage values. It depends on the root surface areas of the teeth. Different teeth in the oral cavity have different size, shape, length and number of roots. Thus they have different values of root surface areas. The anchorage value of a tooth depends on the RSA. Bigger the RSA, more is the anchorage value of the tooth. By incorporating more teeth in anchor unit, the RSA is increased and thus the anchorage value also increases.

Anchorage values of different teeth (Figs 2011 and 2012): Proffit, as modified from Freeman's work, has described that anchorage values of teeth are roughly equivalent to the RSA of each tooth (Table 20.2).

Anchorage savers: Those additional appliances used in conjunction with teeth to increase the resistance to tooth movements are known as anchorage savers, e.g. transpalatal arch, double transpalatal arch, lingual holding arch, Nance's palatal arch, head gear, lip bumpers and modification, using removable appliance with posterior bite plate, etc.

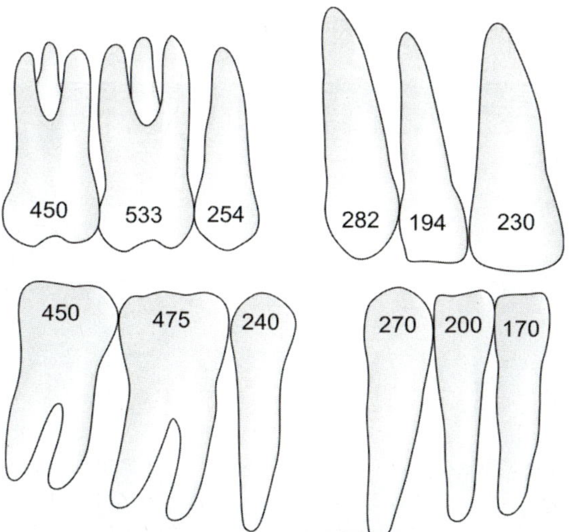

Fig. 20.11: Anchorage values of different teeth as depicted by their root surface areas, as described by Proffit.

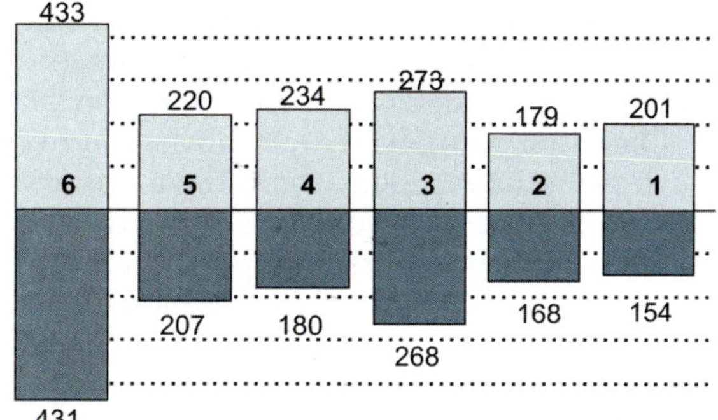

Fig. 20.12: Anchorage values of different teeth as depicted by their root surface areas.

Table 20.2: Anchorage values

Tooth	*Upper*	*Lower*
Second molar	450	450
First molar	533	475
Second premolar	254	240
Canine	282	270
Lateral incisor	194	200
Central incisor	230	170

The **transpalatal arch (TPA)** (Figs 20.13 to 20.15) is made of hard SS wire of at least 0.9 mm size or a bar spanning the palate

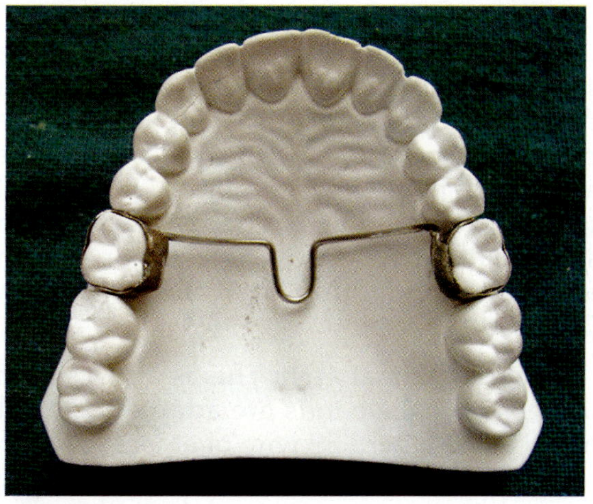

Fig. 20.13: Transpalatal arch for augmentation of anchorage.

transversely, and has a U-loop in the middle of wire. It is kept 2–3 mm away from the palatal tissues, and connects two bands on the maxillary first permanent molars by soldering or using the lingual sheaths. This auxiliary appliance can be used for multiple purposes, e.g. to change or stabilize the position of the maxillary molars in three dimensions, producing molar rotation and uprighting, stabilizing intermolar width during treatment, maintaining leeway spaces during the transition of the dentition. It also is used for additional anchorage during retraction of the anterior segments during extraction treatment. However, with TPA also, some anchorage loss occurs, so alternative methods (e.g. microimplants) should be used if maximum or absolute anchorage is desired. Double TPAs can also be used extending between first and second molars (Fig. 20.14).

Modified form of TPA has been used, in which acrylic button is placed in the region of U-loop. It gives a wider area on which tongue keeps on applying the pressure and prevents the molars from extrusion. It is esp helpful in vertical growth and open bite cases.

Lingual holding arch (LHA): It is the counterpart of TPA used in lower arch. The bands are placed at first molars and a hard SS wire of at least 0.9 mm size is adapted from molar of one side, touching the lingual surfaces of premolars, passing just above the cinguli of the incisors and touching them, to the other side molar. Then, the wire is soldered or passed in lingual sheaths, to both the molar bands and finished. This is the passive form of LHA. It can also be made active, if U-loops are incorporated just mesial to the molars, and then it can be used to gain space in the arch by activated the loops. It can also be expanded to widen the lower arch (Fig. 20.16).

Nance's palatal arch: This is also used in upper arch. The bands are adapted on first molars, and a hard SS wire of at least 0.9 mm size is adapted from molar of one side passing through the rugae area of palate, to the other side and soldered to the molar bands. An

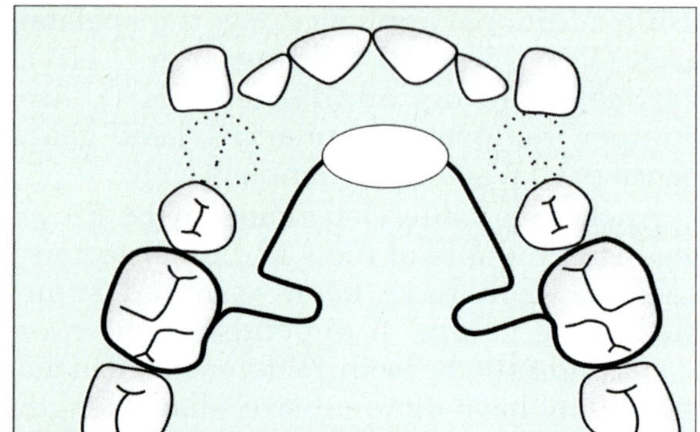

Fig. 20.14: Nance's palatal arch for augmenting the anchorage.

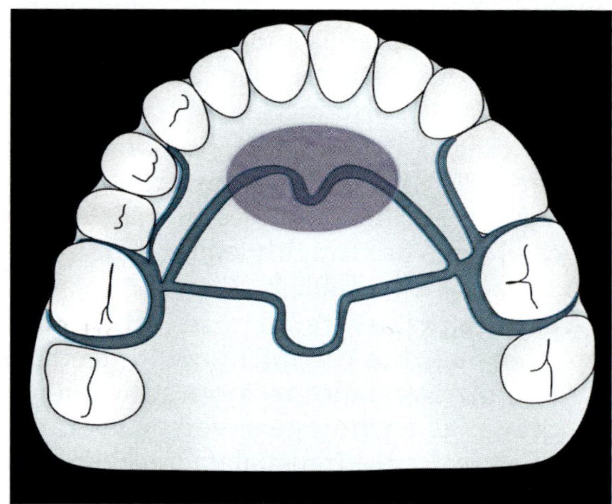

Fig. 20.15: Combination of Nance's palatal arch and transpalatal arch for augmenting the anchorage.

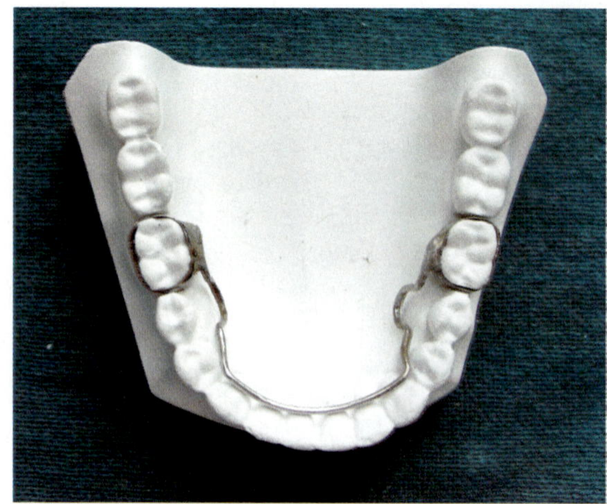

Fig. 20.16: Lingual holding arch for augmentation of anchorage.

acrylic button is placed in the rugae area including the wire in it, and finished and polished. Thus, this appliance obtains the anchorage from molars and the rugae areas. But, it is difficult to clean below acrylic and thus leads to gingival inflammation. It may need periodic removal, cleaning and recementation (Fig. 20.15).

Hamula lingual arch: It consists of 0.045" round stainless steel lingual wire which is attached with Hamula First Fit molar bands. These bands come with mesial and distal occlusal stops. Two segments of 0.022 × 0.028'' SS wire are soldered occlusally to these stops. The band is cemented and the wires are bonded to the occlusal surfaces of the premolars and second molars to give extra anchorage by involving more teeth. The edgewise wire rests on the occlusal surfaces without any interference.

Headgears: They apply a distal force on the first molars and thus prevent their mesial movements. They obtain the support from extraoral sources like parietal or occipital bones, and cervical area of the neck.

Lip bumpers and modifications, Denholtz appliance, augmentor, reverse lip bumper: These appliances incorporate the forces of upper or lower lip muscles, which are then directed to first molars in the distal direction, thus preventing their mesial movements. They help in preventing anchorage loss, may cause distal movement of molars, cause distal tipping/uprighting of molars, and also help in increasing the arch width by keeping the cheek muscles away from labial surfaces of the teeth. Hooks can be incorporated in them so that elastics can be used for moving the teeth. The acrylic part of lip bumper also helps in stretching the periosteum of bone and thus bone remodeling in these regions (Fig. 20.17).

Posterior bite plate appliance: Acrylic covers the occlusal surfaces of the posterior teeth, beyond the free way space, which then prevents the extrusion of the molars during treatment. It may also apply some intrusive pressure on the posterior teeth.

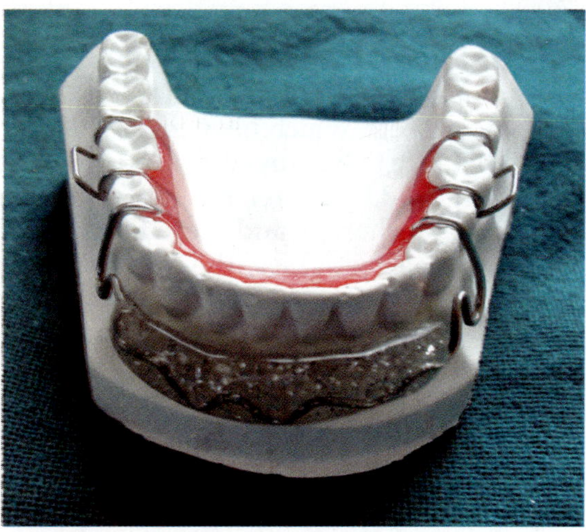

Fig. 20.17: Lip bumper is also used for augmentation of anchorage.

Anchorage planning: It is a very important aspect of treatment planning for the success of treatment and for achieving the treatment objectives. Various factors are considered to assess the anchorage demands of a case so that proper mechanics can be used during the treatment. Anchorage requirements are assessed by a number of factors which are briefly mentioned below:

1. **Number of the teeth being moved:** The more the number of teeth to be moved, greater is the demand for anchorage, e.g. in an extraction case, retraction of 6 anterior teeth as a unit will need more anchorage as compared to the retraction of only 4 incisors. It depends on the total RSA of the anchor units and the unit being moved. So, to put less strain on the anchors, generally the canines are retracted separately. Then the canines are included in the posterior segment to augment the anchorage, which is then used to retract the 4 incisors as a unit. But, with the use of micro-implants, all the 6 anterior teeth can be retracted en-masse. It helps to reduce the total treatment time.
2. **Type of the teeth being moved:** The smaller teeth, e.g. incisors, which have less RSA, can be moved easily, without

causing much strain on anchors as compared to the bigger and multi-rooted teeth, e.g. premolars, canines, molars, etc. which have more RSA.

3. **Distance to be moved:** If the distance to be moved by the teeth is more, it needs more anchorage and more time, e.g. in large overjet cases, the anterior teeth need to be moved by 6–7 mm, which needs maximum anchorage requirement.
4. **TSALD:** If TSALD is more, then anchorage requirements are maximum, as compared to the cases in which TSALD is lesser.
5. **Type of the tooth movement to be achieved:** Tipping of tooth requires lesser force and less anchorage requirement, while bodily movement requires more anchorage, as it causes more strain on the anchorage unit.
6. **Duration of OTM:** If the treatment is prolonged, it puts more strain on the anchors.
7. **Growth pattern:** It plays a very important role in anchorage. Anchorage is better in horizontal growth pattern cases as compared to the vertical growth cases. Vertical growth cases have more anchorage requirements than the horizontal growth cases. It is because the trabecular pattern of mandible is approximately perpendicular to the direction of applied orthodontic forces in horizontal growth cases, as compared to in vertical growth cases.
8. **Extraction cases:** Since they require space closure and the teeth have to move for a greater distance, the anchorage requirement are more in such cases as compared to non-extraction cases.
9. **Age of the patient:** In adult patients, the bone is denser, the teeth take more time to move. Also, due to periodontal disease, the bone support around the anchor teeth is decreased, thus the anchorage demand in such cases is more esp in extraction cases requiring retraction of canines and incisors.
10. **Periodontal support:** Teeth with decreased PD support being used as anchorage require reinforcement to avoid anchorage loss.

Based on these factors, the anchorage requirement of every case is individually determined. Cases requiring high anchorage need reinforcement of anchorage by various means, e.g. by including more number of teeth in the anchorage unit; by using appliances like TPA, LHA, NPA, HG, microimplants, etc. However, some unwanted movement of anchor teeth always occurs during treatment, this is called as anchorage loss. It leads to loss of space, which was to be needed for teeth retraction.

BONE ANCHORAGE DEVICES IN ORTHODONTICS

Screws made of biocompatible material are placed in jaw bones which are used as anchors either solely or in association with other teeth and anchorage appliances.

Limitations

The conventional anchorage systems have some limitations, like:

- Patient compliance
- Relative number of dental anchorage units
- Periodontal support
- Iatrogenic injuries
- Unfavorable reactionary tooth movements.

Requirements of an Orthodontic Anchor Implant

The main requirements for implants are that they should be:

- Small and affordable
- Easy to place, and remove
- Resistant to orthodontic forces
- Able to be immediately loaded
- Usable with familiar orthodontic mechanics
- Biocompatible.

Types of Skeletal Anchorage

Nanda has described it in two types:

1. **Direct anchorage:** Which utilizes force from the actual implant that takes the place of a missing tooth and eventually supports a dental restoration.
2. **Indirect anchorage:** They are placed solely for orthodontic purposes and is generally removed once its anchorage duties have been fulfilled.

Indications

Orthodontic bone anchorage is indicated in:

1. Large amount of tooth movements
2. Dental anchorage is insufficient because of absent teeth or periodontal loss.
3. Asymmetric tooth movement
4. Intrusive mechanics
5. Intermaxillary fixation/traction
6. Orthopaedic traction.

Definition

Skeletal anchorage system (SAS): These are those devices fixed to bone to increase orthodontic anchorage (Fig. 20.18).

Temporary anchorage devices (TAD): these are those devices, e.g. implants/screws/pins/plates, etc. which are placed for orthodontic anchorage and are removed when treatment is completed.

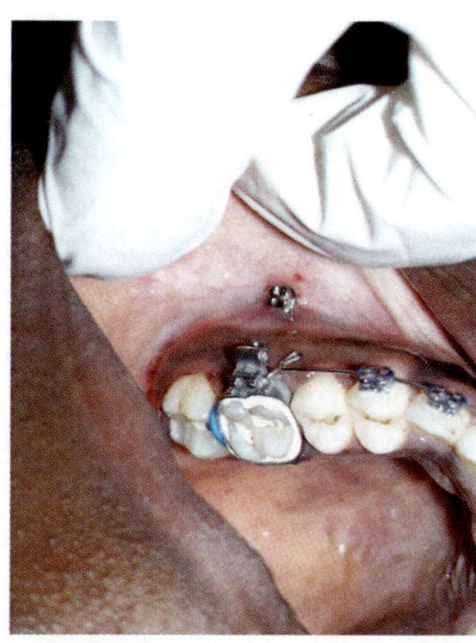

20.18: Microimplant placed in upper molar area for absolute anchorage.

Skeletal anchorage: It can be defined as the anchorage which is directly taken from intraoral bone, without involving the teeth. The term skeletal anchorage can include all kinds of skeletal anchorage devices including miniplates, prosthodontic implant, onplant, etc. It has been variously termed, such as, skeletal anchorage system, miniscrew, microimplant, microscrew implant, temporary anchorge device (TAD), etc.

Classification of bone anchorage devices: Implants are of two types:

- **Osseointegrated implants:** Dental implants; palatal implants
- **Non-osseointegrated implants:** Miniscrews; microscrews; surgical plates, etc.

On the basis of principal design element:

- Screw (mini-implant)
- Plate (miniplate).

Types of Miniscrews

- Self-drilling
- Self-tapping.

Head Types of the Microimplants

- Small head SH
- Long head LH
- No head NH
- Circle head CH
- Bracket head BH
- Fixation head FH.
- Dual top anchor screws: they have 0.0 22 × 0.0 25" cross-section slot.

Sites of placement (Figs 20.19 to 20.21): There are specific sites for placement of these implants for best results depending on the availability of bone, divergence of roots, etc. which are

1. Maxillary and mandibular interproximal areas
2. Maxillary subnasal spine
3. Mandibular symphysis
4. Paramedian and midpalate
5. Retromolar
6. Infrazygomatic
7. Maxillary tuberosity areas.

For miniplates, recommended sites are:
1. Zygomatic process of maxilla
2. Mandibular body distal to first molar
3. Maxillary buccal plate above premolar/ molar root area.

Site of miniplates placement:

In maxilla-zygomatic buttress, Y-plate is used; in piriform rim, I-plate is placed.

In mandible, in anterior border of ascending ramus, in mandibular body, the T-plate or L-plate is used.

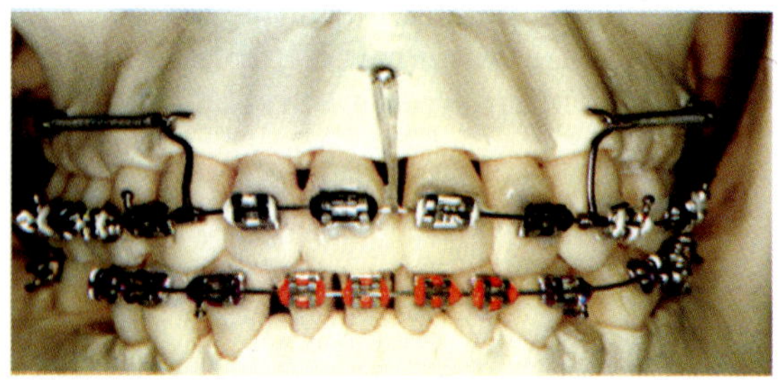

20.19: Microimplant in place in upper arch in incisal region for intrusion of incisors *(Courtesy: Internet for academic purpose only).*

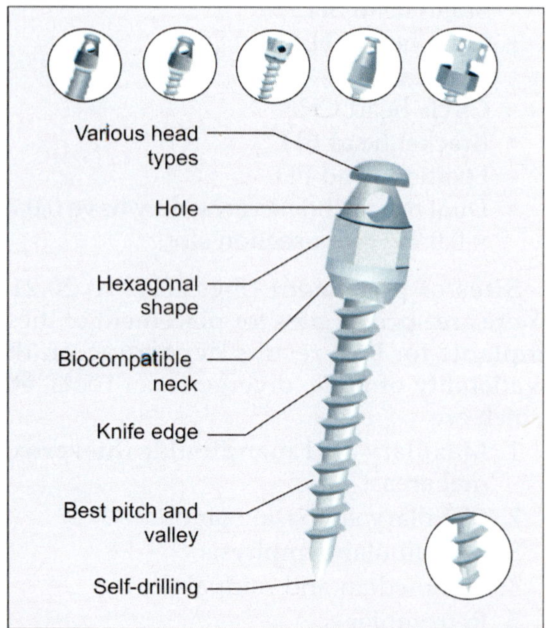

20.20: Parts of microimplant *(Courtesy: Internet for academic purpose only).*

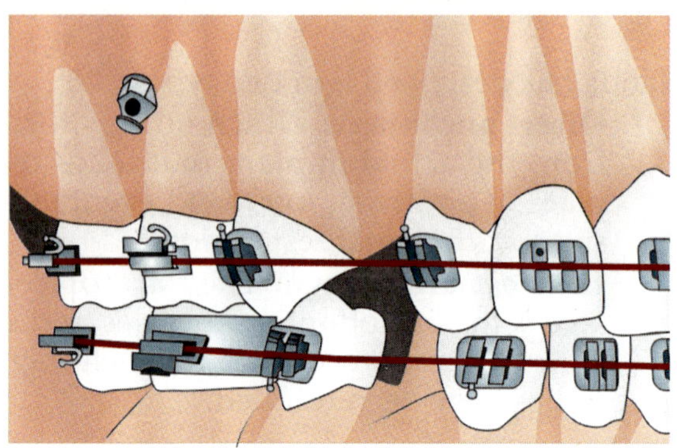

20.21: Microimplant in place in upper arch in molar area *(Courtesy: Internet for academic purpose only).*

Parts of miniscrew (Fig. 20.2): It has three parts:

1. Head: Long head, bracket head, hole head
2. Neck: Short, long, should be placed in thick mucosa
3. Body: Tapered shape is more common and safer than parallel shape; has threads to be screwed in the bone.

Advantages of Mini-implants

- They can be loaded immediately or after a healing period of 2 weeks.
- It can withstand force upto 250 gm.
- No patient co-operation is needed for anchorage and tooth movements.
- Anchorage loss is zero or very minimal, so most of the space can be used for retraction of the teeth maximally.
- There are no reactionary forces on the posterior teeth, and hence the side effects like molar extrusion, etc. are eliminated.
- The treatment is fast and hence time is saved. The retraction of 6 anterior teeth can be done in one step, without taxing anchorage.

Clinical applications of microimplants (Fig. 20.22): Implants can be used for facilitating any type of the tooth movements during orthodontics. They help to reduce the treatment time, minimising the anchorage

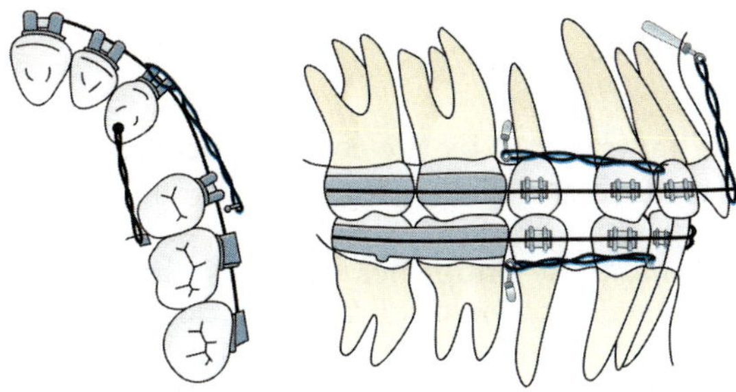

Fig. 20.22: Line diagram showing the use of implants for absolute anchorage for retraction and intrusion of anterior segment of the arch *(Courtesy: Internet for academic purpose only)*.

loss and thus helping to use the extraction spaces to the maximum. Following are some of the clinical conditions in which implants can be used.

- En-masse anterior retraction
- Intrusion of anterior teeth: For correction of deep bite.
- Posterior intrusion: For correction of open bites.
- Molar uprighting/distalization: For correction of molar relations and to gain space in extraction cases.
- They can also be used for maxillofacial protraction.
- Forced eruption for further prosthetic treatment, etc.
- For periodontally compromised patients.
- For correction of canted OP; asymmetries of the dental arches; midline corrections.
- Adult orthodontic treatment who have multiple missing teeth, or who need comprehensive orthodontic treatment for retraction of anteriors in bimaxillary protrusion cases.

Conclusion

Anchorage is one of the most important aspects of orthodontic treatment. A proper diagnosis and treatment planning helps to determine the anchorage requirement. It helps to determine the mechanics and appliance selection. Different methods of anchorage reinforcements have been devised by the clinicians to take maximum benefit of the extraction spaces and to achieve the desired treatment objectives.

Microimplants have been a boon in orthodontics to provide an absolute anchorage. Many cases which needed surgical options have been treated with orthodontics only using micro-implants, which helped to provide acceptable orthodontic results. Factor of patient's cooperation is minimized to zero, and the treatment time is also reduced with the help of implants in certain cases. These days, numerous types of implants designs are available to the orthodontist and should be the part of routine practice of any orthodontist.

VIVA VOCE QUESTIONS

1. **Define anchorage?**
   It is the nature and degree of resistance to displacement as offered by an anatomic unit for effecting a tooth movement.
   Classify anchorage; and define simple, stationary, reciprocal, single, compound, multiple/reinforced, inter maxillary/ intra maxillary; intraoral; extraoral; muscular and cortical anchorages.

2. **Why it is not possible to move the ankylozed teeth?**
   Because for a tooth to move, a viable PDL is required so that the biochemical changes can take place. In an ankylosed tooth, a part of PDL gets fused with the bone and so a tooth cannot move.

3. **How does the implant serve as the anchorage source?**
   Implant does not have any PDL, but gets engaged with the bone through osseointegration, similar to an ankylozed tooth and so they cannot move even under heavy force, so the implants are very good anchorage.

4. **What do you mean by muscular anchorage?**
   Perioral ms can be used as a source of anchorage for effecting the movement of teeth, e.g. lip bumper uses force of lower lips to distalize or to upright the lower molars.

5. **What is Baker's anchorage?**
   When anchorage of one arch is used to cause movement in the opposite arch, it is ka Baker's anchorage, e.g. class II, and III intermaxillary elastics.

6. **What is meant by the cortical anchorage?**
   According to Rickettes, when the roots of lower molars are torqued in the buccal cortical plate of mandible under heavy forces, there occurs the hyalinization of PDL, which does not allow the mesial movement or the loss of anchorage due to heavy cortical bone. It acts as the cortical anchorage.

7. **What is the anchorage loss?**
   It is the unwanted movement of the anchor teeth during the orthodontic treatment. It is observed by mesial tilting of the molars, labial movement of the incisors, etc.

8. **What are the anchorage savers?**
   These are the modalities applied during treatment so as to avoid the loss of anchorage under the forces, e.g. head gear, transpalatal arch, lingual holding arch, Nance's palatal arch, etc.

SELF-ASSESSMENT QUESTIONS

1. What are the signs of anchorage loss?
2. What are the anchorage values as provided by the upper and lower teeth?
3. What do you mean by Group A, B and C anchorage?
4. What do you mean by extraoral anchorage?
5. How do you obtain anchorage in treatment a removable appliance?
6. What factors/methods can be used for preserving the anchorage during orthodontic treatment?

21

Age Factor in Orthodontics

INTRODUCTION

Orthodontic patients are from different age groups. Previously, most of the patients belonged to adolescent and early age. With increased esthetic concerns, better facilities, tooth-colored braces and increased affordability, now the late adult group patients also seek orthodontic treatment. Age of the patient is a very important consideration during orthodontic treatment planning, esp the biologic/skeletal age of young patients. It helps to decide the treatment modality, mechanics, and the prognosis.

Diagnosis

Diagnosis is the most important step during treatment planning. To differentiate the abnormal conditions requiring treatment, the knowledge of normal developmental sequence or conditions of that particular age is of paramount importance. Certain developmental stages are normal for a particular age, but they appear abnormal features to the anxious parents. These features are called self-correcting anomalies or the transient malocclusion. These features appear during normal development of dentition and should not be disturbed, as they disappear themselves with future development. Some of such features of transient malocclusion have been discussed in details in the Chapter 8 on Development of Dentition. These are:

a. Anterior open bite in gum pad stage
b. Physiological spacing in primary dentition
c. Primate spacing
d. Ugly-duckling stage
e. Anterior deep bite
f. Mild lower incisal crowding
g. Flush terminal plane relation, etc.

Determining the age of the patient: Age can be determined by the chronological age, i.e. from the date of birth; the dental age, i.e. status of dental development; the skeletal age, i.e. the stages of various bone development or skeletal markers. The chronological age is misleading and does not give exact growth status of the patient. Also the dental age does not significantly match with the growth status of the patient, since some patients have delayed dentition while others have fast dentition. It is calculated by studying the stage of calcification and root development of teeth. The stage of calcification of mandibular second molar and canines have been found to be a reliable marker of skeletal age. The best method to determine the growth status of the patient is the skeletal age or bone age or the biological age. It is determined by studying the various stages of development of certain bones and the ossification centres, which develop according to a particular pattern. The common methods to study skeletal age are certain bones of wrist; the CVMI status; and certain phalangeal stages from hand-wrist X-rays, which have been discussed somewhere else in the book.

Correlation of Age and the Treatment

Growth modulating appliances, e.g. FJO, headgear, reverse facemask and chin cup, and expansion appliance work best during active growth for stable results. The knowledge of growth status of the patient is very important for treatment planning and success of treatment. Ensuing growth can be used beneficially to provide the best treatment. The growth modification can help to achieve normal skeletal relationship of the jaws. Benefits can be enumerated as follows:

1. **Role of age in expansion:** Expansion of upper jaw is stable when it is achieved during growth phase. It is generally during the age range of 9 and 11 years in females and males respectively. Since the growth of face in transverse dimension gets completed at an early age, thus any intervention should be done during the active growth spurt phase. During early age, the midpalatal suture is soft and not much interdigitated, which can be opened easily with lighter forces, and stable results can be achieved. Even the tooth movement achieved is bodily at young age. But with increased age, mostly the tipping occurs due to expansion which leads to relapse.
2. **Preventive and interceptive treatment:** Abnormal growth can be redirected to achieve a more favorable jaws relation. It helps to reduce the severity of the condition, and further complex orthodontic and orthognathic surgical interventions, e.g. skeletal class III due to mandibular prognathism can be intercepted at an early age by chin cup appliance to redirect the mandibular growth. It helps in reducing the severity of this condition by inhibiting the excessive growth and thus the requirement of future orthognathic surgery.
3. **Proper dentition development:** The normal direction of dental eruption in mesial and occlussal direction can be used for proper guidance of erupting teeth to a more factorable position, e.g. during the use of functional appliances, certain areas of acrylic are relieved so that the teeth can be guided to proper direction and position.
4. **Growth modification:** Certain skeletal conditions resulting due to abnormal direction and amount of growth can be improved by modifying the future growth. Functional appliances can be used to redirect mandibular growth in skeletal class II cases due to mandibular retrognathism. However, such interceptive treatments should be started during the active growth periods. Other procedures are reverse face mask to treat maxillary deficiency; chin cup to control excessive mandibular growth; and headgear to control excessive maxillary growth.
5. **Self-esteem:** Malocclusion leads to disturbed esthetics and psychological distress, an early treatment can help in improving the self-esteem of the child.
6. **Late treatment:** If the treatment is taken after the growth is over, the skeletal improvement is limited, and only the dental improvement can be achieved. It involves following disadvantages:

(a) Role of growth: One of the most influential factors during treatment is the presence or absence of growth. Mild to moderate orthodontic and orthopedic changes can be achieved during active growth period since the young bones and soft tissues are more adaptable to changes and the results achieved are more stable. But, certain severe skeletal problems should be treated only by surgery after the growth has ceased. Because if they are treated by surgery during growth period, then the ensuing growth can lead to its reappearance needing another surgery after growth has ceased.

Active growth helps to attain a more normal skeletal relation. During active growth, the soft tissues also get better adapted to new position of basal bones and teeth, and help in stability of results. But, certain malocclusion can only be treated when growth is over, e.g. conditions requiring extensive orthognathic surgery like severe skeletal class III cases due to excessive mandibular prognathism or maxillary deficiency, should be treated after growth is over, otherwise continuing growth can lead to re-appearance of pre-treatment condition, which may require re-surgery.

(b) Limited treatment options: During active growth, different modalities can be used for intercepting the malocclusion and redirecting abnormal growth, e.g. functional appliances, dentofacial orthopedics, expansion and eruption guidance. But after growth is over, only dental movement and surgical options remain to be given to the patient, e.g. a skeletal class II with increased overjet can be treated with FA during growth, but after growth only options remaining are either reducing overjet by extraction of teeth and retraction of anteriors or by orthognathic surgery with maxillary set back or mandibular advancement.

(c) Compromised treatment objectives and non-ideal results: Since in adult patients, the growth has ceased, the ideal objectives of treatment, i.e. function, esthetic and stability cannot be fully achieved. So compromise has to be made during the treatment. A fully comprehensive orthodontic treatment cannot be given to the adult patients. In adult patients, orthodontic treatment helps to achieve reasonable, realistic goals to achieve best possible esthetic and functional results. However, if orthognathic surgery can be combined with orthodontic therapy, better esthetic, functional and stable results can be achieved in adults.

EFFECT OF AGE ON THE OTM

With age, various changes appear in the tissues of body. Growth of the bones decreases and later ceases completely to unappreciable quantity. Bone density increases with age, leading to decreased vascularity of the periodontium. So, the OTM is also affected.

Bone density: Bone density increases due to increased calcification, and number of osteogenic cells decreases with age. The tooth movement is slower in adults as compared to adolescents. It is due to slow start of biochemical changes and thus initiation of tooth movement is slow due to changes in periodontium, but once the OTM starts in adults, it progresses at a rate almost equal to the adolescents. Special care is taken regarding the level of forces. Lighter forces are used with larger intervals between activation in adults. Chances of root resoprtion are more in adults than youngs.

Tissue vitality: Since the young patients have more vascularity and cellularity of the periodontium, the initiation of biochemical changes is faster in adults. Thus, the rate of OTM is more in youngs.

Apical foramen: Apical foramina of adult teeth are small as compared to youngs, the orthodontic forces can cause damage to neurovascular bundles, root resorption, etc. of such teeth more commonly as compared to the teeth with wider foramina. There are also more chances of recovery of any damage occurred to the pulp or root of tooth in young patients as compared to adults.

Comparison of Young Patient to Adult Patients

Adult patients seek orthodontic treatment for various purposes, e.g. to improve esthetics, function, to achieve better relation of teeth to have better prosthesis; and better maintenance of oral hygiene. But, there exist many differences among young and the adult patients.

Absence of appreciable growth: Since in adults, there is no appreciable growth, there are limited treatment options available for adults. In youngs, the functional and orthopedic appliances can be used to achieve better skeletal relations. But in adults, the treatment options are OTM and surgical only.

Periodontal conditions: Adults have generalized periodontal disease leading to compromised bone support in certain areas of dental arches. Lighter forces are used in adults, as heavy forces can lead to bone loss and mobility of teeth. Presence of active periodontal infection makes the bone more susceptible to resorption, leading to rapid bone loss. Also anchorage loss is more in such teeth.

Diagnosis: Adults may show various problems like impacted teeth, some pathological conditions, wear and tear of teeth, bone loss and faulty restorations. These factors affect the treatment plan and the results. They may also have multiple missing teeth, with changed axial inclination and occlusal levels of the teeth. Treatment may involve RCT, occlusal reduction, bone grafting, etc.

Appliance design and selection: In young patient, advantage of growth can be taken by using functional and orthopaedic appliances for skeletal changes. But in adults, only OTM and surgical options are feasible. Since lighter forces are required in the adult patients due to increased bone density, the lighter wires are used, with increased gap between appointments.

Esthetic consideration: Generally, the adults come with a complaint of esthetics. So they do not approve the metallic braces and thus require tooth-colored braces and/or lingual appliances.

Cooperation and motivation: Adult patients are more cooperative and are self-motivated for the treatment as compared to children.

Tissue vitality: There are more chances of loss of vitality of tooth in adults than the youngs, due to increased bone density and decreased cellularity and vascularity of the tissues.

Treatment objectives: Ideal objectives are difficult to achieve in adults by simple orthodontics, since there is no growth. But better results can be achieved by surgical treatment.

Treatment appreciation: Adults appreciate the treatment results more than youngs.

Conclusion

Age at the time of treatment holds a particular importance during the treatment planning of the patient. Due to increased demand on esthetics, the adult patients also seek orthodontic treatment. But, there is no appreciable growth in them. Treatment in young age takes advantage of active growth and helps in skeletal improvement. Growth consideration is taken during treatment and it helps in treatment planning. Surgical options for severe skeletal conditions are reserved for postgrowth periods to avoid relapsing of condition due to ensuing abnormal growth.

22

Methods of Gaining Space

INTRODUCTION

Most of the problems in orthodontics are related with space deficiency due to many reasons. These conditions, e.g. unraveling the crowding, leveling the curve of Spee, retraction of proclined teeth, derotation of anterior teeth, etc. need spaces during treatment. Depending on the TSALD, soft tissue and growth factors, the clinician evaluates the space requirement of the case. Depending on TSALD, the case can be non-extraction type, borderline type or extraction type. A non-extraction type case may need some space in the dental arches for alignment of teeth. The borderline case may fall in extraction or non-extraction category depending on its skeletal and soft tissue factors.

There are various procedures through which a clinician can gain the space during the orthodontic treatment, which can be grouped as:

A. **Conservative methods:** For example, expansion, molar distalisation, uprighting of the molars/premolars; derotation of posterior teeth; proclination of incisors.

B. **Non-conservative methods:** Extractions; proximal stripping/slicing.

These methods are described below.

I. Expansion

Arch expansion is the method of increasing the transverse dimension of the dental arches. Arch augmentation is another term which is used when the dimension of the arch is increased in saggital dimension by proclination of the incisors. Both the procedures help us to gain the space. However, a proper indication should exist to perform the procedure, so that the stable results can be achieved.

Expansion is usually done in the narrow, constricted V-shaped arches. It is most stable when done during the period of growth. It is mostly indicated in upper arch, and then the lower arch is articulated to the upper arch during treatment. Best age of arch expansion is during the mid- and late-mixed dentition period, when the maxilla is undergoing transverse growth, e.g. in maxillary arch, it can be done at around 9–11 years age to achieve skeletal changes. In females, it should be done earlier than males. During this age, the growth of maxillary intercanine width, and erupting canine helps to achieve skeletal effects. It can also be done till late ages but then dental changes are more as compared to skeletal changes, e.g. till the interdigitation and fusion of midpalatal suture.

But in mandible, skeletal effects cannot be achieved since there is no patent suture. Any attempt of expansion leads to dentoalveolar expansion. It should be avoided as it is not stable if intercanine width is increased esp after 9 years of age. If an increase in width or intercanine width is needed in mandible, then it needs a permanent retention to stabilize it.

In adult patients, the skeletal effects can be achieved by RME/SARPE in which the palatal suture has already interdigitated. Dentoalveolar effects can be achieved by slow expansion, which will need prolonged retention. Recently, methods, like distraction osteogenesis and surgical splitting of palate, etc., have been used successfully for expanding mandible, maxilla, etc. even after growth has ceased, but these methods always need prolonged retention period for stability and for reorganization of soft tissues.

Types of expansion: Expansion can be of three types: (1) slow, (2) rapid and (3) semi-rapid.

Slow expansion: As the name suggests, it is a method of attaining expansion slowly over a period of time. As Proffit has described, it results in dentoalveolar changes and skeletal changes in the ratio of 1:1, especially if it is done when active growth is taking place. But, in adults, the changes are mainly dental. Expansion helps to gain different amount of space in the different segments of dental arches. Studies have shown that it helps to gain 1 mm, 0.5 mm and 0.25 mm space per mm of expansion in canine, premolar and molar region, respectively. There are various methods of expansion used in orthodontics, the details have been described in the chapter of expansion.

Active Plate with Jack Screw

It is the most commonly used removable appliance having an expansion screw as active element, with clasps for proper retention. Screw is opened with a key which separates the sections of the plate. Amount of movement is controlled but force is heavy that decays rapidly. Screw opens 0.8–1.0 mm per complete turn or approx. 0.2 mm in a single quarter turn (i.e. 0.1 mm per side). This activation is within the limits of the width of PDL and thus the PDL remains viable. For SME, the screw should be opened 2–3 times in a week and single quarter turn each time. The rate of active tooth movement should not exceed 1 mm per month (expansion 1 mm per month bilaterally). The plate can be modified by designing the splits for anterior expansion, transverse expansion, and anteroposterior expansion (Y-plate).

Coffin springs: It was designed by Walter Coffin. It is an omega-shaped loop made of 1.0–1.25 mm thick SS wire, adapted on the palate. It extends from the mesial half of first premolar to the line joining the distal surfaces of first permanent molars, opening mesially. It is activated by expanding the sides out with the help of a three-pronged pliers. It can be used as fixed or removable design.

Quad helix: It is made of hard SS wire of 0.9–1.0 mm diameter. It has four helices (2 anterior and 2 posterior) for the flexibility of wire. Its parts are anterior bridge, i.e. the wire between anterior helices, the palatal bridge, i.e. the wire between anterior and posterior helices. Outer arms are the free wire ends adjacent to the posterior helices adapted on the palatal aspects of premolars and canines on both sides, and is soldered to the lingual aspect of molar bands. It can be modified with the outer arms extending to opposite sides of lateral incisors, thus causing expansion and anterior proclination of incisors. It helps in expansion as well as correction of rotation of molars.

It is activated for anterior expansion by opening posterior helices, and for posterior expansion by opening anterior helices.

Arch expansion by fixed appliances: Expanded archwires are used thus causing dentoalveolar expansion. Quad helix or TPA can be used in association with fixed mechano-therapy.

II. Molar Distalization

It is the movement of molars especially the upper molars in a distal direction. Molars are distalized for improvement of the relationship of upper and lower molars. It is generally done when maxillary first molar has migrated mesially after premature loss of primary second molars, thus causing a mild class II molar relation. It also helps to create space especially in upper arch, which is used for alignment of premolars or canines. Best time to achieve this movement is usually before eruption of permanent second molars, as the movements are easier and faster due to soft bones and non-interference of second molars; and there is less anchorage taxing.

It can also be done in patients with erupted second molars, but there it takes a lot of anchorage preparation; and more time is needed. Microimplants can be used for such a purpose. It can help to gain approx. 4–5 mm space per side, i.e. molar can be distalised by a full cuspal width.

Methods and Appliances of Distalization

There are various methods of molar distalization. These can be extraoral or intraoral methods. The appliances can be removable of fixed type. Distalizaton can be done on one or the both sides of the arch. In mandible, the bodily molar distalization cannot be achieved, but only the uprighting can be achieved to gain some space. It is due to cortical bone and the external oblique ridge of mandible, that bodily distalization of lower molars is difficult.

i. Extraoral methods: Head gears (head cap or neck strap) are attached to the outer bow of face bow, inner bow of face bow is attached to the buccal tube on the molars. Intermittent force is applied. Patient cooperation is essential. Also, J-hooks with headgear can be used with intervening open coil spring on a full fixed orthodontic appliance, to apply the distalizing force on molars.

ii. Intraoral methods: They can be removable or fixed type of appliances.

1. Removable split pate and jack screw.
2. **Magnets:** Distalization can be done by using repelling magnets. Magnets are placed on tooth to be distalized and on the mesial tooth with facing the same polarities, thus causing a repulsive force. Anchorage on the mesial tooth is reinforced by using a Nance holding arch.
3. **NiTi open coil spring:** A sufficient length of NiTi OCS is compressed between tooth to be distalized and the mesial tooth. Whole arch is bonded with fixed appliance and the anchorage is reinforced with Nance's holding arch or with microimplants.
4. **Pendulum appliance:** A lingual sheath is welded on the palatal aspect of band on the tooth to be distalized. The spring with a helix is made of 0.032" TMA wire and is inserted in the acrylic button placed in the rugae area. The bands are also made on the first premolars and wires are welded and included in the acrylic button. Active arm of spring is forcefully engaged in the sleeve.
5. Distal jet appliance; Jones jig; K-loop distalizer; Keles slider; multi-distalizing arch (MDA); titanium twin force appliance; Lokar's appliance; Carriere's distaliser, etc. are other appliances used for distalization, the details of which are out of the scope of this book.

III. Uprighting of Molars

During the space loss, the molar gets mesially tipped. By uprighting the molar, certain amount of space can be recovered. It can be done by uprighting spring of regainer; by T-loop in the archwire; or by including anchor or tip-back bends in the arch wires.

IV. Derotation of Posterior Teeth

During space loss after the loss of adjacent tooth or premature loss of a primary adjacent tooth, the adjoining teeth shift in the extraction space and get mesiolingually rotated, which reduces the arch length. It is due to the trapezoidal shape of molars/premolars, thus the width at its diagonal is more as compared to that between mesial and distal contact areas. The rotated posterior teeth occupy more space thus creating TSALD, because their hypotenuse is longer than their MD or BL dimension. Space can be gained by derotation of posterior teeth. It can be achieved by using a force couple; by using TPA/LHA, NiTi palatal expander; quad helix, etc.

V. Proclination of Anterior Teeth

Incisors can be proclined so that they can be arranged along an increased arch circumference, thus providing the extraspace. This can be done in case of retroclined incisors, e.g.

in class II division 2 cases; and in cases of upright anteriors and concave profile. Judgment should be made that proclined incisors do not encroach on the lips/soft tissue, otherwise that position is unstable due to a continued lingual force by lips on the incisors, thus needing a permanent retention. Also, the labial alveolar plate thickness should be considered to avoid any gingival and alveolar recession on the labial side during proclination.

VI. Proximal Stripping

It is the process of removal of enamel from the proximal surfaces of the teeth. It is also called disking/slenderization/reproximation/proximal slicing. It is used to reduce MD dimension of those teeth which seem to be wider than the normal dimensions. Wider teeth create a space discrepancy, which can be best judged by Bolton's analysis and Peck and Peck ratio. It can be done in any segment of the dental arch but mostly it is done on lower anteriors.

Incisor irregularity of 3–4 mm is often present in early mixed dentition. Procedures like preservation of leeway space, selective disking and extraction of primary teeth are used to gain some space to help correct a shortage of space for the permanent incisors. Disking of primary teeth is generally used during early dentitional development for improved alignment of erupting teeth, and may also be used before a decision is made to either initiate a serial extraction or nonextraction therapy. Mesial stripping of the primary canines provides space for lateral incisors; and the maintenance of primary canines in dental arch aids in the natural expansion of the intercanine width during eruption of permanent canines. Interproximal enamel reduction may be used in adult patients with crowding, where extraction of teeth is not an option.

Indications

- It is indicated when there is minimal space requirement for alignment of teeth. So, it helps in avoiding the extractions.
- It also helps in lower anteriors as an aid to retention, since the contact areas become flatter and thus do not slip away.
- It helps to achieve better alignment or to maintain the corrected alignment after treatment over a long time.
- It is also done in cases of tooth material discrepancy between upper and lower arches (based on Bolton's analysis). So, it helps in determining the amount of stripping required in upper and/or lower arches to create mutual proportional balance.
- Any discrepancy in the ratio of MD and BL diameter of lower incisors as determined by Peck and Peck ratio, may also be helpful to determine requirement of stripping of lower incisors.
- It can help to improve the incisal relations. In some cases, the buccal occlusion is in excellent intercuspation, but the maxillary anterior teeth need to be retracted slightly to establish incisal contact. Some space in the upper anteriors can be gained by stripping, in which the maxillary anterior teeth can be moved distally to an acceptable incisal relationship.

It needs to be done to improve the shape of incisors. In some cases, the MD width of incisors is wider at contact areas. Also the contact areas are present more incisally which leads to creation of black triangles, which are not adequately filled by gingival papillae. By slicing, these contact areas can be brought slightly cervically thus decreasing the size of black triangles and giving better shape to incisors and better esthetic effects. It also helps to gain space and may be used for minor relocation of incisors.

Contraindications

- It is generally not indicated in severe arch length-tooth size discrepancy, where extractions are required.
- It should not be done in patient with increased susceptibility to caries.

- It should not be done in young patients having large pulp chambers.

Advantages of Proximal Stripping

- In minor TSALD cases, it helps in avoiding the extraction in the borderline cases, as some of the space can be gained by other means also for alignment.
- It also helps in flattening the contacts of anteriors and thus helps in retention by preventing the slippage of contact points.
- With proper alignment and eliminating TSALD, it may help in establishing favorable overjet and overbite.

How to Diagnose for the Requirement of Stripping

Arch length analysis: TSALD of upto 2.5 mm as done by Carey's method is an indication of stripping.

Peck and Peck ratio: Peck and Peck developed their index of the ratio of MD/FL dimensions of lower incisors, to determine whether a lower incisor is favourably or unfavourably shaped to achieve good lower anterior alignment. The following ranges were given by them for MD/FL index values for the lower incisors: 88% to 92% for the mandibular central incisor and 90% to 95% for the mandibular lateral incisor. Enamel reduction of lower incisors helps in adjusting sizes and values to within these ranges.

Bolton's analysis: Overall ratio and anterior ratio help to calculate the excess of tooth material in upper or lower arches. Minimal discrepancy can be corrected by stripping. Bolton's ratios are the anterior ratio (mean 77.2 ± 1.65%; range 74.5–80.4%) and the overall ratio (mean 91.3 ± 1.9%; range 87.5–94.8%) of tooth-size differences between the mandibular and maxillary mesiodistal sizes. Interproximal enamel reduction helps to correct the ratio to ensure well-aligned and properly occluding dentitions. Also, it may even indicate the feasibility of extracting one lower incisor.

IOPA and bitewing views: They help to find the enamel thickness and a rough estimate of the enamel that can be removed on each surface of the tooth without exposing the pulp chamber. It also helps to evaluate the proper orientation of the proximal surfaces of teeth, to maintain the interproximal bone and papilla in healthy condition.

Guidelines for Stripping

In literature, the guidelines for stripping have been published, which help to guide the clinician to achieve best effect. These are:

- The interdental reduction is limited to 1mm per contact point.
- Proper diagnosis and planning is done, and thus the clinician should measure and chart the accruing space.
- Enamel walls should be parallel.
- Proximal walls should be finished as smoothly as possible.
- The original contour and morphology of the teeth should be obtained.
- The new enamel should be treated with concentrated fluoride solution to replenish it in the newly created surface enamel.

Enamel Thickness Available for Reduction

Approximately 50% of interproximal enamel can be safely removed. Bitewing radiographs provide good information for the thickness of interproximal enamel. Stroud and others found that the enamel on second molars is thicker (by 0.3–0.4 mm) than enamel on the premolars. Also the distal enamel is thicker than mesial enamel. Assuming that 50% enamel reduction leaves adequate protection for the tooth, applying this procedure to the premolars and the molars should yield 9.8 mm of additional space for realignment of mandibular teeth.

Amount of proximal stripping: Amount of the enamel removal should be equally distributed among all the teeth in a segment requiring stripping. As a general rule, not more than 50% of enamel thickness or upto 0.25 mm of enamel should be removed from one surface.

How to Do It

It can be carried out with the help of mechanical method or chemical method:

1. Metallic abrasive strips.
2. Safe-sided carborundum disks.
3. Long thin tapered fissure burs.
4. Air rotor stripping (ARS)
5. Chemical stripping using 18% HCl or 37% o-phosphoric acid.

Arch length—tooth size discrepancy should not be more than 2.5 mm (arch perimeter analysis). Interarch tooth material discrepancy is assessed by Bolton's analysis. IOPA X-rays are taken to gauge the thickness of enamel.

Proximal stripping is done to reduce the enamel thickness not more than 50% of the total enamel thickness. To be on safer side, not more than 0.25 mm of enamel should be removed per surface of the tooth. It should be done in a segment of the arch involving multiple teeth equally distributing the amount of slicing. Under LA, a segment of 0.8 mm brass wire is inserted below the contact area to avoid injury to the dental papilla during slicing with a bur, under copious irrigation with water to avoid thermal pulp injury.

Spontaneous remineralization of the enamel has been found to occur after approximately 9 months. A mechanical stripping procedure combined with the chemical action of 37% phosphoric acid produced enamel surfaces that encouraged "self-healing" on the basis of remineralization enhanced by the application of fluoridating or remineralizing solutions.

Fluoride varnish should be applied on the teeth to replenish the newly created enamel surface with fluoride to make is caries resistant. Patient should be advised to use fluoridated tooth paste or mouth-wash for at least 3 months.

Drawbacks

- It alters the morphology of teeth, which gives unesthetic appearance.
- If not done properly especially in lower incisors which have less width, it may lead to sensitivity or pulpal irritation.
- It may also lead to loss of contacts if not done properly, leading to food impaction and further caries or gingival problems.
- It creates the roughened proximal surfaces also result in plaque accumulation thus causing caries and periodontal disease.
- It may also cause sensitivity of teeth.
- It leads to loss of surface layer of enamel which is rich in fluoride, thus the new surface is more susceptible to caries.

Fluoride application after stripping: It is very important since removal of surface layer rich in fluoride leads to increased caries-susceptibility. So, fluoride varnish should be applied immediately after stripping and the patient should be advised to use fluoride tooth paste and mouth wash for at least 3 months.

VII. Extractions in Orthodontics

It is a very common method to gain space during orthodontic treatment for alignment and leveling; and retraction of proclined teeth. Extraction of one or more teeth may be required during treatment. Such extractions are called as therapeutic extractions. It is generally used in cases of high TSALD. It can be used in borderline cases which have vertical growth, very little growth, abnormal soft tissue morphology.

During orthodontic treatment, the most common teeth extracted are first premolars; and sometimes single lower incisor. Third molars are removed because of their impaction or space discrepancy in posterior region. Other teeth may be needed to be extracted depending on the condition and prognosis of the tooth.

Serial extraction is an interceptive procedure to create spaces in the dental arches for the erupting permanent teeth, so that they can naturally align themselves during eruption. It is done in mixed dentition having a severe expected TSALD, and helps to reduce the severity of a potential developing condition.

Details of extractions in orthodontics, and the serial extraction have been discussed in separate chapters.

Conclusion

The pendulum of orthodontic treatment had swung from non-extraction philosophy of Angle, to the extraction philosophy of Tweed. However, recent trend is again toward the non-extraction methods of treatment as far as possible. Certain methods as described above can be used conservatively to gain spaces for alignment of teeth and correction of inter-relationship of the teeth, and thus avoiding the extractions.

23

Expansion in Orthodontics

INTRODUCTION

The malocclusion cases have a combination of features like crowding, protrusion, increased overjet, posterior cross bite, narrow dental/ skeletal bases, etc. To treat such conditions, mainly three methods are used to gain the spaces viz. extraction, interproximal reduction, and expansion, depending on the space requirements. Expansion is a conservative method of space gaining and it is an increase in the transverse dimension of jaw bases, the dental arch or a combination of both. The prime objective of expansion is to coordinate the maxillary and mandibular arches. Besides gaining the space, it is used to treat as an adjunctive procedure during face mask therapy also.

Historical Background

Various expansion techniques were employed by early dental practitioners like Fauchard (1728), Bourdet (1757), Fox (1803), Delabarre (1819), Robinson (1846), White (1859) with different rates of success. Emerson C Angell has been called as the father of rapid maxillary expansion (RME). The procedure originated in United State with Angell (1860) who placed a screw appliance between maxillary premolars of a girl age 14.5 years and widened her arch one quarter inch in 2 weeks. But, his findings could not be substantiated.

In 1877, Walter Coffin introduced coffin spring for arch expansion. This spring was believed to cause separation of midpalatal suture in young children. Angle was a proponent of non-extraction treatment, and hence he used the heavy expanded arch wires to expand the dental arches to align the teeth. According to him, all the teeth are needed in the dental arch for a normal occlusion.

Around the beginning of 20th century, ENT surgeons showed interest in this technique of orthopedic expansion of maxilla. In the late 1940s, Graber advocated RME for the treatment of cleft lip and palate patients. After demonstration of its potential in experimental animals, the method was reintroduced in the United States in the early 1960s by AJ Haas.

Indication for Expansion

1. It is done to widen the dental arch especially the upper arch if they are constricted.
2. It is also done to gain some space in the arches for alignment of teeth in mild discrepancy case.
3. It is done in cleft palate cases to achieve a normal arch shape and it also helps to find the exact defect in palate before the bone graft placement.
4. It is indicated in cases having active growth potential with patent midpalatal suture, in horizontal/normal growth pattern cases.

Contraindication

1. Patients having vertical growth pattern are not good candidates for expansion. It is because during expansion, the palatal cusps hang down, which lead to D and B rotation of mandible, leading to worsening of profile and increased face height.

2. Patients in whom active growth is not there, they get more dental effects rather than skeletal effects.
3. Some uncooperative patients are not good candidates for the appliances.

Advantages

1. It helps to gain the space in arches for teeth alignment.
2. It helps to increase the nasal volume thus decreases the resistance to respiration.
3. Fixed appliances help to derotate the molars, thus achieving better alignment and gaining the space.
4. RME helps to activate the circum-maxillary sutural system before reverse face mask therapy, and thus helps in better response with ful mask.
5. Helps in treatment of crossbite and thus prevents the functional deflections of lower jaw during closure. Thus, it helps in maintaining the health of TMJ.

Diagnosis and Treatment Planning for Cases with Transverse Discrepancy

A proper diagnosis is important before taking the decision of expansion. A visual examination is performed to determine the shape of arches, which generally gives a fair idea of need of expansion (Fig. 23.1). The facial and cranial patterns are also noted, since face width, cranial width, and dental arch width are positively correlated. A proper history is also taken to establish the cause, e.g. genetic, habits, trauma, etc. There are certain cast analyses which help us to determine the requirement and the amount of expansion needed. These are Pont's analysis, Linder Harth analysis, Ashley Howe's analysis, etc. PA cephalometric analysis by Rickett can be performed to determine the width of skeletal bases and any constriction of dental arches.

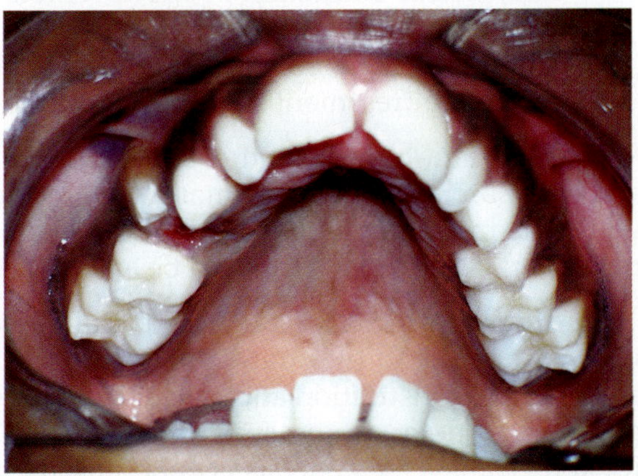

Fig. 23.1: V-shaped upper arch.

1. Pont's Analysis

Pont's analysis helps in determining whether the upper dental arch is narrow or normal; and whether there is a need for arch expansion. It is done by calculating the arch width in premolar and molar regions.

Method: MD size of four maxillary incisors is used to determine the ideal arch width in PM and molar areas. The steps are:

- Determination of sum of upper incisors (SI)
- Determination of calculated PM value (CPV)

$$= \frac{SI \times 100}{80}$$

- Determination of calculated molar value (CMV)

$$= \frac{SI \times 100}{64}$$

- Determination of measured PM value (MPV) which is measured from distal pit of first premolar of one side to distal pit of first premolar of other side.
- Determination of measured molar value (MMV) which is the width from mesial pit of first molar of one side to mesial pit of first molar of other side.

Results: The above values are compared. If calculated value is greater than measured value, then the expansion is required. If measured value is greater than calculated, then no expansion is required. The difference between these two values can determine how much expansion is needed. However, there exist racial differences and thus the same values cannot be used in every patient. It has been found from studies that Pont's analysis gives overestimation of the expansion needed.

2. Linder Harth Analysis

It is essentially the same procedure as Pont's analysis with a slight modification of Pont's analysis.

- Determination of CPV

$$\frac{SI \times 100}{85}$$

- Determination of CMV

$$\frac{SI \times 100}{65}$$

Results: If calculated value is greater than measured, expansion is required. If measured value is greater than calculated, then no expansion is required.

3. Ashley Howe's Analysis (1954)

It is done in maxillary arch only. It is a method to correlate the total tooth material with arch width in maxillary molar and premolar regions. The discrepancy is calculated to determine the need for expansion and treatment planning is done using this information.

Steps

- Determination of total tooth material (TTM): It is the sum of MD widths of 12 teeth from permanent first molar of one side to that of other side in maxillary arch.
- Determination of premolar diameter (PMD): It is the distance between the distal pits of first premolars.
- Determination of premolar basal arch width (PMBAW): It is measured intraorally, as the distance between the canine fossae just distal to the canine eminence / roots. If the canine fossa is not easily identifiable, then the measurement is done at a point 8 mm apical to the interdental papilla distal to canine. This gives the width of dental arch at the apical base, i.e. basal width of the maxillary jaw.
- These two values, i.e. PMBAW and PMD are compared.

Inferences: If PMBAW is more than PMD, the arch expansion is possible. It means that the dental arch is narrow and thus can be expanded within the limits of its skeletal base. This will give stable results and buccal teeth will not lose the torque.

If PMBAW is less than PMD, the arch expansion is not possible. It means that already the dental arch is of more width over a narrow skeletal base, and further attempt to widen the dental arch may lead to loss of torque. Here, the attempt may be done to achieve a skeletal expansion of the jaw bases with surgical procedures if needed absolutely depending on the case.

PMBAW ratio: It is called as the premolar basal arch width percentage. The ratio between the apical base width at the premolar region and the total tooth material is called the PMBAW percentage. According to them, to achieve a normal occlusion with full complement of teeth, the basal arch width in premolar region should be 44% of the TTM, i.e. MD size of 12 teeth.

$$\text{PMBAW \%} = \frac{\text{PMBAW} \times 100}{\text{TTM}}$$

a. If PMBAW% is 37% or less, it indicates a basal arch deficiency and there is need of extraction of teeth for correction.
b. If PMBAW% is 44% or more, then it is a non extraction case.
c. If PMBAW% is 37–44%, it is a borderline case, where extraction of first premolar is decided based on other factors of growth pattern, soft tissues, etc. Here, subjective treatment planning required.

If there is a crossbite and measurement across the arch show that the mandible is wide while the maxillary arch is normal, a skeletal mandibular discrepancy should be evaluated.

Radiographic analysis: PA cephalometric view can help to evaluate the symmetry, asymmetry, constriction and size of jaw bases and help in determining suitability for RME. Ricketts transverse analysis is generally used for this purpose.

Space gained by expansion: Arch expansion is done to create space during treatment of mild to moderate TSALD cases. If the upper arch can be considered roughly as a half circle till the first molar region, then approx 0.78 mm space can be gained with one mm of expansion. 1 mm of expansion of dental arch roughly leads to an increase of 0.5 mm space in canine region, 0.33 mm gain in premolar region and 0.2 mm gain in molar region. 1 mm increase in the arch width leads to a gain of 0.78 mm in the arch perimeter. (Formula of perimeter of circle is 2 πr. The dental arch can be considered as a half circle, so its arch perimeter will be πr. Now, an increase in the arch width, i.e. the expansion achieved, by 1 mm leads to gain of 0.78 mm arch perimeter, as r will be ½ of the expansion amount to calculate the arch perimeter by formula πr).

CLASSIFICATION OF EXPANSION

It can be classified as:

Depending on the rate of expansion: It is of three types: (1) slow expansion, (2) rapid expansion, and (3) semirapid expansion.

According to need of surgery for expansion: It may be surgically assisted RME (SARME/SARPE) in adult cases where the midpalatal suture has mostly intedigitated.

Depending on the type of appliance/force used: It may be active expansion and passive expansion.

Depending on the results achieved: McNamara has described the types of expansion produced can be divided arbitrarily into three categories, viz. orthodontic expansion; passive/physiologic expansion; orthopedic expansion.

1. Orthodontic Expansion

It can be produced by conventional fixed appliances and by various fixed or removable expansion appliances, etc. which usually results in lateral movements of the buccal segments. It is primarily dentoalveolar in nature, with lateral tipping of the crowns of the involved teeth and a resultant lingual tipping of roots. The resistance of cheek musculature and other soft tissues may lead to a relapse of the achieved orthodontic expansion.

2. Passive/physiologic Expansion

Here, no active forces or appliance is applied on the dental arches. When the forces of the buccal and labial musculature are shielded away from the dental arches, e.g. with the lip bumper, oral screen or FR-2 appliance of Frankel, bionator, etc. a widening of dental arches often occurs, due to physiological/intrinsic forces produced by tongue. Breiden, et al in an implant study demonstrated that bone deposition occurs primarily along the lateral aspect of the alveolus rather than at the midpalatal suture. A similar type of spontaneous arch expansion is also observed after lip bumper therapy, in which the lower anterior teeth come forward under the forces of tongue, thus helping to gain the space in anterior arch.

3. Orthopedic Expansion

Here, changes are produced primarily in the underlying skeletal structures rather than by the movement of teeth through alveolar bone. RME appliances are the best examples of true orthopedic expansion. RME separates the midpalatal suture and also affects the circumzygomatic and circummaxillary sutural systems. The new bone is deposited in the area of expansion and thus the integrity of the midpalatal suture usually is reestablished within 3 to 6 months .

Differences between Orthopedic and Orthodontic Forces

Orthodontic forces: These forces are lighter in nature which mainly leads to movement of teeth. Adaptive changes are seen in specific alveolar bone adjacent to moving teeth.

Orthopedic forces: These are heavy forces and result in major skeletal change occurring in basal structures of mandible and maxillae. It involves interaction between basal bone and alveolar bone.

Classification of Expansion Appliances

They can be broadly classified into:

I. **According to appliance attachment:**
   1. **Removable appliances**, e.g. active plate with jack screw, and functional appliances.
   2. **Fixed appliances:** They are of following two types:
      a. Tooth borne, e.g. Isaacson, Hyrax, Minn expander
      b. Tooth/tissue borne, e.g. Derichsweiler type, Haas type.

II. **According to the rate of expansion:**
   1. **Slow** (e.g. W-arch, quad helix, Coffin spring)
   2. **Rapid** (e.g. Hyrax, Minn, Isaacson)
   3. **Semi-rapid**

III. **Surgically assisted RPE.**

Differences between RME and SME: The main differences between RME and SME are given in Table 23.1.

SME is considered a better procedure as seen from the above table, because the end-result of both the procedures is the same, i.e. 1:1 achievement of dental and the skeletal effects. But, SME forces are within the safe and physiological limits without damaging the investing tissues and are comfortable to the patient. Thus, SME is better than the RME except under exceptional circumstances, e.g. where surgical splitting of palatal suture is required.

SLOW MAXILLARY EXPANSION

Slow expansion as the name suggests is the slow process for expanding the maxillary arch using lighter forces applied for a longer duration. A number of appliances have been used for this purpose. These appliances are removable appliance with Jack screw, quad helix, bihelix, W-arch, Coffin spring, NiTi palatal expander, etc. The objective of expansion is to widen the maxilla and not just to expand the dental arch by moving the teeth relative to the bone.

Originally RME was recommended to meet this goal. It was based on the theory that heavy forces applied to the teeth lead to development of hyalinized zones due to necrosis of PDL and thus do not give enough time for the tooth movement. Thus these forces would be transferred to the suture, and the suture would open up while the teeth move only minimally relative to their supporting bone. But, clinical experience and studies show that this procedure is painful and leads to more tissue damage.

Storey and Ekstrom suggested that slow expansion allows physiologic adjustment and reconstitution of sutural elements over a period of about 30 days. McAndrews

Table 23.1: Differences between RME and SME

S. no.	*Criterion*	*RME*	*SME*
1.	Opening/activation	0.5–1 mm /day 3.5–7 mm/week	1 mm/week
2.	Frequency of screw opening	90° 2 times/day	90°/2–3 days
3.	Forces generated	10–20 lbs	2–4 lbs
4.	Tissue damage	More	Less
5.	Skeletal : dental effects	8 : 2	5 : 5
6.	After 4 months of retention	5 : 5; relapse is more	5 : 5; relapse is less
7.	Pain during treatment	More	Less
8.	Development of midline diastema	Yes	No
9.	Midpalatal sutural opening (occlusal X-ray)	Seen	Not seen
10.	Active treatment time	Less	More
11.	Retention time needed	Long	Short
12.	Total treatment time	Almost same	Almost same

demonstrated that the application of light, continuous forces in the area of periosteal growth allows normal arch to develop at any age without undue tipping of the abutment teeth.

SME has also been associated with more physiologic stability and less potential for relapse than with RME. The time between subsequent activations is sufficient to maintain and repair the integrity of tissues. In RME, that time is very short. The slow expansion procedures increase the percentage of orthodontic movements because the effect on suture with lighter forces is not direct. The rate of expansion in slow expansion is 0.5–1 mm per week compared to about 0.5–1 mm per day with RME.

Slow expansion is achieved by activating the spring or screw to generate about 2 lbs of force, in contrast to about 10 lbs force with RME. Slow expansion that maintains tissue integrity apparently needs lesser period of retention, which is significantly shorter than for rapid expansion.

Best age of slow expansion is considered to be the early mixed dentition period, i.e. around 8–9 years of age. At that time, the maxilla is undergoing a phase of active transverse growth, the bones are softer, and there is adequate number of teeth in the arch esp permanent first molars, to give adequate retention. The RME can be reserved for the patients in whom the active growth has passed, and those who need a quick response to activate/open circum-maxillary sutural system before the reverse face mask therapy in maxillary deficiency cases.

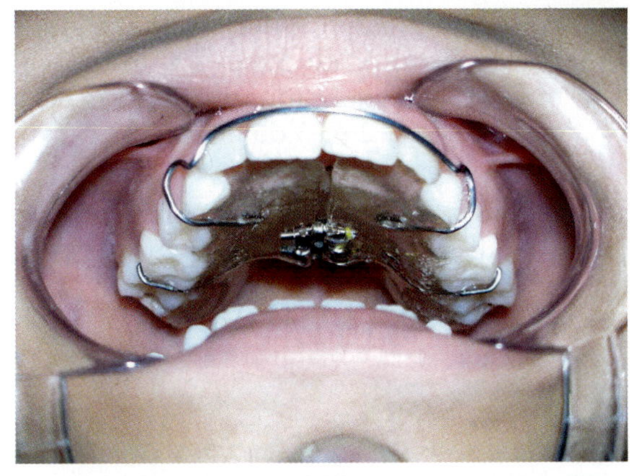

(a)

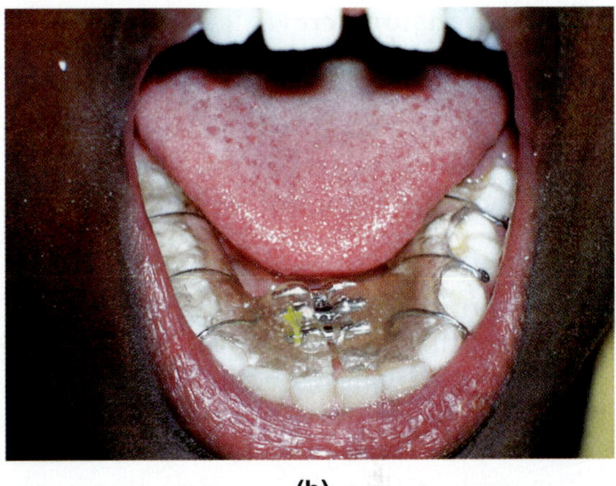

(b)

Figs 23.2a and b: Removable appliance with expansion screw in upper and lower arches.

Appliances Used for Slow Expansion

1. **Removable appliance with Jack screw:** It is a removable appliance made of acrylic, which has a Jack screw/E-screw in the center. The plate is split in two parts, joined together with the screw, so that these 2 parts are free to move on opening of the screw (Figs 23.2a and b). It also has retentive clasps to hold the plate in the dental arch firmly, and a labial bow may also be included which may help in simultaneous retraction of upper incisors. However, acrylic has to be removed from lingual side of upper incisors for that purpose. The screw is incorporated in the acrylic appliance separated in two halves. Multiple clasps are mandatory to provide adequate retention of appliance in the arch so that it does not get displaced during use, otherwise forces will not be applied properly. Because of the instability of the teeth during the expansion process, failure to wear the appliance even for one day requires back-adjustment of the jack screw. Most screws open 0.8–1 mm

per complete revolution, so that a single quarter turn produces 0.25 mm of tooth movement. The patients are advised to activate after 2 or 3 days (Fig. 23.3).

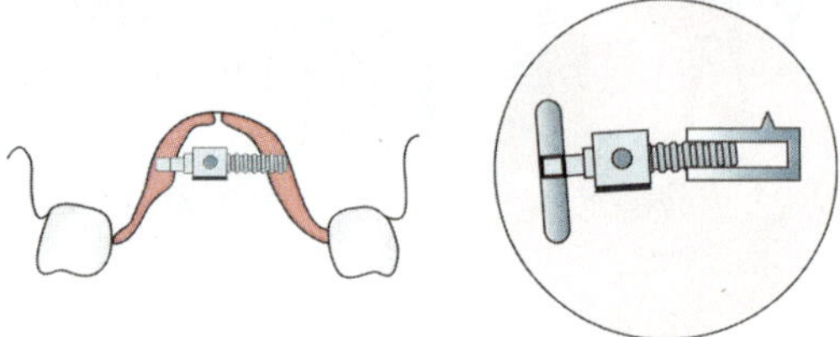

Fig. 23.3: Cross-section of the appliance and the screw. Note that the expansion screw is positioned parallel to the OP.

Expansion screw: It is an assembly made of stainless steel having 2 or 3 pins with sleeves and a screw. The screw has a neck in the centre, with 4 holes oriented at 90 degrees to each other. On activation, the pins and sleeves slide onto each other. There is a plastic arrow which determines the direction of opening/activation of the screw. Different designs and sizes of jack screws are available for specific purposes. The jack screw can be oriented in various fashions in the plate to achieve desired expansion (Figs 23.4 to 23.8). It may also be used to move the incisors labially to increase the arch length, e.g. in class II division 2 cases. Other uses of Jack screw can be distalisation of molars, or canines, expansion of lower arch, asymmetric widening of arches to correct cross bite, expansion in canine region only by putting a lock in distal end of the cut. 3D expanders are also available. Modified screws can be used to move single incisor labially, etc. (Figs 23.9a to c).

Pitch of the screw: It is the amount of opening achieved with full one turn/ 360° of the E-screw. It is approx. 0.8 mm. So with 90° turn, we achieve the 0.2 mm opening of the screw, i.e. 0.1 mm/side of the arch. Since the normal width of PDL is approx 0.22–0.25 mm, so with 90° opening, only 0.1 mm/side of the PDL is compressed and thus the health of the tissues is maintained under light forces. This activation produces forces which get quickly dissipated in the tissues and do not cause injury to the tissues (Figs 23.10a and b).

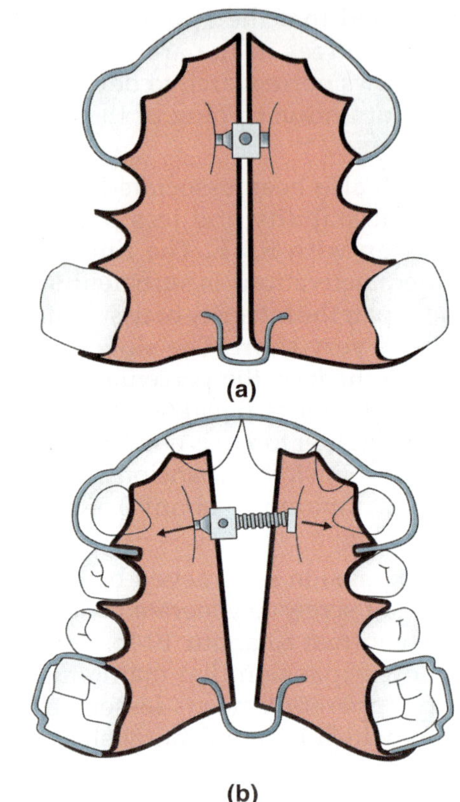

Figs 23.4a and b: Removable expansion appliance with a posterior stop, thus directing all the expansion force in the anterior region only.

2. **W-arch appliance:** It is a fixed appliance, and was designed by Porter, hence also called as Porter's appliance. A 0.032–0.036" hard s.s wire is bent in a W-shape and is soldered at bands placed on permanent first molars. Long length of the wire reduces the forces making them lighter and physiological. The appliance is activated enough before cementing. It works at an ideal force when 8–12 mm of activation is done to obtain dental and/ or orthopedic effects in deciduous and mixed dentition. It is kept 1–1.5 mm away from the palatal tissues and gingival tissues. It is activated by opening the

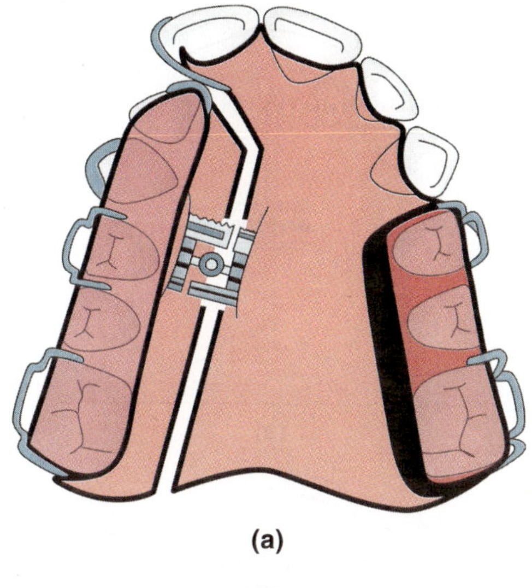

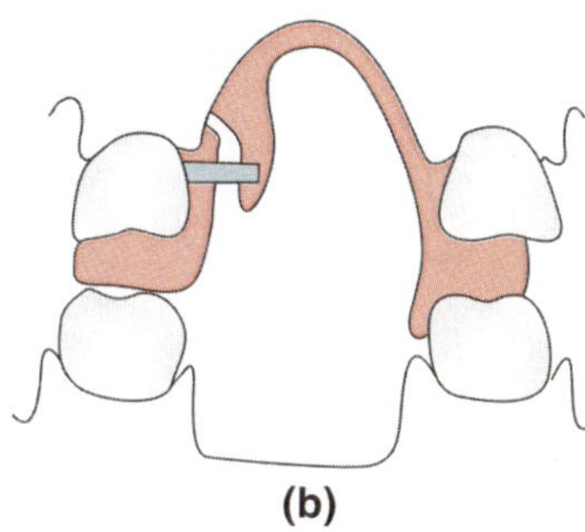

Figs 23.5a and b: Expansion of the buccal segment on one side. The bigger part of plate acts as anchorage and small part is the active part. In second fig, the interdigitated occlusal acrylic helps to block the movement of normal part from expanding, while on the treatment side, the acrylic has been smoothened to allow free buccal movement of segment to be expanded. However, occlusal acrylic is kept on both side to prevent the supraeruption of buccal teeth.

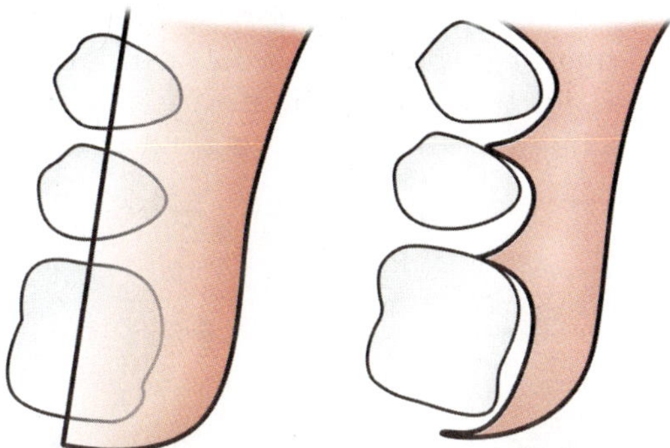

Fig. 23.6: Acrylic cover on the occlusal surfaces, while second figure shows the trimming of the acrylic in such a way so as to allow the distal tipping/shifting of the buccal teeth, thus gaining some space in the anterior segment.

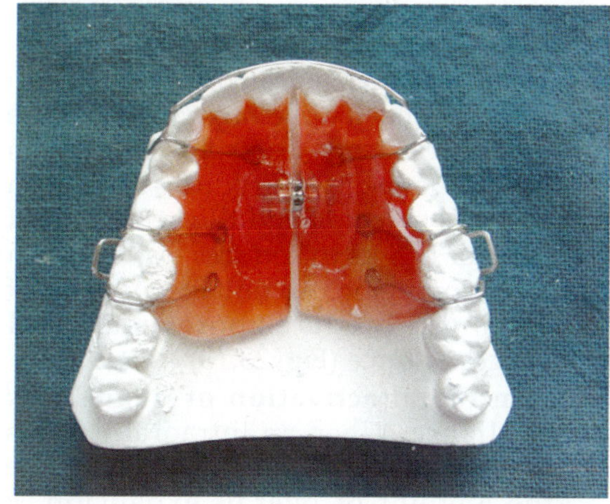

Fig. 23.7: Removable appliance for transverse expansion.

apices of the W-arch and can be easily adjusted to provide more anterior than posterior expansion or vice versa (Fig. 23.11).

3. **Bihelix appliance:** It is a modification of W-arch appliance in which two helices have been incorporated in the posterior region. They help to increase the length of wire to provide an increased range of activation and further reducing the forces. Also, they help in achieving a better activation by opening (Fig. 23.12).
4. **Quad helix appliance:** It is a modification of bihelix appliance in which 2 more helices have been incorporated but now in the anterior region. They also help to increase the length of wire and further reducing the forces. They help to increase the range of activation and yield more flexibility. It has been designed by Ricketts. Historically, Farrar and Coffin (1875) had suggested such appliances. The appliance is constructed of 0.40″ Blue Elgiloy wire. It is soldered to bands which are cemented to either the maxillary first permanent molar or the deciduous second molars, depending on the

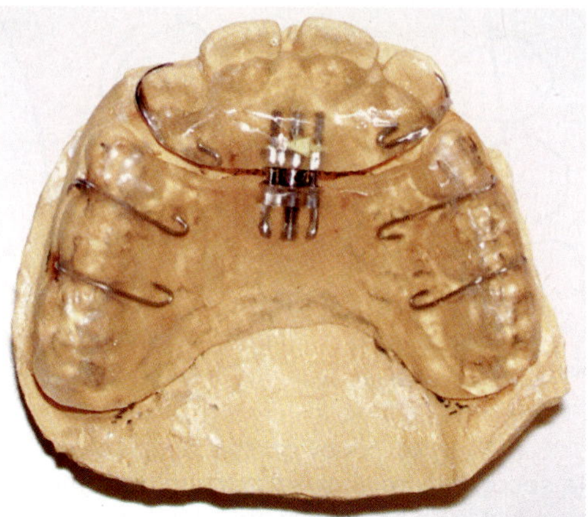

Fig. 23.8: Removable appliance for sagittal expansion or labial movement of upper incisors.

age of the patient or can be bent to fit into a lingual sheath. The lingual arm of the appliance extends to cuspids. Activation of posterior helices introduces expansion in anterior region and the activation of anterior helices introduces expansion in posterior region. An initial expansion of 8 mm will produce approximately 14 ounces of force (Fig. 23.13).

Intraoral activation of quad-helix appliance: When an intraoral bend is made in the anterior segment to increase the amount of overall expansion, a reciprocal bend must be made in the posterior section in order to compensate for the tendency for mesial rotation of the upper molars. Therefore, three intraoral adjustment bends are usually made at each activation.

5. **Coffin spring:** It was designed by Coffin and hence the name. It is an omega-shaped loop bent with a hard s.s wire of 1.25 mm thickness and is incorporated in a removable appliance. It is made extending from first premolar region to the mesial surface of permanent first molar, and kept 1–2 mm away from the soft tissues. The appliance is retained by means of Adam's clasps. Activation is done by using three prong pliers, by pressing the distal most area of the loop

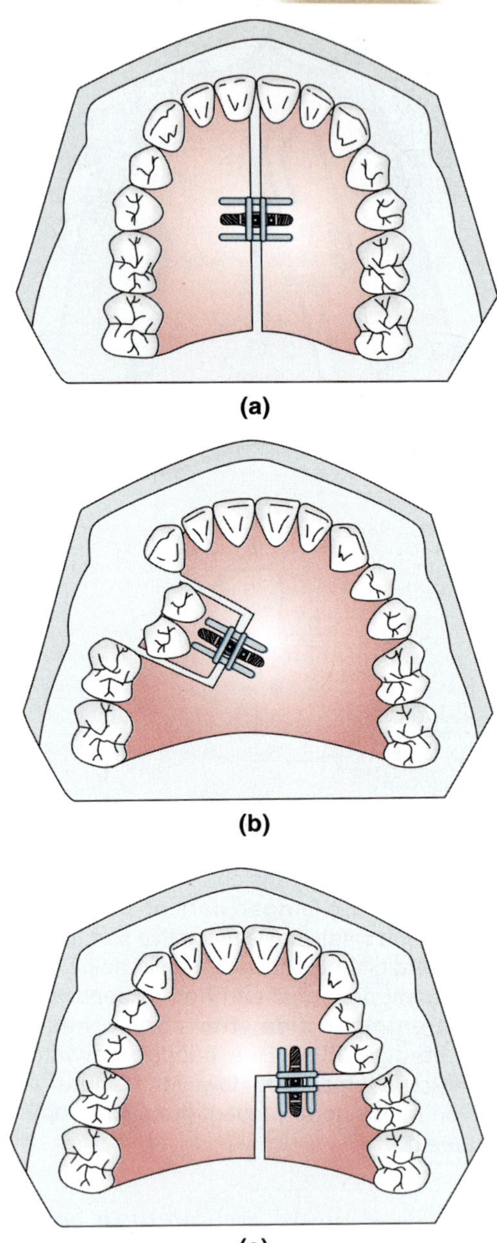

Figs 23.9a to c: Expansion appliances for: (a) Transverse expansion of the upper arch; (b) For buccal movement of premolar segment; (c) For distal movement of molars to gain space and to correct the molar relationship.

to open it laterally, thus widening the loop (Fig. 23.14).

6. **NiTi expander** (Figs 23.15 and 23.16): This is one of the recent advancements

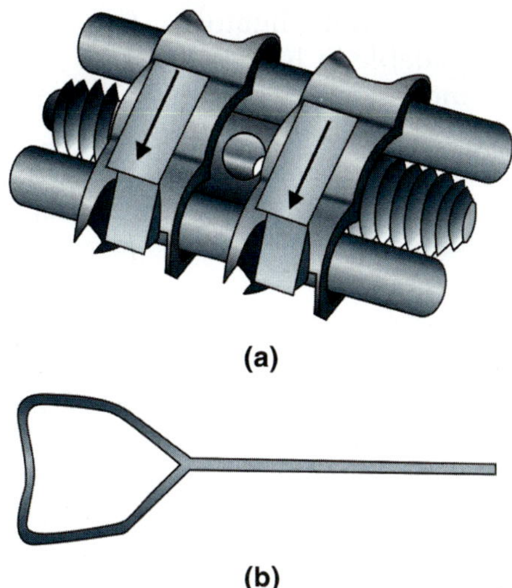

(a)

(b)

Figs 23.10a and b: Expansion screw and activation key. Note the hole to receive the activation key; and the arrow in which direction the screw has to be opened.

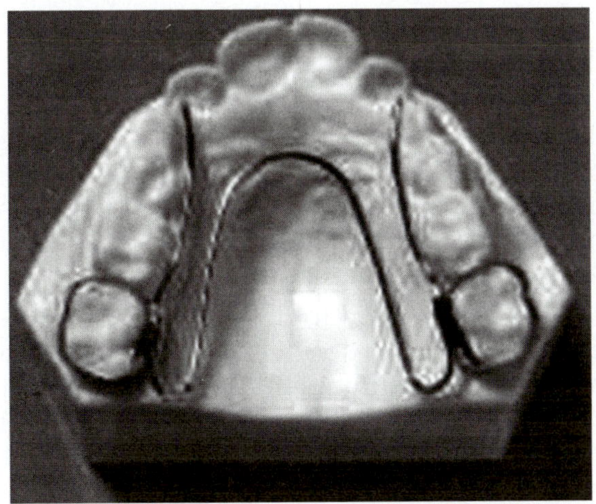

Fig. 23.11: W-arch appliance (Porter's) for slow expansion of upper arch *(Courtesy: Internet)*.

for expansion. It was designed by Arndt using nickel titanium's properties of shape memory and transition temperature to apply slow, continuous forces for maxillary expansion. This appliance expands at a rate that maintains tissue integrity during repositioning and remodeling of teeth and bone. It delivers a force of 350 g in 3 mm increments. Because the force of

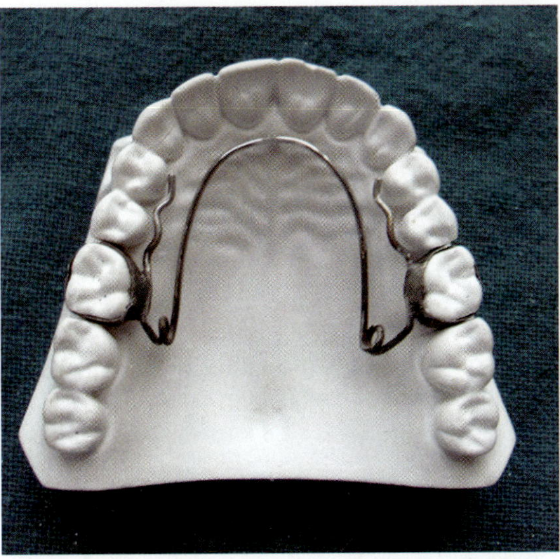

Fig. 23.12: Bihelix fixed expansion appliance.

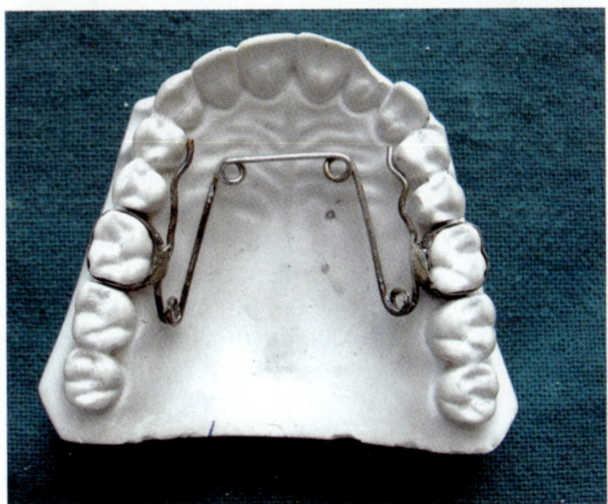

Fig. 23.13: Quad helix fixed expansion appliance.

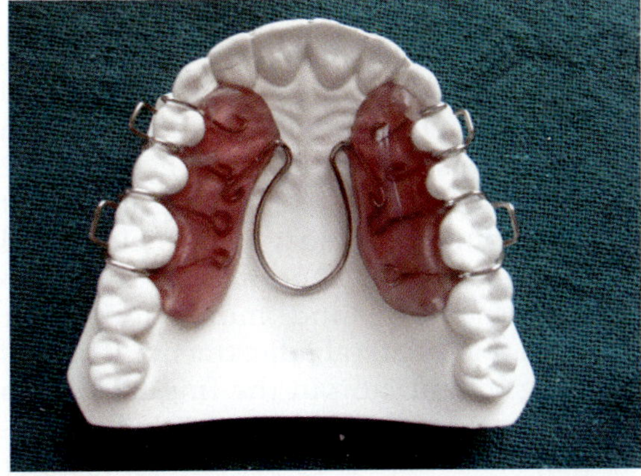

Fig. 23.14: Expansion appliance with Coffin's spring.

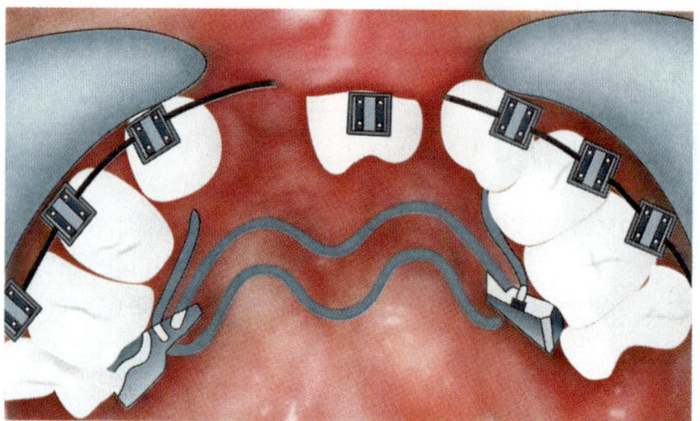

Fig. 23.15: Fixed NiTi palatal expansion appliance, NPE-1, in a case of cleft palate.

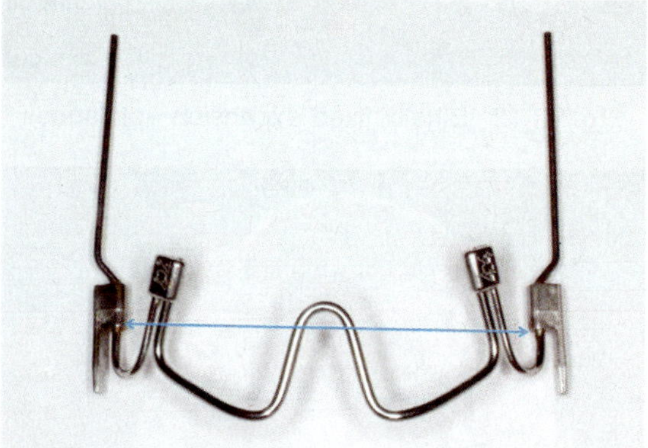

Fig. 23.16: NPE-2 appliance. Blue arrow shows the intermolar distance between the palatal surfaces *(Courtesy: Internet for illustration purpose only).*

appliance is pre-programmed, it is self-limiting. Nevertheless, slight adjustment can be made by the clinician at any time to constrict the appliance or add further expansion.

Design of NPE: It is available as two types: (1) NPE-1 and (2) NPE-2. It has 1–2 palatal springs made of NiTi which extend between the first molars (NPE1 has 2; NPE 2 has 1); 2 lateral arms made of SS extending form first molar to canine region adapted to their lingual surfaces; a lingual sheath attachment to receive assembly; and molar loops for unilateral and bilateral adjustments. There is a locking indentation in the lingual sheath which fastens the appliance securely to maxillary first molar bands. To prevent removal or accidental dislodging, the appliance should also be tied with the ligatures. The appliance, NPE is available in 10 sizes from 26 to 44 mm in 2 mm increments. A size that is 3 mm wider than the required width is selected. It also helps in derotation of molars to correct the molar relationship from mild class II to class I relation; and thus helps in gaining the space.

It generates optimal, light, uniform, continuous expansion forces. Its central part is made of thermally activated nickel titanium alloy. The rest of the appliance, including the anterior arms, is made of stainless steel. It can be used alongwith the fixed appliances. NiTi part has a transition temperature of 94°F. At room temperature, the expander is very stiff to bend for insertion. Chilling the expander with ice, or refrigerants like ethyl chloride or tetrafluoroethane, softens it, allowing easy manipulation. After placement, the expander regains its original shape under the influence of body temperature. A 3 mm increment of expansion exerts only about 350 g of force.

How to determine the needed size: As described by Arndt, the distance between the lingual grooves on the palatal side of permanent first molars at the gingival level is noted. To it, 3–4 mm for expansion and 2–3 mm for overexpansion is added.

Another method to determine the appropriate size as described by Nanda, is to measure the mandibular intermolar width at the central fossae. Because the mesiolingual cusps of maxillary molars occlude in these fossae, expansion to the mandibular intermolar width will provide optimal occlusion. If the mandibular molars are lingually inclined as a dental compensation for a skeletal posterior crossbite, as often occurs, it is appropriate to add another 1–2 mm to the expansion requirement. In any case, 2–3 mm should be added for overexpansion. In very narrow arch, 2 NPEs should be used, i.e. step wise expansion is done.

The rate of expansion depends on the age of the patient, because of interdigitation of midpalatal suture affects the response with increasing age. Patients in the primary or early mixed dentition take lesser time, depending on the severity of the case. Expansion in adolescents can take longer time, upto three months, while even longer time is needed in adults.

Mandibular Williams expansion appliance: It was introduced by Dr Jeff Williams in 1994. It is mostly used for mixed dentition treatment with crowded lower incisors. It uses two long stainless tubes soldered to each of the lower primary second molar bands with extensions back to contact the lingual of the 6-year molars. An expansion screw is secured to the molar bands by wire extensions extending to transverse the anterior portion of the mandible. An arc of .016 NiTi archwire inserts into the forward ends of the stainless tubes and, as the expansion screw is activated the NiTi wire is moved forward to automatically uncrowd the incisors. The .016 NiTi archwire is bonded with a small bit of composite, to the most lingually positioned incisor. It may be replaced monthly with a slightly longer length of .016 NiTi to maintain positive pressure against the lingual of the incisors. In cases where the mandibular 6 year molars are fully erupted, they may be banded instead of the primary second molars.

Indications for use of Williams expansion appliance: A narrow mandibular arch needing transverse correction. In such cases, a developing mandibular anterior crowding is present.

It is activated by turning the screw one turn every 3 days. Each turn of the screw is equivalent to ¼ mm of expansion. The expansion is continued until the proper intercanine width is achieved. The appliance can be left in place for some time and later on replaced with retentive LHA fitted to permanent first molars for retention. This should stabilize the teeth and bone for a period of up to 12 months.

Other Methods

Functional appliances: Generally, the FAs are needed to bring the retrognathic mandible forward to have a balanced relationship with maxilla. In such cases, the mandible arch width is found to be lesser. So, the component to expand the maxillary arch is also incorporated in functional appliances. It can be done either by using expansion screws/ springs or by incorporating buccal shield to relieve the abnormal buccal soft tissue pressure on the dental arches. It leads to changes in the arch dimension and arch circumference. Few examples are bionator, twin block, FR-II, oral screen, etc. It leads to passive expansion if tongue forces are used.

Magnets: Darendeliler used two repelling samarium cobalt magnets to achieve maxillary expansion. Pins and tubes were placed in the appliance to guide the separation of palate. The midpalatal magnets (each 10 mm × 5 mm × 5 mm) produced 500 g of force, which declined to 250 g during the three weeks between activations.

Transpalatal arches (TPA): It is attached at the first permanent molars. It is an important auxiliary used in fixed appliance therapy esp to boost the anchorage in upper arch. It incorporates a U-loop in the middle and can be expanded / modified to cause small amount of expansion or constriction of inter-molar width since it is directly attached to molars only; to derotate molars to correct the molar relation and to gain some space by derotating them; to keep an intruding or anti-extrusion forces on the teeth on which it is attached.

Rapid Maxillary Expansion

As the name suggests, RME is a procedure to obtain expansion of maxilla rapidly. It uses heavy forces for shorter duration to achieve mainly skeletal effects. So, RME is essentially a dentofacial orthopedic procedure. The forces range from 10–20 pounds per day and the active phase is of around 2–4 weeks followed by a retention phase of 3–4 months. Heavy forces and that too applied rapidly through the teeth, lead to development of areas of necrosis and hyalinisation in PDL around the teeth. So these teeth do not move and hence all the force is transferred to the skeletal base and circummaxillary sutures, leading to disarticualtion of sutures. It also causes a relative reduction in the nasal airway resistance by disarticulating the maxilla from other bone particularly septal and palatine bones and thus helping to increase the area of nasal passage, and helps in improving the breathing. Timms in 1960s had given a comprehensive review of RME in his book. But, now a lot of modifications have taken place in the types of appliances and introduction of surgical interventions for maxillary expansion.

Anatomical Considerations

Maxilla is a pyramid shaped bone with a body and zygomatic, frontal, alveolar and palatine processes. It is attached by various sutures to surrounding bones, which are oriented obliquely in upward and forward direction, and are almost parallel to each other. Body of the maxilla articulates with the following bones:

- Cranially:
  1. Frontal
  2. Ethmoid
- Facially:
  1. Nasal
  2. Lacrimal
  3. Inferior nasal conchae
  4. Vomer
  5. Zygomatic
  6. Palatine.

Morphology of the midpalatal suture: It is formed by the junction of three opposing pairs of bones namely (Fig. 23.17).

1. Premaxillae,
2. Maxillae and
3. The palatine bones.

Melsen, (1975) in a histological study found the maturation pattern of midpalatal suture at different developmental stages.

- **First stage:** Infantile period. The suture is very broad and Y-shaped.
- **Second stage:** Juvenile period, the suture is found to be more wavy.
- **Third stage:** Adolescent period, the suture is characterized by a more tortuous course with increasing interdigitations.

Indications of RME: As discussed above, the SME is physiologically better than RME, but in certain cases, RME may also be needed.

1. Marked narrowing of the arches: Clinically, it may be presented as increased buccal corridors; paranasal hollowing; or narrow alar bases suggest maxillary constriction.
2. Unilateral or bilateral crossbite.
3. Maxillary deficiency: There the maxilla is treated by reverse face mask therapy to bring it forward. Before that phase, a phase of RME is given which helps to activate and loosen the circummaxillary sutural system for an easy pull of maxilla.
4. Nasal septal deviation and mouth breathing due to enlarged adenoids.
5. Cleft lip and palate.

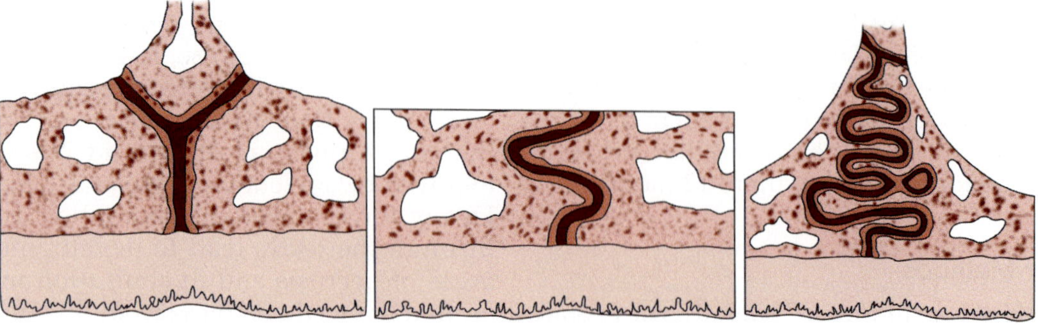

Fig. 23.17: Diagram showing increasing interdigitation of midpalatal suture with increasing age *(Adapted from Timms).*

6. Adult cases with little growth potential having narrow arches, where it can be combined with surgical palatal splitting.

According to Gray and Brogan, medical indications for RME are:

1. Poor nasal airway
2. Septal deformity
3. Recurrent ear, nasal or sinus infections
4. Allergic rhinitis
5. Asthma.

Contraindications of RME

- Midpalatal suture synostosis. However, it is a relative contraindication, as adjunctive surgical procedures can be used.
- Patients who have anterior open bites, steep mandibular planes, with vertical growth patterns and convex profiles are generally not well suited to RME. It is because the expansion leads to buccal tilting of teeth and thus prematurities between the maxillary palatal cusps and mandibular buccal cusps appear. It leads to a downward and backward rotation of mandible. Instead of a banded appliance, the use of a bonded acrylic appliance with occlusal coverage will minimize this effect by distributing force throughout most of the maxillary teeth.
- Uncooperative patients, who do not activate the appliance or those who break it.
- Patients who have a single tooth in crossbite, as generally in them, the dental arch is normal. Correction of such a crossbite needs only little space and a simpler appliance.
- Patients who have skeletal asymmetry of the maxilla or mandible.
- Adults with severe anteroposterior and vertical skeletal discrepancies are not good candidates for RME.
- Patients with periodontally weak dentitions, that will not be able to sustain the heavy forces of RME and may further lead to loss of PD tissues.

Drawbacks of rapid expansion: Orthopedic maxillary expansion was first described by Angell in 1860. The side effects which have been reported in adult patients are:

- Buccal tipping of posterior teeth
- Extrusion and bite opening
- Buccal root resorption
- Alveolar bone bending
- Buccal cortex fenestration
- Buccal gingival recession
- Loss of buccal cortex
- Palatal tissue necrosis
- Inability to open midpalatal suture
- Pain
- Relapse of the results.

These effects are all due to the change in bone density and sutural articulation with increasing age of the person.

Heavy forces are generated with RME which lead to pain and necrosis of PD tissues. Isaacson and Ingram showed that single activations produce forces ranging from 3–10 pounds and that multiple daily activations can cause cumulative residual loads of upto 20 or more pounds.

Histological studies have shown free-floating bone fragments, bleeding, micro-fractures, vascular disorganization and connective tissue inflammation in suture site. Research show that (Ekstrom and co-workers) slowly expanded suture becomes well organized in about 30 days and is established within 3 months. Storey suggested that slow expansion allows "physiologic sutural adjustments" with less trauma, more reparatory reaction and better sutural stability than rapid expansion of sutures. It requires a lengthy period of rigid stabilization/retention to allow sutural readjustment and dissipation of accumulated residual forces at different sutures of the maxilla.

Regulation of Expansion

Various factors considered important are:

1. **Rate of expansion:** The patient is asked to open the screw 2–4 times by one

quarter turns per day. The rate of expansion of 0.5–1.0 mm per day is done and the active expansion is completed in 2–4 weeks. Here, the arch is widened partly by tilting the teeth buccally and partly by moving the maxillae apart. The effect of expansion of the dental arch on the maxillary base increases as the rate of expansion is increased.

2. **Form of the appliance:** Thrust is delivered to the teeth at the inferior free borders, i.e. alveolar processes of the maxilla and it must reach the basal portion. The rigidity or flexibility of the appliance plays an important role in this effort, the effect of expansion of the dental arch on the maxillary bases increases as the rigidity of the appliance (anchorage) is increased.
3. **Age of the patient:** With the increasing age, rigidity of the facial skeleton and sutures increases which restricts bony movements. In general, the effect of expansion on the maxillary base is best during 8–11 years of age when we can expect the skeletal changes, after which there are more chances of dentoalveolar changes. Studies have questioned the efficacy of expansion during primary dentition period, but it has been documented that if arches are expanded for treatment of posterior cross bite in primary dentition, there are chances that the developing permanent teeth also follow the expanded position of primary teeth and then erupt in a correct position.
4. **Midpalatine suture:** It plays a key role in RME. With age, the interdigitation of suture increases. The shape of suture in Infancy is Y-shaped. At juvenile age, it is T-shape; while at adolescence, it achieves a Jigsaw puzzle shape due to increased interdigitation.

Appliance Design and Construction

A number of factors are duly considered during the RME appliance fabrication which are:

- Rigidity
- Number of teeth included in appliance
- Load distribution
- Appliance retention
- Expansion
- Economy
- Material
- Hygiene.

Requirements of an RME Appliance

Rigidity

The appliance should be rigid so that it leads to nearly parallel opening of the suture. A flexible appliance is not stable and it causes the tilting of dentoalveolar elements too far buccally and consequently skeletal effects will be minimized. It is because the expansion is desired at the level of the maxillary base but the force is applied to the teeth near their free lower border. The removable appliances are not suitable to achieve RME and so the fixed appliance is required to achieve the desired results. The fixed appliance can be of two types, i.e. banded or bonded. These can also be modified by adding the acrylic cap splints to cover the occlusal and part of buccal aspects of posterior teeth. The cap splint helps preventing the extreme buccal tipping of the crowns of teeth. Thus, the premature contacts between upper and lower teeth are not created, and maxillary teeth show more of a bodily movement of teeth. Advantage of such appliance is that the mandible also does not show negative side effects, like D and B rotation, increase in facial height and convexity of face, etc. The acrylic cap splint may also help in converting the occlusal forces to the intrusive forces acting on upper and lower teeth, which will at least prevent extrusion of the teeth. It also helps in dissipation of the forces to wider area.

Tooth utilization: It is best to incorporate as many teeth as possible as the entire lower portions of the maxilla are to be moved laterally. It helps in wider distribution of forces and reduces the load on individual teeth and resulting periodontal damage. Involving more number of teeth also provides better retention of the appliance. Generally,

4 teeth are banded, and the acrylic splint is used to involve other teeth in the appliance as a single unit.

The active component: It can be a spring or a screw but a spring reduces the rigidity and control. Thus a screw is better for expansion, which should have a thread of sufficient length to complete the expansion without interruption and replacement. Changing the screw in between treatment leads to relapse, endangers the rigidity and wastes time and material.

Economy of time and material: The appliance which makes least intrusion into the oral space is best tolerated by the patient. Here the banded appliances have a distinct advantage over the bulky cap splints. However, the cap splints reduce the clinical time and also prevent the buccal tilting and extrusion of buccal teeth, as compared to the only-banded appliances. With banded only appliance, only band adaptation and impressions are needed. But for splint type appliance, the chair-side work increases, which involves band adaptation, impression, and bite registration, acrylic adjustment while fixing the appliance. Laboratory work also increases. But, this work and time invested to make splint appliance helps the clinician and patient by reducing the total treatment time and the side effects of buccal tilting and torque loss of the teeth.

Hygiene: A fixed appliance leads to increased stagnation of food and plaque; reduces natural and artificial massage and cleansing. Banded appliances with the lesser amount of interconnecting material produce minimal covering of the dental and palatal mucosa. But this appliance has much inherent flexibility. In spite of being less hygienic, cap splints are considered to be the appliance of choice as any deleterious effect of improper hygiene are superficial and reversible in the well-managed patient.

RME appliances (Figs 23.18 to 23.22): These can be divided into banded or bonded appliances. The commonly used banded appliances are:

Hyrax appliance: It is an RME appliance where the screw is welded to the bands on first premolars and first molars. The RME screw called as Hyrax is the trademark of Dentaurum. Its full name can be expanded as Hygienic rapid expander. The screw has four long arms made of hard SS wires, which are adapted to the bands and soldered (Fig. 23.19).

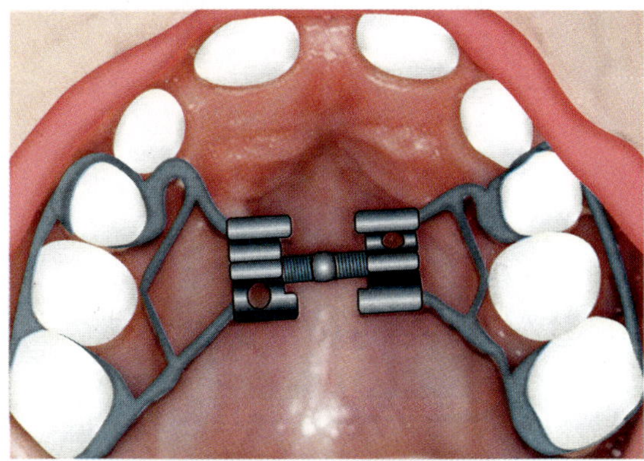

Fig. 23.18: Fixed rapid maxillary expansion appliance.

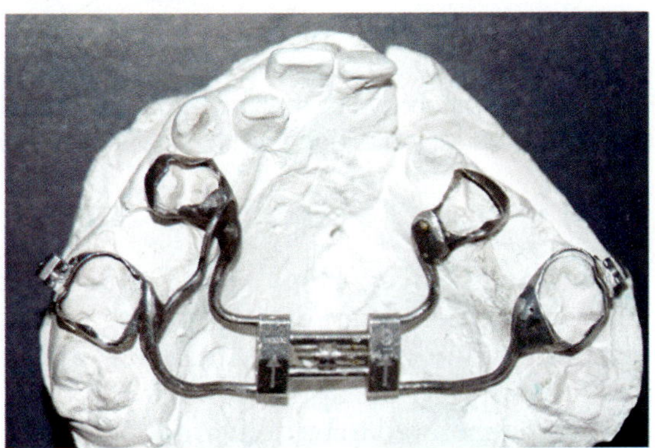

Fig. 23.19: Hyrax appliance for RME.

Isaacson type: This appliance uses a special spring-loaded screw called Minne expander which is adapted and soldered directly to the bands, and no acrylic is used. Minne expander is a heavy caliber coil spring that is expanded by turning a nut to compress the coil. Spring-loaded screws and Minne expander may continue to exert expansion forces after completion of the expansion phase unless they are partially deactivated.

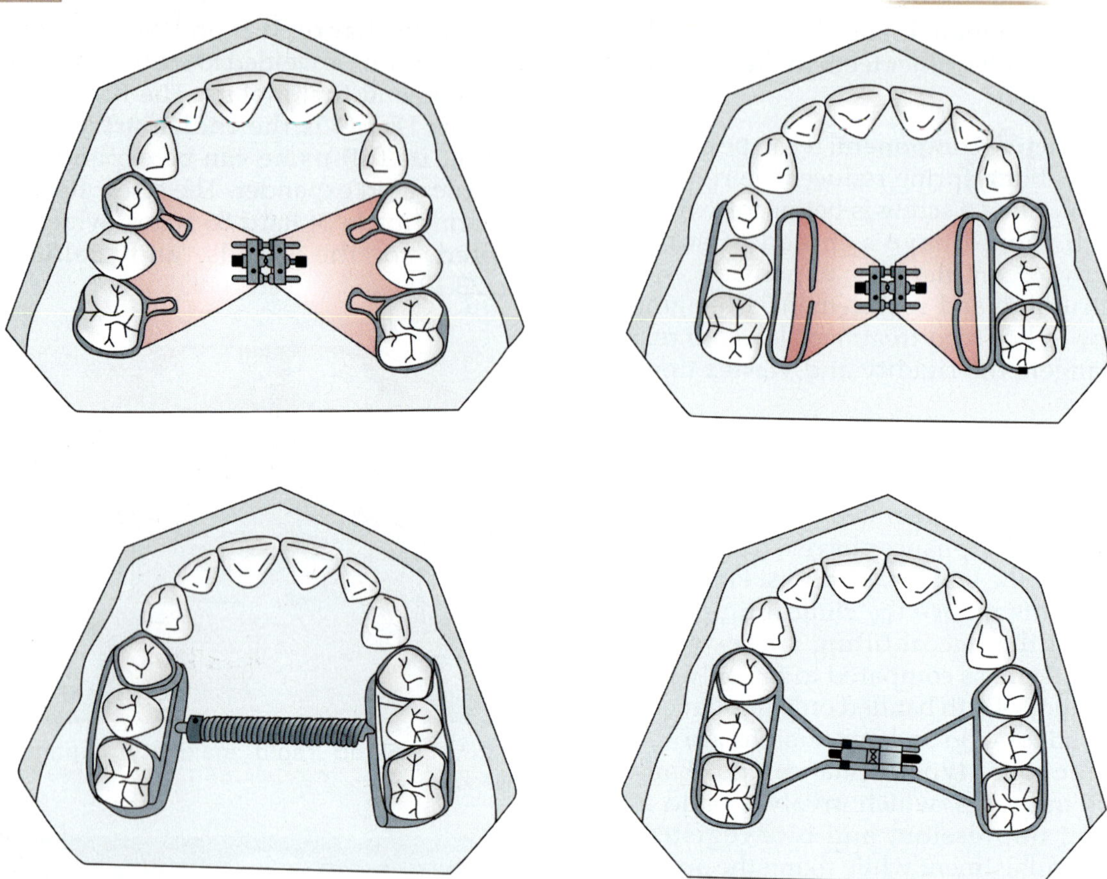

Fig. 23.20: Different types of fixed expansion appliances for RME: **Derichsweiler type; Haas appliance; Isaacson type** Minne expander; Hyrax appliances in that order.

Haas appliance: Haas stated that more bodily movement than dental tipping can be obtained when acrylic palatal coverage is added to support the appliance. It will permit the forces generated to be delivered to both the teeth and the underlying skeletal tissues. However, inflammation of the palatal tissues generally occurs due to improper cleaning under the acrylic. The appliance consists of bands placed on maxillary first premolars and first molars. A midline jack screw is incorporated into the acrylic pads that closely contact the palatal mucosa. The acrylic does not cover the occlusal surfaces of the involved teeth. Support wires may be adapted around the buccal and lingual surfaces of the posterior teeth, to add rigidity to the appliance.

Derichsweiler type: Tags are welded and soldered to the bands to provide attachment to the acrylic which is extended to palatal aspects of all the non-banded teeth except incisors.

Bonded rapid palatal expander (Fig. 23.21): This is fixed to the teeth by acid, etch technique. The posterior occlusal coverage by acrylic acts as a posterior bite block, inhibiting the eruption of the posterior teeth during treatment and making possible the use of this appliance in patients with long facial heights. The acrylic occlusal coverage also opens the bite posteriorly, facilitating the correction of anterior cross bites if required. This appliance has been widely publicized by McNamara.

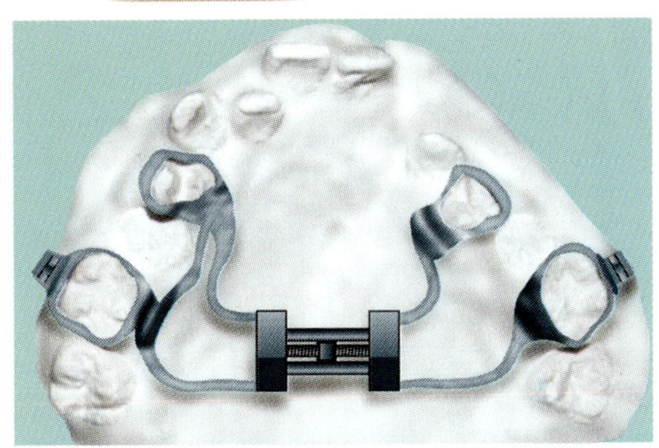

Fig. 23.21: Fixed RME appliance as designed by McNamara. It is a bonded type of appliance, having the posterior bite blocks which are then cemented/ bonded to the teeth.

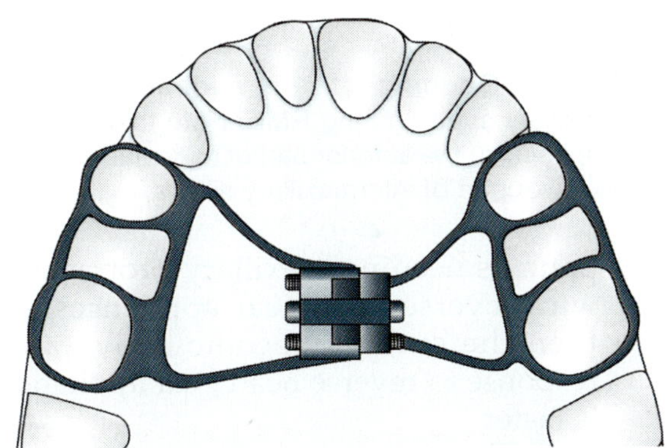

Fig. 23.22: Bonded type of fixed appliance for RME.

Hilgers pendex: This is a fixed appliance which helps to produce orthopedic expansion of the maxilla, as well as rotate and distalize maxillary first molars. Patient's cooperation is not required. It has an expansion screw inserted in the acrylic button, and .032 TMA springs produce a light and continuous force for distalising the molars. Hilgers T-Rex appliance is a modified Hilgers pendex where additional anchor arms are soldered to the molar bands. Thus the expansion is completed before molar distalization, which is then effected by cutting the anchor arm connection from molar bands.

DeLuke contoured expander (DCE): It is similar in appearance and function to a bonded rapid maxillary / palatal expander, but does not have metal framework. This makes the DCE easy to insert and remove, improving patient comfort. The DCE is fabricated on Biostar® using Splint Biocryl to ensure uniform thickness. The natural anatomic contour at buccal and gingival margins eliminates plaque trap and reduces inflammation, making the DCE extremely hygienic.

Instructions on how to expand: The patients are classified into three age groups:

1. **Upto age of 15 years:** An activation of 180° per day is done divided as 90° in the morning and 90° in the evening.
2. **15–20 years:** Due to increased resistance in midpalatal suture, the separation is difficult and painful due to force build up when a turn of 90° is given. So overall rotation of 180° is done by splitting the rotation into 4 turns of 45° each separated by equal time intervals.
3. **Age over 20 years:** In this age, there can be substantial build up of tension and pain due to increased interdigitation of midpalatal suture. So, only 45° turn in the morning and 45 in the night is advised initially to start the bio-mechanical response in the tissues. Later on, it can be increased to 4 turns of 45° each with adequate division between them.

Zeibe in 1930 advocated 180° rotations/ day which is within limits. He stated that more than 0.5 mm expansion per day causes rupture of blood vessels. With this 180° turn per day the expansion screw will provide upto 10 mm expansion in 4 weeks. that is 2.5 mm per week or 0.36 mm per day. The regime for the rotation of screw is prescribed according to following classification. Zimring and Isaacson in 1965 recommended the following turn schedules:

- Young or growing patients: two turns each day for the first 4–5 days and one turn each day for remainder of RME treatment.

- Adult patients: two turns each day for the first two days and one turn each day for the next 5–7 days and one turn each other day for the remainder of the RME treatment.

How much to expand: Studies by various authors, e.g. Kerbs (1964), Stockfisch (1976) and Linder Aronson et al (1979) show that almost 30–40% relapse occurs after RME before stability eventually was reached. Extent of this relapse is largely unpredictable. So an overcorrection is incorporated during expansion. A general guideline about how much to expand is to stop when the buccal inclines of maxillary palatal cusps are in contact with the lingual inclines of buccal cusps of the mandibular teeth. After that, the RME screw is fixed with acrylic or composite to avoid its reverse movements. The same appliance is used as retainer for 3–4 months to give time for tissue organisation and sutural stabilisation. A new fixed transpalatal retainer is fixed after this period for a prolonged time. Mew (1983) suggested that one should over-expand the molars 2–4 mm beyond the required distance to allow for the expected relapse.

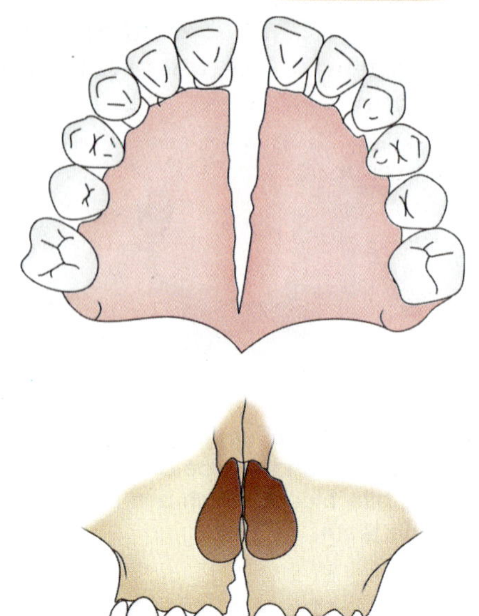

Fig. 23.23: Opening of the midpalatal and intermaxillary suture during RME. Note that there is more opening in the anterior part of midpalatal suture and in lower part of intermaxillary suture.

Changes after RME Therapy (Fig. 23.23)

- Changes in bone: Due to the application of forces across the palate, the maxilla will move apart with a breakdown of midpalatal suture, opening like a fan, the most anterior and inferior points moving the greatest distance with a fulcrum somewhere within the nasal airway. Since maxilla is connected with many bones on superior, lateral and posterior aspects, the opening of midpalatal suture is more in anterior region as compared to posterior region, opening in a V-shaped fashion. The midpalatal suture after force application opens earlier in juveniles (1–2 days) and later in adults (3–4 days). In young children, the fulcrum of opening of sutures may be as high as the fronto maxillary suture. It is beneficial to have a phase of RME in patients needing maxillary protraction with reverse head gear appliances, as then the sutures become active and response to reverse head gear appliance is faster.
- In one week, the dental arch width increases by 2–3 mm and the suture gets opened approx 50% of this amount. But further occlusal expansion does not maintain this ratio, as an element of relapse gets introduced, and the dentoalveolar effect increases.
- A rigid appliance exerts a parallel opening and produces expansion at a greater distance from the appliance as compared to flexible appliance, which produces expansion mainly in lateral inclination.

Changes in the dentition: The teeth move buccally under forces of expansion, and their buccal inclination increases. A force component is also generated along the axis of teeth resulting in a slight extrusion. A midline diastema is created due to rapid separation of midpalatal suture. If central incisors are not incorporated in the appliance, they will return to their original position after some time due to the recoil of the trans-septal fibers. Appearance of midline diastema is the sign of a positive response of RME therapy. During the initial period, the teeth may become slightly loose and often tender to percussion.

Effects of RME on mandible: Due to RME, buccal tipping of teeth occurs which leads to extrusion of maxillary palatal cusps. It causes premature contacts with lower teeth and thus the mandible may rotate downward and backward, leading to increase in anterior face height and convexity of the face.

Effect on nasal volume: It helps to increase the palatal width, the nasal base and thus nasal volume increases. The resistance to nasal breathing is reduced and thus the patient starts breathing through nose. He gradually stops the mouth breathing habit, and its side effects get controlled.

Hazards of RME: Since RME applies heavy forces on teeth and bone, it may also lead to certain side effects. They may be following but are not limited to them.

- Oral hygiene problem as the appliance is fixed one.
- Tissue damage (limit rate of expansion by 0.5 mm)
- Infection and gingivitis.
- Root resorption of teeth
- Failure of suture to open if it is fused, interdigitated, etc.
- Dislodgment and breakage of appliance
- Pain.

Retention after Expansions

Retention helps to hold the bones and dentition in new position while all other forces generated by appliance have decayed. The screw in the fixed appliance is blocked with resin to prevent its reverse-turning itself which may lead to loss of expansion. The appliance is itself-modified to act as retention appliance during the first 3 months. Always an overcorrection is done during expansion to provide a leeway for the inherent relapse. For overcorrection, the maxillary palatal cusps should be held occluding with the mandibular buccal cusps with a retention appliance. After the removal of fixed appliance, the mouth is left without any appliance for a few days to permit the recovery of palatal mucosa. Then a new removable or fixed retainer should be given to the patient for few more months, to give time for the reorganization of tissues. After some months when the stress and strain get eliminated, the retention plate can be discarded and the teeth can be allowed to tilt inward, settling into their natural occlusion.

Surgical Assisted Rapid Palatal/Maxillary Expansion (SARPE/SARME)

SARPE is the procedure of expanding the maxilla where palate is surgically splitted before starting the expansion. It is used in cases where normal expansion procedure is not successful and there is increased interdigitaiton of midpalatal and circum-maxillary sutures with advancing age. The main indications are:

1. Increased age of the patient, with increased interdigitation of midpalatal suture.
2. A severe skeletal maxillomandibular transverse discrepancy.
3. Extremely thin, delicate gingival tissue or presence of significant buccal gingival recession in the buccal region of maxilla
4. Significant nasal stenosis.
5. It is used to increase maxillary arch perimeter for alignment; and to correct posterior crossbite.
6. To widen maxillary arch in cleft patients.
7. It can also be used in adult patients to reduce wide buccal corridors for esthetic improvement.

Surgical procedures have been devised to help to achieve maxillary expansion in skeletally mature patients, which are of two types:

1. Surgically associated RPE (SARPE)
2. Maxillary segmentation and individual repositioning during Le Fort I surgery. Procedure choice depends on the surgeon operating and requirements of the orthodontist.

Medical history: Medical condition of the patient should be thoroughly evaluated as certain conditions can influence the result of expansion. Conditions leading to synostosis and extreme calcification of sutures are the roadblocks in the path of successful results, e.g. hyperthyroidism, hypophosphatemic vitamin-D-resistant rickets, mucopolysaccharoidosis, and mucolipidosis, etc. Also patients on certain drugs, e.g. zoledronic acid, which is an antineoplastic drug also hampers/stops bone remodeling processes.

Areas of resistance to lateral expansion are:

a. Anterior support (piriform aperture pillars)
b. Lateral support (zygomatic buttress)
c. Posterior support (pterygoid junctions)
d. Median support (midpalatal suture).

The areas of resistance are relieved during surgery. The appliance should be fitted immediately after surgery and activated so that a patent gap is created at osteotomy site. Then latency period of 5 days is followed so that a callus is formed, after which RME schedule is started till overcorrection is achieved.

Distraction osteogenesis (DO) has given a new dimension to orthodontics, as it can help us to achieve better skeletal improvements which were previously not possible with orthodontics only. The SARPE is a form of DO where the expansion appliance acts as a distractor device. Other uses of DO has been to gain mandibular length and maxillary protrusion in cases of deficiency; correction of asymmetry of mandible, treatment of CLP case, etc.

Conclusion

Expansion is a very useful procedure in orthodontics, especially during growth period. As there is a pendulum swing toward the non-extraction treatment plans keeping in view the soft tissue and profile considerations, expansion has emerged a valuable adjunct to gain space to treat a wide variety of clinical cases. However, to achieve successful results, the proper diagnosis and case assessment is very essential. Consideration of age and growth pattern of the patients is of utmost importance in treatment planning.

VIVA VOCE QUESTIONS

1. **What are the various appliances for the fixed expansion procedure?**
   Fixed expansion by—Coffin, Haas, Hyrax, quad helix, w-arch, bihelix, NPE

2. **What are the main differences between RME and SME?**

	RME	*SME*
1. Opening	0.5–1 mm/ day (3.5–7 mm/ week)	1 mm/ week
	90° BD	90°/ 2–3 days
2. Force generated	10–20 lbs	2–4 lbs
3. Tissue damage	More	Less
4. Skeletal : dental expansion.	8:2	5:5
5. After 4 months of retention	5:5	5:5

3. **Which of the above-said procedures is considered better, i.e. RME or SME?**
   SME is definitely better as seen from the above table, because the end-result of both the procedures is the same, i.e. 1:1 achievement of dental and the skeletal effects. But, SME forces are within the safe and physiological limits and comfortable to the patient.

4. **What is the pitch of the E-screw?**
   It is the amount of opening achieved with full one turn/360° of the E-screw. It is approx 0.8 mm. So with 90° turn, we achieve the 0.2 mm opening of the screw, i.e. 0.1 mm/side of the arch.

5. **What is the width of PDL?**
   Normal width of PDL is approx 0.22–0.25 mm. So with 90° opening, only 0.1 mm/side of the PDL is compressed and so the health of the tissues is maintained under light forces.

6. **Which of the following is better-SME or RME and why?**
   SME is better than the RME except under exceptional circumstances. It is because, SME applies the forces with in the physiological range without damaging the investing tissues.

7. **How much space can be gained by expansion?**
   If we consider the upper arch as half circle till the first molar region, we can gain a space approx. 1.56 mm/mm of expansion.

8. **What modalities are available for expansion?**
   Coffin spring, porter's appliance, bihelix, quad-helix appliance, NPE, i.e. Ni-Ti palatal expanders, fixed expansion appliance, TPA, etc. besides removable jackscrew appliances.

9. **Why this name has been given to the quad helix appliance?**
   It contains four helices in the design so it is called by this name.

10. **Why Coffin appliance is called so?**
    It was first designed by Coffin.

11. **What is the role of the helices in the quad helix appliance?**
    Helices increase the length of the wire in the appliance. So lighter forces are applied by the appliance.

12. **What is the advantage of NiTi palatal expanders?**
    Since it keeps on applying a light continuous force on the tissues, it is tissue-friendly. Also there is no need of repeated removal of this appliance for activation as the Ni-Ti wire has shape memory property.

13. **What are the main contraindications of expansion?**
    It is not indicated in vertical growth pattern cases, as it tends to worsen the facial pattern. Also, it is not indicated in the patient who are past their growth age.

14. **How does the expansion improve the respiration pattern?**
    It increases the area of nasal passage and so reduces the resistance to air flow. So, the pattern can change from mouth to nasal pattern.

15. **What are the other uses of E-screw?**
    It can be used for distalization of molar to gain space; to move the incisors anteriorly in case of class II division 2 m.o; to gain space for correction of cross bite of maxillary canine; to

expand arches in CLP patients; to widen the arches in case of treatment with myofunctional appliances in class II division 1 m.o.

16. Till what age, the midpalatal suture is not ossified?

It ossifies at approx 12–14 years of age. After this, only dental effects come in effect with least skeletal effect with expansion.

17. Till what age, the skeletal effects can be gained by expansion?

Most of the skeletal effects can be achieved at approx 8–9 years of the age, however decrease amounts of skeletal effects are still achievable till 12–14 years age.

18. What is the pattern of expansion?

Opening of the midpalatal suture is fan-shaped, i.e. maximum opening at the incisor region decreasing progressively posteriorly. Similarly, it is there in the superoinferior direction, with maximum opening towards the oral cavity. Also, with expansion, maxilla rotates in a downward and forward direction. So, it helps in correcting the maxillary hypoplasia. It is also indicated before starting the Delaire's face mask therapy. It leads to proclination of maxillary incisors.

19. What is the best age for expansion and why?

8–9 years is the best age for expansion, as it is an approx time for a growth spurt to come and also, the mid-palatal suture is also viable and not interdigitated.

20. If a patient of 25 years age comes to you with narrow maxillary arch indicated for expansion, what will you do?

Palatal expansion with surgical splitting will be done.

21. What is the difference between arch expansion and arch augmentation?

Arch expansion is the widening the arch in the transverse direction, while the arch augmentation is the lengthening the arch by moving the teeth in anterior/labial direction, e.g. in class II division 2 cases.

SELF-ASSESSMENT QUESTIONS

1. Why expansion is contraindicated in vertical growth pattern cases?
2. Till what relationship of upper and lower cusps, the expansion should be done during RX?
3. Why overexpansion is done while expanding and till what limit?
4. Which analyzes/indices give indication for requirement of expansion in a particular case?
5. What are the chances of stable results in expanded mandibular arch?
6. How does mandibular intercanine width affect the expansion decision in mandibular arch?
7. Why there are great chances of relapse of expansion in a surgically treated case of cleft palate?
8. What is the advantage of posterior bite plane in expansion appliances in case of vertical growth pattern?
9. What is Porter's appliance?

24

Extractions in Orthodontics

INTRODUCTION

Extraction is a common procedure used during orthodontic treatment to make space for alignment, levelling and retraction of proclined teeth. During developing years of dentition, some primary and permanent teeth are removed to make way for eruption and better alignment of remaining teeth in dental arches having tooth size–arch length discrepancy (TSALD). This interceptive procedure is called serial extraction or guidance of eruption. During corrective therapy when comprehensive orthodontic treatment is being instituted, extraction of one or more teeth may be required for treatment. Such extractions are called therapeutic extractions. The type and severity of malocclusion, age, growth pattern, and soft tissue morphology of patient, etc. are some of the major factors guiding the decision of extraction. Different types of extractions used in orthodontic treatment are as follows:

- Serial extraction
- Therapeutic extractions
- Compensating extractions
- Balancing extractions
- Wilkinson's extractions.

Definitions

Serial extraction: It is the procedure where sequential removal of some primary and some permanent teeth is done to provide space for other teeth to erupt and align in the dental arches. It is generally started in 8–9 years of age, in the patients having severe TSALD.

Therapeutic extractions: These are the extractions needed during comprehensive orthodontic treatment to align, level and retract the teeth. Mostly, first premolars are extracted.

Compensating extractions: This is the removal of a corresponding tooth in the opposite arch to preserve the buccal occlusal relationship. It is generally recommended in class I cases. It is done to minimize occlusal interference because it then allows the teeth to maintain occlusal relationships as they drift. However, it is more difficult to justify compensating extraction than the balancing extraction, especially when it involves extracting a tooth from an intact arch.

Balancing extractions: This procedure is the removal of teeth from the opposite side of the same dental arch, designed to minimise the midline shift. Generally, if the extraction is the done on one side, then there are chances that the teeth mesial to the extraction space start moving in the space, leading to midline shift and asymmetry of the dental arch. It generally happens in the incisor region due to lip pressure. To avoid this, the corresponding tooth on the other side of arch is removed. In the mixed dentition, when the primary tooth of one side gets exfoliated while other side is retained, then it should be removed, so that the permanent teeth do not move to the other side and midline is maintained. Even during serial extraction, the extractions of teeth should be on both sides of the dental arch simultaneously, so that midline shift does not occur.

Wilkinson's extractions (Figs 24.1a to d): Permanent first molars are very sensitive to the

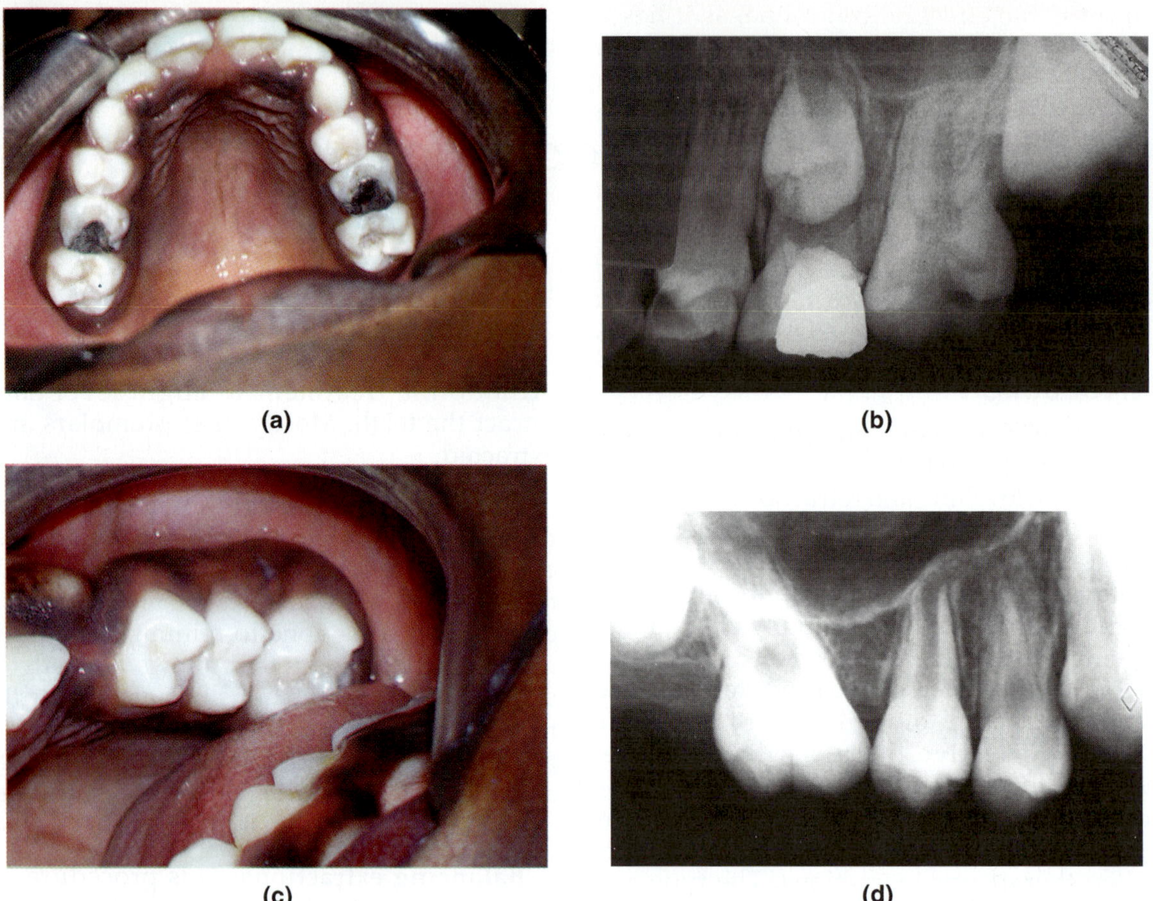

(a) (b) (c) (d)

Figs 24.1a to d: A case of Wilkinson's extraction: I/O view of caries damaged upper permanent first molar; IOPA showing deep caries exposure of upper permanent first molar; I/O view showing mesial eruption of upper permanent second molar in contact with premolar after some months of extraction of upper permanent first molar; IOPA showing mesially erupted second molar;

caries, leading to gross caries destruction or caries exposure. If it happens, then the first molars can be extracted, and then wait is done for eruption of second molars in that space. But this procedure is best if done at 8½–9½ years of age. Its advantage is that it helps to provide space for eruption of third molars and their chances of impaction are minimized. But disadvantages are that second premolar and molar can rotate in the space; and orthodontist does not get adequate anchorage unless second molar erupts. Care should be taken that this procedure is done only if third molar is present.

Early loss of primary incisor/s has little effect on the permanent dentition except esthetic problems. It is not necessary for balancing or compensating extraction in case of the loss of a primary incisor. But the early loss of a primary canine leads to midline shift in all cases except the spaced dentition. The more is the crowding present in the dentition, the more is the need for balancing extraction to avoid midline problem. If balancing is not done, the force of the erupting canine on one side leads to shifting of the incisal segment and hence midline to the other side. In case of loss of a primary first molar, a balancing extraction may be needed in crowded arches. If the primary second molar is lost, then there is no need to balance because this will have no appreciable effect on centreline, as it lies far away from the midline. But, it may lead to space loss due to forward movement and tilting of the adjacent or erupting first permanent molar. In such cases, a space maintainer should be inserted.

Philosophy behind Extractions

There are two schools of thought regarding extraction decision. EH Angle advocated that all cases should be treated as "non-extraction". According to him, a full complement of 32 teeth is required for an ideal occlusion. So, he resorted to expansion of the arches to align them. However, this later on led to relapse of treatment results. Calvin advocated extraction, as he discussed that the alignment of teeth in high TSALD cases by expansion leads to unesthetic and unstable results.

Tweed followed Angle's finished case as "non-extraction cases" initially, and then found that the results were unesthetic and relapsed, and thus required extractions. After extractions of bilateral first premolars and retreatment, he showed improved results of aesthetic and stability. He devised his famous "Tweed's triangle of cephalometrics" based on which he discussed that the lower incisors should be upright on their basal bone, i.e. IMPA angle should be approx 90°. Later on, he refined his research to find that FMIA angle which defines the facial esthetics, should be in the range of 65°. He found that the extraction decisions are also based on the growth pattern of the jaws. He used these three angles to calculate the total arch discrepancy in the lower arch which included COS, and head plate correction (HPC). His mechanics were based on the lower arch, with the upper arch fitted to the lower arch during the treatment.

Beggs' philosophy of extractions: Beggs was an Australian orthodontist and was in favour of extractions. According to him, the extraction of teeth compensate for the lack of natural tooth attrition in civilized man. Stone Age man showed proximal attrition and the growth of jaws, leading to mesial migration and creation of space for alignment of the teeth. But modern people diet is soft, which does not stimulate the growth of jaws and enamel loss, thus the jaws of the modern society are smaller. This evolutionary trend leads to less space in the dental arches and thus 3rd molar impaction and crowding of teeth. To correct the irregularity, since the arch length or the jaw size cannot be increased much, the only way to gain space is extraction of some teeth to reduce the total tooth material.

Indications of Extractions

Extraction of some teeth is required in case of severe teeth size–arch length discrepancy to provide the space for alignment of other teeth. TSALD is mostly seen due to space loss in improperly managed dentition. Other cases may be due to improper growth of jaws, some syndromes, etc. Space loss may occur unilaterally or bilaterally. The degree of space loss also depends on factors like the arch affected, site in the arch, and time elapsed since tooth loss. The amount of space loss is also dependent upon the adjacent teeth present in the dental arch and their status. The space loss is generally due to following causes:

1. Interproximal caries of primary molars
2. Loss of primary molars without proper space management
3. Alteration in the sequence of eruption of permanent teeth
4. Congenitally missing teeth
5. Traumatic loss of tooth
6. Ectopic eruption of teeth
7. Ankylosis of a primary molar
8. Impacted tooth
9. Transposition of teeth
10. Abnormal resorption of primary molar roots
11. Premature and delayed eruption of permanent teeth
12. Abnormal dental morphology, e.g. peg lateral are smaller which may lead to mesial shifting of the canines during eruption.

Decision of extractions depends on various factors involving soft tissue, growth pattern, anchorage requirement, etc. for correction of interarch relationship (sagittal). In orthodontics, there are some indications to extract the teeth as given below:

1. **TSALD:** For proper alignment of teeth in jaws, the total tooth material should be in consonance with the arch length available. The size of teeth and the dental arch size are genetically determined, the latter also somewhat affected by environmental factors. More tooth material leads to crowding or proclination of teeth. If crowding is moderate to severe, the size of arches or jaws cannot be increased beyond certain limits, only way to get space for alignment is extraction of one or more teeth.

   Contemporary extraction guidelines: According to Proffit, TSALD can be divided in following 3 categories.

   - If less than 4 mm arch length discrepancy, then extraction is rarely indicated.
   - If it is 5–9 mm, it is a borderline case, which can be treated both by extraction and non-extraction basis, depending on other factors like growth pattern, soft tissue esthetics, growth status, etc.
   - Ten millimeters or more, then extraction is almost always required to obtain enough space.

2. **Correction of sagittal interarch relationship:** Extraction decision depends on the sagittal relation of teeth also. It helps to achieve a normal sagittal interarch relation, normal incisor and molar relationship. For example, in Angle's class I cases, the AP relation is normal, but there may be crowding or bimaxillary proclination, etc. The extraction is done in both arches to maintain molar relation.

   In Angle's class II malocclusion with increased overjet but normal lower arch, needs only upper first premolar extraction. It helps in reduction of overjet by anterior retraction, and maintaining molars in class II relation. But, if there is crowding in lower arch also, with increase overjet, and molars not in proper class II relation, it requires first premolar extraction in both arches to correct molar to class I and incisors relations.

   In mild Angle's class III relation, often extraction is limited to lower first premolars or single incisor with lower anterior retraction to correct crossbite relation. Upper incisors may need some proclination to correct the crowding and cross bite relationship.

3. **Abnormal form and size of teeth:** Some conditions, e.g. fused teeth; hypoplastic teeth beyond salvage; traumatized teeth; caries damaged and pulpally involved teeth, abnormal morphology, etc. warrant the removal of such teeth rather than normal teeth. The extraction of such teeth may increase treatment time, cost and anchorage burden, and complicate the mechanics.

4. **Abnormal relation of skeletal bases:** Severe skeletal problems are not treated by orthodontics alone, but they require orthognathic surgical procedures for achieving normalcy of skeletal relations. But, they also need a presurgical phase of orthodontics to prepare the dental arches for surgery. During orthodontics, the extractions are generally needed for proper arrangement of teeth on their basal bones and to resolve the irregularities. These extraction combinations are generally different from those needed for only-orthodontics, e.g. during the treatment of a skeletal class II with bimaxillary proclination, the incisors need to be uprighted on their basal bones, and this may need extraction of bicuspids.

Extraction Choice

Choice of extraction is based on the requirement of the case. Most commonly, the first premolars are extracted for orthodontic treatment. It is because their position is between anterior and posterior quadrants. Also, they are not generally useful during masticatory functions. Since most malocclusions have anterior crowding and increased overjet, the first premolars are strategically located nearest to the areas of discrepancy. Their removal also does not jeopardise the anchorage settings, since the 6 smaller anterior teeth are pitted against larger posterior teeth having more root surface area. They are removed when maximum retraction of anterior teeth is needed, and maximum anchorage is required.

In cases which have a lower arch almost normal, while there is an increased overjet with full class II, then only upper first premolars are extracted for retraction of anterior teeth to correct overjet. The case is a maximum anchorage case.

In certain situations, second premolars need to be extracted. It is generally needed when the anterior discrepancy is less, and no much retraction of anterior segment is needed. The facial balance is not much disturbed due to malocclusion, and major discrepancy lies in the buccal region. The case is treated as moderate anchorage. The space is closed from both the sides, i.e. by slight anterior retraction and by anchorage mesialisation. It also helps to provide the space for erupting third molars. Also, if second premolars are impacted or blocked out of arch or badly-rotated, then they can be extracted.

In some cases, a combination of first and second premolars maybe extracted. It is needed when there is major discrepancy in upper anterior region, e.g. crowding and increased overjet; while in lower arch, there is mild discrepancy in anterior part, and the molars are in half-cusp class II relation. The upper first premolars and lower second premolars are removed. The space in lower arch is mainly used to mesialise the posterior segment to correct molar relationship.

Conditions which need removal of upper second premolar and lower first premolars are generally having a class III molar relation, with lower anterior crowding. Upper space is used to correct molar relation to class I by mesialisation of molars.

A single lower incisor extraction is needed in cases of moderate crowding in lower incisor segment, when the upper arch is normal. But if increased overjet is there with lower incisal crowding, then it will need removal of upper first premolars also.

Sometimes first or second molars also need to be removed. First molars are removed when they are badly damaged by caries. Second molars are generally removed when the distalisation of first molars is needed, especially in upper arch. It is done carefully only if third molars are of normal shape and positioned favorably.

Upper lateral incisors are many times congenitally absent, in which case the canines can be reshaped to lateral incisors; and first premolars can be reshaped to somewhat canines. In case of class II division 2, the lateral incisors may sometimes be removed instead of first premolars, especially in adults, to decrease the treatment time and mechanics.

But upper central incisors and canines are least common tooth to be removed, as they affect the esthetics the most. Upper central incisor being of bigger size can never be duplicated in oral cavity by reshaping the other natural teeth except when a PFM crown is placed. Canines have the longest and strongest rots and they support the modiolus and lips, and contribute to better smile by supporting the lips and cheeks. However, if they are impacted, malformed and they cannot be aligned, then they have to be sacrificed.

Indications for extraction of different teeth for orthodontic purpose:

A. Maxillary central incisors: These teeth contribute to esthetics, smile, and facial balance. They are rarely chosen for extraction except in rare situation where they are not salvageable, e.g. if it is an unfavorably impacted position and cannot be aligned; if it is badly carious or traumatized, and its prognosis is poor; if inverted / dilacerated and cannot be properly aligned. Then, the lateral incisor needs to be brought in its position, with certain space left on its mesial and distal sides, so that a proper sized PFM crown of central incisor shape can be placed. The canine is reshaped to lateral incisor, and first premolar is shaped as canine.

B. Maxillary lateral incisors: These are also important for the proper balance of anterior segment of dental arch, and contribute to the smile and esthetics. They hold a golden proportion in the width with central incisors, and canines for a proper balance. This golden proportion is 1: 0.618. Extraction of lateral incisors is also avoided to maintain the esthetics. But in certain situations, it may need extraction, e.g. if central incisor is impacted or blocked out, and the lateral incisor and canine have migrated mesially in its space, then to bring central in, we have to remove either first premolar or lateral incisor. If lateral incisor is removed, then canine is reshaped in the form of lateral incisor and the first PM is shaped to canine to achieve a better esthetics and balance.

Sometimes, if lateral incisor is missing on one side which may be congential or due to avulsion after trauma, then it may need extraction on the other side to maintain the symmetry of the arch, and to correct the midline. The canines are reshaped in the form of lateral incisors for esthetics.

Certain other conditions, e.g. gross caries/ pulp involvement/discoloration/trauma/ malformation of any incisor which cannot be restored/repaired, may warrant the extraction of incisors in the extraction cases.

C. Mandibular incisors: They are also major contributor to the esthetics and smile. They hold a proper proportional relation with the upper anterior teeth (Bolton's anterior ratio) to create a proper anterior relation and guidance with the upper anteriors. Their extraction is also avoided generally. But in certain cases having lower anterior crowding, where upper arch is well-aligned, and there is good occlusal interdigitation, with normal overjet and overbite, then a single lower incisor can be removed. It is done to reduce lower anterior crowding which is approx. 5 mm. Other indications can be: If one of the incisors is completely out of arch, and there is good interdental contact between rest of the teeth; If a lower incisor has poor prognosis due to caries/trauma/gingival recession/ bone loss. In mild class III cases with lower incisor crowding, it may be needed.

Its extraction should be avoided as far as possible in cases of retroclination of lower incisors, and deep bite cases. It leads to reduction in the lower intercanine width which leads to secondary reduction in upper intercanine width, and thus the crowding may appear in upper arch, or overjet discrepancy may appear.

D. Canines: Extraction of canines should be avoided as far as possible, unless they are unfavourably impacted and cannot be aligned in the arches. Canines provide support to the corners of the mouth (modiolus), its extraction results in flattening of face and thus poor esthetics. Maintenance of canines is very important to maintain or achieve canine-guidance occlusion. Also, canines have longest roots in the teeth and provide a canine-eminence to give esthetic effect. It is with the help of canine tips that people are able to eat and tear hard foods, etc. The forces of mastication are distributed to the basal bones through one of the force-trajectories through the canine roots. Contact between first premolar and lateral incisor is rarely satisfactory. Premolar cannot be used properly for esthetic effect and for canine-guidance occlusion. Also the palatal cusp of 1st premolar has to be reduced which may lead to sensitivity, caries-susceptibility, etc. Canine is generally removed only if is unfavourably impacted; if it is damaged due to trauma/caries beyond repair; or if it is erupted completely out of arch with good contact of lateral incisor and 1st premolar, when the parents do not want to take the treatment due to financial reasons and insist on extraction of canine which is abnormally placed, however a written consent should be obtained in such cases.

E. First premolars: First premolars are the most common choice of extraction as part of orthodontic treatment because of its strategic location. Due to their location, the space available due to extraction can be utilized for correction in anterior region, while having enough teeth to provide good anchorage in posterior region. They lie in the middle of anterior and posterior segments, and can be used in correction of crowding of both anterior and posterior segments easily. If the crowding is concentrated in anterior segments or there is increased overjet, it is the best tooth to remove. Rest of the buccal teeth are used for a better anchorage to pull anteriors backwards. Canine and second premolars make proper contact. It is indicated in cases of moderate to severe crowding, or in moderate to severe proclination of teeth.

F. Second premolars: They are not very common to extract but they may be indicated in mild crowding in anterior region (with minimum anchorage) where mesialization of posterior segment is required to correct the molar relationship and to close the space by anchorage loss, e.g. in Angle's class II case, where the lower arch has minimal crowding. The second premolar is removed to resolve the anterior crowding. Rest of the space is used to bring molars mesially in class I relation. Sometimes, combination of upper first and lower second PM is used for extraction, if overjet is increased and upper crowding is more in anterior region. In other situations, upper second / lower first combination is used when crowding is concentrated in lower anterior region. Other situations which warrant the removal of these teeth are:

- If it is unfavorably impacted or in blocked out position.
- If it is damaged due to caries / trauma and is beyond repair.
- In the treatment of anterior open bite, the extraction of the tooth as posterior as possible is done as such an extraction helps to close the bite. In fact, removal of the posterior tooth and then the mesialization of remaining posterior teeth helps in closing the bite. It is because the area of occlusal contact moves mesially. A 1 mm reduction in posterior contact leads to 3 mm closure of anterior bite.
- Also it should be removed in an extraction case, if it is deeply filled and has a poor future prognosis.
- If it is located completely out of arch, and there is a good contact between 1st premolars and 1st molars or that contact can be established easily, and there is minimal anterior crowding.

G. First molars: Extraction of first molars is avoided since they are the main teeth in the dental arch. It is used to classify the occlusion, and the one of the main goal of orthodontic treatment is to achieve class I relation. It provides the major occlusal table for mastication as it is having larger occlusal surface area. Its extraction is avoided as it reduces the occlusal table and occlusal efficiency. Almost 50% of occlusal efficiency is due to proper health of first molars.

Also, its extraction leads to improper anchorage, since only second molars are not able to handle the anchorage requirements in certain cases.

Also, the space closure becomes difficult and the teeth adjacent to extraction space become tilted and rotated during treatment, correction of which needs a prolonged treatment time and efforts. It is more problematic in lower arch due to denser bone.

Its extraction provides minimal space for correction in anterior region.

It deepens the bite, as the occlusal contact is reduced and moves mesially so it helps in correction of open bite.

It is extracted if it is grossly decayed / filled with poor future prognosis.

In case of impacted second premolar due to inadequate space in the arch, then first molar can be extracted so the premolar may erupt in the arch either spontaneously or by orthodontics. But in such cases, it should be confirmed that the second and third molars are healthy and favorably situated in the jaws.

Factors to Consider for Extraction of First Permanent Molars

Following factors should be considered before planning extraction of first permanent molars: dental age of the patient; amount of crowding in buccal and anterior part of dental arch; the restorative state / carious or endodontic status of the tooth; the occlusal relationship; presence and condition of the other teeth.

Restorative state of the first molar: First permanent molar/s during the mixed dentition are extracted when these teeth have gross caries; large restorations; irreversible pulpitis; periradicular pathology / infection; or severe hypoplasia. But if patient has good oral hygiene, and restorative treatment may have a good long-term prognosis, then hypoplastic molars should be conserved. However, hypoplastic molars should be considered for extraction rather than healthy teeth if space is needed for correction of malocclusion.

Dental age of the patient: Ideal time for the extraction of diseased first molars is before the eruption of second molars, usually at the age of 8–9 years. Since the upper molars face disto-occlusal direction while developing, and then straighten up while erupting, it helps to achieve a spontaneous space closure if extraction is properly timed. Timing is more crucial in mandible than in maxilla, since in mandible the developing teeth face mesially and also erupt in a mesio-occlusal direction. Delayed extractions result in tilting of teeth, incomplete space closure and thus poor contacts are established.

The presence of crowding: Due to early loss of the second deciduous molar, crowding in premolar region occurs due to mesial migration of first molars and space loss, which may lead to impaction of second premolars. Extraction of first molars may result in spontaneous resolution of buccal segment crowding in such cases, but it should be avoided unless first molars have poor prognosis. Extraction of first molars does not resolve crowding in labial segments spontaneously as it is very far behind the area of problem.

Wilkinson's extraction: Permanent first molars at the age of 8½–9½ are extracted if they are grossly carious, and carious broken with a poor prognosis. At this age, the second molars are expected to move mesially with proper axial inclination to fill the space. But if extraction is delayed, then axis of second molar will need orthodontic treatment for proper contacts and positioning. Other benefits are it leads to minimizing the crowding in buccal segment. Impaction of third molars may be avoided as they also get space and move mesially. According to Wilkinson, all the permanent first molars should be removed at 8½–9½ age, since they are the most caries prone teeth in mouth. The second and third molars take that place and chances of impaction of third molars are minimised.

Drawbacks: It provides limited space to relieve the crowding anteriorly. It leads to rotation and tipping of second premolars and second molars into the extraction space. While doing orthodontic treatment, inadequate anchorage is obtained (due to absence of 1st molars).

H. Second molars: It is not a common tooth to be removed, as it reduces the posterior anchorage. But, there may be certain indications which may guide for its removal.

- It is usually avoided, but if third molars are of good shape and position, then it can be done. It helps to avoid third molar impaction (by extracting before eruption of third molars), as they also get space and move mesially.
- If the distalization of first molars is required to gain space in the arch, then it can be removed to put less strain on anchorage. But, third molars should be in proper shape and position to take place in the arch.
- It is also indicated in treatment of open bite since extraction of buccal teeth has a bite-deepening effect. Extraction of second molars does not help to minimize the anterior crowding.
- If it is grossly decayed and the third molars are developing and are healthy,

then it can be removed and third molars can be aligned in the arch, especially in upper arch.

I. Third molars: It has no role in space gaining during orthodontic treatment. They are extracted if impacted or malformed. Also due to small jaws, there is usually crowding in posterior segment of jaws, which can be calculated by total space analysis, which warrants extraction of third molars also. They are also removed prophylactically in cases of lower anterior crowding, since a mesially directed force has been established as a mild cause of lower incisor crowding. They may be removed when the distalization of upper arch is needed.

Balancing Extractions

Removal of another tooth on the opposite side/contralateral tooth in the same arch to prevent midline shift which is likely to occur due to unilateral extraction-space occurring due to shifting of teeth to that side. It generally occurs when there is premature loss of primary mandibular canine or first premolar on one side, the permanent incisors shift to that side under the forces of lower lip.

Compensating Extractions

Compensating extraction refers to extraction of an antagonistic tooth in the opposite jaw on the same side. It is done to prevent the over-eruption of the tooth, and thus preserving the occlusal relation. It also helps to preserve the molar relationship on that side. It is generally done in class I relationship so as to preserve the molar relation.

DRIFTODONTICS

As the term suggests, it is the natural drifting of teeth to correct the problem. When the teeth are removed and space is left without maintenance or no appliance therapy is instituted, there is a natural tendency of teeth to drift in the spaces. Although this drifting is considered problematic in the mixed dentition leading to space loss where we need to preserve the space for permanent teeth to align. But, it is a blessing in disguise in that condition where this drifting helps in spontaneous resolving of the crowding. This phenomenon is better seen in lower anterior region after extraction of first premolar, and less frequently in upper anterior region. It is because of the fact that lower lip pressure is more constant augmented by mentalis m on lower teeth as compared to upper lip pressure on upper teeth. Also the maxillary canine has a stronger bone trajectorial pattern around that area of canine eminence and more root surface area, which may resist this spontaneous correction.

Driftodontics depends on a number of factors, e.g. age of the patient, amount of crowding, circumoral and buccinators muscles, etc. Generally, it occurs in the mesial direction, i.e. mesial migration occurs after the extraction. It is more common in young age when teeth are erupting and the jaws are growing.

It is also seen that when all the first premolars are extracted at the same time, but the braces are placed only in upper arch, while lower teeth has no braces. Now under the influence of retraction forces on the upper incisors, the lower anteriors start shifting, aligning and retracting spontaneously and thus space closure occurs. This reduces the time for which the braces are placed in the lower teeth. It can also be seen when the teeth have been extracted but patient does not return for the treatment for a long time, or the patient is not suitable for fixed appliance treatment at that point of time, e.g. during guidance of eruption or serial guidance. Such shifting helps in reducing the irregularity and thus fixed appliance is used for a lesser time. It may lead to deepening of bite due to uprighting of the teeth, which is a favorable response in open bite cases. Also, the crowns of teeth get tilted distally, and roots mesially, thus creating root crowding, which will need orthodontic correction.

When such extraction is to be planned, it should be done in a balanced manner, i.e. on both the sides. It helps to maintain arch integrity and midline matching. If unilateral extraction is done, then midline shift is seen on the side of extraction. Also, the tipping of teeth on the side of extraction is seen, as the crowns get distally tilted and roots go mesially causing root crowding in incisor region. It also leads to asymmetry of the anterior arch form. Also the mesial migration leads to disturbed molar relation on that side and unusual tipping of the buccal teeth in mesial direction.

Factors to be Considered for Treatment Planning in Borderline Cases

Borderline cases are those which may be treated by extraction or non-extraction basis, based on TSALD. But this decision, i.e. the choice of non-extraction approach or the method needed for reduction of tooth material depends on a number of factors. These factors are:

1. Facial esthetics
2. Soft tissue factors
3. Arch length discrepancy
4. Direction, pattern and status of growth
5. Facial pattern
6. Functional requirements
7. Ease of treatment; treatment time; and risk/benefit consideration
8. Patient cooperation
9. Post-treatment stability of the denture.

Arch length discrepancy: According to Proffit, TSALD in 5–9 mm range is the borderline case, and all effort should be made to treat them on non-extraction basis. But growth pattern, facial esthetics and soft tissue balance may modify decision in certain cases.

Facial esthetics and soft-tissue factors: Patients having a straight profile, and competent lips can be treated by non-extraction methods by gaining space and aligning the teeth, since any proclination will not affect the esthetics much. But cases already having a fuller profile, non-competent lips will show a poor change post-treatment if treated by non-extraction approach. A less than normal nasolabial angle also tends to decrease in such cases and contributes to poor esthetics.

Growth pattern: Space gaining methods, e.g. expansion, distalization, etc. in a vertical growth pattern case and skeletal open bite cases further lead to D and B rotation of mandible, leading to increase in vertical height and worsening of the profile. Extractions done in such cases help to close the bite, and U and F mandibular rotation, contributing to a betterment of the profile. Horizontal growth cases should mostly be treated by non-extraction methods.

Facial pattern: Long face cases should be treated by extraction approach as mentioned above. Short face cases are generally treated by non-extraction methods.

Patient cooperation: If patient is cooperative in the methods required for space gaining (e.g. Headgear, Myofunctional appliances, etc.), then non-extraction methods can be used in favorable cases, otherwise extractions may be needed if patient does not cooperate.

Ease of treatment and time: Some space gaining methods need a lot of time, mechanics and efforts; costlier treatment, and make the treatment complicated. Prolonged treatment may lead to burn-out of patient cooperation. Heavy forces used with headgear, expansion appliances, etc. and prolonged treatment may also tax the anchorage; may lead to root resorption; and development of caries/ WSLs/gingival or periodontal problems, etc. These side effects should also be evaluated to decide the treatment approach.

Post-treatment stability: It should be evaluated in non-extraction cases, since if the teeth or dental arches encroach the soft tissues, then the relapse potential increases, e.g. while expansion, the arches may encroach the buccinators muscles; and the proclined incisors encroach the lips, which in turn apply counteracting forces, leading to relapse. Because the lower arch is more constrained, the limit of expansion and stability is less for it than the maxillary arch. Moving lower incisors forward more than 2 mm leads to instability, because teeth get thrust into the lower lip and the pressure seems to increase sharply on teeth. Increasing intercanine width in lower arch is not stable. Expansion of mandibular arch can be done upto 9 years age since after that the mandibular intercanine width does not increase. In such cases, prolonged fixed retainers are needed. Otherwise, extraction decisions are taken to treat such cases.

Conclusion

During orthodontic treatment, the cases may fall under three different categories depending on TSALD. Some cases are treated purely without extraction; while some definitely need extractions. In between, there lies a category which needs a thorough evaluation of certain factors of esthetics, growth and soft tissues, etc. to decide whether it needs extraction or not. Certain methods of space gaining can be used without adversely affecting the esthetics and stability, and can be treated without extraction. With the advancing knowledge, better mechanics and anchorage methods available, the recent era has seen the pendulum swinging toward non-extraction approach to treat the cases as far as possible. However, the choice of extractions in the cases needing extraction is quite variable depending on the requirements and indications, and thus a thorough diagnostic analysis should be done before doing any extraction.

25

Molar Distalization

INTRODUCTION

It is the process of pushing the permanent molars distally. It is done to gain some space in the dental arches having mild discrepancy for alignment of teeth, and/or to achieve Angle's class I molar relation. It is easily and mostly done in the upper arch because the bone of maxilla is more spongy as compared to mandible. In maxilla, the tooth movement is bodily, while distal tipping of molars occurs in mandible. It is because the compact bone and the oblique ridge of mandible do not allow a bodily movement of roots of molars.

Correction of a Rotated Molar

There are two types of class II molar relationships. The first is due to a rotated class I molar, where the mesiobuccal cusp of the maxillary first molar comes in a class II relationship. The second type has the mesiolingual cusp of the maxillary first molar anterior to the marginal ridge of the mandibular first molar.

Before planning the molar distalization, a proper evaluation of the first molar position and rotation should be done. Generally, the upper first molar rotates mesiolingually around the apex of palatal root. A mesiolingually rotated upper first molar gives the effect of class II or mild class II relation. Also a rotated molar occupies more space in dental arch as compared to non-rotated molar due to its shape.

Rotation of upper first molar can be checked by Ricketts' method by examining the dental cast. If a line joining the disto-buccal and mesiolingual cusps of the upper first molar passes through the tip of upper canine, then the position of the molar is normal. In pseudo class I relation, the molar is found to be rotated. A correction of rotated molar leads to improved relation of molars and gives some space also. After this judgement, the planning of molar distalization is done.

Factors to be Considered for Molar Distalization

Following factors should be considered for planning the treatment by molar distalization.

- Age of the patient
- Dental eruption status and growth status
- Periodontal status of the patient
- Presence of second molar
- Cooperation of the patient
- Growth pattern
- Facial profile
- Bite depth
- Cost
- Amount of the distalization needed

Indication: Following are the conditions which may need molar distalization:

- It can be used to correct Angle's class II molar relation to class I relation in patients who have a horizontal growth pattern, are in actively growing stage; are having deep bite and flat facial profile.
- It is done in cases of mild class II molar, half cusp class II, etc. to achieve class I molars relation.

- To gain space in the dental arch for alignment of teeth anterior to molars, especially in mild to moderate discrepancy, where nonextraction treatment is possible.
- In growing children with only first molars erupted.
- To help in opening the deep bite, since molar distalization has an extrusive effect and thus mandible goes D and B. These cases should have horizontal or normal growth pattern and should be in active growth stage.

Contraindications

- It is not indicated in open bite cases. Molar distalisation leads to extrusion/ hanging of molar cusps which can further lead to increase in open bite, as the hanging cusps create premature contacts in the posterior region. A 1 mm of extrusion in molar region leads to approximately 3 mm bite opening.
- It is not done in patients with convex profile. With extrusion of molars, the mandible gets rotated in the D and B direction, further increasing the convexity of the facial profile and the anterior face height.
- It is not indicated in the vertical growth pattern cases, because the extrusive effect of distalization leads to D and B rotation of mandible and increases the anterior face height.
- In growing cases, the extrusion of molar can be compensated by the vertical growth of ramus, and it does not have negative effect on face height and face profile. But in not growing cases, this advantage is not available.

Anchorage Planning

Best time to distalize the first molars is before the eruption of second molars, when the crown of second molars is near the middle of root of the first molars. If the second molars are erupted, then more anchorage is needed, because of increased number and root surface area of teeth to be distalized. During molar distalization, reciprocal forces are generated directed in anterior direction (Newton's third law). A proper anchorage planning is done to distalize the molars to avoid any proclination of anterior teeth.

METHODS OF MOLAR DISTALIZATION

The literature is replete with the different methods but discussing all the methods in details is beyond the scope of this book. A brief discussion has been presented here. They can be broadly divided into following two categories:

1. Appliances needing patient cooperation
2. Appliances needing no patient cooperation

They can also be classified according to the type of appliances:

- Removable appliances
- Fixed appliances
- Intraoral appliances
- Extraoral appliances
- Appliance using the muscular force, i.e. lip bumpers.

A. Appliances which Need Patient Cooperation

1. Removable appliances: They can be removed by the patient and thus are dependent on patient cooperation. Modified Hawley's appliances can be used which includes finger spring and expansion screws, with posterior bite plane (PBP). Since patient cooperation is needed, they are not much effective. Also they lead to tipping molar.

a. **Cetlin's appliance:** It is a removable appliance, in which a finger spring is made mesial to the molar to be distalized. Spring is made of 0.6–0.7 mm SS wire. A posterior bite plate is generally incorporated to relieve the occlusion for unhindered movement of tooth (Fig. 25.1).
b. **Removable appliance with expansion screw:** A 2-pin expansion screw is placed near the tooth to be distalized, and cuts are placed in the acrylic plate. The larger

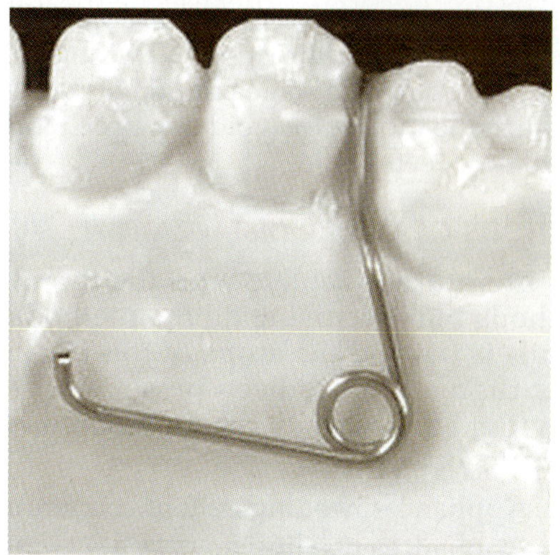

Fig. 25.1: A spring for distal movement of molar.

part of acrylic serves as anchorage while the smaller part serves as active part. Proper retentive components are placed in the appliance. A regular activation schedule of screw is prepared, generally 90° every alternate day. A posterior bite plate is generally incorporated to relieve the occlusion for unhindered movement of tooth.

Disadvantages of removable appliance:
- Patient cooperation is needed
- It leads to tipping of the teeth
- Longer time is needed
- Bulky appliance is a problem in cooperation
- Speech and adaptation problems with the removable appliance.

2. Headgear: It is an extraoral appliance. It is one of the oldest and good appliance for molar distalization, as no intraoral reciprocal forces are generated during its use. But it entirely depends on the patient cooperation.

Method: The teeth to be distalized are banded and round buccal tube of 0.045" size is welded/soldered on them. The bands are cemented in place. The inner bow of the face bow is adjusted so as to stay away from labial surfaces of teeth by at least 2 mm. The small U-loops are bent in the inner bow just mesial to the molar tubes which act as molar stops and they are used for further activation and adjustment of inner bow. The outer bow is adjusted in length and angulation according to the patient's growth pattern, facial profile and bite depth, e.g. a high-pull headgear is used in patients having vertical growth, and open bite or shallow bite cases. Intermediate headgear is used in normal pattern cases. Cervical headgear is used in cases with horizontal growth and deep bite cases, where molar extrusion during distalization is beneficial for correction of deep bite (Fig. 25.2).

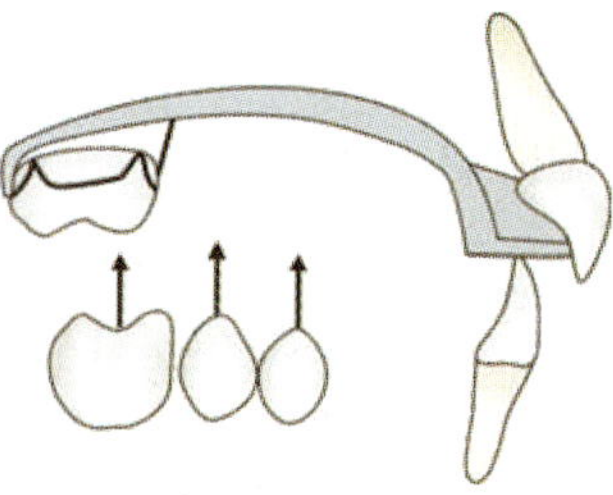

Fig. 25.2: Anterior bite plane is needed in many cases to open the occlusion so that molars can be distalized unerupted of occlusal interdigitation.

If patient is having a full bonded fixed appliance in the mouth, then the J-hook head gear is used for molar distalization with open coil spring in between. A force of approx 250 gm per side is used. An expected rate of tooth movement is 1 mm per month, if patient cooperates.

B. Appliances which do not Need Patient Cooperation

To eliminate the need of patient cooperation, the clinicians have developed many fixed appliances for molar distalization.

Advantages:
- Patient cooperation is not needed
- Continuous forces are applied.
- Due to non-interrupted movement, the rapid movements are achieved, so less treatment time is needed.
- Bulky appliances are not required.
- Helps to achieve bodily movement of teeth.

Disadvantages:

- Costly
- They are fabricated in laboratory, thus needing another patient visit, and some special instruments, e.g. soldering, acrylization, etc.
- Can be placed by a trained clinician only.
- Need regular check-up for maintenance.

Types of molar distalizers: Some of the fixed appliances used for this purpose are given below, but the list is not complete and many other appliances/modifications have been discussed in the literature.

- Pendulum appliance
- Jones jig
- Distal jet appliance
- K-loop molar distalizer
- Nance arch and NiTi coil spring
- Magnets
- Open coil spring
- Using implants
- Carriere appliance
- Multi-distalizing arch
- Distal screw: Distal jet with miniscrews
- NiTi palatal expansion appliance
- TPA
- Derotation of molars
- Frog appliance: JCO 2011
- Lokar appliance.

Mechanical principles: Certain principles, as suggested by clinicians like Burstone, must be borne in mind when designing such an appliance:

- Magnitude of forces
- Magnitude of moments
- Moment-to-force ratio
- Constancy of forces and moments
- Bracket friction (frictionless appliances are generally more predictable and efficient)
- Anchorage
- Ease of use
- Cost.

During molar distalization, two major effects are of particular concern. These are tipping of the molar, and anterior movement of the anchorage teeth (i.e. anchorage loss as seen by proclination of front teeth; appearance of rotations/crowding; increased overjet). If the first molar is tipped back rather than moved bodily, it will lead to occlusal problems, because of the hanging of mesial cusps and creation of premature contacts. Also, it will not provide sufficient anchorage for retraction of the teeth anterior to it, as it will have a tendency to get upright and thus move mesially again under the influence of the retraction forces. Effective control and manipulation of the moment-to-force ratio can help to achieve bodily movement, controlled tipping, or uncontrolled tipping, as the individual case dictates.

A brief discussion of some of the commonly used molar distalizing appliances follows.

1. K-loop molar distalizer (Fig. 25.3): This appliance was designed by Kalra V, 1995, hence the name "K". It consists of a K shaped-loop to provide the forces and moments and a Nance button to resist anchorage. The K-loop is made of .017" × .025" TMA wire, which can be activated twice as much as stainless steel before it undergoes permanent deformation, and produces nearly half the force as

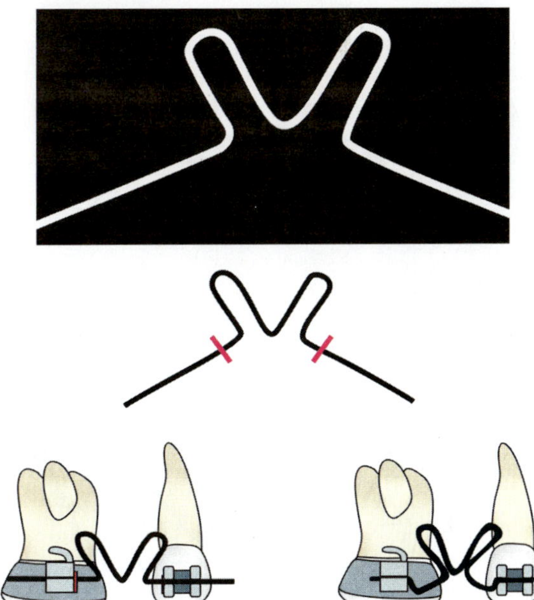

Fig. 25.3: K-loop for molar distalization *(Adapted from Varun Kalra, JCO).*

compared to the one made with stainless steel. Each loop of the K is 8 mm long and 1.5 mm wide. The legs of the K are preactivated by 20° and inserted into the molar tube and the premolar bracket. These 20° bends produce moments that counteract the tipping moments created by the force of the appliance. Thus, the molar moves bodily instead of tipping. The palatal Nance button is fixed on the first premolars or first deciduous molars to provide anchorage. The button should be large enough to provide adequate anchorage. The acrylic can be modified as a bite plane in some cases.

2. Jones' jig appliance (Fig. 25.4)**:** It was designed by Jones and White 1992. It is a prefabricated appliance which has an open-coil nickel titanium spring to deliver a force of 70–75 g, when compressed for 1–5 mm. It can be used simultaneously with the fixed appliance. A Nance palatal arch appliance is used for anchorage, which can be attached to first or second premolar or primary molars. The Jones Jig is inserted in the molar tube and is activated with the help of ligature wire thus compressing the NiTi spring. The ligature wire is attached to the first or second premolar or primary molars bearing the Nance palatal arch.

3. The pendulum appliance (Figs 25.5a and b): Hilgers in 1992 described this appliance. It has a large Nance acrylic button for anchorage with bands at first/second premolars. The first molars are fitted with bands having lingual sheath to receive the spring. The lingual sheaths on the upper molars should be .036" so that the .032" wire fits loosely. 0.032" TMA wire is used to make the springs which apply a light, continuous force to the upper first molars. The Pendulum springs consist of a recurved molar insertion wire, a small horizontal adjustment loop, a closed helix, and a loop for retention in the acrylic button.

The springs are made close to the center of the palatal button to maximize their range of motion, to allow for easier insertion into the lingual sheaths, and to reduce forces. Thus, the appliance produces a broad, swinging arc or a pendulum of force from the midline of the

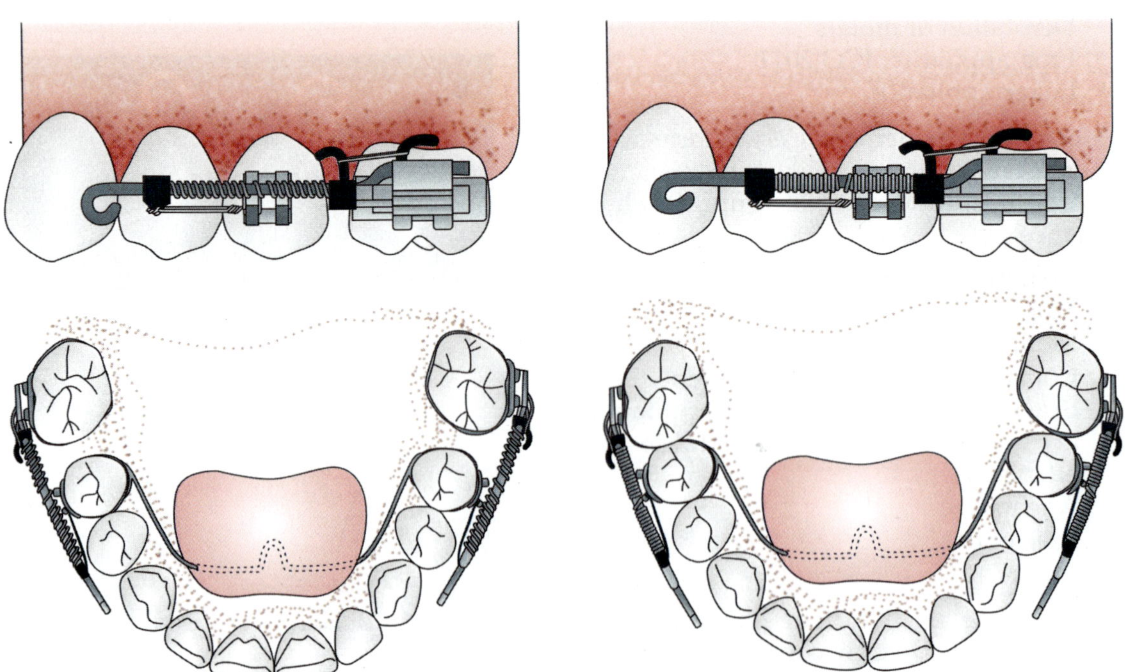

Fig. 25.4: Jones' jig for molar distalization *(Courtesy: Internet for illustration purpose)*.

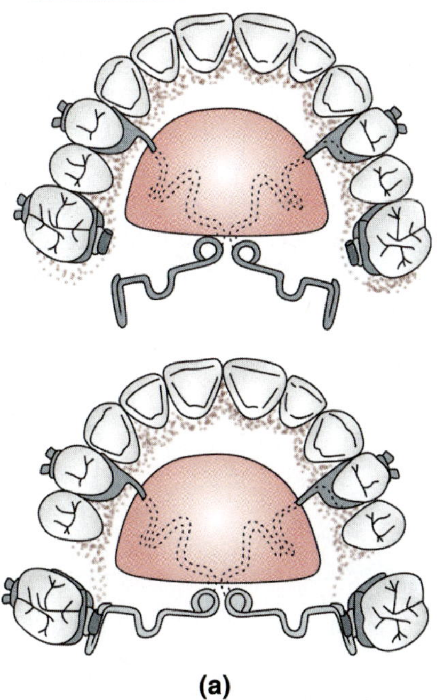

(a)

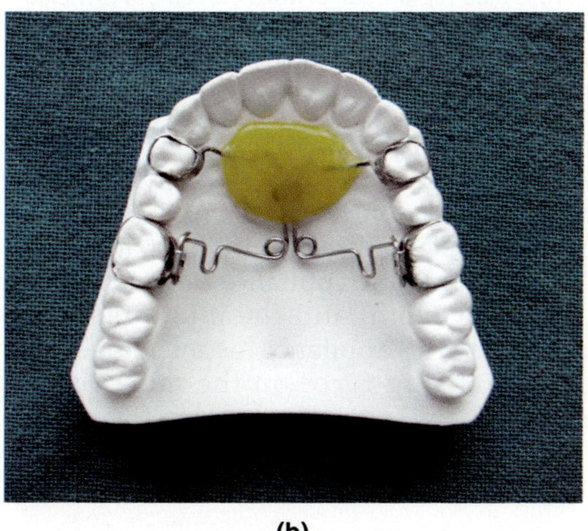

(b)

Figs 25.5a and b: Schematic diagram and model of a pendulum appliance for molar distalisation.

palate to the upper molars. Since the swinging arc tends to bring the molars palatally also, so the spring is expanded by opening the adjustment loop before inserting in the lingual sheath. Also the end of spring to be inserted in lingual sheath is adjusted so that the molar does not rotate. Pendulum springs are preactivated before appliance placement the springs are bent parallel to the midline of the palate. After cementation of the appliance, the mesial end of the recurved loop is inserted in the lingual sheath. The small horizontal adjustment loop allows for some lingual compression of the spring during placement. This appliance can be used to gain the lost space due to mesial molar movement; to correct the class II molar relation; to derotate the molar, etc. A variation of this appliance is a bonded-type of appliance where the wires from Nance palatal arch are bonded to the first/second premolar rather than banding.

4. Pend-X appliance: If expansion of the upper arch is needed, a midpalatal jackscrew can be incorporated into the center of the Nance button.

5. Distal jet appliance: The distal jet is a fixed lingual appliance which can be used bilaterally or unilaterally for molar distalization. It consists of a bilateral piston and tube system. The tubes are embedded in Nance acrylic button supported on maxillary second premolars. The tube is extended distally, adjacent to the palatal tissues and is aligned parallel to occlusal plane upto the molars. A bayonet shaped wire is inserted into the lingual sheath on the permanent first molar bands, and it extends into the tube like a piston, with nickel titanium open coil spring in this tube and piston arrangement. Spring can be activated by using a lock that is used to compress the spring distally. 180 gm force is recommended for distalization during mixed dentition, while 240 gm force is used during permanent dentition with erupted second molars. The activation lock is pushed distally to compress the spring and locked on the tube. After distalization is complete, the appliance can be converted to Nance holding arch by removing the coil spring and locking the activation collar over the junction of tube and piston wire. The supporting wires are then cut from the premolars and Nance button so that the premolars move distally by driftodontics. The distalization of maxillary molars takes place with less distal tipping and without lingual movement than occurs with the pendulum, and the distal jet can be easily converted into Nance holding arch to maintain the corrected molar position.

6. Carrier distalizer: It is made of mold-injected, nickel-free stainless steel. It has two parts, i.e. canine pad and molar pad, which are bonded to the canine and first molar. The canine pad allows distal movement of canine along the alveolar ridge without tipping, has a hook on which class II elastics is attached to apply distal force. This pad is having an arm, whose posterior end is in the shape of a ball which articulates in a socket on the molar pad like a ball and socket joint. It can be used to accomplish three types of molar movement, i.e. uprighting of the crown, distal rotation around the palatal root, and distal displacement without concurrent distal tipping of the crown.

It is available in three different sizes: 23 mm, 25 mm and 27 mm. The appropriate size is determined by measuring from the midpoint of the maxillary first molar's buccal surface to the midpoint of the maxillary canine crown, using a calliper. The anchorage is created in lower arch to receive the class II elastics. It can be attained by using LHA; full fixed appliance; microimplant; Hamula arch, etc. Heavy elastics of ¼" size, 200 gm force are used in class II fashion.

7. Magnets: Two magnets are placed in repelling mode. The magnets are just placed near the mesial surface of the tooth to be distalized. This method can be used with full fixed orthodontic appliance in upper arch, or if partial appliance is placed, then a Nance palatal arch is needed for anchorage. Initial force of distalization is adequate, but with tooth movement and thus increased distance between the magnets, the force level decreases.

8. NiTi coil spring (Fig. 25.6): Open coil spring is placed squeezed between the second premolar and the mesial to the molar to be distalised, in a full fixed appliance in upper arch. The anchorage is augmented with Nance palatal arch or headgear. NiTi spring provides a constant continuous force, and it has low decay rate.

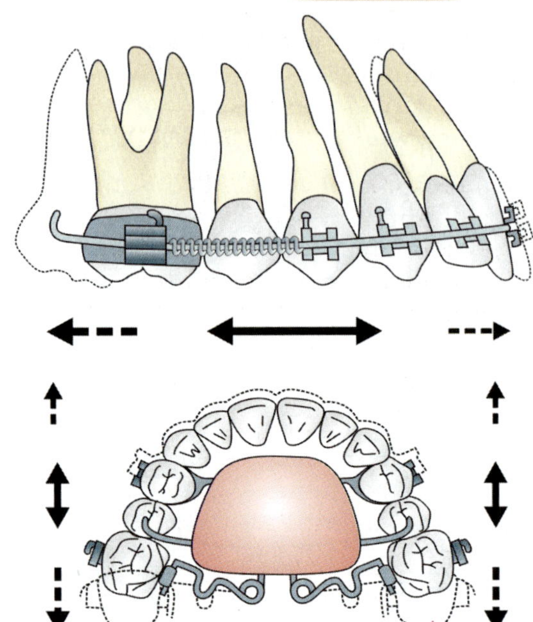

Fig. 25.6: Open coil spring for molar distalization. But, there is also reciprocal forward movement of incisors. Another figure of molar distalization by pendulum appliance also depicts the anchorage loss by forward movement of incisors.

9. Microimplants: They are being used widely these days to provide anchorage during orthodontic treatment. They can be used to provide direct or indirect anchorage. A full orthodontic appliance can be placed on the upper teeth, and the microimplant is attached to this appliance for anchorage. Then the distalising force on the molar can be applied by NiTi open coil spring (Fig. 25.7).

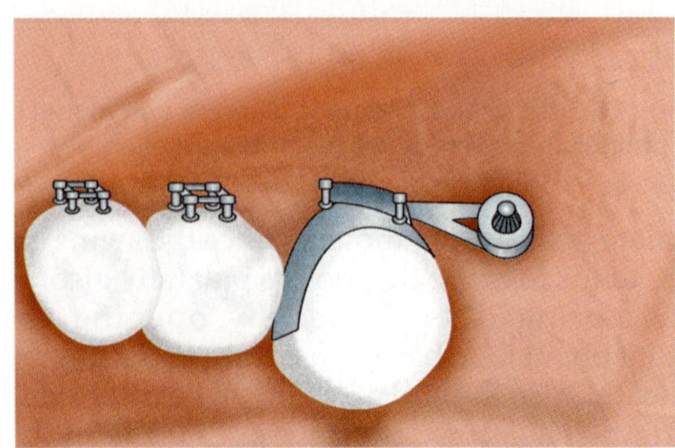

Fig. 25.7: Microimplant for distal movement of molar, and can also be used for anchorage.

10. NPE NiTi palatal expander: It is attached to the molars with the help of bands. It helps to correct the molar relation by derotating them while expanding the upper arch.

11. Transpalatal arch (TPA): Can also be used for minor distal movement of upper molar but for unilateral movement only, as the other side molar or the dental arch is used to provide the anchorage for its movement. It also derotates the molar thus correcting its apparent class II position. But, it is not a widely preferred modality due to its doubtful effect.

12. Simplified molar distalizer or frog appliance: This molar distalizer has been described by Ludwig, Glasl, Kinzinger, et al in 2011. It is a modified pendulum appliance. It is called as the "Frog appliance" due to its design. It has a special distalizing screw which has special slots to receive the TMA springs. One end of these TMA springs is attached to the molars in lingual sheath while other end is inserted in this special distalizing screw, which is activated intraorally with a special key for distal movement of a palatal arch connected to the molars. This screw is inserted in the Nance palatal button fixed at first premolars. A modification have been designed which is called as the Skeletal Frog, which has mini-implants placed in the palatal region in the region of first premolars. Mini-implants are placed just behind a line connecting the first premolars at the mesial contact point or about 6 mm behind the incisal papillae. The miniscrews should be less than 3 mm away from the midpalatal suture to ensure adequate bone thickness. An 0.032" TMA wire is used to make the pendulum springs with uprighting, expanding and toe in bends placed in the spring. These bends help to counteract the molar tipping and rotation moments. The spring arms are activated distally to provide about 200 gm of force.

The distalizing screw is reactivated every 4 to 5 weeks, with three to five full turns at each appointment, which is enough to achieve 1–2 mm of distalization per month. Each 360° activation opens the screw body 0.4 mm. Alternatively, the patient or parent can activate the appliance by rotating the screw a quarter-turn every 3 days, because the screw is easily accessible intraorally with the help of hex key.

13. Distal propeller: This design has been proposed by Jena and Panda 2009. The distal movement mainly occurs due to tipping and rotation of the crown, which is undesirable. It is be cause the force is applied coronal to the center of the resistance; flexible nature of the appliances; and loose joint between distalization appliance and the attachment on molar contributing to the tipping and rotation. Therefore, a more rigid appliance with a solid joint between appliance and the attachment on molars could cause distal movement of the molars with minimal tipping and rotation. Thus, the rigid "Distal Propeller' appliance has been designed with the aim to distalize the molars bodily and without rotation (Figs 25.8a and b).

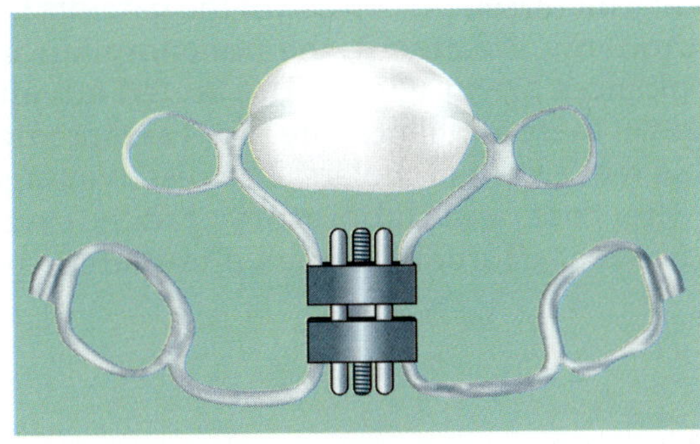

(a)

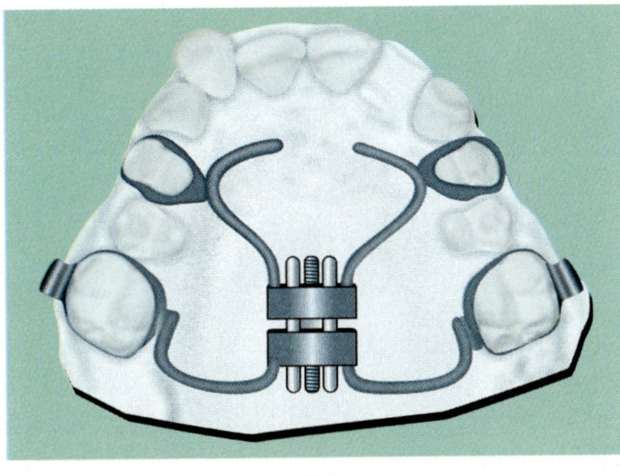

(b)

Figs 25.8a and b: Molar distalizer called as distal propeller by Jena.

Design: Bands are adapted on the maxillary first molars and first premolars on both the sides. An 11 mm Hyrax screw is adapted such that the four legs of the screw are adapted near the four bands, and the screw is oriented to open in AP direction. The arrow marks on the Hyrax screw serves as the guide for intraoral activation of the screw. The distal legs of the screw are soldered to the molar bands. The mesial legs of the screw are soldered to the premolar bands and also incorporated in the acrylic for the palatal anchorage, as a Nance palatal arch. The appliance is cemented in place with GIC cement.

Conclusion

Molar distalization is a method to gain space in the dental arch for alignment of teeth, and to correct the molar relation to class I. Many methods have been described in the literature. Due to increased perception of the patients for orthodontic treatment, the noncompliances appliances are in vogue. The added advantages of these appliances are rapid and predictable movement of molars. The disadvantage is the cost and laboratory procedures. However, affordability has eliminated the cost factor to a large extent. In our views, the Pendulum appliance is one of the most used appliances because it is custom-made, involves less cost, can be easily fabricated, does not prefabricated components and can be easily activated. Later on it can be used for retention purpose of the distally moved molar. However, all the other appliances have some advantages and disadvantages which should be considered before selecting the appliance for a particular patient.

Further Readings

1. James J. Hilgers: The Pendulum Appliance for class II Non-Compliance Therapy Volume 1992 Nov (706–714).
2. Jena A and panda. S. Distal Propeller: Innovation in Molar Distalization Appliance Design. Cyber journal orthodontics. Jun, 2009.
3. Jones, & White, Rapid class II Molar Correction with an Open-Coil Jig-Volume 1992 Oct (661–664).
4. Ludwig, Glasl, Kinzinger, Walde, and Lisson. The Skeletal Frog Appliance for Maxillary Molar Distalization. JCO 2011, VOLUME XLV NUMBER 2; 77.
5. Valrun Kalra, The K-Loop Molar Distalizing Appliance. Volume 1995 May (298–301).

26

General Concepts of Orthodontic Appliances

INTRODUCTION

Malocclusion conditions are due to abnormal position of teeth and jaws. Positional changes of teeth and jaws are needed to correct these situations. Forces are applied on teeth and dentofacial structures to move them from one position to other position in the bone, and/or to redirect the jaw growth during orthodontic treatment. These forces are applied by using special active devices which are called orthodontic appliances. Also, some appliances are used to keep the teeth in the new treated position, which are passive in nature and are called retentive appliances.

Classification of the Orthodontic Appliances

They can be divided in the following types:

a. Removable appliances/fixed appliances/semifixed appliances
b. Active/passive/retentive
c. Mechanical/myofunctional appliances: Myofunctional appliances can also be removable or fixed appliances. They can be group I/group II/group III appliances.
d. Tooth borne/tissue borne/tooth–tissue-borne
e. Myotonic/myodynamic
f. Orthodontic/orthopedic.

Definitions

These terms can be defined as follows:

Removable appliances: These are the appliances which can be removed by the patient for cleaning, etc. They are made of acrylic and wire components. However, **all wire retainers** have been described by GK Singh, which minimizes the discomfort of use by removing acrylic components. Recently, they have been also made of thermoforming materials especially retainers and TMD appliances, e.g. night guards, etc. Invisalign technique also uses the removable appliances made of special material and techniques by CAD CAM process.

Fixed appliances: These appliances are directly fixed on the teeth surface by banding or bonding. They cannot be removed by the patient, but by the doctor only. They are versatile in nature and are mostly used in practice. They help in moving the teeth in three dimensions and have better control on their movement.

Semifixed appliances: These are the appliances, a part of which can be removed by the patient but not the whole appliance.

Mechanical appliances: These are the appliances which can apply pressure on the teeth and supporting tissues by active components for the purpose of tooth movement.

Myofunctional appliances: As the name suggests, these are the appliances which derive their force by activating the muscles for correction of dental and skeletal relationships. They can be active, passive or loose fitting appliances depending on the design and underlying philosophy of designing. They harness the natural forces of orofacial muscles and transmit them to basal bone through teeth and alveolar bone. They transmit, eliminate or guide these forces and direct them in proper direction to achieve proper muscular balance and growth redirection. They are mainly used to treat the jaw discrepancy.

Active appliances: These are the appliances which exert the forces by their active components for effecting the tooth movement.

Passive appliances: These appliances do not apply forces on the teeth and their investing tissues. These are given as adjunctive modalities during the active treatment, e.g. bite plates.

Retention appliances: These appliances are passive in nature, and are used to maintain the corrected teeth in their new locations after orthodontic treatment is over. So, they function to avoid the relapse. All retentive appliances are passive in nature, but all passive appliances are not retentive. They may be removable or fixed. Removable retainers are made of acrylic or Essix thermoforming materials.

Tooth-borne appliance: It is the appliance which is totally supported by the teeth.

Tissue-borne appliance: This is the appliance which derives its support from the soft tissues surrounding the teeth.

Tooth–tissue-borne appliances: These appliances derive the support from both the teeth and the tissues.

Myotonic appliance: Myofunctional appliances which depend on the muscle mass for their action.

Myodynamic appliance: Myofunctional appliances which depend on the muscles activity for their action.

Orthopedic appliance: An appliance which applies heavy, intermittent forces for the purpose of causing changes in the skeletal relations of the jaw bases.

Orthodontic appliance: An appliance which applies lighter, continuous forces for causing the movement of teeth in the alveolar bone, without causing any skeletal changes.

Group I myofunctional appliances: These appliances transfer their forces directly to the teeth for correction of malocclusion.

Group II myofunctional appliances: These appliances reposition the mandibular base and the resulting forces are then transmitted to the teeth and the supporting tissues for correction of malocclusion.

Group III myofunctional appliances: These appliances also cause repositioning of the mandible, but their area of operation is vestibule of the mouth, e.g. Frankel appliance.

Advantages of Removable Appliances

1. They can be easily removed by the patient for cleaning purpose and thus a better oral hygiene can be maintained.
2. They are easy to fabricate.
3. Easy tipping movements can be done by them.
4. They are cheap and cost-effective.
5. They require less chair side time for fabrication and adjustment.
6. Fabrication of these appliances require less sophisticated instruments.
7. They can be used by general dental practitioner for treatment of simple conditions.
8. They are less complex than the fixed appliances.
9. They are used in many cases with fixed appliances also to augment the treatment progress, e.g. during correction of cross bite, a removable appliance with posterior/anterior bite plate can be used to open the occlusion.

Disadvantages of Removable Appliances

1. Patient cooperation is a major factor for the success of the treatment.
2. They can be lost or damaged.
3. They get broken easily if not handled carefully. The breakage is a problem in epileptic or spastic patients.
4. They can only be used for the movement of one or two teeth at a time, while

fixed appliance can be used for moving many teeth at the same time. So, it takes a lot of time with removable appliances.

5. They can only perform tipping movement, so they cannot be used to do bodily movement or rotation or torquing.
6. They cannot be used for treating the abnormal root inclination of the teeth.
7. The finishing results are poor than fixed appliances.
8. They cannot be used in extraction cases since it is difficult to close spaces.
9. They cannot be used for treatment of cases with unfavorable growth.
10. Patient can have allergy to acrylic. Thermoforming material can be used in such cases, but they do not hold wire elements properly and thus are not much effective. Only, certain elevations can be created in the thermoformed appliances to apply forces on the teeth but they can only be used for minor adjustments in dental positions.

Advantages of Fixed Appliances

1. They are fixed on teeth and cannot be removed by patients, so patient cooperation factor is largely eliminated. However, still a component of cooperation is needed so that patient does not damage or break the attachments.
2. They can be used to perform multiple movements of teeth at the same time, e.g. tipping, torquing, rotation, etc.
3. They have better control on the teeth in all the three dimensions.
4. Since multiple teeth can be controlled and moved at the same time, the treatment time required is less. Thus the results are better.
5. They can be used simultaneously with Myofunctional or orthopedic appliances.
6. They can be used to treat all types of cases from mild to severe ones. They are versatile in nature.

Disadvantages of Fixed Appliances

1. They are complex in nature and can be used by trained person only.
2. They are costly.
3. Maintenance of oral hygiene is difficult as they are fixed on the teeth. Plaque and food debris get accumulated around the attachments and thus cleaning is difficult.
4. Gingival problems especially swollen gums are seen since the attachments are near to gums and there are more plaque deposits.
5. Some patients may be allergic to nickle component of the appliances.
6. They take more chair side time when patient comes for adjustments, as time is needed to remove the old wires and either to modify them or to place newly fabricated wires with required bends, etc. and then ligated back in the brackets.
7. Patient has to come on regular visits to the clinician. If the gap of follow-up becomes longer, then it may also lead to abnormal tooth movements, e.g. it may lead to over-retraction of upper incisors leading to cross bite development; loss of torque; over-tipping, etc.
8. If appliance gets damaged, it may apply mis-directed forces on the teeth.

Advantages of Myofunctional Appliances

1. They are used during growth period and help in achieving skeletal correction.
2. They also help in redirecting the growth of jaws in proper direction.
3. They help in elimination of abnormal habits.
4. They can be used in conjunction with fixed appliances.
5. They harness the natural forces and thus do not apply abnormal forces on the teeth.
6. They help to physiologically develop the dental arches and jaw bases.

Disadvantages of Myofunctional Appliances

1. Removable type of appliances depend on patient cooperation.
2. They are bulky and can lead to adjustment problems.
3. Single piece appliances, e.g. bionator, activator, etc. cause speech problems and patients stop using them properly due to discomforts.
4. They are difficult to make.
5. They need precision in fabrication and frequent adjustments.
6. They need a lot of chair time and laboratory time.

Ideal Requirements of an Orthodontic Appliance

Orthodontic appliances used for treatment should satisfy certain requirements which can be discussed under following broad headings:

a. Biological requirements
b. Mechanical requirements
c. Esthetics requirements
d. Hygienic requirements.

Biological Requirements

Appliances apply forces on the teeth and supporting structures leading to biochemical changes in the tissues. These appliances should satisfy following biological requirements.

1. They should apply forces within the physiological limits so as not to injure the investing tissues.
2. They should be able to produce desired OTM.
3. They should be able to produce physiological changes in the tissues.
4. They should not produce pathological changes, e.g. devitalisation of pulp, root resorption, etc.
5. They should be biocompatible.
6. They should not interfere with natural growth and function.
7. Appliance should not disintegrate in the oral fluids.

Mechanical Requirements

Some of the mechanical requirements are:

1. They should be simple to fabricate.
2. They should apply physiologically light forces to the teeth and supporting structures. They should apply forces of desired intensity, direction and duration.
3. Appliances should be strong enough to bear functional forces.
4. They should not be bulky and should be universal in nature.

Hygienic Requirements

Appliances should be simple so as not to interfere with oral hygiene. It should ideally be self-cleansing or should be easy to clean. Oral hygiene should be well-maintained because the attachments act as niche for plaque harbouring and lead to gingivitis and caries lesion. Caries can be initially seen as white spot lesions (WSL), which is subsurface mineralisation around the brackets and gingival to the band margins. WSL should be controlled as soon as possible by maintaining oral hygiene and using fluoride-containing tooth paste and chlorhexidine mouthwashes, as they have tendency to revert back to normal structure before frank cavitation of enamel occurs.

Esthetic Requirements

One of the major objectives of orthodontic treatment is better esthetics, so the appliance should not be lead to a compromised esthetics. Removable appliances are more esthetically favorable by patients as compared to fixed ones, because they can be removed at will by the patients at certain occasions. The appliance should be less conspicuous, and esthetically acceptable. With the introduction of tooth colored plastic or ceramic brackets, the esthetics of fixed appliances has improved considerably over the metallic braces. Lingual brackets have added a new dimension to the fixed appliance therapy and thus more adult patients are being attracted toward the orthodontic clinics.

Conclusion

Orthodontic appliances help to move the teeth in new position and then to keep them there. There is a wide variety of appliances which can be selected by clinicians depending on the requirements. One of the major point to be remembered that the forces applied by them should be within safe physiological limits, to avoid any injury to the teeth and tissues. Also they should satisfy the esthetic needs of the patients.

27

Removable Appliances

INTRODUCTION

These appliances can be removed and reinserted in oral cavity by the patient. Historically, they have been in use in dentistry since 19th century, much before the advent of fixed appliances. In their initial days, they were crude, bulky, and were made of precious metal wires and vulcanite plate. With continued quest for better options, the modern day removable appliances came into the foray. The modern day appliances are made of stainless steel hard wires and acrylic and are better in design, esthetics, mechanics and efficiency.

They are used to treat malocclusion conditions which require simple tipping movements. They can move the teeth in mesiodistal and labiolingual direction. Since they can apply single force only, they cannot be used for complex movements, like torquing, rotations, translation, etc. Also, they cannot move multiple teeth at the same time, and thus after the role of one appliance is finished, a new appliance may be needed for another tooth movement in the same patient. They are also used during fixed appliance therapy to augment the treatment (e.g. bite plates) and then as retention appliances.

Another variety of removable appliances are the removable myofunctional appliances which harness forces of muscles. They help in redirecting the jaw growth and achieving a normal relation of jaw bases, but they will be discussed in another chapter.

Uses of Removable Appliances

Since they only move the teeth by tipping, they can be best used.

1. For retraction of incisors which are proclined and have spaces between them.
2. For closure of midline spaces between central incisors by moving them mesially.
3. By pulling the canines back in their own space or the space created by extraction of first premolars in case, if canines are labially blocked-out.
4. Some other conditions in which they can be used will be subsequently discussed in this chapter.
5. They can be used during fixed appliances for various purposes, e.g. to augment anchorage, to open the bite during crossbite correction, to apply intrusive forces on molars with the help of posterior bite plates, to expand the maxillary arch, etc.
6. They are also used as retainers.
7. They are used for habit breaking, control of mouth breathing, etc.

Advantages and disadvantages of removable appliances: *See* Chapter 26 General Concepts of Appliances

Mechanical principle: Main principle during the use of RA is the apex position of the affected tooth. RAs are capable of only tipping movements.

Position of the apex of the tooth: The main point to be considered during tooth movement with removable appliance is the initial position of the apex of the tooth to be moved. Removable appliance causes only the tipping movement, with more movement of crown in the direction of force, and minimal movement of apex of root opposite to the force direction. The teeth with their apices in normal position but crowns shifted in abnormal direction are best treated by tipping movements achieved with removable appliances.

Since the force is applied at the single point on the tooth, they cannot be used for causing bodily tooth movements, torquing and rotations. However, judicious cutting of acrylic and activation of labial wire can be used for labial root movement of incisors in some cases, but there, the patient-cooperation and regular check up is needed to avoid over torquing/torque loss/root prominence, etc.

However, intrusion and extrusion can be effected through removable appliances often mediated by using the forces of eruption. The acrylic ramps known as bite plates are incorporated in the appliances which can help in selective intrusion or extrusion of the teeth. This mechanism will be discussed later in the chapter.

Tendency to rotate the teeth: Since the force applied by RA is away from the Crot of tooth, it leads to tooth rotation in some cases, e.g. when canine retractor spring is used to retract the canine, then the tooth may rotate mesiolabially. It happens because the force lies labial to the crot of canine, thus producing a moment.

Interrupted force application: The force applied by RA is not of continuous nature because it abruptly falls to zero when appliance is removed. Also there is rapid force decay rate.

Amount of force: Amount of force applied should be light, so the active components should be made of lighter wires. Also the activation should be adequate to generate lighter forces so that they compress the PDL upto its half width, and does not crush the PDL.

Components of a Removable Appliance

It has following three basic components, i.e. retentive components, active components and acrylic base plate.

- **Retentive components:** They help in retaining the appliance in place.
- **Active components:** They help in applying forces for the movement of the teeth.
- **Base plate:** It binds all the components into a single functional unit.

A. Retentive Components

They help in keeping the appliance in place and resist its displacement. A well-retained appliance is necessary for proper application of force to achieve adequate tooth movement, and for a better cooperation from the patient. If an appliance is loose or uncomfortable, the patient stops using it and thus the treatment does not progress.

The retention is obtained by using special wire components known as clasps which engage the undercuts on the tooth surfaces below the height of contour. These undercuts lie below HOC on all the four surfaces, i.e. buccal, lingual, mesial and distal surfaces of the tooth (Fig. 27.1). The undercuts on buccal and lingual surfaces of teeth are more near to gingival margin of the tooth, they are shallow because the HOC lies at the junction of middle and cervical third of the tooth and have lesser retentive ability. They can be seen from the proximal aspect. Some clasps which are made to use this undercut are half clasp, three-fourths or C-clasp, Jackson's clasp, Southend clasp (on anterior teeth). Since these clasps need the undercut lying in cervical third of tooth, they can be made only on those teeth which are fully erupted.

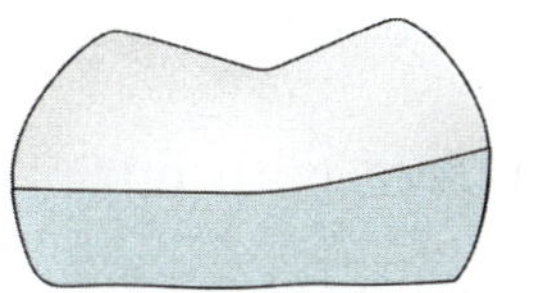

Shaded area on buccal aspect in molar shows the undercuts which receive arrowheads of the Adam's clasp

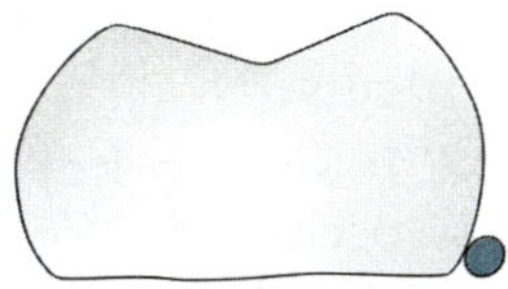

View from proximal aspect, showing undercut below HOC, which receive clasps during adaptation and helps in retention of the appliance)

Fig. 27.1: Undercut area below the height of contour, which is the ideal area to receive the clasps for retention of an appliance.

Undercuts which lie on mesial and distal surfaces of the tooth, are more prominent and have better retentive ability. It is because the proximal surfaces of teeth converge from their widest dimension at contact points towards the cervical side and the HOC lies in the middle third of the surfaces. They can be seen from the buccal or lingual aspect. Clasps using these undercuts are pin-head clasp, Adams clasp, triangular clasp, ball-end clasp, twin block (Clarks's) delta clasp, modified ball-end clasp, etc. (Fig. 27.2).

Requirements of an Ideal Clasp

1. It should be easy to fabricate.
2. It should have an adequate retentive ability.
3. It should be strong, sturdy and should not get distorted under masticatory forces and under the forces when appliance is removed from the mouth. That is why it is made of hard, heavy SS wire, e.g. of 0.7 mm or more size wire (21 gauge or less).
4. It should be easily adjustable during follow-up visits and should be universal to use.
5. It should be passive on the teeth, i.e. should not apply any force on the teeth they are engaging, otherwise this may lead to movement of these teeth and thus anchorage and stability of appliance is affected.
6. It should be able to be used on partially and fully erupted teeth.
7. It should not impinge on soft tissue and should be able to engage shallow undercuts.
8. It should not interfere with normal occlusion.
9. It should not break during the use otherwise it should be reparable or modifiable to other form of clasp, e.g. Adams clasp, if breaks, can be modified to a pin-head clasp easily. If there is not proper retentive ability of the clasps, then the appliance has to be refabricated.

Types of clasps: Different clasps have been mentioned in literature, e.g. half clasp; three-fourths or circumferential or C-clasp; pin head clasp; ball end clasp; Adams clasp; triangular clasp; Jackson's clasp; Crozat clasp; delta clasp, Duyzing clasp, etc. Some of them have been briefly described below. The detailed fabrication can be seen in books dedicated to removable appliances (Figs 27.3 and 27.4).

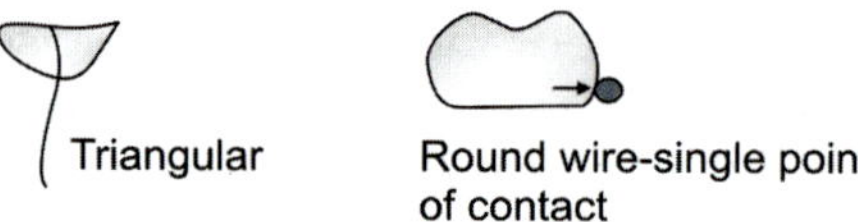

Fig. 27.2: A round wire used for clasp fabrication achieves a single point of contact with the tooth surface due to its round cross-section.

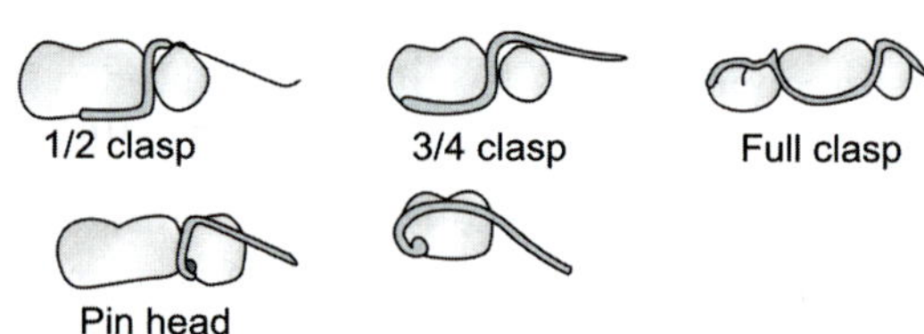

Fig. 27.3: Different types of retention clasps.

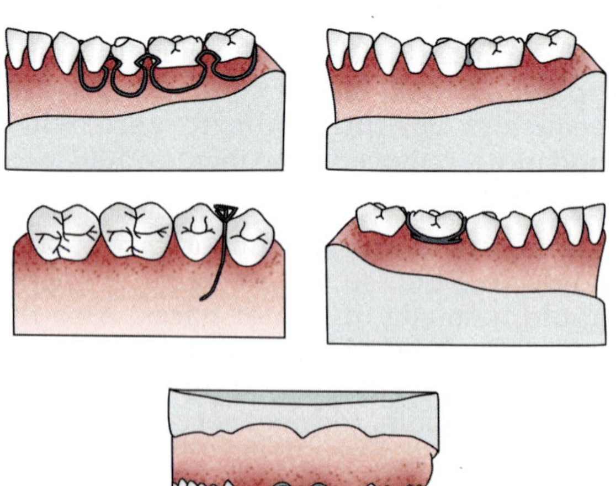

Fig. 27.4: Different types of retention clasps: Schwarz clasp; ball-end clasp; triangular clasp; Crozat clasp; Southend clasp.

Half clasp: It is adapted on the buccal cervical undercut below the HOC parallel to free gingival margin. The free end of the wire starts at approx midpoint of the tooth's buccal surface and then adapting parallel to gingival margin, is adapted in one of the proximal undercut mainly buccodistal, and carried over to the occlusal embrasure. Then it is adapted on the palatal/lingual aspect where it is engaged in the acrylic. It is simple to fabricate. Disadvantage of this clasp is it that it cannot be made in partially erupted tooth because the cervical undercut is not available. Also, it has a single point of contact on the tooth surface, i.e. along the margin of round wire, thus limiting its retentive capability. During adjustment, generally it gets displaced, loosing its adaptation on the tooth surface and thus starts touching at a premature contact. In that condition, the appliance starts dislodging from the dental arch. At this point of time, it is better to modify it in a pin-head clasp. It has a single retentive arm.

C-clasp (Fig. 27.5): It is also known as three-fourths, three-quarter or circumferential clasp. It is an extension of half clasp. Its free end starts from the one proximal undercut, generally mesiobuccal, is adapted parallel to the free gingiva, then it is adapted in the other proximal undercut mainly buccodistal, and carried over to the occlusal embrasure. Then it is adapted on the palatal/lingual aspect where it is included in the acrylic. Thus it also has only one retentive arm. Its advantages and disadvantages are same as half clasp.

Jackson's clasp or full clasp: It is also a modified C-clasp. It is also called U-clasp due to its shape. It engages the cervical undercut and both the mesial and distal-proximal undercuts. The wire is adapted in cervical undercut parallel to gingival margin, and then both the free ends are engaged in proximal undercuts and carried on to the occlusal embrasures, and then adapted on palatal side. It has better retentive ability and has two retentive arms to engage acrylic. It is also simple to construct, but it cannot be used in partially erupted teeth.

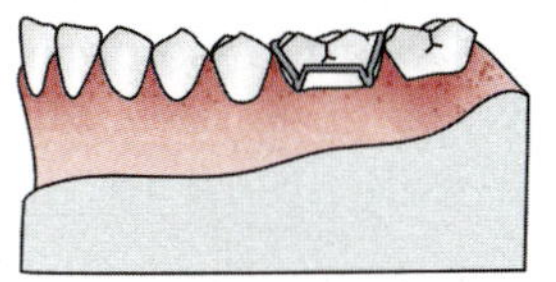

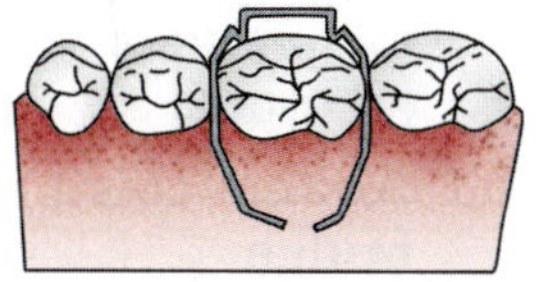

Fig. 27.5: C-clasp; full clasp.

Pin-head clasp: It is one of the simplest clasps. One end of the wire is bent on to itself in the shape of small helix or awl-pin-head, which is engaged in the buccal embrasure between two adjoining teeth just below the contact area. This head is oriented at approx 45° to the occlusal plane or the buccal surface of the tooth. It should be slightly prominent so that it can be used for removal of the appliance with finger pressure. The free end of wire is adapted in occlusal embrasure and then adapted onto the lingual surface, to be engaged in acrylic. It is simple to construct. Disadvantage is that it displaces/traumatises the gingival papilla. Overactivated clasp can apply separating forces on the adjoining teeth. The free end of the helix/head may irritate the soft tissues.

Ball-end clasp: A 1.5–2 mm diameter bead of solder material is soldered on one of the free end of the wire. It is then adapted engaging the buccal embrasure between two adjacent teeth. The contact of ball with the two teeth gives point of contact and thus the retention. The free end is adapted on lingual side to be inserted in acrylic. It also helps in additional retention. Advantage over pin head is that its free end will not be irritating to the soft tissues due to its smooth contours. Disadvantage is that it needs solder material and soldering procedure which may cause weakening of the wire and the breakage at the soldered area.

Triangular clasp (Fig. 27.6): It is a modified pin-head clasp. It is a small clasp having a triangular head. It is placed between two adjacent teeth in the buccal embrasure. It can be of two types, i.e. with hook and without hook. One end of the wire is bent in the form of an equilateral triangle, which starts in the centre of one side of the triangle. It is adapted in the buccal embrasure below contact area of two adjacent teeth. It gains its retention form both the adjoining teeth. The triangle is kept

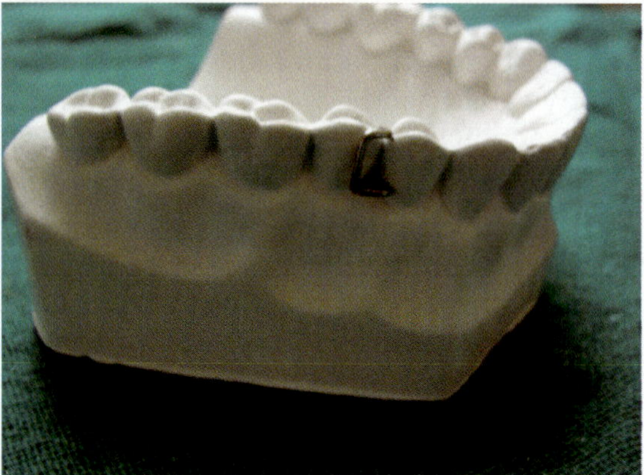

Fig. 27.6: Triangular clasp.

parallel to OP. A hook can also be incorporated in it opening in distal side to engage the elastics if required. It can be used to gain additional retention, along with Adams clasp.

Adams clasp (Figs 27.7a and b): It was designed by C Philips Adams, and opened the gates for better retention of the appliances. It is also called as Liverpool clasp, universal clasp, Modified arrowhead clasp, etc. This engages the buccoproximal undercuts below HOC on the same tooth and offers maximum retention or undercuts.

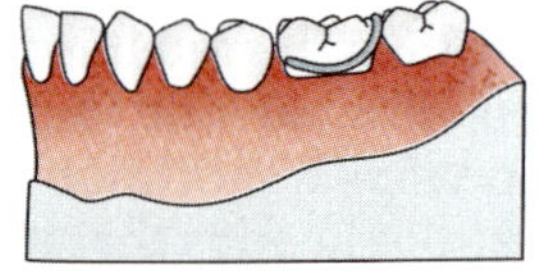

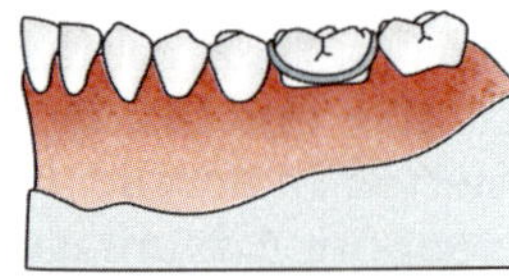

(a)

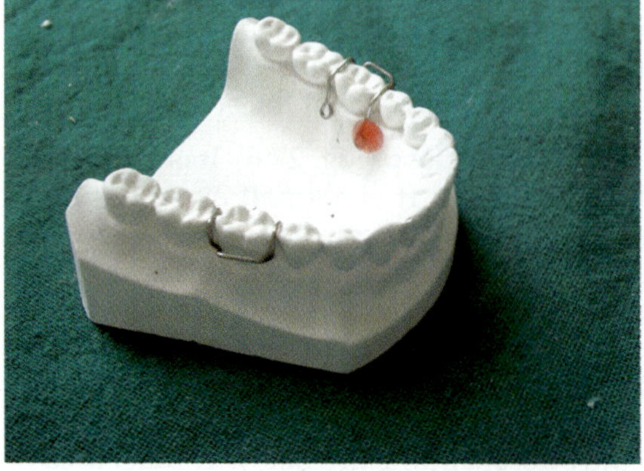

(b)

Figs 27.7a and b: Ideal Adams clasp.

It is generally made of 0.7 mm hard SS wire. It has following parts: 1 bridge, 2 arrowheads, 2 occlusal segments and 2 retentive arms.

The bridge is made of the length equal to or slightly more than the distance between the buccal cusps tips if made on molars, or approx two-thirds the mesiodistal dimension of the tooth it is being made on. The arrow heads are made in V-shape, which are oriented at 135° to the bridge, and they engage the mesial and distal buccal undercuts. The bridge is oriented at 45° to the buccal surface, approx in the middle of the crown and away from the buccal surface of the tooth. The free arms are adapted in occlusal embrasures and then on the palatal side to be engaged in acrylic as retentive arms. Its figures and details can be looked in the book on removable appliances.

Advantages of Adams Clasp

1. It engages the two undercuts on the same tooth and offers maximum retention.
2. It has two points of contact and thus is more stable.
3. It is rigid.
4. It can be made on the partially erupted teeth.
5. It can be made on primary and permanent teeth.
6. It can be made on two adjacent teeth as long bridge.
7. It can be made for anterior teeth also.
8. If broken, it can easily be converted in the pin head clasp.
9. It can be modified in various shapes.

Modifications of Adams Clasp (Figs 27.8 to 27.11)

1. Adams clasp with soldered buccal tube: It can be modified as the buccal tubes can be soldered on bridge
2. Adams clasp with soldered hook: It can be modified as a hooks can be soldered on bridge
3. Adams clasp with helix bent in the bridge
4. Adams clasp with distal extension hook.

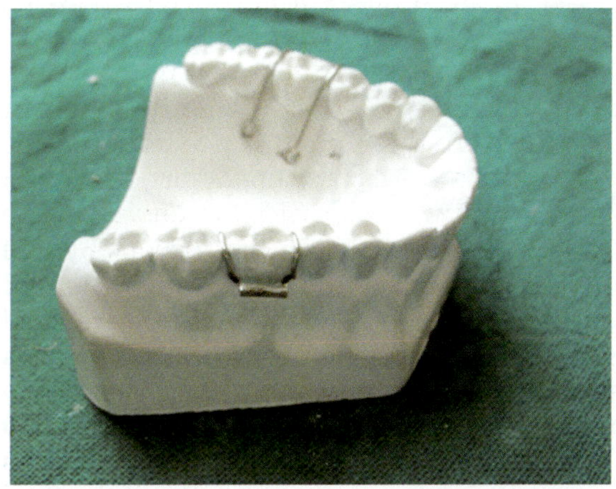

Fig. 27.8: Adams clasp with soldered buccal tube.

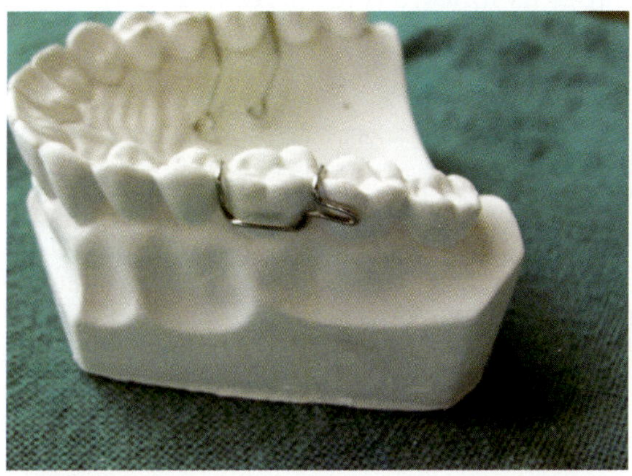

Fig. 27.9: Adams clasp with distal extension.

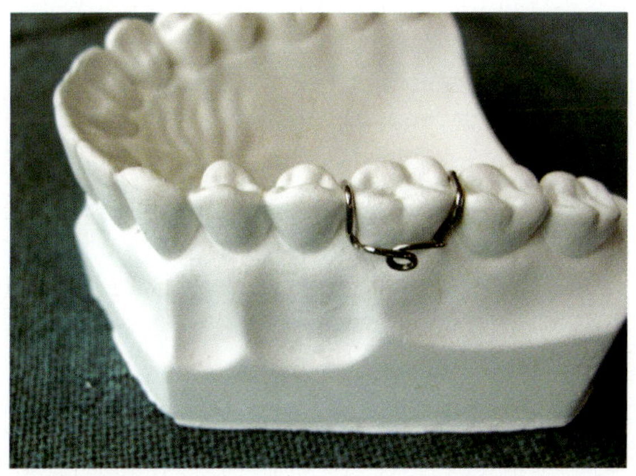

Fig. 27.10: Adams clasp with helix.

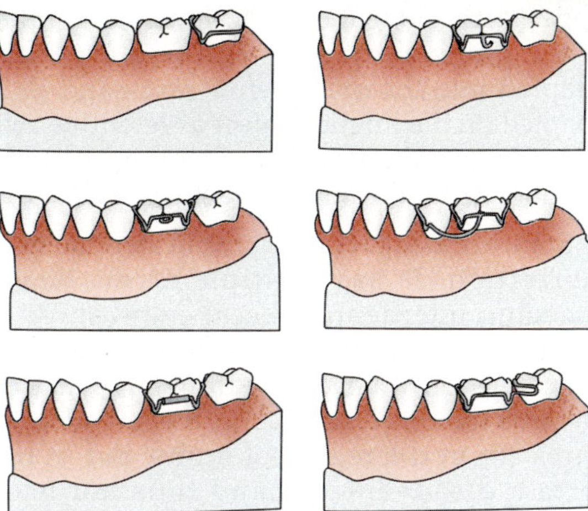

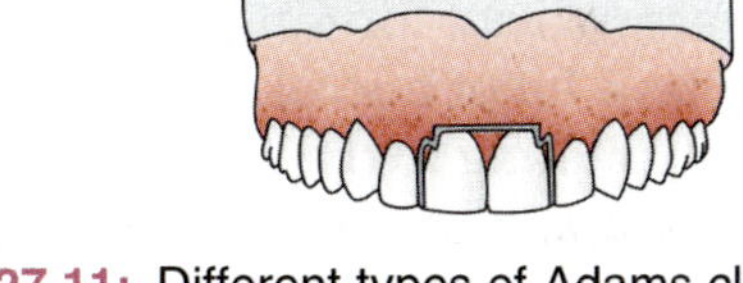

Fig. 27.11: Different types of Adams clasps: Adams clasp with single arrowhead; Adams clasp with soldered hook; Adams clasp with helix; Adams clasp with additional arrowhead; Adams clasp with soldered tube; Adams clasp with distal extension; Adams clasp on incisors.

5. Adams clasp with additional arrowhead: For gaining additional retention, another arrowhead can be bent on adjacent tooth, and its free arm is soldered to the bridge of main Adams clasp.
6. Adams clasp with single arrowhead: It can be made on partially erupted teeth or distally tilted teeth.
7. It can be modified in to form spiral of wire on the bridge to form a tube in which inner bow of headgear face bow can be engaged.
8. Adams clasp on incisors, canines and premolars can also be made in the same way, and help augmenting the retention.

Disadvantages: Its construction is complex and more time-consuming as compared to other discussed clasps.

Southend clasp: It is the clasp which is made in one-piece on two central incisors especially upper teeth, along the cervical margin parallel to the gingival margin. The free-arms are adapted into the incisal embrasure and then adapted on the lingual aspect as retentive arm to be inserted in acrylic. It helps to gain retention from the anterior teeth as well.

Schwarz clasp: It is a complicated clasp in fabrication. It has multiple arrow heads engaging interdental-buccal embrasures of many adjacent teeth. This is the only clasp in which the arrow heads rise from gingival side towards the cervical area, i.e. the arrowheads wires are in the region of gums. But, it has certain disadvantages and thus not used anymore.

1. Its fabrication is difficult and needs special arrowhead forming pliers.
2. It occupies a lot of buccal vestibule.
3. It can be irritating to the soft tissues.
4. Since it is made of single long wire, it may be more flexible and may get distorted with use.
5. Its adaptation is difficult.

Crozat clasp: It is a modified form of Jackson's full clasp. A wire is adapted parallel to gingival margin of the tooth below the HOC on buccal side which engages the mesial and distal undercuts also. This is soldered to the full clasp. It provides additional retention, but needs soldering procedure and instruments. It is also obsolete nowadays.

Modified Adams clasp by Clark: It is called **delta clasp**. Clark modified the Adams clasp in his landmark article on Twin block appliance. He removed the arrowheads and replaced them with the loops which may be triangular, ovoid or circular in shape. According to him, it has better retention, reduced metal fatigue, less fracture of clasp during use, and needs lesser adjustments.

ACTIVE COMPONENTS OF THE REMOVABLE APPLIANCES

Active components are those components which are used to apply forces on the teeth to cause tooth movement. They are broadly divided in four categories:

1. Labial bows
2. Springs
3. Expansion screws
4. Elastics

A. Labial Bows

They are adapted on the labial/buccal surfaces of teeth with U-loops incorporated for activation and adjustment. They are used generally for retraction of proclined incisors having spaces in between them. Since they have to apply light forces on the teeth, they should be made with round, light, hard s.s wires of 0.5–0.6 mm diameter. But if the total length of labial bow is more, then 0.7 mm wire can be used. They are also used in passive form for making retainers. They are of various shapes as follows (Figs 27.12 to 27.23):

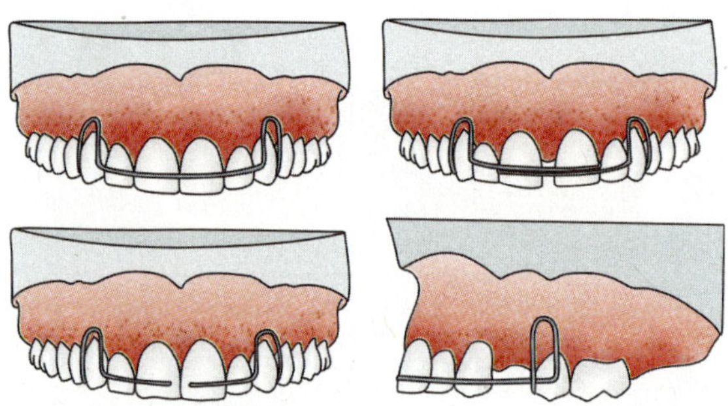

Fig. 27.12: Different labial bows: medium labial bow; modified split labial bow; split labial bow; reverse labial bow.

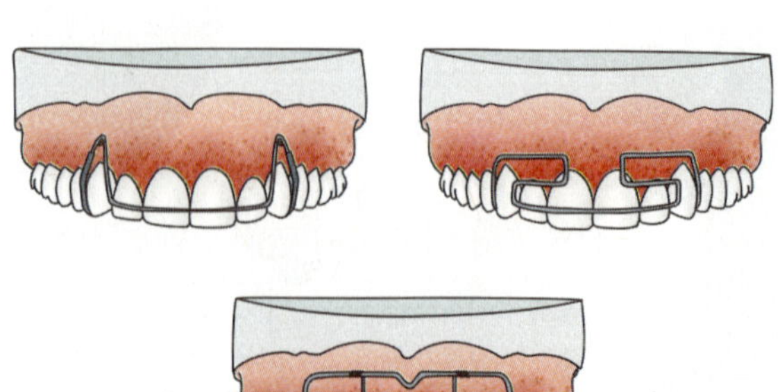

Fig. 27.13: Different labial bows: Robert's retractor; mills retractor; high labial bow with apron spring.

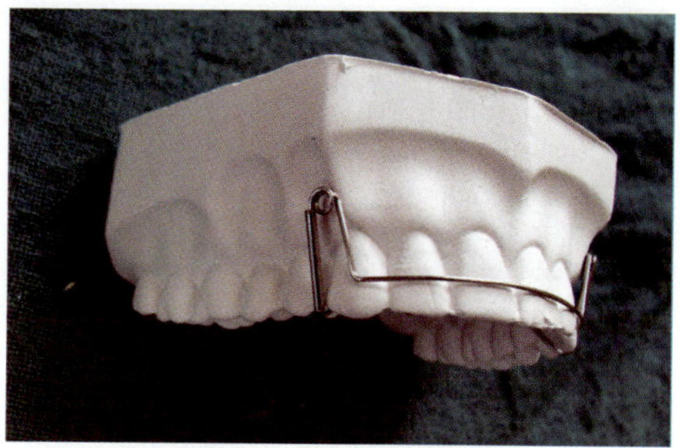

Fig. 27.14: Robert's retractor.

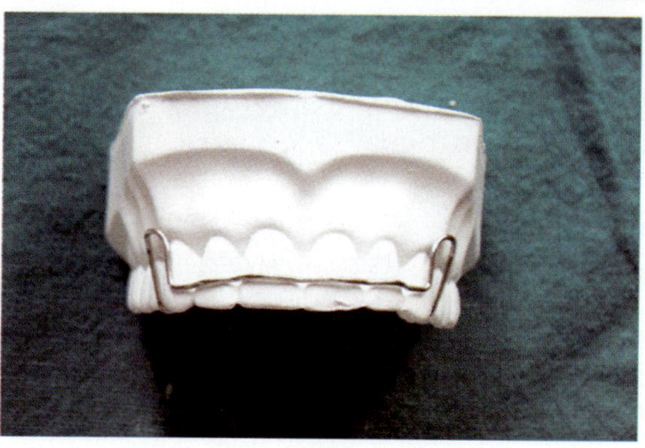

(a)

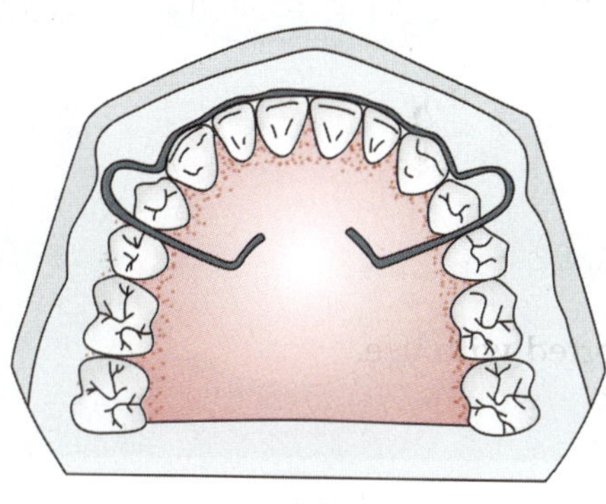

(b)

Figs 27.17a and b: Fitted labial bow.

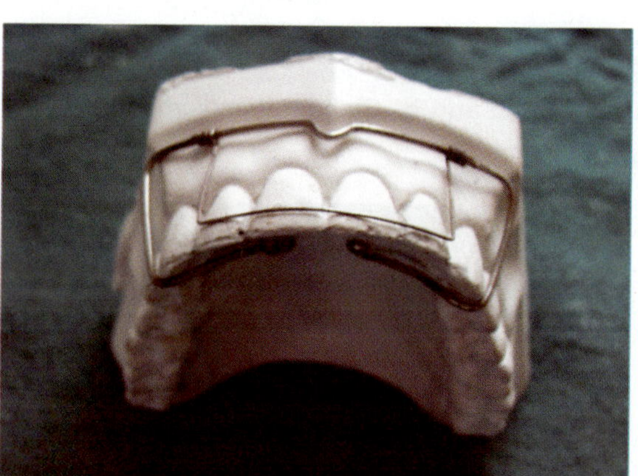

Fig. 27.15: High labial bow with apron spring.

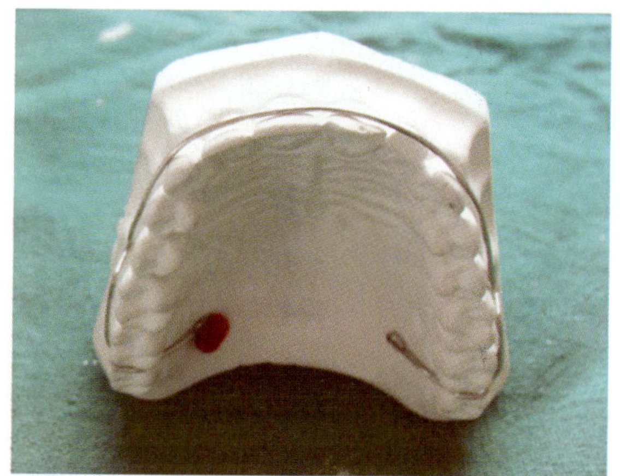

Fig. 27.16: Beggs retention bow.

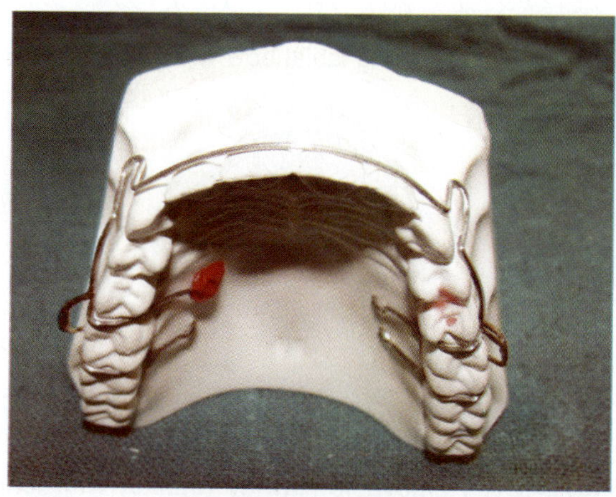

Fig. 27.18: Soldered labial bow.

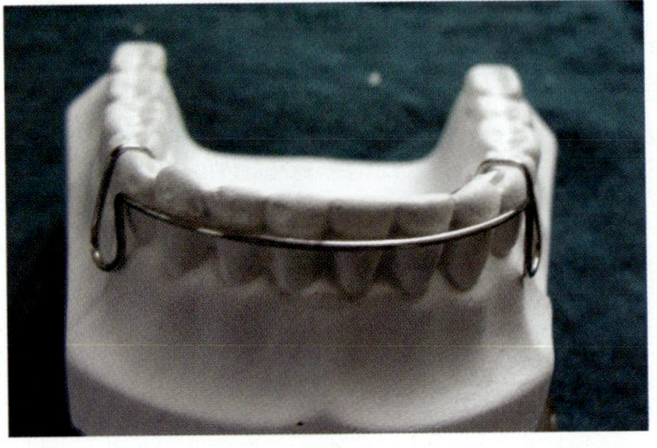

(a)

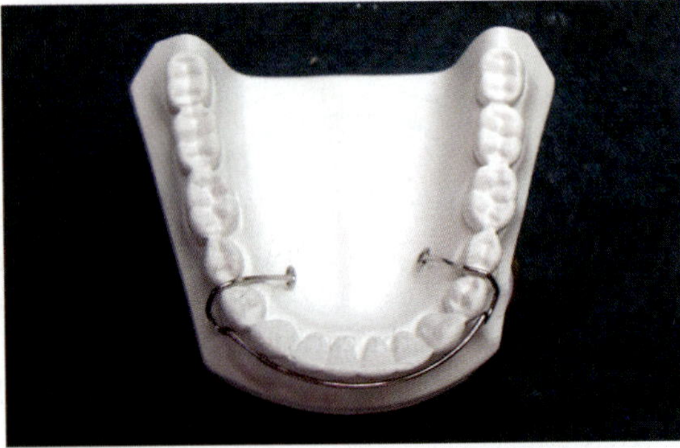

(b)

Figs 27.19a and b: Long labial bow.

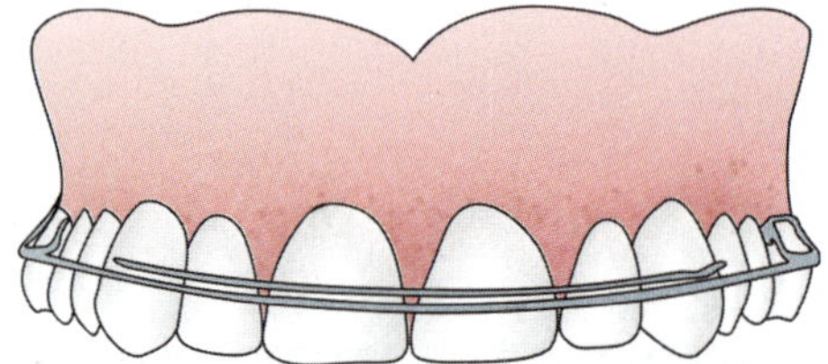

Fig. 27.20: Long labial bow with elastics.

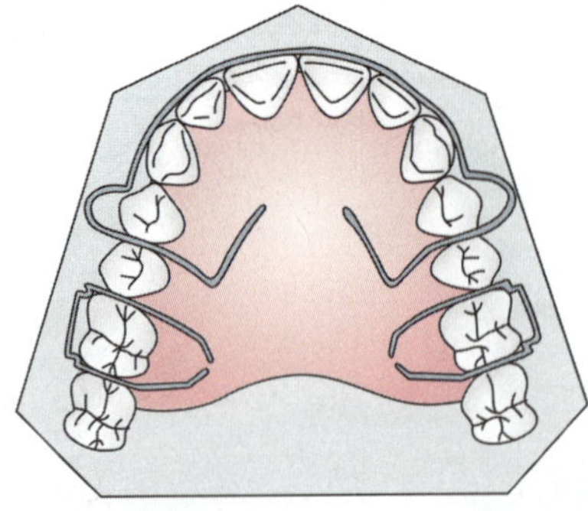

Fig. 27.21: Removable Hawley retainer with long labial bow.

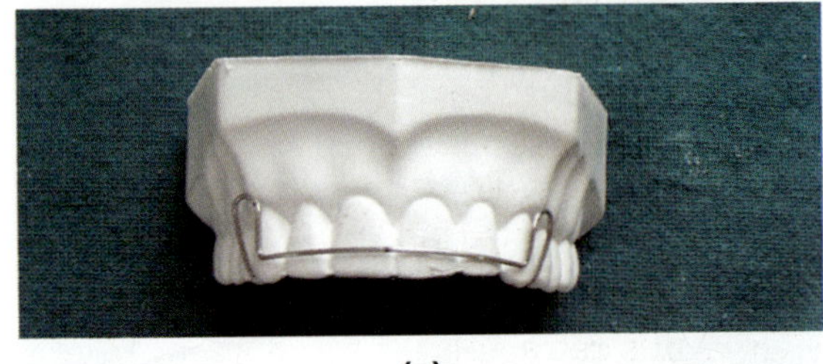

(a)

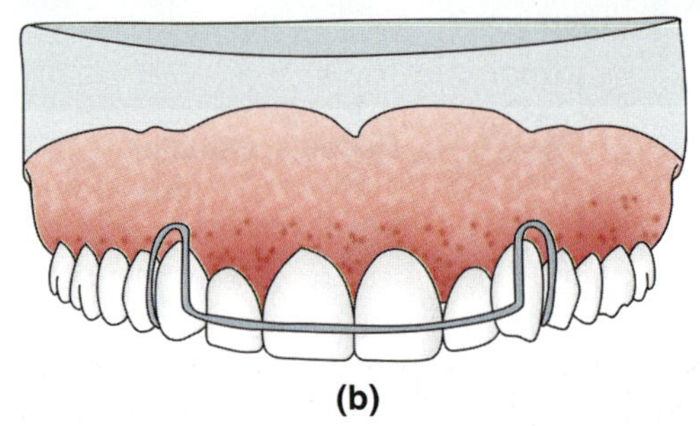

(b)

Figs 27.22a and b: Standard/medium labial bow.

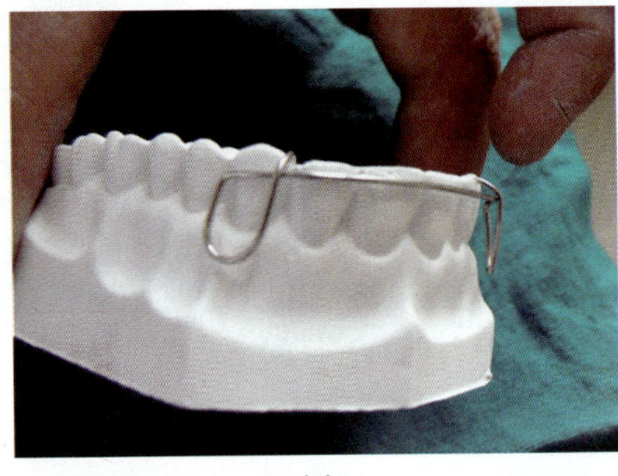

(a)

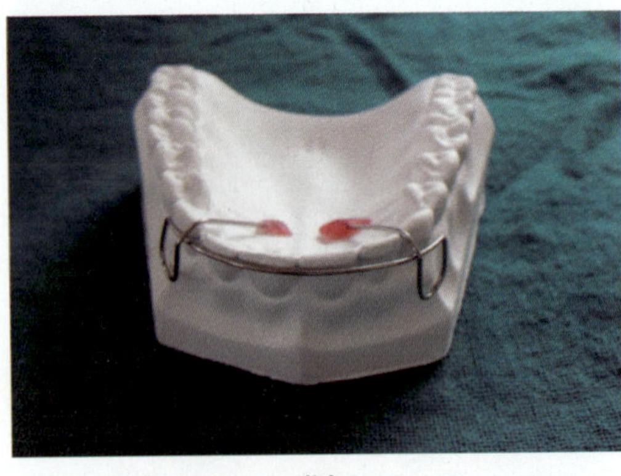

(b)

Figs 27.23a and b: Reverse loop labial bow.

a. Short labial bow
b. Medium labial bow
c. Long labial bow
d. Split labial bow
e. Fitted labial bow
f. Reverse labial bow
g. Roberts retractor
h. Mills retractor
i. Labial bow soldered to bridge of Adams clasp
j. High labial bow with apron spring
k. Labial bow with canine spur
l. Beggs type labial bow
m. Labial bow for retention purpose.

General design and fabrication of labial bow: Hard SS wire of adequate size is taken, and is shaped in the form of arch form. It is adapted at the junction of incisal and middle third of the teeth, touching the most prominent teeth. Since it is made of round wire, they maintain single point of contact with the tooth surface. The marks are placed to incorporate the U-loops. The loop's mesial leg starts at mesial third of the last teeth to be incorporated in the labial bow and it extends 2 mm below the free gingival margin. A U-turn is given and the distal leg of loop is made parallel to the mesial leg and is adapted in occlusal embrasure and then carried to the lingual side as retentive arm. The U-loop should not be at the level of gingival margin where it can injure or irritate the gingiva. The bow is activated by squeezing the two legs, such that only approx. 1 mm palatal displacement of the wire occurs. This is important because 1 mm displacement of wire will lead to shifting of teeth in their PDL space by approx. 0.5 mm or less, and thus PDL will not be crushed.

Mechanism of action: The bow has a single point contact with the labial surface of the teeth. The fulcrum or Crot lies usually at about 40% of the length of the root from the apex. It leads to generation of moment of force which produces tipping of teeth.

Short labial bow: It is made from lateral incisor to lateral incisor, engaging four teeth. Since it span is short, it is made of 0.5–0.6 mm wire. The wire is shaped in the form of anterior arch, and 2 U-loops are incorporated at lateral incisors. It is generally used for retention purpose since its span is less and hence it is less flexible. Or it should be used when there are minor spaces between teeth.

Medium or standard labial bow: It extends from canine to canine. It is more flexible than short bow due to increased wire length. It can be used for moderate space closure. It can also be used for retainer appliance when it is made of 0.8 mm or more diameter wire and its level is maintained at the middle of the middle 3rd of the teeth (Fig. 27.22).

Long labial bow: It extends between premolars. It is also used for retention purpose esp in extraction cases, to avoid opening of the extraction spaces. It can be used for minor anterior space closure. It can help in guidance of the erupting canines. A long bow is made when canines are erupting, so that it does not interfere with eruption of canine by engaging the space meant for canines (Fig. 27.19).

Split labial bow: The bow is splitted in the centre resulting in two separate labial arms with U-loop on each. It has great flexibility and can help in minor retraction. But, its efficiency is not that good. A modified split bow is used for midline space closure, when it is extended and hooked distal to the tooth to be moved mesially. The U-loop helps in activation. But, it may lead to rotation of the tooth disto-labially since the force is passing labial to the centre of rotation of the tooth.

Reverse labial bow (Fig. 27.23): The loops used in it are closed loops rather than open type of U-loops. The loops are placed distal to the canines, while free end passes between canine and premolar. Since the wire length is more in this loop, it is more flexible and thus capable of applying lighter forces due to increased flexibility. This loop is activated differently as compared to the open U-loop. The loop is opened first to move the labial wire towards the palatal side to put pressure on the teeth. It leads to shifting of the labial wire incisually. Then compensatory bend is given in the loop's distal bend to bring the wire at its original position. It is also used for incisors retraction.

Robert's retractor: It is made of 0.5 mm s.s wire. A helix of about 3 mm diameter is incorporated in the V-shaped loops which tends to increase the wire length and hence flexibility. The thin wire and helix make it highly flexible and thus vertical stability is less. Thus, the distal arm of the loop is passed through a steel tubing of 0.5 mm diameter to support it and to avoid distortion during use. It is used in treating severe anterior proclination and esp in adult patients and in periodontally-compromised teeth, where very light forces are required (Fig. 27.14).

Mills retractor: It incorporates a very long wire as the boot-loops/L-loops are incorporated in the bow. The loops have a vertical and a horizontal component. The horizontal component extends till the middle of the central incisors on both sides. This bow is highly flexible and provides light forces over a long range. Its disadvantage is that its fabrication is difficult and it is esthetically unacceptable. It is more prone to distortion during use, and thus needs a regular follow up. If patient keeps on using distorted bow, then abnormal forces may be generated.

High labial bow with apron spring: It is made of hard heavy SS wire of 0.9 mm or more diameter, which extends in the labial vestibule of upper arch, and it is adapted so as to avoid the maxillary labial frenum. An apron spring of lighter wire of 0.4 mm size is wound around this high labial bow adapted to 1 or more teeth and both the ends are soldered to the wire. It approaches the tooth from gingival side. Since it is very flexible wire, so it is used to generate very light forces to move the teeth palatally. It can be used in adult patients and periodontally involved teeth. It is used to treat very large overjet due to extreme proclination of the front teeth, where the usual labial bow wire gets slipped gingivally upon activation and thus no forces come into play.

The apron spring is activated by bending it towards the teeth. Since it is very flexible, it can be activated for upto 3 mm at one time. Its range of action is long and force decay is less. Only disadvantage is that construction is difficult, needs soldering, and may cause soft tissue injury.

Fitted labial bow (Fig. 27.17): This is made of hard wire of approx 0.7 mm or more size. The wire is adapted on the labial surfaces of the front teeth, and is used mainly in retainers. It cannot be used for any active movements. Its construction is difficult since finer bends are needed to adapt them to contours of teeth.

Soldered labial bow: The labial bow is made with U-loops in the region of canines-premolar, and then its free ends are extended back till the bridge of Adams clasp, where they are soldered. It is given after active orthodontic treatment in a retention appliance. It allows for a better settling of the occlusion as no wires cross the occlusal surface. Its drawback is that it needs soldering and its equipments. Also soldered points tend to break. It is flexible as the point of soldering is far behind, and thus the patient may distort is while removing the appliance. Generally, such bows should be supported by additional wires wound around them and engaged in the acrylic in lateral incisor-canine regions.

Labial bow with elastics: A hook can be soldered on the distal arm of the loops. It is used to engage elastic which crosses on the labial surfaces of incisors, thus applying lighter lingually-directed forces for their retraction (Fig. 27.20).

Beggs retention bow: This is made to have U-loops in the embrasure region between canine and second premolar in extraction cases. The distal ends pass distal to last erupted tooth, are adapted on the palatal region to be engaged in acrylic. It serves the purpose of active and retentive component of the appliance. It can be activated if extraction space opening is observed during retention phase. Due to length of wire, it is flexible and can be used to apply lighter forces. It allows for settling of the occlusion as no wires cross the occlusal surface. It is flexible as the point of retention is far behind, and thus the patient may distort it while removing the appliance. Generally, such bows should be supported by additional thinner wires wound around them and engaged in the acrylic in lateral incisor-canine regions.

B. Springs

They are the active components used for movement of 1 or more teeth, mainly in labial direction or mesial or distal direction.

Ideal Requisites of a Spring

1. It should be easy to construct.
2. It should apply light forces in the desired direction.
3. It should remain active for a longer range and time.
4. It should be easy to adjust/activate.
5. It should be easy to clean.
6. It should be strong enough not to get distorted during use.
7. It should not dislodge or slip during use.
8. It should not irritate the soft tissues.

Factors Considered during Designing the Spring

- Deliver optimum force
- Longer range of action
- High degree of elasticity
- Force generated by a spring can be summarized as:

$$F \alpha EDrtDl^3$$

F=force, E=modulus of elasticity, D= deflection

r=radius of wire, l=length of wire

Diameter (D) and length (L) of the wire: Flexibility of spring depends on the properties, length and diameter of the wire used to construct them. More flexible is the spring, the lighter are the forces; and it will remain activated for a longer distance/range.

The force generated by a spring is calculated by formula D^4/L^3. It implies that if thicker wire is used, it will increase the applied force and decrease the flexibility of spring. So by doubling the diameter of wire, the force is increased by 16×. The activation of spring is difficult and it applies more force for a given deflection of active wire.

An increased in length increases the flexibility and thus decreases the force applied, the wire can be deflected for a greater distance. So, by doubling the length of wire, the force is decreased by 8×. That is why, to increase the length of spring, the coils, loops and helices are incorporated in the wire.

Load-deflection rate: Ideal spring should have an almost flat load/deflection curve so that the force applied remained constant as tooth moved. Load-deflection rate (LDR), means that the amount of load applied leads to how much deflection of active arm of the spring. LDR should be small so that lighter loads lead to more deflection of the wire. Conversely, during the movement of teeth, a loss of deflection of wire leads to minimal amount of force loss, and thus the applied force remains almost constant over a longer range for a longer period of time and does not need frequent activation. Higher LDR means that more load applied leads to lesser deflection and thus heavy forces act on the teeth.

Load-deflection rate signifies the flexibility of the wire. It means the amount of deflection of wire under a specific load. If we compare two wires of different length and/or diameter, the thinner wire/longer wire is deflected more than the other one under the same load and hence it applies less force under the same distance of activation. It also signifies the loss of force/force-decay during the tooth movement for the amount of deflection of wire. A low L-D rate is required for the active orthodontic appliance.

Force to be applied: Force produced by the spring depends on the number of teeth to be moved, the type of tooth movement, the characteristics of bone, and root surface area. Since according to the **optimal force concept**, a 26 gm/cm^2 of force is required for the tooth movement. The spring should not apply heavy force.

Patient comfort: Lighter forces should be used for tooth movement. Heavy forces cause discomfort, pain, root resorption and devitalisation of teeth. Spring should not cause soft tissue irritation or trauma. It should be positioned and activated in such a manner that it should not dislodge the appliance.

Direction of the applied force: Force should be perpendicular to the surface and the long axis of teeth. Since the spring provide the point contact on the tooth, they lead to tipping movement only. If the spring slips or slides on the tooth surface, a proper force will not be applied, the appliance may get dislodged, and there will not be any tooth movement and correction. When the active arm contacts the tooth surface, it will move perpendicular to the point of contact. When the force acts on an inclined surface, the force is split into horizontal and vertical forces. These forces will tend to displace the appliance. Care should be taken to prevent slippage of the spring on lingual surfaces of anterior teeth while correcting the cross bite or lingually positioned tooth. To prevent dislocation of appliances, the retentive clasps should be of good quality.

Force: Force should be lighter and within physiological limits. Forces get converted to pressure, i.e. force per unit area (P = F / A). So the applied forces depend on the root surface area (RSA) of the tooth. More the area, more force can be applied so that the pressure lies within physiological limits. Force applied gets distributed along the RSA. Single rooted teeth have less RSA while multirooted teeth have more RSA. Lower forces are required for teeth with shorter root and single-rooted teeth. For a single rooted tooth, a spring should deliver a force in range of 25–40 gm. Multirooted tooth needs more force for tooth movement to be distributed on wider RSA so that pressure comes in optimal range.

- **Deflection:** More deflection leads to a longer range of movement, and thus lighter forces can be delivered. With a smaller deflection of the spring, the force applied will decrease rapidly and so it will require activation more frequently. The expected rate of tooth movement is 1–2 mm a month, so an activation of 3 mm is used.
- **Bauschinger effect:** If the spring is deflected in the same direction as previous bending, its elastic recovery is better than if it is deflected in the opposite direction.
- **Direction of tooth movement:** There should be a single point contact between the spring and the tooth.
- While making a spring, its active arm should be towards the tissue and the retentive arm away from the tissue. This design helps in preventing any displacement of the active arm and keeps the force near the centre of resistance of tooth.
- **Coil:** It is made so that it lies close to the emergence of active arm from base plate. This increases the length of active arm and thus helps to apply lighter forces and increased range of action. It should be adapted as close to the centre of resistance, so that there is less tipping of the tooth. The internal diameter of the helix should be at least 3 mm for better flexibility.
- A wire of lesser diameter should be used, as it has a low load / deflection ratio, i.e. for a lesser load, the deflection should be greater. Such a spring applies a lesser force, will have a greater deflection and a longer range of action. Also the force decay per unit of deactivation will be less.

Classification of Springs

Springs can be classified as follows:

A. Based on the nature of stability of spring:

- **Self-supported spring:** It is made of thicker wire. It can support itself.
- **Supported spring:** It is made of thinner wire. It lacks adequate stability. So, the wire can be encased in a metallic tubing to give it support. A wire guide can be incorporated to avoid the sliding or

lifting of active arm away from the tissues. These are called guided springs. Alternatively, the spring can be boxed under acrylic to avoid coming in contact with teeth or occlusal forces directly to avoid breakage, etc.

B. Based on the presence or absence of helix:

- **Simple:** Without helix
- **Compound:** With helix

C. Based on the presence of loop or helix:

- **Helical spring:** Springs which have a helix. They can be single-helical or double-helical springs.
- Looped spring: This has a loop.

D. Based on the support of the terminal ends:

- **Cantilever:** One end of the spring is free, e.g. finger spring, etc.
- **Noncantilever:** When both ends are in the acrylic, e.g. labial bow.

E. Based on the presence of helix:

- **Single cantilever spring:** Which has one helix and one active arm, e.g. finger spring.
- **Double cantilever spring:** Which has two helices separated by a wire and thus has more flexibility and range of action, e.g. Z-spring.
- **Kinked cantilever spring:** The terminal part of active arm is bent to avoid any interference during the movement by the palatal surface of a premolar during the movement of a palatally displaced canine into the arch. This is overcome by kinking the spring, which still behaves as a lever pivoting on the coil.

Parts of a spring (Fig. 27.24): A spring has generally three parts, i.e. active arm, retentive arm, and helix/coil. Coils can be 1 or more than 1 depending on the design. The active arm helps to apply the force, while retentive arm is engaged in the acrylic. The helix helps to generate the force, helps in increasing the wire length, and range of action, and thus decreasing the force. The retentive arm should be made longer than the active arm so that it does not loosen from the acrylic. Terminal end of the retentive arm is bent over or made wavy so that it does not slip out of acrylic. The terminal end of active arm is bent over itself so that its sharpness does not irritate the soft tissues.

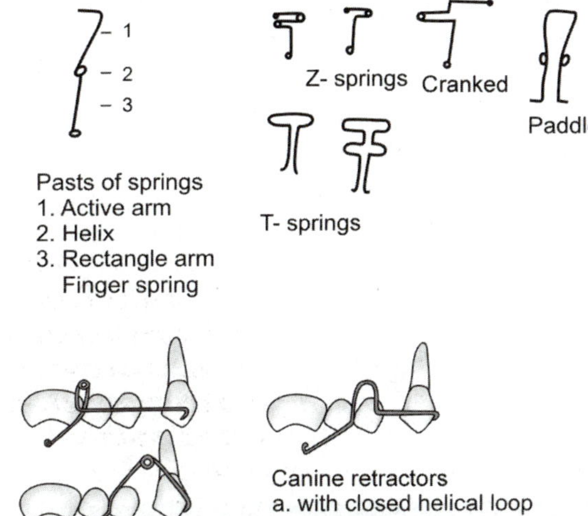

Fig. 27.24: Different parts of spring, and different types of spring.

Examples of some springs: Some of the springs used in the orthodontics are:

- Finger spring
- Z-spring
- Canine retractors
- Paddle spring
- Coffin spring
- T-spring.

Description of some springs: Below, we describe briefly some of the springs for general idea. The details can be seen in books dedicated to removable appliances.

Finger spring (Figs 27.25 to 27.28): It is a type of single cantilever spring, i.e. one end is free and the other is fixed in acrylic, and it has one helix in it. It is used for mesiodistal movement of teeth esp to close the midline diastema, or to move the tooth overlapping on the other tooth to resolve the crowding. It is called finger spring because of its shape, as it engages the tooth like a bent finger. It is made of a 0.5 mm stainless steel hardwire. It consists of three parts:

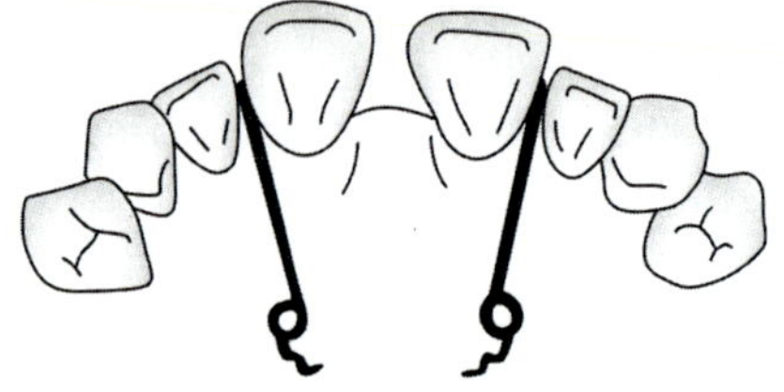

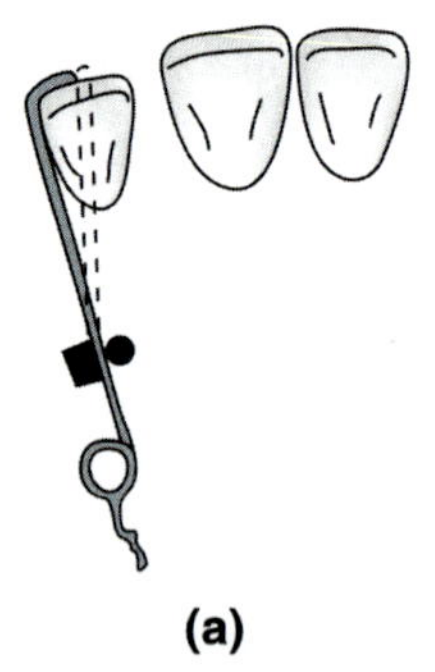

(a)

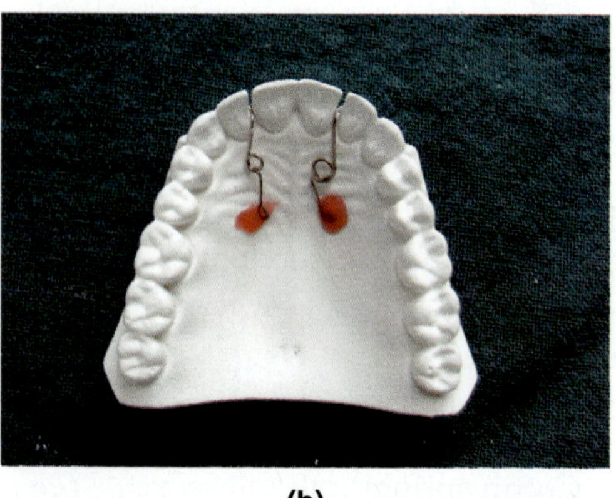

(b)

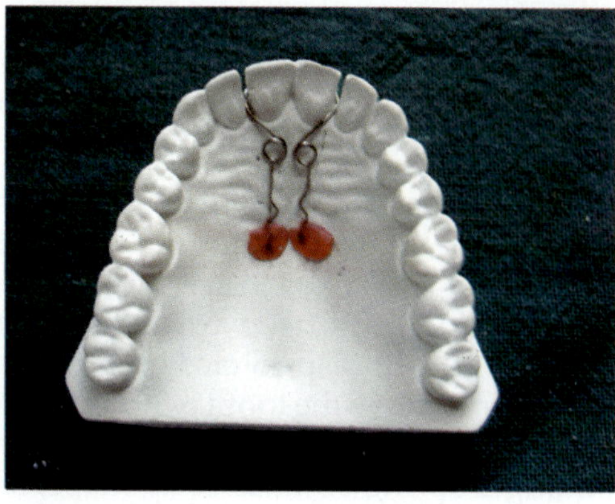

(c)

Figs 27.25a to c: Finger springs for mesial movement of central incisors.

1. **An active arm:** It is adapted toward the tissue and is 12–15 mm long. A guide/ guard wire can be used, if deep bite does not allow the thickness of acrylic in the region. Boxing of active arm needs to be done in order to protect it from damage in some cases. The active arm should be perpendicular to the tooth surface, so that the force is applied in the direction of tooth movement needed.

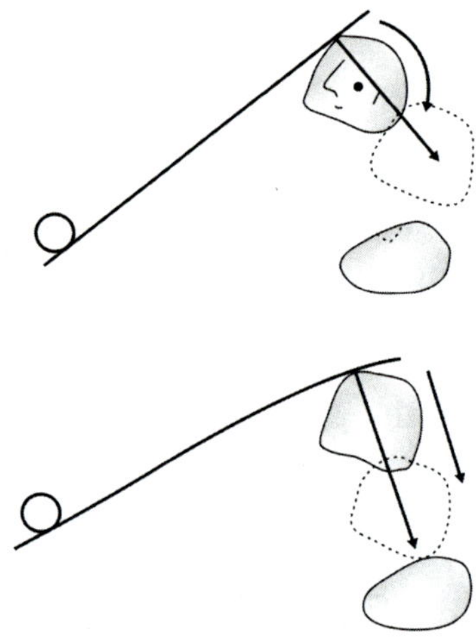

Fig. 27.26: Active arm of the finger spring should be adjusted so that the applied force moves the tooth in the arch as shown. by 2nd picture, rather than out of the arch as shown by 1st picture.

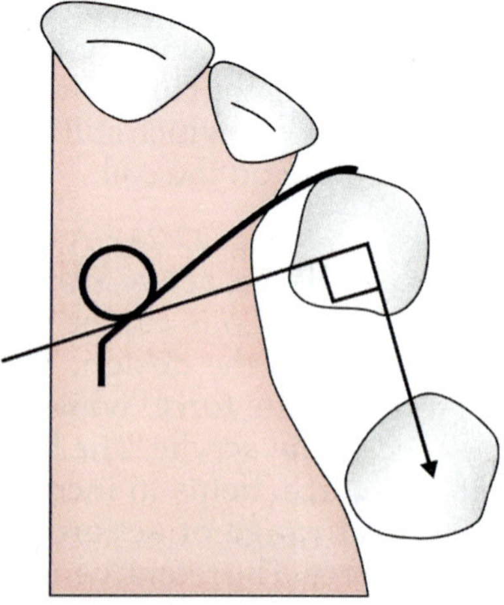

Fig. 27.27: Direction of force should be at right angle to the long axis of the tooth directing the tooth in the arch.

2. **Helix:** It is placed close to its emergence from the base plate. It is the point where force is generated. It helps to increase the length and flexibility of spring. The coil should have an internal diameter of 3 mm. Since during activation of the spring, the coil should close for maximum resilience and generation of proper force (Bauschinger effect), the coil should be placed on the opposite side of the direction of the tooth movement. Generally, the helix is positioned approximating the Cres of the tooth.

   Position of the helix: First, the final position of the tooth is imagined. The long axes lines of the pretreatment and post treatment positions of the tooth are drawn on the model. The point of intersection determines the position of helix.
3. **Retentive arm:** It is inserted in the acrylic to provide the anchorage. Its length should be equal or more than active arm. There should be 0.5–1 mm gap between wire and tissues, so that acrylic can flow in that space to engage the wire properly. The active arm and coil are boxed under wax before acrylisation. It helps to prevent flow of acrylic and clogging of the coil; protects them from occlusal forces from distortion; helps in guiding the active wire; and prevents the slippage of the active arm away from the tooth.

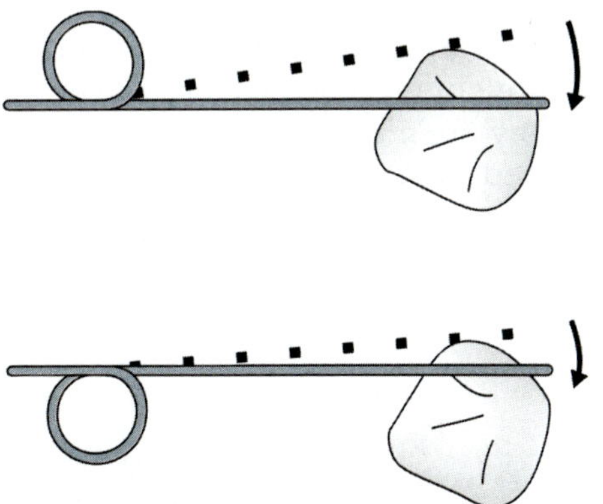

Fig. 27.28: For good efficiency of the active arm of finger spring, the helix is made such that the helix closes when the active arm is activated or you can say that the helix is made in the opposite direction to that of movement of the tooth. Dotted line shows the position of active arm of spring after activation, and arrow shows the direction of movement of tooth.

Adjustment: To activate the spring, adjustment of the free/active arm of spring is done as close to coil as possible. The active arm is moved toward the tooth to be moved to apply the force. An activation of 3 mm is appropriate to apply optimal forces.

Z-spring: This is also a cantilever spring. It is constructed in the form of letter-Z, that is its name. It is adapted on the lingual surface of tooth to be moved labially, e.g. crossbite of upper incisor (Fig. 27.29).

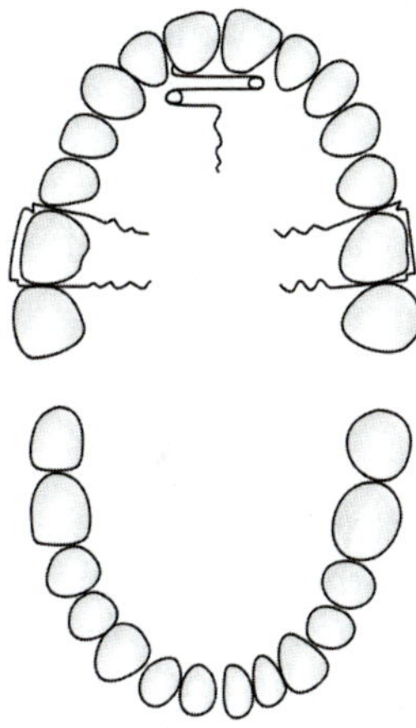

Fig. 27.29: Z-spring mostly used for labial movement of tooth.

Single arm Z-spring: It is used for labial movement of the tooth where the active arm is bent to rest on lingual surface of the tooth. It has a single helix only. It can be modified to be adapted to lingual surfaces of four incisors to move them labially. In that case, generally, 2 criss-crossing springs are used and are made of 0.6 mm wire.

Cranked single cantilever spring: It is made when palatal surface of adjacent tooth interferes with the movement of wire. The active wire is kinked to avoid that interfering tooth and thus is adapted on the tooth to be moved.

Double cantilever spring (Z-spring): It is made with two helices which are separated with a segment of wire. The free end of spring rests on the lingual surface of the tooth. Since it has longer wire, it is more flexible, more range of action, and applies lighter forces. It is used to treat the retroclination of incisors. It can also be used for correcting the minor rotations of incisors. Incisor tooth is supported by labial bow on the labial side which provides another point of contact and thus helps to generate a couple (Figs 27.30 and 27.31).

Construction: It is made by a 0.5 mm SS wire. It can be made for 1–2 teeth. It has two coils of small diameter, with intervening wires in the active arm. The free end is adapted on the lingual surface of the tooth just above the cingulum. It is slightly inclined towards apical side so that it does not slide along the slope of lingual surface during activation. For correction of minor rotation, the free end touches the palatally-rotated edge of the tooth.

The two arms of the spring have two helices in between them. The arms are crossed over to each other before acrylisation so as to give more range of activation. They are kept perpendicular to the lingual surface of the tooth. The free end of the wire should not slide along the lingual surface of the tooth, otherwise the force is wasted. The spring can be boxed in wax prior to acrylization. Activation is done by opening the helices thus moving the free arm labially, it increases the distance between two wires. It can also be activated by a single movement by grasping its outer arm and pulling it outward.

T-spring: It is made in the form of T. It is generally used to move the lingually minor-displaced premolar or canine in the labial direction. These teeth need more forces due to their increased RSA and thicker surrounding bone. The usual Z-spring cannot apply the required forces (Figs 27.32 and 27.33).

It is constructed with a 0.5 mm wire in the form of T, adapted to the lingual surface of the tooth. It has smaller length but its range action of spring can be increased by incorporating loops in the vertical arm.

Coffin spring: It was designed by Walter Coffin. It is used for dentoalveolar expansion of the upper arch if it is narrow or has cross-bite. It is made of a 1.2 mm wire. It is adapted in the midpalatal region extending from center of first premolar to distal of first molar. It is omega-shaped and it stands 1 mm away from the palatal tissues. Generally, the open end of the omega loop faces forward. The retentive arms engage the acrylic and the appliance is retained by using clasps on the teeth. It can be activated by pulling the both arms laterally or by pressing the distal curve of the omega to open it. Activation of 1–2 mm per session is required. It is also used in bionator where it helps to control or train the tongue (Figs 27.33 and 27.34).

Paddle/flapper spring: It is used for the labial movement of especially lower incisors when they are more lingually tilted. The wire is adapted on the lingual surface from just below the incisal edge, with two vertical arms extending cervically. The helices are bent on

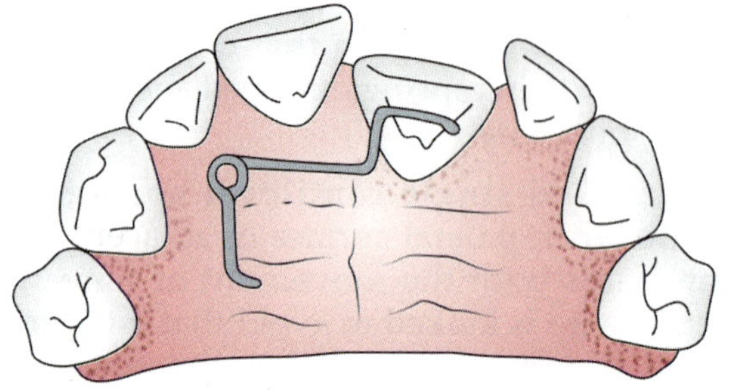

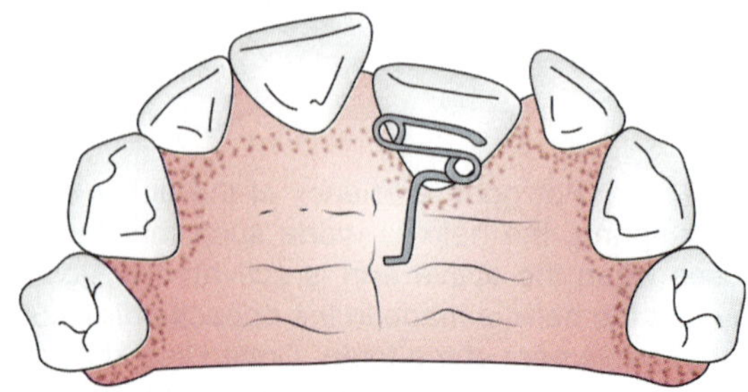

Fig. 27.30: Cranked cantilever spring; double cantilever / Z-spring.

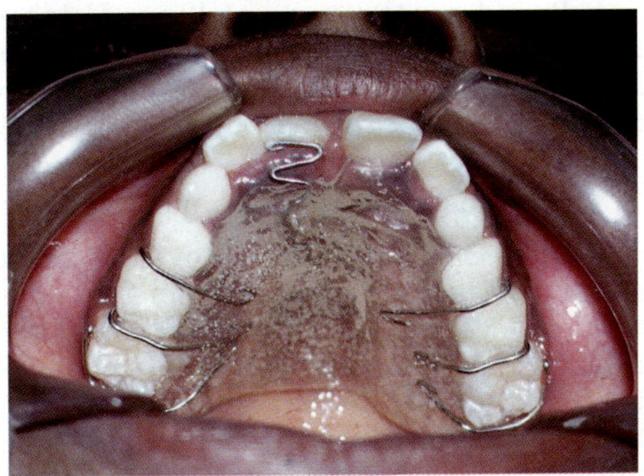

Fig. 27.31: Double cantilever/Z-spring in a removable plate to correct cross bite of central incisor.

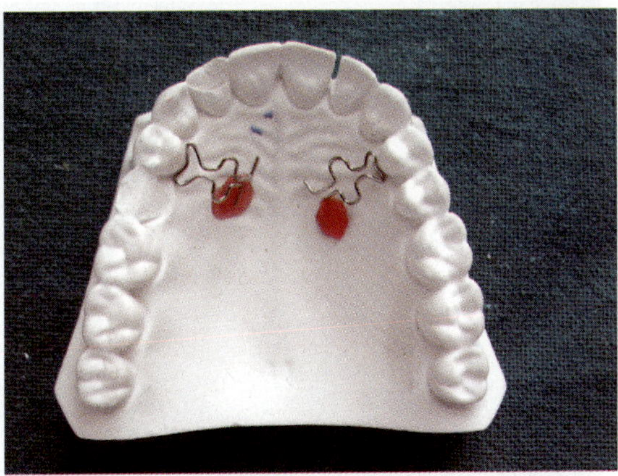

Fig. 27.32: T-springs for individual tooth labial movement.

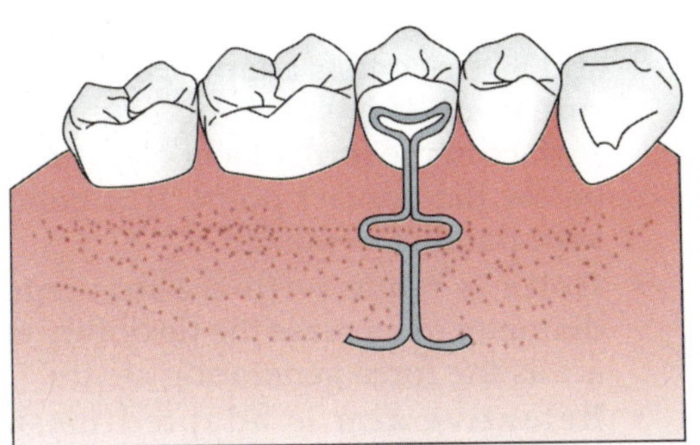

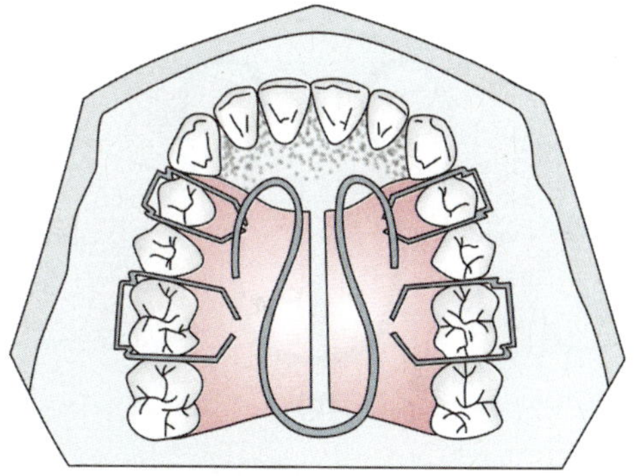

(a)

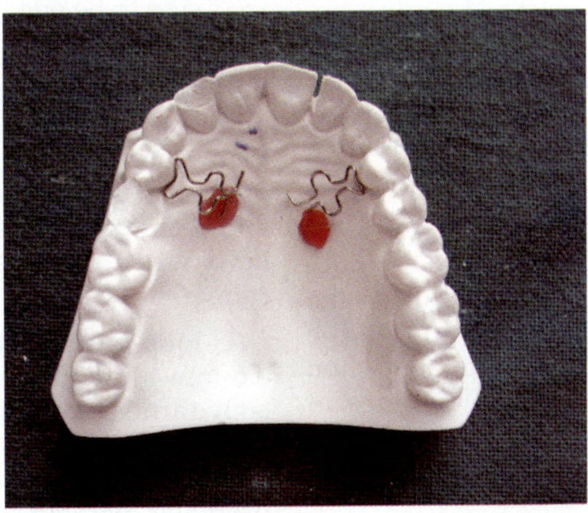

(b)

Figs 27.33a and b: T-spring; Coffin spring.

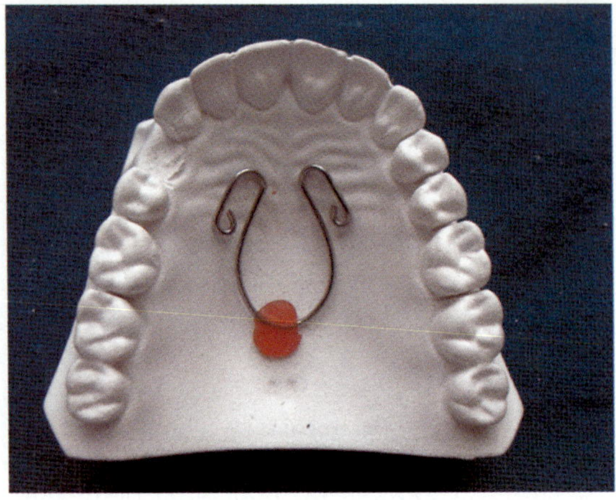

(a)

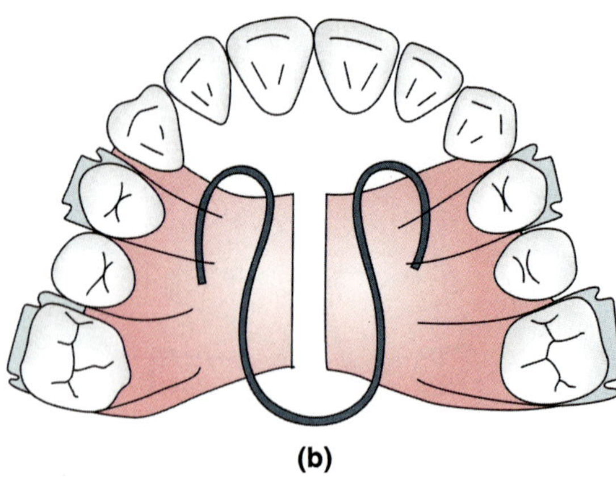

(b)

Figs 27.34a and b: Coffin spring, spring in a removable appliance.

both the vertical arms. The terminal ends act as retentive arm which are engaged in acrylic. It is a flexible spring and has a snap-fit when appliance is placed in the oral cavity. It is activated by bending the active part toward the labial side.

Canine retractors (Figs 27.35–27.40): As the name suggests, they are used to move the canine distally or sometimes lingually when canines are erupted labially. They are of following types:

- **Based on the position:** Buccal CR; palatal CR
- **Based on the presence of loop or helix:** CR with helix; CR with loops
- **Based on the type of loop:** U-loop; closed helical loop; open helical loop, Reverse loop canine retractor
- **Based on support:** supported; self-supported
- **Based on the action:** push type; pull type:

Uses of CR: They help to move the canine distally when the canine is within the line of arch and needs to be distalized. CR may also be used to pull the canine in the arch when it is erupted labially, this action is supported by the labial bow. Since the springs cause the tipping of the teeth, thus those canines which have their apices in a normal position while crowns are mesially directed, are the best candidates to be retracted.

Construction: It is made of 0.5 mm hard SS wire and it has following parts.

- **Active arm** is placed towards the tooth and its free end is adapted on the mesial side of canine wrapping to the palatal surface in the form of a hook to engage it below the contact point. It is generally kept parallel to the OP.
- **Helix** is made with a 4 mm internal diameter to increase the flexibility and to act as the force generating centre.
- **Retentive arm** is adapted mesial to second premolar passing in the occlusal embrasure and adapted on the palatal side to be engaged in the acrylic.

Activation is done by opening the coil and thus shifting the end of active arm distally. It deflects the active arm occlusally which is then readapted parallel to the OP. Another method of activation is by cutting the free end and readapted. This will help in closing the helix when the free end is engaged on the canine.

U-loop canine retractor: It is made of 0.5–0.6 mm hard SS wire. It has three parts, i.e. active arm, U-loop, and the retentive arm. The U-loop is made in the region of first premolar and its free distal end passes distal to the first premolar, passing on to the palatal surface as retentive arm. The U-loop is made like in a labial bow in the region of canine, with free

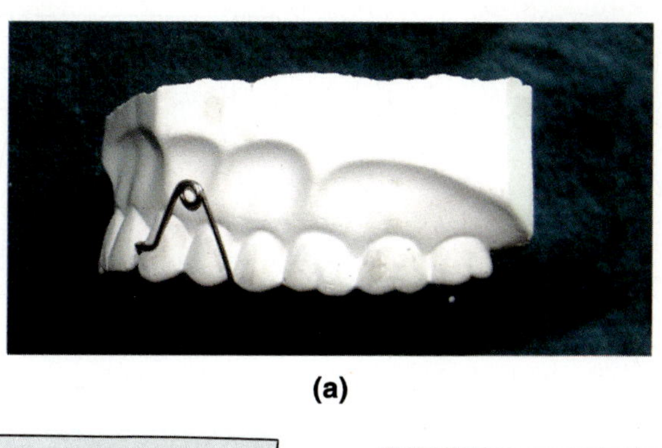

(a)

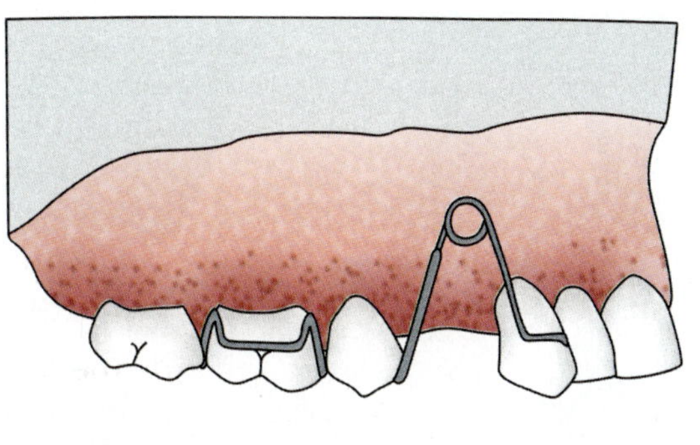

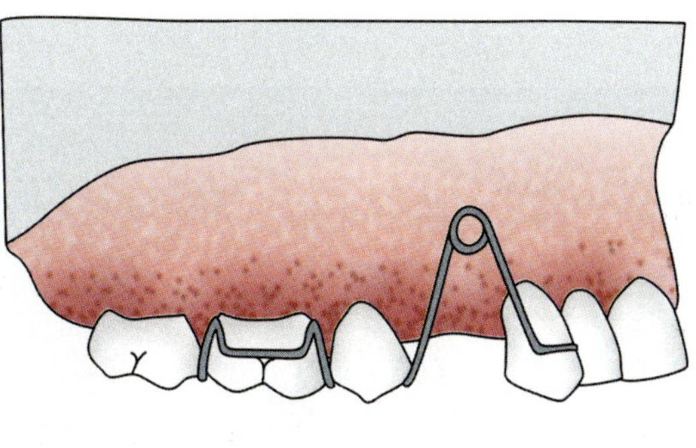

(b)

Figs 27.35a and b: Buccal canine retractor. Sleeve on the distal arm of the spring is to support the thin wire, it is a supported canine retractor.

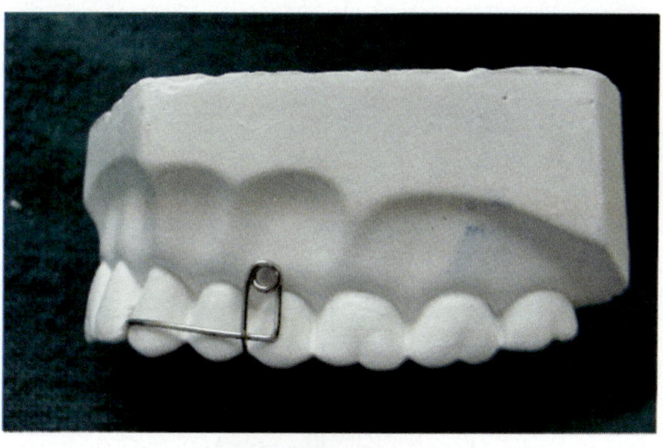

(a)

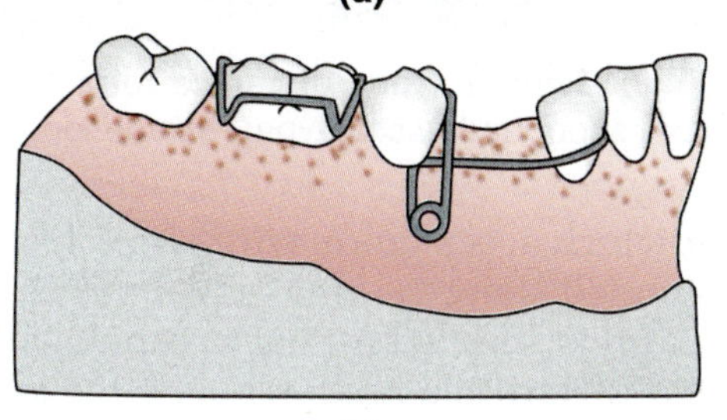

(b)

Figs 27.36a and b: Closed vertical loop canine retractor.

end of active arm bent around the mesiolingual aspect of canine to be retracted. It is activated by compressing the loop and readapting the active arm almost parallel to OP. It can also be activated by cutting the free end by 1 mm and then readapting it. Since the active arm is small, the activation should be small for lighter force. It can only be used if only small retraction of canine is required. It is simple to make and is less bulky.

Helical canine retractor: It is also called ***reverse loop canine retractor*** as a closed vertical loop with helix is used. It is made of 0.6 mm s.s hard wire. Parts of this CR are an active arm, a closed vertical loop with helix, and a retentive arm. The helix is positioned 3–4 mm below the free gingival margin. The mesial arm of loop is bent to pass mesial to second premolar onto the occlusal embrasure and then adapting on palatal surface to act as retentive arm. The distal arm is bent at right angle, passes below the retentive mesial leg of the loop, is adapted along the middle third of

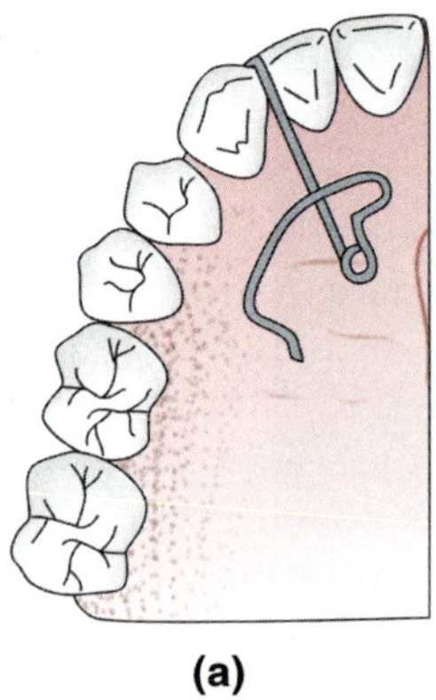

(a)

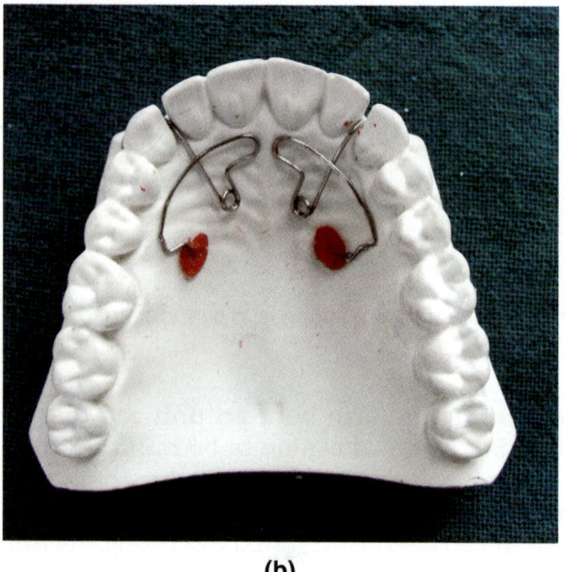

(b)

Figs 27.37a and b: Palatal canine retractor with a guide wire.

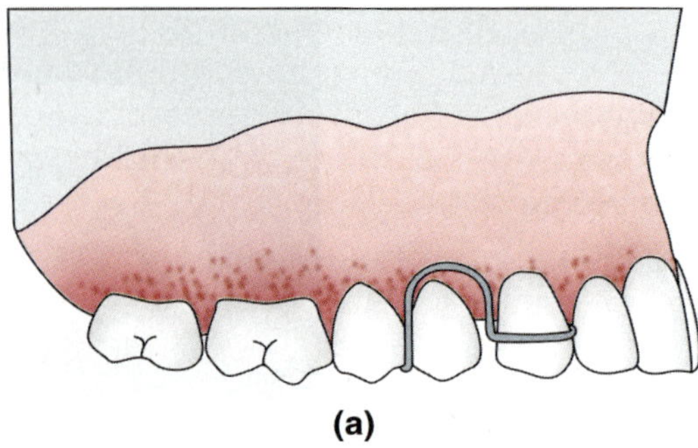

(a)

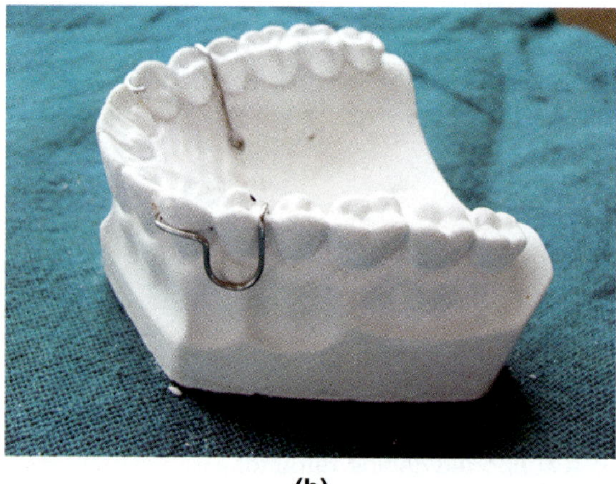

(b)

Figs 27.38a and b: U-loop canine retractor.

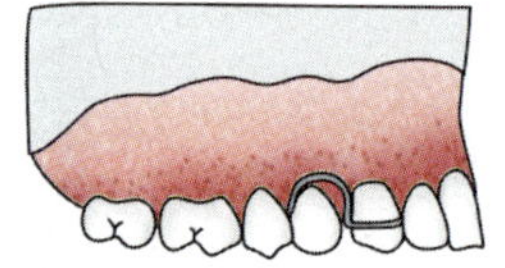

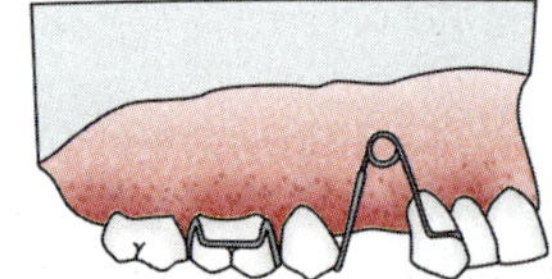

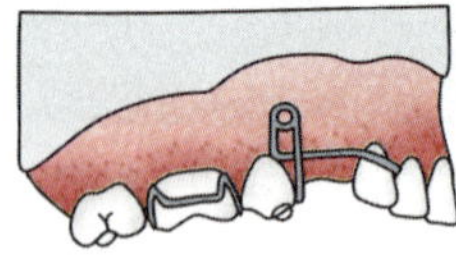

Fig. 27.39: Different types of canine retractors: U-loop type; supported buccal type; reverse loop type.

the buccal surfaces of the teeth parallel to the OP and is engaged around the mesial surface of the canine. It can be activated by cutting the free end by 1mm and then readapting it or by opening the helix and readjusting the active arm. Since the length of wire incorporated is longer, it is more flexible with more range of action and lighter forces.

Palatal canine retractor: It is adapted on the palatal surface of maxilla. It is made of 0.6 mm s.s hard wire. Parts of this CR are an active arm, a helix of 3 mm internal diameter, and a crossing-over retentive arm of sufficient length which acts a guide wire also. The helix is positioned along the long axis of canine. The active arm is adapted mesial to canine, and is adapted toward the tissues, below the guide-retentive arm. Retentive arm extends upto mesial aspect of first molar. It should remain straight as it determines the path of movement of the canine. It is used when the canine is palatally placed. The activation is done by opening the helix by 2 mm or enough to apply a light force on the canine. It should be wax-boxed before acrylization.

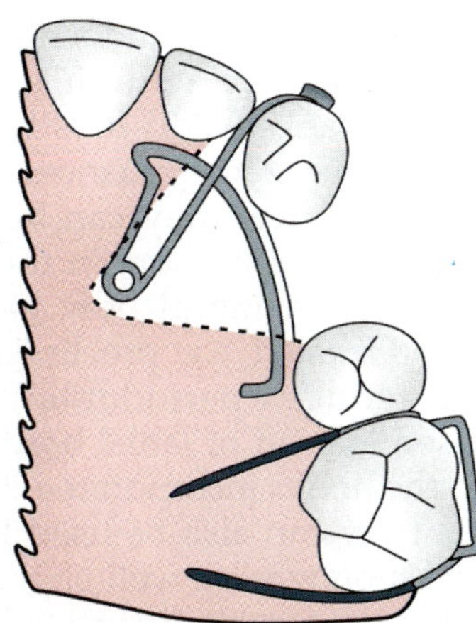

Fig. 27.40: Palatal canine retractor.

Buccal canine retractor: It is used when canine is buccally placed or is high in vestibule. It is adapted on the buccal side of the arch. It consists of an active arm, an open V-shaped loop with helix and a retentive arm. The helix is of 3 mm internal diameter. Coil lies distal to long axis of canine midway between the initial and the final position of the canine. The mesial leg of loop acts as active arm and is kept away from the tissues to prevent soft tissue injury. It is bent at approx half the crown length of canine and is adapted to the mesial surface of canine below its contact point. The distal leg is adapted mesial to the second premolar over to the occlusal embrasure and then adapting on palatal surface to act as retentive arm. It can be of two types, i.e. supported and self-supported. Self-supported CR is made of 0.6 mm wire, while the supported CR is made of a thinner size 0.5 mm wire. To strengthen the supported CR, its distal leg is passed through a sleeve of 0.5 mm SS tube.

Activation is done by closing the helix by 1 mm in case of self-supported CR as it is made of thicker wire, while in the supported CR, the helix is closed by 2 mm.

C. Expansion Screws

Screws are the active components which can be incorporated in the removable appliances for different types of tooth movements, e.g. expansion of arch; distal/mesial movement of canine or premolar; labial movement of incisors, etc. The appliance is split in two parts, which may be equal or unequal in size. Equal sized parts are done for bilateral expansion of the arches by reciprocal anchorage, while unequal splitting is done to move a tooth or a segment of teeth, while the larger part acts as anchorage. The acrylic incorporating the screw is split to make a small active part which moves with the opening of the screw, and a larger part which acts as anchorage. It is activated by the patient at regular intervals by a special key. It applies intermittent heavy forces which decrease with the movement of the tooth. Different uses and types of appliance can be studied in chapter of expansion.

Classification of Screws

They are of two types, i.e.

- Skeletal expansion screw: It is fixed to teeth by bands. It brings about rapid expansion, e.g. Hyrax.
- Dental expansion screw: It is used for slow tooth movement. It may be used for bilateral arch expansion or for movement of single tooth/segment of teeth.

Some of the different types of expansion screws:

- Bilateral symmetrical expansion screw for maxillary arch
- Mandibular bow screw
- Encased expansion screw
- Sectional expansion screw—moving a single tooth or a group teeth
- Trapezoidal—used in narrow maxillary arch
- Radial-anterior region is expanded more
- Three-dimensional—movement in three direction
- Spring loaded
- Expansion screw used with activator
- Traction screw—closure of extraction spaces

- Telescopic screw—moving a single tooth or a group of teeth in labial direction
- Piston spring screw
- Anterior transverse expansion only: It is a modified Hawley appliance with expansion screw. Here, a wire of 0.8 mm or more size is bent in the form of a V with a helix and is incorporated at the distal end of the midline cut in the plate. It prevents opening of the plate in distal area while all the force is directed in the anterior canine to canine area for expansion.

General guidelines to use E-screw: Proper position of the E-screw is necessary for the better results. Some of the common practical aspects should be followed as given below:

- Axis of the expansion screw should be parallel to the occlusal plane
- It should be placed as low as possible in the palatal vault so that the force is near to the Cres of the tooth or segments of teeth. It helps to achieve more bodily movement.
- For bilateral symmetrical expansion, the screw is placed in the canine–premolar region.
- For distalizing a posterior tooth, it is placed mesial to the tooth to be moved.
- Appliance should seat properly and the retention should be good. A loose appliance is uncomfortable and patient does not use it. Improperly fitted appliance does not stay in the arch and gets displaced on activation, thus the forces are not applied properly, and no results are seen.
- Monitor expansion by the use of holes drilled into acrylic in each half of appliance.
- The patient/parent should be trained how and in which direction the screw is to be rotated, which is generally directed by an in-built arrow.

D. Elastics

These are the active components made of latex, and apply forces when they are stretched between two specific points. For proper force, they should be stretched 3 times the internal diameter. Elastics are available in various sizes, i.e. thickness and diameter, and force range. They are seldom used with removable appliances, and mostly used as part of fixed/semi-fixed appliances. With the removable appliance, they can be used to retract the proclined incisors in those cases where forces from labial bow cannot be controlled and trusted, e.g. proclined teeth in adults with reduced periodontal support. They are used instead of labial bow, and are attached to the hooks incorporated in canine-PM region. They can also be used for inter-maxillary traction when a well-aligned lower arch is present. A well fitting removable appliance can provide an anchorage point for either class II or class III elastic traction. They can help for localized tooth movement, e.g. occlusal movement of partially erupted tooth; treatment of a single tooth crossbite by using it in cross-elastic fashion. Drawbacks with use of elastics are the gingival trauma; and the flattening of the arch. Patient cooperation is needed for the proper use of elastics. Some patients may show allergy to latex. Nowadays, latex-free elastics are also available.

Various elastic products are available these days to be used during orthodontic treatment, but mostly are used during fixed orthodontic treatment. These components can be studied in the chapter on components of fixed appliances.

BASE PLATE

It is made of cold-cure or heat-cure acrylic and is used to hold the active and retentive wire components in one piece. It also helps in distributing the forces to the wider area of tissues, thus providing the anchorage. The appliance is a tooth–tissue based appliance, gaining its retention through clasps on the teeth, and also form the adhesive forces between tissue and plate. It can be modified to incorporate the bite planes of acrylic in some specific situations. Since the base plate encroaches the area of tongue in the oral cavity, it leads to the initial adjustment problems. It should be of minimal thickness so as to provide adequate strength and also not interfering in the tongue function. It should be comfortable to the patient to gain his co-operation. Generally 1.5–2.0 mm thickness is adequate (Fig. 27.41).

The upper base plate generally extends upto the distal of the first molars, thus giving an adequate strength. But in expansion appliances, it is extended to the last erupted tooth. The mandibular plate is adapted on the lingual surface only and thus due to less bulk, it is prone to breakage, so it should be made thicker (and especially in anterior region) to give strength. Its height should be adjusted to prevent irritation of lingual sulcus. It can be reinforced by incorporating a hard SS wire in the plate, contoured along the lingual alveolar surface of mandibular arch. The acrylic should be well adapted with no gaps around the necks of the teeth which are not to be moved. It gives proper retention, avoids food impaction and helps in better anchorage. The acrylic can be trimmed judiciously during the tooth movement so as not to interfere during treatment, e.g. during retraction of proclined incisors, the acrylic should be removed at least 2–3 mm away from the lingual surfaces. The acrylic is trimmed judiciously during bite plates and myofunctional appliance treatment to allow eruption and other needed movements of teeth.

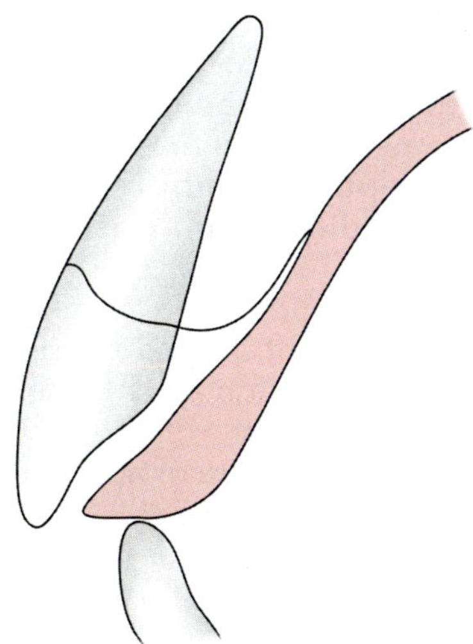

Fig. 27.41: Anterior bite plate where lower incisors occlude on the bite ramp to raise the bite. The acrylic may be relieved lingual to upper central incisors to provide space for their palatal movement.

Management of Removable Appliances

Delivery of appliances:

1. The appliance should be well polished, without sharp edges and nodules especially on the tissue surfaces, and should be non-irritating to the tissue.
2. It should be snugly fitting without applying unnecessary pressure on the teeth to be used as anchorage.
3. It should not dislodge during use, so the clasps should be well made.
4. Active components should not irritate the tissues and should be well fitted for the area where they are needed.
5. Patient should be educated regarding care of appliance, so that he does not distort the active and other components during use.

Instructions to the patient:

1. He should be told about the various components of the appliance and how to take care of them.
2. He is told about the number of hours to use the appliance; whether to remove during eating or not especially bite plates should be used during eating also.
3. Information should be given as how to remove and insert the appliance in the mouth.
4. He is advised to clean the appliance at least 2–3 times per day with tooth brush with light strokes to avoid any distortion and breakage, and wash in running water.
5. He should keep appliance dipped in water, when not in use, otherwise distortion of acrylic and misfit of appliance can occur.

6. Any sharp points or problem, he should visit the doctor for adjustment.
7. Tooth brushing should be done after every meal to clean the oral cavity and then appliance should be placed. Chlorhexidine mouth wash should be used.
8. Appliance should be placed once a week overnight dipped in antiseptic/ cleansing solution or chlorhexidine/ betadine solution.
9. He should take care of appliance so as not to drop and break it.
10. If it is lost or broken or irritating, then he should immediately come to the doctor for its refabrication or repair.

Follow-up:

1. Signs of appliance usage in the oral cavity, e.g. pressure lines on the mucosa of plate and cheeks, etc. give a fair idea whether patient is cooperating with the use of appliance or not. An unused appliance looks cleaner.
2. The appliance should be inspected for any sharp edges or spots and should be adjusted.
3. The active components should be adjusted minimally so as to apply light forces, and they should not irritate the soft tissues.
4. Retentive components should be adjusted to keep the appliance firmly in place, without applying any force on anchorage tooth, and they should not irritate the soft tissues.
5. The acrylic should be removed/adjusted if it is interfering in the path of tooth movement.
6. Cooperation, oral hygiene and cleaning of appliance instructions should be reinforced.

Problems encountered during removable appliance therapy:

1. Patient cooperation: If patient does not use it properly, then no results can be expected. He may break it or loose it.
2. Oral hygiene problems: If not cleaned properly, it may lead to development of gingivitis, gingival hyperplasia, bad breath, etc.
3. Problems with speech and excessive salivation: Since it encroaches on the tongue area in oral cavity, the patient has difficulty in proper and clear speech during initial days. Even salivation increases.
4. Soft tissue problems: If the appliance has sharp edges or nodules, it may lead to trauma of soft tissues and ulceration.
5. Caries: If oral hygiene is neglected, it may also lead to caries.
6. Pain: If undue force is applied, it may lead to pain, mobility and devitalizaton of the tooth.
7. Tooth mobility: excessive force can lead to undue trauma or traumatic occlusion with the appliance can lead to tooth mobility of teeth.

Conclusion

Removable appliances are integral part of orthodontics. They can easily be used for treatment of certain malpositions of teeth without any problem, and they are inexpensive. They are also required in conjunction with the fixed appliance for helping during the treatment. A proper knowledge of indications and use of removable appliance helps in smooth treatment of malocclusion. If they are comfortable, the patient's cooperation is very well achieved. However, their use is contraindicated if patient is having the allergy to acrylic. Orthodontic literature has numerous removable appliances used for treatment of various malocclusion conditions, which have been mentioned at appropriate places in the text. However, an attempt will be made to compile them in one chapter for the convenience of reader.

VIVA VOCE QUESTIONS

1. **What are the basic components of a removable appliance and their functions?**
There are three basic parts, i.e. retentive components, active components and acrylic base plate.
Retentive components = help in retaining the appliance in place.
Active components = help in applying forces for the movement of the teeth.
Base plate = binds all the components into a single functional unit.

2. **What are the various active components?**
These are labial bows, springs, screws and elastics.
Labial bows are = short and long labial bows; split labial bow; reverse labial bow; high labial bow with apron spring; fitted labial bow; Robert's retractor and Mill's retractor.
Active labial bows are generally made in 22 or 23 gauge SS wire.
Passive/retentive bows are made in 21 gauge SS wires.
Bows used in functional appliances are made in 19 or 20 gauge SS wires.
Springs can be = simple/compound; helical/looped; self-supported/supported springs.

3. **Which are the factors on which the force of the spring depends?**
It depends inversely on the cube of the length of the wire; directly on the fourth power of the diameter of the wire (since force = D^4/L^3). The heavier is the wire, more is the force and lesser is the flexibility; and vice versa.

4. **What is the load-deflection rate of a wire?**
It signifies the flexibility of the wire. It means the amount of the deflection of the wire under a specific load. If we compare two wires of different length and/or diameter, the thinner wire/longer wire is deflected more than the other one under the same load and hence it applies less force under the same distance of activation. It also signifies the loss of force/force-decay during the tooth movement for the amount of the deflection of the wire. A low L-D rate is required for the active orthodontic appliance.

5. **What are various retentive components?**
These are Adams clasp; pin-head clasp; C-clasp; southend clasp; crozat clasp; Jackson's clasp; triangular clasp; ball-end clasp, etc.

6. **What are the various common appliances used in the orthodontics with their main functions?**

Coffin spring	Expansion
Quad helix	Expansion
Jack screw	Expansion
Porter (W-arch)	Expansion
Bihelix	Expansion
Schwarz App	Expansion
NPE I, II	Expansion
TPA, LHA, NPA	Space maintenance, anchorage savers
Distal shoe appliance; aka Roche's appliance	For guiding mandibular Permanent first molar to erupt after premature loss of primary mandibular first molar
Anterior bite plate	Bite opening
Posterior bite plate with Z-spring	Treatment of anterior crossbite
Reverse bite plate	Bite opening and mandibular forward displacement
Catalan's/(L) inclined plane	Treatment of anterior cross bite
Bionater, twin-block	Myofunctional
activator, FR, etc.	Myofunctional
Herbst, Jasper Jumper	Myofunctional, fixed
Chin cup, Petit's/and Hickham appliance, Delaire's face mask	For treatment of Skeletal class III
Oral screen	For treatment of protruded incisors with spacing, and for expansion of arches.
Cetlin appliance, pendulum app., distal jet	Molar distalization

Lip bumper	For hyperactive mentalis m, lip sucking; anchorage
Tongue blade	Treatment of Anterior crossbite
M-spring	Closure of midline diastema
Hewley's appliance	For retention (also known as dental crutch)
Clip on retainer	For retention
Kesling tooth positioner	For retention
Nakamura's	Treatment of class III
Jackson's clasp	U-shaped
¾ circumferential	C-shaped
Southend clasp	M-shaped (anterior region)
Triangular clasp	
Ball-end clasp	
Schwarz clasp	Also known as Arrowhead clasp with a number of arrowheads
Crozat Pin head	U-shaped with wire soldered

Finger spring—for MD OTM

- Z spring—for labial OTM
- T- spring, paddle/flapper for labial OTM
- M spring = closure of midline diastema

7. Which is the most basic removable appliance?

Hawley's appliance is the most basic removable appliance and so other appliances are the modification of this appliance. It is known as dental crutch also. It is a passive appliance. The main purpose of this appliance is the retention.

8. Which appliance is used for the mesiodistal movement of the teeth?

A removable appliance with finger-spring incorporated in the appliance is used. This helps to close the diastema b/w the teeth. The finger spring is made of 22 or 23 gauge SS wire.

9. What are various features of a finger spring?

1. The active arm touches the tooth.
2. The helix is made in the direction opposite to the direction of the tooth movement. Helix helps to generate the light forces. A rule of thumb is that the helix should close on activation for application of the proper force.
3. The helix is placed generally midway between the initial and the final position of the tooth.
4. Internal diameter of the helix is 3 times the diameter of the wire.
5. Helix is placed at least 5 mm beyond the free gingival margin, near to the c. res of the tooth, and it should be parallel to the palatal surface.
6. The active arm should be placed towards the palatal tissues.
7. The activation should be approx 3 mm, such that it is able to produce a movement @ 1 mm/month.
8. The length of the retentive arm should be longer than the active by at least 1.5 times.
9. The retentive arm should not cross the midline.

10. Which appliance is used for the labial movement of the tooth?

Various components can be used, e.g. Z-spring; E-screw; paddle spring and T-spring. It is generally used for the treatment of the cross-bite relation of the incisors and/or tooth in linguoversion, e.g. in class II division 2 cases.

A posterior bite plane is incorporated in the appliance to create a gap between the incisal edges.

Z-spring is made of 22 or 23 gauge wire. It is made with 2 helices; the active arm should be towards the apex of the tooth and force applied by this spring is perpendicular to the long axis of the tooth.

11. What is the prerequisite for the alignment of any tooth in the arch?

Adequate space should be present/created for the proper alignment of the tooth in the arch, e.g. during the treatment of crossbite; during the retraction of the incisors, etc.

12. Which appliance is used for the lingual movement of the teeth?

Mostly, labial bow is used for this purpose. The bow is made active, in 22 or 23 gauge wire. The level is generally placed at the junction of incisal and the middle third of the crown. It should be parallel to the incisal edges of the anterior teeth. The length of the U-loop should be such that it should extend only 2 mm below the free marginal gingiva of the canine.

13. What is the main disadvantage of the removable appliance?

It causes the tipping of the tooth, e.g. with crown moving lingually, the root moves labially.

Also, only simple tooth movements can be done.

The success rate depends on the cooperation of the patient.

Finishing of teeth positioning is poor.

14. What is the role of the canine retractors?

It helps to move the labially/mesially erupted canines in the arch. If space is not there, it is created by removal of first premolar.

Disadvantage of this appliance is the mesio-labial rotation of the canine, due to the force being applied labial to the center of rotation of the tooth.

15. What is an anterior bite plate appliance?

- It is a modified Hawley's appliance, which has got a ramp extending from canine to canine in maxillary arch appliance.
- It is used for opening of deep bite; it is best in average/horizontal growth pattern cases;

16. Why it is contraindicated in vertical growth pattern cases?

- C/I in vertical growth cases since with the eruption of molars, the mandible moves in a downward and backward direction, which further increases facial height and profile becomes more convex.

17. What is the mechanism of action of anterior bite plate?

- It mechanism of action is that it allows the supraeruption of mandibular molars for opening of the deep bite.
- 2–3 mm interocclusal gap in the first molar region is created for supraeruption of mandibular molars. The plane of the plate is kept parallel to the OP.
- Further opening of the bite can be accomplished stepwise.

18. If the interocclusal gap is more than 2–3 mm, what problem can be encountered with anterior bite plate?

If gap is > 4–5 mm = Tongue interferes with molar eruption and bite does not correct

19. What is the side effect of anterior bite plate appliance?

Causes anterior force on (U) incisors leading to flaring of these teeth. So, it is good for C2D2 m.o.

20. What is deep bite and how it is classified?

It is the vertical overlap of upper incisors to the lower incisors more than the normal, i.e. 2 mm. It can be classified as skeletal/dental; complete/incomplete, etc.

21. How can we treat a deep bite case?

It depends on the growth pattern of the patient; and upper lip relation of the incisors. In case of horizontal growth pattern, the molar extrusion should be done for it, as it leads to the down and back rotation of the mandible. But in case of vertical growth pattern, the molar extrusion should not be done, as it may deteriorate the facial profile and increase the face height.

Also, if upper lip length is normal but there is gummy smile or increased visibility of upper incisors, the upper incisors should be intruded.

22. What is the normal relationship of upper lip to the incisal edges of upper teeth?

At rest, the incisal edges of upper incisors are exposed by only 2–3 mm.

23. What is the normal relationship of upper lip to the upper teeth in full smile?

If the length of upper lip is normal with the normal inclination of upper incisors, the upper lip in full smile lies at the level of the gingival margin of the upper incisors.

24. What is a reverse bite plate appliance?

It is modified Hawley's appliance which has got a ramp extending from canine to canine, but its plane is kept at 45–60° angle to the OP (Fig. 27.42).

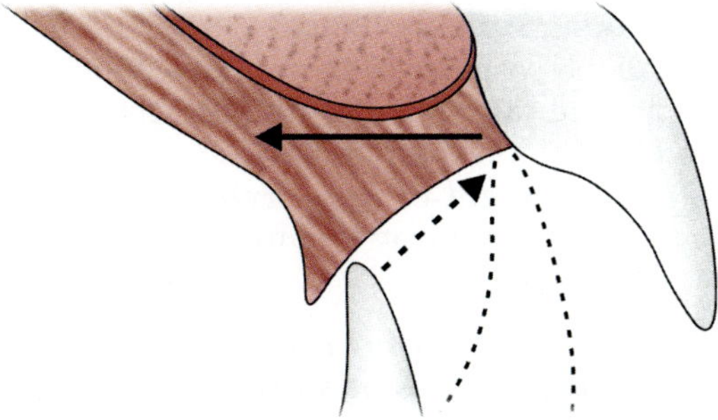

Fig. 27.42: Reverse bite plane which has a 45° ramp which leads to forward positioning of the lower jaw, as shown by dotted outline of lower incisors.

25. What are the indications of this appliance?

It is mainly used for the opening of the bite; and brings the mandible forward in cases of the mandibular retrognathism cases. It is best used during the growth phase of the child.

26. What is the mechanism of action of this appliance?

It helps to open the bite; it also shifts the mandible forward along the incline especially in Class II div 1 cases; as the plane is kept at 45–60 degrees to OP. Interocclusal gap should be 2–3 mm in the first molar region.

27. What is the side effect of this appliance?

It causes an anterior force on (L) incisors and hence their flaring, as the mandible, which has been slid forward on the ramp tries to go back to its original position under the influence of its attached ms.

28. What is a posterior bite plate appliance?

It is a modified Hawley's appliance, either in upper or lower arch, having acrylic covering the occlusal surfaces of the posterior teeth, so that the teeth of the opposing arch are in even contact with it.

29. What is the use of this appliance?

It helps to create a gap between incisal edges of U/L teeth, i.e. incisal clearance during the treatment of anterior crossbite with the help of Z-springs, etc.

It also helps to treat the anterior open bite by causing intrusive forces on the molars.

It also helps to create a gap between the occlusal surfaces of one side of the teeth, if the other side is in crossbite and needs expansion of the arch.

30. What precaution should be taken while making such appliance?

All the posterior teeth should be touching the acrylic ramp evenly on both the sides for efficient mastication.

The height of the acrylic should not be excessive as it may lead to fatigue of the ms of mandible.

31. How it is helpful during the expansion therapy in cases of vertical growth pattern cases?

It is used in the expansion appliances to avoid the extrusion of the molars during expansion in such cases.

32. What are the important features of a Hawley's retention appliance?

It is the most basic of the removable appliance.

It contains Adams clasps, labial bow and the acrylic base plate.

The acrylic should be touching all the teeth of that arch on the lingual surfaces just above their height of contour/HOC. It helps to avoid the movement/relapse of the teeth on lingual side/or of rotations.

Labial bow should be made passive, made in 21 or 20 gauge SS wire; should be evenly touching the teeth to avoid their labial displacement.

Level of the labial bow should be in the middle of the crown of the teeth. It helps to avoid the relapse of the torque corrections.

Can be modified with cribs in case of habits and in other cases.

33. What is a habit breaking appliance?

Used for those patients who themselves want to leave the habit.

These are not the punishment appliances but the reminder appliances.

Main component is the cribs made of 21 gauge SS wire.

Cribs are made on the lingual side of the maxillary anterior teeth in the canine to canine region, their height adjusted so that they do not injure the lingual tissues of lower arch when mouth is closed; and also does not allow the anterior movement of the tongue or easy entry of finger in the mouth.

The levels of the cribs should be the same, parallel to the incisal plane, and should be 1–2 mm beyond the incisal edges of maxillary incisors. It should not injure the lingual tissue of mandible.

Position of the cribs = are usually placed in line with the lingual embrasures of upper teeth.

Help to break the seal of the finger with the tongue, lips and cheeks during the digit sucking habit, and does not allow the build up of the vacuum, and so does not give the psychological satisfaction to the child.

34. What is an expansion appliance?

It is a modified Hawley's appliance, which has got an expansion screw place in the midline. It is use to increase the transverse dimensions of the arch. It is a very good appliance for the interception of the malocclusion.

35. What is the position of the E-screw, and why?

E-screw placed on the line joining the upper canines, so that force of the expansion is mainly directed in this area.

It is because the main narrowing of the arch occurs in this area because 8 ms are attached at the corner of the mouth/modiolus, which overlies the upper canine area. When the balance of intraoral and extraoral ms is disturbed, the arch narrowing mainly occurs in this region. Similarly, in CLP cases, the main narrowing is in this region only, with the intermolar width being normal.

36. What are the other uses of E-screw?

It can be used to gain space during the teeth alignment; it helps to increase the nasal passage area and so in the treatment of the mouth breathing habit.

It acts as a reminder also to a patient of digit sucking habit.

It can be used to treat the anterior crossbite if more teeth are involved or if maxillary canine is involved. Maxillary canine being a strong tooth and having the longest root, is least affected by Z-spring.

It is also used to labially incline the central incisors in cases of class II division 2 pattern.

37. What is an oral screen/vestibular screen?

It is an appliance which is placed in the labial vestibule of the mouth, i.e. between labial surfaces of the teeth inside and the lips and cheeks on outside.

38. Why is it known as the vestibular screen?

Because it occupies the vestibule of the mouth.

39. What is the extension limit of oral screen?

It extends posteriorly covering the mesial half of the last erupted molars, i.e. the mesial half of the maxillary first molar if given in the age range given below.

40. Which is the best age for the use of oral screen?

Best age = early mixed dentition period, i.e. 8–9 years, as it is the time of palatal width increase.

41. How does it help in expansion of the upper and lower arches?

It helps in the expansion of arches, when spacer of wax is placed during fabrication of this appliance, extending from the canine to last molar region. Expansion occurs with the help of the tongue pressure.

42. What are the other uses of oral screen?

Retraction of upper anterior teeth, by the help of the lip forces.

Treatment of mouth breathing, tongue thrusting; digit sucking habits.

43. What is the use of ring and where it is kept?

It is kept at the junction of middle and incisal third of upper C.I. (which is the normal level of the lower lip), Used for lip exercises. It should be made of 20 gauge or thicker SS hardwire.

44. What is the use of spacer placed in the oral screen?

Spacer provides space for expansion of arches by tongue pressure

Modified with holes, cribs, lingual screen, etc. for specific purposes.

45. What is an inclined plane appliance?

It is an appliance having an acrylic covering the lower incisors at an angle to the occlusal plane and touching the lingual surface/s of the upper incisors. It is used to treat the upper incisors which are erupting in the cross bite relationship, i.e. in developing crossbite.

It is not successful in treating a tooth, which has completely erupted in the crossbite.

Proper space must be there in the arch for alignment of the tooth in crossbite.

46. How do you obtain the anchorage for the treatment of the crossbite?

At least one tooth on each side of the culprit tooth are involved in the appliance to make the anchorage surface area more than the tooth being treated.

47. What is the angle of the incline plane?

The angle of the incline is made at approx 45–60° to the occlusal plane so that the culprit incisor slides along this incline.

48. What is the maximum time for which it should be used and why?

It should be worn only for 2–3 weeks, as the prolonged wear may cause overeruption of molars and may lead to open bite.

49. What is a lip bumper appliance?

It is a removable or fixed appliance; a sort of myofunctional appliance.

The acrylic button is fabricated in the lower anterior vestibule.

50. What is the mechanism of action of lip bumper?

It helps to keep the lower lip away from lower incisors and prevents their lingual tilting. It is indicated in lip sucking habits.

It also transfers the force of lower lip to the molars and causes their distal tipping. It helps to increase the anchorage.

51. What should be the position of the acrylic button in this appliance?

The acrylic button should be about 5–6 mm high. It should extend from mesial of one canine to the mesial of the other canine.

Its acrylic button should be kept 2–3 mm away from the labial surfaces of the lower incisors. This space also allows the incisors to move labially under the tongue forces.

The acrylic button is placed at the level of the marginal gingiva of the lower incisors region, somewhat towards the vestibule, causing a stretch of the periosteum also.

52. What are the effects of this appliance?

This appliance helps to avoid lip trap, helps labial tipping of incisors, help increase the arch length by distal tipping of molars and labial tipping of incisors; avoids the lip biting habit and controls the hyperactive lower lip and mentalis m.

It stretches the periosteum in the lower incisor region and helps in the deposition of the bone in that region.

Its modification in the upper vestibule is ka Denholtz appliance.

Its other modification is Augmentor appliance, which is used to treat a case of maxillary hypoplasia. It obtains its anchorage from the lower molars.

53. How will you treat the following conditions by removable appliances?

Condition	Treatment
Anterior cross-bite	Z-spring in a maxillary appliance with posterior bite plate
Posterior cross-bite	Z-spring or E-screw or T-screw with anterior bite plate, to create gap
Midline diastema	Finger spring. Remove the cause also.
Generalized diastema in incisor region	Labial bow only if adequate overjet present. Acrylic has to be relieved on lingual side to provide a space for lingual movement of the teeth.
Habits	Cribs in the maxillary appliance; but is normal till 3–4 yrs of age and should not be disturbed
Mesially placed canines	By canine retractors after creating space distal to canine, e.g. by extraction of first premolar
Contracted arch maxillary	Expansion appliance especially during the growth period
Deep bite	By anterior bite plate to allow the posterior teeth to erupt
Open bite	By giving posterior bite plane, which does not let the posteriors to erupt; and may apply the intrusive force on them.
Lingually inclined incisors	By giving z-spring lingually to push them labially, followed by retention
Mandibular retrognathism	By myofunctional appliance if the child is in growing phase;
Maxillary retrognathism	By Delaire's face mask especially during 8 yrs age;
Mandibular prognathism	By chin cup; apply orthopedic forces; should be retained till the growth period is over till 18 yrs age.
Maxillary prognathism	By head gear to restrict forward growth of maxilla
Mouth breathing	By oral screen; also helps in expansion of the arch and lingual tipping of the upper incisors
Developing cross bite	It is due to erupting incisors when its deciduous tooth is not shed; is done by inclined plane used for 2–3 weeks only.
Ugly-ducking stage	Should not be disturbed as it is a normal developmental sequelae.

Supernumerary tooth	Extraction; otherwise may lead to deflected path of eruption of other teeth and so malocclusion.

SELF-ASSESSMENT QUESTIONS

1. What are the various sizes of elastics available for orthodontic RX?
2. Classify deep bite condition?
3. What is the role of RAKES in RX of habits?
4. What are the modifications of oral screen?
5. Lip bumper appliance in upper arch is also known by what name and what are its functions?
6. What is the pitch of E-screw?
7. What are the different designs of E-screw available in market?
8. What are the differences between SME and RME?

General points of importance during wire bending:

1. The retention tag should be adapted at least 0.5 mm away of the palatal tissues so that acrylic engages the wire all around, and also the length of retentive arm should be at least equal to or longer than the active arm.
2. Proper wire size should be used
3. Sharp edges should be smoothened
4. Avoid incorporating stress during bending.
5. Try to bend around the round beak of the pliers so as to distribute the forces on wire during bending, If bending is done on sharp beak, it leads to concentration of stresses at that point and can lead to breakage in future.
6. Heat the s.s. wire to relieve stresses of bending till it is straw colored by passing on a flame.
7. Do not bend the wire many times at same point, as it will lead to fatigue and breakage later on.

28

Fixed Appliance and Components

INTRODUCTION

An appropriate fixed appliance should be chosen for the particular patient from a wide variety of appliances available. Removable appliances can be used for minor tooth movements only, the conditions requiring more comprehensive tooth movements can only be treated with fixed appliances. Fixed appliances are those appliances which are directly fixed to teeth and cannot be removed by the patients. These appliances can help in achieving multiple tooth movements in three dimensions. The patient cooperation factor is largely reduced, and the applied forces act continuously on the teeth.

Advantages of Fixed Appliances

1. They are fixed on teeth and cannot be removed by patients, so patient co-operation factor is largely eliminated. However, still a component of co-operation is needed so that patient does not damage or break the attachments.
2. They can be used to perform multiple movements of teeth at the same time, e.g. torquing, translation, tipping, rotation, etc.
3. They have better control on the teeth.
4. Since multiple teeth can be controlled and moved at the same time, the treatment time required is less.
5. They can be used to treat all types of cases from mild to severe ones. They are versatile in nature.

Disadvantages of Fixed Appliances

1. They are complex in nature and can be used by trained person only.
2. They are costly.
3. They need costly and special instruments for management and fixation.
4. Maintenance of oral hygiene is difficult as they are constantly fixed on teeth. Plaque and food debris get accumulated around the attachments and thus cleaning is difficult. It may lead to development of localised areas of enamel decalcification.
5. Gingival problems especially swollen gums are seen since the attachments are near to gums and there are more plaque deposits.
6. They take more chair side time.
7. Patient has to come on regular visits to the clinician. If the gap of follow-up becomes longer, then it may also lead to abnormal tooth movements, e.g. it may lead to over-retraction of upper incisors leading to cross bite development.
8. If appliance gets damaged, it may apply forces in abnormal direction on the teeth.

Instruments used: Special instrument and different types of pliers are needed for the modification and fixation of these appliances. Some of the pliers, etc. are: Howe pliers; pin and ligature cutter; distal end cutter; bird beak plier; Tweed's ribbon arch plier; bracket positioner; bracket holding forcep; hard wire cutter; Young's plier; torquing plier; band forming pliers; spot welding machine; soldering instruments, etc. the list is endless.

Components/materials used in fixed appliance: A number of components are used during fixed appliance therapy. Let us divide the components according to use:

1. Separators
2. Band material, preformed bands; preformed bands with prewelded buccal tubes.
3. Brackets: Types of brackets, material, standard edgewise/preadjusted; Beggs; MBT; Roth; Combination; lingual, etc.
4. Buccal tubes
5. Bonding material
6. Arch wires: SS, NiTi, TMA, Australian, etc.
7. Components for ligating the wire, e.g. ligature wire; Elastomeric modules; ligature rings, etc.
8. Elastics
9. Pins and ligature
10. Ortho wax (Figs 28.1a and b)
11. Lingual button, cleats, sheaths,
12. Hooks
13. Coil springs.

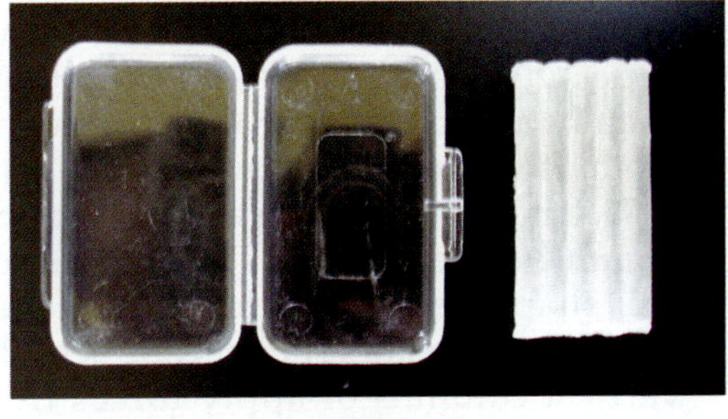

(a)

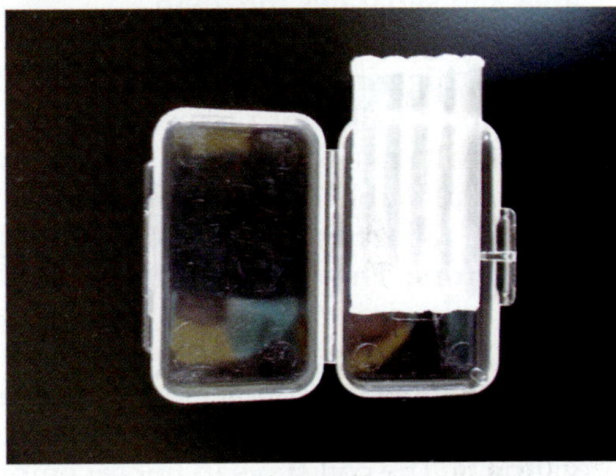

(b)

Figs 28.1a and b: Orthodontic wax which is used to prevent soft tissue laceration by sharp edges of bracket or wires.

Separation

It is the process of creating the space between the teeth to be banded esp molars and premolars, by separating them through conservative methods. Since the contact areas are tight, it is difficult to push the band material between the teeth, or it needs a lot of pressure and sometimes injury to soft tissues if inadvertent pressure is applied. In adults, the contact areas become flat due to proximal attrition and flattening of the marginal ridges; and hence it becomes more difficult to put the band material across. In young children, however, the contacts may be not tight and can accommodate banding without separation. The separators shift the adjacent teeth within the confines of PDL and create enough space to push band material with much ease.

Types of Separators

To achieve separation, there are several methods as detailed below:

1. **Brass wire separators:** Brass wire of 0.5–0.6 mm diameter is tightened around the contact area to separate the teeth. The force applied on the contact area leads to shifting of teeth within the PDL, thus creating the space.
2. **Elastomeric or ring separators:** They are made of latex elastic and are thicker in size with small diameter. One strand of ring is slipped below the contact area while other remains in occlusal embrasure, thus encircling the contact area. When it contracts around the contact area, it separates the teeth. They apply an initial high pressure and the many patients feel lot of pain. It is placed with a special plier called as separator–placing pliers.
3. **Jumbo separators:** They are used for treating partial molar impactions especially second molars. They are

slipped between the teeth, thus deflecting the partially impacted tooth distally and facilitating the eruption of tooth. It was designed by Robert Cerny 2003. It is 6 mm diameter and 2 mm thick.

4. **Dumb-bell separators:** They are dumb-bell shaped elastic which is stretched between the teeth. When it contracts, the vertical columns of apply forces from buccal and lingual sides on the contact area and separates the teeth.
5. **T P spring or Kelsing spring:** It comes in 2 sizes, bigger for molars made of 020 inch, and smaller for premolars made of 018 inch. It has a occlusal leg, one gingival leg and a double loop activating coil.
6. **Beggs' separating springs; Kesling's separators:** They are made of 0.018 or 0.020 inch wire. It contains a coil and two arms crossing each other. One arm is passed below the contact area and other on the occlusal embrasure, thus activating it. The coil stays in buccal embrasure. When the two arms come toward each other, they separate the teeth. It applies less force and thus is better tolerated by patients.
7. **Nickel titanium separating spring:** 1991 by McGann.

Details are described in chapter of separation.

Banding

It is the procedure in which the band material of adequate size is wrapped and adapted around the tooth at proper height and contour, and the welded. It is used to receive other molar attachments (Figs 28.2 and 28.3).

Procedure of Band Adaptation

A proper size of the band material is selected. About 2.5 inch long strip of band material is taken and its ends are welded together to make a ring. After separation, this ring is wrapped around the tooth to be banded and then adapted to the contours of the tooth with the help of band pusher. The occlusal edge of band should be parallel to the occlusal surface of the tooth.

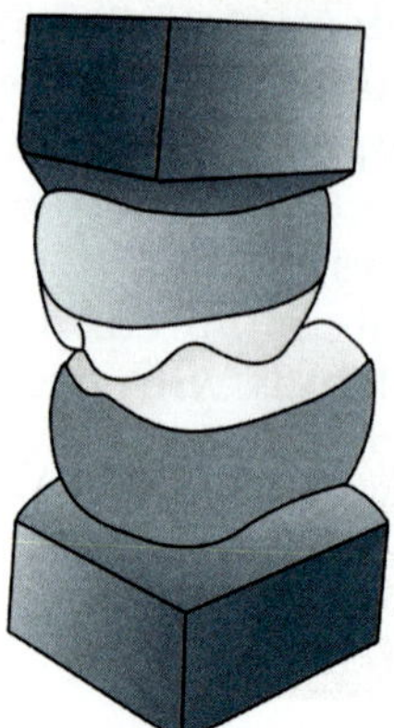

Fig. 28.2: Adapted molar bands.

After adaptation, it is removed from the tooth and weld-tacks are placed on it at the junction near the tooth. The extralength of the band material is cut away leaving about 2 mm, which is then readapted to the contour of the tooth by bending in the mesial direction. It is again welded with the main body of the band to make a seam. The sharp margins of the band are smoothened and gingival and marginal contours are placed in proximal areas.

Since canines are long, there a small piece of band material is welded on the occlusal margin to make an apron, so that the bracket can be properly and fully positioned on the band for welding. The band is cemented with the fluoride-containing cement under proper isolation.

Different-sized band materials are used for different teeth. The width and thickness of the band materials generally used in orthodontics are:

0.0180 × 0.005" and 0.0180 × 0.006" for molars;

0.0150 × 0.004" for premolars and canines; and

0.0125 × 0.003" and 0.0125 × 0.004" for incisors.

Preformed bands (Figs 28.4 and 28.5): Preformed bands of different sizes are available for molars. They are passive components and are made of soft stainless steel material. The attachments like brackets, buccal tubes, lingual sheaths, etc. can be

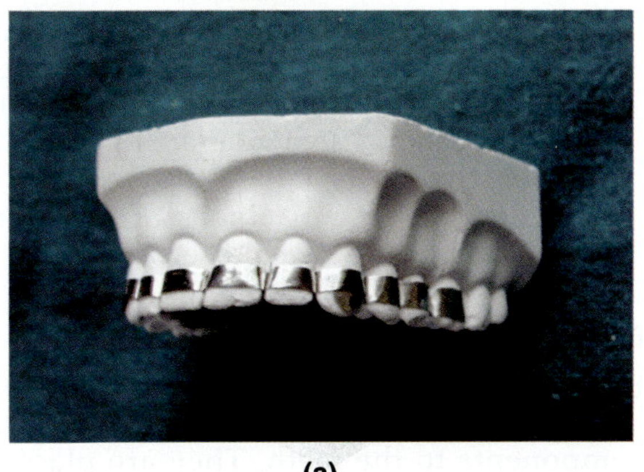

(a)

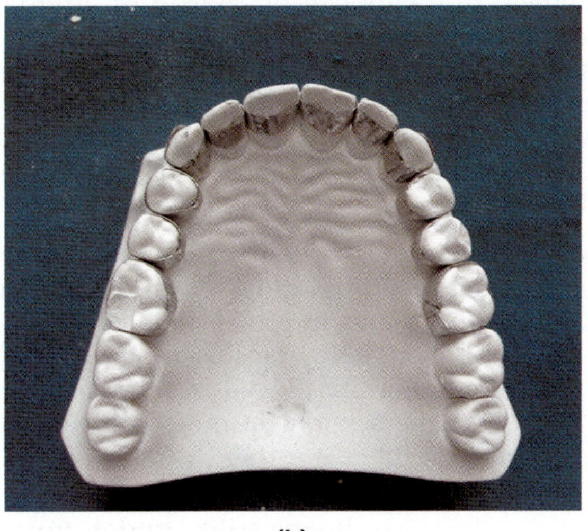

(b)

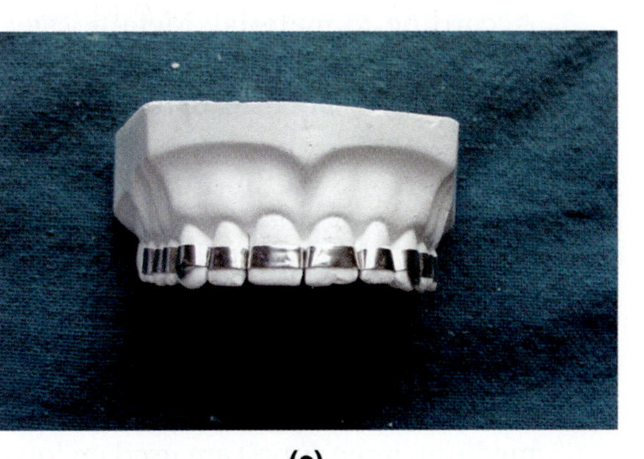

(c)

Figs 28.3a to c: Bands adaptation on different teeth as seen on the casts.

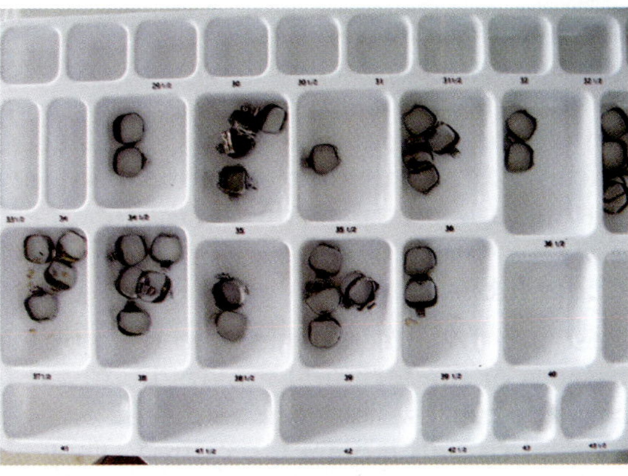

Fig. 28.4: Preformed molar bands of different sizes in the box.

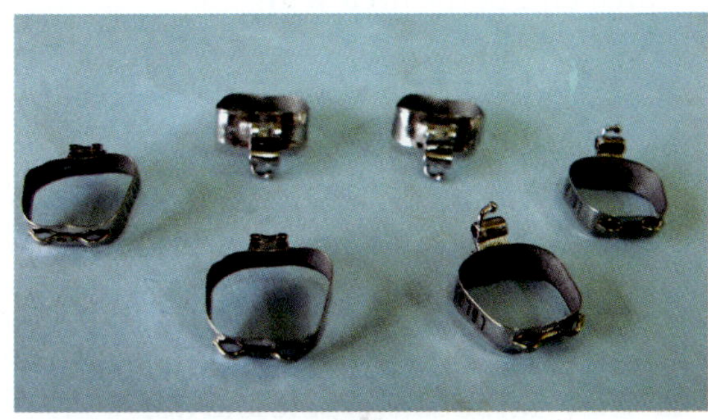

(a)

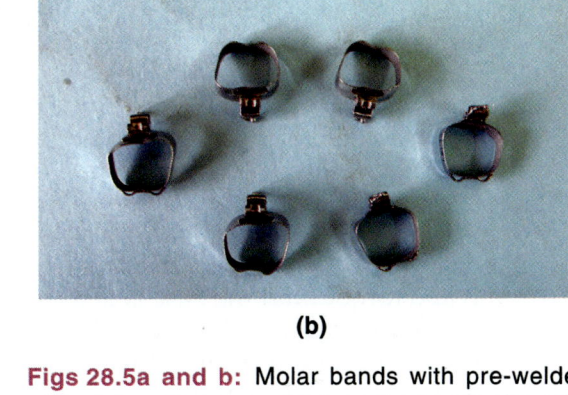

(b)

Figs 28.5a and b: Molar bands with pre-welded molar tubes. Laser marking on the bands show the size and the tooth for which they are. The laser marking is always on the mesial side of the band.

soldered or welded on them, which are then cemented on teeth with fluoride containing cements, e.g. GIC. They are also available with prewelded molar tubes and/or lingual sheaths/lingual cleats. So, the effort of adapting and welding the bands and attachments are highly reduced. The prewelded attachments are laser-welded and thus are stronger as compared to chair-side electric welding, and their failure rate is very low, thus minimizing repairs during the treatment.

Buccal Tubes

These are the attachments placed on buccal surfaces of the terminal molars involved in fixed appliances. They can be placed on both first and second molars if required. They are made of steel and are wider mesiodistally for a better mechanical advantage. They receive terminal end of the arch wire.

Types

They are of different types:

1. They can be weldable and bondable. Weldable tubes have extended base which receive the weld on the bands, while bondable tubes have mesh which can be directly bonded on tooth surface.
2. They can be convertible and non-convertible.
3. According to slot size: They are 0.018" or 0.022".
4. Tubes can also be: Round slot or rectangular slot. Round slot tubes are generally used in Beggs' appliance, while rectangular slot are used in edgewise appliances.
5. Tubes can be further classified as: Standard slot or preangulated/pretorqued slot. Standard slot has zero degree of tip and torque; and the base is of even thickness. Preadjusted slots have inbuilt features of tip and torque in them; and their base is not flat but of variable thickness. The base is thin mesially and thicker distally, thus giving the molar inset-effect.
6. Tubes can also be: Single, double with one rectangular and one round slot, double rectangular, triple with 2 rectangular and one round slot. Double tube with one rectangular and one round slot is used when headgear with face bow is to be used or some other intraoral appliance like lip bumper, etc. has to be used along with fixed appliance. Double rectangular is used when 2 archwires are to be used during treatment at the same time.
7. Tubes can be with hooks or without hooks, to receive elastics, etc.

Brackets

Brackets are the attachments which act as handles to transmit the forces of active components to the teeth. They are placed generally on the labial surfaces of teeth, but with the advent of lingual technique, the special brackets can be placed on lingual surfaces also. Brackets have mainly horizontal slot which receive the archwires. But modified brackets have vertical slots also to receive various types of hooks, springs, accessories, etc. Various types of brackets are available. They can be classified as follows:

1. They may be weldable or bondable. Since banding leads to lot of soft tissue trauma and gingival problems, now only bondable brackets are used. They are generally placed from incisors to premolars, while the molars receive the buccal tubes.
2. According to the technique: Standard edgewise; Beggs (ribbon-arch type); preadjusted edgewise SWA; Roth; MBT; combination; lingual, tip-edge, etc.
3. According to material: Metallic/steel; ceramic; plastics; composite;
4. According to slot size: 0.018" or 0.022"; combination
5. According to method of placement: bondable, weldable
6. According to hooks: With hooks; without hooks. Hooks can be used to engage elastics, springs, e–chains, etc. during treatment.
7. According to size/width: Small; medium; large. Small are used on lower incisors; medium on maxillary lateral incisors, all canines and premolar; large on maxillary central incisors and molars;

8. According to the base: Flat or curved. Flats are used on incisors since they have flat surfaces. Curved are used on canines and premolars since they have curved surfaces.
9. According to number of slots: Single slot; double slot; combination. Generally, they have main horizontal slot. Double-slotted brackets have a horizontal and a vertical slot. Combination brackets may have two horizontal and one vertical slots. Tip edge brackets have slot which have been cut at the corners to widen/narrowing the slot when the tooth moves during the treatment.
10. According to ligation: Self-ligating; bracket which need ligation
11. According to number of wings: Single or twin brackets.
12. Self-adhesive brackets.

Bonding procedure: Attaching the bracket on labial/lingual surfaces of teeth directly on enamel with the help of composite material is called bonding. The bondable brackets have meshed-surface where the bonding material gets impregnated and the brackets get mechanically attached with the enamel. Two main types of orthodontic bonding materials are used, i.e. self-cure/chemical-cure material, and the light-cure material. Bonding can be done by two methods, i.e. direct bonding and indirect bonding. The direct bonding is most commonly practiced. It involves the following steps:

1. The teeth surfaces are cleaned and polished to remove any plaque or other deposits.
2. Proper isolation is achieved by using cotton rolls.
3. Etching: The 37% orthophosphoric acid is applied at the surface of teeth for 15–30 seconds at a predetermined position. Initially, the etching time was recommended to be 60 sec. It is done for longer time in primary teeth or fluorosed teeth (Figs 28.6a and b).

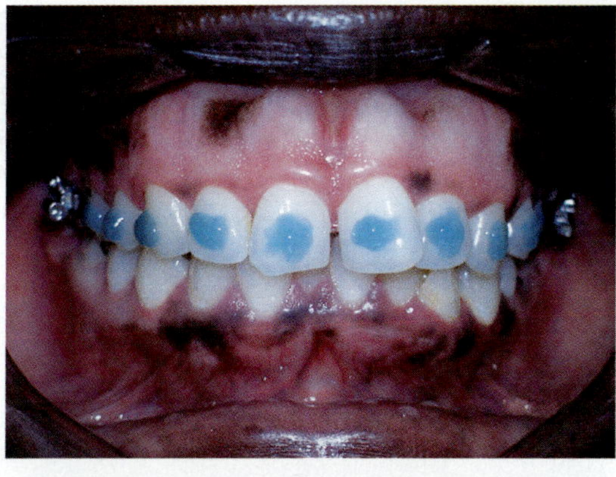

(a)

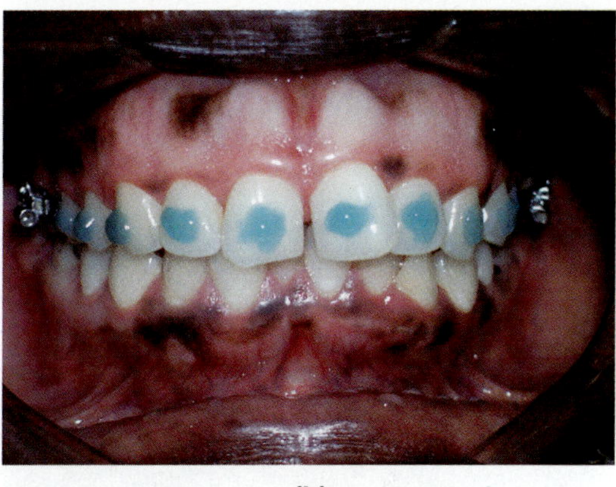

(b)

Figs 28.6a and b: Placement of etchant on the enamel surfaces.

4. Washing: Etchant is washed under a continuous stream of water for at least 30 seconds under proper high-power suction. The water should be free of any oily things (Fig. 28.7).
5. Drying: The surface is dried with a continuous lighter flow of dry air to remove any water from the etched enamel. This should be done for 15 seconds or till the frosty appearance of the etched enamel surface appears. The etching creates microporosities in enamel. Proper isolation is of utmost importance since any contamination with water or saliva leads to the bond failure. If contamination occurs with salive, a 15 sec etching is done again (Fig. 28.8).

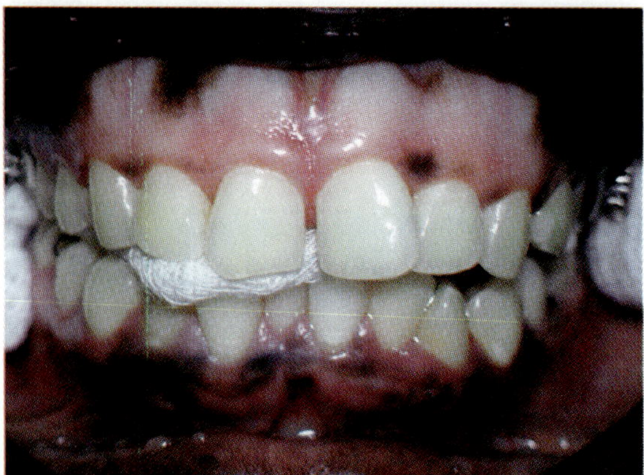

Fig. 28.7: Enamel surface after application of bondingagent after etching.

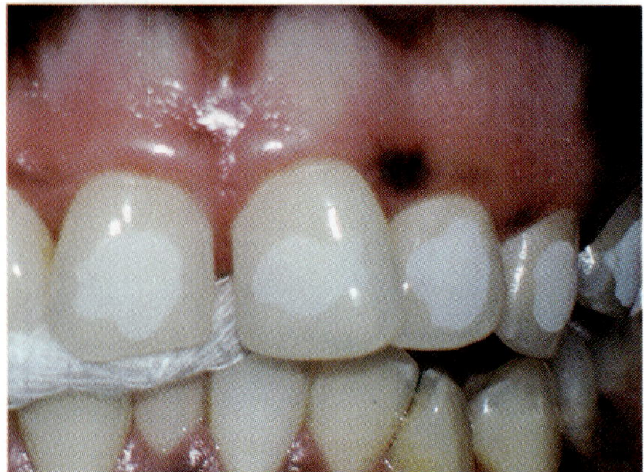

Fig. 28.8: Surface appearance of enamelafter acid etching, washing and drying. Frostappearance shows that the surface is ready forbracket bonding.

6. Primer: The primer is applied on the etched surface. This is unfilled resin which gets incorporated in the etched enamel by capillary action. If light cure material is being used, then it is to be cured by visible light for 10 sec.
7. Adhesive and bracket application: Small amount of orthodontic adhesive is taken and applied on the mesh surface of the base of bracket. It is fixed on the etched surface of tooth under pressure at the exact location. The flash, i.e. extra-material escapes around the bracket which is removed with a sharp explorer before curing.
8. Curing: Chemical-cure material starts curing when primer and adhesive come in contact. Light-cure material starts curing when exposed to visible light in blue range under 430–470 nm. It is cured for 40 seconds (Fig. 28.9).
9. Self-etching primers (SEP) precoated adhesive brackets; light cure for 5 seconds; argon light, etc. are other modifications used in bonding.
10. Strength of bond material: The bond strength achieved after proper bonding is around 6–8 MPa, which is much higher than the usual forces applied during the orthodontic treatment.

Edgewise type of brackets: Standard edgewise; preadjusted edgewise; MBT, etc. brackets have horizontal rectangular slot opening labially. These brackets receive rectangular wire. The horizontal dimension of wire/slot is larger than the vertical dimension. These brackets provide at least 2-point contact with the wire and thus greater control over the tooth movement leading to bodily movement of teeth and preventing extreme tipping of the teeth.

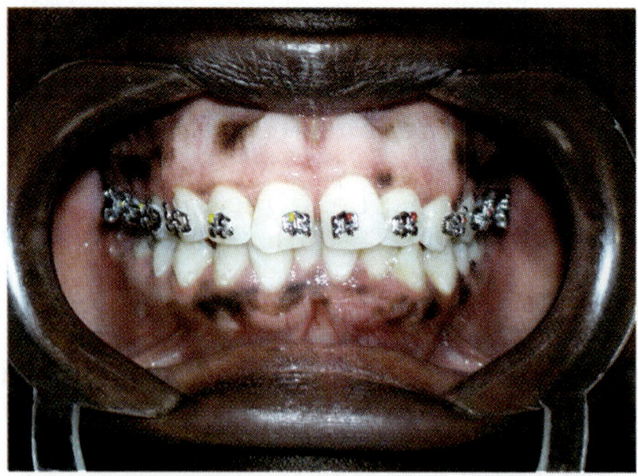

Fig. 28.9: Bonded brackets on the tooth surfaces.

Ribbon arch brackets: They are brackets which have vertical slot which opens on gingival side when placed on the tooth, and receive the brass pins to hold the arch wire. The horizontal slot is very small in MD dimension, through which the arch wire passes. These brackets are used with round wires mainly which provides the single-point contact, which leads to uncontrolled tooth tipping in labiolingual and mesiodistal direction. However, modified techniques using ribbon arch brackets also. Use rectangular wire in ribbon arch form for better control of the tooth movement.

Metallic brackets: Initially, noble metal brackets, e.g. of gold were available, but they were expensive and soft, so now, steel is used to make them. Brackets have evolved through a lot of hard work and clinical research of various authors, e.g. Angle, Andrews, Roth, etc. Angle in 1920s designed his standard edgewise brackets which was having no tip-no torque in-built in the bracket. Andrews in 1970's designed brackets having in-built tip and torque; later on modified by Roth, Ricketts, MBT, etc. having different values of tip and torque. Another breakthrough is introduction of lingual brackets (Figs 28.10 and 28.11).

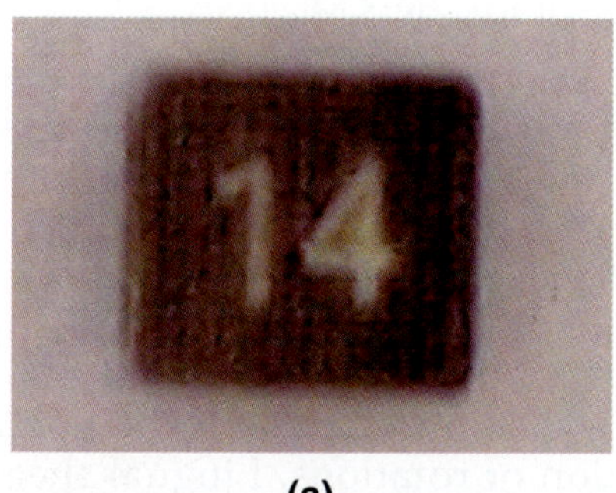

(a)

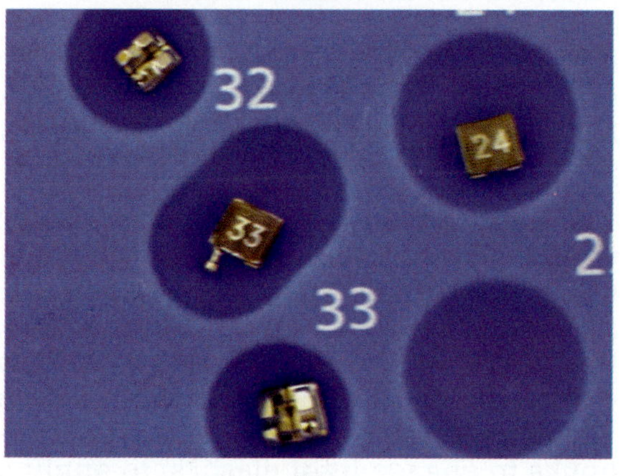

(b)

Figs 28.10a and b: Base of a bondable bracket, e.g. the number 14 shows that this bracket is for # 14 tooth.

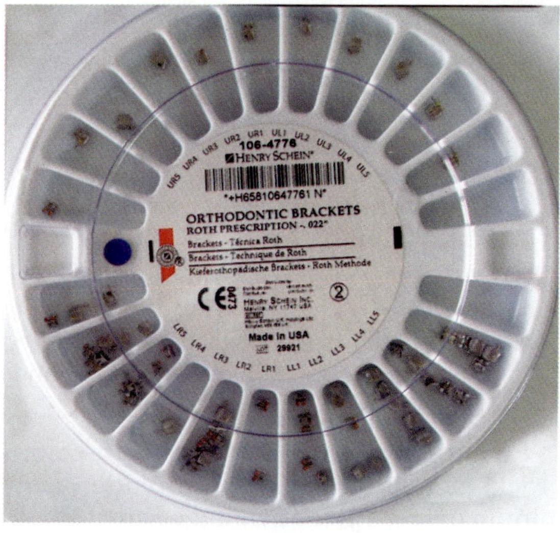

(a)

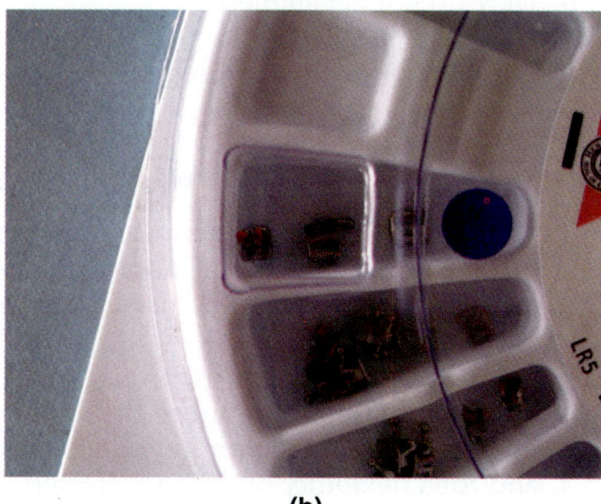

(b)

Figs 28.11a and b: Brackets in the kit box.

Advantage

Metallic brackets have following advantages:

a. They are hard and stronger and thus do not get distorted and wings do not break during use.
b. They are cheaper.
c. They can be recycled.
d. Friction is less at bracket–wire interface, so treatment is faster, and lesser forces are required.
e. Their removal after treatment is easier and less damaging to the enamel.

f. Can be welded or bonded.
g. They can be sterilised by autoclaving.

Disadvantages

a. Due to metallic color, they are less esthetic. Adult patients generally do not prefer them.
b. Corrosion can occur and staining of teeth can occur.
c. Some patients may exhibit some allergy to brackets, especially nickle, but chances are very rare.

Ceramic brackets: They are tooth-colored brackets, made of zirconium oxide or aluminum oxide. Their advantages are:

a. They are esthetic and more acceptable.
b. They do not get stained.
c. They are biocompatible.
d. They are durable and dimensionally stable.

Disadvantages

a. They are brittle and generally get fractured esp the wings and hooks during use. Thus they cannot be used in high-stress area.
b. To give them strength, their size is increased so they are more bulky, and thus inter-bracket span gets decreased and thus flexibility of wire is affected.
c. More friction is generated at bracket-wire interface.
d. Cannot be recycled and reused.
e. During ligation, if more force is applied, they can break, or get debonded, because their mesh is not as good as metallic brackets. It is seen especially during rotation correction of anterior teeth.

Plastic brackets: They are made of polycarbonate material. They are also esthetic as compared to metallic ones. They are available in different colors and fluorescent color. But, they have some disadvantages:

a. They are weaker in strength.
b. They are manufactured to have single wing to avoid wing-distortion during ligation, this feature reduces ligation effectiveness.
c. They are not effective for rotation correction.
d. They do not hold ligation better.
e. They get stained during use.
f. They get distorted and have poor dimensional stability.
g. Friction at wire-bracket is high.
h. Get loose easily during use and ligation.

Lingual brackets: They are specially designed to be used on lingual surfaces of the teeth, thus they are behind the teeth and are not seen. They are very esthetic. But they are costly, irritating to tongue, cannot be used in every patient and also special training is required to do this technique. The wire bending, etc. is more complicated as compared to labial techniques, e.g. Incognito braces, known as ibraces, made of gold for lingual orthodontics, invisible braces by 3 M.

Lingual attachments: They are placed on lingual surface of teeth or bands to assist during the treatment. They can be of various types, e.g. lingual cleats, lingual buttons, lingual sheaths; lingual ball end hooks. They are generally used to engage elastics or e-chains for applying forces from the lingual side or to help in couple formation during correction of rotations. Lingual sheaths are placed so that the additional heavy wires can be placed to augment anchorage or for rotations, expansion or torquing the tooth, by using TPA, LHA, etc. They can also be used for engaging the active springs for distalisation of the molars from the palatal aspect.

Ligature wires: They are dead soft thin SS wires of 0.009–0.012 inch size. They are used to ligate the archwires to the brackets. The process of tying wire to bracket is called ligation. They can also be used to activate elastic chains or elastic modules to apply lighter forces on teeth. Other uses are to make hooks to engage light elastics; to apply in figure of 8 fashion to make units of multiple teeth or to prevent opening of spaces; to retain the rotated tooth; to make spiral wire

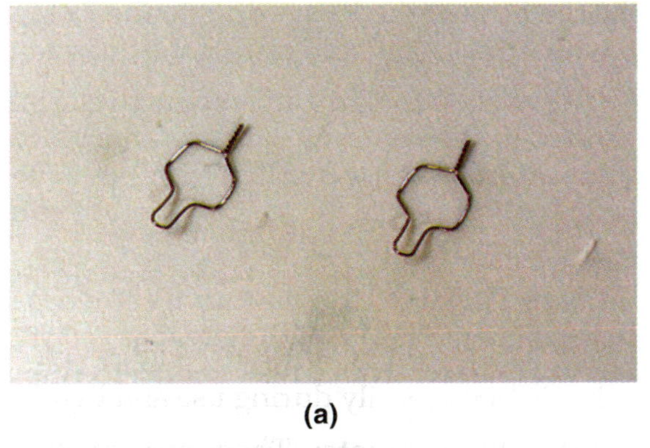

(a)

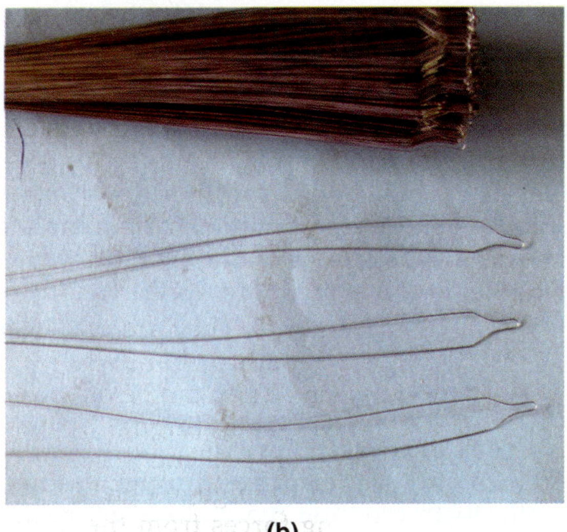

(b)

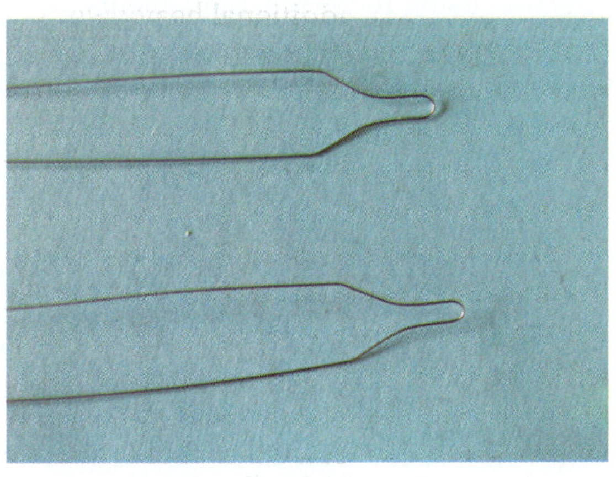

(c)

Figs 28.12a to c: Ligature wires for individual tooth ties, and lengths for full arch – ties.

retainers, etc. They are available as spools or as long length wire to be used in full arch. They are also available as preformed pieces to tie single tooth (Figs 28.12a to c).

Lock pins: They are made of brass and are used to ligate archwire to the bracket in Beggs appliance. They are inserted in the vertical slot from the gingival aspect and curved on the incisor aspect. They are also of different shape and sizes, depending on their use during the different stages of treatment. One type has its head shaped as a hook to receive the elastics during treatment.

Elastic Products

Various elastomeric products are used as active components during treatment, e.g. elastics; elastomeric chains; elastomeric ligating modules, elastic thread, etc. (Figs 28.13 and 28.14).

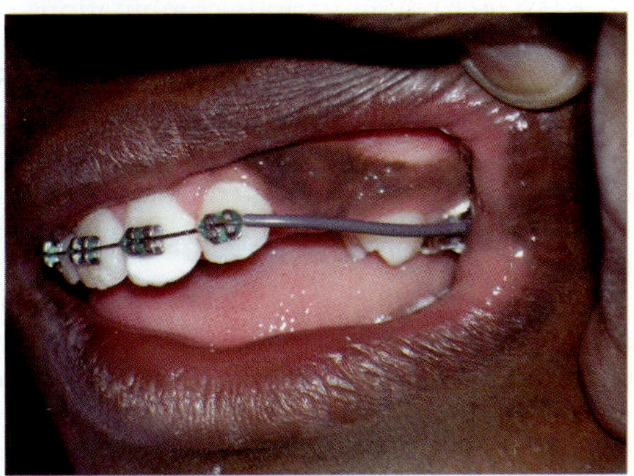

Fig. 28.13: Elastic archwire tubing/sleeve on the wire which helps in preventing soft tissue trauma due to long span of non-ligated wire.

Elastics

Various sizes of elastics are available according to their internal diameter and the thickness, which apply different levels of forces. They can be used to apply light, medium or high forces. So, they are judiciously used during the treatment for specific purposes. They resemble like rubber bands and made of latex. But, now latex-free elastics are also available which can be used in

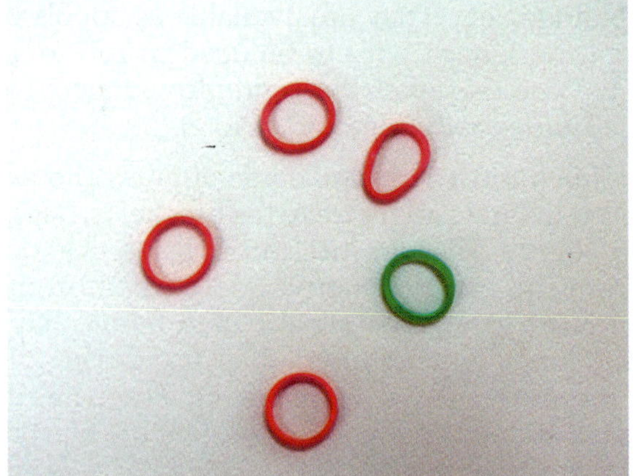

Fig. 28.14: Elastics/rubber bends used in orthodontic treatment.

patients having latex-allergy. They can be color-coded for easy identification. Common sizes available are 1/8, ¼, 5/16, and 3/8 inch diameter, etc. (i.e. 1/16, 2/16, 3/16, 4/16, 5/16, 6/16 inch); with various combinations of small, medium and large thickness of the rubber material. The force indicated by manufacturer is estimated to be generated when the elastic is extended 3 times its original diameter. Very heavy elastics are used for applying orthopedic forces with headgear, chin cup, etc.

During treatment, they can be used for many purposes, e.g. treatment of crossbite; treatment of open bite; to close spaces; to retract the incisors; to correct molar relation; for use with headgear for skeletal effects in dentofacial orthopedic treatment; etc. Their use can be classified according to the fashion in which they are placed during the treatment.

Class I elastics: They are intra-arch elastics, i.e. used in the same arch, and they are placed between molar and incisors/canines. They can be used to close the spaces; for retracting the teeth; for anchorage loss.

Class II: They are used to treat class II malocclusion. They are intermaxillary elastics and are placed from lower molar to upper incisors. They help in retraction of upper incisors/anteriors and mesialisation of lower molars. They are also used during torquing of upper incisors to prevent labial flaring of them.

Class III: They are used to treat class III malocclusion. They are intermaxillary elastics and are placed from upper molar to lower incisors. They help in retraction of lower anteriors and mesialisation of upper molars. They are also used during anchorage preparation in lower arch (Fig. 28.15).

Baker's elastics: They are the intermaxillary elastics used in class II or Class III fashion as described above.

Cross elastics: They are intermaxillary elastics and are used from upper to lower tooth/teeth crossing the occlusal plane and help in correction of cross bite esp of posterior teeth. They tend to tip the teeth in opposite direction using reciprocal movements.

Triangular: They are generally used in buccal segment as intermaxillary elastics to

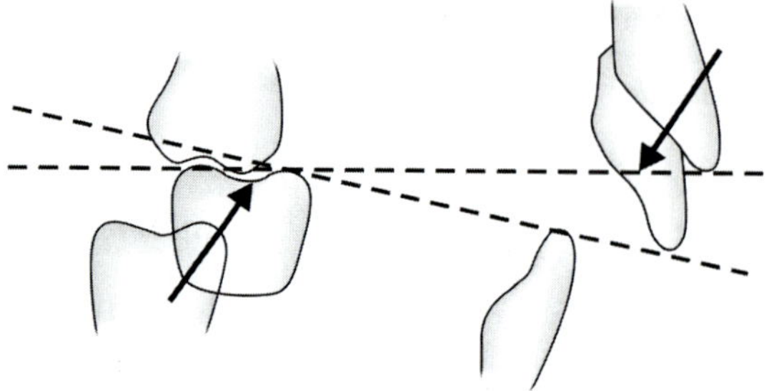

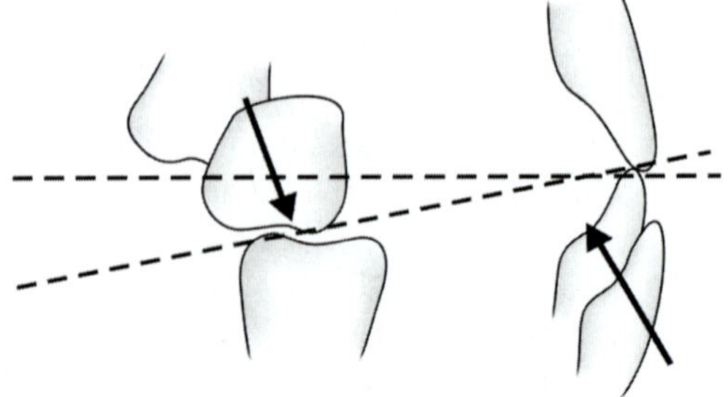

Fig. 28.15: Figure shows the change in orientation of occlusal plane with the use of class II and III elastics. With class II force, the OP moves down anteriorly and up posteriorly, while with class III elastic, the direction of OP is movement is reversed *(Redrawn from Proffit & Fields for academic purpose).*

close the open bite or to help in settlement of occlusion.

Box elastics: They are intermaxillary elastics used to treat open bite in anterior and/or posterior segments. They help in extrusion of upper and lower teeth towards each other to close the open bite. The choice of extrusion of teeth depends on the position of the teeth in relation to occlusal plane, lip line, incisal exposure, lip length, etc.

W with a tail and M with a tail fashion: They are intermaxillary elastics used in buccal segments, to refine the molar relationship and to help in occlusal settling.

Check elastics: They are also used for occlusal settling during the finishing stages of occlusion. They are named as check, as they are attached as "the right tick-mark".

Oblique elastics: They are intermaxillary elastics used to help in treatment of midlines and molar relationship and occlusal interdigitation. They are used in combination of class II and Class III fashion at the same time. It is also supported by another intermaxillary elastic in anterior region extending between canines of opposing sides. Thus these three elastics run parallel to each other during use.

Elastic chains: These are the elastic material which is available as long chains of small interconnected rings. They are available as different colors and are of different types based on the distance between the rings. Thus they can be short, medium or long. They help in space closure by attaching them from molar to molar and for retraction of teeth by putting them between molar to the hooks between incisors. Small pieces can be cut and ligated by ligature wires between the active and reactive units. They can also be used to apply couple of force to derotate the tooth. It can be used for other purpose during treatment as the demand for force arises, e.g. crossbite correction, correction of molar's buccal flaring; to ligate the arch wire in brackets by cutting individual rings, etc. However, they should be used so as to apply lighter forces, as their forces are unpredictable. When applied from molar to molar for space closure, they lead to contraction of dental arch, so the arch wire should be expanded during this phase. Initially they apply high forces but with time the force degrades as they absorb saliva, etc. and thus the force drops very rapidly after 7 days. So, their force is not reliable and continuous (Fig. 28.16).

Elastic thread: It is a thread form of elastic, where the core is made of latex and the covering sleeve is of silk. It is available as spool and a desired length can be cut during its use. It helps in closure of mild spaces; to apply couple of force for derotation, etc. It also absorbs water and gets degraded and thus looses its force.

Elastomeric modules: They are two small rings separated by variable length of rubber between them. They are short, medium or long, and are applied between teeth to help in space closure, derotation; retraction, etc. Force applied varies based on its length.

Ligating rings: They are small rings used to attach archwire to the brackets. They are available in different colors, and are attached to a common elastic base in the numbers of 10 or 20, thus to be used for a single patient or single arch. They are made of elastic and thus absorb water and swell and loose elastic property with time.

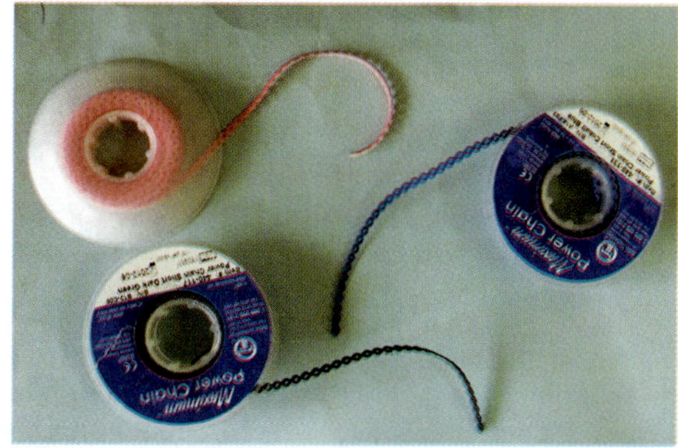

Fig. 28.16: Elastomeric chains, called as E-chains for applying space closure forces and for other used during fixed orthodontic treatment.

Springs (Fig. 28.17)

They are the active components used in orthodontics to achieve various types of movements. They are formed of SS; and NiTi materials. In orthodontics, following springs are generally used, i.e. open coil spring, closed coil spring, uprighting spring, torquing spring, etc.

Uprighting spring: It is made of very small diameter wire like 0.010" SS, and it is used to move the roots to mesial or distal direction to upright them in the basal bone. They are used in Beggs appliance.

Torquing spring: It is used to move the roots of teeth in labial or palatal direction to bring them in the centre of spongy bone. They are generally used in Beggs appliance. Other variation of torquing spring is MAA appliance.

Coil springs: They are made in the form of a continuous spiral and are available in lengths or individual form. They are of two types, i.e. open and closed. They are made of either SS or of NiTi material.

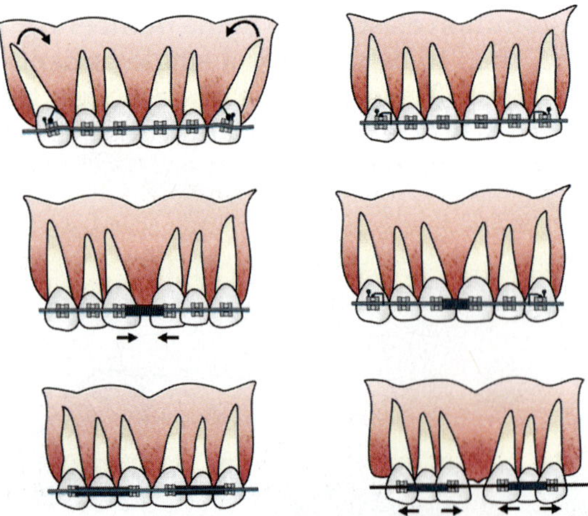

Fig. 28.17: Mesial root uprighting force on the roots of canines; root-uprighting springs on canines; closed coil spring between central incisors to close midline diastema; open coil spring between central incisor and canine to open space for the instanding lateral incisors. Arrows show the direction of movement of teeth.

Open coil spring is placed in between two teeth by compressing it to open the space between them. They also help in pushing the premolar, molar or canine distally. **Closed coil springs** are placed to close the space between the teeth. Closed springs are available with hooks which can be stretched from molar tube hook to canine bracket hook or intermaxillary hook distal to lateral incisor to pull them back. They are available in various lengths to apply adequate forces when stretched depending on the distance between molar hook and the other hook in incisor region. SS springs loose their force with time, while NiTi springs apply a continuous force.

Archwires

They are the active components of fixed appliance. They are ligated in the bracket slots and lead to various tooth movements by applying forces on teeth or acting as a medium of force application. They are also used to augment the anchorage, to expand the arches, to give proper arch form, etc. Also, the wires act as the channel on which the teeth slide during the movements. They can also be used to form various types of springs and loops for effecting the desired tooth movements. Initially, the archwires were made of pure gold, but they were expensive. Then with the advent of stainless steel in 1940s, the arch wire of SS came in use, they have better strength, less flexibility, cheaper, as compared to the gold. In 1970s and 80s era, the archwires made of NiTi, TMA, elgiloy, etc. were introduced in orthodontics. They are very flexible as compared to SS and better elastic properties. Multi-stranded arch wires, Australian wires, etc. are also used in the clinical settings.

Types

1. Based on cross-section: round; rectangular; multistranded;
2. Based on the material: Gold; SS; NiTi; Co-Cr-Ni; TMA/beta-Ti; optiflex
3. Based on formability: SS are formable; while NiTi are not formable.

Ideal requirements of archwires: Several features are desirable for optimum performance of wires during treatment. These are large springback, low stiffness, high formability, high stored energy for initial arch wires for leveling and alignment phase. During the retraction phase, the wires needed should have higher stiffness, with lesser springback so that they do not get distorted during the major tooth movements, and are able to maintain the arch form and anchorage. They should also show biocompatibility, environmental stability, low friction, and the weldability or solderability. Three main properties of orthodontic wires are strength, stiffness and range. A brief description of these desirable characteristics is as follows.

1. **Springback:** This is also referred to as maximum elastic deflection, maximum flexibility, range of deflection, or working range. It is the ratio of yield strength to the modulus of elasticity of the material (YS/E). It determines the range of action of the wire. Higher springback means the ability to large activations with lesser applied force with a resultant increase in working range and time. So, fewer archwire changes or adjustments will be required. Springback is also a measure of how far a wire can be deflected without causing permanent deformation.
2. **Stiffness or load-deflection rate:** This is the force delivered by an appliance and is proportional to the modulus of elasticity (E). It is the amount of load (force) required to achieve the desired amount of displacement. Low stiffness or load deflection rate means (1) the ability to apply lower forces, (2) a more constant force remains over-time, as there is less degradation of forces over a range of deactivaction and (3) greater ease and accuracy in applying a given force.
3. **Important relation** between them is shown as

   Strength = stiffness x range

   Springiness = 1/stiffness
4. **Formability:** It means that the wire should be able to withstand permanent deformation when bent in the form of loops and bends. High formability provides the ability to bend a wire into desired configurations, such as loops, coils, and stops without fracturing the wire.
5. **Modulus of resilience or stored energy:** This property represents the work available to move teeth. It is reflected by the area under the line describing elastic deformation of the wire.
6. **Resilience** is amount of force the wire can withstand without permanent deformation. High resilience means high working range.
7. **Biocompatibility:** Wires should be biocompatible, and the tissues should be tolerant to elements in the wire, i.e. non-allergic.
8. **Environmental stability** means that the desirable properties of wire are maintained for extended periods of time after manufacture, i.e. shelf-life of the product should be long. This ensures a predictable behavior of the wire when used. They should be resistant to corrosion.
9. **Joinability:** It is an important requirement so that the clinician is able to attach auxiliaries to orthodontic wires by welding or soldering, it helps to incorporate modifications in the appliance. NiTi wires don't allow soldering or welding, while SS wire has both properties.
10. **Friction:** While using sliding technique for space closure and canine retraction, the bracket has to move over the wire. Frictional forces come into play since the surfaces of wire and bracket are not perfectly smooth. To overcome excessive amount of friction, heavy forces are applied, which may result in loss of anchorageor binding accompanied by little or no tooth movement. The

preferred wire should be one that produces the least amount of friction at the bracket/wire interface.

Mechanical Properties and Their Clinical Implications

Stainless Steel Wires

The large modulus of elasticity and high stiffness of SS wires indicates the use of smaller sized wires for alignment of teeth. To reduce stiffness or to increase flexibility, loops are placed in wire during alignment phase. High stiffness is helpful in resisting deformation by the applied forces.

The yield strength to elastic modulus ratio (YS/E) indicates a lower springback of stainless steel than titanium-based alloys. The stored energy of activated stainless steel wires is less than beta-titanium and nitinol wires. This implies that stainless steel wires produce higher forces that dissipate over shorter periods of time than either beta-titanium or nitinol wires, thus requiring more frequent activations or arch wire changes. More load is required to attain the deflection, and during deactivation, there is drastic force loss. Thus the forces applied do not remain of constant or continuous nature.

Cold working contributes to the high yield strength and modulus of elasticity of stainless steel. Residual stresses are generated in the wire after bending which markedly affect the elastic properties of the wire. These stresses are relieved by heat treatment which helps to enhance the elastic properties of wire. The recommended temperature-time schedule for stress-relieving stainless steel is 750°F (399°C) for 11 minutes. Funk recommends that a straw-colored wire indicates that optimum heat treatment has been attained.

Cobalt–chromium Wires

Cobalt–chromium (Co–Cr) alloys or Elgiloy wires are manufactured in four tempers: soft (blue), ductile (yellow), semiresilient (green), and red (resilient) in increasing order of resilience. Blue Elgiloy is the softest and can be bent easily with fingers or pliers. It is used in case where considerable bending is required. Heat treatment of blue Elgiloy increases its resistance to deformation. Yellow Elgiloy is relatively ductile and more resilient than blue Elgiloy, and can be bent easily. Heat treatment helps to further increase its resilience and spring performance. Green Elgiloy is more resilient than yellow Elgiloy and can be shaped with pliers before heat treatment. The most resilient Elgiloy is marked red and provides high spring qualities. But it withstands only minimal working. Heat treatment makes red Elgiloy wire extremely resilient by causing **precipitation-hardening.** But this wire fractures easily after heat treatment, all adjustments should be made before this **precipitation-hardening process**.

With the exception of Red Elgiloy, non-heat-treated Co–Cr wires have a smaller springback than stainless steel wires, but it can be improved by adequate heat treatment at the temperature 900°F (482°C) for 7–12 minutes. This causes precipitation-hardening of the alloy, increasing the resistance of the wire to deformation. The advantages of Co–Cr wires over stainless steel wires are greater resistance to fatigue and distortion, and more resilient spring.

Nickel-titanium Wires (Figs 28.18 and 28.19)

They were introduced in orthodontics by Andersan in 1971. Nitinol (its full from is Nickle Titanium Naval Ordinance Laboratory), has a stochiometric ratio of 45 : 55 of nickel and titanium. It has high ***springback,*** low stiffness, high working range and high flexibility, leading to large elastic deflections super elasticity. They help to deflect the wire with less force and thus can be ligated easily in crowded teeth. Due to these properties, the wire applies lighter and constant forces over a long range of deflection. Fewer arch wire changes or activations are required, and they produce more constant forces on teeth than stainless steel wires. A rectangular wire can be inserted early in treatment which helps to

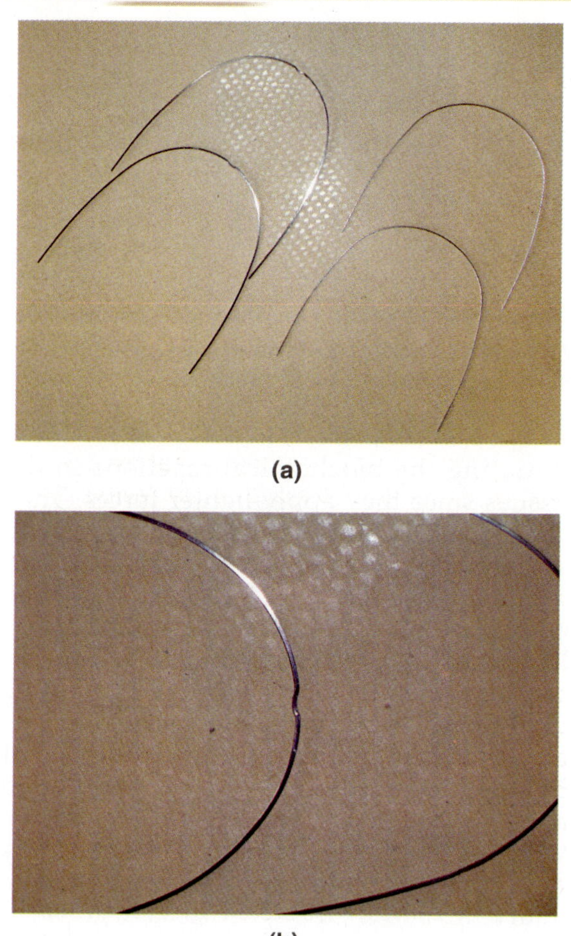

(a)

(b)

Figs 28.18a and b: Preformed NiTi wires: rectangular and round. The midlines of the wire are either marked with laser or an indentation/dimpled in the wires.

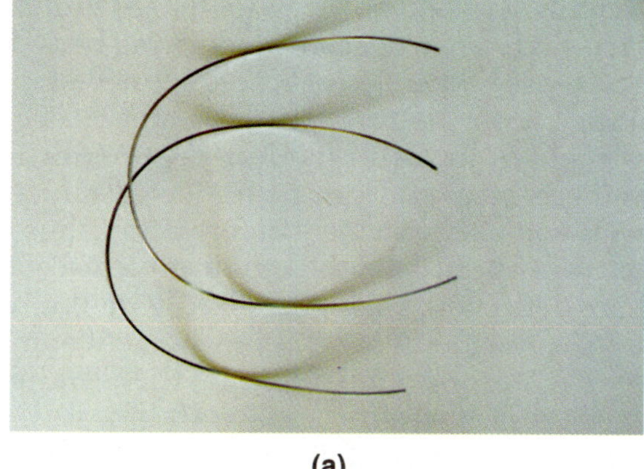

(a)

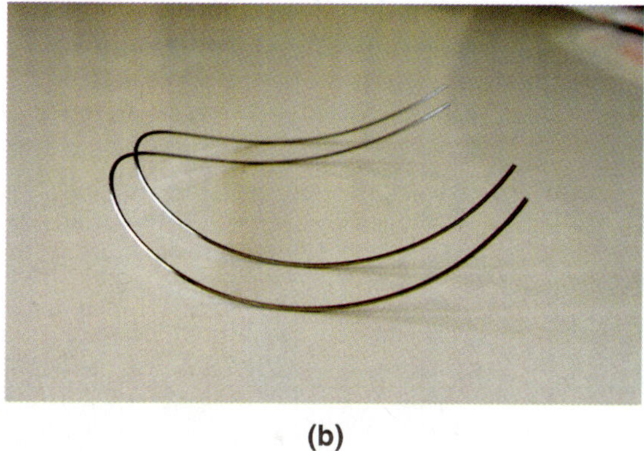

(b)

Figs 28.19a and b: Reverse curve of Spee NiTi wires which are preformed and are used for bite opening.

attain simultaneous levelling, torquing, and correction of rotations.

Another property is the "***shape memory***" phenomenon, i.e. the wire can return to its original shape after distortion, thus applying the forces on teeth and bringing them in line. Nitinol wires need fewer arch wire changes, less chairside time, lesser time to accomplish rotations and leveling, and less patient discomfort. But it has poor formability; cannot be soldered/welded, and it fractures readily when bent over a sharp edge. Crimpable hooks and stops only can be used. Also, friction is generated with nitinol wires is highest, while friction with stainless steel wires is lowest. Friction depends on the amount of titanium present in the alloy, thus Beta-titanium wire has less friction than NiTi but more than SS. These wires can be recycled and reused as there is no appreciable loss in properties of nitinol wires after as many as three recycles.

HANT wires are heat activated NiTi wires, which are very flexible, have shape memory. They get activated intraorally under the body temperature to apply the forces on the teeth, after they have been ligated even in extremely out-of-arch teeth.

Beta-titanium Wires

It was introduced by Burstone and Goldberg. Beta titanium or titanium-molybdenum alloy (TMA) has a modulus of elasticity less than stainless steel and about twice that of nitinol. It has high range of action and spring back. It can be used when lesser forces are necessary along with better stiffness need. The springback for beta-titanium is superior to stainless steel and can be deflected almost twice without permanent deformation; thus it delivers about half the amount of force at more deflection. So, bigger sized wire can be used leading to full bracket engagment and a greater torque control than the smaller stainless steel wire.

It has good formability so stops and loops can be bent. It is also weldable, thus the hooks, etc. can be attached to them (Fig. 28.20). But it has higher levels of friction than stainless steel or Co–Cr wires during sliding of teeth.

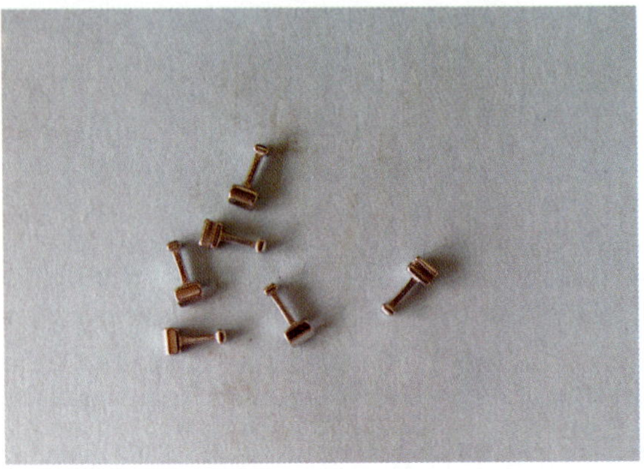

Fig. 28.20: Crimpable hooks which can be crimped on the archwires with the help of plier and are used for attachment of elastics. They eliminate the need of soldering the hooks on the wires.

Multistranded Wires (Fig. 28.21)

Multistranded wires are multiple thin stainless steel wires which are coiled around each other or around a common axial wire, to make a round or rectangular form. They are more flexible, and more deflection can be attained to ligate in badly deflected teeth. Stiffness is less than the normal stainless steel wire of same size. They have larger springback than solid stainless steel or beta-titanium wires. They are generally used in the most initial stage of treatment in cases having extremely deflected teeth and help in

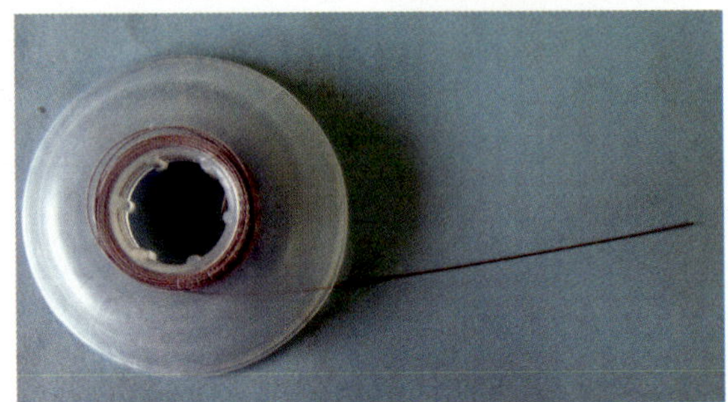

Fig. 28.21: Spool of multistrand wire, generally used in the very initial stages of treatment.

initiating the biochemical reactions in the tissues since they apply lighter forces. They are also used in the last stages when occlusal settling and a physiologically-balanced arch forms are needed before debonding. When occlusal settling elastics are needed, they are ligated so that reciprocal tooth movements can be achieved. However, they cannot be used to achieve full alignment, bite opening, etc. since they are not that stiff. They cannot be used to maintain the arch form, or to augment anchorage, etc. Other disadvantage with them is that the terminal ends generally gets frayed/opened and cause soft tissue injury.

HISTORICAL PERSPECTIVE OF FIXED APPLIANCES

The orthodontic treatment was provided to the patient with removable appliances, which could not help to attain multiple movements and the results were not good. So, clinicians started developing the fixed appliances for greater control of tooth movements. EH Angle is considered as the ***father of modern orthodontics***, since his untiring efforts and constant innovations led to the birth of widely used edgewise appliance. The brief history is depicted as follows.

Development of the Edgewise Appliance

The E-Arch Appliance

It was the first prototype appliance where a heavy, ideal expansion arch was attached to first molar bands. Other teeth were also banded which were ligated to this expansion arch. It employed crown movements of teeth and simple anchorage and the dentition was expanded in all dimensions (Fig. 28.22).

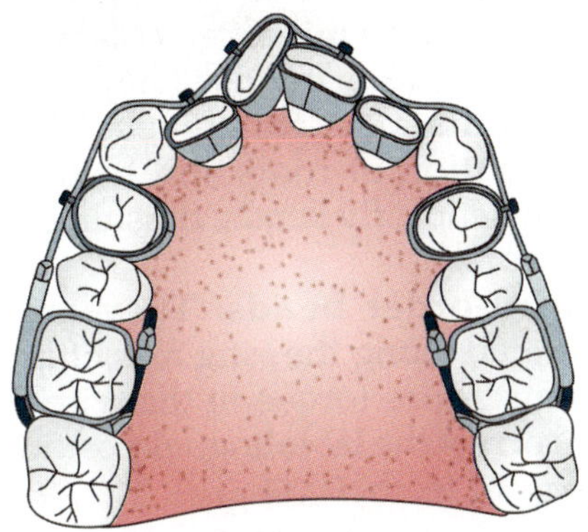

Fig. 28.22: E-arch appliance: the very first fixed appliance by Angle for correction of malocclusion.

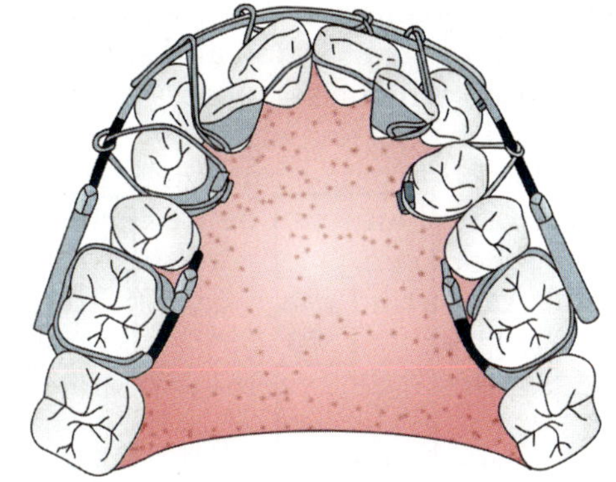

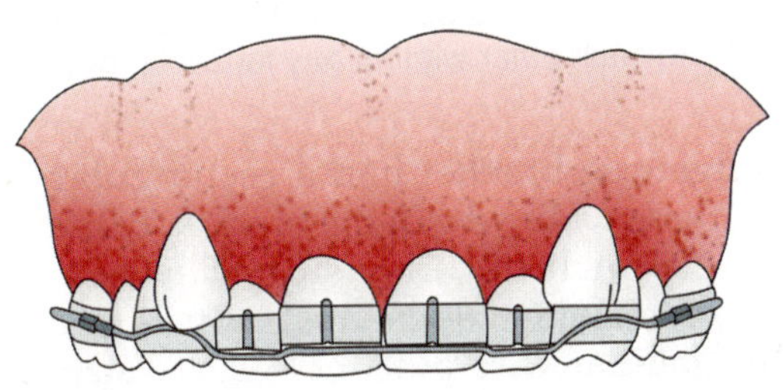

Fig. 28.23: E-arch appliance in the figure shown above shows the crude nature of appliance. Note that banding of all teeth was done at that time because bonding was not invented. The teeth were ligated with ligature wires. The figure below shows the pin and tube appliance given by Angle at a later date, whose modified form became famous as Beggs appliance later on.

The Pin and Tube Appliance, 1912

Angle developed the pin and tube appliance for bodily movement. But this was difficult to make since it needed perfect soldering and alignments of the pins on the archwire to the tubes placed vertically on the bands placed on the teeth. Archwire changes involved similar exercise. The pin and tube appliance was very difficult appliance to manipulate. But, it was the first appliance with a mechanism for root movement (Fig. 28.23).

The Ribbon Arch Appliance, 1925

Because the pin and tube appliance was difficult to use, Angle in 1925 developed the ribbon arch appliance. Brackets with a vertical slot facing occlusally were used. It was a simpler appliance to manipulate. Gold archwires were used and they were held in the slots of brackets by lock pins. It helped to achieve better control in rotation, buccolingual and incisogingival movements. But, mesial and distal tipping could not be achieved with them because of no mesiodistal dimension of the slot, and thus the teeth could not be moved bodily and root uprighting was difficult. It provided only one-point contact of wire to the slot. The Begg technique is the modified form of this appliance in which the brackets are placed upside down, i.e. slot of the bracket opening gingivally, rather than occlusally as in original design.

The Edgewise Appliance, 1928 (Fig. 28.24)

Angle changed the brackets by placing the slot in the center and in a horizontal plane rather than a vertical plane. Wings were introduced to hold the ligation. Intitally, only 2-winged bracket were formed, thus the bracket has a small MD width. It was not giving better control. Then Angle placed 2 brackets side by side on the same band separated by a distance, thus increasing MD width of the slot and resultant bracket and thus a better tooth control was achieved. The wings were now 4, and this bracket came to be known as **twin-bracket**.

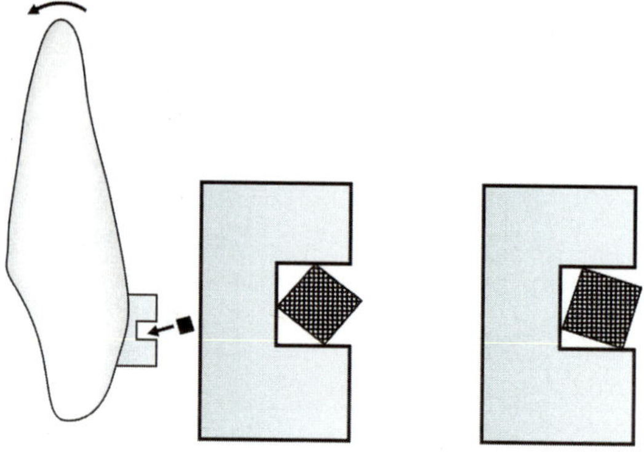

Fig. 28.24: Slot of an edgewise bracket as seen from the front and from lateral side. The slot edges are parallel to each other without any inbuilt tip or torque.

Edgewise bracket had a rectangular slot with three walls within the bracket, 0.022 inch by 0.028 inch in dimension. The slot was horizontal, which opened labially. It received a rectangular wire of 0.022 × 0.028" size. The narrow dimension of the wire is vertical, while larger dimension is horizontal. It provided 2-point contact of wire to the slot thus giving more control of OTM in all the 3D. It provided more accuracy and thus a more efficient torquing mechanism. To achieve better positions of teeth, bends in 3D were introduced in the arch wire which are known as first-order, second-order and third-order bends (Fig. 28.25).

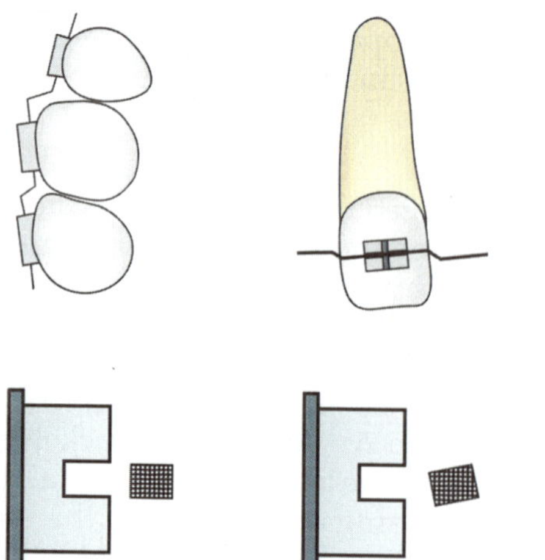

Fig. 28.25: Order; second-order; and third-order bends.

1. **First-order bends:** They are those bends which are placed in labiolingual direction, and are also called in-out bends. They are placed to compensate the labio-lingual thickness of the crowns of the teeth, e.g. upper lateral incisor inset, canine eminence; molar offset, etc.
2. **Second-order bends:** They are placed mesiodistally to correct the axial inclination of roots and teeth, e.g. tip back bends, fly bends, finishing bends in incisors;
3. **Third-order bends:** They are incorporated along the long axis of arch wire to introduce torque in the wire. It helps to correct the labiolingual position of the roots of teeth.

Advantages of Edgewise Appliances

(Figs 28.26 to 28.31)

1. They can move teeth in all the 3D of space.
2. Can attain all types of tooth movements.
3. Have better control of the teeth.
4. They help to attain bodily OTM.
5. Good finishing of results.

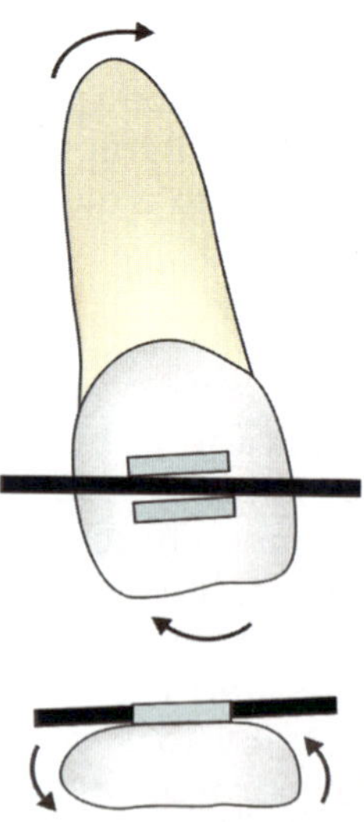

Fig. 28.26: Archwire crossing the bracket slot obliquely will lead to application of root uprighting forces as shown by the arrows, It is called as second order bend. Similarly, the wire activated in the slot will help to correct the minor rotation as shown by arrows in second figure, through first-order bends.

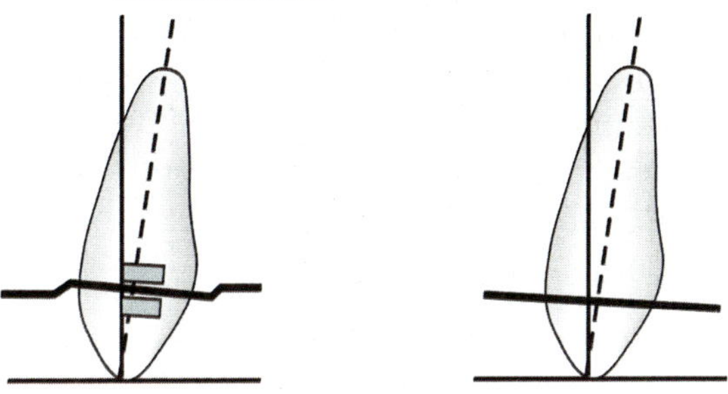

Fig. 28.27: Second order bend leads to correct the axial inclination of the root of the tooth.

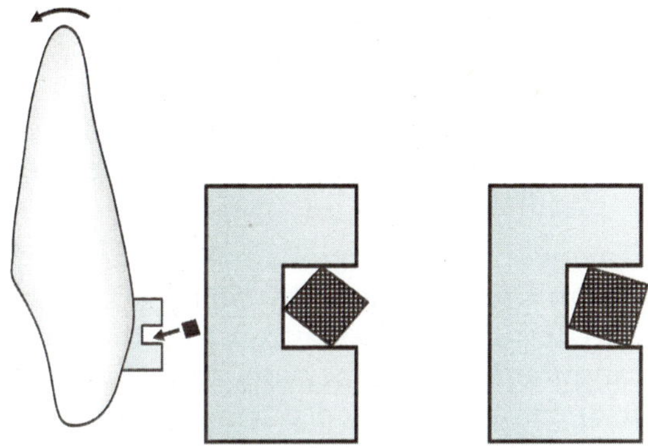

Fig. 28.28: A torque wire when inserted in slot of bracket applies the forces when it comes in contact with the slot walls. A smaller sized wire will be having more "play" and will not be much effective for torquing. So, proper size wires with minimal play should be used during torquing.

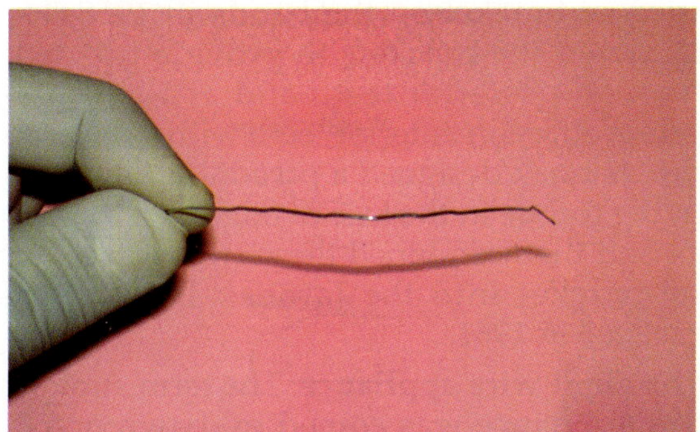

Fig. 28.29: Archwire showing second-order bends in incisal region for root uprighting to place them slightly distally as compared to crowns, and in molar region which are called as anchor bends to create the anchorage by distally tilting the molars.

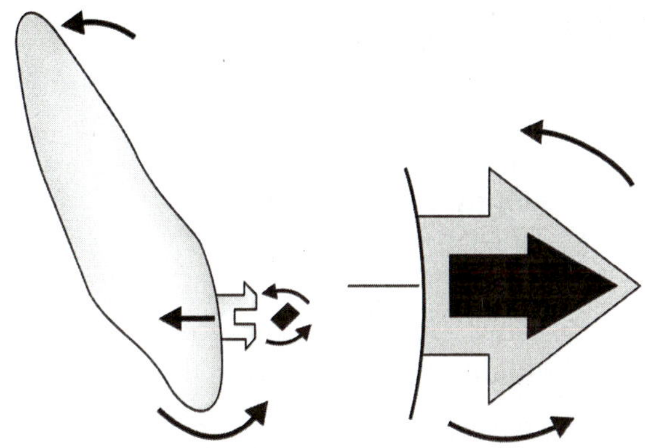

Fig. 28.30: When a torqued archwire is inserted in bracket for moving the roots palatally, there is a labial crown movement generated leading to labial movement of crown, which should be counteracted by a reciprocal force so that the controlled palatal root movement is affected.

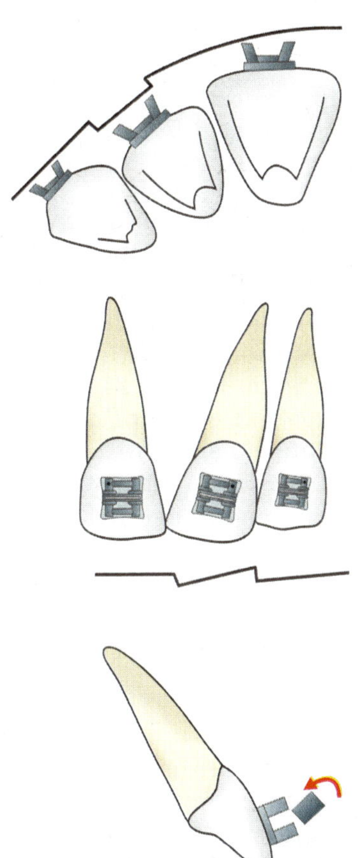

Fig. 28.31: First-order, second-order and third-order bends in the archwires.

Disadvantages

1. Complicated wire bending is required
2. More time taken
3. Expensive
4. Heavy forces are needed
5. More friction is there
6. More anchorage requirements
7. Extraoral appliances may be needed
8. Show difficulty in treating the deep bite.

Angle was in favor of nonextraction of teeth for treatment, he expanded the arches to treat the crowding. He was of the opinion that full complement of teeth is needed to achieve the occlusion. But his results started to relapse. His technique was modified by Tweed who introduced the concept of extraction of teeth to achieve better stability. He also introduced concept of anchorage preparation. However, now many modifications have been introduced in this technique.

Beggs' appliance: Beggs was a student of Angle. He introduced ***light wire differential force technique***. He used ribbon arch appliance of Angle, by placing the bracket upside down, i.e. the slot opened gingivally rather than occlusally. The teeth are moved by tipping using the lighter forces. Bodily movement cannot be achieved. The roots are then uprighted by root-uprighting springs and torquing springs. It uses high strength SS wires, Australian wires of different sizes depending on the stage of treatment. The treatment is divided in three stages:

Stage 1: alignment, decrowding, rotation correction

Stage 2: retraction of incisors, space closure bite opening, anchorage loss, molar correction

Stage 3: torquing and root uprighting.

Advantages

1. Lighter forces are used, which are within physiological limits.
2. Less chances of root resorption
3. Tipping is achieved and en masse retraction of anteriors can be done.
4. Less time is needed.
5. Minimal friction is generated, since buccal tubes are round and 0.036" diameter.
6. There is no strain on anchorage
7. Extraoral forces are not needed
8. Better deep bite correction.

Disadvantages

1. No bodily movements
2. Torque loss in initial stages of treatment
3. Patient's cooperation is required for use of elastics and regular follow-up visits.
4. Complicated torquing mechanics are needed.
5. Causes tipping of roots of buccal teeth which needs uprighting to make them parallel.

However, modifications have been introduced in this technique by many clinicians, e.g. Jayde VP, who has introduced the use of rectangular wires in the slots so that a better control can be achieved during movements. Modified torquing auxiliaries, e.g. MAA have been introduced for better control.

CONTEMPORARY APPLIANCES

Concept of the Fully Preadjusted Appliance

Holdaway first attempted to eliminate the need of wire bending by altering the orientation of bracket on the bands in 1958. He angulated the brackets to provide tip-back effect on posterior teeth and artistic positioning effect on anterior teeth with a flat arch wire. Jarabak designed a preadjusted bracket having torque in the face of edgewise bracket slot and then combined these two features in one bracket into the Jarabak Light Wire Brackets, in 1961.

Straight wire appliance: The term straight wire appliance was coined by Lawrence F. Andrews as it eliminates or minimizes bending of archwires to detail tooth positions. Andrews in 1972 incorporated the values of tip, torque and variable thickness of bracket base in the brackets, which is based on his **six**

Keys to normal occlusion. Thus he eliminated the need to place the bends in the arch wires, thus only straight wire was placed in brackets. These special features differ for different teeth. But these values were based on the values obtained from non-orthodontic normal subjects, and there was no consideration for overcorrection and relapse. **Roth** introduced excess values of tip, torque in his appliance, and also modified the bracket positions. It helped to introduce an overcorrection factor in the appliance. Later on, **PAE and MBT** appliances have been introduced with modified values and features. But the basic concept is the mixture of Angle's and Andrew's ideas.

Tip-Edge Brackets

The tip-edge bracket is designed as a modified edgewise bracket, with option of free tipping. It is made by removing diagonally opposed corners from the edgewise slot which has been cut at its ends to give an effect of ***trapezoidal form***. It then helps to achieve the desired distal crown tipping during differential tooth movement. It is a preadjusted system, as the slots have incorporated tip, torque, etc. in them. So, the preformed arch wires can be used in them to achieve second order changes, mesiodistal crown tipping, etc. with light intraoral forces. Brackets have a vertical slot also, which receives the auxiliaries. Root uprighting, tip and/or torque, etc. can be achieved by using torquing and root uprighting auxiliaries. When the teeth are in tipped position, the slot is in the open/ broader dimension; and the arch wire is free to move. These auxiliaries help to upright the roots. It is done on the full dimension arch wires. As the roots upright, the slots dimension decreases, which then close-in on the main arch wire. Thus the clearance between the slots and the main arch wire is reduced considerably which then activates the torquing features incorporated in the brackets.

Segmented Arch Technique

As the term suggests, the segments are used in the anterior and posterior segments of the dental arch to move particular groups of teeth. The anchorage is augmented by using TPA, LHA and second molars. Also lighter arch wires are used for treatment, which do not apply abnormal reactive forces. It has been propagated by Burstone, where the segmented arch wires and appliances are used for treatment. They are claimed to have better mechanical advantages and better anchorage planning.

Lingual Appliance

It is placed on the lingual surfaces of teeth to give an **invisible orthodontic** effect. It had started in mid 80's and with continued refinements it has become comfortable treatment option. Many companies have manufactured the lingual brackets with special features. Incognito, iBraces by 3M is made of gold. The brackets are bonded on the teeth surface using specially formed individual trays by indirect method of bonding. The positioning and tray formation is done in special labs using specific software and the machines. The arch wire template is also formed which helps to guide the clinician to fabricate the arch wires depending on the progress stages of treatment. Prefabricated arch wires can also be designed in lab to be used in patients.

Invisalign Treatment (Fig. 28.32)

Align Technology developed the Invisalign system for the orthodontic movement in 1998. This method was the first one to be exclusively based on a 3D digital technology 3D. 3D (virtual) images of individual malocclusions are obtained and fed in the computer. A series of stages is designed to move the teeth into 0.15 to 0.25 mm successive precise movements using the computer programs and recorded data. Stereolithographic casts are produced for each stage, and then ***0.7 mm thick*** transparent appliances (aligners) are formed using these casts. These aligners are numbered properly according to the treatment stages, and patient is advised to use them sequentially for an average of ***2 weeks (14 days)*** each.

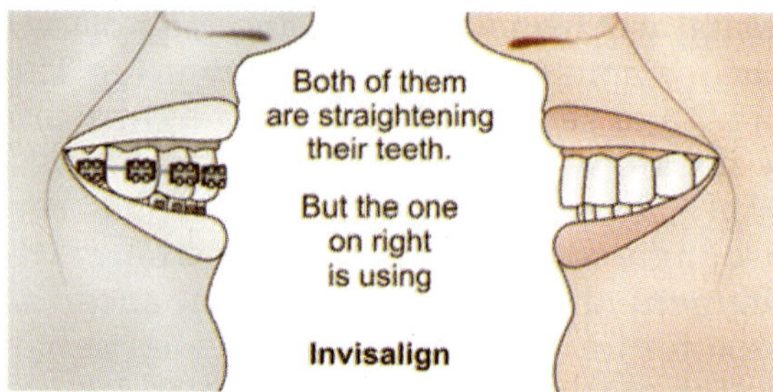

Both of them
are straightening
their teeth.
But the one
on right
is using
Invisalign

Fig. 28.32: Figure showing metallic braces and invisalign.

Its advantages are that these are transparent and removable; provide better esthetics; and are hygienic as they can be removed for cleaning.

It is used in treatment of mild crowding and spacing from 3 to 6 mm. They have limitations in the treatment of complex malocclusions, e.g. deep bites, extraction cases, molar distalization, dental extrusions, open bites, and patients showing periodontal problems, difficulty in moving teeth to larger distance like in extraction cases, extrusion and rotation, and also the cases involving impacted teeth or during the mixed dentition. Auxiliaries can be used to aid in treatment, e.g. attachments bonded to enamel, partial cuttings in the aligners, bonding of buttons to the tooth or to the aligners, and the application of intra- and intermaxillary elastics, etc. for controlling the undesirable effects and achieving some other mild-tooth movements.

SureSmile* technology: This concept is the brain child of Dr Rohit Sachdeva. It is a computer based treatment planning and appliance fabrication, where the arch wires are designed in the laboratory according to the patients' original malocclusion. These arch wires are fitted in the patients' mouth progressively with the ongoing treatment. It has been designed keeping in mind to reduce the errors due to appliance management during the treatment. It involves an image-capturing, 3D visualization tool for diagnosis, monitoring, and regular communication with the patient for the progress of treatment. It also helps to fabricate precision appliances to deliver truly customized orthodontic care to the patients.

SureSmile (Orametrix) is a computer aided treatment concept, which came in market in 2005. It is a method used to facilitate the orthodontic finishing. In this process, the digital method is used to record the 3D images of teeth and brackets. Then a computer software is used to make a 3D treatment model of the patient's teeth, and to develop a **virtual treatment plan** (VTP). It helps to guide the computer to make preprogramed NiTi wires, which help to move the teeth in desired positions. So this philosophy is a "**patient-centered practice**". It delivers the high quality care and decreases discomfort, cooperation demand, chair time and treatment time.

Clinical Procedure

The dentition is prepared for scanning by applying a thin white film and the dental arches are scanned with OraScanner. OraScanner uses structured white light to take images in rapid succession. A full OraScan is taken, which is then integrated with conventional photographs and X-rays, to be stored as electronic record. OraScan image Processing software arranges the captured images into a 3D ***representation of dentition***. The treatment planning done. When the orthodontist is satisfied with the final target positions/occlusion, the automatic digital bonding of the chosen bracket prescription for ***bracket positioning*** is started. Then the ***digital archwires*** are created. The archwire requirements are determined in 3D for the refined and finalized bracket positions using the software. Features, like curve of Spee, expansion, and asymmetric arch forms can be incorporated into the archwire. After the finalization of geometry of digital archwire, then appropriate cross-section, material, and force output required from the archwires are selected from the computer menu.

It helps to give an ***electronic prescription of the archwire design*** and customized bracket positions on the image of the original malocclusion. This treatment plan is used for computerized fabrication of archwires and precision bracket trays at the SureSmile Precision Appliance Center. The trays are fabricated with a Biostar** vacuum former over solid models generated by stereolithography from the OraScan images. Brackets are then positioned in the precision trays and are bonded using ***indirect bonding technique***, e.g. Reliance Maxi-Cure Sealants A and B can be used for indirect bonding. Complete bonding of both arches is accurate and fast using indirect bonding.

At subsequent visits, the OraScanner can be used to evaluate the progress, which helps in communicating to the patient. New OraScans are used to make finishing wires and fixed lingual retainers before debonding. Final records can be taken with OraScan and stored digitally for future reference, thus eliminating the need to store plaster models.

Conclusion

Fixed appliance is a brilliant innovation and result of untiring efforts of its pioneers. It has been modified and redesigned in subsequent years. The experienced clinicians have always strived to provide the best treatment to the patients. The fixed appliances have matured from the crude form to the digitized format. Contribution of Angle to the science of orthodontics can never be forgotten, who has been rightly called as the father of modern orthodontics. The research and development in the field of orthodontics have given us the state of art component, e.g. SWA, NiTi and HANT wires, ceramic brackets, lingual brackets and the digital orametrix system to mention a few. The constant search for convenient methods has led and still leading the development of various components and techniques for fixed treatment.

29

Myofunctional Appliances

INTRODUCTION

As the name suggests, these are the appliances which activate the orofacial muscles and take their force from the activity of the muscles to bring about desired changes in dentoskeletal tissues. They are also called functional appliances (FA). They are different from active appliances where the force is supplied by active components like springs and elastics, etc. In myofucntional appliances, the force is obtained by activation of the surrounding muscles. These appliances help in redirecting, eliminating or transmitting the natural forces to the adjacent tissues. Since most of the malocclusions are created by imbalance in the muscular forces leading to disturbance in the growth and hence improper denotskeletal balance, the myofunctional appliances help to achieve a normal skeletal pattern by redirecting the growth. Since they help in proper skeletal relationship, this process is also a functional jaw orthopedics, and the appliances are called function jaw orthopedic (FJO) appliances.

FAs are a variety of removable and fixed appliances which help to alter the arrangement of various muscles influencing the function and position of the mandible and to transmit the muscular forces generated by altering the mandibular position sagittally and vertically to teeth and the basal bone, resulting in orthodontic and orthopedic changes (Fig. 29.1).

Functional appliances have been used since the 1930s. There are a number of functional appliances based on the philosophy, their use, method of action, and effectiveness.

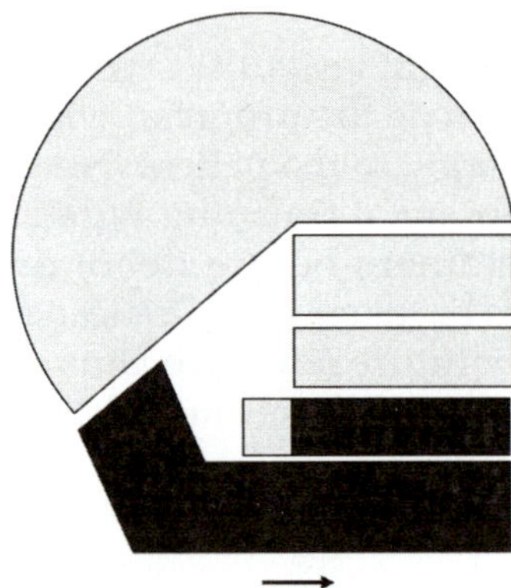

Fig. 29.1: Normal relation of upper and lower skeletal jaw bases and dentoalveolar segments.

Definition

They can be defined as those appliances which are passive and loose fitting, if removable; (fixed functional appliances are fixed to the teeth by banding/bonding and attaching to fixed orthodontic appliances), and they harness the forces from orofacial muscles, which are then redirected to the adjacent teeth and alveolar bones through the appliance. Functional appliances can be removable or fixed appliances that are held in contact with both upper and lower dental arches. These appliances hold the mandible in a desired postured position away from the rest position of the patient.

Classification

FAs can be classified in various categories as follows:

1. Removable or fixed.
2. Myotonic and myodynamic appliances

3. Tooth borne and tissue borne appliances.
4. Group I, group II, group III FAs.
5. Appliances for treatment of class II, class III malocclusion.

Removable appliances can be removed by the patient, e.g. activator, bionator, Frankel appliance; twin block, etc.

Fixed-appliances cannot be removed by patient, e.g. Jasper Jumper appliance, Forsus, MPA 1, 2, 3, etc.

Tooth-borne passive appliances are those which have no intrinsic force, but depend on the soft tissues and muscles to produce the forces which are directed to the tissues for the desired results.

Tooth-borne active appliances are those appliances which include active components like expansion screw, etc.

Tissue-borne passive appliances are those appliances which are located in vestibule and have little or no contact with the teeth.

Myotonic appliance: Myofunctional appliances which depend on their muscle mass for their action.

Myodynamic appliance: Myofunctional appliances which depend on the muscles activity for their action.

Group I myofunctional appliances: These appliances transfer their forces directly to the teeth for correction of malocclusion.

Group II myofunctional appliances: Appliances reposition the mandibular base and the resulting forces are then transmitted to the teeth and the supporting tissues for correction of malocclusion.

Group III myofunctional appliances: These appliances also cause repositioning of the mandible, but their area of operation is vestibule of the mouth, e.g. Frankel appliance.

Changes achieved by FAs: FAs are used for redirecting and modification of the growth to intercept and treat the jaw discrepancies. They can help to achieve following changes:

- Orthopedic changes
- Dentoalveolar changes
- Soft tissue/muscular changes.

Orthopedic changes are:

1. Change the growth direction
2. Accelerate the remaining growth, e.g. in mandibular condyles
3. Help in remodeling of glenoid fossa.
4. They can also restrict the growth of jaw, e.g. in treatment of skeletal class II, they activate mandibular growth but restrict maxillary growth. This effect is called head gear effect.
5. Change in the spatial relationship of jaws
6. May help in increasing or decreasing the jaw size.

Muscular changes:

1. Achieve a better muscular balance and tonicity.
2. Eliminate the abnormal activity of muscles, e.g. lips, cheeks, tongue, etc.
3. Help in proper functioning of the muscles.

Dentoalveolar changes: FAs can achieve dentoalveolar changes in 3D.

1. They help in achieving expansion of dental arches by eliminating buccal forces.
2. The appliances used for treatment of skeletal class II cause labial tipping of lower incisors and palatal tipping of upper incisors.
3. To achieve the proper relationship of upper and lower dental arches.
4. To achieve proper arch shape.
5. To redirect the erupting teeth in a better position and can help in increasing the dentoalveolar height and facial height.

Indications and Advantages of Functional Appliances

1. Functional appliances can be used to treat all types of skeletal malocclusion, but they are most effective in treating skeletal class II malocclusions due to mandibular deficiency.

2. They can be used for prevention and correction of oral habits, like thumb/lip sucking, mouth breathing, etc.
3. They are used to reduce the skeletal discrepancy during growth phase, and may help to improve facial and muscular balance.
4. They eliminate abnormal muscle function and thus help in normal development.
5. They take advantage of growth, thus treatment can be started in early age.
6. Psychological problems associated with malocclusion can be avoided at an early age.
7. Since they are removable, oral hygiene can be well maintained.
8. They involve less chair side time as they are made in laboratory.
9. Visits to orthodontist are less and they are less expensive as compared to fixed appliances.

Limitations of Functional Appliances

1. They cannot be used in adult patients since active growth is not there.
2. FAs lead to maxillary and mandibular molar extrusion. Although this is helpful in eliminating a skeletal deep bite esp in horizontal growth cases, but in vertical growers, it leads to an unfavorable increase in lower anterior facial height and downward and backward rotation of mandible. Therefore, functional appliances are contraindicated in backward mandibular rotators with minimal overbite.
3. Since they cannot be used for individual tooth movements, so fixed appliance therapy is also required to achieve final finishing and optimal functional occlusion.
4. Patient cooperation is required esp with removable appliances.

Timing of Treatment

Since active growth is very important to achieve good results, the age at which functional appliance therapy is instituted is of major importance for the successful correction of skeletal malocclusions. Functional appliance treatment should be coincident with periods of active growth. However, since timing of growth spurts in females is early as compared to males, the FA in females should be started at an earlier age.

Growth spurts occur nearly 2 years earlier in girls than in boys. So, the treatment must be done earlier in girls than in boys to take advantage of the adolescent growth spurt. If treatment is delayed too long, the opportunity to utilize the active growth gets missed. In early-maturing girls, the adolescent growth spurt often comes before the late mixed dentition period, so that by the time the second premolars and second molars erupt, physical growth is all but complete. So, most girls should receive FA/orthodontic treatment while they are growing rapidly during the juvenile growth spurt, i.e. during the mixed dentition rather than after all succedaneous teeth have erupted. In slow-maturing boys, the dentition can be early permanent dentition and even then a considerable amount of physical growth remains. In the timing of orthodontic treatment, clinicians should treat girls earlier than boys, keeping in mind the considerable disparity in the rate of physiologic maturation. The FA treatment should be timed such that it is started before achievement of peak height velocity (PHV) because after PHV, the growth rate starts declining.

Possible Mechanisms for the Correction

There are several possible mechanisms through which functional appliances help in class II correction. These include:

- Encouragement of mandibular growth (including condylar growth) as a secondary response to its anterior dislocation from the articular fossa
- Encouraging mesial and vertical mandibular dentoalveolar growth
- Remodeling changes in the temporomandibular joint, and remodeling of glenoid fossa.

- Retardation or redirection of the mesial and vertical growth of skeletal maxilla
- Retardation of the mesial and vertical maxillary dentoalveolar growth
- Overjet correction through a combined maxillary and mandibular orthopedic effect with maxillary incisor lingual tipping and mandibular incisor labial tipping.

There is a lack of consensus regarding the relative orthodontic/orthopedic correction by functional appliances. Some believe that the changes are primarily dentoalveolar, others believe that the changes are primarily dentoalveolar with some maxillary orthopedic effects. Still others think that functional appliances result primarily in orthopedic changes, particularly increased mandibular length and limited tooth movement. Generally, functional appliances obtain the average 6 mm of correction needed for the resolution of class II malocclusion through a combination of orthopedic (30–40%) and dentoalveolar (60–70%) effects.

Functional appliances and mandibular growth: The influence of functional appliances on mandibular growth is a controversial issue. Some researches show that functional appliances stimulate mandibular growth leading to an increase in mandibular length (in the range of 1–2 mm) and condylar/glenoid fossa remodeling, but these changes are not large. Since the increase in mandibular length is not that significant, the changes by FA therapy are a combination of skeletal and dentoalveolar effects. During active growth and favorable (horizontal/normal) growth pattern, more skeletal changes are expected, while if the growth is in terminal stages, most of the effects are dental effects. Removable FA should be best used during active growth period for skeletal effects. In late stages of growth, the fixed FAs are used to take advantage of remaining growth, as they act full-time on the tissues. But, most of the time, the changes are a combination of skeletal and dental effects, the percent age of dental effects increases with increasing age, as the growth potential gets reduced with age.

Mechanism of action of FA: The basic concept of FA is that a new pattern of function is created by them, which leads to development of new morphologic pattern. So the functional matrix theory comes into play. Mostly, the FAs are used to treat skeletal class II pattern due to mandibular retrognathism. When mandible is advanced and held in this position by the appliance, the orofacial matrix increases and the related muscular function comes in play. It can refer to different **functional components**, like lips, tongue, cheek, masticatory muscles, facial and hyoid muscles, etc. Since the activated muscles apply forces on their attachment areas, the process of bone remodeling starts, leading to development of new functional and morphogentic pattern. It leads to a different arrangement of teeth, improved relation of teeth in 3D, and an improved occlusion, a change in facial balance, etc.

Mechanism of action of functional appliances: concept of creating a "new pattern of function":

Andresen's activator was supposed to activate the masticatory, facial, lip, and tongue musculature, especially the protractor muscles of the mandible. With its large forward bite registration, the **Herren activator** is also called as H-activator, as it is the appliance with more horizontal advancement, so the masticatory muscles are in a forced lengthened or shortened condition compared to their rest length. This change in muscular tonicity tries to bring the mandible to its original position during rest, but it is restricted by the activator's forced guidance. Thus, the force generated by this action of muscles gets transferred to the maxilla and the maxillary dentition in a distal direction. It helps to restrict forward growth of maxilla and also applies distal force on the teeth. This force may be adequately utilised for retraction of upper incisors, and distal guidance/movement of premolars/molars.

The **Harvold-Woodside activator** is also called as V-activator, because it has more vertical opening to stretch masticatory muscles and to control the eruption of teeth.

The muscles are stretched due to their elastic properties and the isometric contractions come in play in them. Elasticity of the muscles tries to move the mandible toward the rest position, which is inhibited by the appliance in place. The isometric contraction thus changes the muscle matrix and strengthens the facial muscles, particularly the buccinators and the lips. Activator thus induces changes in the musculature supporting the mandible relative to the maxilla and finally a rearrangement of the muscle attachments occurs.

Bionator is one of the less bulky appliances. According to Balters, the equilibrium between the tongue and circumoral muscles is responsible for the shape of the dental arches and intercuspationof teeth. Balter's philosophy is based on tongue function. According to him, the position of tongue is at fault leading to a skeletal problem. In mandibular retrognathism, the tongue is posteriorly placed, thus keeping tongue in a distal position. In mandibular prognathism, the tongue is forward placed. Coffin spring used in bionator helps in activating the dorsum of tongue in forward direction and thus stimulating anterior mandibular positioning for correction of class II problem.

Fränkel's functional regulator uses the vestibule as the operational base in contrast to all other functional appliances. The labial, lingual, and buccal pads and shields affect the postural activity of facial and masticatory muscles by means of a training effect. The buccal and labial shields placed highly in the vestibule also put traction onto the periosteum which stimulates bone growth in the apical subperiosteal areas and provide a guidance of eruption for the teeth.

The **combination of activator and headgear** (Teuscher's appliance) is used in certain cases. The functional part helps in inducing additional condylar growth and freeing the mandible from its habitual position. The distal and upward force from headgear results in inhibiting abnormal nasomaxillary growth.

Treatment principles: FAs work on two main principles: (1) force application and (2) force elimination.

1. **Force application:** With the insertion of FAs in oral cavity, the muscles get activated and these forces are transferred to the adjacent tissues. These lead to compressive stresses and strain on these tissues and lead to development of new morphologic and functional pattern of bone and tissues. Most of the FAs work on this principle.
2. **Force elimination:** It is the elimination of abnormal forces of adjacent tissues falling on the dentition and supporting bone. It then leads to normal development of jaws and dentition. A change in function leads to development of new morphogentic pattern. Most of the FAs have certain components which prevent the abnormal forces to fall directly on the dentition, e.g. abnormal activity of the muscles involved in buccinators mechanism lead to abnormal development of the dental arches. Abnormal forces of these muscles can be eliminated by using oral screen. Such components used in FAs are in the form of bite plates, shields or screens, and the construction bite helping in repositioning of the mandible.

Case selection: For a successful treatment results, the cases should be carefully selected. Following considerations should be followed.

General and dental considerations: In general the criteria used for case selection are similar to those proposed by Trenouth:

1. A well-aligned lower arch.
2. A well-aligned upper arch. Patients having mild irregularities in upper and lower teeth require a short phase of fixed appliances to eliminate the crowding before FA treatment.
3. A class I to mild class II skeletal pattern.
4. Forward posture of the mandible by the patient will give a satisfactory soft tissue profile, i.e. a positive visual treatment objective (VTO).

5. A person who is undergoing active growth.

Visual treatment objective: It is an important chair side diagnostic test to decide for using the FA. It helps to forsee the future profile and facial muscle balance. The patient is asked to bring the mandible forward in a desired position. This position is judged by bringing the molars and canines in class I/ superclass I position, with reduction of overjet and overbite, and improvement of profile and lips relationship. An improved profile is considered a positive indication for FA treatment. Worsening of profile indicates that some other treatment should be considered (Figs 29.2a and b).

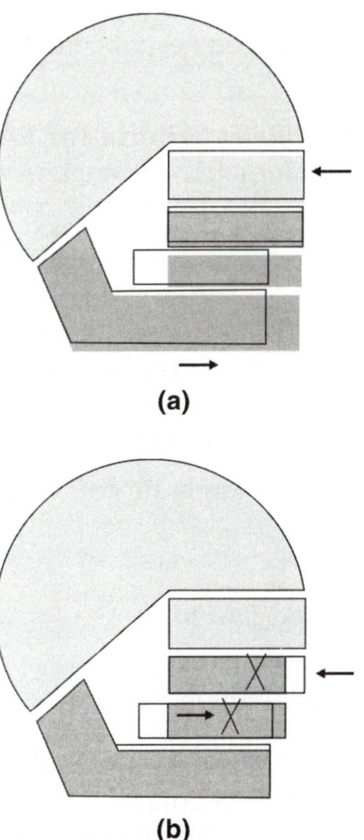

Figs 29.2a and b: Line diagrams showing that maxilla is in a normal position as related with the anterior cranium, while the lower jaw is placed in a distal position. It can be clinically visualized as corrected by bringing the mandible forward with myofunctional appliances especially during active growth stage. This is called clinical VTO. Also there is a distal force comes into play on maxilla during FJO therapy.

Study model VTO: VTO using upper and lower pretreatment models: Upper and lower models are aligned in normal molar and canine relationship to judge the outcome. If these relations appear normal, with a normal overjet, then FA can be planned for that patient.

Age: Since FAs lead to growth modification, so the best time for using them is during the active growth period. The optimum time for using FA treatment is after 10 years age when there is timing of the adolescent growth spurt. The growth status of patient should be evaluated by hand wrist X-rays or CVMI status. Appearance of adductor sesamoid of thumb generally corresponds to the beginning of pubertal growth spurt, i.e. onset of PHV, equivalent to stage 2 of CVMI. MP3 cap stage heralds the peak of pubertal growth spurt, which is equivalent to stage 3 of CVMI; or Fishman's SMI 6. Best age for starting FA treatment is considered when the patient's growth is in acceleration phase of growth curve, just before PHV.

Appearance of secondary sexual features indicates the slowing/finishing stages of growth, e.g. in females, growth of breasts, appearance of pubic hair, and onset of menstruation are indicators of almost completed growth. In males, appearance of facial and pubic hair, growth of penis, change of voice, etc. are such physical pubertal signs.

Growth modification must be done before the adolescent growth spurt ends. It can be contended that since there is rapid growth during primary dentition, why not to do treatment during that age. But although most of the anteroposterior and vertical jaw discrepancies can be corrected during primary dentition, relapse occurs due to continued growth in the original disproportionate pattern. This will need another second phase of treatment during adolescence.

But if treatment is delayed till permanent dentition, then there may not be enough growth remaining for effective modification, especially in girls; and the psychosocial benefits to children gets denied.

Treatment during the preadolescent years should be given if the child is having esthetic and social problems; is trauma-prone, or some other specific indications exist. On the other hand, it is not desirable to routinely begin treatment for many skeletal problems until the adolescent growth spurt.

Sex: Since the timing of growth spurt in females is earlier than males, FAs in females should be started before males. Generally, in females the growth spurt comes at around 10 yrs while in males at around 12 years age.

Growth pattern: Children with horizontal to normal growth pattern are best suited for FA therapy, since molar extrusion should be compensated by vertical growth of ramus for stable results.

Skeletal considerations: Mild to moderate skeletal Class II cases are best suited for FA therapy. Severe cases may require surgery, distraction osteogenesis, etc. Cases having normal maxilla and mandibular retrognathism with normal mandible are best candidates. However, mandibular deficient cases in skeletal class II pose special problems.

Since the main role of FAs is to reposition the mandible in normal saggital position, the normal sized mandible which is retrognathic can be easily repositioned. But small sized mandible may not be brought in normal relations since FAs may not lead to increase the growth potential of mandible. However, literature has conflicting results. Some research shows that FAs can increase the mandibular length, stimulate condylar growth, etc. while other reports show that a significant growth and increase in length cannot be achieved.

High angle/vertical growing cases can be present as deep bite or open bite cases. Deep bite cases can be treated with good results in active growth phase by repositioning the mandible forward, by using high construction bite and not grinding it so as to avoid buccal teeth eruption. It also applies an intrusive force on the teeth, thus preventing their further eruption.

But open bite cases are difficult to treat. It is difficult to apply intrusive forces on the posterior teeth and close the bite. Such cases either need comprehensive mechanotherapy using microimplants and intrusive forces, or surgical intervention is needed.

Class II division 2 cases can be treated with them after correcting the axial inclination of incisors.

Mild class III cases can also be treated by modifying the construction bite, and repositioning the mandible distally. However, since the posterior repositioning of mandible is less as compared to the anterior direction, they can be used for mild class III cases only. Literature shows that the changes achieved are mainly dento-alveolar, with very little skeletal changes. Reverse bionator, class III twin block, etc. have been described in literature for this purpose.

Cephalometrics criteria for FA therapy: Certain cephalometric parameters which help to determine the favorable cases for FA therapy are as follows.

- SNA: normal
- SNB: small
- ANB: 4–8
- Active growth phase
- Growth pattern: Horizontal/normal
- Basal plane angle PP-MP angle
- FMA
- IMPA
- Decreased LAFH
- Bjork's sum
- Nasolabial angle.

Rakosi-Jarabak analysis is one of the best cephaloemtric analysis for deciding FA case.

Saddle angle, NSAr angle: It is the angle between anterior and posterior cranial bases. Posterior cranial base houses the glenoid fossa and thus this angle denotes the position of glenoid fossa.

- A large saddle angle indicates a posterior position, a small saddle angle indicates an anterior position of the glenoid fossa.

- If this deviation in position of the fossa is not compensated by the length of the ascending ramus, the facial profile becomes either retrognathic or prognathic.
- The mean value is 123° ± 5°.

Articular angle (SArGo angle): It is the angle between posterior cranial base and the posterior border of ramus. It is affected by downward and backward rotation of mandible, and thus the growth pattern. In vertical growth, it is more. If the bite is opened by extrusion or distalization of the posterior teeth, the angle increases, while the mesial movement of the teeth will make it smaller. A large articular angle has a retrognathic effect on the profile, while a small angle on the other hand prognathic changes. The mean value is 143° ± 6°.

Gonial angle: The Ar-Go-Me angle indicates the form of the mandible, with reference to the relation between body and ramus. The gonial angle also plays a role in growth prognosis. A large angle indicates more tendency to posterior rotation of the mandible, with condylar growth directed posteriorly. A small gonial angle on the other hand indicates vertical growth of the condyles, giving a tendency to anterior rotation with forward growth of the mandible. The mean value is 128° ± 7°.

Upper and lower gonial angles: The gonial angle is divided by a line drawn from nasion to gonion. This gives an upper and a lower angle. The upper angle is formed by the ascending ramus and the line joining nasion and gonion.

Growth of ramus in anterior direction leads to upward and forward rotation of mandible and thus the prognathism of the lower face.

- If the upper angle is greater (58–65°), the direction of mandibular growth may be expected to be sagittal, i.e. horizontal, providing the lower angle is smaller (60–70°). This is a favorable pattern for FA treatment.
- If the upper gonial angle is small (43–48°), the direction of growth is likely to be caudal, i.e. vertical. The lower gonial angle is larger.
- A large upper angle suggests horizontal growth changes, whilst a large lower angle indicates vertical growth; a small upper angle relates to caudal, and a small lower angle to sagittal growth.

Sum of posterior angles: It is also called **Bjork's sum**. It is the sum of the three angles (saddle, articular and gonial angle) is 396° ± 6° (Bjork).

If it is greater than 396°, the direction of growth is likely to be vertical; if it is smaller than 396°, growth may be expected to be horizontal.

Basal plane angle: It is the angle between palatal and mandibular planes. PP-MP. It defines the relation of mandible to the maxillary base. It also determines the rotation of the mandible.

If the basal angle is large, the mandible is usually rotated backwards (vertical growth type), if it is small, the mandible is rotated forwards (horizontal growth type). The mean basal angle is given as 25°.

There is a definite decrease in the angle with age, from 30° at 6 years old to 23° at 16.

Upper occlusal plane angle (Pal-Occ) and lower occlusal plane angle (Occ-MP): The basal plane angle is divided in two parts by the occlusal plane. The upper angle (between palatal and occlusal plane) is 11°. The lower angle between occlusal and mandibular plane) is 14° on average.

Angle of inclination: The angle of inclination is the angle between the Pn line (perpendicular at Se-N from N') and the palatal plane. Its value is 85°. A large angle signifies anteinclination, a small angle retroinclination of the maxilla face. The angle is also used to assess maxillary rotation.

SN-MP:
- This angle gives the inclination of the mandible to the anterior cranial base. Mean value is 32°. It also helps to predict the growth pattern of the face. Increased angle is seen in vertical growth pattern and decreased angle is seen in horizontal growth pattern.
- According to Schudy, the posterior and anterior inclination of mandible is studied based on this value. If the angle is greater than 32°, inclination is posterior; if it is less than 32°, then it is anterior.

N-S-Gn (Y-axis): Growth of face is considered to take place in D and F direction, along the Y-axis, S-Gn line. This angle also determines the position of the mandible relative to the cranial base. Its mean value is 66°.

- If it is greater than 66°, the mandible is in a posterior position, with growth predominantly vertical. If the angle is less than 66°, the mandible is in an anterior position relative to the cranial base, and growth is predominantly anterior.

Anterior and posterior face height: Anterior face height (AFH) is N-Me distance and the posterior face height (PFH) is S-Go distance. These values also indicate the growth pattern of the face. Ratio of PFH: AFH is called Jarabak's ratio. The mean value for this is 62–65% (Jarabak ratio). A higher percentage means a relatively greater posterior face height or smalled AFH, and a horizontal growth pattern. A small percentage means a relatively shorter posterior face height or increased AFH and thus the vertical growth.

Extent of anterior cranial base (ACB), sella entrance-nasion: The ACB, Mx base and Md base are related proportionality in a balanced face. The ACB distance is used to assess the proportional lengths of the maxillary and mandibular bases.

Extent of posterior cranial base, sella-articulare: The extent of the posterior cranial base relates to the position of the mandibular fossa and, therefore, has a major effect on the profile. A short posterior cranial base denotes a shorter distance between sella and articulare; the mid-face appears more prognathic, with a secondary reduction in anterior face height. The mean value is 32–35 mm.

Extent of mandibular base: This is determined by measuring the distance gonion–pogonion (projected onto the mandibular plane). The mean value is 68 mm at age 8, with an annual increase of 2 mm for boys and 1.4 mm for girls (up to age 16).

Extent of maxillary base: The points A and PNS are projected perpendicular to the PP and distance is measured.

Ramal height: The distance between Ar and Go points.

The ideal length of mandibular base as compared to anterior cranial base is 3 mm more than the Se-N distance. Ratio of upper and lower jaw bases is 2:3, and of ramal height to mandibular base is 5:7.

Components of Functional Appliances

In this chapter, mostly the removable FAs will be discussed, while fixed FA will be briefly mentioned. The FAs generate forces by changing the mandibular posture, and the soft tissue pressures against the teeth, or both. The functional appliances consist of various components of wires and acrylic, depending on the design and the philosophy of the treatment/appliance. Almost all the FAs are tooth–tissue-borne appliance except Frankel appliance which is the only tissue-borne functional appliance. It occupies the vestibules of oral cavity. However, a combination of several components can be used in modified FAs based on the patient's needs. Such appliances are called as **hybrid appliances**.

The basic concept of all FAs is same, i.e. mandible is advanced to be in a normal skeletal relation with maxilla. The skeletal midlines are matched (rather than dental midline) so that skeletal asymmetry does not develop during treatment; or if any asymmetry is present, then it is treated by matching skeletal midlines while taking the construction bite.

The **components approach** to functional appliance design is followed for treatment of asymmetric growth. Proper knowledge of components and their treatment effects help to plan the treatment by combining the appropriate components.

General components of a removable FA are active, retentive, and plastic components. Specifically, the FAs can have following components:

- Functional components
- Retentive/stabilizing components
- Arch development components
- Vertical control components
- Orthopedic components.

Functional components: Effective growth modification occurs when the musculature is used to posture the mandible forward, rather than by external pressure, i.e. with Class II elastics. Functional components help in changing the function of associated tissues by activating the muscles or by relieving the abnormal muscular pressure from the dentoalveolar tissues. These can be lip pads, lingual pads/flanges, buccal shields, ramps/bite plates, etc.

1. In most FAs, the flanges in mandibular lingual vestibule provide preprioceptive stimulus to posture the mandible to a new position. But if the appliance contacts the lingual surface of the mandibular incisors, it produces a labially directed force on these teeth as the mandible attempts to return to normal resting posture. Thus, the activators, bionators, twin block, etc. should be relieved behind the lower incisors.
2. In FR appliance, the buccal shields and lip pads reduce soft tissue pressure on the dentition; and the lingual pad stimulates the mandible in new position. Lip pads force the lip musculature to stretch during function, presumably improving the tonicity of the lips.
3. Lip pads keep the lips away from teeth, thus the lips stretch to achieve an oral seal, e.g. lip bumper.
4. **Buccal shield** holds the cheek away from the dentition and, helps in arch expansion under tongue forces by altering the buccinators-equilibrium. This shield extended in vestibule depth helps in periosteal stretching that facilitates deposition of bone, e.g. oral screen.
5. **Ramps** in the appliance help in posturing the mandible forward, e.g. reverse bite planes; inclined planes of twin block appliance, etc. It is better to have two ramps in contact, as in the twin block appliance, than to have the lower anterior teeth contact a ramp only on the upper appliance.
6. If an extraoral force is needed, then a facebow can be fitted into headgear tubes attached to almost any type of tooth-borne functional appliance except a Frankel appliance.

Arch Expansion Components

1. Acrylic buccal shields and hard wires like the buccinator bow in bionator; buccal shield in FR/oral screen, etc. help to keep the buccal soft tissue away from dentition, which disrupt tongue-cheek equilibrium, and leading to buccal movement of teeth and arch expansion. The plastic buccal shield is more effective in producing buccal expansion than wires to hold the cheeks away from the teeth.
2. A combination of lip pads and buccal shields will result in an increase in arch circumference, i.e. flaring of anterior teeth also.
3. Expansion screws, Coffin's springs, etc. can be used to actively expand the arches. But as a general rule, the passive expansion achieved from changing soft tissue pressures is preferred over active expansion.

Vertical Control Components

1. With FA, the vertical dimension is opened beyond the freeway space, which stretches/activates the soft tissues which exert an intrusive force on the teeth. Intrusion usually does not occur, but the eruption is impeded. Thus the occlusal or incisal stops, bite blocks, etc. can be used to control the vertical position teeth, by allowing teeth to erupt where desired and preventing it where it is not. Posterior stops can be constructed of wire, e.g. in FR appliance. Complete bite block touching upper and lower teeth prevents both maxillary and mandibular eruption and thus are extremely useful in controlling vertical dimensions.
2. Lingual shields or cribs prevent the tongue; fingers, etc. from coming between the teeth and thus enhancing tooth eruption.

Stabilizing Components

Clasps can be used to retain the appliance in position, e.g. Adams clasp, delta-clasp, ball end clasp, etc. The upper labial bow in many functional appliances is considered a stabilizing/passive component which helps to guide the appliance into proper position, but not to apply any pressure on upper incisors. If upper incisors tip lingually, then it leads to reduction in overjet, reducing the chance of further mandibular advancement, if required.

Orthopedic and torquing components: Some cases need extraoral forces to control the maxillary growth.

1. The Stockli-type activator is used in conjunction with high-pull headgear and incorporates torquing springs to control lingual tipping of the upper incisors.
2. The vertically oriented springs contact the incisors near the cervical line, while the incisal edge of these teeth is prevented from moving lingually by the acrylic. This creates the couple needed for bodily movement or torquing of the incisors.
3. A headgear-facebow assembly augments horizontal restriction of maxillary growth and controls descent of the maxilla.

Various common FAs: Some of the common removable FAs used are:

- Oral/vestibular screen
- Lip bumpers
- Activator
- Bionator
- Twin block
- Frankl appliances.

VESTIBULAR SCREEN (Figs 29.4a to c)

It is a simple FA in the form of a curved shield of acrylic occupying the buccal/labial vestibules of upper and lower arches with teeth in occlusion. It was designed by Newell in 1912. It is also called oral screen.

Mechanism of action: It helps in changing the muscular equilibrium, and helps either in redirecting and applying the forces of some muscles on some teeth or by eliminating the forces of certain muscles falling on the teeth; or by both (Fig. 29.3). Thus it acts by both **force**

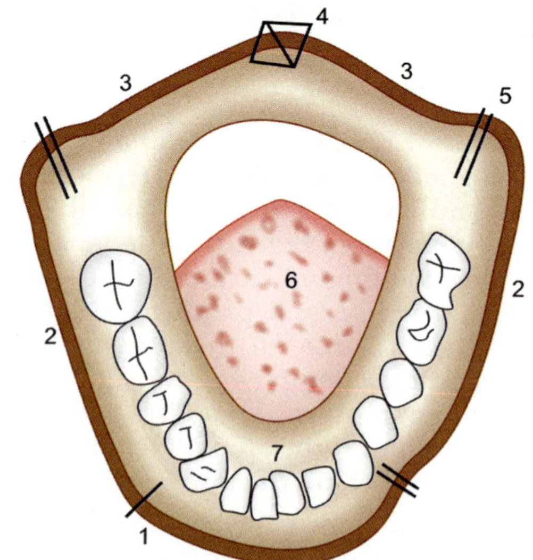

Fig. 29.3: Buccinator mechanism: the associated muscles remain in equilibrium and help to shape the dental arch.

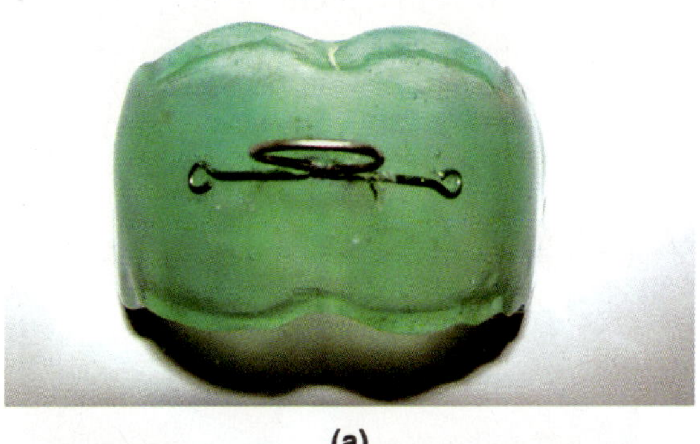

(a)

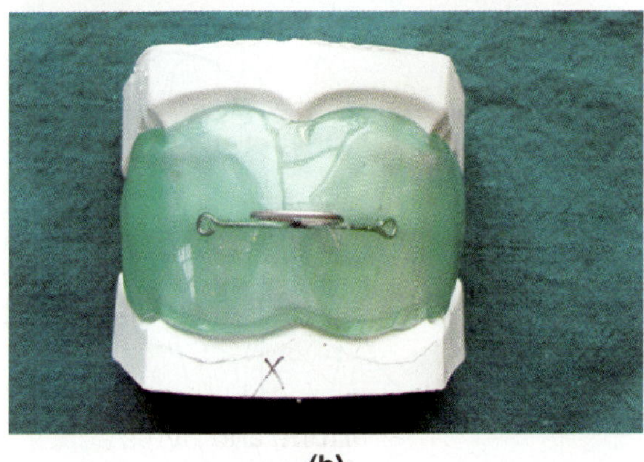

(b)

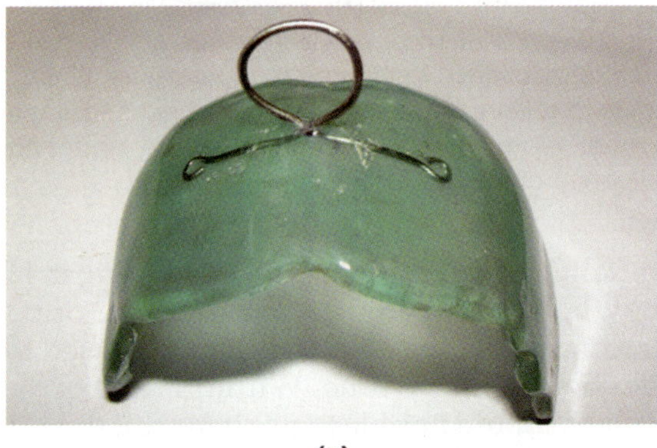

(c)

Figs 29.4a to c: Oral/vestibular screen application.

application and **force elimination.** It relieves forces of cheeks from buccal surfaces of posterior teeth, while the tongue continues to apply the force on palatal/lingual surfaces of teeth (buccinator mechanism) leading to dental arches expansion. Similarly, the forces of upper and lower lips are directed on proclined upper incisors to move them lingually.

Indications:

1. The patient should be in growing period. Middle mixed dentition period is better since that time the transverse growth is also taking place. With the buccal movement of primary teeth, the buds of permanent teeth also move buccally and then erupt in a better arch form.
2. It can be used for treatment of mouth breathing habit. It can also be modified to intercept other habits like tongue thrusting, lip and cheek biting, finder sucking, etc.
3. It can also be used for treatment of mild proclination of upper incisors which have spacing between them.
4. It can be used for muscle exercise especially if upper lip is short.
5. It can be used for passive expansion of the dental arches as explained above.
6. Mild Class II can also be treated with it when it is made with construction bite with mandible displaced anteriorly.

Fabrication:

1. Upper and lower impressions with proper vestibular depths are taken and casts are made.
2. Upper and lower casts are occluded and sealed with plaster. A construction bite is used to occlude and seal if mild disto-occlusion has to be corrected.
3. Wax spacer: The 2–3 mm thick wax is adapted on the labial/buccal surfaces of teeth and the alveolar bone to provide relief, in which the teeth will move buccally during expansion under tongue forces.
4. If upper incisors are proclined, the wax is removed from their labial surfaces so that acrylic is in direct contact with them, and force is directly applied to them.
5. Wax is adapted till the distal half of the last erupted molars. Since this appliance is used during mid-mixed dentition, usually last erupted molars present in oral cavity are the permanent first molars only.

6. Original design did not have this ring. A hard SS 0.9 mm wire is used to make a ring which is adapted on the labial surfaces of the front 6 teeth. The diameter of the ring is generally made of the size of little finger. Its level is kept at the middle of upper central incisors, since generally the lower lip extends upto this level. If it is kept at a more incisal level, the appliance will be uncomfortable to patients (Fig. 29.5).
7. The acrylic is extended in the depth of vestibule till the point where the mucosal tissues reflect outwards. This helps to provide a stretch at the periosteum and thus remodeling of bone (Frankel philosophy) (Fig. 29.6). A modified oral screen design can be made where acrylic is kept upto canine region only, while buccal acrylic is replaced with hard thick wire components to keep the cheek away from the posterior teeth (Fig. 29.7).
8. Posteriorly, acrylic is extended upto the distal margin of the last molar.
9. Appliance is finished, and polished. It should not have sharp edges.
10. The frenum areas should be relived to avoid any trauma.

Appliance delivery: The patient is advised to use the appliance during day and night. Initially, he will be uncomfortable using it. He may be advised to increase the time of use gradually. In the beginning, it can be used for few hours in day time. Within 2 weeks, the patient should be able to use it for full time, 24 hrs a day. He is told to remove it during eating and brushing, etc. He is instructed to maintain the lip seal during use. The ring helps as an exercise device when the lips are stretched towards the ring. Advice of proper cleaning, and maintaining it is also given.

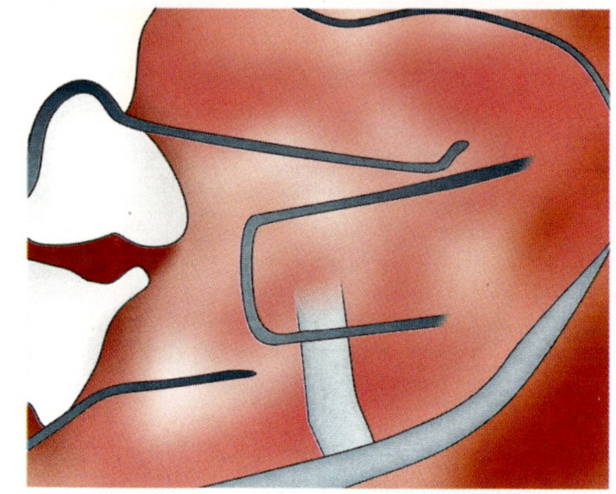

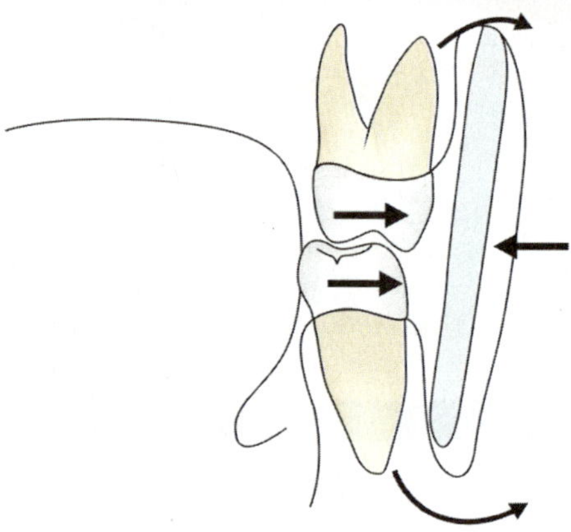

Fig. 29.6: Location of oral screen, or acrylic pad of Frankel appliance in the depth of buccal vestibule. It helps to relieve the active forces of cheeks falling on buccal teeth, which then can expand under the influence of tongue forces.

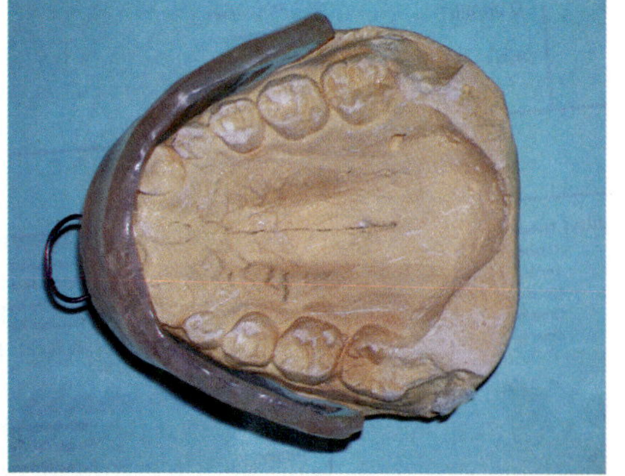

Fig. 29.5: A vestibular/oral screen on the maxillary cast. Note the gap between oral screen and the buccal surfaces of teeth, which help in physiologic expansion of arches under the influence of tongue forces.

Modifications: It can be modified by including various features.

a. **Hotz modifications:** A metal ring is included in the screen as explained above (Fig. 29.8).

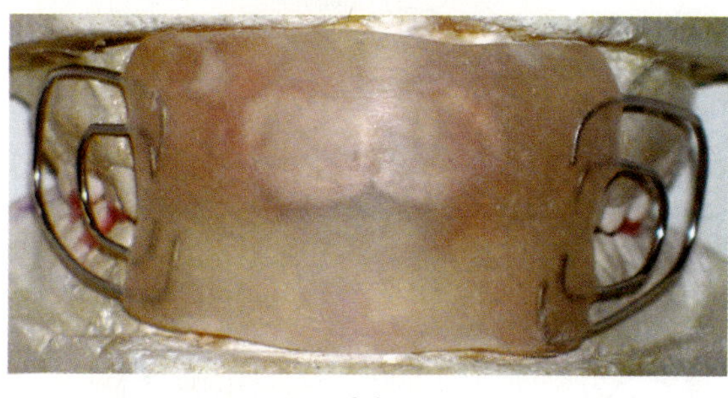

(a)

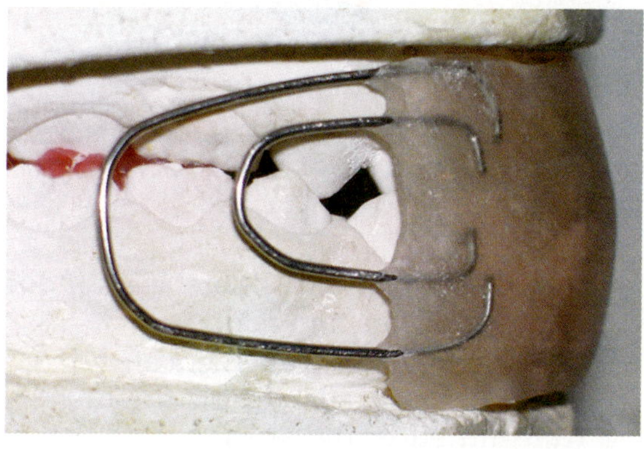

(b)

Figs 29.7a and b: A modified oral screen in which buccal acrylic is replaced by sturdy wires, which will help to keep buccal musculature away from dental arches. Its action will be the same as the buccinator – loops of bionator appliance.

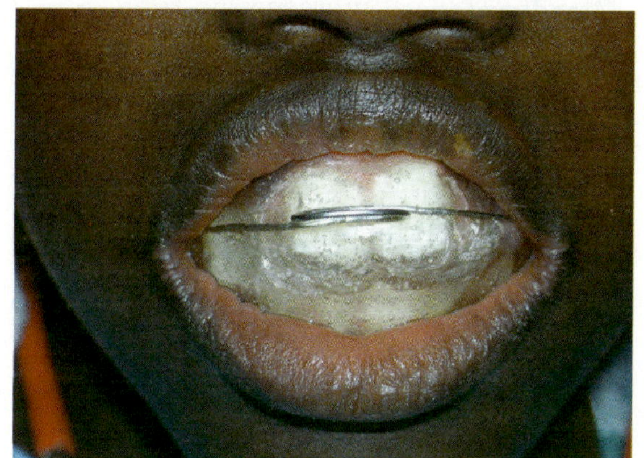

Fig. 29.8: Oral screen in the mouth of a patient. The ring is used to activate the upper lip by stretching towards the ring, and helps in lip lengthening.

b. **Lingual vestibular screen:** Patients who have tongue thrust habit, a lingual screen can be incorporated which is attached to main screen by a thick wire passing between lateral incisor-canine region through the occlusal embreasure (Fig. 29.9).

c. Alternatively, a crib can be placed on lingual aspect of teeth to prevent anterior tongue thrusting.

d. **Breathing holes:** Mouth breathing patients will find it difficult with oral screen. So many holes are placed in anterior region for breathing. These holes are gradually closed when the patient starts breathing through the nose. However, this screen cannot be used if patient is having obstructive type of mouth breathing unless obstruction form nasal passage is removed.

e. For patients having only mouth breathing problem, but having normal arch width, etc. then wax spacer is not given.

LIP BUMPER (Fig. 29.10)

It is also called lip plumper. It can be removable or fixed type. It acts by force elimination and force application/redirecting the muscular forces. It is situated in the labial vestibules at the marginal gingival level. It can be used both in upper and lower arches. Various modifications have also been devised to be used in skeletal class II or III cases.

Uses:

1. It is used in patients with lower lip sucking habit. It keeps the lip away from coming between the teeth.
2. Treatment of **lip trap:** It is also used if patient is having hyperactive mentalis muscle. Lower lip applies pressure on lower incisors and pushes them lingually, causing flattening and crowding of segment. Lower lip may also apply force on lingual aspect of upper incisor causing their flaring and thus increase in overjet. The lip bumper used in lower vestibule keeps the lower lip away, breaking hyperactivity of mentalis. It

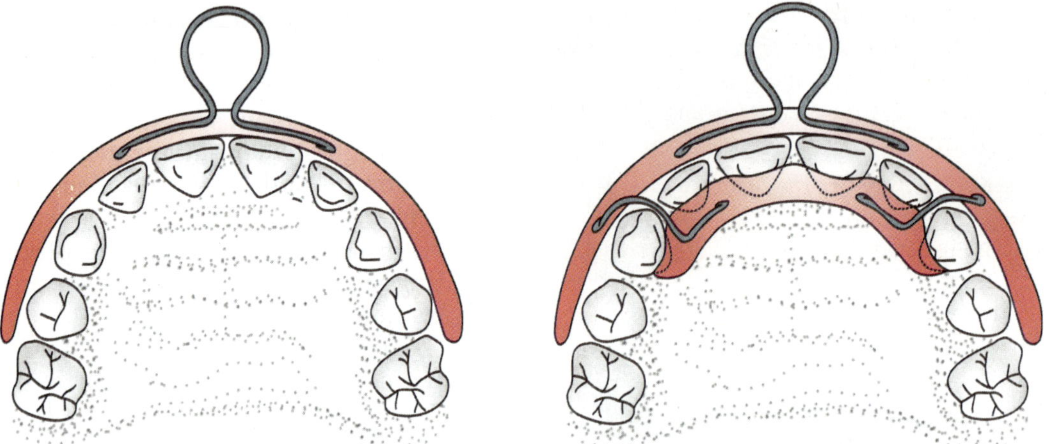

Fig. 29.9: Schematic diagram of oral screen: first figure shows a normal design, while second figure is a modified form in which a lingual screen is also added to prevent tongue-thrusting habit, especially in anterior open bite cases.

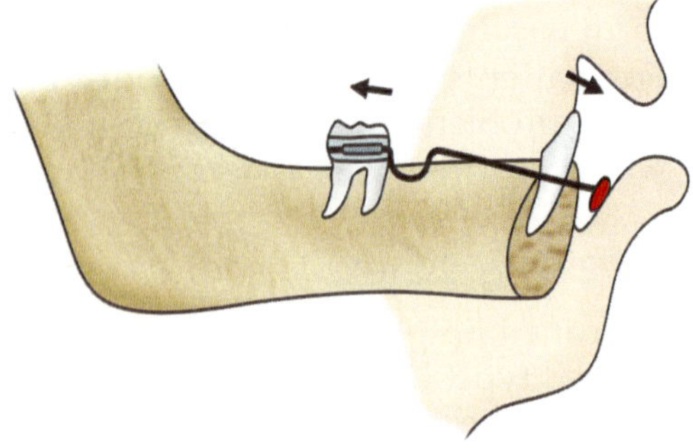

Fig. 29.10: Lip bumper helps to keep lower lip away from incisors, thus they move forward under tongue forces, while forces of lower lip are directed to the lower molars for their uprighting.

helps in breaking the lip trap, and thus upper and lower lips try to approximate each other to make a seal. The lower incisors move labially under tongue forces and upper incisors go lingually under upper lip and lower lip (if lip competency is normalised) forces, thus reducing the overjet. It also increases arch length of lower arch, and reduces crowding.

3. Lip bumper is placed in deep vestibule of anterior region which applies stretch on the periosteum of that area and thus help in bone remodelling. An adaptation can be seen in FR II appliance. Thus they can be used in mild skeletal class II due to deficiency in chin region.
4. They can be used to augment anchorage, when the muscular forces are distally transmitted to the anchor teeth, generally permanent mandibular first molars, which prevent the forward movement of anchors.
5. They may distally tilt or upright the molars, or sometimes distalize them. But, the degree of movement is very less. Thus, they can be used for space regaining by applying distal force on the molars.

Disadvantages:

a. They are uncomfortable for patients, and pose problems in speaking and eating by keeping lower lip away from tongue and upper lip.
b. They are difficult to make. Fixed ones require banding of the molars and then soldering. Alternatively, buccal tube of 0.045" size is welded on the bands to receive the lip bumper.
c. Removable ones depend on patient cooperation for proper use.
d. Fixed ones have problem of proper cleaning and oral hygiene.
e. Fixed ones have problems, if adjustment is to be done. The whole assembly is to

be removed and recemented. Sometimes, the solder joints break, needing full exercise of repair.

f. The buccal wires can cause irritation of buccal mucosa.

Appliance design: For fixed appliance, the permanent first molars are banded and they are lifted in impression to be casted in POP. The thick 1.0 mm hard s.s wire is adapted from molar to molar. It may have U-loop just mesial to molars for future adjustments. The distal end can be activated to achieve molar derotation/uprighitng, and also prevent sliding of lip bumper through the molar tubes. The legs of U-loop are generally made of equal length of 5 mm. A modification has also been suggested by Greenfield, 2011, where the distal leg of the loop is longer than mesial leg which is used in hyperdivergent cases. In some forms, instead of U-loop, the molar offset bends. But the advantage of U-loop is that it can be adjusted to extend the lip bumper further by opening it, which may be required when the lower incisors flare under the influence of tongue forces, and come near to the labial shield. The wire is adapted around the dental arch and is kept away from the labial surfaces of incisors, and zig-zag bends are placed to hold the acrylic. A 2–3 mm wax spacer is placed in anterior region and then acrylic is poured to make a lip shield which incorporates this wire. The acrylic is extended from canine to canine, and the upper margin is kept at the level of marginal gingival and lower margin extending in the vestibule, causing a stretch on the periosteum.

This assembly can be directly soldered on the molar bands. It can be also inserted in the 0.045" round tube which is soldered/welded on the bands. The buccal parts of wire generally irritate the buccal mucosa, so the sleeves can be used there. This part also helps to keep the cheeks away from the teeth and hence a passive expansion occurs in premolar area.

Modifications (Figs 29.11a and b):

1. **Denholtz appliance:** It is the lip bumper which is used solely in upper arch, supported at upper molars (Fig. 29.12).
2. **Augmentor:** It was designed by Sharma, JIOS 1998. It is used in skeletal Class III cases due to maxillary deficiency. The appliance is supported in lower arch at molars, with its lip shield extending in upper labial vestibule. It helps to keep upper lip away from the teeth and causes periosteal stretch. Hooks also can be soldered to its arms to use class III elastics. It can be uncomfortable as it crosses from lower to upper arch.
3. **Acrylic-free modification:** Bagga has suggested a modification in which the acrylic is not used to make a lip pad in

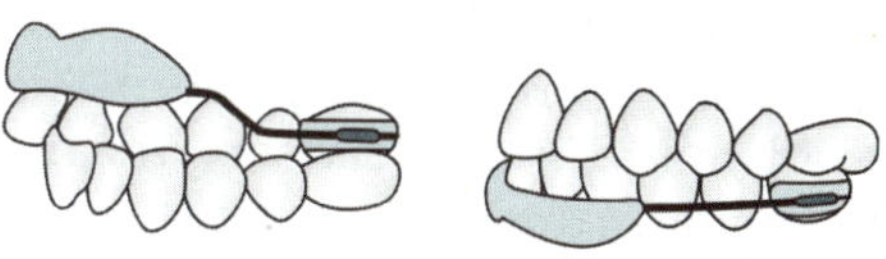

Fig. 29.12: Denholtz's appliance; standard design of lower lip bumper.

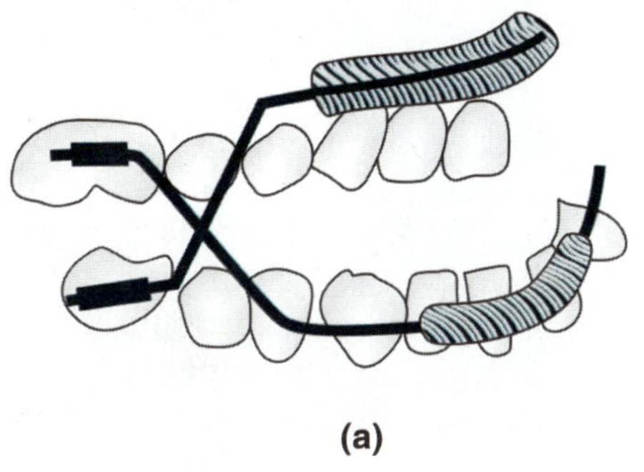

(a)

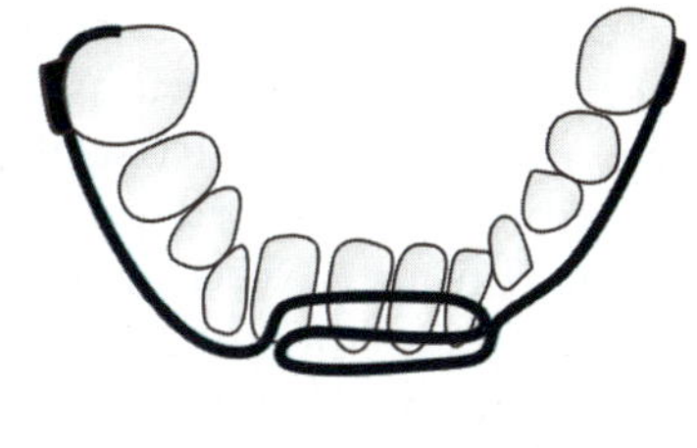

(b)

Figs 29.11a to b: Modifications of lip bumpers: Denholtz's appliance; reverse lip bumper (Malhotra), and Augmentor (Sharma); All-wire lip bumper (Bagga).

the anterior portion, but it is made of a thicker wire with wire bent in the form of cribs in the labial region to keep the lower lip away from teeth.

4. **Greenfield's modification:** He has suggested to make distal legs of the U-loop longer than the mesial legs, to be used in hyperdivergent cases.
5. **Modified lip bumper** by Rakesh malhotra: It is supported on upper molars, with the lip shield in the lower anterior vestibule, causing a periosteal stretch, and a distal force on upper molars. Using this appliance, the patient tries to keep mandible in forward position to avoid extreme pressure on the lip and thus growth modification effect sets-in. Hooks also can be soldered to use elastics. It can be uncomfortable as it crosses from upper to lower arch.
6. **Preformed lip bumpers:** They are also now commercially available.

ACTIVATOR

It is an FA which is used to position the mandible in the forward position. Since it activates the muscles, that is why it was called activator. It was one of the first FA described in the literature. The history of FAs is very long. Kingsley, in 1879 used a vulcanite plate in the upper arch of the patients having retruded mandible. He used an anterior inclined plane in this plate to guide the mandible in forward position when the patient closed.

Pierre Robin used an appliance called **monobloc** made of vulcanite. He used it in patients of Pierre Robin syndrome who have small retruded mandible and glossoptosis, to keep the mandible in forward position. It helped to open the airway. It was called monobloc since it is a one-piece appliance involving both upper and lower arches.

Andresen 1908 designed a **loose-fitting appliance** for use in his daughter who was under fixed appliance treatment, but was going for vacations. He made a modified Hawleys retainer in upper arch to which a lower lingual shield was added in such a way to keep mandible in forward position. When his daughter came back, he noted marked improvement of dental relation in sagital dimension and improved facial profile. He called it as **biomechanical working retainer**. Later on with the help of Haupl in Norway, he modified his appliance. They called this process as **functional jaw orthopedics**. Other names of this appliance are **Norwegian appliance** and activator (since it activates the muscles) (Figs 29.13a and b).

Indications of activator: It is mainly used in growing children with favourable growth pattern, having retruded mandible. It can be used in following conditions.

a. Class II division 1
b. Class II division 2

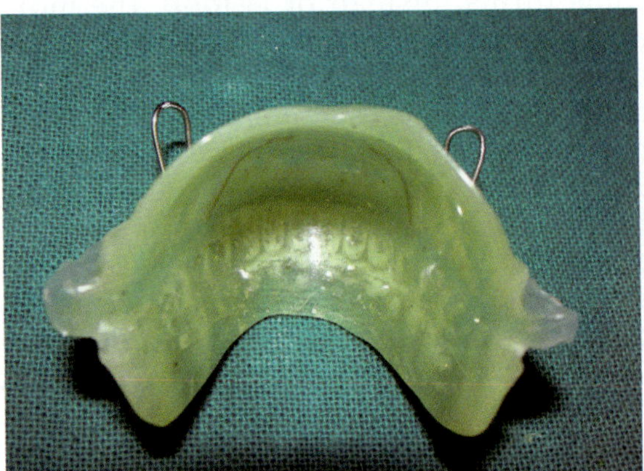

(a)

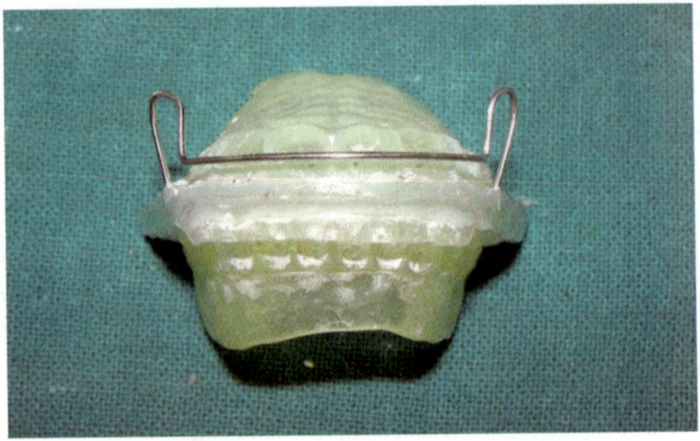

(b)

Fig. 29.13a and b: Activator.

c. Class III
d. Class I open bite
e. Class I deep bite
f. As a first phase of treatment to improve skeletal relation for patients who need major fixed appliance.
g. It can be used as retainer also
h. Patients having decreased lower facial height due to lack of dento-alveolar development.

Contraindications

1. Patients having vertical growth pattern with long face and convex profile.
2. Non-growing patients
3. If lower incisors are severely proclined, since it causes proclining force on the lower incisors.
4. Cannot be used in class I cases having crowding due to TSALD.
5. Patients having nasal obstruction/ stenosis until it is corrected, since then breathing will be problematic.
6. Uncooperative patients

Case selection: Following criteria should be kept in mind while selecting the case for successful results.

1. Actively growing patient with horizontal to normal growth pattern
2. Well aligned lower and upper arches.
3. Lower incisors upright on their basal bone.
4. Normal or mild deficient mandible, which is posteriorly placed.
5. Improved facial profile and muscular balance when VTO is done.
6. Cooperative patient.

Advantages

1. Ensuing growth can be redirected to achieve better skeletal relation.
2. It is inexpensive.
3. The treatment can be started at early age, so it gives psychological benefits to the child.
4. The interval between follow up appointments are long. Also chair side time needed is less.
5. Patient has not oral hygiene problems, as it is removable.
6. After this phase, some patients may not need fixed appliances.
7. Better and stable results can be achieved by redirecting the growth.

Disadvantages

1. Patient cooperation is needed.
2. Fabrication of appliance involves construction bite and articulation. Also, an experienced person is needed to fabricate the appliance.
3. It does not move the teeth individually so precise detailing cannot be done with it.
4. It may cause proclination of lower incisors.
5. It may cause downward and backward rotation of mandible and thus increases facial height. So, it should not be used in vertical growth cases.

Mechanism of action: When the activator is placed in the mouth with mandible in forward position, it leads to activation of the muscles of mastication. These activated muscles contract to bring the mandible back in the original position, but that is prevented by the appliance. This force is then redirected in forward direction to the lower teeth, and backward force on the upper teeth. Activator thus induces the **musculoskeletal adaptation** and new pattern of mandibular closure and morphogenetic pattern. Following effects are seen during the FA therapy for skeletal class II cases (Fig. 29.14).

Headgear effect: The backward force on the upper jaw and teeth leads to restriction of forward growth of upper jaw. It also leads to distalisation of upper dentition. The teeth are directed to erupt distally under the influence of this force and selective cutting of acrylic is needed from the appliance to guide the eruption. This effect of FA is called as headgear effect.

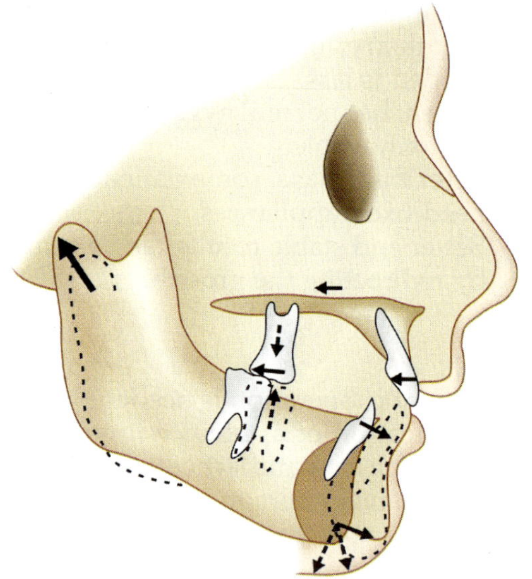

Fig. 29.14: Effects of a myofunctional appliance for treatment of skeletal class II condition due to mandibular retrognathism. Note that mandible has come D and F, with compensating growth in condylar region. The maxillary dentition moves distally, called as "Headgear effect". Lower incisors flare labially, which is called "class II elastic effect".

Class II elastic effect: The force component directed forwards on lower teeth causes flaring of the lower incisors. It is called Class II elastic effect. Selective trimming is done to direct the eruption of lower molars in U and F direction. The reciprocal force which gets directed on maxilla leads to lingual tipping and thus some extrusion of upper incisors. These effects lead to rotation of OP in the clockwise direction. To prevent flaring of lower incisors, the acrylic should be trimmed so that it does not touch the lingual surfaces of incisors, and thus the force is distributed to the alveolar region.

Pterygoid response: With continuous use of FA, the muscles get adapted to the new position. The inferior head of lateral pterygoid muscle gets shortened and adapted in new position. When after some time, the clinician tries to push the mandible backward, he is not able to do that and patient feels pain. It is called pterygoid response. It is a favorable sign during FA treatment. A compensatory condylar growth occurs in upward and backward direction.

Viscoelastic property: With the use of FA, the force is also generated due to swallowing and during sleeping. Passive tension is generated in muscles, tendons and soft tissues, etc. which is responsible for action. It is called viscoelastic property.

Construction bite: It is a very important step. An intermaxillary record is taken in wax to relate the mandible to maxilla in a new desired position in 3D. It involves the repositioning of mandible in a forward and downward direction. Generally, the mandible is advanced by 4–5 mm and opened vertically by 2–3 mm beyond freeway space in premolar region. Freeway space is the space between upper and lower teeth at rest position when the muscles are in least tonic-clonic contraction state. The vertical opening is done beyond the free way space to activate the muscles. The maximum anterior displacement recommended is 3 mm behind the maximum anterior displacement possible.

Types of construction bites: Construction bites have been classified as small/medium/high, depending on the amount of vertical opening done. It depends on the philosophy of the appliance; the growth pattern of the patient, and vertical facial height, e.g. more sagittal displacement is done for H-activator, while more vertical displacement is done for V-activator. Depending on the extent of opening, different types of reflexes are generated in the muscles of mastication, which are clasp knife reflex; myotactic reflex; and viscoelastic effects, but the details are beyond the scope of this chapter.

Rule of ten: For taking the construction bite, a **"Rule of 10"** is followed as a general guide. The total displacement in sagital and vertical direction should be approx 10 mm, e.g. if sagital advancement is 6–7 mm, the vertical opening should be 3–4 mm.

Steps to take construction bite (Fig. 29.15):

1. Impressions of upper and lower arches are taken with proper anatomical records

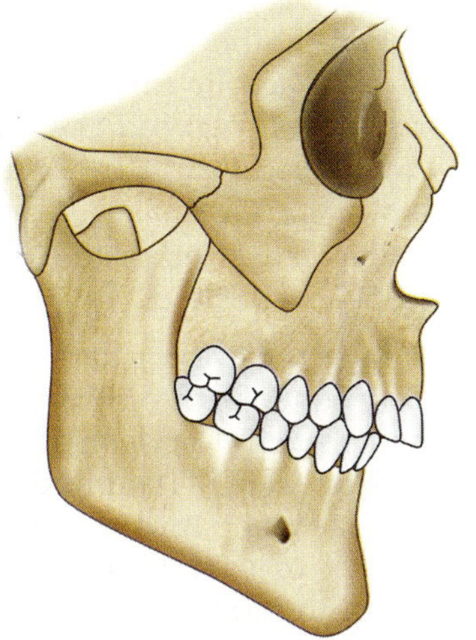
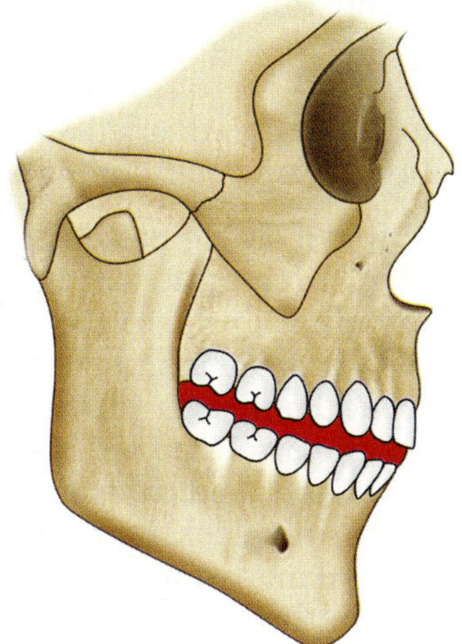

Fig. 29.15: Registration with wax where the mandible is moved in a D and F direction to achieve skeletal class I relation of upper and lower jaws.

and depth of vestibule. They stone casts are made in pairs. First pour are used for working model, while second pour are used for record purpose.

2. The desired advancement and opening is planned for the patient. It is generally based on the free-way space and VTO. The marks can be placed on the working models of the patient to check later on the accuracy of the bite.
3. The wax sheet is taken and rolled and shaped in horseshoe shape. Its thickness should be 2–3 mm more than the planned opening.
4. The roll of wax is placed on the lower model and pressed to obtain indentations of teeth on it. The midline of lower arch, the MB grooves of first molars and the contact point between mandibular canine-first premolar is marked on the wax.
5. The patient should be seated upright in the dental chair and in unstrained position.
6. The patient is asked to practice the desired position few times before taking the bite to bring the mandible in new position. The wax bite is placed in the mouth of patient and the mandible is guided lightly in the desired position. The patient is asked to bite in the wax till the required opening.
7. The skeletal midlines of upper and lower jaws are matched to maintain the symmetry. Dental midlines should not be matched as they can be deviated due to local factors.
8. The molars and canines should be brought in a super class I position. The overjet and overbite are reduced.
9. It is then checked on the casts for accuracy. If not accurate, then it should be repeated.

Articulation of models: Construction bite and models are assembled accurately and are articulated in free-plane articulator with POP. The lingual side is faced anteriorly for easy working of acrylic on the palatal and lingual side of the casts if it is a one-piece appliance, e.g. activator, bionator. For twin block appliance, the articulation is done with labial surface facing the front.

Wire bending for activator: Activator has simple wire elements in the form of a short labial bow of normal design in the upper arch only. It is made of 0.8–0.9 mm hard s.s wire from canine to canine. It is generally kept away from the labial surfaces of the teeth by a thickness of a dime. If it touches the incisors, then under the forces generated by the appliance, it leads to lingual movement of upper incisors; decrease of overjet; and hence limits the further advancement of mandible.

Acrylic part: It is a single piece appliance having connected three parts of acrylic, i.e. maxillary plate, mandibular plate and the interocclusal bite. It can be made of cold-cure or heat-cure acrylic. For heat cure, the wax up of exact form of the appliance is made and then it is acrylised. Care should be taken about the labial bow during flasking and acrylisation. The lingual flange of mandibular part is extended deep in the vestibule. It helps to keep the mandible forward by irritating the lingual mucosa and thus the patient tries to avoid the pressure and trauma.

Delivery and management of the appliance: The appliance is properly finished and polished before delivery. A comfortable appliance is must for getting proper patient cooperation.

The patient should be told about the benefits of using the appliance properly. Patient can be motivated by showing him the photos of other patients who have benefitted with FA. He can be shown photos of himself without and with construction bite to show him the changes.

He should be taught how to insert, remove and clean the appliance. He is also told about initial problems, like increased salivation; speech problems; tension in muscles and headache, etc. for few days.

He is advised to use the appliance for full day and night. Initially, to get used to it, he is advised to use it for few hours in day time, and then gradually increasing the time and even extending to night wear also. When the appliance is not in the mouth, he should keep it in water to avoid distortion. As a general rule, he should be able to use it for full time within 2 weeks. He should be told about speech problems, etc. during initial days.

He should be advised to come to clinic after 24 hrs to see any trauma on the mandibular lingual tissues in incisor region, since the force of appliance is applied there. To avoid it, the wax relief can be given there during fabrication. Also acrylic can be relieved from the lower incisors to avoid the forces there and thus avoiding labial inclination of lower incisors.

To achieve desired results, a trimming plan should be established.

Trimming of the appliance (Figs 29.16a and b): A proper selective trimming of acrylic is planned to achieve desired dento-alveolar relationship in 3D. Trimming can be done to achieve lower molar eruption, distal movement of molar, incisors intrusion or extrusion, incisors lingual movement, etc. It depends upon the requirement whether you

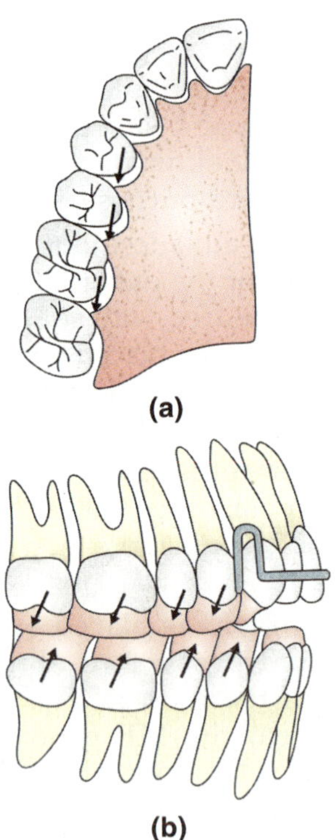

Figs 29.16a and b: First figure shows how the acrylic is trimmed in upper part of an activator or bionator so as to apply a distal moving force on the buccal teeth. Second figure shows trimming of acrylic on the bite blocks so as to allow a mesial and upward eruption of lower teeth, while upper teeth move downward and backward, if allowed to erupt. However, generally, only lower teeth are allowed to erupt during FJO treatment.

are treating class II or class III malocclusion. Selective trimming is planned, where some part of the acrylic is removed to make space for tooth movement and other part is kept in touch with the teeth to act as **guiding planes**. Mainly, the activator is used for aiding the eruption of upper and lower molars in proper direction to achieve normal dentoalveolar relation.

During treatment of class II relation, generally, the upper molars are not allowed to erupt (as they erupt in mesial and occlusal direction further increasing the class II relation). Here, the lower molars are relieved in such that they erupt in mesial, buccal and occlusal direction to achieve class I relation. The molar height is increased in those cases only where patient has skeletal deep bite and horizontal/normal growth pattern.

The upper molars are relieved such that they move in distal and buccal direction to aid in expansion. The acrylic on distolingual aspect is relieved and on mesiolingual aspect is maintained to act as guiding plane to apply a distalising force on upper molars. Similarly, the lower molars are relieved on mesiolingual aspect while loaded on dsitolingual aspect to aid in their mesial movement.

The trimming is reversed for treatment of class III relation. There the upper molars are allowed to erupt while lower molars are held not to erupt.

Modifications: Various modifications of activator have been suggested by different clinicians as below but their details are out of the scope of undergraduate study.

The bow activator of Schwarz: It is split along the OP such that maxillary and mandibular parts are separate and mandible can be advanced stepwise without making a new appliance. These 2 parts are joined by horizontal U-loop in distal area to control and advance the lower part.

Wunderer's modification: It is used to treat Class III malocclusion, and an anteriorly opening expansion screw is used to move maxilla forward.

Cybernator of Schmuth/the reduced activator: Palatal acrylic is removed to make the appliance less bulky, and having a palatal wire as in bionator.

The propulsor: It is hybrid appliance having an oral screen and a lower lingual flange to keep mandibular forward.

Cutout or palate free activator: It is having very less acrylic in maxillary arch.

Karwetzky modifications: It is split in the OP such that maxillary and mandibular parts are separate and mandible can be advanced stepwise without making a new appliance. They are joined by a vertical U-loop in first molar area to advance the mandibular part. It has been modified in three types for treatment of class II, III and asymmetry.

Herren's modification: He used maximum anterior displacement of mandible, i.e. 3–4 mm beyond the normal Class I molar relationship, while the vertical opening is kept only 2–4 mm. By more advancement, more mesial force is expected to come in play on mandible and a reciprocal distal force on maxilla. The appliance is retained in upper arch with the help of clasps and lower lingual flanges are extended deep in the vestibules to keep mandible in forward position. Herren predicted that with every 1 mm increase in mandibular advanced position, an extra sagital force of 100 gm comes to be applied on mandible.

BIONATOR (Figs 29.17a to d)

It was designed by Balters during 1950s. It is also a single piece appliance as activator, but with very less bulk as compared to activator.

Indications

1. It is used for treatment of class II division 1 case which has well aligned lower arch with lower incisors upright on the basal bone; a horizontal to normal growth pattern; actively growing child; retruded normal-sized mandible, etc.
2. Class III cases when reverse bionator is used.
3. Cases with open bite.
4. Class II division 2 cases after alignment.

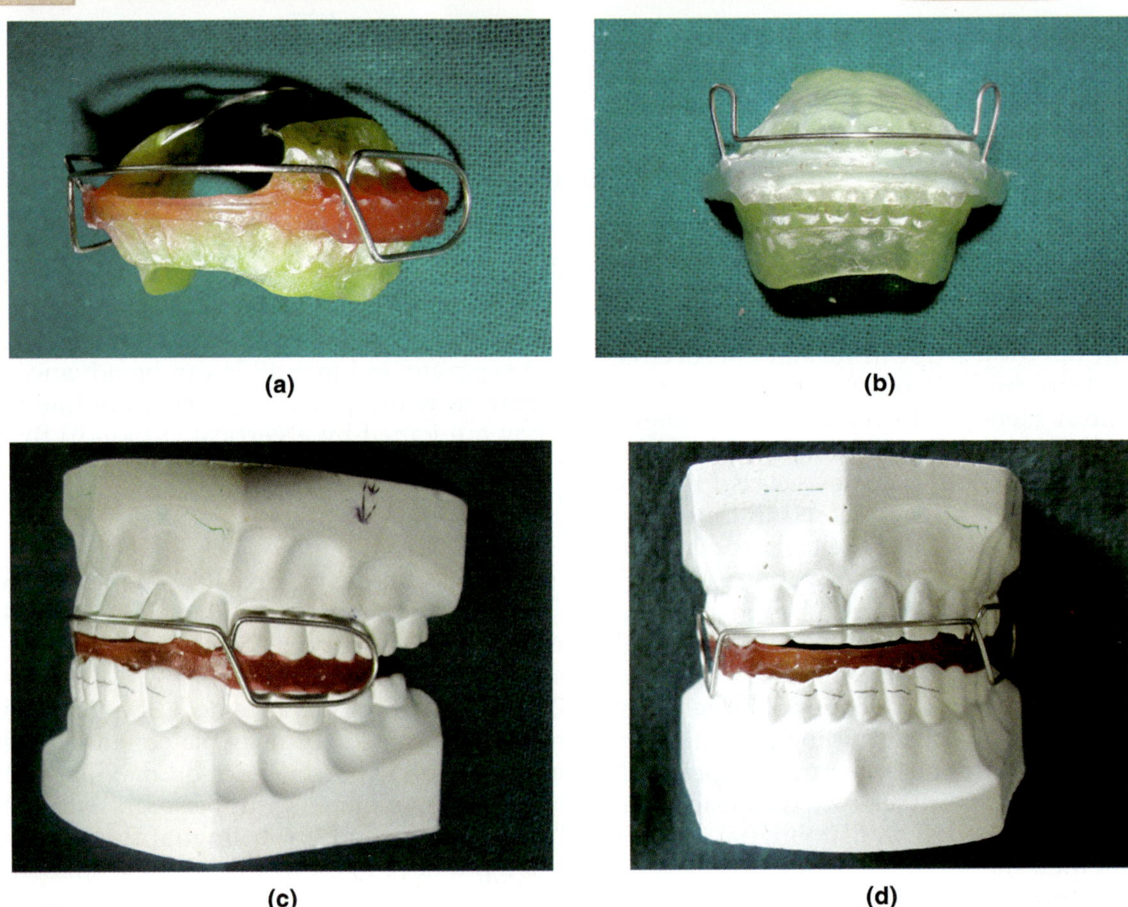

(a) (b) (c) (d)

Figs 29.17a to d: Bionator

Philosophy of bionator: Balters considered that the tongue plays an important role in development of dentition and skeletal relations. In class II cases, the tongue has a backward position, and thus the mandible gets retrognathic. Bionator helps in repositioning the tongue forward and thus helping to achieve a normal skeletal relationship.

Types of bionator: It is of three types:

Standard appliance which is used for treatment of class II cases (Fig. 29.18).

Class III bionator: It is also called **reverse bionator**. It is used to treat class III case.

Open bite bionator: For treatment of open bite.

Construction: Here, we will discuss the standard appliance for class II treatment. It is a single piece appliance with a lower part, an occlusal bite part, and small acrylic part on the palatal sides; and the wire components.

The mandibular part is a horseshoe-shaped acrylic plate on the lingual side of lower arch extended till distal of the last erupted molar, generally the permanent first molars (since such patients are generally in mixed dentition period). It extends upto 4 mm gingival to the free marginal gingiva.

Incisal capping is done upto incisal third level of the lower anterior teeth. It helps in prevention of flaring of incisors during the treatment.

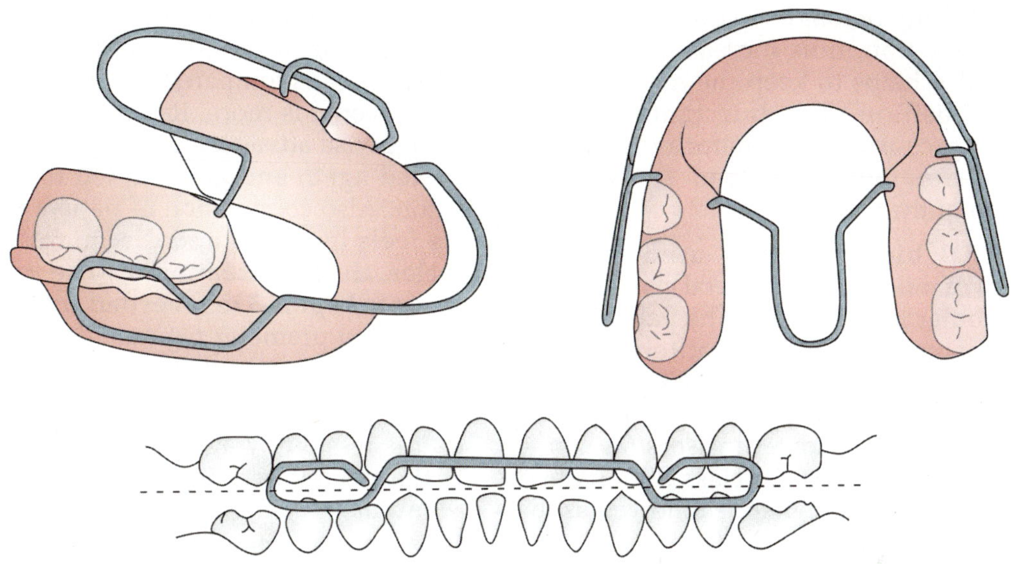

Fig. 29.18: Standard bionator: note the Coffin spring, buccinator loops in the appliances.

Maxillary part: It is limited to the first premolar to first molar region only on both sides. The anterior part is kept open. It is also extended upto 4 mm below the free gingival margin. It helps to house the terminal ends of wires.

Occlusal part: It lies between upper and lower OP in the space provided by the construction bite. It is trimmed to cover only palatal half occlusal surfaces of upper teeth and extended distally to mesial half of the last erupted molar.

Wire components: There are two major wires in bionator which are palatal arch and the vestibular wire. They are made of 1.2 mm and 0.9 mm size hard s.s wire respectively.

The palatal arch: It is adapted as **Coffin spring** shape, extending from the half of the first premolar till a line joining the distal surfaces of permanent first molars. It is adapted 1–2 mm away from the palatal tissues. In class II bionator, it is kept open anteriorly so that the distal part activates the dorsum of tongue to bring it forward. When tongue is stimulated D and F, it brings the mandible alongwith, increases the oral space and functional matrix attached. In class III bionator, the loop is kept open distally, while the anterior closed end stimulates the tongue to move backwards and downward, thus shifting the mandible D and B. Thus a new pattern of functions is created, affecting the functional matrices in that area.

Vestibular wire and buccinator loops: It is made of 0.9 mm wire bilaterally symmetrical. It is adapted in the form of a labial arch in upper incisors region till middle of canines. Then it is bent downward to reach lower 3–4 region, till the level of gingival papilla. It is bent distally parallel to papilla levels, and a curved bend is placed extending to the mesial half of the last erupted molar (generally first permanent molar). It is again bent forward running at the level of marginal gingival (thus completing the buccinators loops) and is inserted in upper 3–4 region to go palatally, adapted there and inserted in acrylic. The buccinator loops help to keep the cheeks away from the dental arches and thus help in passive expansion and development by buccal eruption of these teeth.

Mechanism of Action of Bionator

With bionator, the mandible is displaced downward and forward in cases of class II therapy. The palatal arch activates or stimulates the dorsum of tongue in downward and forward direction, thus increasing the oral space. It also helps to keep the mandible in forward position. The buccinator loops release the pressure of buccinator as falling on the posterior teeth and lead to passive expansion of the arches.

Class III bionator: It is used for the treatment of mild form of skeletal class III due to mandibular prognathism. The palatal arch opens posteriorly, and its anterior part stimulates the dorsum of tongue in D and B direction. The vestibular wire is adapted on the labial surfaces of lower incisors (as compared to upper incisors for class II bionator) and then the same designed is followed as in standard appliance.

Open bite appliance: It is same as standard appliance, but the anterior part of maxillary plate is closed so that tongue cannot get thrusted in incisor region during swallowing. The acrylic is adequately relieved not to hamper the natural eruption of upper and lower incisors, thus helping in reducing the open bite (Fig. 29.19).

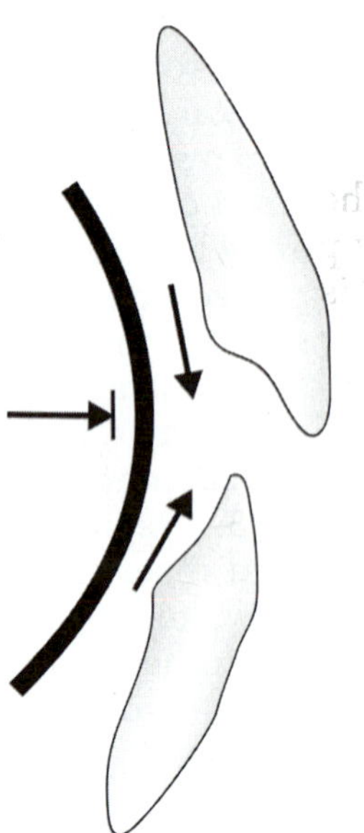

Fig. 29.19: Myofunctional appliance which is used in anterior open bite case. The lingual plate prevents the anterior tongue thrust, while the upper and lower incisors are free to erupt and reduce the open bite.

Bite registration: Procedure is same as for activator. Stepwise advancement is considered better as compared to single advancement if overjet is more. Researchers say that with stepwise advancement, the muscles get activated again and get adapted to a better position. Also cooperation of patient is more as he feels less pain and discomfort in the muscles during treatment. The vertical opening is kept 2–3 mm beyond the freeway space in first premolar region.

Advantages of Bionator Over Activator

a. It is less bulky and lighter in weight as the palatal acrylic is reduced to minimum.
b. More comfortable to use.
c. Helps in relieving the muscular pressure from the dental arches by buccinators loops.
d. Better development of the dentition, as the teeth expand passively under tongue force.
e. Controls and stimulates tongue movements by palatal loop.
f. Does not encroach on the tongue space as much as activator since the palatal acrylic is very less. So, speech clarity is better.
g. Less acrylic material consumption.
h. Less traumatic to vestibular mucosa since it is not extended in mandibular lingual vestibular depths.
i. Cleaning is better and hence oral hygiene is good.

Disadvantages

1. Since it has less acrylic, so it is weaker in midline and prone to breakages.
2. The wire components are more prone to be distorted if not handled carefully by patient.
3. Wire components are difficult to make as compared to activator.
4. Modifications, like incorporation of expansion screw, etc., are not possible with it.

TWIN BLOCK APPLIANCE (Figs 29.20 and 29.21)

It was introduced by WJ Clarke in1980s. Since it is in two pieces, it is called twin block appliance. Upper and lower appliances are separate plates, articulated by inclined planes to reposition the mandible.

Philosophy

Clark believed that the proper inclined plane relationship of cusps of upper and lower teeth is important for proper occlusion and growth of jaws. Occlusal forces are transmitted through dentition and they provide a constant proprioceptive stimulus to influence the growth and trabecular pattern of supporting bone. Malocclusion is frequently associated with discrepancies in underlying skeletal and soft-tissue structures resulting in unfavourable occlusal function. The proprioceptive sensory mechanism controls muscular activity which leads to functional stimulus for or deterrent to the full expression of bone growth. The unfavourable cuspal contacts of class II molar occlusion guide the mandible in a distal direction when teeth come in occlusion. This mechanism acts as an obstruction to normal forward mandibular translation, and thus restricts the mandible to achieve its optimum growth potential in a forward direction. The result is that mandible remains small and/or retrognathic.

The occlusal inclined planes are the functional mechanism of natural dentition. With the help of the intermaxillary inclined planes incorporated in twin block appliance, the distally-directing inclined planes of teeth are avoided. The acrylic inclined planes of the appliance guide the mandible in forward direction and the forces of occlusion thus help in correcting the mandibular position, muscular adaptation and the malocclusion. These forces are then directed in the proper direction and thus the mandible is guided forward by the occlusal inclined planes.

In skeletal class II cases, the transverse maxillary development is also restricted due to a distally occluding mandible. In this situation, the narrower bicuspid part of lower arch is in relation to the wider molar area of upper arch. Thus, the lower dentition does not support the maxillary arch, therefore the maxillary intercanine width and inter-premolar widths get reduced. The constricted maxillary arch has the effect of locking the mandible in a distal occlusion and prevents normal mandibular development.

When the mandible is advanced and relieved of the restricting effect of upper arch, the mandible responds by a favourable growth in anterior and downward direction, with readpatation of soft tissue matrix. During advancement, since the wider molar parts comes forward in relation with somewhat narrower molar–premolar area of maxillary arch, so to prevent the chances of buccal cross bite, an expansion screw is incorporated in upper arch to achieve active expansion.

Design of the Appliance

This appliance contains two appliances which are modified Hawley's appliances. They occlude at the inclined planes in interocclusal area which help to keep the mandible guided in the forward direction (thus breaking the distally guidance of class II molars).

Upper appliance: It has a labial bow from 4–4 region, an expansion screw in midline for transverse expansion, and retention clasps. Clark modified Adams clasp and named it Delta clasp, which can be used on first permanent molars and premolars. It has basic elements of Adams clasp, i.e. bridge, retentive loops and retention tags. The retentive loops are the modified arrow heads, that they have round or ovoid loop rather than open arrow head loops. This clasp does not get early fatigue and is subject to less breakage. The ball end clasps can be placed on other teeth to get extra retention.

The labial bow is kept passive in the incisal region to avoid any premature retraction of the incisors. If incisors are retracted prematurely, it reduces overjet and then limits the provision of further advancement of the mandible.

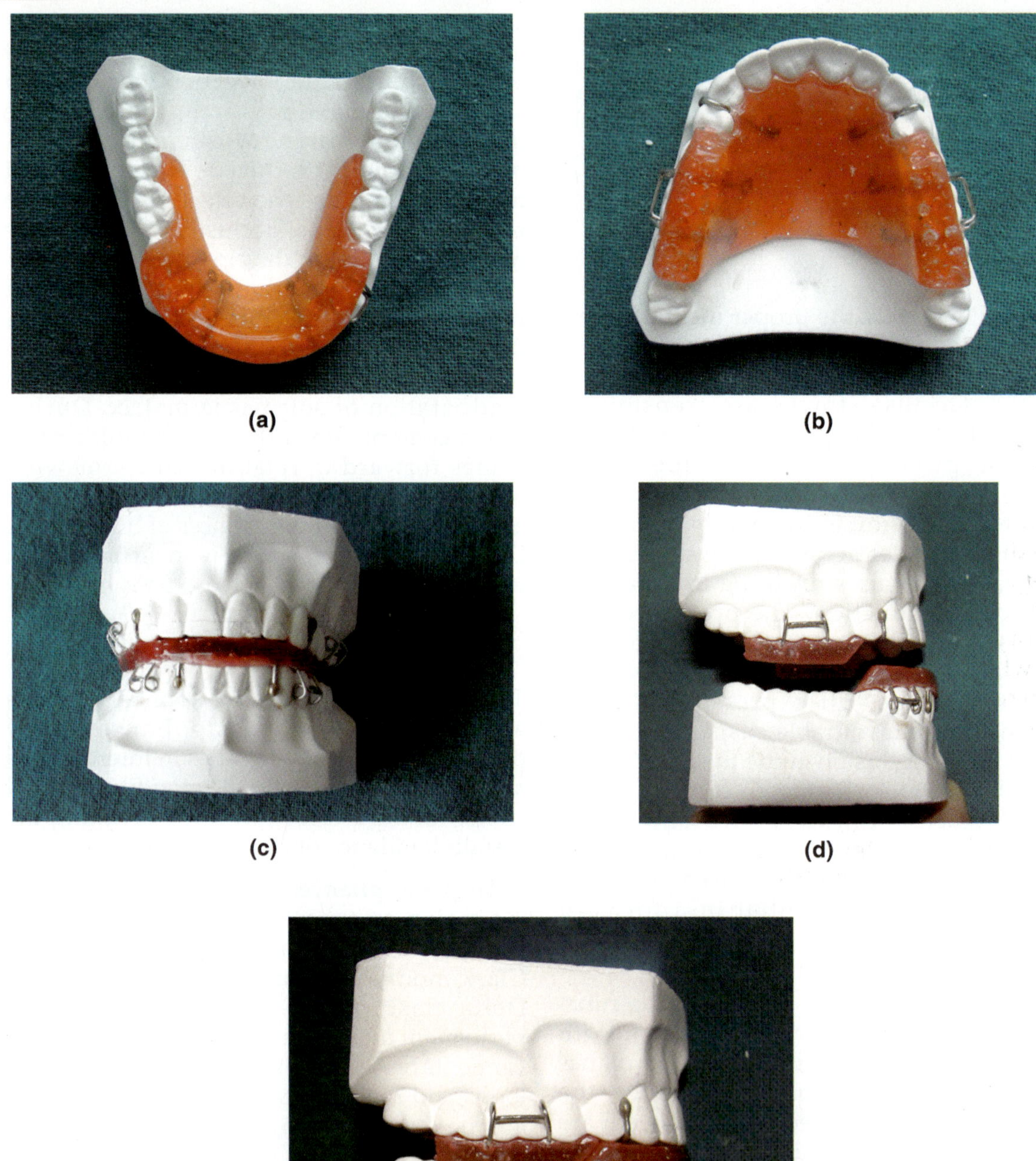

(a) (b) (c) (d) (e)

Figs 29.20a to e: Twin block appliance.

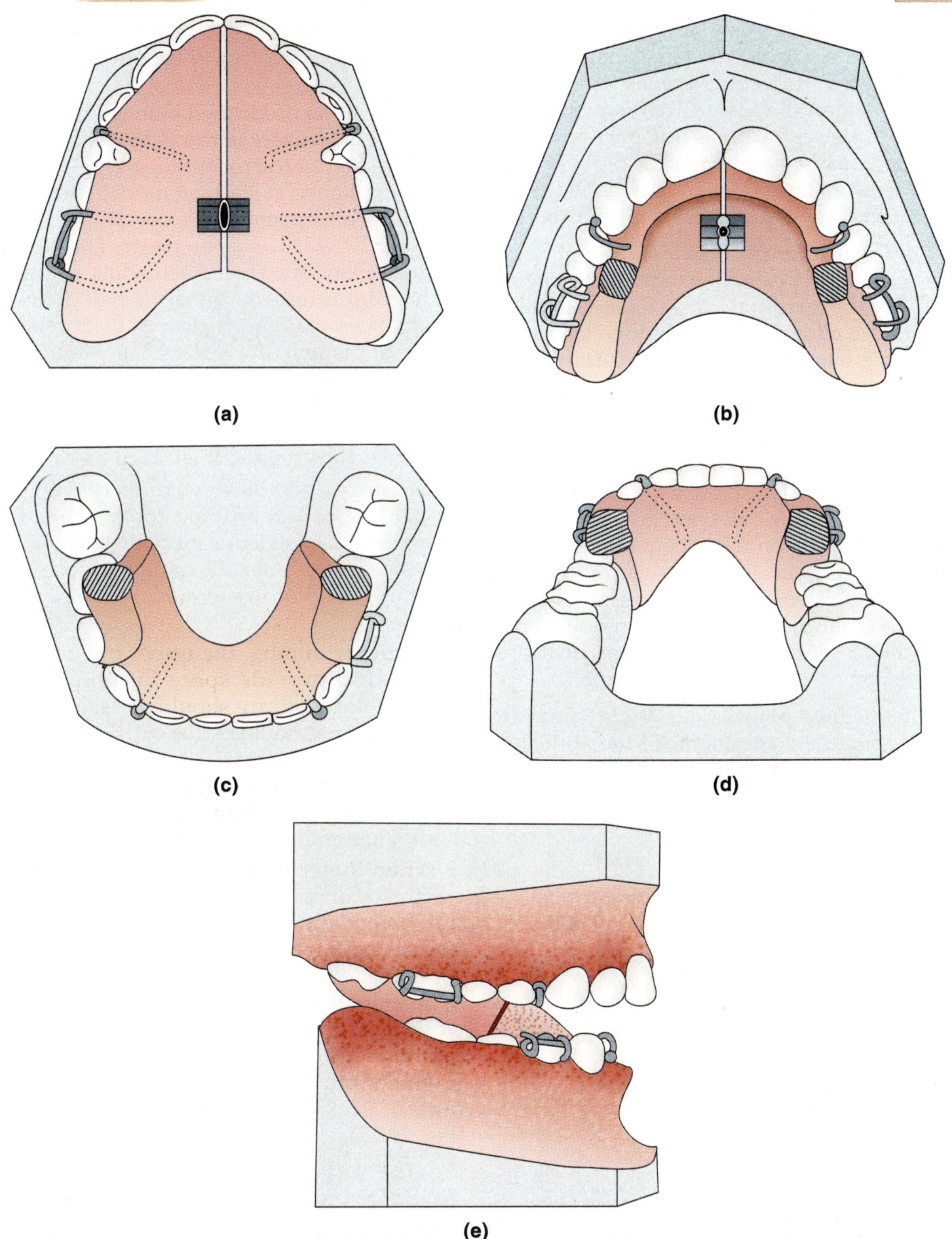

Figs 29.21a to e: A twin block appliance: upper appliance with expansion screw and buccal occlusal coverage; shaded areas in the figures show the direction of inclined planes on upper and lower plates; upper and lower plates in occlusion. The inclines keep the mandible in a forward position.

Expansion screw is placed as active component to help in transverse expansion. It is activated ¼th turn once a week. It is placed because when the lower arch is positioned forward, its wider posterior part comes in relation with the narrow middle part of upper arch. To avoid development of cross bite in this region, the active expansion is introduced.

Lower appliance: It is a simple Hawley type plate. It was extended to premolar region only in the original design, but clinical experience allow it to be extended upto first molar region to distribute the forces to wider area; to strengthen it, and to avoid accidental swallowing of the appliance. However, it should be kept away from the first molars so as not to interfere with its eruption. The retentive delta-clasps are placed on first premolars and the ball-end clasps are placed in the incisor region. They help to prevent the labial flaring of lower incisors. **Incisal capping** may be placed instead of ball end clasps. Labial bow and expansion screw have also been placed in some modifications depending on patient's requirements.

The inclined planes (Fig. 29.22): These are very important components of the appliance which help in guiding and keeping the mandible in forward desired position. They are generally located in the second premolar region.

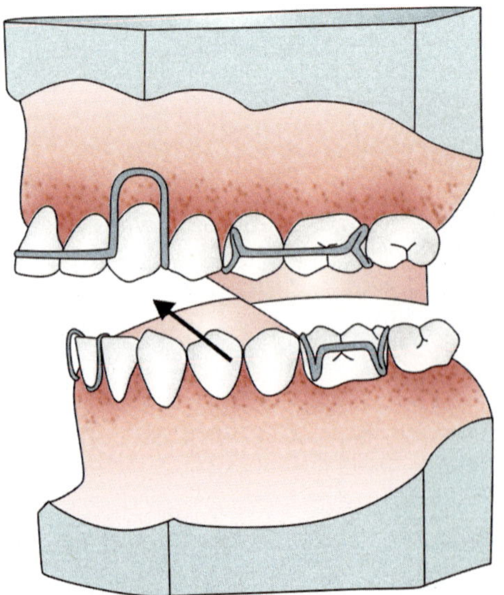

Fig. 29.22: Inclined planes of twin block move the mandible in forward position.

The position of inclined plane is kept clear of the mesial surface of lower first permanent molars so as not to prevent their eruption. On lower appliance, it starts at mesial surface of lower second premolar, goes at 70° to OP mesially towards upper teeth. The upper inclined plane is adjusted according to lower, such that it is rests on the distal half of lower second premolar and is clear of the mesial of lower permanent first molars. This way, it can be imagined that the direction of inclined plane in twin block appliance for class II treatment is in the same direction as the class II elastics, (it is reverse in class III cases).

The upper bite block extends distally till mesial half of last erupted tooth, while the lower bite block extends mesially to cover 1st PM and gets thinner till canine region. This trimming helps to give maximum space to tongue.

During trimming, the upper bite block is trimmed to provide space for eruption of lower molar, but care should be taken so the inclined plane should not be cut. Some part of the inclined plane remains in touch with distal half of second premolar for support. If inclined is cut, then the mandible will not have a guidance and can move distally.

When lower molars have erupted sufficiently to come in contact with upper molars, the lower appliance is removed while the upper appliance is modified to include a reverse bite plane. It helps to keep the mandible guided anteriorly in corrected position, while providing space for eruption of lower premolars to come in occlusion with upper premolars to close the occlusal gap in that region. It also acts as retainer later on (Fig. 29.23).

Advantages

a. **Function:** Inclined plane follow the principle of natural inclined planes of teeth, guiding the mandible in forward direction. The force generated is better

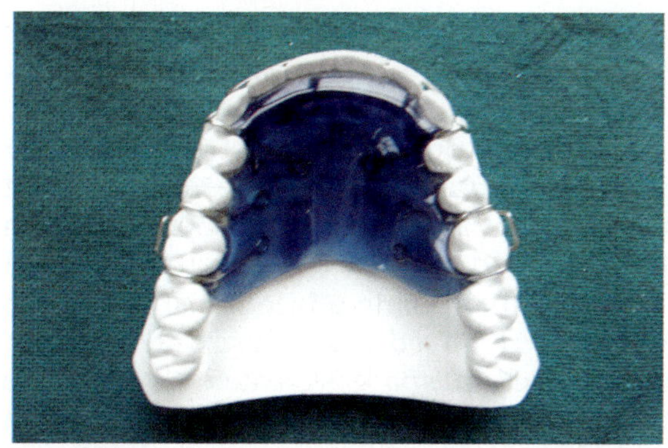

Fig. 29.23: Reverse bite plate appliance. Note the anterior slant on the bite plane in anterior region.

distributed. The **dual-force** from muscle activation and occlusal function comes into play. Since patient can eat with it, there is better distribution and regular activity of the muscles of mastication. It helps to better adjustment of function and new morphogenetic pattern.

b. **Comfort:** One of the most comfortable since it is in two pieces and patient can eat, speak, laugh with it, as there is no restriction of mandibular movements.
c. **Expansion and arch development:** Expansion screw helps in active expansion of upper arch. Screws can also be inserted for sagittal expansion to bring incisors forward.
d. It is easy to fabricate in lab and easy wire bending.
e. **Faster results:** Since patient is comfortable, he can use it for 24 hours and thus results are rapid.
f. **Re-activation:** If stepwise advancement is required, then the same appliance can be modified by adding acrylic on the upper inclined plane. No new appliance is required at that time.
g. **Esthetics:** It is more esthetic as any objectionable wire component, like labial bow, can be removed. Improvement in facial appearance of the child is immediately noticed, giving a positive boost to cooperation.
h. Clinical adjustment is easy and less chairside time is required.
i. It can also be used with fixed appliances.
j. It provides better sagittal and vertical control and fast treatment results.
k. It can be activated asymmetrically and thus helps in asymmetry treatment. It can also be used for TMD treatment as a splint.

Modifications: Due to its comfort and wide incorporation of this appliance in orthodontics, it has been modified in many designs to achieve the desired treatment objectives. Its fixed variety has also been designed. Magnetic blocks, twin blocks for open bite and class III treatment and for TMD treatment has been designed. The details are beyond the scope of this book.

FRANKEL APPLIANCES (Figs 29.24 to 29.26)

This appliance was designed by Frankel of Germany. It is also called functional regulator FR or oral gymnastic appliance. It is a type of tissue-borne appliance. The design of this appliance is very different from activator. It acts mainly by force-elimination. It shields the abnormal buccal and labial forces of musculature from the dental arches, and helps in proper development of the basal jaw bone. Thus it also provides an atmosphere for normal development of muscular balance.

Philosophy behind FR: According to Frankl, the dental arch and dentition develop by proper balance of perioral muscles. Abnormal forces from these muscles create a barrier for proper growth of the jaws. This appliance helps to shield away these abnormal forces from the dentition on bucco-labial side, so that they are free to develop under the influence of lingual forces. Also, since this appliance is loose, the patient keeps it in place by playing with it deliberately. This helps in exercise of the muscles and thus their functional correction.

The periosteal pull and activation of remodeling: The lip pads and buccal shield components of FR apply an outward stretch on the buccal periosteum which helps in bone formation and remodeling on the apical base.

Maxillary anchorage: As compared to activator, FR is firmly anchored in maxillary arch with the wires passing through the occlusal grooves made in primary first molar region. Lingual pads are made in lower incisor region, which helps to keep the mandible in forward position by acting as proprioceptive trigger. As the patient tries to bring the mandible back, the lingual mucosa is irritated by this pad and this patient is forced to keep mandible forward.

Differential eruption: The permanent upper first molars is fixed in position by occlusal stop made by a wire resting in its central groove, but the lower molar is free to erupt since they are kept free of any appliance element. The differential eruption of lower teeth helps in correction of vertical dentoalveolar height, deep bite and class II molar relation when lower molars erupt in mesial and occlusal direction.

Effect on maxilla: Since there is very little contact of appliance with maxilla and palate, there is no appreciable retrusive force on maxilla, while most of the force helps in mandibular advancement. This appliance is very well suited for patient having normal maxilla, in mixed dentition period, with horizontal growth pattern and deep bite cases.

Effects of FR: Following effects are seen with FR.

Improvement in sagittal position of mandible: Mandible is retrognathic in skeletal class II cases. FR brings it D and F to skeletal class I position.

Increase in sagittal, vertical and transverse dimension: Buccal shields and lip pads eliminate abnormal labial and buccal forces acting on dentition. Due to change in equilibrium, the forces from tongue lead to development of dental arch width and form. The shields and pads also apply outward stretch on the periosteum and thus help in deposition of bone in apical base areas.

The lingual pads in lower lingual region act as proprioceptive guide to keep mandible in forward position. The forward positioning of mandible helps to increase the volume of oral cavity and thus adaptation of new dento-skeletal and morphologic relations. A new mandibular positioning is achieved by gradual adaptation of muscles of mandible and condylar adaptation in U and B direction in the glenoid fossa.

Since while taking a bite registration, the mandible is moved downward and forward, an interocclusal space is created, in which the lower teeth are free to erupt, while upper teeth are held back by wire components. It helps in increase in vertical dentoalveolar height and bite opening. This is aided by the ongoing vertical growth of ramus, adaptive growth of condyles and simultaneous adaptation of associated muscles to new morphogenetic pattern.

Muscle function adaptation: FR helps in overcoming the abnormal perioral muscles activity and helps in their readaptation. The buccal shields and lip pads eliminate abnormal labial and buccal forces acting on dental arches. They also lead to periosteal stretch and bone formation in basal area. Lip pads keep lips away from the teeth, prevent hyperactivity and lip trap, etc. and aid in development of lip seal and apical bone growth.

Types of FR: Based on the use, FR has been designed in the following types:

- FR-1: is used to treat class I and mild Class II division 1 cases.
- FR-1a: used for class I with mild crowding, and class I deep bite cases.
- FR-1b: for class II division 1 with upto 5–6 mm overjet.
- FR-1c: for class II division 1 with overjet more than 7 mm.
- FR-2: for class II division 1 and division 2 cases
- FR-3: for treatment of class III
- FR-4: for treatment of open bite and bimaxillary protrusion
- FR-5: This has headgear also and used for treatment of vertical growth cases with long face height.

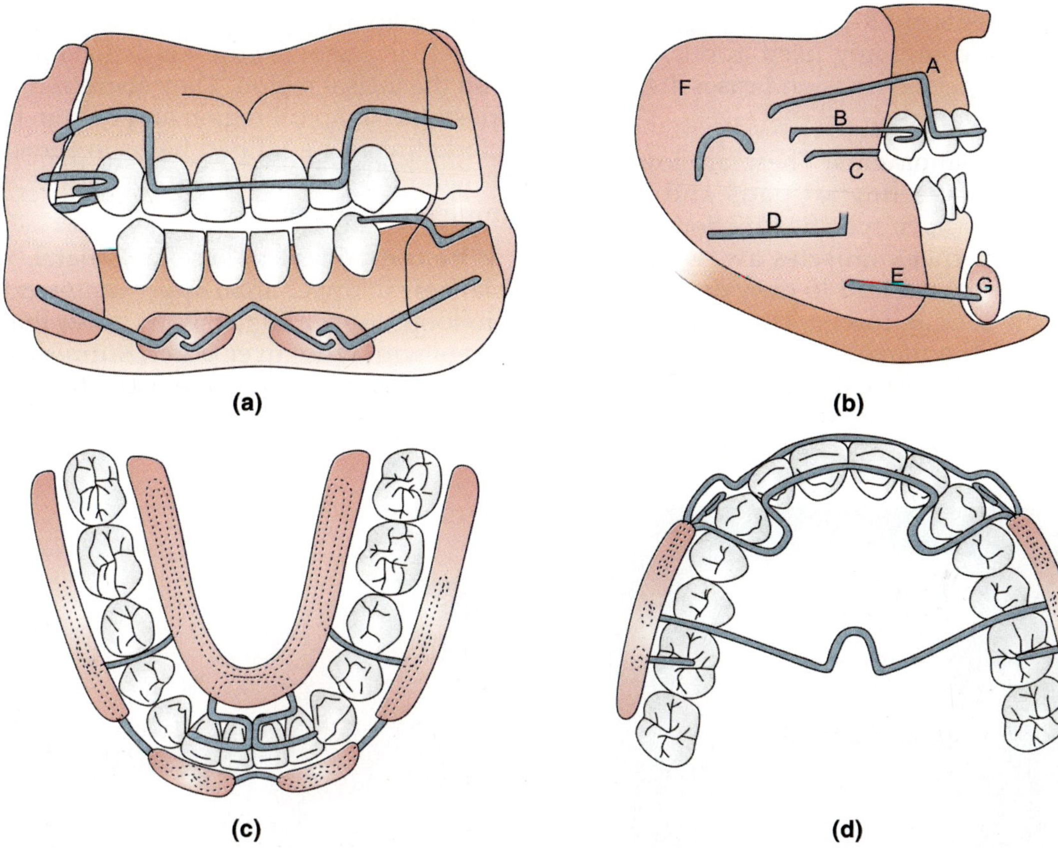

F A B C D E G

(a) (b)

(c) (d)

Figs 29.24a to d: FR-2 appliance and its various components from different aspects.

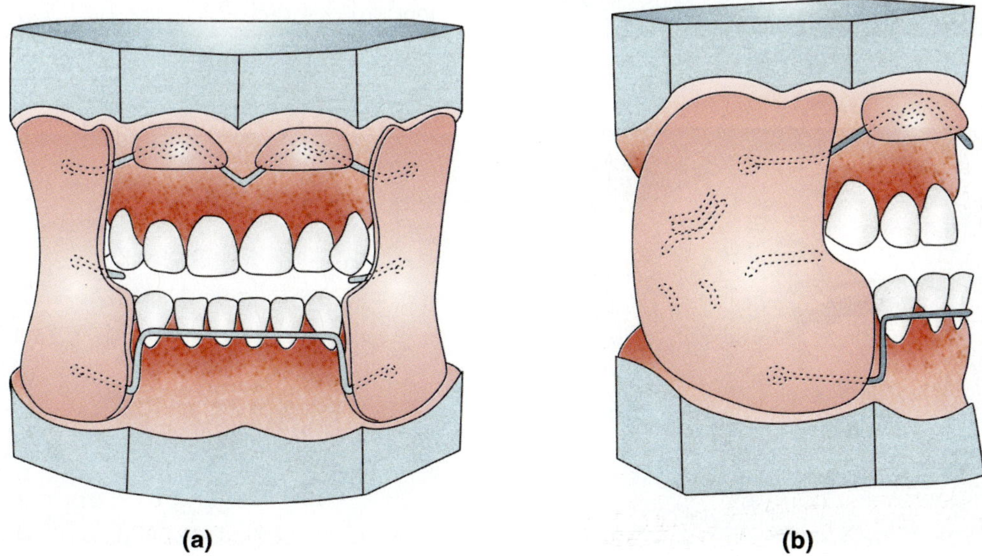

(a) (b)

Figs 29.25a and b: FR-3 appliance for class III correction. Note the position of anterior lip pads which are located in upper arch as compared to FR-2.

Components of FR-2: F-R2 appliance is one of the most commonly used appliances for treatment of class II division 1 cases. It has following components.

Acrylic components: These are lower lip pads and lower lingual pads and buccal shields. They have specific functions. Buccal shield keep cheek muscles away from the dental arches, and lead to their development under the tongue forces. Thus they help in expanding the narrow dental arches. They also stretch the periosteum in apical region and help in bone remodelling. Lip pads keep the lower lip away from incisor region. Thus they help in removing the restriction of lower lip on the incisal region. They also stretch the periosteum in apical region and help in bone remodelling. Lingual pad helps in directing the mandible forward due to proprioceptive stimuli on lingual mucosa.

Wire components: These are palatal bow, labial bow in upper arch, upper canine extension/loops; upper lingual bow, lower lingual springs with cross over wires; support wire for lower lip pads. They are made by 0.8–0.9 mm hard SS wire.

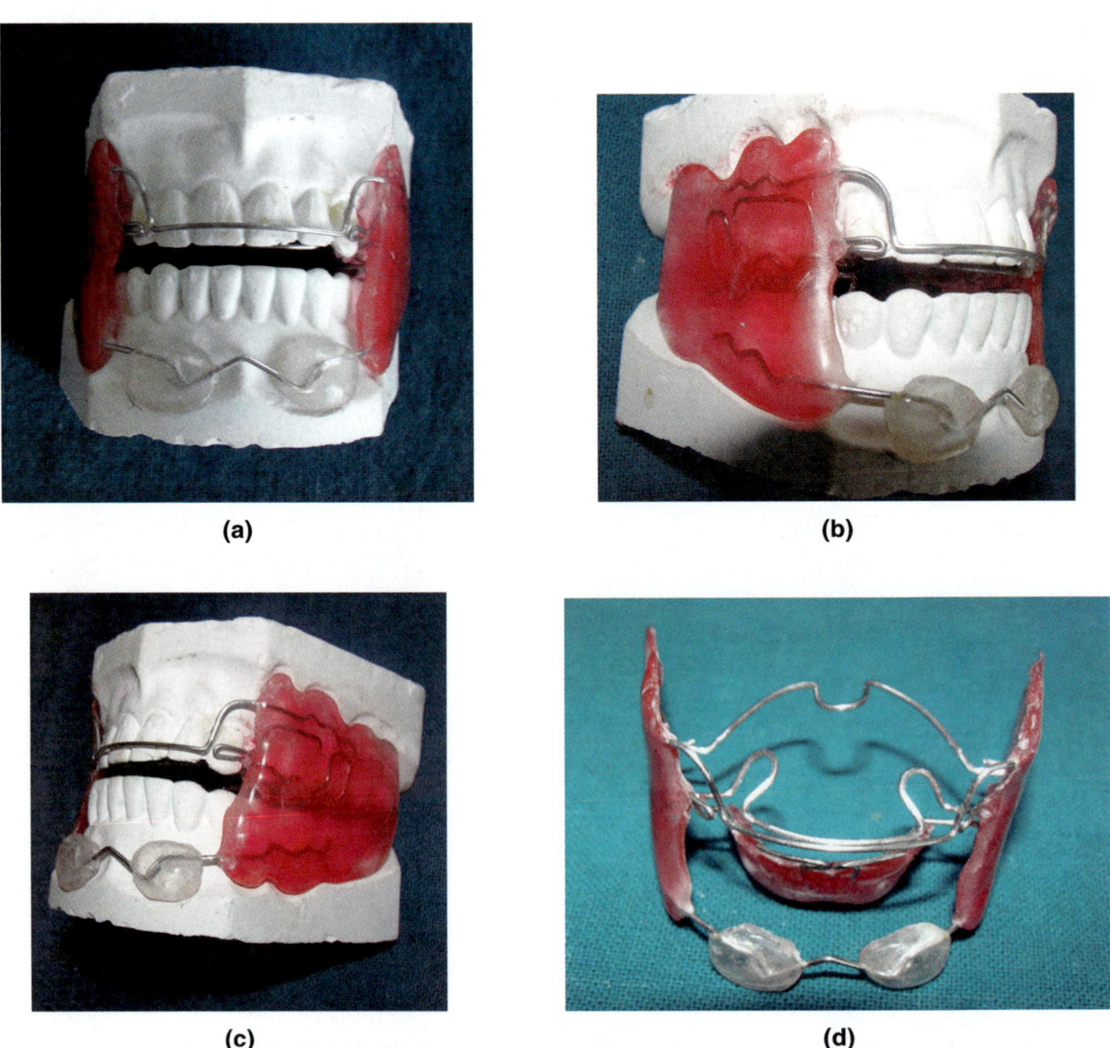

(a) (b) (c) (d)

Figs 29.26a to d: FR-2 appliance.

Lip pads: They are two in lower anterior vestibule one on each side of midline; extending deep in the vestibule. They keep lower lip away from the teeth, help in lip seal, prevent lip trap and creating periosteal stretch, thus helping in bone development in this area and contributing to mandibular growth (increase in length, and reducing the mandibular prognathism). They eliminate hyperactive mentalis activity. In FR-3, the lip pads are in upper vestibule for these same functions (reducing the maxillary retrognathism by removing restrictive effect of upper lip).

Buccal shields: They are extended deep in the buccal vestibules. They are kept away from the dentition and alveolar area with the help of wax relief during fabrication. They help in eliminating the abnormal buccal forces falling on dentition and also cause periosteal stretch in the basal region.

Palatal bow: It is a transpalatal wire with a U-loop in midline and it crosses the OP through the embrasure mesial to first permanent molar. Its terminal ends are bent to be brought back to rest in the central fossa on occlusal surface of first permanent molar. They stabilise the appliance and prevent molar eruption.

Canine loops: These wires are attached to buccal shields and stand away 2–3 mm from canines. It helps to eliminate the effect of muscles of modiolus from the canine region and thus aids in **development of intercanine width**.

Labial bow: Upper labial bow is adapted in middle third of upper incisors in the ideal form and is kept passive and away from the teeth. In lateral incisor region, it is bent so as to insert it in buccal shields. In FR-3, this is made on lower incisor region.

Lingual stabilising bow: It is made in upper arch with U-loops in canine region, with its terminal ends crossing between canine–first premolar to insert in buccal shield. It is adapted to lingual surfaces of incisors and prevents their lingual tipping during the treatment.

Lower lingual springs: They rest on lingual surfaces of lower incisors. They prevent their supra-eruption, help in their proclination if retroclined. They are inserted in lingual pads.

Lingual crossover wire: It is made of 1.25 mm wire, adapted on lingual side of lower arch 3–4 mm below the marginal gingival and crosses the OP between 3 and 4 region to insert in buccal shields. It helps to support the appliance.

Labial support wires: They are three small components in lower labial vestibule which connect the labial pads together and to the buccal shield. The labial frenum is avoided during fabrication. They are inclined gingivally to keep the pads deep in vestibule.

Construction bite: Bite is taken in **minimal sagittal advancement** so that there is no obvious strain on mandibular muscles. For minor sagittal problem, the bite is taken in edge to edge relationship. Frankel recommended that the maximum advancement and vertical opening should not be more than 2.5–3 mm. This vertical opening is enough for the wires crossing the OP. For FR-3, the mandible is retruded minimally to be in most comfortable retruded position.

Separation and seating grooves: Before taking impression, heavy elastic separators are placed in upper C-D region and 6-E regions to create space through which the cross over wires pass which help to keep the appliance anchored to upper teeth. If separation is not enough, then seating grooves are created in primary teeth by slicing the distal contacts of these teeth.

Appliance management: Appliance should be comfortable to patient. He should be advised to increase the wear time gradually to full time wear so as to get used to it. Patient is also taught how to remove and insert it in oral cavity, and advised to handle it carefully and clean it daily. He is also instructed to perform oral exercises, e.g. talking, reading, etc. to train the muscles.

FIXED FUNCTIONAL APPLIANCES

Removable appliances have problem with patient cooperation. Also they are not effective when patient is near end of growth phase. At that time, for best response, the full time wear of FA is required. It can be used alongwith the fixed appliances to prevent the loss of treatment time. Some fixed FAs have been designed to overcome these problems. Papiadoupolas in his book has explained them very descriptively but detailed discussion is not being considered in this book. Some examples are (Figs 29.27 to 29.30):

- Herbst appliance
- Jasper Jumper appliance
- Forsus
- MPA 1, 2, 3, 4, etc.
- Eureka spring
- Adjustable bite corrector
- Saif spring
- MARA
- Klapper spring I and II types
- Sabbagh super spring SUS
- Biopedic appliance.

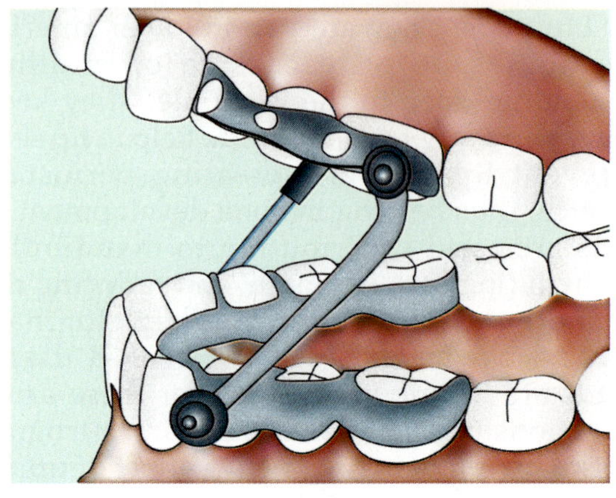

(a)

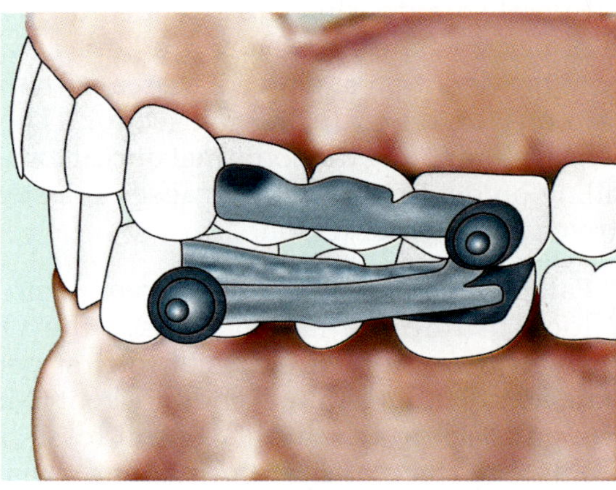

(b)

Figs 29.27a and b: Fixed rigid myofunctional appliance.

Herbst Appliance (Fig. 29.28)

It was introduce by Herbst in early 1900s but was not widely used. It was reintroduced in 1979 by Hans Pancherz.

Indications

It can be used for following cases.

1. To treat class II cases in post-adolescent cases where residual growth can be used. It is used for 6–8 months in such cases.
2. To treat class II cases due to mandibular retrognathia.
3. Can be used in mouth breathers where removable appliances are uncomfortable.
4. Can be used in uncooperative patients.
5. Can be used in patients with TMD.

Design: It consists of a telescopic mechanism which is attached to maxilla and mandible to keep the later in the forward position. It acts as an artificial joint. It consists of a tube which is attached to distal of upper first molar, and a rod/plunger which is attached to mandibular first premolar. The rod is measured to the required length according to mandibular advancement required and it is inserted in the tube. Herbst appliance is of two types, i.e. bonded and banded types.

Bonded type: It has acrylic splints covering the buccal, occlusal and lingual aspects of the posterior teeth in upper and lower arches. They are reinforced by the heavy wires for strength. The pivots are fixed in the splints

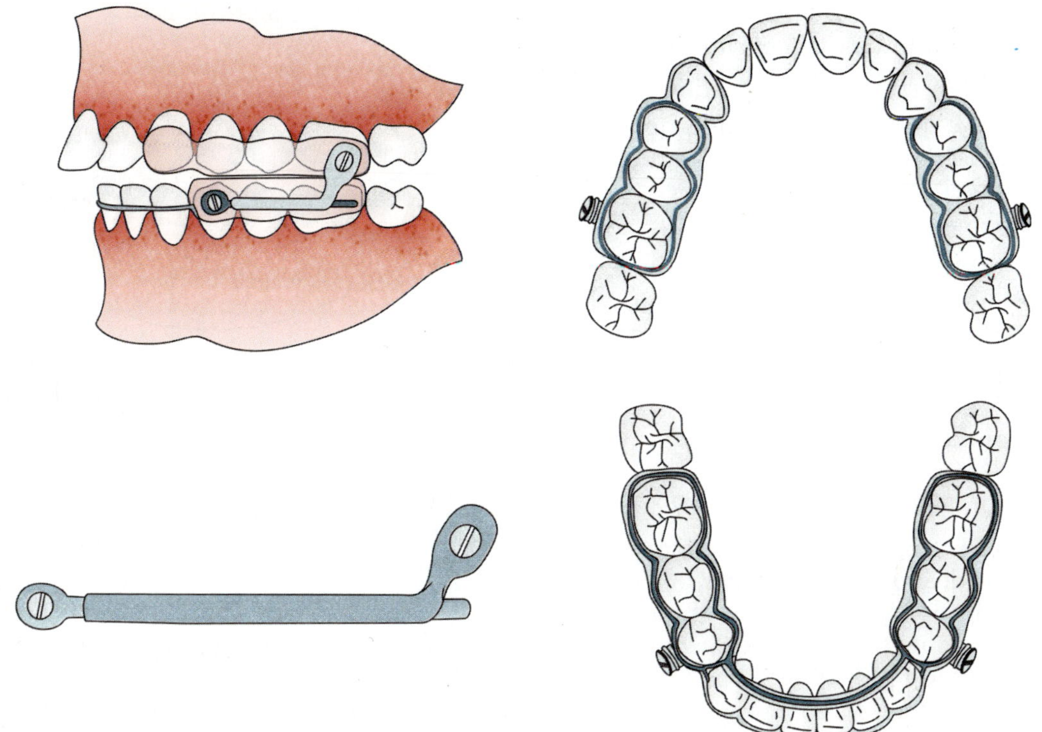

Fig. 29.28: Herbst appliance: a rigid fixed myofunctional appliance and its parts, and how it is attached to the arches.

distal to upper first molar and at lower first PM, where the terminal ends of the assembly will be attached.

Banded types: Bands are fabricated at upper first molars and at lower first premolars, and pivots are soldered to them at required locations where the terminal ends of the assembly will be attached.

Advantages

a. Patient cooperation is eliminated.
b. It is fixed so is used for full time, the treatment effects are rapid.
c. It can be used with fixed orthodontic therapy also.
d. It can be used in later stages of growth and can help in gaining advantages from the residual growth.
e. It can be used in patients having mouth breathing habit due to nasal obstruction.

Disadvantages

a. It is a rigid assembly, so patient has difficulty in mandibular movements.
b. It can lead to temporary functional disturbances.
c. Repeated loosening and breakage is seen especially lower premolar area.
d. In splint bonded type appliance, enamel decalcification and plaque accumulation is seen.
e. It may lead to development of dual bite with TMD problems.
f. During closure, sometimes the assembly can pose problems as it may come in between the teeth.
g. There is tendency of posterior open bite at the termination of treatment.
h. It leads to flaring of lower incisors, and mainly dentoalveolar effects are achieved.
i. Patient feels initial discomfort.

Treatment effects: During treatment of class II case, following effects are seen.

a. Class I or super class I relation
b. Decrease in overjet which occurs by increased mandibular length and flaring of lower incisors.
c. Bite opening
d. Increased in mandibular length
e. Distal movement of upper molar which also helps in treatment of class II relation.
f. Applies inhibitory forces on maxillary growth.
g. Glenoid fossa remodeling

JASPER JUMPER (Figs 29.29 and 29.30)

It is a fixed, flexible tooth borne appliance which was designed by JJ Jasper in 1980. It is not a rigid appliance and thus is more comfortable to patient. It is called Jasper Jumper as it helps to jump the bite.

Design

It is **spring module** made of SS which is covered by a polyurethane tubing, and is flexible. The ends of springs have SS end caps which are fitted distal to upper first molar and distal to lower canines. It is generally used with fixed appliance. On upper arch, a ball-end pin is passed through its end cap, and then pin is inserted through the head gear tube of the molar tube. It is thus attached distal to first molar band. But, it is not closely brought to the tube and a gap is left between distal end of the molar tube and end-cap of JJ for sufficient clearance during movements. It also helps in further activation of the JJ during the treatment if step wise advancement is desired, by pulling the pin mesially and bending it.

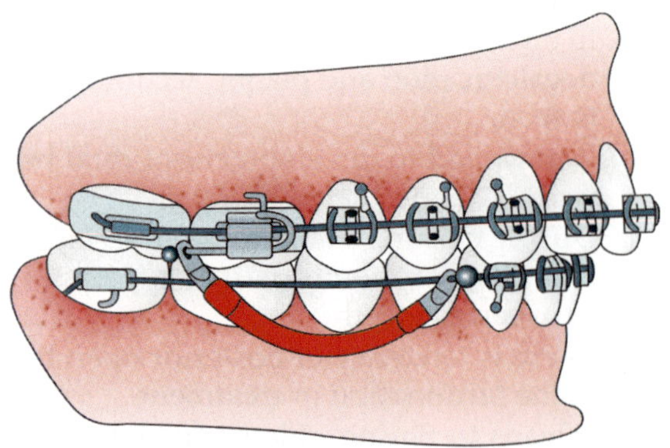

Fig. 29.29: A fixed myofunctional appliance, e.g. Forsus: it has a spring module in it which helps to keep mandible in forward position.

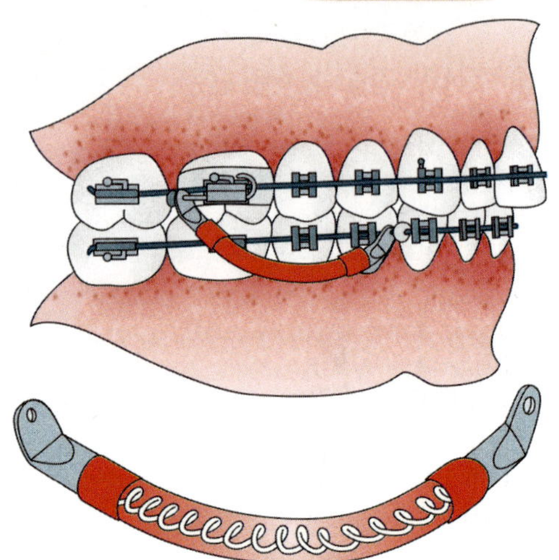

Fig. 29.30: Jasper Jumper: A flexible fixed myofunctional appliance. Note that there is a spring module enclosed in the rubber tubing.

The required length of the appliance is chosen depending on the advancement required. The lower end is passed on the lower base arch wire distal to canines. A bead; loop or a bend is placed in wire to keep this end away from the canine bracket to prevent its breakage. The arch wires should be heavy, rectangular wires with adequate amount of lingual crown torque in the lower incisor region. Sometimes, the brackets of lower premolars are removed to help in sliding of lower end on the arch wire during function. A polyurethane tubing helps in prevention of plaque accumulation and avoids the trapping of buccal mucosa in the spring during action. This appliance is available in 7 sizes ranging from 26 to 38 mm, in an increment of 2 mm.

Indications: It is indicated for skeletal class II cases with mandibular deficiency or/and retrognathia.

Mechanism of action: Required length of the JJ is calculated by measuring the distance from mesial end of upper molar tube to distal of the bead placed distal to lower canine after desired mandibular advancement. 12 mm are added to this distance to get exact size of JJ required. This covers the curvature of JJ module when the mouth is closed, the length of the molar tube; and its attachment distal to upper first molar with a clearance there. When mouth is closed, the JJ module being longer, tends to curve and produces mesial force on the mandibular arch and a reciprocal distal force on the maxillary arch.

Effects of JJ: Research shows that it leads to both skeletal and dental effects in the ratio of 40:60. Following effects can be observed.

a. Flaring and intrusion of the lower incisors, due to D and F force on the mandibular arch. Flaring of lower incisors is controlled by sufficient lingual crown torque in the incisal region of the base arch wire.
b. Distal tipping and intrusion of upper molars, and backward tipping of upper incisors: due to a backward reciprocal force component on the upper arch.
c. Mandibular clockwise rotation: The mandible is displaced D and F under the influence of FA.
d. Forward movement of condyles and point B. The mandible is displaced D and F under the influence of FA.
e. Restraining of maxillary growth: due to a backward reciprocal force component on the upper arch.

Advantages

1. It is flexible so functional problems during mandibular movements are lesser.
2. Produces continuous force
3. No patient cooperation required
4. Better oral hygiene
5. More comfortable to patients.
6. Greater degree of mandibular movements as compared to Herbst.

Other appliances: There are many other fixed appliances described in literature, e.g. Forsus, MARA, MARS, MPA 1,2,3 etc. but their description is beyond the scope of this book.

Summary: FAs are very effective interceptive modality to redirect the growth and to achieve a balance of skeletal and soft tissues in dentofacial region. They should be used during the active growth phase for best and stable results. A proper diagnosis, selection of patient and treatment planning is necessary for successful results.

VIVA VOCE QUESTIONS

1. **Define a myofunctional appliance?**

   It is defined as an appliance which causes activation of ms attached to mandible when placed in the oral cavity. And obtains its effects on the dentofacial tissues by the forces from these ms. It is also called functional jaw orthopedics (FJO).

2. **What is the best age for the treatment with a functional appliance (FA) ?**
   - Best age for treatment with FA extends from 10 years to pubertal growth phase.
   - M =12–14 years ± 1 year
   - F =10–12 years ± 1 year,
   - 2–3 years earlier in girls than boys.

3. **What are the main indications for use of the myofunctional appliances?**
   - The patient should be in the actively growing status.
   - Best in horizontal growth pattern cases with a normal sized but retrognathic mandible.
   - VTO should be +ve, i.e. an improvement of the facial profile should be evaluated before giving the appliance.

4. **What do you mean by the biphasic treatment?**

   It is the combination of the early treatment, i.e. during the active growth period; and the late treatment. The skeletal problem is treated during the active growth phase. Then after some time, the treatment of dental malpositions is done after the eruption of permanent teeth.

5. **What is the symptomatic treatment?**

   It is the treatment of the symptoms with which the patient reports in the dental clinic.

6. **What is the mechanism of action of the functional appliance?**

   With the help of a functional appliance, the mandible is placed in a forward position. This activates the muscles attached to the mandible. These ms try to come back to their original position and so apply a backward pull on the appliance. But being engaged in the upper section of the appliance, the mandible is not able to return to its original state. A downward and forward force comes into play acting on mandible.

   But in turn, that force is transferred to the maxillary arch in an backward and upward direction, producing redirection of maxillary growth and the retraction of maxillary incisors; it may also cause the distalization of the maxillary molars.

7. **Explain the satisfaction of the theory of functional matrix concept with the help of myofunctional appliance therapy?**

   When the mandible is placed forward with the help of the functional appliances, there is an increase in space of oral cavity. Also, the tongue is placed more forward and downward. Thus the functional matrix related with this stretch of the ms of tongue and the mandible gets activated and adaptation of the bony tissues takes place according to this new position of the soft tissues.

8. **What do you mean by pterygoid response with the functional appliances?**

   Pterygoid response = Lateral pterygoid m. (inferior head) is affected. Checked at 6-8 weeks after start of FA therapy. When the mandible is manipulated forcefully backward, a pain is felt in this muscle, which signifies the +ve response and a successful treatment. This muscle gets adapted to a new position and its length is shortened with FA R_X.

9. **What is meant by the headgear effect of the functional appliance?**

   Headgear effect = An upward and backward force on maxilla is applied, as the mandible tries to go back to its original position under the influence of the stretched musculature. This force also prevents the maxilla from growing downward and forward. It leads to retraction of proclined incisors and distalisation/distal tipping of molars.

10. **What is the class II elastic effect with functional appliances?**

    When the mandible is placed forward and downward with the help of a functional appliance, the mandible tries to go back to its original position, as the ms attached to it get activated. That reciprocal force gets transmitted to the mandibular teeth in a forward direction and to the maxillary incisors in a backward and upward direction. This force causes the flaring of lower incisors and also helps the lingual tipping of upper incisors. This is called as the class II elastic effect.

11. **What is the approx. amount of the force generated with a myofunctional appliance?**
    Approx. anteroposterior force is 315–395 gm; and the approx. vertical force is 70–175 gm depending on the vertical and the horizontal displacement of the mandible.

12. **What should be the vertical opening with a myofunctional appliance?**
    It depends upon the amount of free way space and on the anterior facial height of the patient. With construction bite, bite is opened 2–3 mm beyond free way space.
    It helps to activate the ms of mandible for proper effects.

13. **How do you determine the amount of forward placement of mandible for the correction of class II malocclusion?**
    It depends on the overjet values of the case. **"The rule of ten"** is followed. According to it, the total amount of vertical opening and horizontal displacement should be 10 mm. So, if vertical opening is more, the horizontal displacement should be less and vice-versa.

14. **For the correction of overjet with the help of a functional appliance, which is better, i.e. single-step advancement or partial-displacement followed by a second appliance with remaining correction?**
    If overjet is less than 10 mm, single-step correction is indicated, with the vertical opening 2–3 mm beyond the freeway space to activate the ms.
    If overjet is more than 10 mm, a two-step advancement is indicated, since single advancement may jeopardize the health of the soft tissues and may be uncomfortable. According to some studies, it is better to proceed in 2-step as it helps to activate the ms once again during the treatment.

15. **How do we achieve correction of class II molar relation with activator?**
    The upper teeth are allowed to erupt in the downward and backward direction, while the lower teeth erupt in upward and forward direction to allow the correction of the class II molar relation.

16. **Why the overcorrection is justified with the functional appliance therapy?**
    Always overcorrection is done to allow for some relapse after completion of the treatment phase, so that the required amount of correction may be achieved.

17. **Why activator is called so?**
    Because it activates the ms attached to the mandible. It is also called monobloc and Andresen's appliance or Norwegian appliance.

18. **What is a bionator?**
    It is a modification of activator in which the palatal acrylic has been replaced with coffin's spring. It also incorporates the buccinator loops to keep the cheeks away from the buccal side of the posterior teeth to help the expansion.

19. **What is the philosophy of bionator?**
    Bionator is based on philosophy of tongue.

20. **What is the mechanism of action of bionator?**
    With bionator, the mandible is displaced downward and forward in cases of class II therapy. The Coffin spring activates or stimulates the tongue in downward and forward direction, thus increasing the oral space. The buccinator loops release the pressure of buccinator ms falling on the posterior teeth and lead to expansion of the arches.

21. **What is the main function of the Coffin spring used in the bionator?**
    Main function of Coffin spring in bionator is to stimulate the tongue and to bring in effect FM theory concept of growth.

22. **What is the area of the operation of Frankel appliance?**
    FR appliance functions in vestibule of oral cavity, stretches the periosteum and causes bone growth and adaptation.

23. **What is the twin block appliance and why it is called so?**
    It is a myofunctional appliance. It is a 2-piece appliance separately for upper and lower arches, that is why it is called twin block appliance.

24. What is the advantage of twin block on other functional appliances?

Twin block is better because it is a two piece appliance, is comfortable, allows complete mandibular movements without any discomfort, proper speech is possible and can be worn for 24 hours for faster and better effects.

25. On what philosophy, twin block appliance is based?

It is based on the inclined plane relationship of the upper and lower posterior teeth.

26. At what age, the appliance therapy for controlling the oral habits should be advised?

Appliance therapy to control oral habits is not recommended for children less than 8 years age.

27. What are the few examples of fixed functional appliances?

Jasper-jumper, Herbst appliance, MARS appliance, etc.

SELF-ASSESSMENT QUESTIONS

1. How much time is normally required for R_X with FA?
2. What dento-skeletal changes can be expected with FA?
3. What is the effect of AGE during FA R_X?
4. Which FA is better—the activator or the twin block?
5. What is a twin block appliance and why it is called so?
6. What is a construction bite?
7. What are different types of crossbites?
8. What is "Rule of Ten" in crossbite formation?
9. What is clasp-knife reflex?
10. What is Biphasic R_X?
11. What is free way space and what is its average value?
12. How do you calculate FW space?
13. How do we achieve expansion with bionator?
14. Why activator is also called Monobloc?
15. Which are different types of FR?
16. What is the area of operation of FR?
17. What is the mechanism of action of FR?
18. What is the role of lip pads and buccal pads in FR appliances?
19. What is the philosophy behind bionator appliance?
20. What is the difference between activator and bionator appliances?

30

Dentofacial Orthopedics

INTRODUCTION

Most of the malocclusion problems are combination of dental and skeletal components. The skeletal class II and III conditions have skeletal malrelationships of mandibular and maxillary jaw bases in various combinations. The simple orthodontic appliances, whether removable or fixed, cannot treat the skeletal components, so special appliances are used for the treatment.

Various combinations of skeletal problems can be classified as below:

A. Skeletal Class II

It can be due to:

a. Maxillary prognathism
b. Mandibular retrognathism
c. Combination of above.

B. Skeletal Class III

It can be due to:

a. Maxillary retrognathism
b. Mandibular prognathism
c. Combination of above.

Skeletal class II problems due to mandibular retrognathism components are treated with myofunctional appliances in the favorable cases which are having positive VTO, horizontal growth pattern, patient in growing phase, etc. while rest of the other problems require the dentofacial orthopedic appliances. Skeletal problems due to abnormal growth become evident at an early age especially around 7–8 years, and the interceptive methods of treatment are needed to control/redirect the abnormal growth. Since the patient is actively growing during this time, the orthopedic appliances are very effective to control/redirect the dentofacial growth during this time.

The appliances which are used to correct the skeletal relationships of the jaw bases are called dentofacial orthopedic appliances and the procedure is called dentofacial orthopedics. The fundamental principle of dentofacial orthopedics is to optimize the development of the craniofacial structures, i.e. to remove restrictions or retardations in the accomplishment of a favorable growth pattern.

Basis of orthopedic appliances: The appliances used should lead to maximum skeletal changes and the least dental changes. There is no system to apply forces directly to the bone, but they are applied through the teeth, which act as handles to apply the forces. When lighter forces are applied on the teeth, they lead to biochemical changes in PDL and supporting alveolar bone and lead to tooth movements. However, if the forces are of heavy nature, they lead to crushing and the hyalinization of PDL, and thus no immediate bony remodeling takes place. These heavy forces are then dissipated to the basal bones of jaws and nearby skeletal structures, leading to skeletal changes. Thus orthopedic appliances use the teeth as mere handles to transmit the heavy loads to the skeletal structures. For orthodpedic appliances to be effective, the two factors should be controlled, viz. amount of the force and the duration of the forces.

Amount and duration of the forces: Heavy forces of more than 400 gm per side are applied to crush the PDL and cause hylinasation thus minimising the tooth movement. The duration is 12–14 hours per day, i.e. intermittent forces are applied for minimizing dental effects.

The approximate recommended extraoral forces per side (in gm) in different stages of dentition are:

- Full mixed dentition: 250–300 gm
- Mixed dentition during exfoliation: 150–250 gm
- Full permanent dentition: 400–500 gm
- Retention in full permanent dentition: 150–400 gm.

Orthodontic and Orthopedic Forces

Forces are the important requirement for any orthodontic/orthopedic appliance to work. There is a difference in the level of forces used for different purpose. Generally, for causing tooth movements, the lighter forces in the range of 50–100 gm/side are recommended, which are called as orthodontic forces. But heavy forces of over 400 gm/side are required for skeletal changes, which are called orthopedic forces. According to Proffit, there exist some differences in these forces as described in Table 30.1.

Biomechanics of orthopedic appliances: For the required results, the applied forces should be applied in the proper direction. The applied forces are related to the centre of resistance of the parts of dentofacial complex. The direction of forces and their distance from the Cres determines the treatment changes needed. Knowledge of the position of various centres of resistance of different parts of dentofacial complex is important. They are given a below.

1. Cres of single rooted tooth: In mid-root region, two-thirds the distance from apex of the root.
2. Cres of molar: lies in the Bifurcation of the tooth in its midroot region
3. Cres of maxilla: lies in the postero-superior aspect of the zygomatico-maxillary suture
4. Cres of maxillary dentition: it lies in the region between first and second premolars in the inter-radicular bone.
5. Crot for bodily OTM lies at infinity
8. Cres of mandibular teeth lies apical and between the roots of premolars.

Table 30.1: Orthodontic and orthopedic forces

Variables	*Orthopedic forces*	*Orthodontic forces*
Force magnitude	Heavy, > 400 gm/side; 12–16 ounces	Light 50–100 gm
Force type	Interrupted; 12–14 hours per day	Continuous
Effects	Skeletal effects	Dentoalveolar effects
Tissue reaction	Causes hyalinization and the rear resorption	Leads to direct resorption
Direction of forces	Depends on the clinical requirement. But extrusive forces are avoided as much as possible	Can be used in any direction. It should not be extrusive, except in rare circumstances
Treatment time	Long, depending on the growth status and effects on the dentofacial complex	Varies, depends on the severity of malocclusion
Rate of change	3–4 mm per year, i.e. slow progress in skeletal changes	1 mm per month, i.e. fast changes in dentoalveolar effects
Patient cooperation	Very much required	Not required except while using elastics or some removable appliance.

The force is generally passed between the Cres of maxilla and the Cres of maxillary dentition. The force passing below the Cres of maxilla tends to rotate it U and F, while force passing above the Cres of maxillary dentition tends to rotate it D and B. These two effects nullify each other and maxillary complex almost moves in a forward direction.

Diagnosis and treatment planning: This is a very important phase of management of any case. A proper diagnosis needs a thorough history, family history, clinical examination, cephalometric examination, photos and study models. Diagnostic records help to find determine the growth pattern, growth rotation and direction, facial heights, deficient or abnormal growth of the jaws, soft tissue profile and nasolabial angle. The CVMI status helps to determine the amount of expected growth. Based on this information, the mechanics and the appliances are determined. A proper direction of applied force is chosen to achieve the desired effects:

A. Horizontal growth pattern + deficient maxilla + normal mandible (with small/ normal facial height). It is a skeletal class III situation, with concave profile: A downward and forward force is applied on the maxilla with the help of reverse face mask. The maxilla is pulled bodily in the normal direction of its growth, i.e. D and F. It helps to bring maxilla forward; rotates the mandible D and B, i.e. in a clockwise direction, thus increasing the face height, decreasing the concavity of facial profile.

B. In case of vertical growth pattern + deficient maxilla + normal mandible, we cannot afford the mandible rotation in D and B, i.e. in a clockwise direction, and increase in the face height. In such cases, the maxilla is pulled forwards, while its downward component is controlled by using a vertical pull head gear.

C. In case of vertical growth pattern + excess maxilla + normal mandible, the overgrowth of maxilla is controlled by using and U and B force applied on maxilla. The force can be applied directly on the molars or by using a maxillary splint. It helps to prevent the further increase in the face height.

D. In horizontal growth pattern cases with decreased facial height, an occipital head gear is given. It helps to bring maxilla D and B, thus leading to increase in face height, and clockwise mandibular rotation.

E. In horizontal growth cases with normal maxilla and retrognathic/deficient mandible, the myofunctional appliances are given. They help to grow the mandible in D and F direction, increase the face height, and decrease the convexity of the profile.

F. Cases having normal growth pattern, with normal maxilla and prognathic mandible, the chin cup with HPHG is given, the direction of force passing in front of the condyles. It helps to control the abnormal growth of mandible occurring in D and F direction. But cases having a vertical growth pattern need the vertical pull headgear to control abnormal mandible growth and the vertical component of the growth by applying intrusive forces on the jaws and dentition.

EXTRAORAL ORTHOPEDIC APPLIANCES

The dentofacial orthopedics involves mainly extraoral appliances, and/or combination of different extraoral and intraoral appliances. A variety of these appliances have been mentioned in the vast literature of orthodontics. Many appliances have been designed by different authors for making the treatment simple, effective and patient-convenient. Recently, the widespread use of micro-implants has made treatment mechanics quite simpler. We will not be able to describe all such appliances in this chapter due to paucity of space and undergraduate viewpoint.

The most common problems with these appliances are the proper patient cooperation, and long duration of the treatment, with slow treatment effects. But still these appliances have been mainstay for the skeletal treatment of many orthodontic problems. These appliances obtain main anchorage from extraoral sources to apply forces in desired directions. Main basic dentofacial orthopedic appliances are the headgear, chin cup, and reverse face mask, while other appliances are the modifications and combinations of such appliances. Different types of myofunctional appliances have also been described to achieve some dentofacial effects, e.g. reverse twin block, reverse bionators, FR III appliances, etc. but they are used in cases of milder form of skeletal class III problems. With advancement in orthodontic knowledge, various modifications in the form of fixed, removable, combination, implants, etc. have also been described in the literature.

- Headgear:
- Reverse face mask: Petit's, Delaire's, Nanda's, protraction headgear
- Chin cup.

Headgears

Headgears are the most commonly used extraoral orthopedic appliances. They have been used for tooth movements also by using lighter and continuous forces, e.g. for molar distalization, canine and incisal retraction, etc. But for orthopedic effects, a heavy force applied intermittently is used, especially during the active growth period to intercept or correct certain skeletal problems or to redirect the abnormal growth of maxilla. They are used generally during evening and night, because the growth hormones are mostly released in the evening. They are also used to gain anchorage. They are mainly of two forms, i.e. J–hook headgear, Klohen face bow headgear. Best age to use headgears is during 8.5–10.5 years in females; and 9.5–11.5 years in males. Headgears are used to control the abnormal excessive forward growth of maxilla. The headgear face bow assembly is the most commonly used appliance during mixed dentition period to redirect the abnormal growth of maxilla.

Classification of Headgears

Based on the site of anchorage, the headgears can be of following types (Figs 30.1 to 30.3):

1. Depending on the direction of pull and site of anchorage.
   a. High pull/occipital headgear
   b. Medium pull/intermediate/combination headgear
   c. Low pull/cervical headgear
   d. Vertical pull headgear
2. It can be of J-hook type or Klohen's face bow type.
3. According to symmetry: Symmetric/asymmetric

Literature has also mention of following modifications but they are very rarely used due to complex designs and inconvenience.

1. Frontal headgear
2. Chest bone headgear
3. Zygomatic headgear.

High pull headgears apply U and B force on maxilla/dentition. Cervical pull headgears apply D and B forces; while the intermediate pull headgear apply mainly backward pull on the maxilla/dentition.

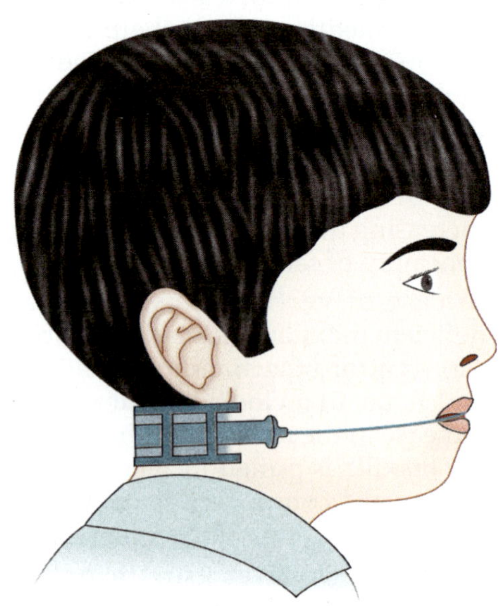

Fig. 30.1: Cervical pull headgear.

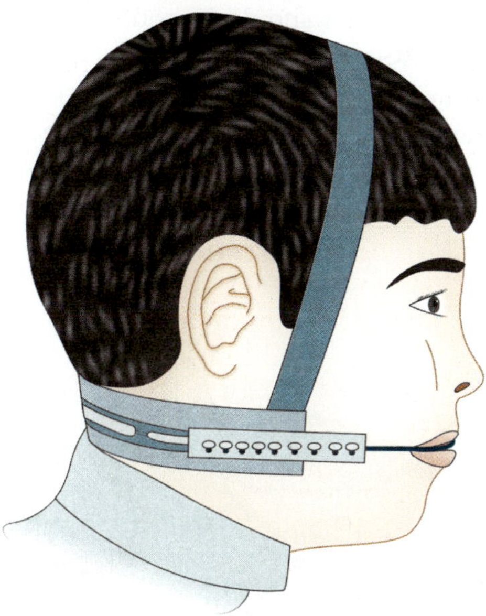

Fig. 30.2: Medium pull headgear.

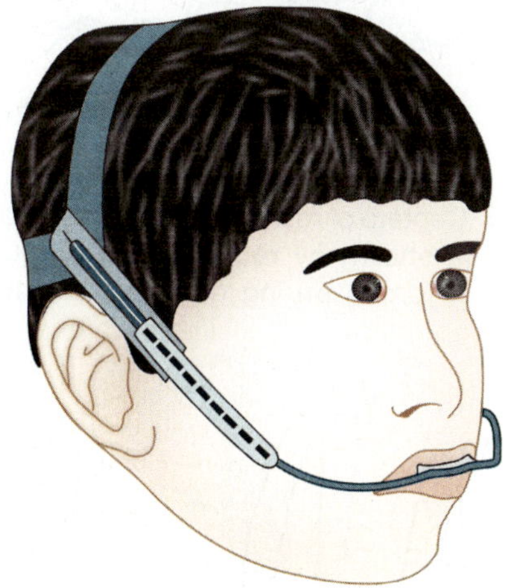

Fig. 30.3: Vertical pull headgear.

J-hook headgear is generally used for applying tooth moving lighter forces, e.g. for molar distalisation, canine retraction, incisor retraction, incisor intrusion, anchorage preparation, molar intrusion/extrusion, etc. The J-hook is made of 0.9 mm hard SS wire. It is then attached to jigs prepared from 022 × 028 SS hard rectangular wire passed through the main arch wire, with the open coil spring at the required location, while the head strap is attached to other end of J-hooks to apply forces for canine or molars distalization. It can also be attached at the soldered hooks on main arch wire in the incisors region for applying intrusive and/or retraction forces.

The headgear used for orthopedic effect is **the headgear–face bow** assembly, which has three main components:

1. Face bow
2. The force element
3. The head cap or cervical strap.

Face bow: The face bow is a bow shaped component made of heavy hard s.s wires which helps in transmitting the applied extra-oral forces on to the maxillary dentition or the posterior teeth. The face bow consists of outer bow, inner bow and the soldered junction. It is generally inserted in the headgear tube (0.045 inches diameter) placed on a banded first permanent molars. In some cases, it may be used with an acrylic maxillary splint to distribute forces on wider area and to apply intrusive forces on whole of maxillary dentition (Fig. 30.4).

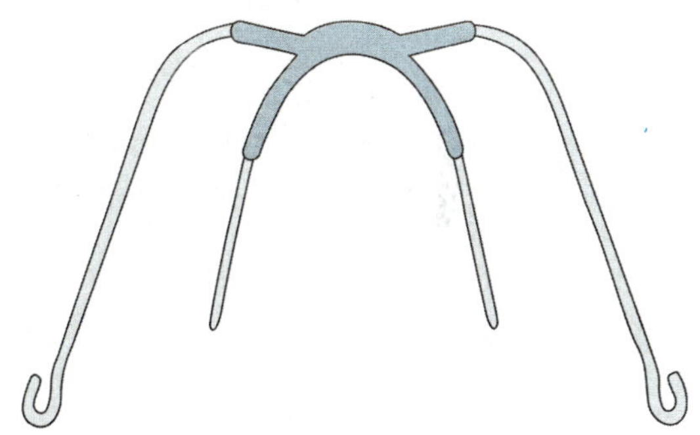

Fig. 30.4: Headgear face bow.

The outer bow is made of 0.060 " or 1.5 mm size s.s hard round wire, which is contoured to fit around the face. It lies 5–10 mm away from the cheeks. The terminal ends are bent in the shapes of hooks so as the elastics/force modules can be attached. The face bows are available commercially made with long outer bows, which can be cut and adjusted for the particular patients. Depending on the requirements and mechanics desired, it can be small, medium or long in length.

- Short outer bow: The outer bow is shorter in length than the inner bow.
- Medium outer bow: The outer bow is equal in length to the inner bow.
- Long outer bow: The outer bow is longer in length than the inner bow.

The inner bow is made of 0.045" (1.25 mm) sized SS hard wire, and is contoured according to the dental arch. The inner bow is inserted in the round headgear tube placed on the first molar bands. It is kept clear of the labial/buccal surfaces of the teeth so as to prevent any direct forces on these teeth. If it is used with fixed appliances, then it should not touch the brackets. The bayonet bends or U-loops are incorporated just anterior to the buccal tubes on the first molar. They prevent in distal sliding of the inner bow in the tubes, help in incorporating molar rotations and uprighting, keeping the inner bow away from the incisor-brackets, incorporating expansion, etc.

Solder joint: Both the bows are joined in the anterior area with solder or welding. It is a rigid joint, placed in midline and is symmetric. But, it can be made asymmetric for certain cases.

Force elements: It is used to apply the forces, and is attached to the head strap and the outer bow. It can be in the form of heavy elastics, springs, or force module strap.

Headgear or strap: This is a prefabricated or commercially fabricated assembly of strong straps, which is worn on the top of skull or around the back of neck or a combination. It takes anchorage from occipital, parietal bones and neck areas. Its selection depends on the requirements of the patient. These can be high pull, medium pull or low pull, vertical pull and asymmetric direction. Various combinations can be made by altering the length of outer bow; the direction of outer bow and the direction of head gear strap/force direction.

Principles in the use of headgears: Headgears apply the forces which can move the teeth and maxilla in all the 3D of space. The following factors should be considered when headgear use is planned.

1. **Center of resistance of maxilla** (Figs 30.5 and 30.6): It lies in the region of postero-superior aspect of zygomaticomaxillary suture. Proper relation of the direction of

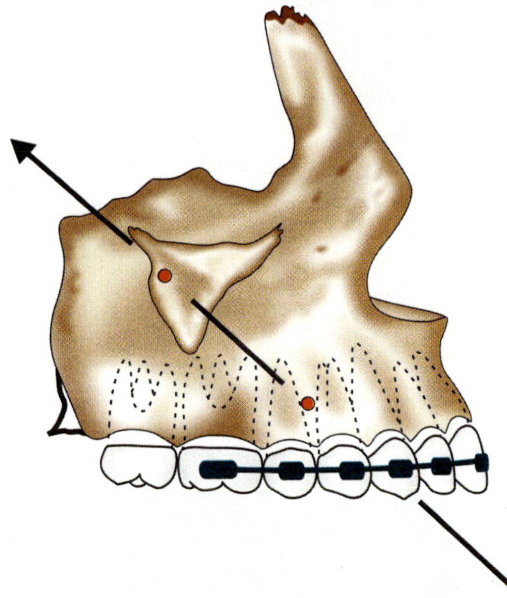

Fig. 30.5: Centers of resistance of maxillary dentition and maxilla shown by red dots, which guide the direction of forces during denotfacial orthopedic treatment.

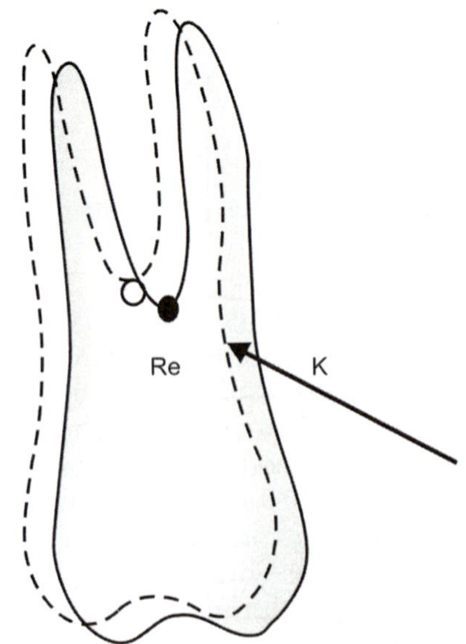

Fig. 30.6: Centers of resistance of maxillary molar.

force should be planned to achieve desired results. The force passing through Cres leads to bodily movement of maxilla in distal and upward direction. But if force passes above or below the Cres, then it leads to anticlockwise or clockwise rotation of maxilla respectively. Such maxillary rotations have a corresponding rotational effects on the mandible, and hence the facial heights and profile.

2. **Center of resistance of maxillary dentition:** It lies in the region of roots of first and second premolars, and is below the Cres of maxilla. Force passing through it leads to bodily movement of maxillay dentition. But if force passes above or below the Cres, then it leads to anticlockwise or clockwise rotation of maxillary dentition respectively. Generally, in clinical setting, the force is made to pass between the Cres of maxilla and Cres of maxillary dentition.
3. **Cres of maxillary first molar:** If the face bow is attached to the molars only, the Cres of molar is important. It lies in the trifurcation area of roots in the midroot level. Force passing through it leads to bodily movement of molar. But if force passes above or below the Cres, then it leads to its anticlockwise or clockwise rotation respectively.
4. **Point of origin of the force and its direction:** The head straps are used to get anchorage from the either occipital region of skull or cervical region of neck. Occipital region has a force direction of upward and backward. Cervical headgears produce backward and downward force. Their effects are thus different. Combination of headgear applies force mainly in backward direction. Thus the direction of force should be carefully chosen for the required treatment effects.
5. **Point of force attachment:** It is the point where the elastic/force element is attached to the outer bow. It can be shifted by changing the length of outer bow; by altering the angle between outer and inner bows; and using high pull or cervical gears. The treatment effects are different.

Placement of facebow: This is a very important step for favorable results. In a correctly fitted appliance, the soldered joint should be comfortably placed between the lips. When the elastic strap is put on the outer bow, it should not stick into the patient's cheeks. The inner bow should fit passively into the headgear tubes.

Buccal tubes: Double buccal tube having a round tube of 0.045" size is welded on the molar band, the round tube may be positioned either gingivally or occlusally. It receives the inner bow of the facebow. In modified appliances, a buccal tube can be inserted in the premolar region of a maxillary splint to receive the inner bow.

The outer bow: Its length and inclination is adjusted according to the needs of the patient. It ends anteriorly to the ears and should be 5–10 mm from the cheeks. Generally, it is kept at 15° to the OP.

Inner bow: The inner bow is adjusted passively in the molar tube such that it is able to slide freely in the tubes when the posterior strap is not attached. It is expanded by 5 mm on each side to provide a snap fit in the molar tubes and to avoid accidental dislodgement. Also, since a contraction force vector also arises when headgear is worn, this expansion will compensate that contraction and prevents the movement of molars in the cross bite situation. The bow is adjusted to a passive position between the two lips. It is positioned at the level of junction of incisal and middle third of upper incisor (which is generally the level of meeting of upper and lower lips). If inner bow is kept at upper or lower level, the lips get irritated.

J-hook headgear: This is used for causing orthodontic movements especially canine retractions and/or incisor retraction and intrusion, or en-masse retraction of anterior teeth. A J-hook is fabricated with 0.9 mm hard SS wire, which is then attached to the hooks soldered to the base arch wires during fixed orthodontic treatment. It is used with prefabricated or conventionally fabricated headgear straps.

The force element: A properly directed force is essential to produce the desired effects. Various attachments like springs, elastics and other stretchable materials can be used to apply the forces. They help to connect the face bow to the head cap or neck strap.

CLINICAL APPLICATION OF HEADGEAR

Headgear can be used for various functions in orthodontics. It can be used for orthopedic changes; anchorage control; tooth movement; controlling the cant of the occlusal plane, etc.

Orthopedic effects: Abnormal maxillary growth in D and F direction leads to maxillary prognathism and increased facial height. It can be controlled / redirected by using heavy forces on the maxilla in upward and backward direction with the help of HPHG. Sometimes, vertical pull headgear is needed to apply more intrusive component on whole maxilla. Forces of approx. 400 gm / side are used for 12–14 hours / day. Better skeletal effects are achieved when the therapy is started during the preadolescent years (Fig. 30.7).

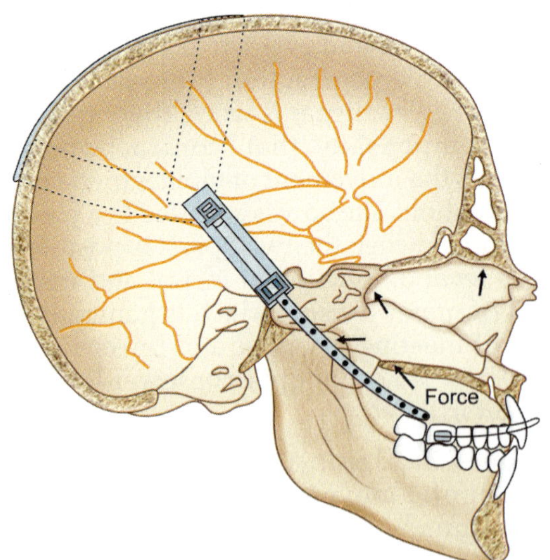

Fig. 30.7: How the forces of HPHG are distributed in craniofacial bones.

Anchorage reinforcement: Headgear can be used to augment the anchorage of molars when intraoral anchorage is insufficient. Forces upto 300 gm / side can be applied, it helps to prevent the mesial movements of the maxillary molars.

En-masse retraction of anteriors or **the whole upper arch** can also be achieved with head gears. The J-hook is used for anterior retraction while face bow is used for dental arch distalisation.

Molar distalization: Upper molars can be distalised to move them in class I relation or to gain space. The force is generally directed in upward and backward direction, especially if the patient has vertical growth pattern. This direction of the forces helps in intrusion of molars also. Unilateral distalization of molars can also be achieved by varying the force level and length of outer bow.

Molar rotation and expansion: Inner bow can be adjusted and expanded to achieve these movements to derotate the molars or to bring them out of crossbite. Derotation of molars also helps to gain space in the arch, and also helps in correction of molar relationship. A mesiolingually rotated upper first molar occludes with lower first molar in somewhat class II relation.

Orthodontic tooth movement: Headgear can be used for movement of canines, incisors, incisor and molar intrusion, en-masse retraction of anteriors and whole maxillary arch, OP rotation, molar extrusion, etc. depending on the mechanics. The force level used depends on the total root surface area of the teeth to be moved. A continuous force is preferred to achieve OTM.

Molar extrusion is achieved by using cervical headgear in D and B direction. It is used in patients having horizontal growth and decreased lower facial height and deep bite.

Molar intrusion is done by using HPHG force in U and B direction. It is used in patients having vertical growth and increased lower facial height and skeletal opdn bite.

Incisor intrusion is required to correct the deep bite, especially in patients with vertical growth, since we do not want molars to extrude. The hooks are placed in lateral incisor–canine regions, and HPHG force in U and B direction is applied with J-hooks. The force should pass through the Cres of upper incisor group which lies on palatal side.

Space maintenance: Headgear is used with a distally directed force to prevent the mesial movement of molars to manage the space mesial to them. Face bow does not have any interfering effect on the erupting teeth.

Protraction Headgear or Reverse Pull Headgear (Fig. 30.8)

Skeletal class III malocclusion due to deficient maxillary growth should be treated as early as possible. The mandible may be normal initially, but if it remains unrestricted (due to anterior crossbite with maxillary deficiency), the mandible can become longer converting to mandibular prognathism also, thus increasing the severity of situation. It is used to treat maxillary deficiency by stimulating the maxillary growth. It pulls the maxilla forward and downward out of anterior crossbite, thus gives an anterior stop to excessive mandibular growth, e.g. in CLP patient, skeletal class III cases due to maxillary deficiency, etc.

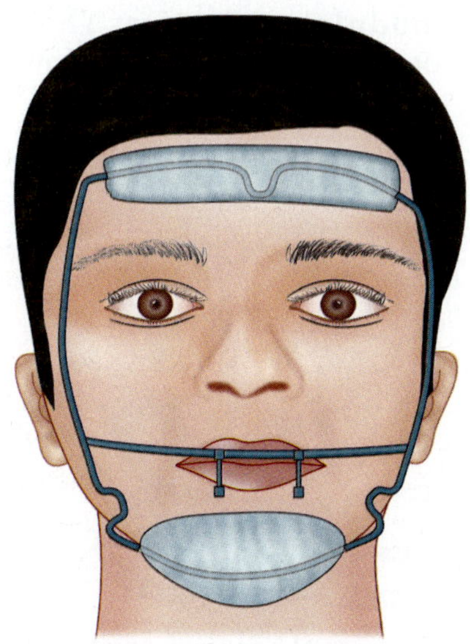

Fig. 30.8: Reverse face mask therapy for a child having maxillary retrognathism.

Best age for use: Normal direction of growth of maxilla is D and F. The main function of this appliance is to pull maxilla in forward and downward direction. To resolve the skeletal discrepancy, the best age is the growing age. For best results, it should be started during the growth spurt stages especially between 8–9 years of age and then continued, since the sagittal growth of maxilla occurs during this time. Generally, a sagittaly deficient maxilla has a transverse deficiency also, so a session of RME before the start of reverse face mask is needed (Fig. 30.9). It also helps in activating the circummaxillary sutures system. At this age, the transverse growth of maxilla is active and the midpalatal suture is patent without any interdigitation, so a proper advantage of growth can be achieved.

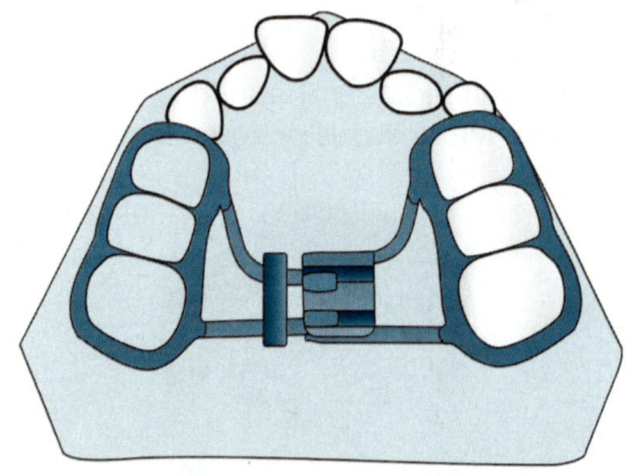

Fig. 30.9: Banded RME appliance which is used as a first step to expand maxilla and activate circummaxillary sutures before reverse face mask therapy is started.

The force direction: Force is directed in downward and forward direction, passing through the center of resistance of maxilla which lies between the roots of premolars in their apical area. Thus the force is kept approximately at 15–20° to the occlusal plane. The amount of force used is in the range of 400 gm per side used intermittently.

Components of Orthopedic Facial Mask

These are:

- Face mask: Chin cup; forehead support; metal frame: A rigid extraoral frame-

work which takes anchorage from the chin and/or forehead
- Intraoral appliance: Bonded maxillary splint
- Heavy elastic: Extraoral elastics, which generate large amount of force.

Chin cup: The protraction headgears take anchorage from chin and forehead. Chin cup is used to take anchorage from chin area. It is usually connected to rest of the face mask assembly by means of metal rods/heavy hard wires. It is available prefabricated or can be fabricated from an impression of the patient's chin region. The inner surface is lined with soft sponge type material to avoid irritation to the skin (Fig. 30.10).

Forehead cap: Forehead support or cap/strap is used to derive anchorage from forehead. It is also available as prefabricated or can be custom made by taking impression of patient's forehead. It is attached to main metal frame with heavy wires or rods. Inner surface is lined with soft sponge type material to avoid irritation to skin.

Metallic frame: It is made of hard heavy metallic rod or thick wires and it connects various components, such as chin cup and forehead cap in a single unit. It also has a horizontal section with hooks to receive elastics from an intraoral appliance. The design of metal frame differs based on the type of face mask.

Intraoral appliance: An intraoral appliance is needed to provide an attachment area for the elastics to provide protracting force on maxilla. The most common type of appliance used is a multibanded appliance with rigid wire. Traction hooks are placed either in the molar or premolar region depending on the need. Since multi-banded appliance is generally not used in mixed dentition period, an acrylic maxillary appliance with posterior bite plate can be used. The traction hook is generally placed in canine–first premolar region extended approximately 6–8 mm apically so that the elastic force passes through the Cres of maxilla. The elastics are stretched from the hooks on the maxillary splint to the cross bow of the facial mask. The direction of pull is about 15–20° in a D and F direction to the OP.

Force module or elastics: The general direction of growth of maxilla is downwards

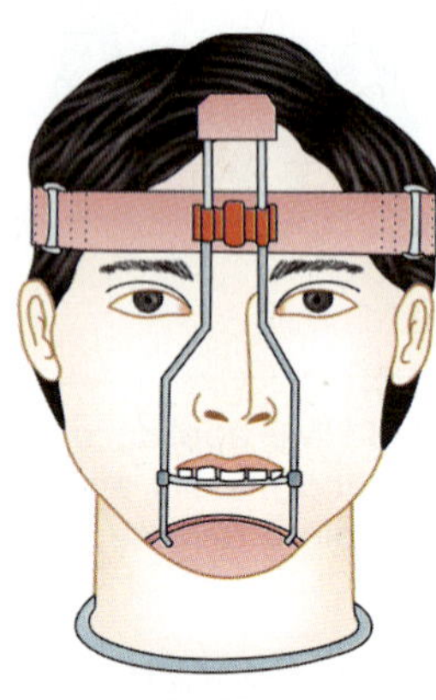

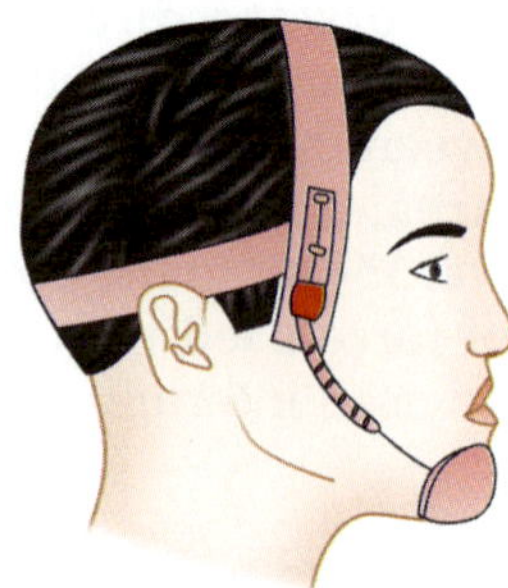

Fig. 30.10: Reverse face mask for treating maxillary hypoplasia; chin cup for control of forward growth of mandible.

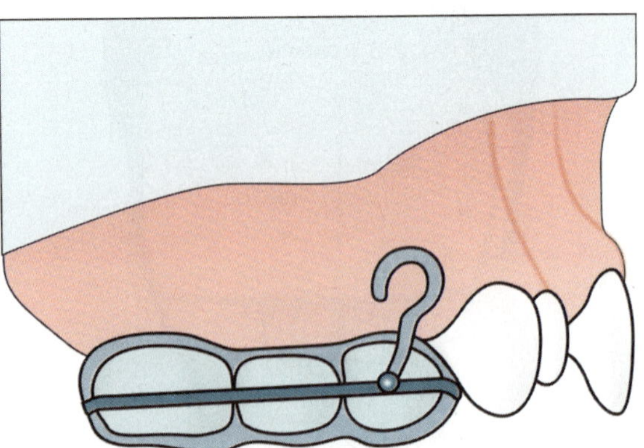

Fig. 30.11: Position of hook is in upper first premolar region from where the elastic is attached for applying a forward force on maxilla with reverse face mask.

and forward, which occurs due to growth in circummaxillary sutures oriented obliquely in the U and F direction. So, a D and F pull of force (15–20° to OP) is applied (450 gm/side for 12–14 hours/day. The best age is approx. 8 years age to attain the skeletal effects, because it is the time of maximum maxillary growth. The force is applied in the region of primary molars so that the force may be directed through Cres of maxilla for maximum skeletal effects.

Types of reverse pull headgear (Figs 30.12 to 30.17):

- Protraction headgear by Hickham
- Face mask of Delaire
- Petit's face mask
- Nanda's modification
- Intentional ankylosis of primary maxillary canines.

Hickham's face mask: It was designed by Hickham in early 1960s and it used chin and

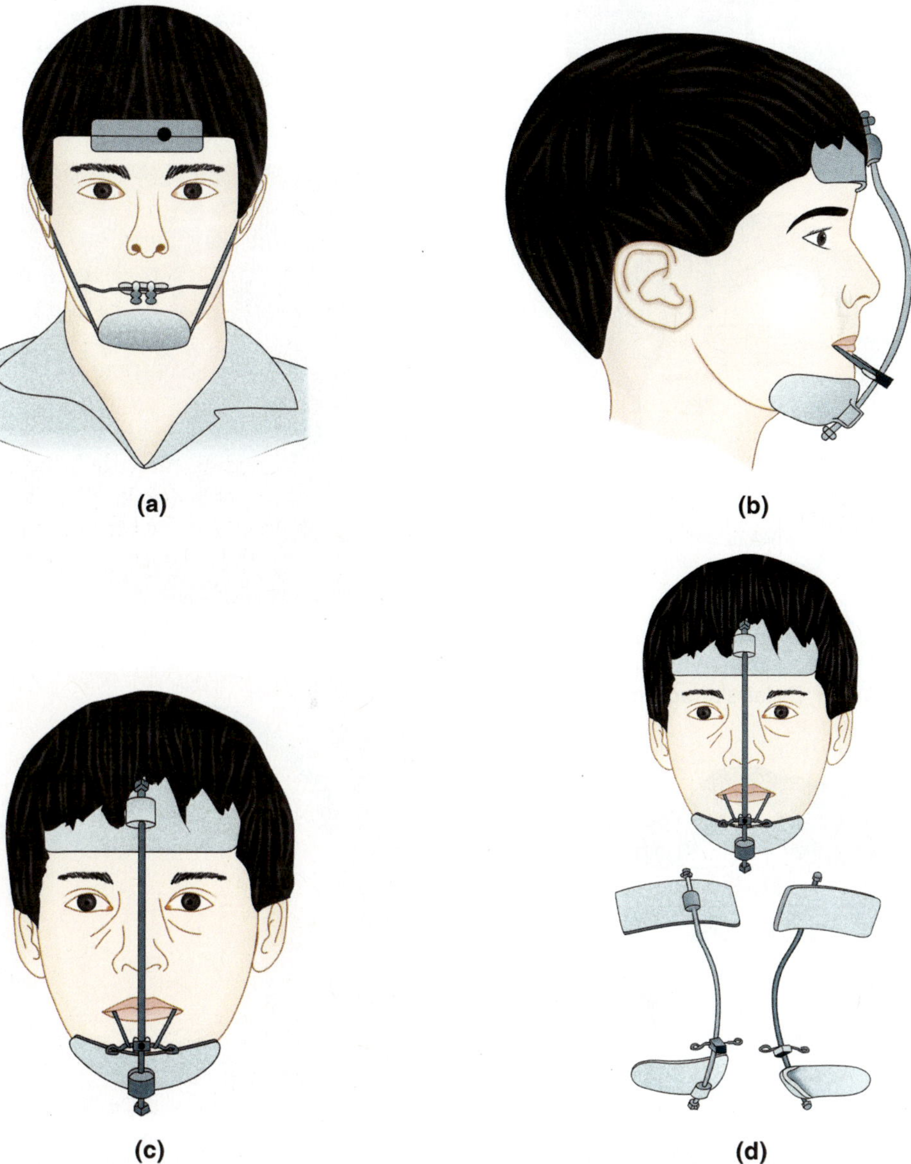

Figs 30.12a to d: Petit type reverse face mask.

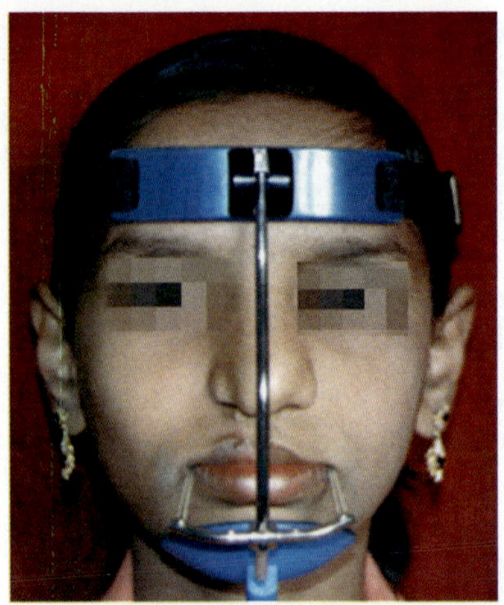

Fig. 30.13: Patient wearing Petit type reverse face mask.

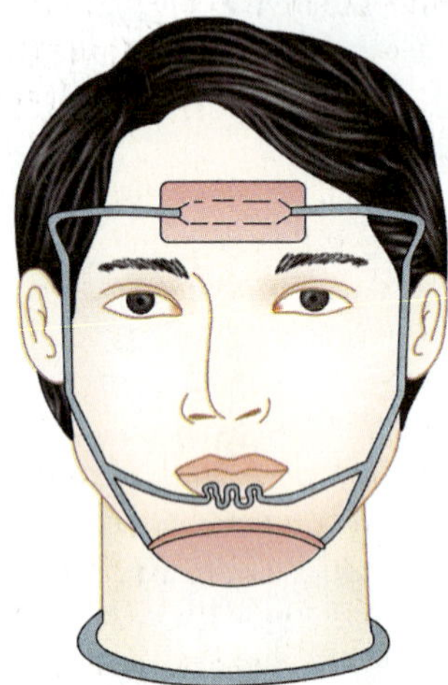

Fig. 30.14: Delaire's face mask.

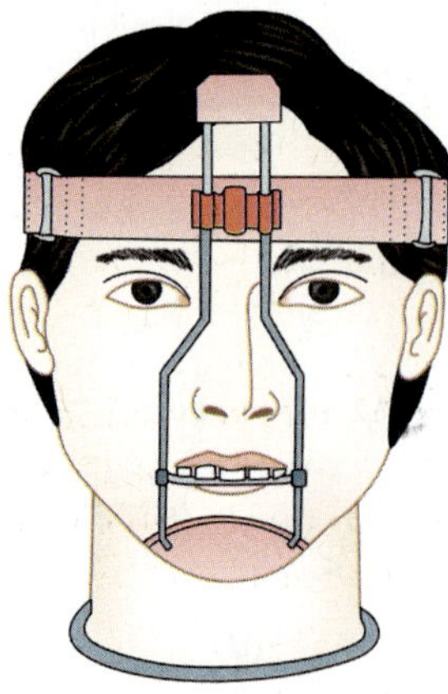

Fig. 30.15: Tubinger model of face mask.

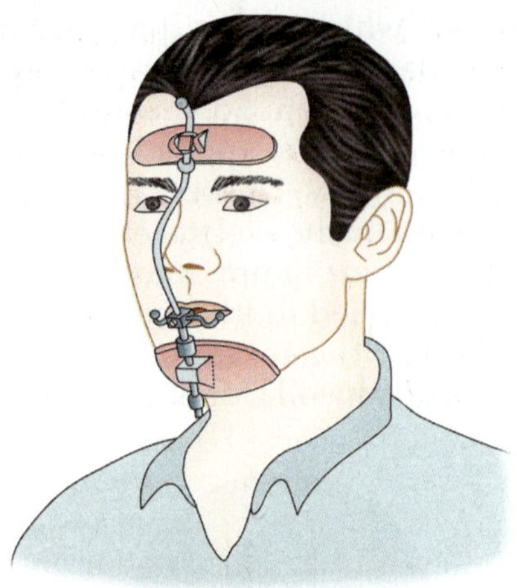

Fig. 30.16: Petit type of face mask.

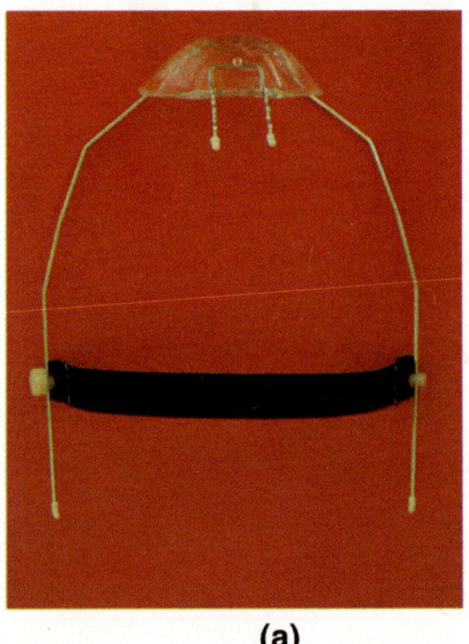

(a)

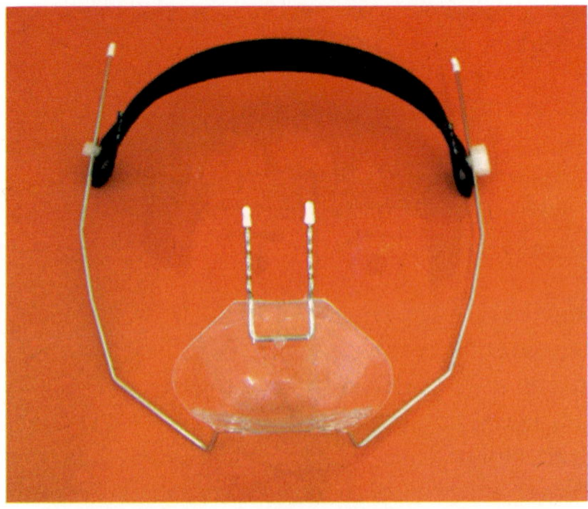

(b)

Figs 30.17a and b: Commercially available Delaire's face masks.

top of the head for anchorage. It has two short arms originating vertically from the chin cup in front of the mouth to engage the elastics for maxillary protraction. These vertical arms should be towards the midline, somewhat away from the angles of mouth so that the elastics do not irritate the soft tissue in angle region. Another two long arms originate from chin cup which run parallel to the lower border of mandible and then go vertically up from the angle of mandible and end behind the ears. There an elastic strap is attached to the end of the long arms to the headgear. This appliance has a better esthetic and comfort than other appliances.

Delaire face mask: It uses chin cup and forehead cap for anchorage and support. It has a rigid wire framework, which is broad and is fabricated according to the face width. This is kept away from the skin so as not to irritate it. It is connected to chin cup and the forehead cap. A horizontal wire running at the level of mouth and having hooks to receive the elastics is attached to the vertical arms.

Tubinger design: It is having a chin cup and then two vertical rigid rods arise from it which have a distance between them slightly more than the mouth width. In the nasal area, these rods are shaped according to nose, and then they pass near the root of nose at the region of mesial canthi of eyes. The superior ends of these rods are housed in a forehead elastic band which encircles the head. At the level of mouth, a horizontal bar having hooks to receive the elastics is attached. The forehead elastic band and this horizontal bar can be adjusted in level by sliding along the vertical rods according to the patient's needs.

Petit type face mask: It has a chin cup and forehead cap, with a single rod running in the midline and contoured according to the face. This is also kept away from the facial structures in midline. It has a cross bar with hooks to receive elastics. These three parts are tightened with screws on the vertical rod and thus can be easily adjusted in height according the patient's needs.

Nanda's modification: In it, the face bow is inserted form the distal side of the buccal tube. It has an advantage of not coming out of the tube accidentally.

Grummons protraction face mask: It is a modification which avoids TMJ loading by excluding the chin cup. In place of chin cup, the cheek pads are incorporated in the appliance to give support to the appliance, along with the usual forehead support. The horizontal bar receives the elastics to pull the maxilla in D and F direction.

Indications

Reverse face mask is used for the following purposes.

- To treat maxillary deficiency. It is best done during active growth phase, esp if treatment is started during 8–9 years of age.
- It can also be used to treat prognathic mandible in a growing patient as it has a restricting effect on mandibular growth due to chin cup. U and B forces applied on the chin cup leads to TMJ adaptation to posterior displacement of chin.
- Selective rearrangement of palatal shelves in cleft patients can be done by applying different forces on the two sides. It helps to treat asymmetry of maxilla and rotation of maxillary OP around a vertical axis.
- It can also be used for retention after maxillary advancement surgery or to correct the postsurgical relapse after osteotomies.

Treatment effects produced by facial mask therapy: Forward traction against the maxilla typically has three effects: (1) some downward and forward movement of the maxilla, the amount depending to a large extent on the patient's age. If the patient is actively growing, more skeletal effects can be achieved; (2) forward movement of the maxillary teeth relative to the maxilla and (3) downward and backward rotation of the mandible because of the reciprocal force placed against the chin. This effect also comes when the maxilla comes D and F, it rotates the mandible clockwise in D and B direction (Fig. 30.18).

Advantages

a. It helps to correct skeletal malrelationship of jaw bases especially maxilla, if treatment is started at an early age.
b. It helps to reduce the severity of malocclusion and thus future surgical intervention may be avoided. Thus morbidity and financial burden is reduced.
c. It provides a psychological advantage to the child and parents.

Disadvantages

a. Patient cooperation is a major factor.
b. Uncomfortable
c. Unesthetic
d. Gets dislodged while sleeping and playing
e. Complicated fabrication.

Chin Cup (Fig. 30.19)

The chin cup / chin cap is an orthopedic device used to treat the skeletal class III / mandibular prognathism condition by restricting / redirecting the abnormal forward and downward growth of mandible. It covers the chin and is connected to a headgear for force application and anchorage.

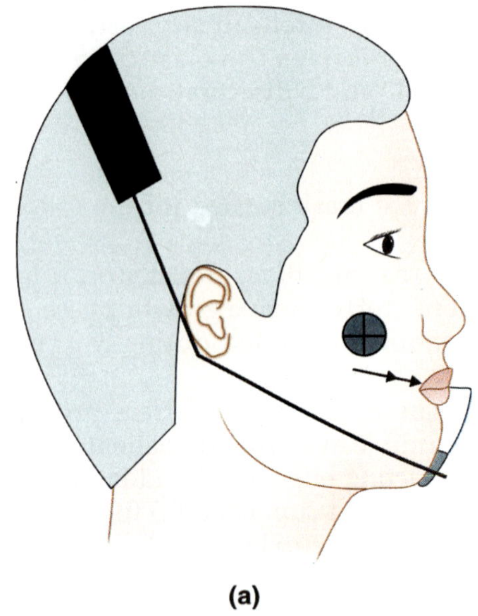

(a)

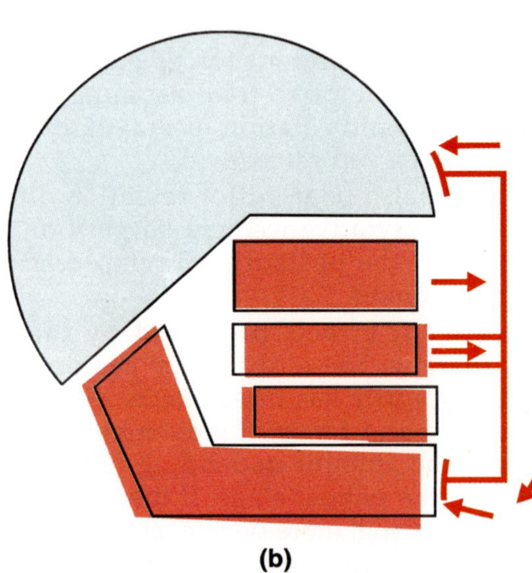

(b)

Figs 30.18a and b: Force components of Petit type reverse face mask; center of resistance of maxilla is shown by a circled cross. Arrows show the direction of effects on different facial components.

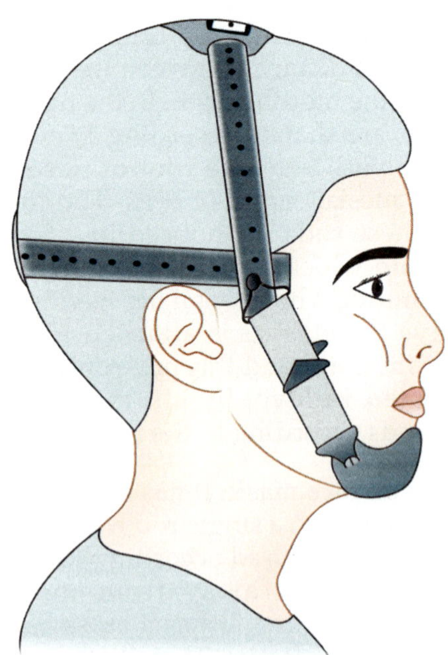

Fig. 30.19: Chin cup assembly with high pull headgear.

Age consideration: The treatment is best initiated at an early age of 8–9 years and continued till at least 16 years of age. Patient with mandibular excess can usually be recognized at an early age despite the fact that the mandible appears retrognathic during early years. Any premature contacts leading the mandibular shifting during mandibular closure, causing anterior crossbite condition should be treated at an earliest. The crossbite should be corrected to normalize the growth of both jaws. Mandible grows in D and F direction, and if growth is left unchecked, the mandible grows fast and leads to increased mandibular length. An anteriorly positioned mandible also restricts the growth of maxilla leading to its deficiency. Since the mandible keeps on growing till 16–18 years of age, the chin cup therapy should be continued till that age of active growth of the mandible. Till that age, the patient is maintained on chin cup as a retainer for night time wear after the active treatment with chin cup is over. It has to be used after the treatment is over, i.e. during retention phase till the growth of mandible is over. Otherwise, the abnormal growth of mandible can again resurface and lead to relapse of the condition. It is also called **Dynamic retention**.

Parts: The chin cup assembly consists of a chin cup that covers the chin, a head cap and an adjustable elastic strap/force module that connects the chin cup with the head cap.

Types: Chin cups can be divided into two types based on the direction of pull: occipital-pull and vertical-pull.

The **occipital pull chin cup** is more frequently used appliance for the treatment of class III malocclusions due to mild to moderate mandibular prognathism (Fig. 30.20).

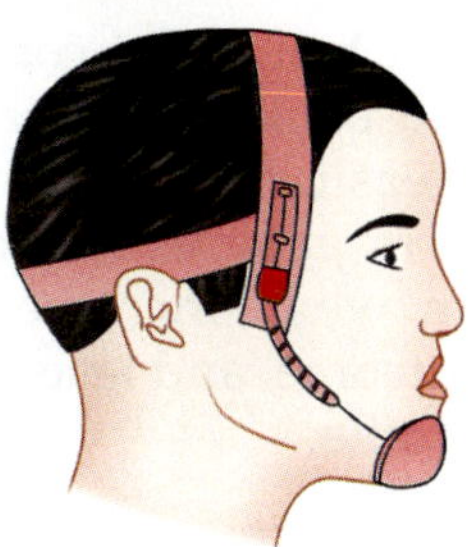

Fig. 30.20: Chin cup with HPHG.

Vertical-pull-chin cups are used for skeletal class III patients with anterior open bite tendencies; and also can be used in patients having increased anterior vertical dimension. Use of a vertical-pull chin cup can result in a decrease in the mandibular plane and gonial angles and an increase in posterior facial height, in comparison to the growth of untreated individuals. It can also cause an intrusive force on the posterior teeth, thus leading to their intrusion or at least preventing the eruption of teeth.

Force application: Initially, a force of 150–300 gm per side is used. Force is gradually increased to 450–700 gm per side over next two months. There are two main approaches to chin cup therapy. The force is aimed directly at the condylar area, thus restricting D and F growth. This force direction is used in cases having normal or vertical growth pattern. In vertical growth cases, a mandibular appliance with posterior bite plate can be used to apply intrusive forces on the upper teeth to achieve closing of MP angle, and decrease in facial height (Fig. 30.21).

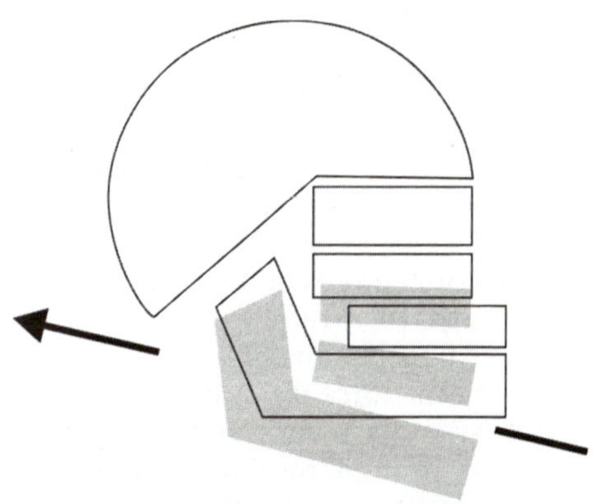

Fig. 30.21: Effect of chin cup treatment in a case of skeletal class III. Note the D and B rotation of mandible and thus improvement in skeletal relation of upper and lower jaws. But, this can only be done in mild cases which have shorter or normal facial heights.

Force passing below the condyle leads to downward and backward rotation of mandible, thus increasing the anterior face height. It can be used in patients having horizontal growth pattern, where increase in face height is a positive outcome, and leads to attaining a better facial profile.

Indications

It can be used in patients having:

a. A mild skeletal class III problem due to mandibular prognathism,
b. Incisors can be brought in edge to edge relation
c. Short vertical facial height
d. Normally positional or protrusive, but not retrusive lower incisors.
e. Pseudo-class III cases can be treated and retained.

Advantages

a. Helps in controlling and redirecting the abnormal growth of mandible.
b. Reduces the severity of skeletal disproportion, and thus need of future surgery.
c. Psychological advantage.

Disadvantages

a. Patient cooperation is required for success.
b. A long treatment time is needed for the appreciable effects.
c. It generally leads to abnormal pressure on TMJ and may lead to development of TMD.
d. A lingual force generated in incisal region cause lingual tipping of lower incisors.
e. Skin irritation on chin area due to sweat or acrylic.
f. Uncomfortable and unesthetic
g. Treatment is started at early age and goes on for many years, so the patient cooperation wears off.

Conclusion

Skeletal effects can be achieved by using dentofacial orthopedic appliances. They should be used during the active growth period of the jaws for maximum benefit. A long treatment period and patient cooperation is needed for proper results.

VIVA VOCE QUESTIONS

1. **What is the direction of force application by reverse headgear/Delaire's face mask?**
   - It is used for the correction of maxillary deficiency. D and F pull of headgear force (15–20° to OP) is applied (450 gm/side for 12–14 hour/day. The best age is approx. 8 years age to attain the skeletal effects, because it is the time of maximum maxillary growth. The force is applied in the region of primary molars so that the force may be directed through' the Cres of maxillary bone for maximum skeletal effects.

2. **What is a headgear and which are the different types of headgear?**
   - It is an extraoral appliance, which obtains its anchorage from head region. It can be cervical/occipital/intermediate vertical type of the headgear; it is also ka low pull/medium pull/high pull headgear.
   - The angle of the pull is + 15° to the OP for medium pull; +45° to OP for high pull and –45° to OP for low pull headgear.
   - It can be used for orthodontic and orthopedic effects depending on the amount of the force and time of wear. For orthopedic effects, it should be used for at least 12–14 hours/day and force used is 350–450 gm/side. It can also be used to increase the anchorage during the treatment.

3. **What is a Delaire's face mask?**
   - It is an orthopedic appliance used for the treatment of maxillary retrognathia, e.g.

CLP, especially during the growth phase. It has a chin cup and forehead support for anchorage.

- Its modified forms are Petit's face mask; Hickham's appliance.

4. **What is the recommended age for the use of Delaire's face mask?**
   - Best age for use of this appliance is 8–9 years, as the growth spurt is in action at that time and maxillary growth is in full swing. It pulls maxilla downward and forward.

5. **What is the placement of the elastics with this appliance?**
   - The elastics are attached from a maxillary appliance from the premolar/primary first molar region to the hooks placed at the level of oral commissure, at least 5–6 mm away from the skin.
   - The force is directed downward and forward (at 15–20° to OP), i.e. parallel to the normal direction of maxillary growth.

   RME is a recommended procedure just before the use of Delaire's appliance, why?

   - A phase of RME before this appliance is favorable as RME helps to activate the circummaxillary sutures.
   - It is also used in CLP patients. Its chin cup helps to control mandibular growth.
   - It also helps in the forward and downward movement of the maxilla, because when RME is done, a force is generated in the backward direction. But, this force is reciprocated by the pterygoid plates and the buttress, which in turn applies a forward force to the maxilla, causing its protrusion.

6. **What is a chin cup appliance?**
   - It is an appliance used to control the mandibular prognathic growth. It is used in skeletal class III cases.
   - It uses high pull headgear, passing just in front of the condyle.

7. **What is the main disadvantage of chin cup appliance?**
   - It causes lingual tipping of lower incisors under its force, which is its disadvantage.
   - It may also cause traumatic changes in the condyle under heavy forces.

8. **Why a long-term retention period is required for the treatment of a prognathic mandible?**
   - It has to be used after the treatment is over, i.e. during retention phase till the growth of mandible is over. Otherwise, the abnormal growth of mandible can again resurface and lead to relapse of the condition. It is also called dynamic retention.

9. **It is said that the corrective jaw surgical procedures/orthognathic surgeries should be done after the completion of the growth phase, why?**
   - If we undertake the surgical procedures during the active growth phase, the condition may recur at a later stage since the growth is taking place according to the same abnormal pattern. The best age for orthognathic surgeries is after the completion of the active growth, i.e. after approx 16–18 years age.

31

Separation in Orthodontics

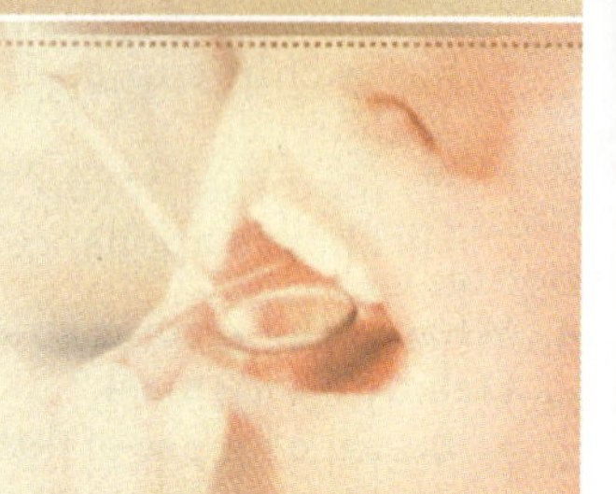

INTRODUCTION

Separation is a conservative process of opening the tight contact areas between the teeth to create mild spaces between them to facilitate the banding of teeth. The tooth is shifted slightly within physiological limits of PDL to create enough space so that the thickness of band material may pass without undue strain on the tissues.

Since the advent of bonding of orthodontic attachments, it is not necessary to band the teeth. Even direct bonding attachments are placed on the molars. However, studies have shown that on molars, the direct attachments have more failure rate as compared to banded ones. Also, in many situations, there is urgent requirement of banding of certain teeth, especially in molar region. It is needed for obtaining proper anchorage with TPA, LHA, etc. and to avoid frequent loosening of bonded buccal tubes mainly from the lower molars.

For proper banding of molars and sometimes other teeth, a sufficient gap is needed between the teeth for proper seating of bands without forcing in and thus ensuring safety of gingiva, and avoiding the pain to the patient. Sometimes, there is no requirement for separation where the contacts are not tight. Tight contacts are generally found in patient with erupted second molars, horizontal growth pattern with skeletal deep bite and strong musculature. Also, in advanced age when there is attrition of interproximal surfaces and the marginal ridges of the teeth, proper passage of band material between the teeth needs separation.

Band Thickness

Generally, the thickness of band materials used in orthodontics are: 0.0180 × 0.005" and 0.0180 × 0.006" for molars; 0.0150 × 0.004" for premolars and canines; and 0.0125 × 0.003" and 0.0125 × 0.004" for incisors. So, there should be sufficient gap between the teeth to accommodate the thickness of band material. The width of PDL is approx. 0.15–0.25 mm. With separators, the tooth shifts within the PDL, causing no damage to periodontal tissues.

Requirements of a Separator

The ideal separating spring should have features like it should be easy to place in any contact, create little or no discomfort during the separation period, and generate enough space for banding, at least 0.006" to accommodate the thickness of band material.

Methods of Separation

To achieve separation, there are several methods as detailed below:

1. Brass wire separation
2. Elastomeric separators
3. Beggs' separating springs
4. Jumbo separators for treating partial molar impactions, by Robert Cerny in 2003
5. TP springs
6. Nickel titanium separating spring in 1991 by McGann

For placing the elastomeric separators, a special separator placing plier is used.

A. Brass wire: In its initial days, the fixed orthodontic treatment involved complete banding of all the teeth for placement of attachments. Soft brass wire of 0.020" size is passed below the contacts of the tooth and brought over the occlusal embreasure and is tightened. The pigtail is tucked in the buccal embreasure. After few days (5–7 days), the separation is achieved. If improper separation was there, the wire can be retightened till proper gap is created to receive the band.

Advantages: It has following advantages:

- Brass wire is self-cleansing.
- It leads to slow separation and hence lesser pain.
- There is no plaque accumulation, as it can be cleansed easily by tooth brushing.

Disadvantages:

- It needs more chairside time.
- More time is required to achieve separation.
- It is painful while insertion as wire may injure gums.
- It may cause bleeding during insertion.
- It may lead to buccal tissue irritation from the pigtail extension if not tucked properly.

B. Elastomeric separation: These separators are made of latex elastic rubber material. They are inserted with the help of a special plier, the separator placement plier (Fig. 31.1). The separator is like a ring, which is stretched with the help of jaws of the plier and one strand of which is slipped beyond the contact area between the teeth and other remains occlusal to the contact. These rings are of smaller diameter which put a pressure around the contact areas of teeth due to elastic recoil and lead to separation (Fig. 31.2).

However, sometimes the elastomeric module may break during placement, leading to injury to interdental papilla due to a high force being used during placement. It may also cause distortion of the module, resulting in insufficient space for banding (Fig. 31.3).

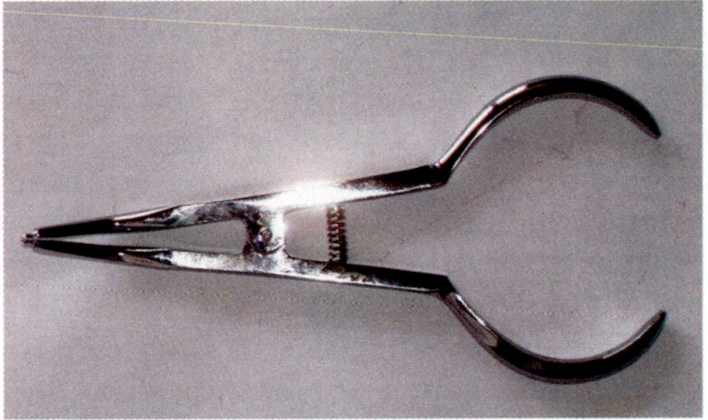

Fig. 31.1: Separator placement plier is used to place elastomeric separators.

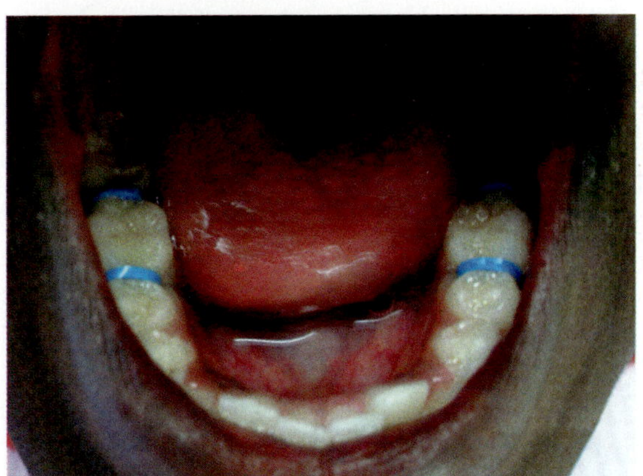

Fig. 31.2: Elastomeric separators.

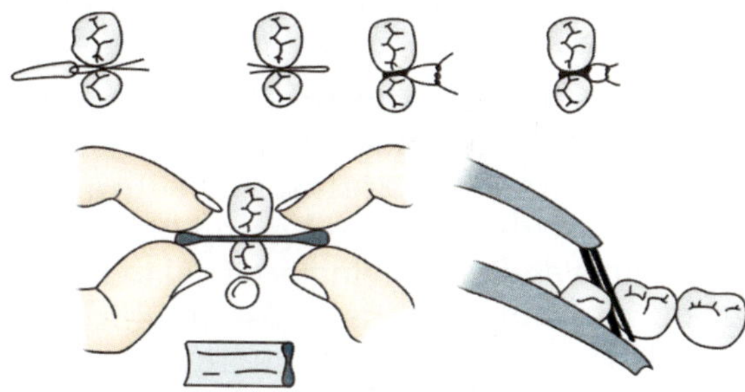

Fig. 31.3: Insertion of separators between the teeth around contact areas. First row shows that a brass wire can be used to pull the elastic separator through the contacts. Another figure shows that placement of jumbo separators with the help of fingers, while last figure shows use of separator placement plier.

To prevent tissue damage, a simple technique can be used. Two pieces of dental floss are passed through the module which is then passed below the contact area. It is then stretched and slipped upward until the occlusal portion of the separator passes through the contact point. If the module breaks during placement, the force is thus directed away from the gingiva preventing the injury. However, it requires more time and patience to thread dental floss through each elastomeric module.

Elastomeric modules can be used comfortably in children and adolescents since they have softer bones, the teeth have rounded contact areas; and are free of restorations or crowns, etc. Adult patients commonly have tight contacts, sharp amalgam fillings, broad contacts due to age-related attrition; flattened marginal ridges which prohibit the slippage of separators from the occlusal side. It may lead to overstretched elastomeric modules or breakage. In these cases, TP springs or brass wire must be used.

Types: Generally, ring type modules are used. Different sizes are available for anterior and posterior teeth.

Advantages: Faster to place; less time consuming; no bleeding; less painful to insert.

Disadvantages: Painful during separation due to heavy forces; more plaque retentive; sometimes may cause latex allergy; need special plier.

C. Beggs' type separator: They are spring clip type separators, made of 0.018" or 0.020" Wilcock SS wire. They are inserted with a bird beak plier, with one strand going below the contact area and other lying occlusal to it. The legs of the spring are criss-crossed which get activated on insertion, causing a tooth separating force (Figs 31.4a to c).

Advantages: Comfortable; lesser time required for insertion; non-painful; does not injure the gums, if placed carefully; less plaque retentive.

Disadvantages: Fabrication is time consuming; costlier; may sometimes rotate around the contact area; may cause tongue laceration, if sharp and longer ends are present. They can lead to problems, if they become loose and swallowed.

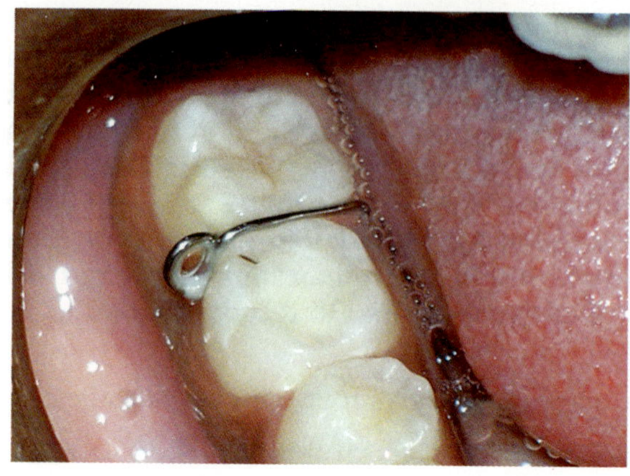

(a)

(b)

(c)

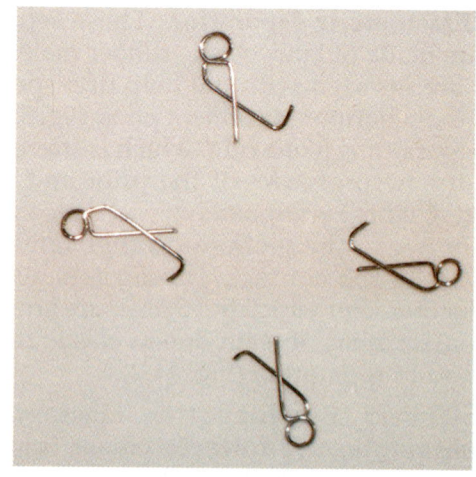

Figs 31.4a to c: Beggs' type/spring clip type separator.

Method of Fabrication

They are generally available as prefabricated but are costly. We can easily make them as a chair side procedure. A length of wire is taken and a helix made around the round beak of a plier. The two ends of the wire are now rebent to come criss-cross to each other. The sufficient length of spring is cut and one end of the wire is bent at around 90°. This wire comes occlusally to the contact area and the 90° bent portion prevents its dislodging. The end of gingival arm is bent over itself at 180° to prevent any sharp points and tongue lacerations.

D. Jumbo separators for treating partial molar impactions: It has been suggested by Robert Cerny in 2003 for facilitating the eruption of molars which get partially impacted due to multiple factors, especially when they get engaged below the height of contour of distal surfaces of the teeth mesial to them.

Conventional elastomeric ring separators come in 2 sizes, viz. **green** which are 3 mm diameter and 0.75 mm thick, and **blue** which are 4 mm diameter and 1.0 mm thick. Jumbo separators are **black** in color and are 6 mm diameter and 2 mm thick. They can be placed with separating pliers and/or slim line needle holders. Sometimes, floss can also be used to insert the elastomeric separators. Local anesthesia may be needed in certain situations.

Advantages: They are inexpensive; require minimum chair time; minor patient discomfort; patient cooperation is not required; and they possess no risk when swallowed on getting loose.

E. TP springs: They are made of tempered stainless steel wire, usually .018" or .020" in diameter. They can be easily placed in difficult contact areas. The hook of spring is inserted into the lingual embrasure, and the shorter segment is opened with a plier to engage the opposite embrasure. But if a spring is very small, it may result in distortion of the spring and thus opening insufficient space for banding. A larger spring will remain loose and rotate around the contact area, which will cause tissue impingement and providing insufficient space.

F. Nickel titanium separating spring: also known as Neet spring, it was designed by Donald McGann in 1991. Nickel-titanium alloys produce light, continuous forces that are especially beneficial in adult patients.

Configuration of the spring: The configuration of spring should be such that it is easy to place, resistant to getting dislodged, and is able to create adequate amount of space. The vertical legs of the spring are divergent, so that the force against the proximal walls of the adjacent teeth would cause the spring to self-seat in a gingival direction. A hook is made at the end of straighter vertical leg for easy engagement in the lingual embrasure. The opposing vertical leg is angled toward the center for engagement in the buccal embrasure. The optimum wire diameter required is 0.018".

Placement: This spring is placed by holding the straighter vertical leg with a small-beak plier with serrated pads to prevent slippage. The hook is inserted into the lingual embrasure, and then stretched over the contact until the other vertical leg seats fully in the buccal embrasure. It can be placed either lingual-to-buccal or buccal-to-lingual. It can be easily removed with a thin beak plier after inserting a curette or scaler under the occlusal part, then holding with plier and taking it out.

Further Reading

McGann BD: Nickel titanium separating spring: *J Clin Orthod,* 1991 May, 25 (5), 315–18.

32

Preventive Orthodontics

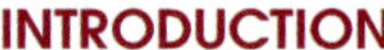

INTRODUCTION

Orthodontics has traditionally been divided in four main branches:

1. Preventive orthodontics
2. Interceptive orthodontics
3. Corrective orthodontics
4. Surgical orthodontics.

With increasing knowledge, surgical facilities, and patients of different age groups seeking orthodontic treatment, two other branches can be added as:

1. Adjunctive orthodontics
2. Adult orthodontics.

The role of orthodontist actually starts from an early age of the child, when he keeps a regular check on his developing dentition, guiding the proper eruption of permanent teeth, saving space for teeth, and preventing the development of malocclusion. A regular check up of child by an orthodontist can help him to avoid a developing condition, as he is able to find out and remove those etiological factors.

Definition

Preventive orthodontics is that branch of orthodontics which includes the procedures undertaken to prevent the development of a malocclusion. Graber has defined **preventive orthodontics as "the actions taken to preserve the integrity of what appears to be normal for that age"**. Since "prevention is always better than cure", an attempt to prevent the developing problem by removal of the causes helps the child in a long run. So, the efforts should be done as early as possible to prevent the development of the malocclusion. Since, the **cause-effect relationship** plays a significant role in development of malocclusion, the timely identification and elimination of the cause can greatly help to prevent development of malocclusion or in reducing the severity of a future malocclusion.

Normal features: Proper knowledge of normal features of dentofacial complex is very important to understand the nature of deviation from the normal occlusion. Diagnosis and evaluation of the case helps in determination of the treatment required.

By diagnosis of the problem and depending on the age of the patient, decision is made whether preventive, interceptive or corrective measures are to be employed. An arbitrary division of such measures has been described depending on the age of the child, but these measures are overlapping depending on the problem. Preventive measures are undertaken in primary dentition period. Interceptive measures are undertaken in mixed dentition, while the corrective measures are taken in permanent dentition. Surgical measures are undertaken in postpubertal period when growth has ceased. Most of these measures generally are used in different age periods depending on the prevailing condition, except major surgical procedures. These measures alone are not always sufficient to control the development of malocclusion and it may require to use a combination of preventive and interceptive, or interceptive and corrective orthodontics measures. Even corrective orthodontics can be divided into:

Limited corrective procedures, which can be provided by a general practitioners (GP) and pedodontist, if they have a knowledge and confidence to perform them.

Extensive corrective procedures, which are to be handled by a qualified orthodontic specialist.

There are some important considerations which must be satisfied to follow the preventive–interceptive orthodontics.

1. The general dentist and pedodontists must have adequate knowledge of growth, occlusion, and normal development of dentition.
2. Patient should be under continual guidance of the dentist.
3. Patient/parental education and motivation should be done on regular basis so that they are able to recognize the developing problem and desire the need for its prevention or correction.
4. Essential diagnostic records should be taken before starting the treatment to help in treatment planning, and to compare the treatment changes.
5. General dentists and pedodontists should refer the patients to orthodontist for management, if the condition of patient is beyond their scope, rather than trying different treatment options for the patient, and thus wasting the valuable time of active growth period of the patient.
6. Regular follow-up of the patient is needed.

Procedures of preventive orthodontics: Certain procedures can be followed during development of dentition depending on the condition of the patient, and these procedures are not limited to primary dentition period only but generally overlap in different phases of dentition:

1. Parent/patient education and counseling.
2. Regular oral health check-up.
3. Caries control especially proximal caries
4. Care of primary dentition
5. Space maintenance
6. Control of oral habits and guidance for muscle exercise.
7. Removal of occsual prematurities.
8. Prevention of damage to occlusion by Milwaukee braces.
9. Management of high attached freni.
10. Extraction of supernumerary teeth.
11. Management of ankylosed tooth.
12. Management of locked first permanent molars, and other teeth
13. Sequential slicing of certain primary teeth to resolve incisor crowding
14. Space maintenance.

Parents' Education and Counseling

Parents' counseling must start before the birth of the child. The expecting mother should be advised to maintain her oral hygiene and take better nutrition, avoid drugs, like tetracycline, smoking, alcohol, steroids, etc. The child should get proper nutrition, and proper nursing. The parents should be advised not to put the child in sleep with milk bottle in his mouth. First visit of the child to dentist should be at around 6 months of age or as soon as the first tooth erupt, with a regular follow up every 6 months. They should clean the teeth of child with a clean cloth or with soft tooth brush at least twice daily. Physiologic nipple should be advised for bottle-fed children. Good oral hygiene maintenance should be emphasized. Correct method of brushing the teeth should be taught. Diet modification; supervision of tooth brushing; and the Pits and fissure sealants should be advised. Fluoride supplements and tooth paste, etc. should be advised to patients living in those areas having deficient fluorides in drinking water. Prolonged use of pacifiers should be prohibited, as it may cause abnormal effect on the bones and teeth of the infant.

Regular Oral Health Check-up

Regular check-up of the teeth of a child is done to look for any caries and to determine the need for any preventive procedure, e.g. in caries prone teeth, pits and fissure sealants should be applied. Proper oral hygiene and brushing should be emphasized. Dietary modification should be emphasized, as to avoid sticky food like chocolates and biscuits, etc. Patients should be prescribed fluoride-containing tooth paste, the dosage prescribed according to their age. In cases of abnormal resorption pattern of the roots, the baby teeth should be extracted when permanent tooth is ready to erupt.

As deciduous teeth are the natural space maintainers for permanent teeth, they should be maintained in healthy condition as far as possible.

Caries Control

Control of caries in primary teeth is of utmost importance. If the proximal caries of the primary teeth is not restored in-time, it leads to loss of arch length. It occurs due to mesial movement of adjacent teeth in the space created by proximal lesion on the tooth. It leads to tooth size-arch length discrepancy when permanent teeth erupt. Also occlusal caries if not controlled, leads to gross loss of crown structure and thus supraeruption may occur. Supraeruption of primary teeth is actually not that alarming as of permanent teeth. Caries may also lead to pulpal involvement needing extensive endodontic procedure and/or removal of teeth and thus requiring space maintenance. Parents should be educated that the primary teeth hold an important role in future development of dentition, occlusion and overall health and psychological benefit for the child and thus should not be neglected. Erupting teeth act as functional matrix for alveolar bone and lead to their growth and increased height.

Maintenance of Tooth Shedding Schedule

A proper knowledge of the schedule and sequence of dental eruption, along with growth of dentofacial complex is very important. The clinician should be aware of **self-correcting/transient malocclusion** conditions during development of dentition, so as not disturb them by mechanical forces. Maintenance of eruption schedule is important to guide the eruption of teeth in proper direction or at least to prevent their eruption in abnormal position, and to reduce severity of the future malocclusion. For this, clinical and radiographic regular check ups are important.

After normal exfoliation of primary tooth, the permanent tooth generally erupts within 3 months. Generally, tooth takes 3 months time to move a distance of 1.0 mm while erupting. There should not be delay of more than 3 months in eruption of permanent tooth after the loss of primary tooth. The primary teeth should not extracted if the tip of permanent tooth is more than 1–2 mm away from the alveolar crest, since most of the space loss after tooth removal occurs within first 6 months. Also, if the primary tooth is removed much before the eruption of permanent tooth, the area, i.e. bone and gingiva become thickened and then the eruption of permanent tooth is delayed or deviated or it may get impacted also. In case of premature extraction of primary tooth, an appropriate space maintainer should be given.

Any obstacle in eruption path should be removed which may be causing the delayed eruption. Some of the common causes are as follows:

1. Over-retained primary teeth or the roots
2. Cyst, granuloma and tumor
3. Supernumerary teeth, odontomes, etc.
4. Fibrosed or thickened gingiva
5. Ankylosed primary teeth
6. Overcontoured or overhanging restorations
7. Tooth stuck below the height of contour of the adjacent tooth
8. Deviated long axis angulation of the tooth

Control of Oral Habits and Guidance for Muscles Exercises

Habits apply abnormal forces on dentofacial structures and lead to maldevelopment. Common habits seen in children are thumb sucking, tongue thrusting and mouth breathing. Thumb or digit sucking habit is considered physiologically normal till 3–3½ years of age. But any prolonged sucking habit should be intervened as it leads to abnormal changes. Parents' education plays a great role in proper nursing. Physiologically designed nipple and pacifier should be recommended. It helps to enhance the normal functional and deglutitional activity. Parents should be educated about the harmful effect of habits and the causes of habits which are generally due to nervous tension in children who feel insecure or neglected.

Muscles exercises: Oral habits are the abnormal functions of the adjacent muscles and soft tissues. To control certain abnormal habits, the retraining of the involved muscles is done to normalize their function. That way, the abnormal forces falling on the adjacent hard tissues are eliminated and the normal growth ensues. Details of the muscle exercises have been discussed separately, e.g. in lip biting, the lip exercises are recommended. For treatment of flaccid perioral musculature, the blowing exercises are advised. For treatment of tongue thrust habit, tongue exercises for proper positioning and swallowing are followed.

Occlusal Equilibration

Functional prematurities are frequently seen during the primary dentition. Most of these are transitory as they appear due to exfoliating primary teeth and eruption of permanent teeth. When the baby tooth becomes loose due to root resorption process, it keeps on paining the child, who then learns to avoid that area during function, leading to deflection in path of closure. Such teeth should be extracted. Functional interferences appearing after the full development of occlusion must be diagnosed and removed. Otherwise they lead to deflected path of closure, abnormal strain on TMJ, establishment of wrong muscular pattern, and thus abnormal growth of jaws and asymmetry of face. Any crossbite in primary dentition should be treated as soon as possible, since crossbite also causes prematurities and associated effects.

The premature contacts can be recognized with articulating paper and the wax bite, and can be grinded away.

Prevention of Damage to Occlusion Caused by Milwaukee Brace

Milwaukee brace is an orthopedic appliance used for treatment of scoliosis. It exerts high force on mandible and the dentition and leads to interference in the growth of mandible, and shifting the teeth. The mandible remains underdeveloped leading to skeletal class II relationship. In such cases, the occlusion should be protected by using functional appliances and regular follow-up is mandatory.

Management of High Attached Freni

In newborn and infants, the maxillary labial frenum is attached to the crest of alveolar ridge, with the fibers of frenum crossing over the alveolar ridge and inserted into incisive papilla. Sometimes, the fibers get actually inserted in intermaxillary suture. It is composed of elastic and collagen fibres, but not any muscle fibres. These fibers retract upwards naturally with eruption of maxillary central incisors and ensuing alveolar growth.

With the eruption of permanent central incisors and alveolar growth, this band of fibres usually gets displaced apical to labial attached gingiva. But in some cases, it does not get displaced and remains inserted in incisive papilla or alveolar crest, leading to creation of midline diastema. In some cases, this band of unyielding fibers is heavier and serves as a barrier to mesial migration of upper central incisors causing midline diastema. Dissecting the frenum fibers from the crest of alveolar ridge in the primary dentition stage may help the diastema to close when the permanent central incisors erupt.

But during mixed dentition, it should not be removed surgically till upper canines have erupted. The erupting canines push the incisors mesially and close the midline space, and pressure atrophy of fibers and retraction. If it is removed surgically at an early time, the scar tissue is formed mainly consisting of elastic fibers which do not allow the closure of space by natural process when permanent teeth erupt.

It can be diagnosed by a strong pull on the upper lip, which causes the appearance of **blanching of the tissue** lingual to the upper incisors, and by displacement of free gingival margin on pulling the lip upward and outwards. Also, notching of the alveolar crest is seen in IOPA view between central incisors due to heavy fibres.

When maxillary midline diastema is diagnosed due to heavy fibres of low-lying frenum in mixed dentition stage, first wait for the eruption of permanent maxillary canines. If the diastema is more than 2–3 mm, then it is expected not to close itself, and thus some other causes of the diastema should be explored and removed. If seen during permanent dentition stage, it should be closed first orthodontically, and then the surgical removal should be done. The process of cutting the frenum is called as frenectomy or **Wanton's clipping**. The entire frenum is surgically removed, with the fibres crossing over the alveolar ridge till their attachment to the incisive papilla.

Scar formed after surgery helps in retaining the closure of space. If surgery is done before the closure, the scar formed which generally consists of elastic fibers, gets bunched up during space closure. It does not let the closed space to be retained and the elastic recoil of scar tissue leads to relapse. Permanent retention should be given in these cases. Sometimes, it may require additional fixed retainer on labial side along with lingual/palatal retainer.

Causes of midline diastema: Such types of freni and midline diastema are generally hereditary. However, before making a final diagnosis and treatment plan, other causes of midline diastema should be ruled out. They are generally microdontia, macrognathia, **midline** supernumerary tooth, peg-shaped lateral incisors, missing lateral incisors, midline cysts, heavy/traumatic occlusion of lower incisors against upper incisors, periodontal shifting and habits as thumb sucking, tongue thrust, lip sucking or nail biting, pin/pen pencil inserting between central incisors, etc. Midline diastema is also seen during the mixed dentition period during ugly-duckling stage.

The lingual frenum connects the base of tongue to the lingual area of symphysis region. If it is long, it may lead to improper speech, improper protrusion of tongue during function and swallowing. It may be called as **ankyloglossia** which may be partial or complete. It may also lead to flaring of lower incisors. It is also seen commonly in infants and new borns, causing problems with suckling. This should be cut as early as possible.

Midline labial frenum in lower arch is rare, but it may also lead to spacing and needs surgical removal.

Extraction of Supernumerary Teeth

Supernumerary teeth are extra teeth other than the usual complement of teeth. They are generally found in permanent dentition. Most commonly they are found in maxillary central incisors region, premolar, distomolar and paramolar region in that order. Supernumerary canines are very rare.

Other odontogenic structures which do not resemble the tooth shape are called **odontomes**. They may be found in any area of dental arches, and may lead to blocking, deflecting or deviating the path of normal eruption of teeth.

It may also cause diastema, e.g. mesiodens lead to midline spacing. To avoid development of malocclusion, they should be extracted at an earliest.

Management of Ankylosed Teeth

Ankylosed teeth are those teeth which get directly joined with the bone with lacking of PDL in some areas. It may happen in primary teeth due to trauma or infection. These teeth do not become loose during normal root resorption process when the permanent teeth are erupting, thus may deflect or prevent permanent teeth from normal eruption path.

They are **diagnosed** by IOPA X-ray; by solid percussion sound as compared to the normal tooth; and by submergence of the ankylosed tooth as compared to the adjacent teeth. **Submerged tooth** has a different level of marginal ridge as compared to normal tooth and is below the occlusal level. This condition should be followed regularly with the help of serial IOPA views to find out the level of root formation of the permanent tooth. They should be extracted at an appropriate time to permit permanent teeth to erupt.

Deeply locked permanent molars: Sometimes, the distal bulge or the height of contour of the distal surface of primary second molars is pronounced, and the permanent first molars get locked below the bulge. It may also happen, if jaw growth is deficient. It prevents the eruption of the molar. In such case, the distal surface should be reduced to relieve the locked tooth. Some cases may require the disimpaction springs or heavy elastic separator to be placed in this area to shift the impacted tooth slightly distally to unlock it. This spring or elastic should be placed under local anesthesia and placement should be confirmed by IOPA view.

Locked erupting tooth: This situation can happen in any part of the dental arch. Mostly first premolars are seen stuck below the mesial contour of primary second molars. Then, the mesial surface is reduced to unlock it. In deficient arch length especially in anterior region, the erupting lateral incisor gets stuck below mesial of primary canine. In such case, the canine should not be extracted but its mesial surface should be grinded to relieve the tooth. Removal of canine at this stage leads to the deficient transverse dimension/inter-canine width.

Locking of the tooth may also occur due to faulty over-contoured filling. In such cases, the over-contoured restoration should be reduced or replaced. Sometimes, the tooth may get locked by the margins of faulty molar bands and thus bands should be recontoured.

Sequential slicing of deciduous teeth to resolve incisor crowding: Many times, the incisors are seen to be crowded while erupting. They require mild spaces to adjust in dental arches. The mandibular lateral incisors are normally seen erupting lingual to the central incisors. Their spontaneous alignment contributes to an increase in mandibular intercanine width. To create the space, the posterior primary teeth are sliced sequentially so that the erupting incisors get in line under the influence of tongue forces. If crowding is mild, then the sequential slicing of posterior deciduous teeth can allow spontaneous alignment of the incisors and also the distal eruption of the canines and premolars, as they distally shift within the alveolar bone during pre-eruption stages during ensuing growth. About 2–3 mm of enamel can be removed from each interproximal surface to be sliced under a water spray.

Space Control/Maintenance

Premature loss of primary tooth may lead to development of malocclusion due to loss/closure of space by shifting of adjacent teeth. It leads to development of TSALD in future. It also leads to changed axial inclination of teeth, shifted midline, spacing, and deviation/impaction of succedaneous teeth. It happens more commonly in posterior quadrants, while in anterior segment, it has only a negative esthetic effect. It becomes important to maintain these spaces to allow proper eruption of permanent teeth in the arch, e.g. if loss of primary second molar occurs, the permanent first molars gets mesially tilted or shifted, leading to partial or complete loss of space for second premolar, which can get either deflected in eruption or impacted. Loss of primary first molar or canine leads to distal shift of anterior segment causing shifted midline, asymmetry of dental arch, and abnormal axial inclination. Loss of incisor generally has no such effect, but leads to speaking problem with escape of air/saliva through the gap, psychological effect and disturbed esthetic effect. To maintain these spaces, the appliances are placed which are known as **space maintainers**, and this procedure is called space maintenance. This topic can be studied in details in the chapter of space management.

Preventive eruption guidance of lower incisors in the 5–7 years old: The most notable characteristics of a malocclusion frequently develop when the deciduous incisors are replaced by the permanent central and lateral incisors. Overbite increases an average of 2 mm, and crowding increases from a 9% incidence in the deciduous dentition to about a 60% incidence in the adult dentition. The increased overbite is probably due to the tendency of lower incisors to erupt lingually, and the upper incisors erupt labially. The increased crowding is due to the bigger MD size of permanent incisors as compared to primary incisors (the permanent lower incisors are 5 mm larger and the permanent upper incisors 7 mm larger than the deciduous teeth, and there may not be enough arch development compensating for this discrepancy. Normally, during eruption, the properly-positioned lateral incisors apply a distal pressure on canines and help in gaining the width esp in mandible. So lack of arch development may be linked to the permanent incisors erupting in rotated or displaced positions, which then minimizes the lateral pressure against adjacent teeth and produces less arch augmentation than would occur if the incisors erupted properly. If some eruption guidance could be provided and if the interincisal width could be increased by only 3 mm, then the subsequent crowding could be eliminated in most of the children.

Nite-Guide appliance: Bergersen (JCO, 1995) introduced prefabricated computer-designed Nite-guide appliance for lower arch, to encourage proper alignment of erupting lower incisors and thereby increase interincisal width. Approx. 3.5 mm of natural arch development during the eruption of incisors is maximized. The two Nite-Guide appliances are based on a normal expectation of 1.5 mm of arch widening as the lower permanent central incisors erupt, and another 2 mm as the lower laterals erupt. The appliance is of two types: the "C" series is used during eruption of mandibular central incisors, and the "G" series is used when mandibular lateral incisors begin to erupt. "C" appliance is 1.6 mm wider than the available space in the incisor segment, and the "G" appliance is another 2.4 mm wider. This appliance is worn only while sleeping. So a total of 4.0 mm of width can be gained with them.

Timing of treatment is critical, particularly for correction of crowding. Postponing appliance wear until the permanent incisors are fully erupted would fail to take advantage of the potential for natural arch development.

Sequential Slicing of Lower Deciduous Teeth to Resolve Incisor Crowding

Lower incisor crowding in the mixed dentition can often be resolved, if treatment is initiated early enough. Some procedures have been recommended for this situation, e.g. serial extractions; extraction of the deciduous canines, followed by use of a lingual space maintainer; lip bumpers; and fixed appliances. The common methods for treating crowding in mixed dentition have disadvantages. Serial extraction decreases arch length and deepens the bite. Extraction of primary canines and cementation of a lingual space maintainer can be time-consuming, costly, involves at least two appointments and laboratory expenses. A removable lip bumper has the same shortcomings as a fixed lingual arch, and needs patient compliance. Sequential slicing of deciduous teeth can help to create some space for the erupting permanent teeth without needing any appliance or patient cooperation. The mandibular lateral incisors normally erupt lingual to central incisors, and their spontaneous alignment contributes to an increase in intercanine width. Excessive enamel removal would prevent the normal intercanine widening. If crowding is moderate (2–6 mm), sequential slicing of posterior deciduous teeth can allow spontaneous alignment of incisors and distal eruption of canines and premolars. The thickness of enamel and health of the teeth to be sliced is judged, the enamel is removed using a copious spray of warm water. To avoid sensitivity, the deciduous tooth should not be sliced until at least half the root has been resorbed. Topical fluoride should be applied, and a fluoride-containing toothpaste should be prescribed after slicing. Sequential slicing of deciduous teeth is simple and only mildly invasive. It requires no patient cooperation and no long-term appliance supervision. When at least half of the deciduous root has been resorbed, there is virtually no dental sensitivity.

Conclusion

Preventive procedures help to prevent the development of an abnormal condition, if diagnosed early. Certain procedures as discussed above but not limited to them, are useful during the development of dentofacial complex. A proper diagnosis and knowledge of growth and development is mandatory so that clinician can timely diagnose and treat, and/or refer the case to appropriate facility.

Further Readings

1. Taken from the JCO on CD-ROM (Copyright © 1997 JCO, Inc.), Volume 1995 Jun(382–395): Preventive Eruption Guidance in the 5-to-7-Year-Old EARL O. BERGERSEN, DDS, M.
2. Taken from the JCO on CD-ROM (Copyright © 1997 JCO, Inc.), Volume 1994 Oct(596–599): **Sequential Slicing of Lower Deciduous Teeth** to Resolve Incisor Crowding - MARCO ROSA, MD, DMD, MAURO COZZANI, DMD, MSCD, GIUS.

33

Interceptive Orthodontics

INTRODUCTION

Certain procedures can be used by orthodontist to intercept a developing malocclusion to reduce the severity of the condition. When exchange of teeth occurs from primary to mixed dentition, certain problems may be seen. Some of these problems may be **self-correcting/transient malocclusion** which should not be disturbed by mechanical appliances. But certain problems are associated with certain causes leading to development of malocclusion. If left untreated, severity of these conditions can increase which later on need comprehensive orthodontic intervention. So to prevent these conditions to develop in severe problems, certain procedures can be used to intercept them and change the course of their development towards normalcy. The causes leading to these conditions are also removed.

Definition

Interceptive orthodontics may be defined as "the procedures employed to recognize and eliminate developing or developed malpositions in the early stages of developing dentofacial complex". In comparison to preventive orthodontic procedures, the interceptive actions are undertaken at the time when the malocclusion is developing or has already developed. These treatment procedures are generally used during mixed dentition period esp during developing dentition and active growth phases.

The parents see the change of teeth from milk to permanent teeth, and see lot of unusual positional and size differences of teeth, and thus get worried. Practically speaking, the majority of patients visiting the orthodontist are of adolescent age group, or in mid to late MDP, it is the main time when the orthodontist sees most of the orthodontic problems. At this age, the active growth of jaws is still undergoing and the growth spurts are expected. Suitable treatment procedures which help in normalising the growth and dentition development and reducing their severity can be employed during this phase. So, interceptive orthodontics is the most important phase of treatment from the patient's and the clinician's perspective. It is the phase when most successful and stable changes can be achieved at the skeletal level, taking advantage of growth. Once the active growth is over, the changes just get limited to dental changes with very little or no skeletal changes.

The preventive and interceptive orthodontic procedures are used during the dentition development; however, preventive procedures are used when dentition and occlusion are normal, while interceptive procedures are followed when the malocclusion starts appearing. Some of preventive procedures can also be used during interceptive phase, because the management of malocclusion is an ongoing process, and certain procedures can be used as overlapping in both phases.

Mechanism of maldevelopment: The growth of dentofacial complex is at its peak during the mixed dentition stage, and the growth spurts appear during this stage. Factors interfering with normal growth lead to development of skeletal problems. Similarly, since the teeth exchange is occurring, the factors which lead to disturbed eruption lead to dental malocclusion. Factors leading to disturbance in muscular patterns and growth disturbance lead to abnormal growth. Factors causing malocclusion can be studied in the chapter devoted to etiology of malocclusion.

Procedures Followed during Interceptive Orthodontics

Certain procedures followed during interceptive phase are as follows:

1. Treatment of developing anterior crossbite
2. Treatment of developing posterior crossbite: transverse problems, e.g. constricted upper or lower arch/ segment.
3. Control of abnormal habits: See Chapter 47 on Oral Habits
4. Serial extraction or guidance of eruption: See Chapter 34 on Serial Extraction
5. Space regaining
6. Muscle retraining and exercises
7. Interception of skeletal malrelation: Expansion, FJO, chin cup, reverse face mask, etc.
8. Growth modification
9. Removal of dental, soft tissue or bony barrier to enable dental eruption
10. Treatment of premature contacts.

Correction of Developing Crossbite

Normally there is a positive overjet all round the dentition, with labial/buccal surface of upper teeth are slightly labial to the labial surfaces of lower teeth. Crossbite is an abnormal relation of teeth in which labial surface of upper tooth is lingual to the labial surface of lower tooth in anterior region. It may be anterior or posterior or combined. In posterior segment, it may vary that buccal surface of upper teeth may be lingual to that of lower tooth, or buccal surface of lower tooth may lie palatal to palatal surface of upper tooth. It may involve single tooth or multiple teeth or full segment or full arch.

Treatment of developing anterior crossbite: Anterior crossbite should be treated as early as possible. It can be classified as follows:

1. Dentoalveolar crossbite
2. Skeletal crossbite
3. Combination of above two
4. Functional crossbite.

Dentoalveolar crossbite (Fig. 33.1): It is the condition involving abnormal relation of teeth only, with skeletal jaw bases in normal relation. In this condition, the one or more upper incisors lie lingual to lower incisor, i.e. in a reverse overjet condition. It generally occurs when the primary tooth/teeth get retained in the dental arch, with the permanent tooth erupting lingual to it. Since the permanent teeth buds develop lingual to the primary teeth, they erupt lingual to primary teeth. But if primary tooth gets retained in the dental arch, the permanent tooth erupts in a lingual relation, thus in the crossbite. Sometimes, the supernumerary tooth or the greater MD width of adjacent teeth especially maxillary central incisors, may also do not allow the erupting tooth to come in the arch and thus they (maxillary lateral incisors) erupt in lingual position. Upper canines are generally the last succedaneous teeth to erupt in oral cavity, since they have to travel a longest path of eruption. If they do not have proper space, they may get deflected either labially or palatally. Palatal eruption leads to their crossbite. Crossbite also leads to gingival and esthetic problems.

Effects of crossbite: Crossbite leads to deflection of condyle on the opposite side, forcing its posterior temporalis muscle to become more active. Due to muscular imbalance, the mandible becomes significantly longer on the non-crossbite side than on the crossbite side. Condyle on non-crossbite side is located forward and downward in the glenoid fossa, while on the crossbite side, it is

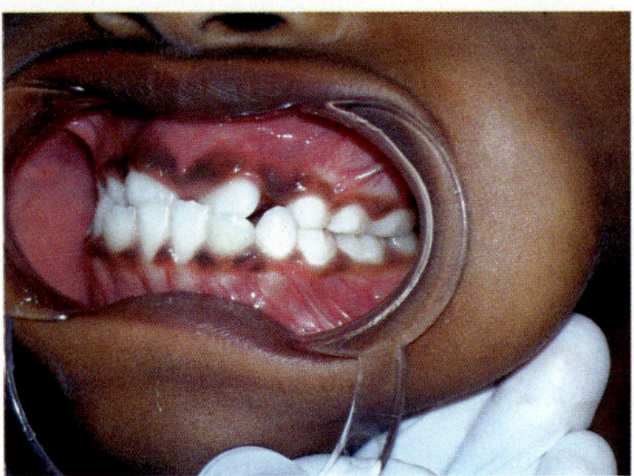

Fig. 33.1: Anterior crossbite in mixed dentition and mesial step, due to maxillary deficiency.

positioned upward and backward, and has a narrower and shorter condyle head. The TMJs adapt to this abnormal displacement of mandible by condylar growth and surface remodelling of the fossae, leading to asymmetry of face and dental arches. Therefore, early crossbite treatment is important to achieve normal growth and development, and but also to help prevent TMD.

Rationale of treatment: Such teeth should be relieved of crossbite otherwise since there is locking of the jaws, the proper growth in the affected dentoalveolar region will be defective. A single tooth crossbite in the incisal region leads to the locking of jaw which may lead to deficient sagittal growth of maxillary region. Also, since the mandible is deflected forward to come in centric occlusion with a crossbite, it comes forward than its normal position, which may lead to an excessive sagittal growth of mandible.

Crossbite in canine region leads to a deficient transverse growth in that region. It also leads to laterally-deflected path of closure and asymmetry developing in face/dental arch and midline shifts. If there is segmental cross bite involving all the incisors/anteriors, then mandible is free to grow sagittaly as it does not have a controlling effect of maxillary incisors, and may overshoot the maxilla; and maxillary growth is inhibited, leading to skeletal class III in long run.

Treatment: The treatment/design of the appliance depends on the level of incisal edge. First of all, the causative retained tooth should be removed. If the incisal edges have not crossed as yet, the tongue pressure is expected to push the tooth in question forwards to a better position in the arch. Otherwise, it can be treated with appliances, like tongue blade; Catalan's appliance; maxillary appliance with Z-spring and the posterior bite plate; an expansion screw appliance; Planas Direct Tracks (PDTs); a sectional fixed appliance, etc. Details will be discussed in future chapter on treatment of crossbites.

In small children, especially in primary dentition, who generally do not use the appliances, the crossbite occlusion can be relieved by bonding composite resin on the occlusal surfaces of the primary second molars, thus unlocking the maxilla, and just relieving the crossbite. The ensuing dental eruption of permanent teeth; growth of jaws and the tongue pressure generally helps in relieving the crossbite.

Developing skeletal crossbite: It is due to abnormal relation or development of upper and/or lower jaws due to their abnormal growth. It can be due to maxillary retrognathism or mandibular prognathism or a combination of both. They can vary in severity as mild, moderate and severe. Mild to moderate forms can be treated or improved by using orthopedic appliances during the growth period. Severe forms need orthognathic surgeries after active growth is over. These appliances help in redirecting the growth in a favorable direction.

Treatment of maxillary retrognathism: If mandible is normal, the deficient maxilla is to be pulled forward and downward to create normal skeletal relation. This condition is generally seen in cases of CLP. In other cases, it is hereditary. The appliance used is reverse face mask (RFM). Since maxillary anterior growth mostly occurs during 8–9 years age, it is the best age to tackle this condition. A phase of RME is given just before RFM therapy to activate the circummaxillary sutural system.

Treatment of mandibular prognathism: If maxilla is normal, but mandible growth is excessive, then it is controlled with chin cup appliance. Chin cup applies an upward and backward force, passing through the condyle and preventing its excessive growth. Since mandible keeps on growing sagitally till 16–18 years of age, the chin cup needs to be used intermittently till that age as a retentive/ maintaining appliance, especially night time wear can be advised. If any surgery is required to correct this condition, it is done only after growth has ceased. Details can be studied in the chapter of dentofacial orhtopedics.

Functional crossbite: It occurs due to premature contacts in incisor region, leading to forward functional shift of mandible in a crossbite situation. This is called as **pseudo-class III** condition. When examined in rest position and at the point of first contact during slow closure, the exact skeletal relation, CR, of jaws and teeth can be found out, which is generally normal. When patient closes in CO position, there is anterior shift of mandible closing in a crossbite. This condition should be treated as early as possible, since this pseudo-crossbite situation will turn in an actual/skeletal crossbite with the ensuing mandibular growth, as there is no anterior check point for the mandible. Treatment can be done first by removal of prematurities. Then the upper anteriors can be pushed labially to overlap the lower incisors, thus locking mandible in normal overbite relation. In cases having spaces in lower incisor region, the lower incisors can be brought lingually to treat crossbite relation while spaces are also closed.

Treatment of developing posterior crossbite: In primary or mixed dentitions, sometimes posterior crossbite is seen, which can be unilateral or bilateral. It can be dental or skeletal. Generally, the skeletal posterior crossbite is bilateral, but appears unilateral in the CO position due to shifting of mandible to one side as patient tries to close in maximum intercuspation. When the patient is diagnosed in rest position or at the point of first contact, the actual crossbite appears bilateral. It is due to narrow maxillary arch or jaw base. The treatment is expansion of upper arch. Since at 8–9 years age, a spurt in the transverse maxillary growth occurs, it is the best time to use expansion appliances.

If lower arch is narrow, then it should be expanded. The intercanine width in lower arch increases by 9 years of age only, after that there is no much change. Any attempt to increase the intercanine width is prone to relapse and needs permanent fixed retainers. Mandible does not have any sutures, so skeletal expansion is not expected but only dentoalveolar expansion is achieved. Studies have shown that when dental arches with primary teeth are expanded, the tooth buds of permanent teeth also follow the primary teeth in new position and later on erupt in a normal relationship with opposing teeth. The details of expansion can be studied in chapter devoted to expansion.

Treatment of Habits

Abnormal habits put abnormal pressure on the teeth and the jaws, thus disturbing the normal muscular balance around the developing dentoskeletal tissues. It thus leads to abnormal growth and development of abnormal relationships. Main habits affecting the occlusion and growth are thumb sucking, mouth breathing and tongue thrusting habits. Along with, the muscular retraining exercises are also advised to patient to change the neuromuscular pattern and assist the mechanical appliance to achieve habit correction. The ENT specialist is also consulted to rule out or treat the nasal or pharyngeal/tonsils problem to treat mouth breathing habit. The details and management can be seen in the chapter on habits.

Trainer appliances: These are the prefabricated single piece appliances made of soft polyacrylic plastic material, the same used to make TMD/night guard appliances. It has been formed by Myoresearch co. It is a single piece appliance, with upper and lower parts fixed in class I relationship. It is used during formative years of dentition, i.e. early-mid MDP. It has many features incorporated to achieve specific treatment goals. It helps to prepare the patients and dental arches for future orthodontic treatment, by reducing the severity of the condition. Thus it acts as an interceptive appliance. Its another modification can be used in conjunction with braces so that the trauma to soft tissues is avoided.

Features of the trainer appliances: Certain features have been incorporated in the trainer appliance to help achieve the treatment objectives:

- **Tongue tag:** It helps in positioning of tongue tip.
- **Tongue guard:** It helps in prevention of tongue thrusting.
- **Lip bumper projections:** They help in reducing the hyperactivity of mentalis muscle.
- **Grooves for braces:** The braces get their place there and thus do not irritate soft tissues.
- **Grooves for the dental arches:** The upper and lower dental arches occupy these grooves and thus help in achieving the class I jaw relation.

Clinical applications: It can be used for many clinical situations:

Open mouth posture and habit correction: Tongue tag helps in active training for positioning of tongue tip in a normal fashion. Tongue guard helps in prevention of tongue thrusting and forces the child to breathe through the nose, thus helping to correct mouth breathing. Since it is a single piece appliance with no opening in the front region, it acts like an oral screen to prevent and to treat the mouth breathing habit. The correction of mouth breathing is one of the most important factors in maintaining maxillary arch expansion. Lip bumpers are small projections on the labial area of lower part of the appliance and they discourage overactive mentalis muscle activity by irritating the soft tissues of lower lip.

Class I jaw positioning: It helps in attaining a class I jaw relation as most functional appliances, and helps in class II correction by forward positioning of mandible. The combination of prevention of tongue thrusting and changing mode of breathing assists class II correction.

Class II correction: A combination of preventing the tongue thrusting and helping to achieve a normal mode of breathing helps in class II correction. It helps to achieve some passive arch expansion, since its shape is somewhat of normal arch form, which applies a low degree of pressure on the dental arches. It is fabricated in an edge to edge class I position, thus making it effective in class II correction, by bringing the mandible in a forward position.

Expansion of arches: Shape of the appliance is in a normal arch form, so it helps in achieving the normal arch form. It also helps in expansion of narrow arches and thus gaining space for alignment of irregular teeth during eruption, by directing them in the buccal direction during use.

Correction of arch form: Since the appliance is fabricated in a natural form, it allows the teeth to align and erupt in a normal arch form. It applies light forces on the teeth which are out of alignment, and moves them in the arch. Also it helps in developing the arches shape, and form, as the forces applied on teeth move them in the arch. For example, in developing class II division 2 case, it can help to move upper central incisors slightly labially and the lateral incisors lingually in the arch by applying light forces on them. Also, the lower incisors align themselves in the lower arch influenced by the lower part of the appliance.

Combine fixed and functional phases: As discussed above, it allows both functional and fixed appliance phases to occur simultaneously. The T4B™ helps to eliminate detrimental forces by myofunctional training during fixed appliance therapy.

Treatment and prevention of TMJ problems: TMJ disorder is generally present in many cases before treatment starts, which can be difficult to treat during fixed appliance therapy. The occlusal changes produced by orthodontic treatment can precipitate acute TMJ symptoms. Evidences show that the orthodontic treatment is not a cause of TMD. The T4B™ has an in-built soft TMJ splint to assist in treatment of this disorder. It has a 3.2 mm thick posterior section, while the anterior section is 2 mm thick, which helps in TM joint decompression.

Bruxism treatment: This appliance has an intervening occlusal bite which helps to control bruxism. It discludes the dentition and decreases abnormal functional forces on dentition and thus prevents the attrition, etc. It also facilitates faster tooth movement by removing the influence of interlocking occlusal forces due to bruxism.

Prevent soft tissue trauma during braces: Trauma to soft tissues occurs during first few days of fixed appliances placement. The T4B™ covers the braces and thus prevents the trauma.

Recommended minimum use: The patient is advised to use them **for at least** 1 hour daily plus overnight during sleeping. With time, he can increase the time of use, depending on the comfort and adjustment to the appliance for better and early results. He should be advised to keep it clean by using a tooth brush 2–3 times a day.

Serial Extraction (Figs 33.2 and 33.3)

Due to decreasing size of the jaws, many children face the problem of developing crowding, which becomes evident at an early age, i.e. around 7–8 years of age. Mostly, the lower incisors are seen erupting in crowded position. The premature exfoliation of primary lower canine is a sure-shot sign of developing crowding. This problem is compounded by deficient growth of the jaws and thus the absence of developmental spaces in dental arches. It leads to development of severe TSALD. If this process is allowed to continue without treatment, then the permanent teeth either erupt in extreme crowding state or some of them may remain impacted in the jaws. In order to reduce the severity of such a condition,

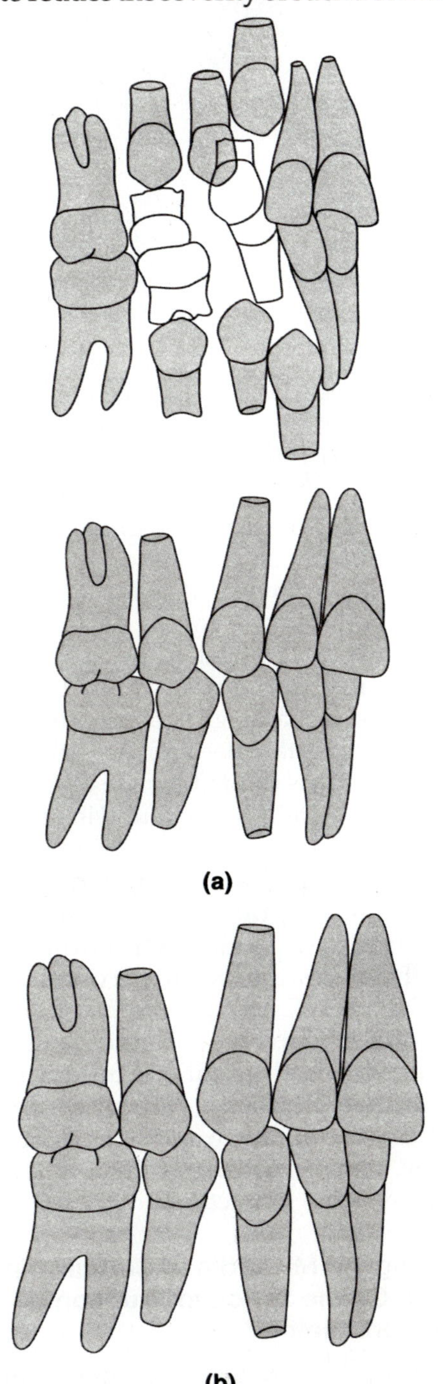

Figs 33.2a and b: (a) Space deficiency during tooth eruption, (b) Alignment of teeth after removal of first premolars as serial extraction treatment.

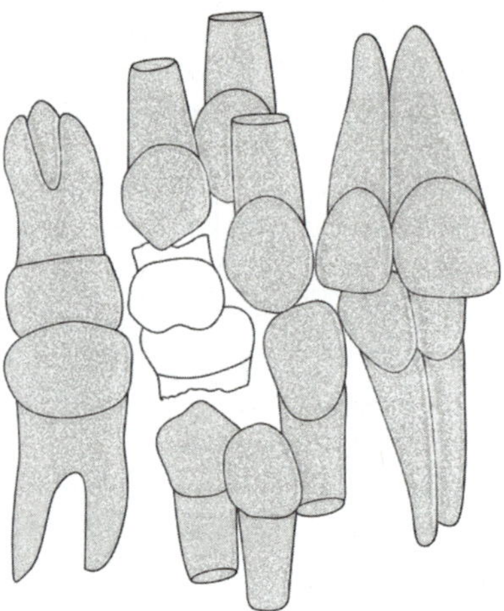

Fig. 33.3: Sever space deficiency in both arches leading to impaction of first premolars which has to be corrected by serial extraction of first premolars *(Redrawn from Graber for academic purpose).*

an interceptive procedure to guide the teeth in the dental arches and to reduce the severity of crowding is followed. It is known as **serial extraction**. It is the process which involves timely and sequential removal of certain primary and permanent teeth to help in alignment of remaining teeth in better position. By removing certain permanent teeth from the jaws, the space is created for the other teeth to come in line. Details can be found in the chapter of serial extraction.

However, it has been redefined as **guidance of eruption** in recent orthodontic literature. Since serial extraction process typically follows the set pattern of extractions, i.e. CD4 or D4C. But guidance of eruption process takes into account other factors, like the stage of root formation; position of the erupting teeth in the jaws; location of crowding, etc. and then decision of extraction is made. It does not necessarily follow the set pattern of serial extraction.

Reducing the MD Width of Certain Primary Teeth to Create Space for Eruption of Permanent Teeth

Due to deficient space in the dental arches, sometimes the permanent teeth are seen as struggling to erupt in the arch. It is mostly seen in the premolar and canine regions, e.g. lower lateral incisor being prevented by mesial of primary canine to erupt due to space deficiency in closed dentition. The erupting tooth is seen as stuck below the curvature/ HOC of the adjacent primary tooth. In such cases, if the space need is mild, then rather than extracting a tooth, the HOC of the proximal surface of the offending tooth is reduced to provide space for the erupting tooth. It helps in prevention of the deflected eruptive path of the tooth, and helps to reduce the severity of the malposition of teeth. In such cases, ensuing growth in transverse and sagittal dimension is expected to overcome future space deficiency also, esp in late-growing patients.

Space Regaining

Primary teeth perform an important function to maintain space for the permanent teeth in the dental arch. But after premature loss of primary teeth and non-maintenance of that space, the ensuing space loss leads to TSALD. It can lead to deflected path of eruption or impaction of permanent teeth. In cases of minor to moderate discrepancy, the space can be regained to align the erupting teeth in the normal arch without extraction of some teeth. The process of gaining the lost space is called space regaining. However, the decision of regaining the space depends on a number of factors, e.g. molar relation, growth status and pattern, soft tissue morphology, patient cooperation, etc. Generally, the major space loss is observed after the ***premature loss of primary second molars*** when the permanent first molars move mesially, and also the first premolars move distally in the space. Some space opening may be seen mesial to first premolars which becomes advantageous while regaining the space. The space regaining cannot be applied in all patients. But if required, it is best to perform at an early age before the eruption of second molars. Once second molars reach a higher level of eruption, it becomes difficult to push both the molars distally. Some of the commonly used space regainers are as follows. For the sake of simplification, they have been discussed in context of loss of primary second molar. They may be of removable or fixed types.

1. **Gerber's space regainer** (Fig. 33.4): A snugly fitted band is fabricated on the permanent first molar, and U-shaped hollow tube is soldered/welded in the mesial aspect of the band. A U-shaped wire which can freely slide in the tube is adapted which touches below the HOC of the distal surface of the tooth mesial to the space. An open coil spring of adequate length and diameter is slid in between the tube and the wire and the assembly is cemented in place, thus activating the spring. The force generated by the OCS helps to regain the space. It mostly occurs by distal movement of the first molar, since the teeth mesial to the space act as anchorage unit. The appliance should be maintained till the eruption of the tooth meant for that area.
2. **Removable appliance with a Jack screw:** A small-sized expansion screw is fitted in the acrylic removable appliance and cuts are placed in such a way that the forces are directed to the first molar to move it distally. The larger part of the appliance acts as anchorage.
3. **Sectional fixed appliance:** This design has been suggested by Goyal (Impressions, 2002). The bands are placed on the teeth mesial and distal to the space. A molar tube is placed on the distal band and an edge wise bracket is placed on the mesial band. The SS archwire of at least 0.018" size is placed in between the bands such that is extends approx. 5 mm beyond the buccal tube. A section of NiTi OCS of 1.5 times the length of the space is placed on the wire. The appliance is cemented in place, thus activating the OCS. The coil spring pushes the teeth away from the space and regains the space. The appliance should be maintained till the erupting tooth comes in line (Fig. 33.6).
4. **Removable appliance with finger springs:** Springs in hard SS wire are adapted on the teeth mesial and distal to the space and acrylised. They are activated on delivering the appliance to the patient and regular follow up is done (Figs 33.5 to 33.7).
5. **Lip bumper:** It can be used when there is hyperactive mentalis, along with some space loss mesial to first molars. It is placed with the bands on molars. The forces produced by lower lip are directed to the molars and thus help to upright the molars, and it also retrains the mentalis muscle to achieve a normal tonicity (Figs 33.8 and 33.9).
6. **Active lingual arch:** A lingual holding arch with U-loops can be used as a bilateral space regainer. The U-loops can be activated and cemented. Further activation can be done intraorally also. The anterior part resting on the cinguli of anterior teeth acts as anchorage, while the first moalrs are distally uprighted.
7. **Active NiTi wire segment:** A longer segment of 0.016" NiTi wire segment is bonded on the 2 teeth mesial to the space. A blob of composite is placed on the etched surface of the tooth distal to space and a notch/canal is created in it. This notch will receive the other free end of the NiTi wire. After curing it, the free end of the segment of wire is inserted in this notch. Since the wire segment is longer, the wire gets activated and applies the forces to regain the space. Negi, and JCO article.

Muscle Exercises or Muscle Retraining

Soft tissues act as functional matrix for growth of face according to Moss' theory. Balance of muscular forces plays a great role in the development of normal dentoskeletal pattern, in consonance with the ensuing growth. The buccinator mechanism, i.e. muscular forces of tongue from inside, and of cheeks and lips from outside, helps in moulding the dental arches in a proper shape. Also, there are masticatory muscles, lingual muscles, pharyngeal and hyoid muscles which all have mutual interaction for developing proper dentoskeletal relations.

Any imbalance in the equilibrium of the forces of muscles leads to abnormal shaping of dental arches and abnormal relation of jaw bases, e.g. abnormal oral habits. Growth pattern of the patient is also affected which further leads to deterioration of muscular balance. If this abnormal muscular pattern is not controlled by retraining the involved muscles at an early age, the pattern becomes fixed in the neuromuscular circuits, and then it becomes difficult to establish the new pattern as the age advances.

Muscles exercises for masseter muscle: To strengthen the masseter, the patient is asked to clench the teeth and count upto 10. It should be repeated for some duration of time.

Exercises for circumoral/lip muscles: Some patients have small upper lip thus the lips are incompetent. Also, some may have lip biting habits. If the soft tissue growth is still continuing (it generally continues upto 16 years of age), then timely lip exercises can give good results. Following exercises can be taught to the patient:

1. Upper lip can be stretched to maintain a lip seal with the lower lip, especially if upper lip is small or hypotonic. Alternatively, the patient can be asked to hold a piece of paper between the lips. They can be asked to over-stretch the upper lip and then the lower lip is extended above the upper lip to cover it and hold it for count upto 10. This exercise can be repeated many times per day.
2. Patients can improve by playing flute, as it brings both the lips in approximation and thus helps to increase the tonicity and length of the lips. Inflating the balloons is also a good exercise for the same purpose.
3. Patient can be asked to hold water in mouth for 10 sec and then repeat the exercise. He can also be told to pump the water back and forth behind the lips to stretch them.

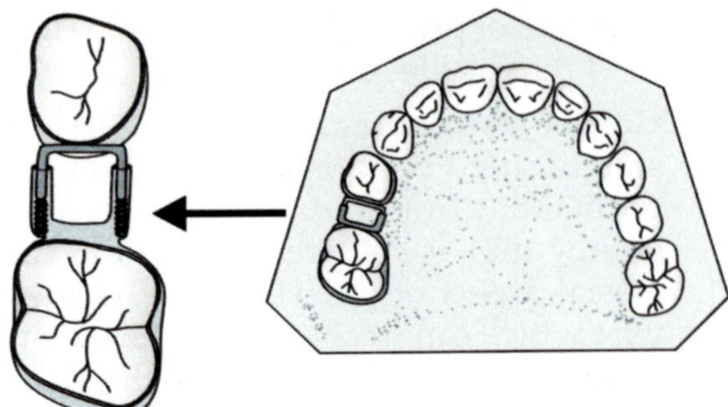

Fig. 33.4: Fixed space regainer: Gerber's space regainer.

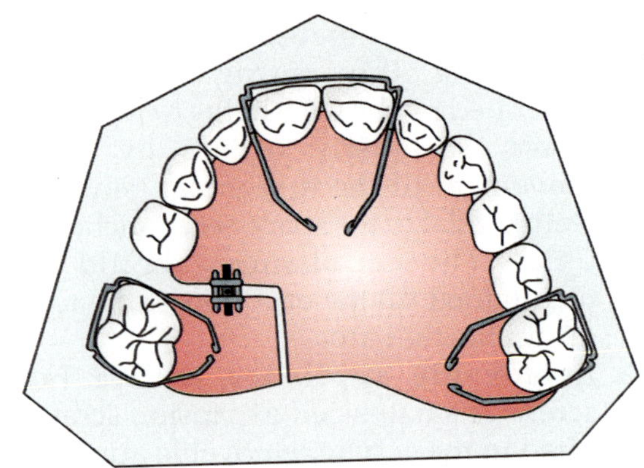

Fig. 33.5: Removable appliance with finger springs at molar region to gain the space by distal movement of molar.

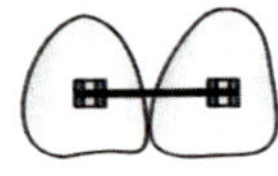

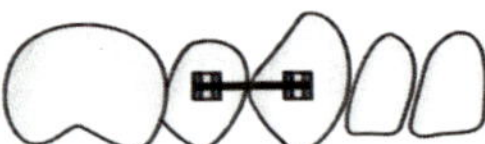

Fig. 33.6: Segmental fixed space regaining appliance with open coil spring to open space for impacted/unerupted second premolar.

4. Patient can be asked to stretch the upper lip towards the chin.
5. Massaging the upper lip in downward direction can also help in stretch.
6. Button pull exercise: A big button of approx 1½ inch diameter with a strong thread through it is used. It is placed behind the lips in the vestibule and hold

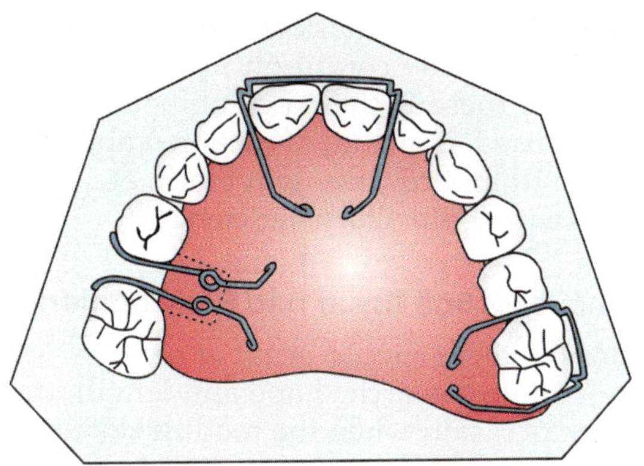

Fig. 33.7: Removable appliance with finger springs at molar region to gain the space by distal movement of molar.

by the lips. The thread is used to pull it outward, while the lips restrain it from being pulled outside.

7. Tug of war exercises: It uses two buttons in the same fashion as above, one button is inside and other is outside for pulling.

Exercises for tongue: Tongue is a very strong and important muscle in oral cavity. It helps in speech, mastication, swallowing, etc. It also helps in molding the dental arches in proper shape, by maintaining equilibrium of forces with extraoral muscles of cheeks and lips. Many habits disturb this equilibrium, e.g. tongue thrust, thumb sucking and mouth breathing habits. Tongue thrust is a habit in which the patient does not keep the tongue in proper position during swallowing and comes sliding between the teeth causing open bite. Sometimes, open bite leads to development of this habit. This vicious cycle goes on till an abnormal position is established. Some of tongue exercises can be used as given below:

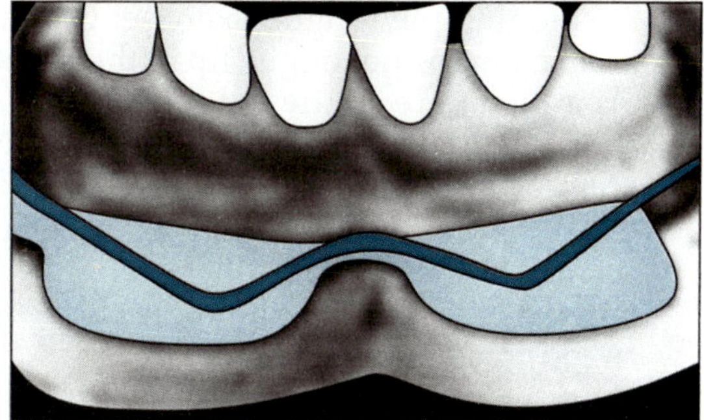

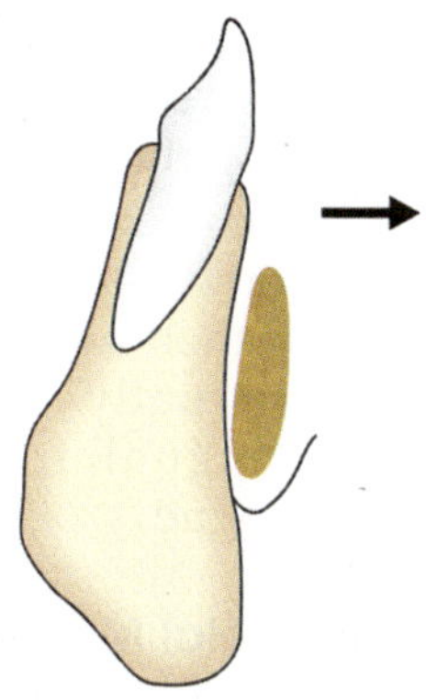

Fig. 33.9: Location of lip bumper in the depth of labial vestibule. It helps to relieve the active forces of lip falling on lower incisors, which then can flare under the influence of tongue forces.

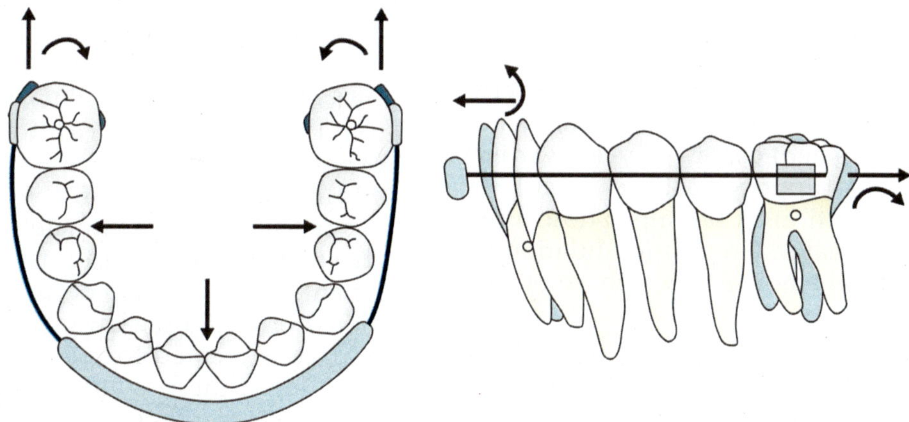

Fig. 33.8: Lip bumper and its effects on the dental arch and the terminal molars.

1. Positioning the tongue exercise: Patient is asked to fix the tongue tip in the rugae area of palate while swallowing. He should attempt not to slide the tongue anteriorly while swallowing.
2. One elastic swallow: It is same as above. A small elastic is placed on the tongue tip and patient is asked to hold the elastic in rugae area and swallow.
3. Two-elastic swallow: One elastic is placed at tip and other in the midline of tongue. Patient is asked to raise his tongue against the palate and then swallow keeping the elastic in position.
4. Hold pull exercise: The patient is asked to keep the tip and mid of tongue against the palate and then he is asked to open the mouth gradually. It also helps to stretch the lingual frenum, beside training the tongue.

Interception of Skeletal Malrelation

An early problem of skeletal malrelation can be intercepted with growth modulation procedures. It helps to reduce the severity of malocclusion and helps in attaining the normal relation of skeletal structures.

Skeletal class II malrelation: It can be due to more growth of maxilla or less growth of mandible or combination of both. Maxillary growth can be restricted by head gear, while mandibular growth can be stimulated with functional appliances. Since the active growth is essential for getting good results, the age at which peak growth is taking place at the time of peak height velocity (PHV), it is the best time to intercept the abnormal growth pattern. Pubertal growth spurts in females (at approx 10 years age) come 2–3 years earlier than the males (at approx. 12–13 years age). So growth modulation in females should be started before males. Growth modulation is started during the acceleration phase of the growth spurt.

Skeletal class III malrelation: This relation is opposite of class II. It can be due to increased mandibular growth or deficient maxillary growth. Chin cup is used for former while reverse face mask is used for the latter condition. If the condition involves combination of these 2, then a combination appliance is used. Some myofunctional appliance, e.g. FR III and reverse twin block, etc. can be used to treat maxillary deficiency.

Removal of Soft Tissue and Bony Barriers

Since the teeth should erupt at a proper time to maintain the arch shape and length, there can be occasion when the tooth is not able to erupt due to certain barriers. Over-retained primary tooth, supernumerary tooth, etc. should be checked. In cases where the primary tooth is lost prematurely, the soft tissue and bony thickening occurs there which act as a barrier to eruption of tooth and delays the eruption. Soft tissue and bony barriers should be removed surgically to stimulate the dental eruption. A surgical opening is made which is larger than the MD size of the tooth. Soft tissue and bone overlying the tooth is removed by surgical excision. Electrocautery can be used if only soft tissue needs removal since there is no bleeding with it. Patient is advised to keep good oral hygiene and he may be prescribed analgesics and/or antibiotics.

Removal of Certain Primary Teeth to Enhance or Redirect Eruption of Permanent Teeth (Figs 33.10 and 33.11)

Most of the times, the problems are seen during the eruption of maxillary canines. Canines develop very high in the jaw near the nasal floor and traverse a long path of eruption. They are mostly the last succedaneous teeth to erupt. Ugly-duckling stage is observed during their eruption. During development, the axial inclination of canine to the midline increases until the maximum angle is reached at approximately 9 years of age. It starts straightening as horizontal movement of its tip/cusp occurs in a distal direction due to ongoing jaw growth and thus more space is created for adjustment in its position. But, if there is an excessive mesial inclination to the midline or the tooth overlaps the root of adjacent incisors, then it is

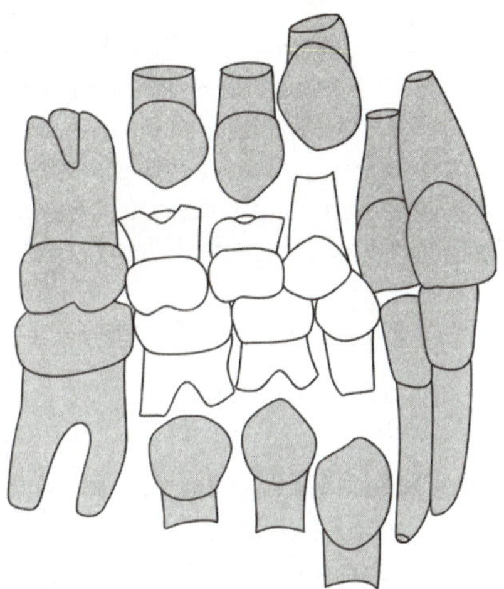

Fig. 33.10: Normal dental eruption in the arches when there is adequate space *(Redrawn from Graber for academic purpose).*

suspected to follow an incorrect eruption path. In such a situation, preventive approaches to re-establish physiologic eruption process is followed to decrease the risk of canine impaction or root resorption of permanent teeth.

Preventive treatment of ectopically erupting maxillary permanent canines by extraction of deciduous canines and first molars has been recommended to promote the eruption of malposed canines, and/or to help in natural uprighting of the canines. Removal of deciduous first molar accelerates eruption and promotes uprighting of first premolar, thus stimulating the correct eruption of the permanent canine by providing more space for the physiologic uprighting of canine crown in a distal direction into alveolar bone.

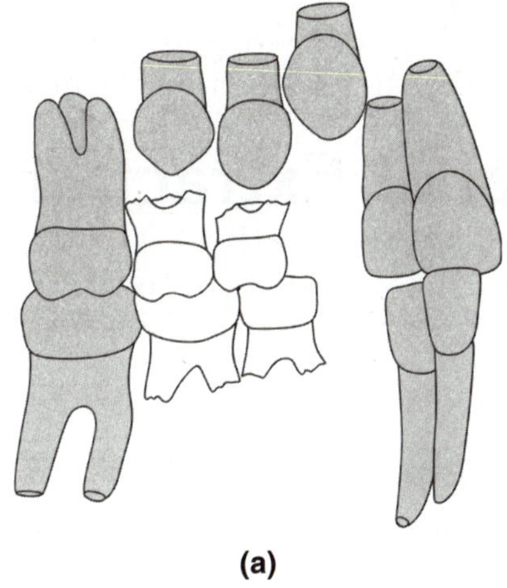

(a)

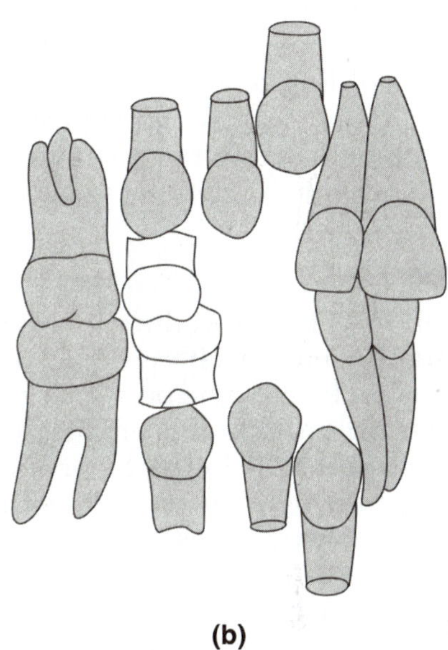

(b)

Figs 33.11a and b: Eruption of canines and first premolars after loss of their counterparts in a dental arch *(Redrawn from Graber for academic purpose).*

Conclusion

During the active period of growth and dentition development, certain transient and developing malocclusal conditions are observed. The transient conditions are self-correcting and should be properly diagnosed and left undisturbed. But, the developing conditions need proper attention and treatment so that their severity can be reduced. The active phase of dentofacial growth gives us a chance to control and guide the developmental sequences. Certain interceptive procedures help to guide the erupting permanent teeth towards their proper place in the dental arches. Others help in attaining or normalizing the skeletal relationships of the jaws; help in correction of abnormal habits and help in redirecting the facial growth in proper direction. Therefore, interceptive orthodontic procedures are very helpful in eliminating or reducing the severity of the orthodontic problems.

34

Serial Extraction

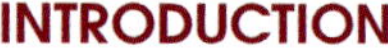

INTRODUCTION

Serial extraction is an interceptive procedure which is started in the early mixed dentition period. It is done in those cases where there are developing irregularities of teeth during eruption. It is due to TSALD in the dental arches. According to Graber, it is indicated when it is found that "an enough space will not be present in the jaws to accommodate all the permanent teeth in proper alignment."

Definition

It is defined as the procedure involving the preplanned, sequential removal of some deciduous teeth and some permanent teeth to facilitate the unimpeded eruption of the permanent teeth. It helps to provide the spaces to guide permanent teeth to erupt in more favourable positions.

History

Kjellgren started this procedure in Europe in the 1930s; where some primary and permanent teeth were removed to pave the way or to guide other teeth into normal alignment. In 1940s, Nance popularized this technique in USA. Hotz in 1970 described it as guidance of eruption. Nowadays, the **guidance of eruption** has been taken up as a better procedure rather than serial extraction, since the main objective of serial extraction is to guide the teeth in proper alignment. However, guidance of eruption does not involve the cook-book approach of extractions of teeth. The decision of extractions is taken based on the situation of dentition of the patient.

Mechanism of effects from serial extraction: Serial extraction takes advantage of the natural process of physiological drifting of the teeth. The teeth always have a tendency to shift toward the extraction spaces, under natural forces of eruption, if not controlled. This drift is especially seen in mesial direction. But when tooth is following its path of eruption within the bone, then it shifts toward the extraction spaces or toward the area of least resistance.

Age of initiating the serial extraction: It is generally started at the age of 8½–9 years of age, if the patient presents at that age. If the patient comes at an early age, then he is placed under observation till the right time comes.

Decision of extractions and sequence of extractions are planned based on the position of permanent teeth in the jaws; expected eruption sequence; and the level of root development. IOPA and OPG views are best source of information for this purpose.

If patient comes at a later stage, then decision is taken regarding extractions, and space management, keeping in view the need of fixed appliance therapy and anchorage requirements.

Indications

Serial extraction can be indicated in following cases:

1. It is most successfully done in cases having skeletal class I relationship.
2. TSALD, tooth-size/arch-length discrepancy: If there is an excess of tooth material as compared to the available

arch length (which may be due to large teeth size or smaller jaw size), then serial extraction is performed to reduce the total tooth material and thus to provide space for the alignment of remaining teeth. TSALD is the main indication to follow this procedure. According to Proffit, serial extraction is done if there are chances of TSALD of 10 mm or greater.

3. There should be having harmonious skeletal and muscular pattern. The profile should be straight and pleasing esthetics.
4. There are least chances that the ensuing growth will help in correction of the crowding of teeth.

Features indicating potential TSALD: Normally especially the lower incisors erupt in a state of some crowding. It is expected that upto 2 mm of crowding gets resolved by natural growth and by forwarding pushing action of tongue on the teeth. But more than 2 mm crowding does not resolve by itself and needs further intervention. If by the age of 8 years, the crowding does not resolve, then it will need intervention procedures. During primary and early mixed dentition stages of eruption of teeth, presence of some of the following features can indicate that there will be TSALD in future.

a. Absence of physiological spacing in primary dentition, i.e. closed dentition.
b. Absence of physiological spacing in mixed dentition.
c. Premature loss of primary canine during eruption of lateral incisors. It indicates that there is less space in the jaws (due to bigger size of teeth or narrow/small jaws), thereby forcing the lateral incisors to cause resorption of roots of primary canines, and premature loss.
d. Moderate to severe crowding of incisors, with no spaces to accommodate them.
e. Ectopic eruption of the teeth, e.g. in crossbite.
f. Space loss after premature loss of the teeth, especially in early mixed dentition period.

Contraindications of Serial Extractions

a. Skeletal disharmony, e.g. skeletal class II and III relations. However, in some cases of skeletal disharmony, this procedure is used as guidance of eruption either in a single or both the arches, depending on the clinical situation.
b. Spacing in the dentitions
c. Congenital absence of teeth, e.g. partial anodontia.
d. Open and deep bite
e. Midline diastema
f. If TSALD is minimal.
g. If there is presence of dilacerated; malformed or caries damaged permanent teeth.

Advantages of Serial Extraction

It is an interceptive procedure and helps to reduce the severity of the developing malocclusion. Some of the advantages are as follows:

a. It helps to guide the teeth towards normal alignment and thus reduces the severity of condition. Thus, the need of future orthodontic treatment is reduced or completely eliminated.
b. The progress of teeth alignment occurs under physiological forces, thus better tissue organization occurs.
c. Psychological advantage is gained when treatment of irregularity is started in early age and that too without using any appliances.
d. Health of tissues is maintained.
e. Oral hygiene is not affected as no appliances are used.
f. If any orthodontic treatment is needed, the duration and cost of treatment is reduced.
g. Lesser retention period is needed after treatment completion.
h. More stable results are attained.

Disadvantages of Serial Extractions

a. Extractions of mandibular primary canines lead to uprighting of lower incisors under the pressure of lip and thus lead to **deepening of bite** and loss of space.

b. Premature extraction of maxillary primary canine leads to impaired increase in intercanine width. It may also lead to impacted or ectopic eruption of canines. Maxillary canines are the last succedaneous teeth to erupt and follow the longest path of eruption. They generally erupt at around 11½ years of age and lead to an increase in intercanine width at that time. So timing of their extraction should be planned judiciously.

c. Extraction of multiple teeth (primary and permanent) may be psychologically traumatic to the children, as they count the total number of teeth extracted.

d. Also, they may count the total treatment time combining the time of serial extraction and observations and then the fixed appliance therapy. Thus the cooperation may be affected.

e. Patient may develop tendency to develop tongue thrust in extraction spaces.

f. Since serial extraction only helps to reduce the severity of developing malocclusion, it is generally always followed by a brief phase of fixed appliance therapy to refine the position of the teeth.

g. If proper planning is not done, then it may lead to loss of spaces by mesial migration of buccal segment.

h. It needs a clinical judgment, since a single approach cannot be used in every patient. Each patient needs an individualized extraction schedule and pattern.

i. Sometimes, misjudgment can lead to removal of some teeth, but later on the jaw growth provides adequate space for alignment.

Diagnosis

Diagnosis is very important phase to plan serial extraction phase. It involves comprehensive evaluation of dental, skeletal and soft tissues. Diagnosis involves following records: Proper clinical examination—intraoral and extraoral.

Dental cast analysis and study. Cast analysis helps to find out the TSALD, and the width of the dental arches.

OPG and IOPA view series is obtained to decide the treatment plan. OPG helps to evaluate the eruption status, stages of dental and root development.

The skeletal relations of jaws should be evaluated by either clinical examination supported by cephalometric evaluation. Skeletal class I relation is the best indication for serial extraction. Growth status of the patient is also helpful to decide the treatment goals. Patient's soft tissues should be harmonious and pleasant. Following features should be evaluated during assessment of dentition: state of tooth eruption and root formation

- Ratio of the size of primary and permanent teeth in dental arches.
- Size of the apical base
- The relation of tooth size, arch width, and supporting bone
- Probable sequence of eruption
- Congenitally missing teeth
- Malformed teeth, dilacerated or caries damaged teeth.
- Positions of unerupted canines, premolars and second molars
- Intercuspation of the first molars.

Procedures of serial extractions: Following points should be kept in mind.

1. Age of start: It is generally started at round 8½–9 years of age. As at that time, the possibility of natural alignment of incisors has already passed. Also, this is the age at which increase in mandibular intercanine width is almost complete

and that is not affected by extraction of other primary teeth. This is the age at which the mandibular permanent canines are in the stage of active eruption and are ready to erupt.

2. Level of root development: The extraction sequence and timing is planned based on the stage of root completion. The primary tooth should not be extracted unless the 50% root of its successor has been formed. If there is less space for eruption of lateral incisors and still the root development is not 50%, then the mesial surface of primary canine is reduced and patient is kept under observation with timely IOPA view of the areas to judge the root status.
3. Sequence of extractions: Extraction sequence is guided by the sequence of eruption of teeth, which is 61234578 in lower arch; and 61243578 in upper arch, e.g. in mandibular arch, generally CD4 is followed, while in upper arch, D4C is followed. It is because the lower canines erupt at an early age, while the upper canines are the last succedaneous teeth to erupt in oral cavity.
4. Distance from alveolar crest: An evaluation of the distance of occlusal/incisal surface of permanent tooth to the alveolar crest should also be made. If that distance is more than 2–3 mm, then the primary tooth should not be removed. An early removal of primary tooth leads to formation of compact bone in that area, which is difficult to resorb under natural forces of eruption and hence the eruption gets delayed rather than enhancing the rate of eruption. The tooth generally erupts at the rate of 1 mm/3 months. The space should be observed during the period of eruption after extraction of primary tooth.

There are three main methods which are generally followed in serial extraction. However, these methods are not always to be followed in every patient. The judgment of sequence of extraction of teeth is decided by the clinician based on the status of dentition of the patient.

Main sequences as described in literature are:

a. Nance's method
b. Dewel's method
c. Tweed's method.

Dewel's method: He proposed the sequence of CD4 esp in lower arch. The primary canines are removed to create space for alignment of incisors. It is done at around 8–9 years of age. After almost 1 year, the primary first molar is removed to accelerate eruption of first premolars. When cusps of first premolars are visible, then it is extracted to provide space for the permanent canine to erupt in a better position.

Sometimes, the first premolar is enucleated at the time of extraction of D. It helps to provide the spaces for permanent canine when they are ready to erupt as per their position near the alveolar crest and root development. However, **enucleation** has its own disadvantage, that since an erupting tooth acts as a functional matrix for alveolar bone, the enucleation leads to a deficient alveolar bone and a ditching in that area.

Tweed's method: It follows the D4C sequence. The D's are extracted at around 8–9 years of age. Then later on, 4 and C's are removed on the same day.

Nance's method: It follows the D4C sequence but there is gap between each extraction.

Conclusion

Serial extraction is a useful modality to intercept the developing irregularity of teeth and helps in guiding the erupting teeth in better position. It helps to reduce the severity of developing malocclusion, and thus reduces the complexity of future orthodontic treatment needed. But, it is not followed as a cook book approach for every patient and an individualized sequence of extraction is planned for each patient. It may sometimes need removal of primary lateral incisors and reducing the proximal surfaces of the primary teeth also to give space to permanent teeth for eruption.

However, with increased experience of clinicians, this procedure has been modified as the guidance of eruption, so as to help in eruption of teeth in better alignment, without sacrificing many teeth; and taking advantage of the growth of the jaws. It involves the maintenance of physiological spaces, by using TPA, LHA, etc. and by achieving expansion of the jaws by using passive or active appliances.

35

Adult Orthodontic Treatment

INTRODUCTION

Past few years have seen an increase in the number of adult patients visiting the orthodontic facilities. This shift has occurred due to favorable factors, like affordability of treatment, awareness, availability of tooth colored orthodontic materials, and availability of the orthodontists. Biochemically, there is little difference in the treatment of adults as compared to the adolescent patients, but certain factors influence the treatment planning and mechanics in adults.

There is no clear-cut line separating the adolescents from the adults. In orthodontic terms, generally the actively growing patients are considered as adolescents, and the patients in which active growth has ceased are considered as adults. So, the males above 18 years and females above 16 years can be considered as adults.

However, the requirement of orthodontic treatment in adult patients can vary depending on the condition. Generally, **young adult patients** who are aware of facial esthetics and good smile take this treatment. In such cases, a comprehensive treatment is imparted to them. These patients generally do not have a periodontally-compromised and mutilated dentition (Fig. 35.1).

There is another group of adult patients who needs this treatment to improve their existing dental conditions to collaborate with restorative work in them. Minor to moderate orthodontics is needed in such cases to help in maintenance and restoration of the remaining dentition and to improve the occlusion by rehabilitation with prosthesis, etc., e.g. some procedures needed to improve the dentition to receive prosthesis and implants, etc. uprighting of molars; forced extrusion of roots or broken teeth; correcting axial inclination of roots to create space for implants, etc.

Adult orthodontic patients generally require a team work and an interdisciplinary approach to deliver efficient treatment, including periodontist, restorative dentist, prosthodontist, endodontist, TMJ specialist, oral and maxillofacial surgeon, implantologist, etc.

Factors leading the adult patients to seek orthodontic treatment: Certain factors have acted as driving force to lead adult patients to seek orthodontic treatment. They are:

a. **Appliance innovations:** Development of ceramic brackets, tooth-colored brackets and wire; invisalign; and lingual/invisible orthodontic tech-

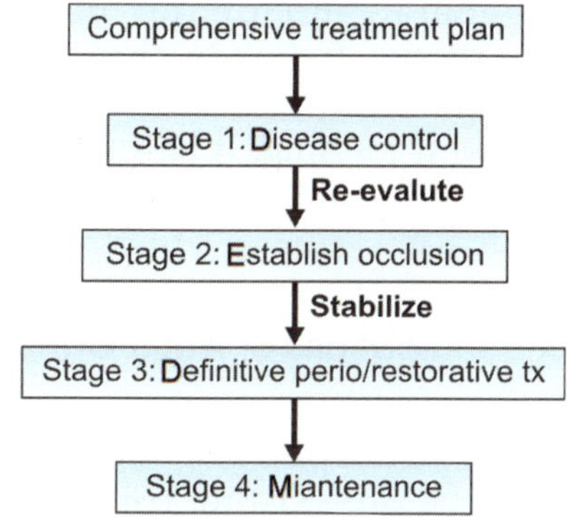

Fig. 35.1: Scheme of treatment plan for multidisciplinary management of an adult patient who needs orthodontic treatment also.

niques have led the adults to seek orthodontic treatment, who otherwise have shunned away from the metallic rail-track braces.

b. **Better placement techniques of brackets:** Due to advent of bonding procedure, and hence discarding of banding, the decision making is easier for the adult patients.
c. **Availability of facilities and orthodontists:** Since the availability of orthodontist has increased in recent past nearby to the residences of the patients, they now need not travel miles to reach the orthodontic clinics.
d. **Improved surgical techniques:** Improved anesthetic and orthognathic surgical techniques and better results have increased the confidence of the patients.
e. **Affordability:** Due to increased income, the affordability for treatment has increased.
f. **Awareness:** Increase in awareness to save the dentition and alongside improved restorative techniques and implants placement has driven the clinicians and patients to think along the lines of maintaining the longevity of the dentition.
g. **Insurance:** Certain parts of the world cover orthodontic treatment under insurance by third party payment.
h. **Desire for esthetics:** Media advertisements, etc. have created awareness for general and dental health and appearance. It needs that the teeth should be aligned, maintained, and replaced if missing. It helps to improve smile and facial balance and boosts the confidence.

Goals and Indications of Adult Orthodontic Treatment

Adult patients especially older adults, generally have pre-existing conditions, like periodontitis, missing teeth, wear facets, etc. that are usually not present in adolescent patients. They want improved esthetics attained by treatment, but function, stability and health of dentition are given more importance in adults. Hence, additional treatment objectives are established at the outset of the treatment. They are:

- To improve the axial inclination of teeth to provide better space to receive prosthesis, and for more favorable distribution of forces along the long axes of abutment teeth.
- To upright and parallel the roots so that there is sufficient bone between roots for good vascular supply and proper contact area. It is also needed for proper placement of dental implants.
- Forced eruption/extrusion of damaged teeth to provide better support at the margin of the prosthesis.
- To achieve parallelism of abutment teeth to have adequate space for fabrication of prosthesis.
- Uprighting and extrusion of posterior teeth to improve vertical osseous defects, axial loading and crown–root ratio.
- To restore functional occlusion keeping in mind existing skeletal relationship.
- Restoring vertical dimension before placing prosthesis in case of collapsed bite and tooth mobility.
- Achieving better lip support by maintaining anterior teeth in slight procumbent position to avert wrinkles around the lips.

Contraindication of Adult Orthodontics

Certain contraindications to adult orthodontic treatment are:

a. Severe skeletal discrepancies which cannot be camouflaged by simple orthodontics.
b. Advanced periodontal tissue loss
c. Local or systemic diseases in advanced stages, e.g. uncontrolled diabetes; sickle cell anemia, etc.
d. Patients on certain drugs, e.g. zoledronic acid for treatment of cancer; hormonal therapy, etc.

e. Unrealistic expectations of patient
f. Lack of patient motivation and co-operation
g. Poor post-treatment stability expectations.

Difference between Adult and Adolescent Patients

Adult orthodontic treatment is almost the same as adolescent orthodontic treatment regarding the tissue changes associated with tooth movement, stages and goals of treatment. Initial tooth movement takes somewhat longer time in adults as compared to adolescent due to more calcified bones in the former. But once the tooth movement gets initiated, it progresses like the adolescent at almost parallel pace. Due to more calcified bone, the lighter forces should be used in adults.

Another difference between these two groups is the lack of active growth in the adult patients. Thus only dentoalveolar changes can be achieved in adults. There are certain issues as mentioned below which need to be considered in adult patients.

1. Psychosocial factors
2. Periorestorative problems
3. Age-related factors:
   - Lack of active growth
   - Age changes in dental, bony and periodontal tissues
   - Increased vulnerability to root resorption
   - Increased vulnerability to TMD.

Psychosocial Factors

Adult patients have high expectations from orthodontic treatment. They inquire and discuss more about the details of treatment, e.g. treatment time, complexity of treatment, number of visits, and treatment outcome, etc. They extend better co-operation during treatment like appliance care and hygiene maintenance, keeping their appointments, etc. but they don't want long-term treatment. So, it is important to discuss with these patients about the limitations and complexity of the treatment, increased treatment time and high relapse potential.

Adult patients hesitate in using the visible appliances, and may ask for esthetic appliance, e.g. ceramic brackets, lingual appliances, invisalign, etc. irrespective of their limitations. They need to be told the benefit and drawback of the appliances.

Periorestorative problems and age related issues: These issues need special considerations in adult orthodontics. These issues also affect the treatment decisions, and the biomechanical planning, as discussed below.

Biomechanical Considerations

It is a very important aspect of adult orthodontic treatment, as it helps to plan the treatment mechanics. It can be discussed under following headings:

a. Periodontal disease and level of supporting alveolar bone
b. Age changes in bone
c. Age changes in PDL
d. Age changes in teeth
e. Age changes in local area
f. Number of teeth present.

a. **Periodontal disease and level of supporting alveolar bone** (Fig. 35.2): Periodontal disease leads to loss of marginal bone and gingival recession, thus decreasing the supporting alveolar bone. It leads to an apical shift of the Cres of the tooth. Normally, the Cres of the tooth lies approx at two-thirds distance of the root length from the apex. The point of force application is thus nearer to the Cres in normal tooth. But with loss of alveolar bone and an apical shift of center of resistance of the tooth the distance from center of resistance to point of force application on the crown gets increased. It leads to increased tipping moment produced by the given force. Therefore, greater counter-moment is required to balance this greater tipping

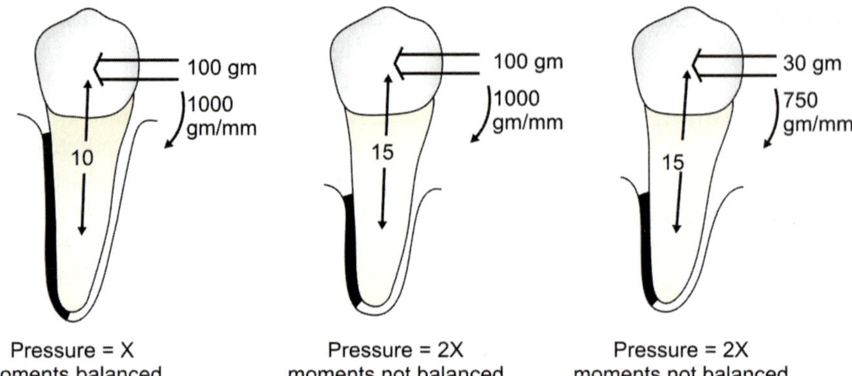

Fig. 35.2: Loss of periodontal tissue leads apical movement of center of rotation of the tooth, thus more pressure is distributed on a smaller area of PDL, and unbalanced moments are created *(Adapted from Graber and Vanarsdall).*

moment to bodily move the periodontally compromised tooth.

Also, due to loss of alveolar bone, the actual root surface area supported by PDL is considerably reduced. The light forces required for a normal tooth are perceived as heavy by such periodontally-compromised teeth. The effective pressure (i.e. force per unit area) is thus increased. So, the periodontally-compromised teeth need even lighter forces and the gap between the activation sessions is also increased to give more time for the readaptation of the tissues.

b. **Age changes in bone:** Due to age changes, the adult bone has increased density of cortical bone, decreased amount of the cancellous bone, and the decreased vascularity of bone as compared to young bone. Such type of bone is less reactive to mechanical forces. The initial tissue reaction takes longer time to start, but once started, it progresses in a normal way as in adolescents. Due to these reasons, there is a delayed response (due to reduced cellular activity in adults) and risk of root resorption (due to dense cortical bone and decreased periodontal width) in adult patients.

c. **Age changes in teeth:** There is decrease in the size of pulp, number of fibroblasts / odontoblasts, and the vascularity of pulp with age. Its effects are increased probability of root resorption and less chances of healing of resorption. The teeth also show wear facets and attrition of occlusal and proximal surfaces, with flattened and broad contacts areas and marginal ridges. It makes banding of molars difficult.

d. **Age changes in PDL:** The tissue reactions start in PDL on application of force. Many types of cells, like osteoclasts, osteobalsts, etc., help in bone remodeling. Due to decreased vascularity and the number of cells in PDL with age, a delayed response to the forces occurs.

e. **Local age changes:** Age-related marginal bone loss around the teeth occurs naturally, which may get exaggerated by periodontal disease. It leads to root exposure and apically-positioned Cres. Loss of teeth due to caries or PDL loss, etc. leads to altered occlusal function. Also, with the loss of occlusal contacts, the supporting bone shows signs of disuse atrophy and the hypercementosis is seen in roots. It influences the mechanics and forces applied.

Following points should be remembered while treating adults:

1. The lighter forces should be used.
2. There should be more time interval between follow-up appointments.
3. Light continuous intrusive forces should be applied. Intrusion of teeth helps to gain the alveolar height.
4. M/F ratio should be increased according to PD status of tooth to achieve bodily movement.

f. **Number of teeth present:** Multiple missing teeth in adults change the anchorage system influencing the treatment plan and extraction decision. Microimplants may be needed for effective anchorage. Intentional RCT and the occlusal reduction of supraerupted teeth may be required in some cases.

Treatment Modalities Available

As there is no active growth in adult patients, so the growth modulation cannot be done. Only dentoalveolar changes can be attained by orthodontic appliances. The possible treatment options remain are orthodontic correction/camouflage and orthognathic surgery. Correction of skeletal anomaly can best be done by surgery involving one or the both jaws as per the requirement.

Extraction Decisions

In adults, mainly mild to moderate orthodontics is done rather than comprehensive treatment. Some teeth may need to be extracted for proper alignment of other teeth and esthetic improvement. Extraction decision depends on periodontal status and the teeth present. Any missing tooth modifies the treatment plan. Absence of molars complicates anchorage planning, and thus a need of microimplants is increased for anchorage, thus increasing financial liability.

Space closure of long-standing extraction spaces is difficult especially in mandibular molar region. Long-standing extraction sites pose mechanical and biological challenges. With the loss of alveolar bone and especially the reduced width of alveolar bone with time in extraction space, only cortical plates, with little or no spongy bone remains. Such structure is highly resistant to tooth movement. Response of cortical bone to orthodontic forces is very slow and anchorage-stressing. In such a situation, it is better to upright the tooth to open the space to receive prosthesis rather than attempting space closure. Maintenance of closed spaces is also very difficult.

Also if there was previous periodontal loss in the extraction site, the tooth should be uprighted to open the space to receive prosthesis, rather than closing the space orthodontically. In such a case, a normal height of alveolar bone cannot be achieved, if tooth is moved into the defect.

There are certain advantages of uprighting the tilted molars:

- Elimination of the vertical osseous defect on mesial side.
- Elimination of plaque harbouring area on the mesial side.
- Parallelism of abutments is achieved and hence less tooth cutting is required for prosthesis.
- Proper sized prosthesis can be formed.
- Decreased treatment time and efforts.

In adult patients having minor to moderate problems, the existing occlusion is maintained. Lower incisor extraction is preferred over bicuspid extraction to relieve crowding, since it will not need tooth movements over a long distance and treatment time is reduced considerably. Proximal stripping is preferred to gain minor spaces. It also helps to attain proper contouring of the teeth in some cases, as the teeth may show triangular interdental spaces due to apical migration of gingival papillae. Occlusal equilibration is done to remove occlusal prematurities and sharp edges, etc.

Appliance Placement in Adult Patients

Since many patients may have heavily restored dentition, special consideration may be required during bonding due to presence of porcelain and metallic restorations. Such restorations require special methods of direct bonding, e.g. HF acid is used to etch porcelain surfaces. Otherwise, such teeth need banding, which will he unsightly in anterior region. The excess adhesive around orthodontic attachments should be removed to prevent any plaque-retentive site. Strict oral hygiene procedures are reinforced to avoid any gingival or periodontal problems. Stainless steel ligatures are preferred to elastomeric modules as they are less plaque-retentive and also cause less friction.

Diagnosis

It is an important part of the treatment since it helps to chart out a blue print of the treatment priorities and the steps. Data is derived from history, clinical examination, study casts, radiological analysis, etc. Other findings different form adolescent patients may be found in adults, e.g. flattened marginal ridges, wear facets, sharp and reduced cusps and thus widened occlusal table; missing teeth; extensive restorations and prosthesis work; periodontal disease, etc.

There are chances of TMD in adults, so the TMJ X-ray films and/or MRI, etc. may be required to diagnose the underlying problem. The findings are prioritized according to **triage concept**, and the planning is done to correct the problem in that sequence. Various possible treatment options should be considered and discussed with the patient. Patient should be involved in the decision making process for his treatment and a consent is obtained.

Orthodontic Treatment in Adults

Proffit has divided the orthodontic treatment of adult patients in following three broad areas:

1. Adjunctive orthodontics
2. Comprehensive orthodontics
3. Surgical orthodontics

Adjunctive orthodontics: It is defined as those tooth movements carried out to facilitate other dental procedures to help in maintaining and improving the function, health and stability of the existing dentition.

It helps to improve a certain aspect of existing occlusion using partial/complete fixed orthodontic appliance, which is used for a period of 6–12 months. Any major change in the existing occlusion is not done.

Goals of adjunctive orthodontics: It helps to improve the accessibility for proper oral hygiene maintenance; increases the efficiency of the dentition; and thus increases the long-term prognosis of dentition and restorative procedures.

Indications of adjunctive orthodontics: It is needed in following situations. The list is not essentially a complete list, and it may be required as per the need and experience of clinician.

- It is needed in long-standing cases of partial edentulism especially in the posterior region, which may have led to mesial tipping of the distal tooth; and formation of pseudopocket on the mesial side of the tipped tooth due to the gingival folding. It also leads to the opened interproximal contacts due to shifting of the teeth in extraction space; and the supraeruption of antagonist tooth.
- It is indicated in cases of the tooth fractured near cervical line, which is not accessible for restorative procedures. Internal or external resorption of the tooth in cervical one-third region may also lead to fracture of tooth at or apical to CEJ. Then, with orthodontics it is extruded to provide proper restorative procedures.
- It is used to improve the poor crown–root ratio of periodontally compromised tooth, where there is loss of alveolar bone leading to shifting of Cres apically.
- It is needed to improve the position of the teeth in the anterior region if there is missing or mutilated tooth, while the adjacent teeth are in malalignment (crowding/spacing/rotation) leading to improper accessibility for restorative procedures.

Procedures undertaken: Following procedures may be needed in adult patients needing adjunctive orthodontic procedures.

A. Uprighting of molars
B. Forced eruption
C. Improving root positioning
D. Alignment of anterior teeth.

A. Uprighting of molars: Distal teeth to the extraction space especially in molar area tip, rotate and drift mesially, leading to loss of space and change in the angulation of the vertical axis. It leads to formation of pseudopocket on the mesial aspect; and narrowing of alveolar ridge at the extraction space due to resorption of the alveolar bone. Maximum space loss occurs within first 6 months of the extraction. It leads to problems in proper prosthesis or implant placement. If this condition is to be treated without adjunctive orthodontics, it will include surgical excision to treat pseudopocket; followed by fixed partial prosthesis with a smaller size of the pontic and over-cutting of abutment teeth. The prosthesis will not be able to transmit forces through the long axes of teeth thereby jeopardizing the long-term prognosis (Figs 35.3 to 35.6).

Best approach to treat this condition is by uprighting of the tilted teeth. It is achieved by distal crown tipping and not by mesial movement of roots. Distal tipping results in extrusion of the tooth, which brings alveolar bone with it occlusally on the mesial aspect and eliminates the osseous defect. Occlusal equilibration of extruded crown is done to remove premature contacts and to improve crown–root ratio. The opening of the extraction space allows fabrication of properly sized pontic, or placement of implant in proper axial alignment. It leads to abutment paralleling, so less cutting of tooth structure is needed and forces are transmitted along the long axes of teeth.

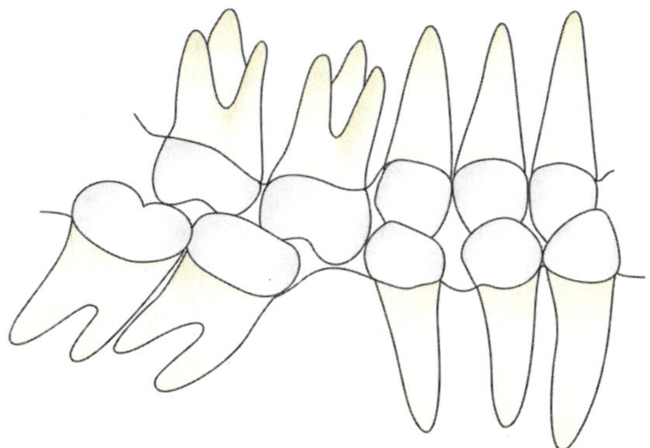

Fig. 35.3: Unattended space left after extraction of a permanent tooth leads to shifting of adjacent teeth in the space; loss of contacts; supraeruption of certain teeth, vertical periodontal defects, etc.

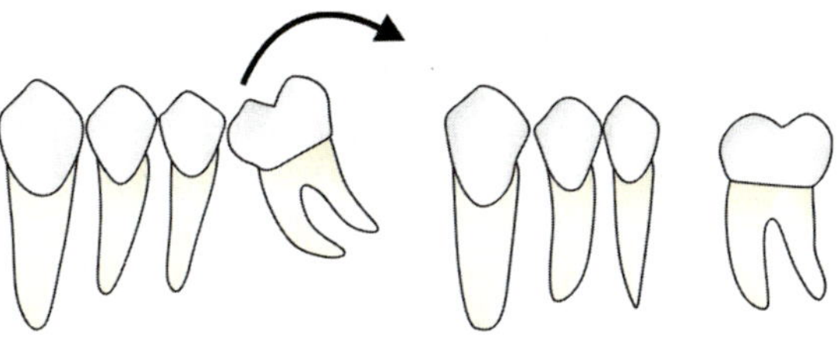

Fig. 35.4: A mesially tilted molar can be uprighted with orthodontic treatment to create the space mesial to it so that proper prosthesis can be placed.

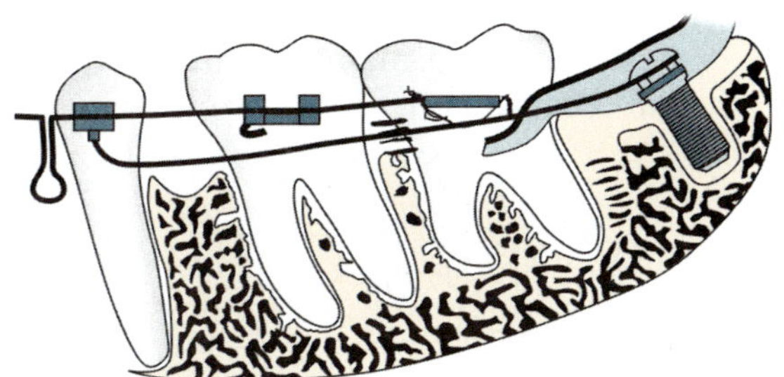

Fig. 35.5: Molar uprighting mechanics can be applied with the help of orthodontic implants in retromolar pad area.

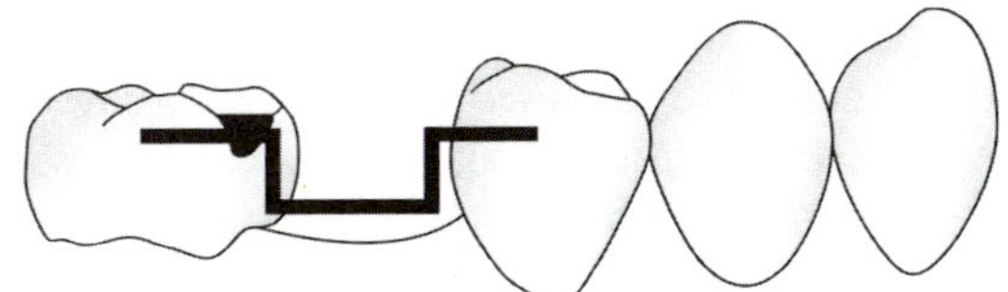

Fig. 35.6: A rigid fixed type of space maintainer should be placed to retain the uprighted tooth till the fixed prosthesis is placed.

B. Forced eruption (Fig. 35.7): A tooth-fracture near the cervical line, or caries in cervical one-third of tooth cause problems during restorative therapy due to inaccessibility, and unavailable sound tooth structure above the gingival line. Such tooth needs extrusion to make it accessible for the restorative procedures. Forced eruption is a controlled orthodontic extrusion of the tooth, which improves endodontic access, permits crown margins to be placed on sound tooth structure, maintains uniform gingival contour enhancing the esthetics.

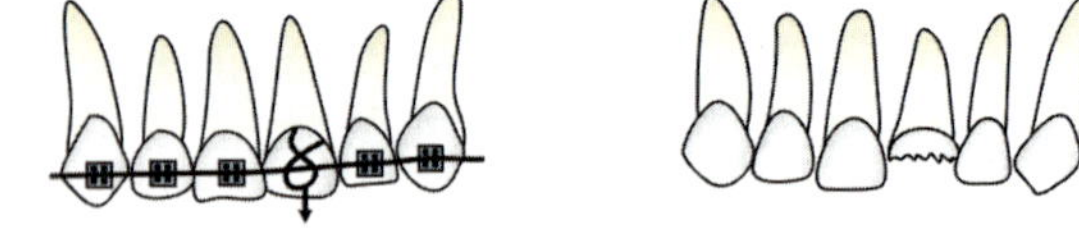

Fig. 35.7: A fractured tooth can be extruded with the help of orthodontics so that it is now easily accessible for treatment with RCT, composite build-up with post and core; or with jacket crown.

C. Teeth with one-wall or two-wall vertical osseous defects can also be treated with forced eruption which leads to bone growth, followed by crown height reduction to remove occlusal premature contact and to improve crown height-root length ratio. But, three-wall defects are not resolvable with orthodontics.

D. Improving root positioning (Fig. 35.8): Due to root proximity / root crowding of teeth, the inter-radicular area is inaccessible for implants placement. Also, the long axes of the roots are not upright, leading abnormal stresses on the PD tissues. There is inadequate blood circulation and a very thin supporting bone, making it prone to periodontal diseases. These roots should be moved away so that bone filling occurs between separated roots and improved bone support and blood circulation. It also provides accessibility for proper restoration and helps in relocating the contacts to proper level. Proper space is created for implants to be placed and for proper prosthesis.

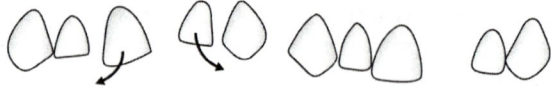

Fig. 35.8: Incisors which got inclined in the space left by extraction of one central incisors can be corrected with orthodontics so that proper space is created to receive FPD or implant in the incisor area.

E. Open gingival embrasure (Fig. 35.9): This is a triangular defect especially between maxillary central incisors. It may be due to divergent roots; abnormal tooth shape, i.e. being much wider at the incisal edges than at the cervical region; and advanced periodontal disease. Root paralleling of divergent roots is done, bringing root apices close to each other. It leads to lengthening of interproximal contact relocating it apically. The interdental papilla gets squeezed and moves incisally towards the contact area to fill the interproximal space. Interproximal reduction of the teeth is required to achieve proper shape.

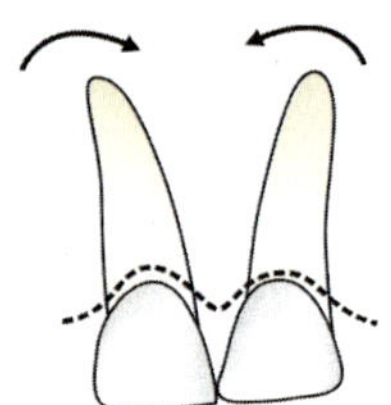

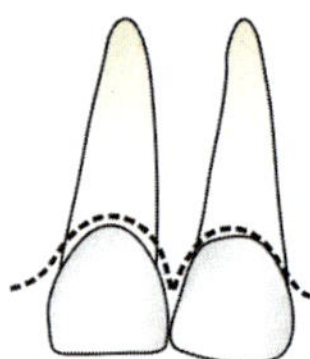

Fig. 35.9: Root uprighting of incisors helps to close the black triangles in interproximal areas of teeth, and also helps to bring the papillary gingiva toward the incisal area of teeth. It gives better esthetic effect.

F. Alignment of anterior teeth: Crowded or rotated teeth do not allow adequate crown preparation and placement of implants, etc. Anterior teeth are aligned to improve access and allow placement of well-contoured restorations. It also helps in maintaining a better oral hygiene.

Treatment time: Initiation of tooth movement takes longer time. This delayed response is suggested to be due to insufficient source of preosteoblasts as a result of reduced vascularization with increasing age. Once the OTM starts, the rate of tooth movement in adults is comparable to adolescents. Since the tissue remodeling is slow in adults, it leads to a slow rate of tooth movement and thus a longer treatment time. Follow-up interval in adults is kept longer, i.e. 6 weeks as against 4 weeks in adolescents, to give time for adequate tissue remodeling.

Tooth movements: Extensive OTM is not done especially in older adults needing only adjunctive treatment. But younger adults need comprehensive orthodontics. As discussed above, due to age changes in pulp and periodontal tissues, the teeth are prone to root resorption and/or devitalization. Therefore, lighter orthodontic forces are used to avoid the root resorption, and moment-control. Light force is used due to less periodontal area for force distribution. The interappointment period is kept at least 6 weeks to give time for tissue repair and reorganization. Certain tooth movements in adults differ from the adolescents, e.g. deep bite in young patients can be corrected by extrusion of posterior teeth, because an encroachment to freeway space is balanced by vertical growth of ramus. But in adults, it is treated by intrusion of anterior teeth. Posterior extrusion encroaches the freeway space due to lack of vertical growth, and stresses the muscles, leading to relapse. Also, the palatal expansion in adults is carefully done to avoid buccal tipping due to extrusion associated with it, or they may need an SARPE. Tooth movements are divided during retraction of anteriors, with proper anchorage management. Light continuous intrusive force should be maintained during retraction. In adult patients segmented arch mechanics is preferred for intrusion.

Anchorage: Headgears are not acceptable to an adult due to esthetic reasons. Hence intraoral anchorage devices, e.g. TPA, etc. should be used to manage anchorage, and the controlled forces are used. Tooth movements can be divided. Microimplants are generally used for augmenting the anchorage, and can help in en-masse anterior retraction in extraction cases.

Vulnerability to root resorption: Adult patients must be informed about the risk of root resorption and thoroughly evaluated for the susceptibility to root resorption. If any sign is seen during treatment, all forces should be withdrawn for about 8 weeks. Orthodontic treatment can be resumed after cessation of root resorption. Use light and intermittent forces. If root resorption still continues, then root canal treatment is done using calcium hydroxide followed by obturation by gutta-percha.

Vulnerability to TMD: There is a higher risk of presence of or development of TMD in adults, hence adult patients need a thorough check up for the signs of TMD before initiation of orthodontic treatment. However, scientific evidence say that orthodontic treatment is not responsible for TMD problems initiation.

Final detailing: Final finishing is done with lighter archwires and then stabilized with immediately placed retainers. Eventual detailing of occlusal relationships needs equilibration, tooth reshaping, incisal edge equilibration and also marginal ridge reduction.

Comprehensive orthodontic treatment: It takes more time to complete. Major changes are done in the occlusion. It is almost similar to adolescent treatment. However, certain considerations are kept in mind:

a. Always use lower force levels.
b. Proper maintenance of oral hygiene
c. Proper planning and management of anchorage
d. Appliance should be simple; comfortable and esthetically acceptable.
e. Follow-up gap is more as to give more time for tissue organization and repair.
f. Prolonged retention protocol is used.
g. Occlusal equilibration for final detailing of occlusion may be needed.

Surgical orthodontics: Severe skeletal dysplasias which cannot be treated/camouflaged by orthodontics alone need orthognathic surgery. Surgery may be needed in maxilla or mandible or both the jaws, depending on the condition. Since there is no active growth left in the adults, the surgery provides better and stable results.

Retention: Retention planning is an integral part of treatment plan. Adults show high relapse tendency, so prolonged retention is required due to reduced cellular activity for tissue remodeling. Patients having abnormal habits need fixed and prolonged retention, assisted by part time removable retainers. Splinting may be needed in periodontally compromised dentition. A regular follow-up is very important.

Further Readings

1. Kahl-Nieke B. Retention and stability considerations for adult patients. Dent Clin North Am 1996;40:961–94.
2. Kalia S, Melsen B. Interdisciplinary approaches to adult orthodontic care. J Orthod 2001;28(3):191–96.
3. Kokich V. The role of orthodontics as an adjunct to periodontal therapy, In: Newman MG, Takei HH, Carranza FA, (eds.) Clinical Periodontology, 9th edn, Philadelphia, WB Saunders Co, 2002.
4. Melsen B. Limitations in adult orthodontics. In: Melsen B (ed). Current Controversies in Orthodontics. Quintessence Publishing Co, 1991.
5. Mirabella AD, Artun J. Risk factors for apical root resorption of maxillary anterior teeth in adult orthodontic patients. Am J Orthod Dentofac Orthop 1995;108:48–55.
6. Norton LA. The effect of aging cellular mechanisms on tooth movement. Dent Clin North Am 1988;32:437–46.
7. Proffit WR, Fields HW, Sarver DM. Contemporary Orthodontics. 4th ed, St Louis, Mosby, 2007.
8. Reitan K. Tissue reaction as related to the age factor. Dental Record. 1954;74:271–79.
9. Reitan K. Initial tissue behavior during apical root resorption. Angle Orthod 1974;44:68–82.
10. Vanarsdall RL, Musich DR. Adult orthodontics: Diagnosis and treatment. In: Graber TM, Vanarsdall RL, Vig KWL (eds). Orthodontics: Current Principles and Techniques. 4th ed, St Louis: Mosby, 2005.

36

Orthognathic Surgery and Orthodontics

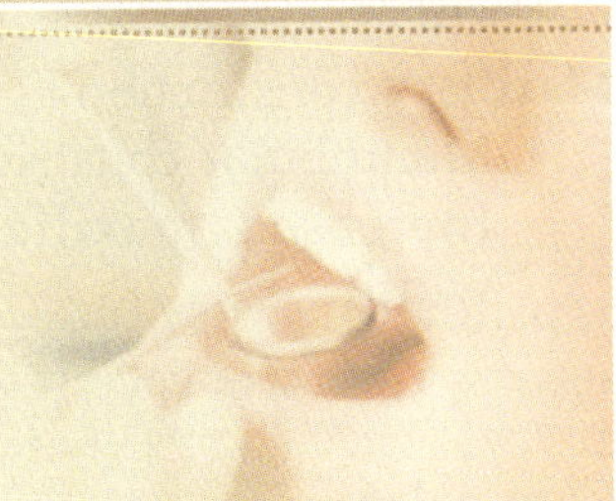

INTRODUCTION

Conventional orthodontic treatment is done to correct the teeth positions and relations; and mild to moderate skeletal imbalances. It involves dental movement, growth modification and camouflage to correct malocclusions and improve facial aesthetics. But if there is a severe skeletal problem which cannot be solely corrected with orthodontics, then the surgery of jaws is needed. Orthognathic surgery is the treatment option used with orthodontic treatment for correction of skeletal problems. Surgery is done to bring the jaws in better relation and/or reposition the dentoalveolar segments.

Definition

Orthognathic surgery is the surgical correction of abnormalities of the mandible, maxilla, or both, which may be present at birth or may become evident with age or may occur due to traumatic injuries.

Dentofacial deformity compromises jaw function and causes psychological distress. Orthognathic surgery is not a substitute for orthodontic treatment, but has to be coordinated with orthodontic and other dental treatments to achieve optimum dentofacial function and esthetics. Improved procedures, materials and anesthesia has helped the clinicians to correct many severe problems.

Goals of Treatment

The overall goal of treatment is to improve function and esthetics by correcting the underlying skeletal deformity.

Timing of Surgery

The jaw surgery should be done after the growth of jaws is complete which is generally 18 years of age, especially mandibular prognathism cases. If surgery is done before that age, there are chances that the ensuing growth can lead to reappearance of the problem. In certain congenital syndromic cases where the skeletal discrepancy provides inhibitory effect for proper growth of jaws, e.g. TMJ ankylosis, cleft palate, growth deficiency cases, etc. an early surgery can be done, but it will certainly need other surgeries later in life to achieve better skeletal relationship.

Patient selection criteria: Proper selection of the patient is necessary for orthognathic surgery procedures for better results. The skeletal problems can involve maxilla, mandible or both jaws, and can be seen in all the three planes of space.

Sagittal Plane

Maxillary retrusion

- Mandibular prognathism
- Maxillary prognathism
- Mandibular retrognathism
- Combination.

Vertical Plane

Short face

- Long face
- Skeletal deep bite
- Skeletal open bite.

Transverse Plane

Maxillary constriction

- Mandibular constriction
- Increased maxillary or mandibular width.

Congenital Problems

Cleft palate

- Other syndromes
- Growth deficiencies

Indications for orthognathic surgery are:

- Moderate to severe class II malocclusions
- Moderate to severe class III malocclusions (maxillary retrusion and/or mandibular protrusion)
- Open bite malocclusions and gummy smiles vertical maxillary excess (VME)
- Severe deep bite with reduced facial heights short face syndrome (SFS)
- Maxillary transverse deficiencies
- Patients with severe chin deficiencies
- Cleft lip and palate and other syndromic patients
- Skeletal asymmetries especially mandibular asymmetry.

Orthognathic surgery procedures: Different types/combinations of surgical procedures can be used depending on the condition of patient. Various procedures are:

- Le Fort I osteotomy: It is one of the most commonly used surgeries of upper jaw. It helps to correct the maxillary problems either by maxillary advancement, maxillary retrusion; maxillary downward movement with grafting; maxillary upward movement, rotation, i.e. in all the three planes of space (Fig. 36.1).
- Bilateral sagittal split osteotomy (BSSO): mandibular surgery
- Transoral vertical ramus osteotomy (TOVRO)
- Genioplasty: Chin advancement/augmentaiton, reduction or recontouring
- Surgically assisted rapid maxillary/palatal expansion (SARME/SARPE)
- Anterior segmental osteotomies
- Dentoalveolar surgeries (Figs 36.2 and 36.3)
- Adjunctive facial procedures, e.g. rhinoplasty; chieloplasty; grafting; botox injections, etc
- Combinations (Figs 36.4 and 36.5)
- Distraction osteogenesis
- Surgery-first concept: Latest concept in certain cases

Steps for combination of orthodontics and orthognathic surgery: a proper treatment planning is very important in these cases. If patient agrees for the surgery, then the orthodontic treatment plan is different as compared to if the patient wants only the

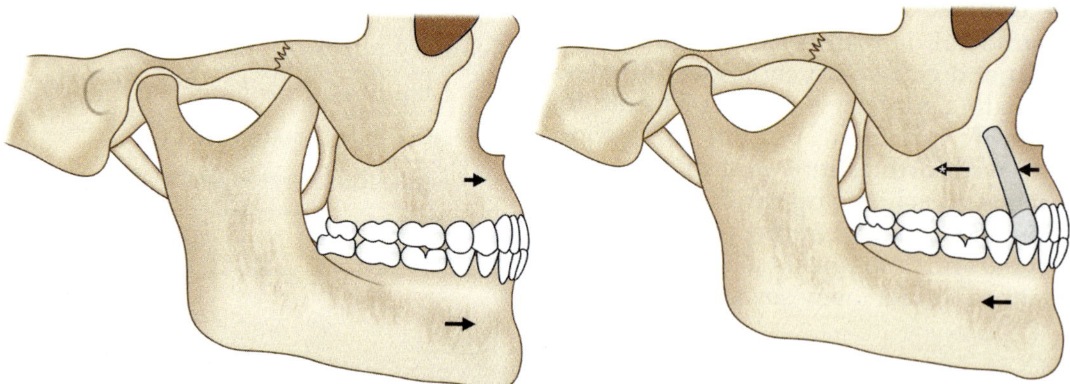

Fig. 36.1: First figure shows segmental osteotomy with forward movement of upper and lower anterior segments in case of skeletal deficiency. Second figure shows that the maxillary anterior osteotomy with backward movement of the segment after first premolar extraction, to treat maxillary prognathism.

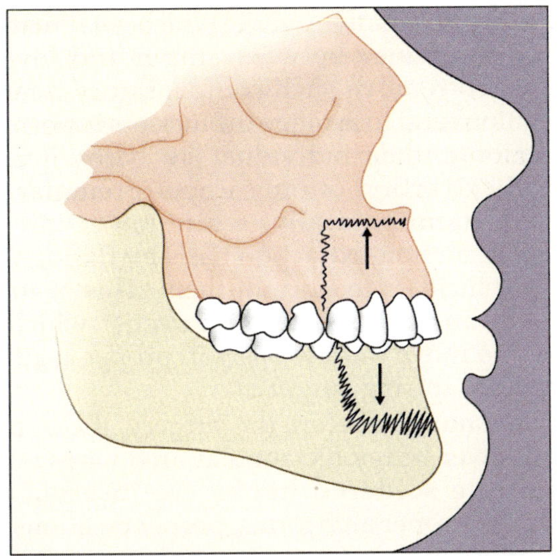

Fig. 36.2: Mandibular and maxillary dentoalveolar osteotomy and their apical movement to treat case of deep bite.

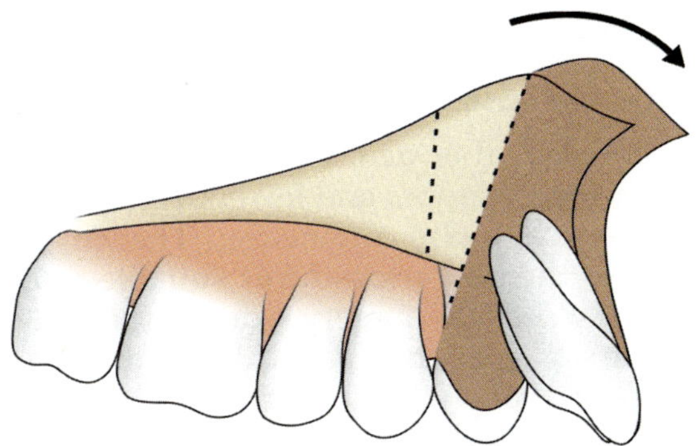

Fig. 36.3: Segmental osteotomy of maxillary anterior part and its forward and downward movement to treat anterior open bite.

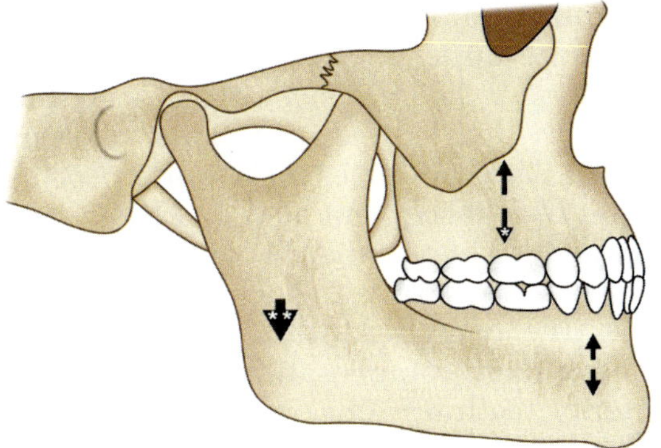

Fig. 36.4: Arrows in the figure show that different segments in maxilla and mandible can be moved in upward and downward directions to treat different problems.

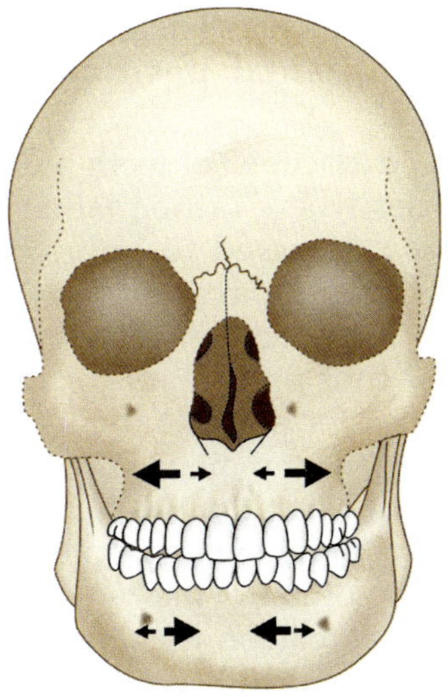

Fig. 36.5: Arrows in the figure show that segments of maxilla and mandible can be moved in lateral directions also. Bigger arrows show that maxillary segments can be moved more laterally than medially, while mandibular segments can be moved medially in a better way than laterally.

orthodontic camouflage of his condition for some improvement of esthetics. The treatment involving jaw surgeries is divided in following three phases:

1. Presurgical orthodontics
2. Surgical phase
3. Postsurgical orthodontics

Presurgical orthodontics: It is the phase in which the dental malpositions are improved and the jaws are prepared for future surgery. Here, the orthodontics is done to achieve decompensations of the dental positions. During development of jaw discrepancies, the teeth acquire positions of compensations influenced by the surrounding soft tissues.

For example, in a skeletal class II case, having an increased skeletal overjet, due to maxillary prognathism or mandibular retrognathism or combination, the lower incisors are generally seen flared/proclined due to forward forces of tongue, while upper incisors may be normally placed. It happens to achieve a normal / near normal dental overjet. In some cases, the upper incisors may get lingually tilted under the influence of upper lip, but it generally does not happen. Some cases may see the flattened lower incisor and proclined upper incisal segment also due to lower lip trap and / or hypoactive upper lip. The arches are generally narrow in such cases. The main objective of orthodontic treatment is to remove these compensations and to arrange anterior teeth upright on their basal bones. When the decompensation is done, the patient finds that his esthetics are worse than before the orthodontics, which may lead to loss of cooperation, psychological concerns and dismay, but it should be explained to the patient before treatment and during treatment that to achieve better skeletal relation during surgery, the dental positions are to be improved.

Also, the extractions of teeth are differently done in cases where orthognathic surgery is planned as compared to only-orthodontic camouflage cases, e.g. a case of class II may need extraction of upper and lower first premolars or only upper first premolars for camouflage treatment. But for patients to be treated with surgery, the patient may need only lower first premolars extraction to upright lower incisors on their basal bone, while upper incisors are either already normal, or they are flared to bring them in normal relation with upper jaw. But if upper incisors are already proclined, then it may also need removal of upper first premolars. In certain cases, upper second premolar may need removal rather than the first, to move the upper molars more mesially so that during surgery, the maxilla may be moved back to proper extent to achieve a class I molar and skeletal relation with mandible.

In skeletal class III cases, which may be due to either maxillary hypoplasia or mandibular prognathism or their combination, the extraction pattern is different for surgical cases as compared to camouflage cases. In such cases, the upper incisors are found to be proclined under the tongue influence, while lower incisors are retroclined under the influence of lower lip. It happens to reduce the severity of negative overjet which gets created by discrepancy between upper and lower jaws. To remove such compensatory dental positions and to arrange the incisors in normal relation to their individual jaw bases, it will need extraction of only upper premolar to move them palatally, while lower jaw is treated on non-extraction basis by flaring the lower incisors to upright them. This in turn creates an increased negative overjet, which is used to move the jaw bases in proper sagittal relations during surgery.

Few months before the surgery, the upper and lower heavy rectangular arch wires with multiple soldered hooks are inserted to achieve proper arch forms, proper positions of teeth, etc. and they also act as splint to stabilize the skeletal components after surgery. The hooks can be used to attach elastics to stabilize the jaws during healing. Rigid fixation of jaw segments is done to stabilize them.

Surgical Phase

After removal of dental compensations and preparing the upper and lower dental arches, the surgical phase commences. The surgeon decides the best procedures suitable to the patient. When the surgery is done in both jaws for the same patient, this is called **bimaxillary surgery**. Following are some procedure commonly used in such cases.

A. Le Fort I Osteotomy (Figs 36.6a and b)

Maxillary surgery using Le Fort I osteotomy is one of the main maxillary surgery. The surgical cuts entirely loosen the maxilla from the adjoining bones allowing it to be moved in all the three planes. The Le Fort I procedure can be used to correct:

1. Anteroposterior discrepancies, e.g. maxillary protrusions and retrusions.
2. Vertical discrepancies: Vertical maxillary excess (VME) with open bites and gummy smiles where the maxilla is reduced in height and displaced upwards to decrease the vertical height. The mandible autorotates in U and F direction, thus giving a component of

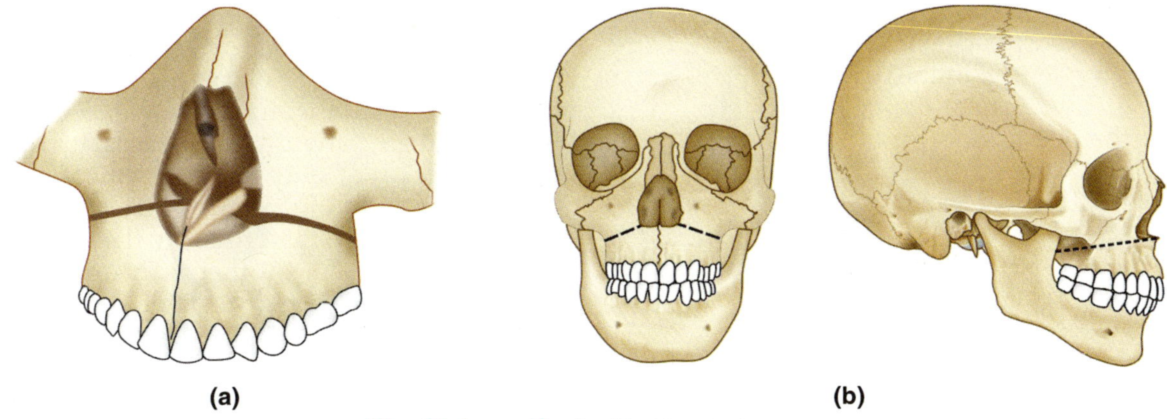

Figs 36.6a and b: Le Fort I osteotomy.

sagittal correction also. To treat skeletal deep bites with little or no incisor display, the maxilla is displaced downwards and graft is placed in that gap and rigid fixation is used. But in such cases, the muscular groups become activated, which may lead to some relapse and pressure on the graft leading to its resorption.

3. Transverse discrepancies: Multiple segmentation of maxilla and midpalatal split helps to treat the maxillary deficiencies with posterior lingual crossbites.
4. Asymmetries producing canted occlusal planes.
5. All of the above.

B. Bilateral Sagittal Split Osteotomy (BSSO)—Mandibular Surgery (Figs 36.7 and 36.8)

Mandibular surgery with the bilateral sagittal split surgical technique is the most commonly used mandibular osteotomy. It involves vertically splitting the ramus by placement of vertical cuts in the ramus on both sides which results in the mandible separating into three pieces, two posteriorly with the condyles and one anterior section. It can be used to move the anterior segment in all the three planes of space to correct various forms of skeletal problems. This form of surgery may be used to correct:

1. Anteroposterior discrepancies: Class II mandibular retrusions and class III mandibular protrusions.
2. Vertical discrepancies associated with anteroposterior discrepancies.
3. Asymmetry and canted occlusal plane.

C. Genioplasty (Fig. 36.9)

Chin advancement, reduction or recontouring genioplasties are cosmetic procedures to correct large or small chins, vertically and/or horizontally, as well as asymmetric chins. In some cases, after orthodontic correction of malocclusion, a residual skeletal discrepancy may compromise facial esthetics, e.g. orthodontic treatment may successfully correct a class II malocclusion but the chin remains retrusive. An advancement genioplasty can be done to correct this problem. Genioplasty can also be used to supplement other procedures to avoid excessive surgical movements. For example, a class II mandibular retrusion may be surgically corrected by a conservative mandibular advancement supplemented by a genioplasty to aesthetically improve the chin position rather than a larger and unstable mandibular advancement. Even the increased anterior facial height can be reduced by genioplasty and removing a part of the intervening bone. To increase the face height, the graft is required with down movement of chin.

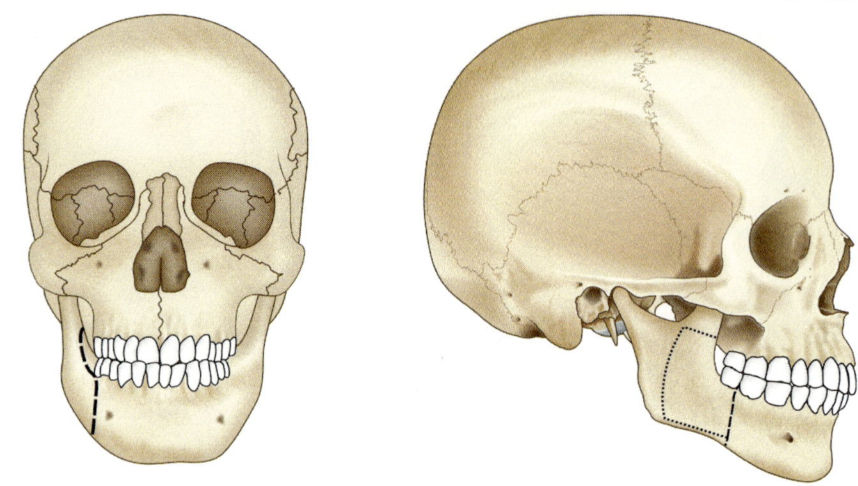

Fig. 36.7: Sagittal split osteotomy.

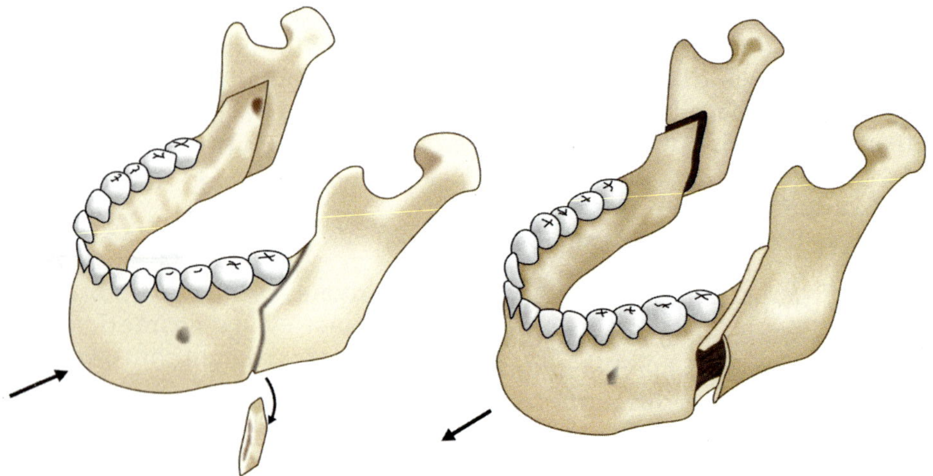

Fig. 36.8: Sagittal split osteotomy with removal of a chunk of bone. It is done to treat mandibular prognathism in case of skeletal class III.

D. Surgically Assisted Rapid Maxillary Expansion

Rapid maxillary expansion (RME) is done in younger patients for correction of maxillary transverse deficiency before midpalatal sutural closure. But in older patients following sutural closure, the widening of maxilla can only be done by surgically assisted rapid maxillary expansion (SARME). The expander appliance is placed prior to surgery. The surgical cuts are similar to a Le Fort I procedure, without the down-fracture but also include a midpalatal split. These cuts release the bony areas which resist lateral expansion of maxilla. The expansion is started 5–7 days after surgery, expanding on average 0.5 mm per day. This procedure is a form of distraction osteogenesis. SARME procedure is also used as phase 1 surgery for skeletal class III patients to correct maxillary constriction before decompensation by orthodontics and the bimaxillary surgery to correct the sagittal skeletal dysplasia.

E. Distraction Osteogenesis (Figs 36.10 to 36.13)

It was introduced by Ilizarov (1988) to lengthen long bones by performing an osteotomy

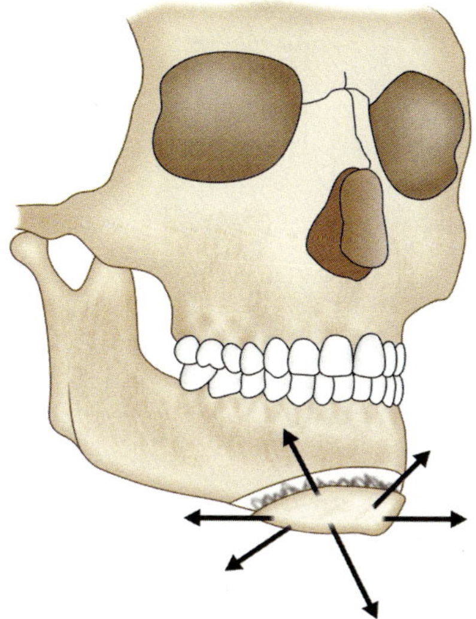

Fig. 36.9: Genioplasty can help to improve the prominence of the mandible in patients having either protrusive or retrusive chin.

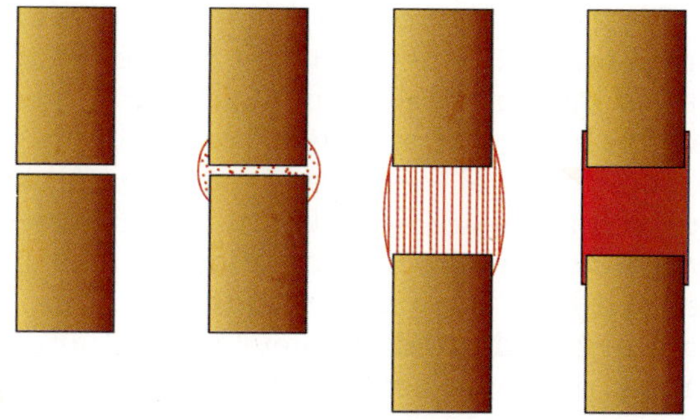

Fig. 36.10: Schematic diagrams showing distraction osteogenesis. A cut is placed in bone, which is then expanded, and callus fills that area, which then calcifies to increase the length of the bone.

or corticotomy followed by progressive separation of the two bony segments with the help of distractors. During this period, bone gets deposited between two bone segments which gradually ossifies. The ideal rate of distraction is approximately 1 mm per day. SARME is a form of distraction osteogenesis. It has also been used to advance and/or widen the mandible in severe mandibular micrognathia cases where surgical lengthening or widening is limited by the difficulty in obtaining adequate soft tissue coverage.

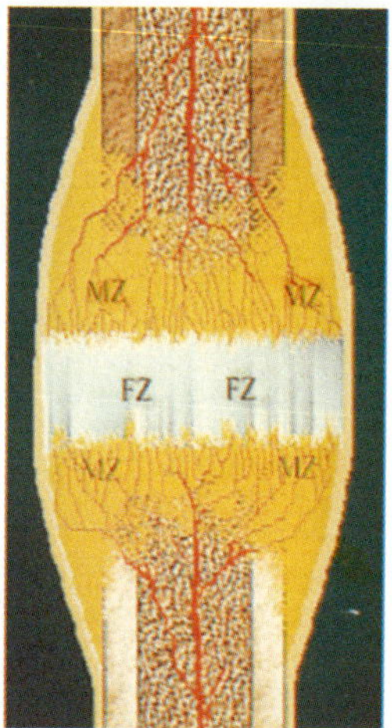

Fig. 36.11: Schematic diagram showing callus formation, and neovascularization.

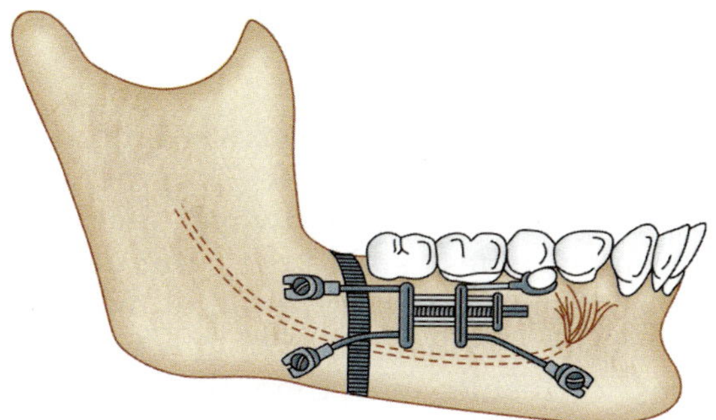

Fig. 36.12: Intraoral distractor fixed in mandible to increase the length of the mandible.

Stabilizing the jaws after surgery: Maintaining the jaws in desired position after osteotomy involves fixation of bony segments. Rigid internal fixation has been mainly used now as compared to the intermaxillary wire fixation due to comfort of mandibular movements. Titanium plates fixed with screws are used to hold the bony segments together rigidly while bony healing takes place. These plates are permanent and do need removal even after healing takes place, unless infected or exposed. Recently, biodegradable plates and screws have been developed.

Limitation in surgical movements: Movement of bony parts during surgery is limited by anatomical constraints and attached soft tissues/muscles. The maxilla can be moved to a greater extent in forward

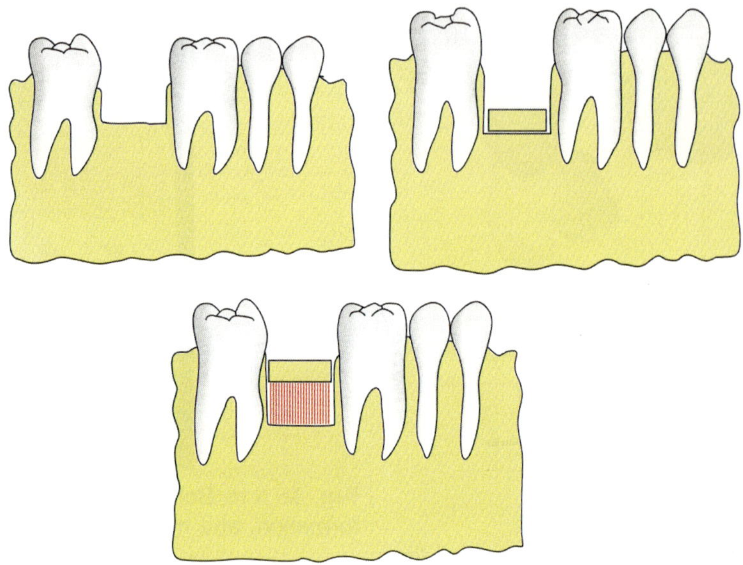

Fig. 36.13: Distraction of dentoalveolar segment to increase the height in that area so that it can receive implant.

direction as compared to backward direction, since the pterygoid plates hamper that movement. Also, downward maxillary movement is less stable than the upward displacement due to activation of masseter-medial pterygoid muscular sling which leads to loss of results with time. Similarly, the mandible can be moved more backward than forward during surgery as the forward movement activates the circumoral muscles. Lengthening of ramus also leads to activation of muscular sling and thus relapse. By surgery, maxilla can be expanded more while constriction of maxilla can be achieved to a lesser extent. Mandibular can be constricted more while expansion of mandible is achieved to lesser extent with surgery. Distraction osteogensis is the procedure which can be used in such cases where the soft tissue does not get activated at once, but gradually gets adapted to the increasing size of the bone, thus achieving a better stability.

Post-surgical orthodontics: After few months of surgical correction, the orthodontic treatment is recommenced to achieve better tooth relations, torque and arch relations, a good occlusion. Finishing is done and retainers are placed during this phase.

Surgery first concept/surgery before orthodontics: A new concept has been suggested by some authors in which the surgery is done before the presurgical orthodontics to reduce the total treatment time. The normal jaw relations are achieved with surgeries, while the dental occlusion and relations are refined later on with orthodontics. But, it cannot be adapted to every patient and a proper patient selection is needed.

Conclusion

Severe skeletal jaw problems cannot be treated with orthodontics alone, and they need the surgical correction. These discrepancies lead to compensations in dental positions during growth and development, which need to be corrected before surgeries. Jaw surgeries help to achieve better jaw relations and esthetics and thus have a positive psychological effect. With improved knowledge of surgeries and better facilities, the OGS is a good option for esthetic-conscious patients. Distraction osteogenesis (DO) has opened new avenues for such treatment, but only side effect of DO is extensive scarring of the areas where extra-oral distracters are used.

37

Surgical Aids in Orthodontics

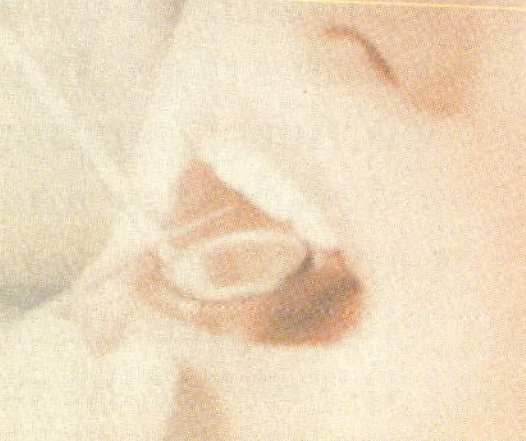

INTRODUCTION

There are certain conditions which require surgical intervention to facilitate the orthodontic treatment. These surgical procedures may be major and minor surgeries. Major surgeries involve orthognathic surgery to establish a normal inter-jaw relationship and the soft tissues; surgical splitting of maxilla for expansion (SARPE); distraction osteogenesis; cleft surgeries, etc. which are beyond the scope of this chapter.

Minor surgical procedures: Certain procedures which are generally used during orthodontics are:

- Extractions for orthodontic purposes
- Serial extractions
- Extractions of impacted and supernumerary teeth
- Surgical exposure of impacted teeth for bonding
- Frenectomy or frenotomy
- Circumferential supracrestal fibrotomy
- Corticotomy
- Dental distraction, Eric JW Liou (1998)
- Wilckodontics
- Placement of orthodontic implants
- Intentional implantation of teeth; by Northway 1980
- Transplantation of tooth
- Ankylosed teeth as abutments for maxillary protraction: Kokich, et al, 1985
- Tooth transplantation with the periodontium intact: Lesar and Cleaton-Jones 1984
- Cryosurgery; cryotherapy
- Electrocautery in orthodontics—Jerrold 1984
- The effect of gingival fiberotomy on the rate of tooth movement; 1986 Tuncay and Killiany
- Reconstruction of alveolar width for orthodontic tooth movement, 1986, Ronald Kaminishi, Howard Davis et al.
- Increasing the width of alveolar crest in prolonged extraction cases
- Lasers
- Gingivectomy/gingivoplasty to facilitate eruption of the teeth
- Gingival grafting
- Reconstruction of alveolar width for orthodontic tooth movement.

MINOR SURGICAL PROCEDURES USED IN ORTHODONTICS

A. Extractions

These are the most common surgical aids as many cases require extractions of some teeth for treatment. They are done to create spaces to align the irregular teeth. They may be of different types like:

i. **Therapeutic extractions:** These are done to gain space during orthodontic treatment to align irregular teeth; to correct the bite depth; to correct axial inclination of proclined teeth, etc. Most commonly, the extraction of first bicuspids is done; but certain cases may need extraction of single lower incisor; extractions of second bicuspids or different combinations of teeth.

ii. **Serial extraction:** It is an interceptive procedure done during mixed dentition stage. It involves the planned, orderly/sequential removal of some deciduous and permanent teeth to overcome developing arch length-tooth size discrepancy, thus allowing the rest of the permanent teeth to align spontaneously in favourable positions. It reduces the time taken and severity of fixed orthodontic phase later on.

iii. **Extraction of supernumerary tooth**, impacted teeth, malformed tooth or carious tooth beyond repair. It is done to remove barriers in normal eruption of teeth, and aid in further orthodontic tooth movements.

B. Surgical Exposure of Impacted Teeth

Certain teeth get impacted in jaws due to non-availability of space for eruption or due to deflected path of eruption. They are then surgically exposed so that clinician can bond an orthodontic attachment to guide it to the desired location. It is done when impacted teeth are present in favorable position and adequate space is available for its alignment. Most commonly, this procedure is done for alignment of maxillary canines. They are found impacted either labially or palatally. Some of the following methods are used for exposure and then bracket placement on the canines.

- **Flap method:** A full thickness flap is raised and bone is removed to expose tip and surface of crown, on which bracket is bonded and traction force with E-chain, gold chain, ligature wire, etc. is applied. The flap is replaced with suturing. It is the most common method used.
- **Tunnel method:** A tunnel is created in the bone ahead of the path of eruption of canine by removal of bone, and then the tooth is guided through it orthodontically.
- **Wire around CEJ:** A wire is ligated around the CEJ of canine after exposure and then it is pulled orthodontically, but this method is not used much.
- **Hole in the cuspid tip:** A hole is created in the crown tip through which wire is passed to apply traction. Later on that hole is filled with composite. But this method leads to loss of natural enamel structure, and thus is not preferred.

C. Frenectomy

It is also called as Wanton's clipping of frenum. It is done in cases of **median diastema** due to low-level attachment of thick fibrous maxillary labial frenum. In infants, the maxillary labial frenum is attached till the incisive papilla with some fibers in the mid-palatal suture. It does not contain any muscle fibers. It gets receeded with the eruption of central incisors and the alveolar growth. But sometimes, it does not receede properly, thus leading to development of midline space. Midline space may also occur due to other factors like it is a normal finding due to growth of jaws and at ugly-duckling stage; due to mesiodens; or due to habits, etc. A proper clinical examination and diagnosis should be done for ruling out other causes and for a proper treatment plan. If frenum is the cause, it is excised and deeply embedded fibrous tissue is removed. However, the timing of excision is controversial. According to Proffit, first orthodontic treatment should be done for space closure and then frenectomy should be done. It should not be done before the space closure. If done before space closure, the scar tissue formed after surgery may prevent the space closure and relapse of the effects. But if done after space closure, the scar formed contracts which help in retaining/maintaing space closed. However, a clinical judgement is also made, if frenum is very thick and creating a space of more than 3 mm, and interfering with eruption or approximation of teeth, then it should be removed at that beginning.

D. Circumferential Supracrestal Fibrotomy (CSF)/Pericision

This method was proposed by Edward (1970) to prevent the relapse of corrected rotations.

Since with the correction of a rotated tooth, the gingival trans-septal fibers and alveolar crest fibers get stretched and they take at least 232 days to reorganize, a long-term retention is required after rotation correction. To reduce this retention period, Edward proposed to sever the stretched fibers till the level of alveolar crest, thus reducing their relapse-causing effect.

During rotation, the fibers of PDL and gingival tissues get stretched and extended. The fibrous elements of periodontal ligaments adapt rapidly to tooth movement by progressive remodeling activity which may help in the shortening of the extended fibers. It also leads to reattachment of new fibers in newly remodelled alveolar bone during orthodontic movement. Such reorganization of periodontal ligament and adjacent alveolar bone is a relatively rapid process, and gets completed in 3–4 months.

But, the supracrestal (gingival and trans-septal) fibers which are attached between the teeth mainly, do not have alveolar bone tissue (which had to be rapidly remodeled) to eliminate their distortions after tooth movement. They remain stretched / tensed and thus lead to relapse of rotational corrected teeth. Reitan reported that the collagenous supporting fibers of gingiva become taut and directionally deviated after tooth rotation, because they remain attached to the tooth during orthodontic rotation, which results in a displacement of the gingiva in the direction of tooth movement.

Thus, due to stretch of these fibers, an elastic force is generated which tends to relapse the rotation correction. It is due to an increase in **oxytalan fibers** during orthodontic tooth movement.

For retention of rotated teeth, following points are taken care of: (1) rotations are corrected by overrotating in the opposite direction; (2) rotated teeth must be retained over a prolong period of time, preferably with a fixed retainer; (3) treatment of rotated teeth must be performed as early as possible so that we may get time for retention; (4) sufficient amounts of osteoid tissue in the root area aids in retention of the rotated tooth because it will not resorb as readily as mature bone; (5) a properly equilibrated occlusion should be attained and (6) it should be aided by CSF. Still, the patient should be made aware of a relapse tendency.

This surgical technique consists of severing all fibrous attachments surrounding the tooth to a depth approximately 3 mm below the crest of the alveolar bone by No. 11 Bard-Parker knife into the depth of gingival sulcus. No excision of attached or marginal gingiva is done. Tissue repair gets completed in 5–7 days. There is no ill-effect on the zone of attached gingiva.

E. Corticotomy

It is done in cases of dental proclination with spacing. Multiple long cuts are made on dentoalveolar region interdentally and joined with horizontal cuts subapically. Teeth are consolidated with fixed orthodontic appliance. The procedure enhances the tooth movement by reducing the resistance of bone and thus decreasing the time taken for movements. Care should be taken not to separate individual units.

F. Dental Distraction

Distraction osteogenesis is a process of growing new bone by mechanical stretching of reparative bone tissue by a distraction device through an osteotomy or corticotomy site of the pre-existing bone tissue. With this technique, new bone is generated in the gap of osteotomy or corticotomy at the approximate rate of 1 mm per day.

To reduce the time taken in orthodontic tooth movement, Eric Liou (1998) described a new procedure for rapid canine retraction in 3 weeks through the distraction of PDL. During orthodontic tooth movement, the process of osteogenesis in the periodontal ligament is similar to the osteogenesis in the midpalatal suture during rapid palatal expansion.

In orthodontic tooth movement, a mechanical force is applied to induce alveolar bone resorption on the pressure side, and alveolar bone deposition on the tension side. On the tension side, the periodontal ligament is stretched (distracted) followed by alveolar bone deposition (osteogenesis). The periodontal ligament is a "suture" between alveolar bone and tooth, which is similar to that of midpalatal suture during RME. Only difference is the rate of osteogenesis. The regular rate of osteogenesis in orthodontic tooth movement during canine retraction is about 1 mm per month, which is much slower than that in distraction osteogenesis, in which movement upto 1.2 mm per week can be achieved.

According to authors, the orthodontic tooth movement is essentially distraction of periodontal fibers (tension side) and transport of the tooth/alveolar bone complex with subsequent osteogenesis. Also, the rapid maxillary expansion is another variant of the distraction osteogenesis concept.

This method is a simple, noninvasive "corticotomy" of alveolar bone at the time of premolar extraction to allow for "bending or transport" of the alveolar-tooth complex into the extraction space. This approach is based on principles of distraction used in the long bones and craniofacial bones, such as the mandible and maxilla.

Procedure: Under local anesthesia, just after the first premolar extraction, a minor surgical scoring of interseptal bone is done. The interseptal bone distal to canine is undermined with a bone bur, grooving vertically inside the extraction socket, along the buccal and lingual sides, and extending obliquely toward the base of the interseptal bone beyond the apical area of canine to weaken its resistance. The interseptal bone is not cut through mesiodistally toward the canine. The depth of the undermining grooves depends on the thickness of the interseptal bone.

An intraoral distraction device is delivered for canine distraction right after the first premolar extraction. It is activated 0.5–1 mm/day without any latency period until the canine is distracted into the desired position and amount. The native interseptal bone distal to canine comes into the extraction socket (transport). It closely follows the canine distraction and eventual contact of canine to the interseptal bone mesial to the second premolar (docking).

Advantages

Minimal loss of the anchorage: The mesial movement/anchorage loss of the first molar is minimal. After the initial tooth movement by an orthodontic force, a lag period persists for approximately 2–3 weeks before tooth movement again proceeds. Here, the canine distraction gets completed while the first molar was still in its lag period or just initiating its mesial movement.

The periodontal ligament is a hydrostatic system maintained by blood pressure of the capillary bed. A force in excess of the **optimum force** level, i.e. 26 g/cm^2 strangulates the periodontal tissues, forcing the tooth into physical contact with alveolar bone and causing hyalinization. This hyalinized tissue has to be eliminated by undermining resorption before the tooth movement starts, which takes 2–3 weeks, i.e. **the lag period**. Any technique that takes longer than 3 weeks to retract a canine may result in loss of anchorage. It is because both, the canine and the anchor unit will move to each other after the lag period. The best way to avoid losing anchorage is to move the canine before the anchor unit moves.

Minimal root resorption: External root resorption starts 2–3 weeks after the orthodontic force is applied and may continue for the duration of force application. The canine distraction gets completed within 3 weeks while the root resorption was just initiating.

Faster distraction of canine: The canine can be distracted fast while the first molar is still in lag period. Since it is started immediately after the premolar extraction, the extraction socket provides no resistance to OTM. The initial filling of osteoid bone in the socket takes place in 3 weeks giving resistance and then solid in 3 months. Here, the canine is distracted into an extraction socket that has not been refilled by solid bone tissue. If the canine is not retracted across the first premolar extraction socket in the first 3 weeks, the rate of tooth movement gets slow down, chances of root surface resorption increase, and the anchor unit starts to move forward. The orthodontic tooth movement is faster and root surface resorption is less in an alveolar bone with loose bone trabeculae and less bone resistance.

Also, the interseptal bone distal to the canine is the only significant obstacle in the way of canine distraction. It is undermined, scored or removed surgically to weaken its strength. It gets bent by the distraction and it closely follows the tooth movement.

Rapid osteogenesis in the distracted periodontal ligament: The radiographic changes of the periodontal ligament on mesial side of the canines can be classified into five stages, from the initiation of the distraction to the complete remodeling of the new alveolar bone, as follows:

Stage 1: During first week after initiating the distraction, the stretching and widening of the periodontal ligament is seen. Bone formation does not become evident in this stage.

Stage 2: During the second week after the initiation to the end of distraction, active growing of striated bone (new bone spicules) in the distracted periodontal ligament occurs. Striated bone grows actively in the distracted periodontal ligament.

Stage 3: Recovery of the distracted periodontal ligament occurs in the first to fourth week postdistraction. The striated bone becomes denser. The distracted periodontal ligament gradually decreases in width and comes back to normal. The radiographic characteristics of the striated bone created by the distraction are similar to a cortical bone.

Stage 4: Remodeling of the striated bone occurs in the period from fourth week to the third month postdistraction. The striated bone eventually becomes the new lamina dura on the mesial side of the canine. The radiodensity of the remodeling striated bone is similar to the cancellous alveolar bone.

Stage 5: Maturation of the striated bone occurs 3 months postdistraction. The new lamina dura achieves a normal thickness.

This new technique can be best used on cases with severely crowded or protruded anterior teeth. The canines can be distracted rapidly, and almost all of the extraction space can be used for retraction with no anchorage loss. After distraction, the anterior tooth retraction can be rapid, while the new bone tissues distal to the lateral incisors are still fibrous. It can also be possibly used to generate new bone and keratinized gingival tissue for treating periodontal disease.

G. Wilckodontics

It is also called as **accelerated osteogenic orthodontics** (AOO). Here, tooth movement is gets accelerated upto three-times by reducing bone density by selective decortications. PDL is bypassed in this process.

Biological principles of AOO: It is based on **regional accelerated phenomenon (RAP).** A large insult to bone, e.g. fracture, or surgery, initiates a localized "burst" of biochemical process to repair the bone. This remodelling induces Ca^{2+} release from adjacent trabecular bone, causing localized osteopenia, i.e. a decreased density of bone. Osteopenia can also be induced in alveolar region by surgically removing selected parts. Osteopenia softens the bone and allows for more rapid tooth movement. Dr Kole introduced this to single-tooth orthodontics in 1959. Drs Thomas and William Wilcko applied this to all the teeth to be moved (1995). Orthodontic treatment is combined with generalized induction of the RAP through the corticotomy of supporting bone in the region of the teeth to be moved.

Advantages of AOO

- It helps to reduce the treatment time. So approx. 3–9 months are taken by AOO as

compared to 12–24 months with the traditional braces.
- There is less chances of root resorption.
- After surgery, there is more bone present to support the teeth and facial profile.
- Lesser chances of relapse.

Disadvantages of AOO

- Cost: It is an expensive procedure.
- Periodontal surgery is invasive and has inherent risks, i.e. risks of anesthesia, postoperative pain and swelling, possibility of infection.
- Regular prescription of medications, e.g. NSAIDs.
- It is not a "pain free" procedure, the teeth still hurt when they are moved orthodontically.
- It is contraindicated for class III patients.

Indications and Contraindications

It should not be used in patients having dental bone loss, periodontal disease, or root damage.

It may be contraindicated in patients with diseases, such as rheumatoid arthritis, that require regular doses of NSAIDs, since they can interfere with production of prostaglandins, thereby slowing down bone growth vital to the success of AOO.

In skeletal class III patients having increased mandibular size relative to rest of the face and the mandible is protruded, there may be anatomical constraints, preventing successful AOO treatment.

Age is not a major factor, as it can be used on children and adults.

Overview of steps:

1. Orthodontics
   A. Conventional orthodontic fixed appliance.
2. Periodontal surgery
   A. Full-thickness flap surrounding teeth to be moved.
   B. Surgical scoring of the area
   C. Bone graft and repositioning of the flap.
3. Accelerated orthodontics.

Description of Steps

Orthodontics: The first step to AOO is conventional comprehensive fixed orthodontic appliance for a few days before surgery.

Periodontal surgery:

A. The next step is a full-thickness flap. Flaps are raised exposing the bone adjacent and around the teeth.
B. Surgical scoring of the alveolar bone is then performed with a bur to induce decortication of the surrounding bone, and the activation of the regional accelerated phenomenon (RAP).
C. A resorbable bone-graft augmentation is then placed over the bleeding area. Antibiotics are mixed with the graft to prevent infection.
D. The soft-tissue flap is then closed.

Accelerated orthodontics: Orthodontic adjustments are made weekly during the period of the RAP, which only lasts three to four months. The accelerated rate of tooth movement returns to normal (preoperative) levels once the bone has healed.

H. Placement of Orthodontic Implants

Orthodontic implants are used to provide anchorage during fixed orthodontic treatment in critical anchorage cases. Implant should be placed in attached gingiva but not in the mobile gingiva. Placement of implant is done under surface anesthesia only, it is important not to give any local infiltration or nerve block to place an orthodontic implant. It is because while placement, if direction or the position of implant placement is wrong, it may enter and damage the PDL space, the pain of which will not be felt by the patient under local anaesthesia. Surface anesthesia is given by the spray just to facilitate the scoring of attached gingiva only for making a guide hole in the bone.

The implant is placed generally approx. 6 mm below the interdental papilla. In maxilla, the direction of placement is approx. 45° directed apically in the centre of interdental bone. In mandible, the implant is directed almost parallel to the long axis of roots of molars.

It should be placed under complete sterile conditions, using proper sterile instruments. Minimal trauma should be done to the investing tissues.

I. Autogenic Transplant Placement

Transplantation is the transfer of tissue or organ from one site to another. Autogenic or autoplastic transplantation is the process where the donor and the recipient is the same individual. Absence of any tooth presents a challenge to the concept of conservative treatment. It can be solved by two approaches, i.e. orthodontic space closure and prosthetic replacement. A new approach has been discussed in which the tooth autotransplantation has been performed in the extraction site.

It can help to eliminate the prosthesis need; orthodontic treatment and associated side effects can be reduced and maximal conservation of tooth tissue can be done. For successful results, certain points must be followed:

1. Cases must be carefully selected; the patient cooperation is very important esp to manage the oral hygiene and avoiding occlusal trauma to transplant during first few days.
2. Better results are obtained, if apex of the tooth is still open, i.e. when the root length of the transplant is between one-half and three-fourths complete. Root apices are open at this time and can easily uptake new blood supply in the recepient area.
3. The recipient site must be healthy, with adequate blood supply, and of adequate size to receive the transplant. The recipient site must be prepared before the placement of transplant to avoid time loss for which the transplant is out of its original site.
4. The length of time from removal to reinsertion should be minimal. It is said that if transplant is out for 30 or more minutes, it is bound to fail. Desiccation of periodontal ligament should be avoided as it can cause resorption, ankylosis, and failure. If you have to hold the transplant at root, a gauge piece moistened with normal saline should be used to hold it.
5. Procedure must be conservative and least damaging. Care must be exercised not to damage the root surface and PDL of transplant. It is better to hold the transplant by its crown.
6. Root-canal procedures are contraindicated with transplant. It should be perfectly healthy.
7. Careful surgical technique is followed and management of soft tissues should be least traumatic.
8. The transplant should be properly stabilised for uptake and kept out of occlusal forces for first few days. It can be done with acrylic splints.
9. Further stabilization can be done through direct bonding from 10 days to 6 weeks, if required. Then the tooth can be treated like any other tooth of similar developmental stage. Circumdental ligation with wires is contraindicated. The chances of a favorable prognosis for a properly prepared autogenic dental transplant are very high.

J. Electrocautery (Fig. 37.1)

Many times, during orthodontic treatment, certain gingival conditions can delay, and/or extend treatment. They can be gingival hyperplasia, hypertrophied gingival margin, thickened gingiva over the long-standing extraction space which inhibits the proper eruption, etc. Such a tissue can be removed by non-surgical means using electrocautery. It is the procedure in which the tissue is contacted and burned via convection as the coagulation necrosis occurs in the range of third-degree burns.

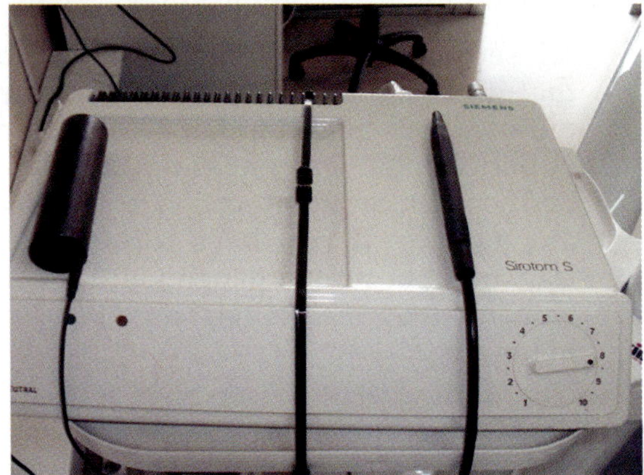

Fig. 37.1: Sirotom S form Siemens for soft tissue electrosurgery:

Indications of Electrocautery

a. One or more teeth showing delayed passive eruption or lack sufficient clinical crown for a correct bracket placement, i.e. the need for clinical crown-lengthening.
b. Waiting for erupting canine or other tooth in oral cavity before it can be bonded and incorporated in fixed appliances.
c. Hyperplastic interdental gingiva which affects the further orthodontic progress, e.g. by improper oral hygiene; due to drugs; due to chronic inflammation, etc.
d. Fibrous gingiva which may interfere with normal eruption. For example, after early loss of primary tooth, the permanent tooth may slow in eruption due to thickening of gums in that area.
e. Hyperplastic/low-lying frenum which may disturb the path of eruption, and also may cause gingival stripping.
f. Long lingual frenum which may interfere with tongue movements and speech.

Advantages of electocautery: Minimum of chair time, patient discomfort and cost.

Precautions with electrocautery: Care must be taken regarding the following:

1. All tissue being treated must be adequately anesthetized.
2. Proper pacing of the instrument should be done during electrocautery; lingering for any prolonged period of time may cause healing problems due to compromise of the hard and soft supporting structures.
3. Constant movement of the unit is a good method to distribute the heat to a wider area and it maximizes cutting potential and efficiency.
4. Hard tissue must be respected, otherwise improper healing of soft and hard tissues may occur as a direct result of improper clinical technique.
5. Prolonged contact with hard tissues should be avoided to prevent any negative pulpal effects.

K. Intentional Implantation

This is a procedure to prepare intentional implant to act as an anchorage site. It is mainly done in maxillary primary canines, which are then used as area of force application to protract the under-developed maxilla with reverse face mask. It is done at approx. 8 years of age when the reverse face mask therapy gives best results as maxilla is growing. Under aseptic conditions and local anesthesia, the canine is extracted carefully avoiding any root fractures and damage to PDL. It is then reinserted and stabilized for few days. It leads to ankylosis of canine, which will not move under the influence of forces. Thus all the forces will be directed to circummaxillary sutures and help in forward movement of maxilla.

Ankylosed teeth as abutments for maxillary protraction (by Vincent Kokich): The maxillary teeth are used as handles to deliver extraoral force to the maxilla. Research has shown that bony remodelling occurs both in the periodontal ligament and at the circummaxillary sutures, which results in tooth movement and repositioning of the maxilla. In some patients the tooth movement is acceptable and often desirable to correct a malocclusion. However, in severe cases of maxillomandibular malrelationships, a maximum amount of skeletal movement is required, which can compromise the periodontal support of the teeth. Here, an immovable object is required in the bone to transmit the extraoral force directly to the sutures rather than the PDL and produce only skeletal effects. One of the methods can be the use of osseointegrated. Other method can be intentionally ankylosed teeth which can be used as anchorage and has been used to expand the intermaxillary suture in monkeys. The use of intentionally ankylosed teeth as abutments can be used for maxillary protraction in a patient with maxillary deficiency, e.g. Apert syndrome, CLP, etc.

Procedure

Extraction: The right and left deciduous maxillary canines were extracted.

Root canal treatment: The root canal treatment is done and is obturated with zinc oxide-eugenol paste. The access cavity is blocked with composite acrylic.

Hook fixation: A hook of 0.040 inch wire is made to allow for attachment of the protraction force. A 2 mm wide hole is made through the crown of the teeth in a labiolingual direction and the wires are secured in position with composite acrylic. The teeth should be kept out of their sockets for at least 30–45 minutes.

Curettage of PDL: The root surfaces should be curetted to remove any remaining periodontal fibers to help in proper ankylosis. For complete reimplantation of teeth into the sockets, 1½ mm of the root apices should be removed.

Stabilization: After careful reimplantation, teeth should be ligated to the adjacent deciduous teeth with 0.008 inch-ligature wire and stabilized with composite acrylic.

Postoperative latent period: The deciduous canines are left unloaded for 8 weeks postoperatively for ankylosis. The teeth get immobile and emit a dull sound with percussion indicating ankylosis.

Start of anterior maxillary protraction: A face mask is fitted to the patient's face. Elastics are used to deliver approx. 16-ounce force to the ankylosed canines in downward and forward direction. The patient should were the protraction appliance approximately 10 hours each day for 12 months till correction and to maintain.

L. Fiberotomy to Increase the Rate of Tooth Movement (Tuncay and Killiany, 1986)

Orthodontic forces are applied for resorption of alveolar bone occurs which is necessary for a tooth to move. Resistance of connective-tissue fibers of gingiva may also play an additional role in determining the rate of tooth movement. It is suggested that the severing the gingival fibers by CSF can help in reducing the resistance. Gingival tissue gets bunched up in the direction of moving tooth and increases the resistance. Removal of this thickened tissue removes the resistance and enhances the rate of tooth movement. But one time severing of gingival tissues is not adequate for elimination of this tissue's resistance to OTM. In the study done on rats, it was found that the teeth that underwent the fiberotomy procedure moved faster (0.63 mm versus 0.51 mm, $P < 0.05$), indicating that the resistance of gingival tissues may be a rate-limiting factor in orthodontic tooth movement. However, routine gingival fiberotomy for the enhancement of tooth movement cannot be recommended.

M. Reconstruction of Alveolar Width for Orthodontic Tooth Movement (Ronald Kaminishi, Howard Davis, 1986, et al.)

Cases of long-standing extraction spaces present with reduction of buccolingual width of alveolar bone. In such a place, there is lack of cancellous bone and so the cortices come in contact with each other, which are very resistant to resorb. An attempt to move teeth in such places may lead to application of more forces and thus the anchorage loss; pain; increased time; gingival recession on the buccal or lingual sides of the tooth; root resorption, etc.

A surgical technique can be used to increase the width of alveolar bone. The obliterated alveolar width can be reconstructed with an autogenous cancellous bone graft, which can be obtained from ramus, symphysis, body or chin areas. Autogenous cancellous bone is placed subperiosteally on the buccal aspect of the constricted edentulous space. The adjacent teeth may be orthodontically moved into the grafted edentulous area in approximately 6 weeks.

Procedure

The surgery is done as an office procedure under LA. An incision is made at approximately a 45° angle posteriorly behind the first tooth distal to the extraction site and carried forward along the neck of the tooth up to the midpoint of the edentulous alveolar ridge. It is extended along the lingual aspect of the crest to the distal aspect of the anterior tooth. It is then carried around the neck of the tooth labially just to the mesial papillae. The mucoperiosteum flap is reflected just to the area of bone into which the tooth is to be moved. It helps to create a subperiosteal pocket to hold the grafted bone. The periosteum is scored only in the area of the mucosa and not in the area of the attached gingiva. The periosteum is relaxed so that an adequate flap can be developed. The area is then covered with a moist gauze sponge.

The 1–3 CC of cancellous bone graft can be removed anywhere from the mandible. The bone is then stored either in buccal vestibule or in a moist saline-soaked sponge. The bone is placed so that the alveolus is slightly overcontoured on the buccal and occlusal aspects. The flap is repositioned and sutured. A 6-week period of healing is allowed. This is the time necessary for bony healing to occur so that the teeth may be moved into the grafted bone in a normal physiologic manner.

N. Autotransplantation of Cryopreserved Tooth in Connection with Orthodontic Treatment (Ole Schwartz, and Christian P. Rank, 1986)

Autotransplantation of the tooth is a valid treatment alternative in cases of tooth loss, aplasia, or ectopia. It often provides an improved result, compared to conventional orthodontic treatment, if an appropriate donor tooth is available and the anatomic circumstances are favorable. But, sometimes it is not immediately possible as a one-step procedure. In such cases, cryopreservation of the extracted tooth is done for many months, before it can be transplanted in the area of need. This extraoral storage period of months or years is needed, because orthodontic treatment is needed to prepare the recipient region. Eg in certain cases, first premolars are removed at the start of treatment, which can be stored to be used later. During this period, sufficient space can be achieved in the recipient region. The thawed graft can be autotransplanted to this position. Endodontic treatment is done 4 weeks after transplantation.

It can also be an alternative to prosthodontic treatment in some cases of tooth loss or aplasia. Techniques for long-term storage of living tissues using cryopreservation have been developed to preserve the vital function of cells. Survival and function of periodontal cells especially seem to be essential for the healing and prognosis of a tooth autograft. Cryopreservation of mature teeth with a vital periodontal membrane is done at (minus) 196° C as devised by Schwartz. Research shows that such teeth are capable of regeneration of a periodontal membrane similar to unfrozen replanted control teeth in monkeys.

Briefly, the cryopreservation technique consists of placing the tooth in a culture medium containing 10% dimethyl sulfoxide (DMSO) and 10% inactivated human serum at room temperature, freezing with a controlled rate of 1.2°C/min to –40°C/min and 6°C/min to –100°C followed by transfer to storage in liquid nitrogen at –196°C. When ready for transplantation months later, the tooth should be thawed at a fast rate of approximately 100°C/min and DMSO is removed after thawing at room temperature, and the tooth is ready for transplantation.

Indications for Cryopreservation of Human Teeth

1. Replantation of avulsed teeth where a period of healing of alveolus is required before replantation.

2. A complicated fracture of jaw through the alveolus, which otherwise would need sacrifice of the involved tooth, but it can be stored during the healing period of fracture, to be replanted at a later date.
3. Cases needing extraction of premolars for orthodontic treatment, which can be replanted in place of a traumatized anterior tooth having unfavorable prognosis (autotransplantation of a frozen premolar to the anterior tooth region could be carried out at a later time, if indicated).
4. Extraction of donor tooth is needed before the orthodontic treatment to create sufficient space at the recipient region.
5. In cleft palate patients, extractions of one or more teeth in the cleft region may be required before surgical closure of the cleft. These teeth can be preserved to be used for later transplantation in the healed cleft area and help to solve orthodontic and prosthetic problems in such patients.
6. It can be used to establish a tooth bank for allotransplantation. Human teeth are potentially available through orthodontic extractions of premolars.

Risks of Cryopreservation of Mature Teeth

Inflammatory and ankysosis/replacement resorption can be a complication. Inflammatory resorption can be controlled by RCT and calcium hydroxide obliteration of pulp cavity.

Ankylosed tooth can be used without further risk for a number of years and thus postponing the prosthetic replacement.

O. Transalveolar Transplantation of Maxillary Canines (Sagne, Lennartsson, and Thilander 1986)

Impacted maxillary canines are one of the most common conditions faced by orthodontists. Their proper alignment depends on their favorable positions. Orthodontic treatment may take a relatively long time, which is generally a cause of rejection by many patients. Such patients may opt for surgical removal and prosthodontic replacement. Transplantation of impacted maxillary canines in many such cases is an alternative to removal by using a modified operative technique called as transalveolar transplantation.

Surgical Procedures

Under local anesthesia and sterile conditions, an incision is made in gingival sulcus buccally or lingually, depending on the position of the canine and a flap is raised. The crown of canine is exposed and bone is also removed near its root. A thin layer of bone should be left close to the cementum to prevent damage to PDL. After achieving proper mobility of canine enough to be transplanted to its new position, the new site is prepared with a bur, taking care not to damage the tooth.

It may be necessary to move the tooth slightly in a buccal or palatal direction to make the preparation possible. The canine should be kept in the alveolar process throughout the preparation. Finally, the tooth is moved through the alveolar process to the most suitable position adjusting in occlusion and articulation. After correction the flap is sutured in its original position. Postoperatively, suitable antibiotics are prescribed for ten days.

Orthodontic Treatment and Fixation

The teeth are bonded and aligned some days before surgical treatment. Immediately after surgery, a bracket is placed on the canine and a square arch wire of suitable dimension is used for fixation to stabilize, but not immobilize, the transplanted canine. The canine is thus finally moved into the exact desired position. It may sometimes require grinding of the antagonist because of its lack of attrition. A postoperative orthodontic appliance and adjustments are done as required for few weeks.

The orthodontic appliance helps to move the transplanted tooth directly into its exact position. The canine is stabilised but not totally immobilized by the orthodontic appliance and there is a possibility that immediate function may stimulate new bone formation.

Endodontic Treatment

Endodontic treatment of the transplanted tooth should be done generally 6–10 weeks postoperatively, to avoid any root resorption.

Precautions: When performing trans-alveolar transplantation:

- Minimize the trauma to the tooth,
- Remove a great amount of bone,
- Leave the tooth in its original position as long as possible
- Prepare a large socket for the tooth.

It is thus essential to avoid trauma from the bur to the cementum and periodontium, to loosen the tooth gently from its impacted position, and not to force it into its new site with hard bone contact. A substantial amount of bone must be removed in most cases to minimize the trauma to the root.

A complete bone healing can be achieved if the cementum of the tooth is not injured. The research also suggests that a normal periodontium with a healthy gingival margin is established parallel to the bone healing and regardless of the preoperative condition of the mucosa at the new site.

P. Lasers

LASER means light amplification by stimulated emission of radiations. It is one of latest methods being used in dentistry for multiple purposes, e.g. RCT, cavity disinfection, soft tissue and hard tissue surgeries, etc. Most of its use has been in the soft tissue surgeries, e.g. gingival contouring, gingivectomy and gingivoplasty, excision of soft tissue tumors, frenectomy, de-epithelialization, soft tissue ablation, removal of large masses of tissue, excisional biopsy, incision, laser deepithelialization for GTR, bactericidal effect in pockets, soft tissue recontouring, treatment of white lesions, apthous ulcer treatment, curettage, hemostasis. In orthodontics, it can be used as an adjunctive tool for some of these conditions, like gingival contouring after orthodontic treatment, removal of pockets, exposing the impacted tooth for bonding, etc.

Advantages: It provides a relatively bloodless and painless surgery; it has a simultaneous ability to cut, coagulate or vapourize; sterilization of wound site; minimal swelling and scarring; little suturing is required; reduced operative time; high patient acceptance; decreased or no post-op pain; reduced stress and fatigue for practitioner and staff.

Limitations: It has certain disadvantages, e.g. it is slower than more traditional methods; no single laser can perform all desired dental applications; cost of equipment is high; specialized training and attention is needed; extra concern for laser safety.

Types:

- ARGON
- CO_2
- Nd:YAG
- Diode
- Er:YAG
- Xe Cl excimer.

Conclusion

Certain conditions can pose problems during the orthodontic treatment. Surgical procedures help in making the course of treatment easy for the patients and clinicians. Minor procedures can be done on the chair under local anesthesia. They may also help to preserve certain teeth, thus preventing/ delaying the prosthodontic intervention; and thus conserving the natural tooth structures; maintaining the esthetics and cutting the cost of treatment.

VIVA VOCE QUESTIONS

1. **What are different types of surgical procedures used in the orthodontics?**
Frenectomy, pericision, extractions, osteotomy and ostectomy, etc.

2. **What do you mean by frenectomy?**
Frenectomy means the incising the low attached labial frenum, which causes midline diastema. It is also called as Wanton's clipping of frenum.

3. **Should the frenectomy be done before the diastema closure or after the closure?**
Frenum should be clipped only after orthodontic diastema closure. If it is done earlier to diastema closure, then scar elastic tissue formed there leads to relapse due to its pressure and does not allow the proper closure of the space.

4. **What is the normal position of the upper labial frenum?**
During the gum pads stage, the frenum is normally attached in the palate near the incisive papilla. It retracts upwards with the eruption of teeth and the alveolar growth. However, in some cases, it does not retract properly and remains attached on the alveolar ridge or palate to a variable degree.

5. **What is blanch test?**
This abnormal attachment of frenum can be tested by the blanch test. When the lip is stretched upward and outward, if the blanching occurs around the incisive papilla region, it is positive for the abnormal around the incisive papilla region, it is positive for the abnormal attachment of frenum.

6. **What is the best age for diastema closure?**
Midline diastema is a normal feature during the eruption of maxillary canines, because the erupting canines slide along the lateral surfaces of roots of lateral incisors (ugly-duckling stage). So, the diastema should not be attempted to close till complete eruption of canines, i.e. till 11 years age approx.

7. **What is the indication of lingual frenectomy?**
Short lingual frenum leading to the stripping of the periodontium from the lower incisors is the indication of this procedure. It may lead to speech problems and the eating inconvenience. However, the tongue tie or the ankyloglossia does not require any treatment in many cases.

8. **What do you mean by pericision?**
Rotational correction and its retention is a difficult procedure. When a tooth is derotated, the transseptal fibers get stretched which lead to relapse. To prevent relapse, these fibres are cut till the level of alveolar crest. This process is a **Pericision or CSF,** i.e. circumferential supracrestal fibrotomy. It was devised by Edward.

9. **What is the minimum retention period required to avoid rotational relapse?**
The minimum retention period required to avoid the rotation relapse is 232 days, which are required for readaptation of transseptal fibers and the alveolar crest group of gingival fibers.

10. **What is the mechanics for rotation correction?**
For correction of rotated tooth, a couple force is required. A couple is a set of two equal forces acting in an opposite direction and separated by a distance. This couple rotates the tooth around its vertical axis.

11. **What do you mean by bilateral sagittal split osteotomy and its indications?**
In cases of mandibular hypoplasia or hyperplasia, this is a recommended procedure. It means that the ramus is splitted vertically on both sides and the mandible is either placed forward or brought backward to correct its relation with maxilla.

12. **What other procedures can be done for the treatment of sagittal problem of mandible?**
- ☐ TOVRO, i.e. transoral vertical ramal osteotomy
- ☐ Reduction genioplasty for treatment of mandibular prognathism
- ☐ Augmentation genioplasty for mandibular retognathism, etc.

13. **Which surgery is mostly recommended for treatment of maxillary sagittal problems?**
- ☐ Le Fort I osteotomy with advancement for maxillary retrognathism.

- Le Fort I osteotomy with backward placement for maxillary prognathism.
- Also, segmental osteotomy in the region of first premolar can be done for both the above problems if indicated.

14. What surgical procedure for treatment of short upper facial height?

Le Fort I with downward placement and fixing a graft in between is the procedure. The graft is fixed with plates.

15. What is the difference in orthodontic treatment planning for a patient agreeing for orthognathic surgery?

For such a patient, the upper and lower teeth are arranged in a proper relation to their respective jaw bases, irrespective to their interocclusal relationship, as compared to the camouflage orthodontic treatment only. Also the extraction pattern differs for both the treatment plans. This phase may make the dental relations more severe than the pretreatment conditions, which later on are corrected with proper surgery. So, patient should be told about this before start of the treatment.

16. How does the osteoid tissue help in maintaining the tooth correction?

Osteoid tissue does not resorb as readily as mature bone, but any retentive effect of an osteoid layer surrounding a tooth is effective for a matter of only a few days, as osteoid is rapidly transformed into new bundle bone—a type of bone more resorbable than mature cancellous bone.

38

Treatment Planning

INTRODUCTION

Treatment planning is the second most important step for orthodontic management after patient examination. Treatment planning is divided into two parts, i.e. treatment aims/ objectives and treatment plan. However, it should be remembered that every malocclusion does not need treatment and thus, the benefits and risks of treatment should be carefully assessed prior to undertaking any orthodontic treatment and explained to the patient.

Treatment planning is the blue print or outline of the procedures to be followed for treatment of patient for the best possible, long term, stable results. A treatment plan is based on thorough examination of patient and his records to reach the diagnosis. Although the malocclusions have been classified in three types by Angle to simplify the understanding of condition, but it should be remembered that every case is different from the other and thus a thorough diagnosis and an individual treatment plan is made for each patient. It is based on several factors and the planning is done in a systematic way. Some easy steps may be followed:

- Setting up the goals
- Setting the treatment objectives
- Assessment of the growth status of the patient
- Assessment of etiology
- Space requirement planning
- Planning the extractions or space gaining methods
- Anchorage planning
- Planning incisors position
- Retention planning
- Appliances selection
- Re-evaluation
- Treatment options planning
- Consent of patients/parents.

TREATMENT AIMS

It has to be tailored according to the individual needs. While planning the treatment, the "**triage concept**" is followed. It means that the treatment sequence is prioritised based on the need of the case and diagnosis.

- Periodontal treatment and treatment of caries lesions
- Removal of etiology
- Orthodontic, orthopedic, surgical or combination planning
- Extraction decisions
- Anchorage planning
- Appliance selection
- Levelling and alignment
- Overbite correction
- Overjet correction
- Finishing and detailing
- Retention planning.

Setting up the Goals

Clinician should aim to provide best possible and stable treatment to the patients. The patients ask for improvement of the esthetics and function mainly. But, the orthodontist has to explain if other changes are needed. The changes which can be achieved by orthodontics should be realistic and clearly explained to the patients. The patients are generally happy when the teeth get straightened and then they ask for appliance removal. Orthodontist should explain them the need of moving the teeth to stable positions by finer detailing. The goals of orthodontic treatment are esthetics, stability, function and health of the dentition. Every clinician should strive to achieve all these goals within the confines of orthodontic treatment.

Need for Treatment

Profit has described six broad reasons that patients seek treatment:

- To remove or reduce the psychosocial handicap due to an unacceptable dental and/or facial appearance
- To enhance dental and facial appearance of individuals to improve their quality of life
- For normal growth and developmental of face, jaws, etc.
- To improve jaw function and correct problems due to functional impairment, e.g. respiration, mastication, speech, etc.
- To reduce the impact of trauma or disease on the dentition
- To facilitate other dental treatment with involvement of other dental specialists, e.g. multi-disciplinary treatment, as an adjunct to restorative, prosthodontic or periodontal therapy.

The orthodontic treatment is now aimed as soft tissue paradigm, i.e. a pleasant, balanced soft tissue relation is to be achieved with treatment. In order to provide maximum benefit for the patient, ideal occlusion as defined by Angle, cannot always be the major focus of a treatment plan. Soft-tissue relationships, i.e. the proportions of soft tissue integument of face and the relationship of dentition to the lips and face, are the major determinants of facial appearance. Soft tissue adaptation to position of the teeth determines whether or not the orthodontic result will be stable. Other goals of treatment are functional occlusion to avoid injury to TMJ and associated tissues; stability of results, and health of associated tissues.

Treatment Objectives

Problems should be listed in the priority order for treatment planning. This is called the triage concept. The problems which need to be attended first are placed at the top. This list will help in deciding the treatment objectives and their possible solutions. A realistic approach should be followed to decide the treatment objectives. Patient's needs and desires, patient's cooperation, doctor's competence, availability of facilities, financial aspects, psychological aspects, etc. should be considered. Generally, patients have the esthetic needs when they come for orthodontic treatment. But if the clinician has some other objective in the priority order to address the patient's present problem, it should be explained to the patient.

Growth Status and Potential

Growth is a very important factor during treatment planning. A thorough knowledge of growth and development of dentition is important to give best to the patient. If patient is in active growth phase, different growth-modulating processes can be used depending on the need of patient. Clinician can use growth modulating treatment, expansion therapy, eruption guidance, etc. during early years of growth. Different modalities can be used to prevent or intercept the developing conditions. In adult patients, where growth has ceased, the treatment options are limited to orthodontic or surgical process.

Assessing Etiology

Assessment of etiological factors is important since many conditions can be controlled or treated by removing the cause. "Remove the cause" should be one of the steps in treatment planning. If the cause is not removed, then it limits the success of corrective procedures, and may lead to relapse, e.g. continued presence of a habit does not allow the correction/stability of the dental positions. If a supernumerary tooth is not removed, it will not allow the tooth movement in the desired direction. However, if etiology is unknown, then it removal of the cause philosophy cannot be followed.

Incisor Relationship Planning

An ideal incisors relation of upper and lower teeth, overjet and overbite has to be determined since it is one of the prime objectives of orthodontic treatment. A proper overbite consonant with the slope of articular eminence is established so as to avoid any incisal interference during protrusive movements (Figs 38.1a to c).

For stable results, the lower incisors should be uprighted on their basal bone, and the upper incisors are adjusted in relation to them. The roots on incisors are slightly flared to distal side to create inter-radicular space, e.g. in class I cases, generally there is crowding with normal incisor relation. But, there may be deep bite which needs to be opened. In some cases of class I molars with increased overjet, extraction of upper first premolars may be needed. In some other situation, the labial flaring of lower incisors may suffice to normalise the relation. In bimaxillary proclination cases, although overjet and bite may be normal, but incisors are proclined and not upright on their basal bone. So extractions are to be done in both arches and then retraction of the anteriors are done.

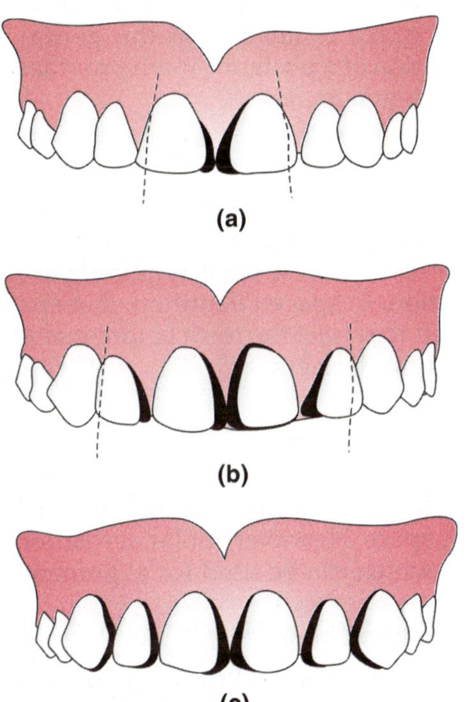

Figs 38.1a to c: The abnormally wide upper anterior teeth lead to crowding. Reshaping of teeth is done to give a better shape and to gain space for alignment. It then also helps to improve axial inclination of teeth.

In class II division 1 cases which have increased overjet, if the incisor retraction is required then space has to be created by extraction of teeth. In some cases, the lower incisors can be flared labially to reduce the overjet. If the patient is in growth phase, then class II division 1 cases can also be treated by myofunctional treatment or headgear therapy as the case may demand.

Class II division 2 cases can be treated by aligning the maxillary incisors either by palatal root torque. Some cases may need aligning them, creation of the overjet and then treating that case either by FA or by extraction of upper premolars or by surgery in adult cases.

Class III cases with anterior crossbite may require either proclination of upper incisors to jump the bite or extraction and retraction of lower incisors. In severe cases of class III cases, it may require surgery of one or both jaws.

Pseudo-class III cases which have incisor interference and forward path of closure, can be treated with flaring of upper incisors in a normal overbite relation. If lower incisors have spaces, they can be retracted also.

Space Requirement Planning

Space requirements are calculated by making measurements on dental casts and also considering the cephalometric criteria, COS, lower incisor position and soft tissue morphology of the patient and growth pattern. Most of the malocclusions require space for correction of teeth, e.g. for treatment of crowding, for decreasing overjet, for bite opening, for levelling of COS, etc.

Correction of Crowding (Figs 38.2a and b)

To align the crowded teeth, space is needed in the dental arches. If crowding is mild, then space can be gained for its alignment. In moderate crowding cases, the treatment can be done by either non-extraction or extraction depending on patient's other factors. The severe crowding cases need extraction. Generally, 1 mm space is required per mm of crowding.

Curve of Spee (Figs 38.3 and 38.4)

To level a deep COS, space is needed. It also needs ½ mm/mm space per side of dental arch or in other word, 1 mm space/mm of COS. Levelling of COS is needed for bite opening. It can be done by either extrusion of buccal teeth or intrusion of anterior teeth or both. Deep COS needs to flattened in lower arch. While flattening COS, the precaution is taken to prevent flaring of lower incisors.

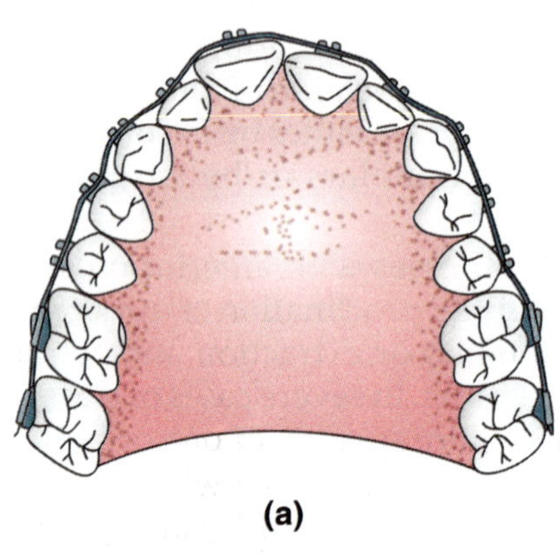

(a)

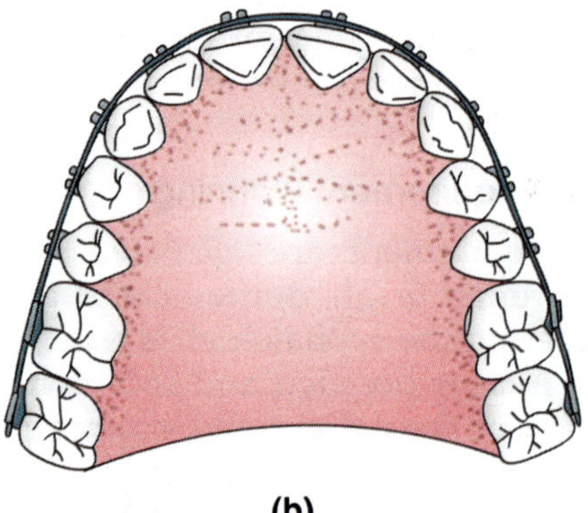

(b)

Figs 38.2a and b: Alignment phase: the wires are used to align the teeth in proper dental arch form.

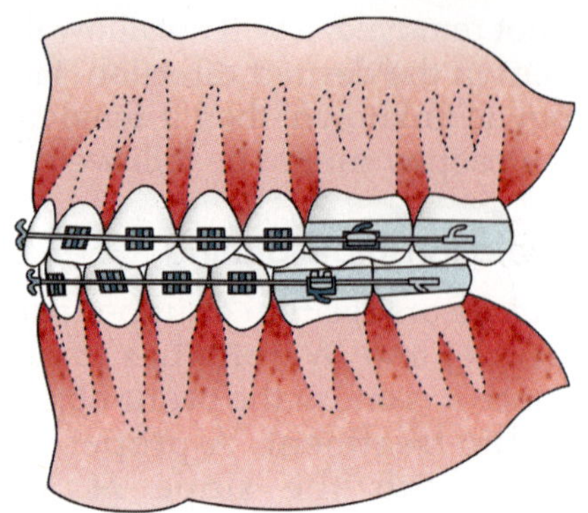

Fig. 38.3: Properly aligned, flat curve of Spee, with proper root angulations of teeth after fixed orthodontic treatment.

Rotation Correction

The teeth should be free of rotations for proper interporximal contacts and embrasures morphology. To correct anterior teeth rotations, space is needed in the dental arch. Derotation of a posterior tooth provides space in the dental arch.

Correction of Proclination and Overjet

Since retraction of incisors is needed in many cases, space is needed to bring them back. Generally, 1 mm space is required per mm of retraction. In spaced dentition, that space can be used to retract the teeth before making any extraction decision.

Molar Relation Correction

To achieve proper interdigitation, the molars are to be moved either distally or mesially. It needs space. However, molar derotation gives space which can be used for alignment.

Anchorage Loss

During retraction and torquing of front teeth and other tooth movements, the reactionary forces come into play at molars, which lead to the mesial movement of molars. Approx 2 mm mesial movement of molars is inevitable whatever anchorage methods are used.

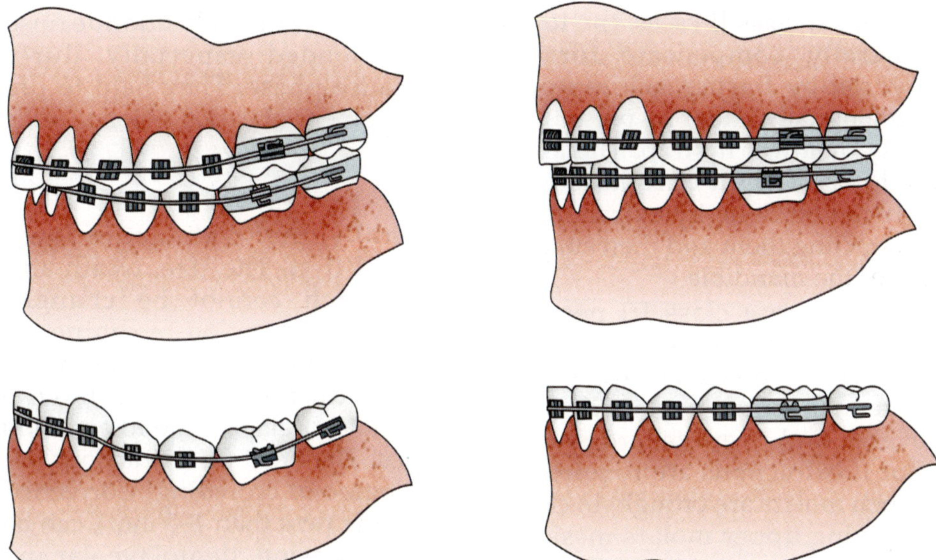

Fig. 38.4: Phase of levelling of teeth using fixed orthodontic appliances. Archwires are used to level the curve of Spee.

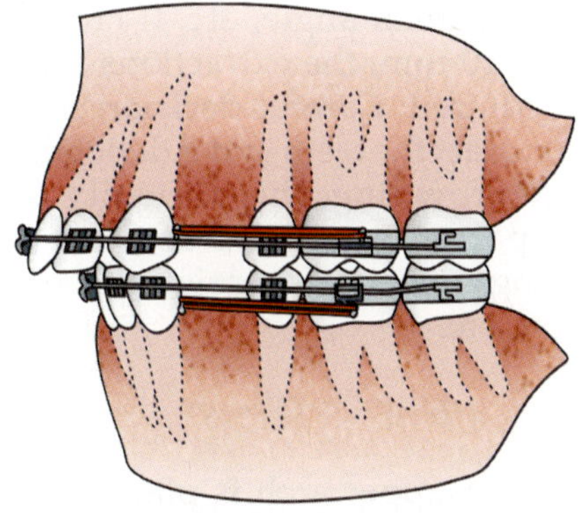

Fig. 38.5: Fixed orthodontic appliance in a case of first premolar extraction, with class I mechanics to retract anterior teeth.

During treatment planning, this factor should always be considered. Nowadays, use of microimplants have increased since they provide absolute anchorage. Extraoral forces also help in anchorage augmentation, but patient cooperation is needed.

Clinician assesses all these factors to plan space requirements and plans various methods to gain the space. Various methods of space gaining have been in discussed in the specific chapter.

Extraction Planning (Fig. 38.5)

Extraction of some permanent teeth is required to achieve treatment objectives. As discussed above, space requirements are assessed and then extractions are planned in the either or both arches. They are generally done to improve molar relation also.

For example, in class I, extractions are done in both arches to maintain molar relation. Some cases may need only one lower incisor extraction depending on the location and severity of crowding, where the buccal occlusion does not need any change.

But in class II, extraction may be done only in upper arch to correct overjet and crowding. In cases of half cusp class II, some of that extraction space can be used to bring molars in proper class II relation. If bicuspid extractions are needed in both arches, then it helps to achieve class I molars. If lower arch is having mild crowding, then extraction of second premolars can be planned. If upper bicuspid and lower one incisor is extracted depending on the severity of crowding, then molars may be in class II.

In severe skeletal class II cases, the lower incisors generally compensate for the increased overjet by flaring, while upper incisor may go lingually under lip pressure or may go labially by lower lip trap. The lower incisors should be brought upright to their basal bone. It can be done by extraction in lower arch, retracting them and then surgical advancement of the mandible.

In mild to moderate class III needing camouflage treatment, the extractions are done in lower arch only and not in upper arch. The molars are maintained in class III only, while the overjet and overbite/crossbite is corrected. But if extractions are required in both arches, then molars are brought in class I relation by moving upper molars mesially. Then it is best to remove upper second premolars and lower first premolars.

If surgery is to be done in skeletal class III cases of severe nature, the extraction planning is done differently. Generally, compensations are seen in upper arch as flared upper incisors, and in lower arch as lingually tilted incisors. When these compensations are removed by bringing them upright on their basal bones, the exact severity is seen by an increased anterior cross bite. To treat such compensations, the upper first bicuspids are removed while no extraction may be needed in lower.

Anchorage Planning

It is a very important consideration since anchorage is required to achieve tooth movements. It depends on a number of factors. Anchorage requirements are calculated while assessing the case and accordingly the mechanics and appliances are planned. Efforts are made to minimize the anchorage loss during the treatment. Anchorage has been discussed in details in its specific chapter.

Oral Health

Generally, before starting orthodontic treatment, the oral cavity is brought in a healthy state. Any caries, gingival and periodotal disease, etc. should be brought under control. Proper tooth brushing and diet advice are given. Daily fluoride rinses are also recommended especially during fixed appliance phase. They help to prevent the development of caries lesions.

Lower Arch

Generally, the treatment of lower arch is planned first. The size, width and form of lower arch cannot be changed much. Excessive expansion in canine and buccal regions; and proclination of lower incisors is contraindicated, as they have a strong potential of relapse due to activation of soft tissues. The need for extractions depends on the degree of crowding. Correction of mild crowding (less than 4–5 mm), can be done by mild expansion, dentolaveolar uprighting, and proclination of retroclined teeth. If crowding is 5–9 mm, the chances for extractions increases as these cases become borderline. Decisions of extraction depends on the factors, like growth status, growth pattern, facial profile, nasolabial angle, etc. If crowding is more than 10 mm, the extractions are nearly always required. Careful decision should be taken to extract the teeth and it depends on the degree of crowding, the difficulty of case, growth pattern and status, soft tissue morphology, need of overjet and overbite correction, etc.

Upper Arch

Treatment of upper arch is planned around the lower arch. Any extractions done in lower arch are generally matched by extractions in upper arch to achieve tooth material ratio (Bolton's).

Overbite and Overjet Reduction

Overbite should always be reduced before overjet reduction is done because deep overbite prevents the incisor-retraction due to the contact of upper and lower incisors. It may also lead to root torquing in labial direction of upper incisors, and thus a root prominence and loss of labial plate, gum recession and root resorption.

Plan the Buccal Occlusion

Proper buccal interdigitation and cusp–fossa relation should be achieved for stable results and proper redirection of occlusal forces along the long axes of teeth. Canines should be brought into a class I relationship to achieve a proper canine-rise occlusion. Molars can be brought either in class I or in full class II relation depending on space and treatment needs. Now, it is not mandatory to bring the molars in class I relation, but the molar interdigitation should be stable. Minimal extractions are planned during treatment since the pendulum of orthodontic treatment is again swung towards non-extraction therapy. For example, in some cases of class II with increased overjet, if lower arch is well aligned, then upper first premolars are removed, the canines and incisors are retracted to reduce overjet.

Suppose, if treatment of crowding in lower arch needs removal of two premolars, then upper premolar extractions are also needed to achieve class I. But if lower arch is well aligned, then space in upper arch can be created by either upper premolar extractions or by distalising the buccal segments. The choice depends on space requirement and the pre-treatment molar relationship. Generally, if full or partial class II molars are present, then premolar extraction is preferred over distal movement, depending on space need. Upper premolar extraction reduces the treatment time and increases patient compliance. If initial molar relation is nearer to class I or needing less than half a unit class II correction, then distalisation is a better choice. But if in such a case, there is increased overjet, and anterior crowding also, then removing upper first premolars to make space, and then retracting upper anteriors in normal relations, and bringing upper molars in full class II relations is good choice. Anchorage requirement of such cases are moderate.

Choose the Appliance

Once the decision for extractions and tooth movements required has been made, the appropriate appliance is selected depending on treatment objectives. The appliances can be chosen from removable, fixed, semi fixed, functional and orthopedic appliances. Some spontaneous alignment of teeth under the natural muscular forces may be allowed after extractions esp in lower arch with moderate anchorage needs. Some self-retraction of lower incisors can also occurs under the retraction forces of upper teeth, but it may lead to deepening of bite needing further correction.

Selection of Appliances

It depends on a number of factors:

- **Growth potential:** Growth modulating appliances are required during active growth phase to harmonise the skeletal relations, e.g. it can be done by using FA or dentofacial orthopaedic appliances.
- **Patient cooperation:** It is an important factor for any successful treatment. Fixed appliances need little or no cooperation.
- **Type of tooth movements:** If simple tipping is required for one or few teeth, then removable appliance can be used, e.g. canine retraction, correction of proclined incisors, correction of single tooth crossbite, etc. Comprehensive, multiple and 3D control of teeth needs fixed appliances. Fixed FAs are needed for uncooperative patients and for patients in late growth stage, and patients needing simultaneous fixed orthodontic appliance.
- **Nature of tooth movement:** If tipping is required for retraction of incisors, then Beggs' appliance can be used. But if bodily movement, torquing, derotation, etc. are needed, then fixed appliance especially SWA, MBT, etc. should be used.
- **Cost:** Removable appliances are cheaper as compared to fixed ones. They need less number of visits to the clinic.
- **Oral hygiene:** Fixed appliances create plaque retentive zones and are difficult to clean as compared to removable appliances.

Retention Planning

It is an inseparable phase of treatment and its duration should be included in total treatment time and told to patients. The patient should be advised and sensitized in the beginning of treatment that retention is a very important phase to keep the teeth in new corrected position after debonding, since if retention is not given, the teeth tend to move to their original position. This relapse depends on many factors which should be judged in the beginning and during the treatment. Some of the factors are described below.

Continued Growth

In skeletal problems, there is tendency to relapse if growth continues in retention phase. Retention is planned to nullify this effect. It is called **dynamic retention**. For example, chin cup is continued till at least 18 years of age as night-time retainer in skeletal class III due to mandibular prognathism. FA can be given in skeletal class II treated cases as retainer. If treatment is done by extrusion of lower molars or intrusion of lower incisors, then upper retainer with anterior bite plate is given.

Growth Pattern

Growth pattern also guides to decide the retention protocol. For example, HPHG may be needed as part-time long-term retainer in vertical growth of maxilla. Reverse face mask is needed in hypoplastic maxilla case. Horizontal growth cases in which deep bite correction is done by extrusion of posterior teeth, the anterior bite plate can be included in Hawley's appliance. Posterior bite plate in appliance is given to keep the posterior dento-alveolar growth in check.

PDL or Trans-septal Fibers

Gingival and PD fibers get activated when rotated teeth are corrected or space closure is done as these fibers are either compressed or stretched. They have a strong tendency to cause relapse due to their elasticity. These fibres should be incised before removing the active appliances and then prolonged/permanent retainer should be planned.

Improper Occlusion

If there is no proper intercuspation of teeth, then abnormal forces are generated on the teeth, which lead to relapse.

Re-evaluation

All these factors should be re-evaluated during the course of treatment to confirm that treatment objectives are achieved or not. If there is deviation, then treatment plan has to changed/modified to achieve the objectives.

Conclusion

Treatment planning phase is the most important step to determine the future course, anchorage, mechanics and retention of the treatment. Various factors should be taken in consideration for a comprehensive plan. The various treatment options should be discussed with patient/parents and an informed consent should be taken. Treatment planning is a very wide concept, but has been discussed briefly in this book due to limitation of space. Interested candidates can study the details in other reference books dedicated to this topic.

39

Informed Consent and Orthodontic Treatment

INTRODUCTION

Informed consent is a written acceptance made by the patient/parents for the treatment, with an understanding of their obligations toward the treatment, the expected results, and associated side effects. Due to legal aspect of the treatment, it has acquired a strategic importance for providing treatment to the patients and is an important requirement of good clinical practice. Dental practitioners must be aware of the principal factors that need to be addressed to ensure that consent is valid.

Orthodontics and dentofacial orthopedics is the dental specialty that includes the diagnosis, prevention, interception and correction of malocclusion, as well as neuromuscular and skeletal abnormalities of the developing or mature orofacial structures. Orthodontic treatment has limitations and potential risks. These are seldom serious enough to indicate that you should not have treatment; however, all patients should seriously consider the option of no orthodontic treatment at all by accepting their present oral condition.

Clinical Relevance

Orthodontic treatment is also associated with certain risks. Thus enough information must be provided to the patients to enable them to perform a risk-benefit analysis, supported by best current scientific evidence, so that an informed decision can be made by them before starting the orthodontic treatment.

Definition of Consent

Consent is defined as: The voluntary and continuing permission of the patient/parents/guardian to receive particular treatments. It is based on adequate knowledge of the purpose, nature, likely effects and risks of that treatment, including the prognosis/likelihood of its success, and possibility of alternative/s to that treatment. There are two main types of consent: **Implied** (e.g. voluntarily opening the mouth to allow examination); or **Expressed** (oral or written to an examination or specific procedure).

However, the more complex the treatment is, there is greater need of obtaining the expressed consent. For consent to be *valid*, the person must be capable of making that particular decision; should act voluntarily and freely (without pressure); be provided with enough information to enable them to make a decision.

What Information should be Disclosed?

There are certain factors which should be discussed with the patient to enable him to do a risk-benefit analysis. For orthodontics, these factors include:

1. The nature and purpose of all viable treatment options
2. The implications of non-treatment
3. What is the success rate/prognosis of each proposed treatment, i.e. what will and will not be achieved and the likelihood of success
4. The proposed benefits, limitations and risks of treatment

5. The degree of patient commitment required.
6. An estimation of treatment time, the frequency of appointments, the need for additional charges and appointments if breakages occur and the need for retention.
7. The cost of the treatment.

Results of Treatment

Orthodontic treatment usually proceeds as planned, and we intend to achieve the best results for every patient. However, we cannot guarantee that you will be completely satisfied with your results, nor can all complications or consequences be anticipated. The success of treatment depends on your cooperation in keeping appointments, maintaining good oral hygiene, avoiding loose or broken appliances, and following the orthodontist's instructions carefully.

Length of Treatment

The length of treatment depends on a number of issues, including the severity of the problem, the patient's growth and the level of patient cooperation. The actual treatment time is usually close to the estimated treatment time, but treatment may be lengthened if, for example, unanticipated growth occurs, if there are habits affecting the dentofacial structures, if periodontal or other dental problems occur, or if patient cooperation is not adequate. Therefore, changes in the original treatment plan may become necessary. If treatment time is extended beyond the original estimate, additional fees may be assessed.

Discomfort: Some discomfort due to the introduction of orthodontic appliances always occurs and even after monthly regular activation of wires, etc. Nonprescription pain medication can be used during this adjustment period.

Relapse: Completed orthodontic treatment does not guarantee perfectly straight teeth for the rest of your life. Retainers will be required to keep your teeth in their new positions as a result of your orthodontic treatment. You must wear your retainers as instructed or teeth may shift, in addition to other adverse effects. Regular retainer wear is often necessary for several years following orthodontic treatment. However, changes after that time can occur due to natural causes, including habits such as tongue thrusting, mouth breathing, and growth and maturation that continue throughout life. Later in life, most people will see their teeth shift. Minor irregularities, particularly in the lower front teeth, may have to be accepted. Some changes may require additional orthodontic treatment or, in some cases, surgery. Some situations may require non-removable retainers or other dental appliances made by your family dentist.

Extractions: Some cases will require the removal of deciduous (baby) teeth or permanent teeth. There are additional risks associated with the removal of teeth which you should discuss with your family dentist or oral surgeon prior to the procedure.

Orthognathic Surgery

Some patients have significant skeletal disharmonies which require orthodontic treatment in conjunction with orthognathic (dentofacial) surgery. There are additional risks associated with this surgery which you should discuss with your oral and/or maxillofacial surgeon prior to beginning orthodontic treatment. Please be aware that orthodontic treatment prior to orthognathic surgery often only aligns the teeth within the individual dental arches. Therefore, patients discontinuing orthodontic treatment without completing the planned surgical procedures may have a malocclusion that is worse than when they began treatment!

Decalcification and Dental Caries

Excellent oral hygiene is essential during orthodontic treatment as are regular visits to your family dentist. Inadequate or improper hygiene could result in cavities, discolored teeth, periodontal disease and/or decalcification. These same problems can occur without orthodontic treatment, but the risk is greater to an individual wearing braces or other appliances. These problems may be aggravated if the patient has not had the benefit of fluoridated water or its substitute, or if the patient consumes sweetened beverages or foods.

Root Resorption

The roots of some patients' teeth become shorter (resorption) during orthodontic treatment. It is not known exactly what causes root resorption, nor is it possible to predict which patients will experience it. However, many patients have retained teeth throughout life with severely shortened roots. If resorption is detected during orthodontic treatment, your orthodontist may recommend a pause in treatment or the removal of the appliances prior to the completion of orthodontic treatment.

Nerve Damage

A tooth that has been traumatized by an accident or deep decay may have experienced damage to the nerve of the tooth. Orthodontic tooth movement may, in some cases, aggravate this condition. In some cases, root canal treatment may be necessary. In severe cases, the tooth or teeth may be lost.

Periodontal Disease

Periodontal (gum and bone) disease can develop or worsen during orthodontic treatment due to many factors, but most often due to the lack of adequate oral hygiene. You must have your general dentist, or if indicated, a periodontist monitor your periodontal health during orthodontic treatment every 3–6 months. If periodontal problems cannot be controlled, orthodontic treatment may have to be discontinued prior to completion.

Injury from Orthodontic Appliances

Activities or foods which could damage, loosen or dislodge orthodontic appliances need to be avoided. Loosened or damaged orthodontic appliances can be inhaled or swallowed or could cause other damage to the patient. You should inform your orthodontist of any unusual symptoms or of any loose or broken appliances as soon as they are noticed. Damage to the enamel of a tooth or to a restoration (crown, bonding, veneer, etc.) is possible when orthodontic appliances are removed. This problem may be more likely when esthetic (clear or tooth-colored) appliances have been selected. If damage to a tooth or restoration occurs, restoration of the involved tooth/teeth by your dentist may be necessary.

Headgears

Orthodontic headgears can cause injury to the patient. Injuries can include damage to the face or eyes. In the event of injury or especially an eye injury, however minor, immediate medical help should be sought. Refrain from wearing headgear in situations where there may be a chance that it could be dislodged or pulled off. Sports activities and games should be avoided when wearing orthodontic headgear.

Temporomandibular (Jaw) Joint Dysfunction

Problems may occur in the jaw joints, i.e. temporomandibular joints (TMJ), causing pain, headaches or ear problems. Many factors can affect the health of the jaw joints, including past trauma (blows to the head or face), arthritis, hereditary tendency to jaw joint problems, excessive tooth grinding or clenching, poorly balanced bite, and many medical conditions. Jaw joint problems may occur with or without orthodontic treatment. Any jaw joint symptoms, including pain, jaw popping or difficulty opening or closing, should be promptly reported to the orthodontist. Treatment by other medical or dental specialists may be necessary.

Impacted, Ankylosed, Unerupted Teeth

Teeth may become impacted (trapped below the bone or gums), ankylosed (fused to the bone) or just fail to erupt. Oftentimes, these conditions occur for no apparent reason and generally cannot be anticipated. Treatment of these conditions depends on the particular circumstance and the overall importance of the involved tooth, and may require extraction, surgical exposure, surgical transplantation or prosthetic replacement.

Occlusal Adjustment

You can expect minimal imperfections in the way your teeth meet following the end of treatment. An occlusal equilibration procedure may be necessary, which is a grinding method used to fine-tune the occlusion. It may also be necessary to remove a small amount of enamel in between the teeth, thereby "flattening" surfaces in order to reduce the possibility of a relapse.

Non-ideal Results

Due to the wide variation in the size and shape of the teeth, missing teeth, etc., achievement of an ideal result (e.g. complete closure of a space) may not be possible. Restorative dental treatment, such as esthetic bonding, crowns or bridges or periodontal therapy, may be indicated. You are encouraged to ask your orthodontist and family dentist about adjunctive care.

Third Molars

As third molars (wisdom teeth) develop, your teeth may change alignment. Your dentist and/or orthodontist should monitor them in order to determine when and if the third molars need to be removed.

Allergies

Occasionally, patients can be allergic to some of the component materials of their orthodontic appliances. This may require a change in treatment plan or discontinuance of treatment prior to completion. Although very uncommon, medical management of dental material allergies may be necessary.

General Health Problems

General health problems, such as bone, blood or endocrine disorders, and many prescription and non-prescription drugs (including bisphosphonates) can affect your orthodontic treatment. It is imperative that you inform your orthodontist of any changes in your general health status.

Use of Tobacco Products

Smoking or chewing tobacco has been shown to increase the risk of gum disease and interferes with healing after oral surgery. Tobacco users are also more prone to oral cancer, gum recession, and delayed tooth movement during orthodontic treatment. If you use tobacco, you must carefully consider the possibility of a compromised orthodontic result.

Temporary Anchorage Devices

Your treatment may include the use of a temporary anchorage device(s) (i.e. metal screw or plate attached to the bone). There are specific risks associated with them. It is possible that the screw(s) could become loose which would require its/their removal and possibly relocation or replacement with a larger screw. The screw and related material may be accidentally swallowed. If the device cannot be stabilized for an adequate length of time, an alternate treatment plan may be necessary. It is possible that the tissue around the device could become inflamed or infected, or the soft tissue could grow over the device, which could also require its removal, surgical excision of the tissue and/or the use of antibiotics or antimicrobial rinses. It is possible that the screws could break (i.e. upon insertion or removal). If this occurs, the broken piece may be left in your mouth or may be surgically removed. This may require referral to another dental specialist. When inserting the device(s), it is possible to damage the root of a tooth, a nerve, or to perforate the maxillary sinus. Usually, these problems are not significant; however, additional dental or medical treatment may be necessary. Local anesthetic may be used when these devices are inserted or removed, which also has risks. Please advise the doctor placing the device if you have had any difficulties with dental anesthetics in the past.

If any of the complications mentioned above do occur, a referral may be necessary to your family dentist or another dental or medical specialist for further treatment. Fees for these services are not included in the cost for orthodontic treatment.

Treatment Failure and Relapse

There exists a high failure rate to complete orthodontic treatment and it may be due to factors like patient non-compliance, incorrect diagnosis or incorrect management (e.g. incorrect choice of appliance). Some percent age of relapse after orthodontic treatment is inevitable and may be due to soft tissue factors (e.g. teeth initially severely rotated); late mandibular growth leading to lower incisal crowding; poor periodontal support; occlusal factors (e.g. insufficient overbite to maintain a corrected class III incisor relationship); non-compliance with recommended retention regime; persistence of habits, etc.

Risks of orthodontic treatment: There are certain risks associated with orthodontic treatment, which have been discussed in another chapter of this book. The patient should be made aware of all the relevant risks associated with treatment, various risk factors, need of patient cooperation and unpredicted growth behavior of the bones. Certain risks associated with orthodontic treatment include but are not limited to the following:

1. Tooth decay, gum disease, or permanent white markings / white spots lesions (decalcification) on the teeth can occur.
2. Roots of some teeth may become shortened during orthodontic treatment. This may also be associated with previous / current trauma, infection of pulp, etc.
3. Disease of bone and gum tissue may occur, particularly if bacterial plaque is not removed daily through good oral hygiene.
4. Teeth have a tendency to change their positions after treatment. Proper wearing of retainers should reduce this tendency. Changes occur throughout life due to various causes, e.g. eruption of wisdom teeth, genetic influences; size of tongue, growth and / or maturational changes, habits, mouth breathing, all of which may be beyond the control of the orthodontist.
5. Problems may occur in temporomandibular joints (TMJ), causing pain, headaches or ear problems. These problems may occur with or without orthodontic treatment.
6. A tooth / teeth having large fillings, traumatized tooth, damaged nerve of the tooth, etc. may see some problems of pain, etc. during orthodontics and may need root canal treatment.
7. Orthodontic appliances could irritate or traumatise the oral tissues. Postadjustment discomfort / pain, etc. occurs the period of tenderness or sensitivity varies with individuals and with the procedure performed. Generally, it may last for 2–3 days.
8. Oral surgery, tooth removal or orthognathic surgery (surgical realignment of jaws) may be necessary in conjunction with orthodontic treatment, especially to correct crowding or severe jaw imbalances. You should discuss the risks involved with treatment and anesthesia with your general dentist or oral surgeon before making your decision to proceed with this procedure.
9. Abnormal growth changes of jaws may limit the ability to achieve the desired results. Growth changes that occur after active orthodontic treatment may adversely alter the treatment results.

10. The total time required to complete treatment may exceed the estimate. It may be due to factors like improper bone growth, poor cooperation, poor oral hygiene, broken appliances, missed appointments, etc. and can adversely affect the quality of the end result.
11. Although exceedingly rare, some patients may have allergies to certain dental materials/gloves/nickel/elastics, etc.
12. Some cases may need restorative dental treatment due to variation in size and shape of teeth, or missing teeth, to achieve ideal result, e.g. cosmetic bonding, crown and bridge restoration and/or periodontal therapy.
13. General medical problems, such as bone, blood or endocrine disorders, certain medications, etc. can affect orthodontic treatment.

Consent to use of records: Consent to use the orthodontic records, including photographs, made in the process of examinations, treatment, and retention for purposes of professional consultations, research, education, or publication in professional journals should also be taken.

40

Early Orthodontic Treatment

INTRODUCTION

Due to increased awareness and financial capability, more parents are concerned about dental health and esthetic needs of their children. The orthodontic clinics have seen an upsurge in the number of young patients. Orthodontic literature is also replete with the ideas, methods and rationale of early treatment. This chapter highlights principle and rationale of providing early treatment to the potential patients to intercept the developing condition.

However, there has always been confusion among clinicians regarding the timing of the orthodontic treatment. Most of clinicians used to treat the patients in late mixed or permanent dentition stage. But due to increased knowledge, a paradigm shift has been seen in the timing of the treatment, with more clinicians now treating the children at an early age.

In a study in Finland seeking the orthodontists' views through a questionnaire, on the timing and indications for early orthodontic care, it was found that the most orthodontists recommended the first assessment of occlusion to be carried out before 7 years of age.

A crossbite (anterior or lateral) was the most frequent indication for treatment in the primary and early mixed dentition. A severe class II division I malocclusion with an increased overjet was mentioned as the other most frequent indication for treatment in the early and late mixed dentition. They found a significant reduction in orthodontic treatment need from 8 to 12 years in a group of Finnish children treated systematically by early intervention.

Timing of Orthodontic Treatment

The orthodontic treatment can be divided into following types depending on the choice of period of treatment:

a. Early treatment
b. Late treatment.

Orthodontic treatment given in the primary or early mixed dentition is regarded as early treatment. **Early treatment** is the treatment of certain conditions of mild nature which need to be resolved at an early age. It may be done in primary dentition period (sometimes) and in early mixed dentition period (mostly). Early MDP is the period when permanent incisors and first molars have erupted. This phase helps to intercept the initial problem, reduces its severity, and leads to normalized development of dentofacial complex. It may be followed by another comprehensive treatment phase in late MDP or early permanent dentition, depending on the nature of condition.

Opinions on timing of orthodontic assessment: American Association of Orthodontists recommends that every child should have an orthodontic evaluation by age 7 or earlier. Although treatment may not be needed at this young age, but an early examination allows the orthodontist to monitor child's dental and jaws development. Early detection and interception can significantly reduce the severity of the condition and hence the need of complex orthodontic/orthopedic treatment in future. Second orthodontic assessment can be done from the early mixed to the late mixed dentition and the third from the late mixed to the permanent dentition.

Late treatment: It can be described as the treatment provided in late MDP or in permanent dentition. It is needed to resolve the condition of severe nature which may be dental and/or skeletal in nature. Severe skeletal conditions which need surgical intervention are treated after active growth has been completed.

Phases of treatment: Depending on the number of phases, the treatment can be divided as:

a. **Single phase therapy:** It is the method of treatment given in one phase only, (i.e. when treatment is started in late MDP and continued in early PDP).
b. **Two-phase therapy:** It involves two phases of treatment, i.e. one initial phase of early treatment of shorter duration (when treatment is given in early MDP); and then the second phase is undertaken in late MDP/early PDP. It may also involve a phase of retention in some cases after phase 1.

Rationale of Early Treatment

The main purpose of early orthodontic intervention is to correct or intercept a developing problem; and thus to prevent the skeletal manifestation of anomalies and worsening of the problem. Early orthodontic treatment will not resolve all potential orthodontic problems or totally inhibit adverse skeletal growth patterns. However, by identifying problems at an early age it is possible to redirect skeletal growth; improve the occlusal relationship; enhance the patient's esthetics and self-image and, perhaps of even greater importance, achieve results that are unattainable later with the eruption of teeth and the cessation of growth. Although there are many orthodontic conditions needing treatment during the early and mixed dentitions, but still there exist certain limitations to early treatment which will be discussed further in this chapter.

The goal of phase 1 orthodontic treatment is to reduce the severity, and to minimize or eliminate the amount of treatment in the second phase of treatment. Phase 1 generally involves an active treatment with simple appliances for a short period of 6 to 12 months, in which skeletodental relation improvement, guidance of occlusion, etc. can be achieved. It is done to remove interferences from the path of normal growth and development. So, it can be merged with interceptive procedures of orthodontics. Phase 2 is started after the eruption of appropriate permanent teeth, and involves the "finishing" process by using a full-fledged fixed appliance.

Early orthodontic treatment is effective and desirable in certain situations of malocclusions. But, there are reports in literature which say that such an approach is not indicated in many cases for which later, single-phase treatment is more effective. Therefore, clinicians must make a decision on a case-by-case basis, when to provide orthodontic treatment.

Indication for and frequency of early orthodontic therapy or interceptive measures: The early treatment of non-skeletal and skeletal orthodontic anomalies in deciduous and early mixed dentition is intended to prevent their conversion to pronounced anomalies, with the ultimate aim of reducing or even eliminating the need for later orthodontic treatment.

Generally in many patients, the orthodontic treatment is best done after eruption of all permanent teeth. In patients with completed active growth having an abnormal growth pattern, the clinician does not face much difficulty because the unwanted changes are minimal. For example, in moderate to severe cases of skeletal class III malocclusion having mandibular prognathism, the definitive orthodontic and surgical treatment should be deferred until the end of active growth period, which is generally considered till 18 years of age for mandibular growth. But, there are certain conditions which need interception during the mixed dentition. It is done to eliminate or modify the developing skeletal and dentoalveolar condition to correct it or to prevent the increasing severity of the condition.

Modification of craniofacial growth: The downward and forward growth of the maxillary complex can be redirected using extraoral appliances and myofunctional appliances. Deficient maxillary growth can be enhanced by using reverse face mask, while excessive maxillary growth can be restricted by using high pull headgear.

Deficient mandibular growth, in growing individuals, can be enhanced at least in the short term with myofunctional appliances, while the excess mandibular growth can be at least restricted or redirected by using chin cup appliance and high pull headgear combination. But, there is little evidence showing that the mandibular growth can be diminished with the use of chin cup, although a redirection of mandibular growth in a more vertical direction can be done. These modalities can be used in combination also depending on the nature of the problem.

Sexual dimorphism: Females are ahead in maturity than males by approx. 2 years. It is very important to be kept in mind during treatment planning. A proper growth status should be evaluated by appropriate SMIs to institute the proper treatment appliance. Eg due to this difference, it is possible that if you plan to give mandibular growth modification treatment at the same chronological age, i.e. late mixed dentition period, in both boys and girls, the boys may be in active period of growth, while the girls have already passed that stage and thus no effect can be obtained.

Patient cooperation: Patient cooperation is the main factor for success of early treatment. It is generally observed that the patient and parents lose interest when the treatment is started at an early age. It is due to the fact that either the treatment needs 2 phases of treatment or the treatment gets prolonged. To prevent it, a proper diagnosis, need of treatment, goals and objectives should be determined. Proper discussion should be done with patient and parents in treatment decision making. They should be explained the benefits of the treatment needed at this time. Milder conditions should be treated at an early age. A shorter, simplified, initial phase of treatment should provided, which is followed by a period of clinical observation during the transition from the mixed to the permanent dentition. Any other condition appearing during transition should be controlled with appropriated method. E-space can be saved by placing a transpalatal arch and a lingual holding arch, which can be used later on for treatment of TSALD with fixed orthodontics.

Ideal time for treatment: Ideal time to start orthodontic treatment in growing patient is a controversial issue. Beginning treatment in primary dentition can prolong treatment over a 10-year span (5–15 years), sometimes requiring three phases of treatment. Delaying treatment in certain cases till late mixed dentition has its own disadvantages in certain cases. It may lead to increased severity of the condition, e.g. females are more advanced in growth than males. If growth modulation is delayed in females, they may have crossed the peak velocity of their skeletal growth, thus the chances of good results by growth modification in females get reduced. If treatment is started in permanent dentition, the problems of poor cooperation by teenagers, little or no growth remaining, root resorption, etc. come into play.

Timing of Early Intervention

The timing of initiation of early treatment procedure depends on the type of malocclusion. Eg for treatment of class I tooth-size/arch-size discrepancy, insufficient space does not allow proper alignment of teeth. Depending on TSALD and arch size, the space maintenance, serial extraction, expansion, or a combination of these can be used.

The treatment of class II with mandibular deficiency is different from class I and class III malocclusions. Treatment of mandibular deficiency/retrognathism with mild to moderate sagittal problems should be started in late mixed dentition period using the functional appliances. The late MDP is the time of active spurt of growth. However, it should be kept in mind that in females, the growth spurt comes 2 years earlier than males. There is a greater mandibular growth response with functional appliances when treatment is given during circumpubertal growth period. Fixed appliances can also be simultaneously started to align permanent dentition in some cases. But, certain patients having severe neuromuscular and skeletal problems should be treated at an early age.

In class II patients with maxillary prognathism, extraoral traction can be employed in mixed dentition to redirect the growth. Headgear is used for best response at around 8–9 years of age when there is active sagittal and vertical growth taking place. Also, at that time, it is easy to distalize maxillary arch as second molars have not erupted.

In class III malocclusion in a child who is at late deciduous or early mixed dentition stage, the treatment has to be started early than other patients. The optimal time for starting an early class III treatment (e.g., by using facial mask, FR-3 of Frankel, chin cup, etc.) is the time when eruption of the upper permanent central incisors occurs, i.e. around 7–8 years age. But, this earlier treatment in class III patients results in an overall longer treatment time.

Efficient orthodontic treatment timing concept: This concept was introduced by Viazis. According to this concept, a malocclusion should be treated as soon as possible if it is expected that the postponement of treatment would lead to severe functional or esthetic problems. Also, the treatment of certain conditions can be deferred to a later stage, when the later treatment is expected to provide the same effects with less overall treatment time and cost.

Indications of Early Orthodontic Intervention

Certain conditions such as dental or skeletal crossbites (which may result in functional shift of mandible) should be treated as early as possible. Habit control, functional crossbite correction, pseudo class III and alleviation of possible crowding, especially in deep bite cases, should be initiated as soon as they are detected.

A deficient maxilla (class III) should be protracted (by facemask) as soon as the upper permanent first molars and permanent incisors have erupted, i.e. around 8 years of age. Mild mandibular prognathism can be effectively addressed at an early age with chin cap therapy or treatment of anterior cross bite. True mandibular prognathism of mild-moderate nature due to excessive mandibular growth should be intercepted by using chin cup and HPHG to restrict/redirect the growth. However, severe cases require surgical treatment after completion of growth.

Finally, any limited treatment (single tooth crossbite, diastema, spacing) can be addressed individually at any age. Any dysfunction and/or pain to the temporomandibular joint should be addressed as soon as it is detected.

Indications for early treatment can include as outlined by Dugoni are:

- Congenitally missing teeth and management of spaces.
- Crowding causing periodontal problems.
- Crowding leading to ectopic eruption of teeth.
- Dental and/or skeletal class II and class III cases.
- Developing midline discrepancies due to unilateral loss of primary teeth.
- Ectopically erupting/chances of impaction of maxillary canines.

- Habits
- Maxillary deficiency
- Moderate incisor crowding
- Posterior and/or anterior crossbites
- Presence of supernumerary teeth leading to deflected path of eruption.
- Proclined incisors with less than 6 mm of overjet should be treated so as to avoid chances of trauma.
- Severe anterior open bite less than 3 mm
- Severe deep bite with palatal impingement.

Benefits of early orthodontic treatment: An early orthodontic intervention can provide following benefits to the patients in which it is indicated:

- It helps to guide the jaw growth.
- It can help to regulate upper and lower dental arches widths.
- Helps in eruption guidance of the permanent teeth into desirable positions.
- It helps to treat the prominent front teeth and thus lowers risk of trauma to them.
- It helps to reduce the chances of iatrogenic tooth damage such as trauma, root resorption and decalcification.
- It helps to control the harmful oral habits such as thumb- or finger-sucking, reduce or eliminate abnormal swallowing or speech problems.
- It helps to improve personal appearance and self-esteem, thus having psychological benefits.
- It helps to simplify or shorten treatment time for later corrective orthodontics.
- It reduces the likelihood of impaction of permanent teeth by removing the blockages and guiding them properly in arches.
- It helps to improve the orofacial environment before the complete eruption of permanent dentition, and the further requirement for complex orthodontic treatment is reduced.
- It provides better patient cooperation, since the children accept treatment without much hassle.
- It provides an opportunity for a decreased or possible elimination of the need for a second phase of treatment by reducing the severity or elimination of the condition.
- There is an increased long-term stability of lower incisor alignment after early correction, as the soft tissues get more time to adaptation.
- There is increased stability of transverse and A-P dimensions changes with phase 1 treatment.
- It helps to reduce the chances of ectopic/impacted canines, by eliminating the restriction in the path of eruption and providing the proper space.
- It helps to reduce the incidence of mucogingival problems by elimination of crowding, and deep bite tendencies.
- With proper development of dental arches, and maintaining the physiological spaces, it helps to reduce the chances of premolar extraction later in treatment.
- With proper growth modulation and correction of skeletal discrepancy, there are decreased chances of future orthognathic surgery.

Disadvantages of Early Treatment

- It needs a two-phase treatment, thus prolonged treatment time.
- Increased cost of the two-phases.
- Patients' cooperation starts burning-out because they calculate the total time since the start of phase 1.
- Some patients may stop taking treatment due to prolonged treatment.

Conditions needing early treatment: Many reports have been published in literature to mention the conditions which need correction as early as possible. Some of them have been described below.

1. Crossbites: All crossbites, i.e. anterior and posterior should be treated as early as possible. Any crossbite leads to deviated path of closure, interference in proper jaw growth, maldevelopment of occlusion, and abnormal forces on TMJs.

Why it is necessary: For example, a single tooth anterior crossbite may inhibit the development of the alveolar bone related to that tooth. A complete anterior crossbite, e.g. in class III or pseudo-class III, leads to interference of maxillary growth, while the mandibular growth is continued uninterfered. It leads to maxillary deficiency or mandibular excess due to abnormal growth.

Advantages: By treatment of crossbite, a functional improvement is achieved, which is healthy to TMJs. It also leads to improved esthetics and thus a psychological boost. Treatment of this condition is easier in mixed dentition as compared to later period as bones are soft, the teeth are in erupting stages, which can be easily redirected to erupt in better position with expansion, etc. If expansion is done in primary dentition to treatment narrow maxillary arch, the permanent teeth follow the new normal position of the primary teeth and erupt in normal relation and arch form.

2. Crossbite in primary canine or incisal region: Sometimes, a mild form of crossbite is present in incisor or canine region, and patient is very young and not cooperative, then the enamel grinding of both the teeth can be done so that they do not come in crossbite relation while in centric occlusion. It will help to prevent the abnormal forces; functional shift, etc. The continuing growth can help in attaining a normal position. The patient should be on regular observation.

3. A complete anterior crossbite in primary dentition, where the major enamel grinding of 8–10 anterior teeth cannot be done, can be corrected by bonding composite blocks on upper primary molars so that patient does not close in crossbite in centric occlusion, thus preventing the other side effects associated with crossbite. The growth will help in attaining a normal relation, as the maxilla grows more than mandible in initial years (cephalocaudal gradient of growth). But, patients should be kept on constant observation.

4. Expansion in primary dentition: Crossbite in primary dentition can be present, mostly due to upper narrow arch, and sometime due to narrow lower arch. Expansion of the affected arch should be done to correct the cross bite. It helps to achieve a normal occlusal relationship, prevents prematurities and deflective path of closure; leads to a normal growth pattern, and achieves symmetry of the face. Also, the permanent teeth buds follow the primary teeth during expansion and it is expected that they will erupt in a normal relationship of the expanded arch later in life and thus there will not be a need to do expansion in mixed or permanent dentition.

Early treatment of transverse discrepancies: Unilateral or bilateral crossbites are due to dental or skeletal discrepancies, or a combination of the two. Correction of transverse discrepancies involves either dental or palatal expansion. The dental expansion is done by simple tooth movement and, generally is best done during phase 2 treatment. But the correction of skeletal crossbite by palatal expansion needs manipulation of midplatal and circummaxillary sutures. So, this procedure must be done before the ossification of these sutures. Once the palatal suture is fused, correction of a skeletal crossbite usually requires surgical intervention.

Ossification of midpalatal suture is extensive, but not complete, in late adolescence. But, in early stages of skeletal maturation (i.e. before adolescent growth spurt's peak height velocity), little-to-no midpalatal interdigitation exists. Therefore, palatal expansion should be started just before the onset of puberty. McNamara has shown that expansion in the transitional dentition is stable.

A patient with a lateral functional shift should be treated with early orthopedic correction. This shift is due to compensatory and habitual deflection of mandible to achieve maximum intercuspation in a case of constricted maxillary arch. When patient closes the mouth, premature contact appears due to palatal constriction, and the mandible shifts to one side to avoid this contact to achieve centric occlusion. Consequently, the condyles are positioned asymmetrically within their respective fossae and the mandible closes asymmetrically, with the lower midline deviated to the shifted side. This gives the appearance of a unilateral crossbite when, in fact, it is bilateral. This condition should be diagnosed properly when the patient is asked to close slowly and the relation of jaws is noted at the first point of contact. If left untreated, this condition can lead to asymmetrical growth of the mandible and uneven remodeling of the glenoid fossa, and leads to permanent facial asymmetry, even if the constricted maxillary arch is corrected at a later date.

Maxillary expansion is the indicated treatment for palatal constriction, which removes the premature contacts, eliminates mandibular shift and allows the mandible to achieve centric relation with coinciding midlines. When this occurs, occlusal symmetry is achieved and symmetrical growth is no longer inhibited. Consequently, a strong argument can be made for early treatment in such cases. Maxillary constriction without a lateral shift does not carry the same urgency and, therefore, can be treated closer to adolescence.

5. Ankylosed teeth: Ankylosis of the tooth is direct joining of root, partial or complete, to the alveolar bone without intervening PDL. It also needs immediate intervention because it cannot self-correct.

Rationale: An ankylosed tooth cannot erupt naturally, and thus a deficiency of the alveolar bone occurs there because a tooth acts as a functional matrix for that part of bone. An ankylosed tooth gets **submerged** as the adjacent teeth keep on erupting. If left untreated then the adjacent and opposing teeth may tilt in this area which leads to occlusal problems.

Treatment: An ankylosed primary tooth should be extracted so that the permanent tooth can erupt in normal position. If it is not done, then the permanent tooth may either get impacted or may erupt in an abnormal position. However, to treat this condition, an appropriate time should be selected. It is best to defer the treatment till the succedaneous tooth development has reached at a level of proper natural eruption. If extracted early then a space maintainer will be required for a prolonged time. The position of permanent tooth should be monitored with the help of IOPA view to see the development of root. Once the root is developed more than 50%, the ankylosed tooth should be removed. It may or may not need a brief period of space maintainer.

6. Developing crowding in incisal region: Due to deficient growth, bigger size of permanent incisors, there may be less space in incisal region, leading to eruption of incisors in crowded state. In such case, the proximal surface of the offending primary tooth can be judiciously trimmed to provide the space for erupting teeth. The primary incisor or canine tooth should not be extracted during this stage, because the erupting lateral incisors are expected to push primary canines laterally and gain some space.

7. Ectopic eruption of teeth: Ectopically erupting teeth should be treated as early as possible, i.e. when discovered. If this problem is not treated early, then it may greatly reduce the arch length for permanent dentition. It may also lead to development of cross bite and deflection of mandible during closure. Simple appliances can be used to treat the cross bite. If a retained primary tooth is the cause of ectopic eruption or crossbite development, then the offending primary tooth should be removed.

8. Blockage of eruption of teeth: Occasionally, the premolars can be found to be stuck beneath the mesial height of contour of primary molars teeth (as they have constricted cervical area and prominent HOCs), thus blocking their eruption. It is a sign of intrabony crowding as seen in OPG. In such cases, the recontouring is done of the culprit tooth to provide the space for erupting teeth. Extraction of primary tooth is not warranted because then a space maintainer will be needed. Many times, the permanent second molar is found stuck below distal HOC of permanent first molars. It should be disimpacted with the help of disimpaction spring to facilitate its eruption.

9. Proclined upper teeth: Excessively proclined upper incisors are prone to trauma and fracture during early school years, as the children push each other or fall while playing. It may sometimes lead to avulsions also. To avoid such mishaps, this condition needs an early treatment. Also, increased overjet due to maxillary incisal proclination leads to lower lip trap, which in turn, increases overjet by proclination of maxillary incisors apart and retroclining the mandibular incisors. The active lower lip also applies a restraining force on mandible and thus interferes its proper sagittal growth. With time, if left unchecked, it becomes a feedback cycle. It also leads to short and hypotonic upper lip.

Treatment: The treatment depends on the condition and etiology of the problem. It can be done with oral screen appliance; or an active Hawley's appliance if there is sufficient space in anterior region; or a modified Hawley's appliance with an expansion screw for gaining the space can be used.

10. Open bites and habits: Anterior and posterior open bites need early treatment. They are often due to digit sucking or tongue thrusting habits. It is a vicious circle when the tongue keeps on interposing in the open bite and does not allow its natural closure (which is expected due to natural eruption of teeth). A continued thumb sucking habit leads to constricted maxillary arch, posterior cross-bite, anterior open bite, deep palate, increased posterior dentoalveolar height, D and B rotation of mandible and vertical face pattern. A continued tongue thrust habit does not allow the teeth to come in normal approximation and thus lead to further development of skeletal problem. If they are not treated early, then the severity can increase and skeletal problems/deficiency set in. Then these conditions cannot be completely treated with orthodontic alone and need orthognathic surgery.

Treatment: Habit-breaking appliances; muscles-retraining exercises, etc. can be used to control habits. Once a normal neuromuscular pattern sets in, the normal growth and development of dentoskeletal tissues can be expected.

11. Early treatment of arch length discrepancies, severe crowding: Due to severe arch length discrepancies in mixed dentition, deflection/impaction of other teeth may occur. It also leads to problem in maintenance of oral hygiene. It can be intercepted by guidance of eruption or serial extraction, where sequential removal of some primary and permanent teeth is done to provide space for other teeth to erupt in line. Early treatment in such cases may be started even when incisors are erupting in crowded position. Mild space problems can be resolved by selective **proximal reduction** of primary teeth in the area of erupting permanent incisors. Reduction of mesial surface of first primary molar can be also done to allow out-of-line canines to start drifting distally and thus erupt in a better position. It helps to reduce the severity of malocclusion and thus makes future orthodontic treatment quicker and more effective. Leeway space is saved by using lingual holding arch, which can be used to resolve crowding and to align lower incisors in the early mixed dentition.

The clinician must have proper knowledge of the normal arch development so that he is able to diagnose and determine the need for appropriate timing of treatment for arch-length discrepancies. During transition from primary to permanent dentition, minor incisor crowding is often seen especially during the eruption of permanent mandibular incisors, i.e. 6–7½ years of age. This crowding of approx. 2 mm gets relieved naturally with the continued growth and development of jaws (refer to Chapter 8 on Development of Dentition) such that there is enough space available for the permanent mandibular canines to erupt. It occurs due to following reasons:

1. With normal growth, a slight increase in arch width occurs across the canines due to increased mandibular intercanine width till 9 years of age. It is also accompanied by labially inclined path of canine eruption. More intercanine width is gained in maxilla than the mandible, and, it occurs more and for longer age in boys than in girls.
2. Permanent incisors erupt in a more labial position than the primary teeth, gaining 1–2 mm of arch length.
3. In the mandibular arch, the primate space is located posterior to primary canines. Consequently, the permanent canines erupt in a more posterior position than their primary counterparts, leaving the gained space of about 1 mm on each side available for the alignment of the incisors.

But in upper arch, a naturally occurring transitional diastema often develops between permanent maxillary central incisors, as compared to the transitional developing crowding seen in mandibular arch. This diastema often causes concern for parents because the teeth appear to be erupting into unfavorable positions. But, this is a natural developing state (ugly-duckling stage) which is self-correcting. This central diastema of 2 mm or less closes naturally with the subsequent eruption of maxillary canines. Larger diastema will require proper diagnosis and the orthodontic intervention to achieve complete closure.

Crowding of anterior dentition can also be controlled by using the leeway space. This space is generally taken up by mesial drifting of permanent first molars if not controlled. But, it can be preserved to relieve crowding of anterior teeth by placing a lingual holding arch, lip bumper, a transpalatal appliance, etc. in the respective arches. Optimal timing for this treatment should coincide with exfoliation of primary second molars.

Arch width expansion is indicated when there is developing crowding which can prevent the natural eruption of certain teeth. For example, the permanent maxillary lateral incisors erupting palatally in crowded position, then the expansion would be indicated at the age of 6 or 7 years. In some situations, malpositioning of teeth leads to unfavorable wear patterns. This also is an indication for early expansion followed by active alignment to prevent continued wear of enamel.

In developing severe crowding, serial extraction is done where sequenced extraction of specific primary and some permanent teeth (generally first premolars) is done to facilitate the teeth to erupt within the dental arch. Ideally, serial extractions begin in the early-transitional dentition.

12. Expansion of lower arch: It helps to gain space in the dental arch which can help to treat mild TSALD cases on non-extraction basis. So an early treatment can be recommended to "develop" the lower arch. It can be achieved by using force systems leading to active and/or passive expansion of the lower arch. It should be remembered that there is no suture in mandible, thus an active skeletal expansion cannot be done. Any arch development is of dental nature, with subsequent adaptation of soft tissues around the new dental arch with time. With oral screen and the Frankel's buccal shields, which activate periosteum lead to development of skeletal tissues and thus help in achieving skeletal effects. Oral screen also helps in arch development by restricting the influence of buccal musculature, while the tongue keeps on applying a buccally-directed force on the arches and thus leads to physiological passive expansion.

Also, the lip bumper in lower arch, and rapid expansion (RPE) of upper arch help to induce passive/spontaneous expansion of lower arch as the maxillary arch widens. The lip bumper helps to gain space in dental arch because it leads to increase in both arch length and width. It occurs by blocking the effect of lips and cheeks on the dental arch, while the tongue keeps on applying outward forces causing lateral and anterior expansion.

Increase in upper intercanine width: Expansion of intercanine width provides more space for alignment than any other transverse change. Germane et al. found that 1 mm of intercanine expansion increases arch perimeter by 0.73 mm, whereas a 1 mm expansion of the molars produces only a 0.27 mm increase in arch perimeter. The actively-increased intercanine width in mandible s not stable as there are no sutures, and always relapses or it needs a permanent retention. So, the intercanine width of mandibular arch should be maintained during treatment. Natural increase in intercanine width occurs till 9 years in mandible in both sexes, while in maxilla, it occurs till 12 years in females, and 16 years in males. A passive increase in intercanine width can be achieved by removing the restricting effects of hyperactive musculature.

13. Cleft palate: Cleft palate patients need timely and phasic orthodontic intervention since very early age. For example, from the time of birth, an obturator may be needed so that they can take proper nutrition without nasal escape of milk. The supernumerary and out-of-alignment teeth need extraction so that other teeth may erupt properly. Expansion of upper arch, alignment of teeth, correction of rotated incisors and crossbite, etc. is needed to aid in surgeries and other restorative needs.

14. Pseudo class III: Pseudo-class III is a condition which is more of dental nature than skeletal, if diagnosed at an early age, and should be definitely treated as early as possible. It occurs due to anterior shift of mandible due to premature contacts in incisal region, thus leading to a complete anterior cross bite. If not treated, it will eventually become a skeletal problem with continued abnormal, unrestricted growth of mandible. It may be seen in primary and mixed dentition. Mild prematurities can be trimmed away to lead a normal closure or to avoid a functional shift. Some premature contacts are relieved by proclining the upper incisor so that the slippage in crossbite condition does not occur while closing.

15. Early class III treatment: Class III skeletal pattern is due to a small and/or posteriorly positioned maxilla, or a large and/or prognathic mandible, or combination of both; or maxilla and mandible that are normal in the sagittal plane of space but underdeveloped in the vertical dimension.

These conditions due to true maxillary retrusion should be treated during the mixed dentition stage for best results. The best age for treatment is generally 8–9 years when the maxilla observes a growth spurt in sagittal as well as transverse dimension. Due to ensuing rapid growth, more skeletal changes can be achieved. The most common treatment for this problem in the growing patient involves the use of protraction headgear, with or without prior palatal expansion. For patients in whom a skeletal crossbite is present, orthopedic expansion is appropriate. Some clinicians suggest that such expansion also facilitates the anteroposterior response to facemask therapy. The transverse expansion can be best achieved during mixed dentition, because midpalatal suture is still patent and is not interdigitated. It is possible to open it easily during this age. Reverse face mask is needed to treat hypoplastic maxilla, while chin cup is used to control mandibular excess.

Approximately 12 ounces force is used for 14 hours a day in a forward and slightly downward direction. The orthopedic and orthodontic responses to this force system include forward and downward movement of the maxilla, with concomitant forward and downward movement of the maxillary dentition, downward and backward rotation of the mandible, and retroclination of the mandibular incisors. All of these changes improve the three skeletal discrepancies contributing to the class III malocclusion. The only class III pattern for which these changes would be contraindicated is one with excessive vertical development.

Face mask therapy is given to patients in the primary to early transitional dentition, because of the patency of the circummaxillary sutures appropriate to this age. Here, the growth modification is based on the premise that applying tension to these immature sutures is a stimulus for new bone formation. As the patient nears the adolescence, more interdigitation of sutures starts which results in less skeletal and more dental response to the protraction forces.

In addition to the presence of patent sutures, the timing of treatment with protraction headgear depends, although to a lesser degree, on the developing dentition. Primary or permanent teeth with adequate roots are required for protraction force application. Consequently, in the late-transitional dentition, the primary teeth do not have full roots and thus present a challenge to face mask therapy, since they may not provide an adequate anchor for headgear.

16. Pseudo-class I described by DeBaets and Chiarini: It is in reality a class II malocclusion perceived as a class I malocclusion. It has characteristics like: deep anterior overbite; Mesial rotation of the maxillary first permanent molars; crowding of the mandibular incisors, etc. It should be treated early to allow the occlusion, dentition and face to develop in a normal and stable manner.

17. Early orthodontic treatment to prevent temporomandibular dysfunction, snoring, and sleep apnea: According to Rondeau, patients having class II due to mandibular retrognathism should be treated early to prevent development of TMD, and OSAS. It should be started before the major growth spurts have passed, so as to take advantage of the active growth.

Oral habits, such as thumb sucking and anterior tongue thrusts, must be treated as early as possible. Blocked airways due to enlarged tonsils or adenoids, should be managed by ENT specialist to normalize the airway, and restore nasal breathing before treatment. The removal of tonsils in children routinely eliminates snoring and sleep apnea. Overjet in class II skeletal patients with retrognathic mandibles is caused by the retruded mandible and, therefore, this should be treated by advancing the mandible with a functional appliance.

TM dysfunction: One of the main causes of TM dysfunction is when the mandibular condyle is displaced posteriorly, causing a compression of nerves and blood vessels behind the condyle. It also causes the disk to become displaced anteriorly, as evident by clicking on opening and closing. When the disk becomes dislocated, the muscles of mastication undergo spasm to protect the joint, which causes headaches, ear symptoms, and pain in the neck and shoulders. Functional appliances help in repositioning the condyle downward and forward in the glenoid fossa. It decompresses the nerves and blood vessels distal to the condyle, and helps in healing of TM joint (TMJ). Many malocclusions frequently have pre-existing TMD, e.g. class II division 2, deep overbite, unilateral crossbite with facial asymmetry, narrow maxillary arch, and class II division 1 skeletal patients with retrognathic mandibles. TMJ health should be evaluated properly, e.g. with the help of a questionnaire, range of motion measurements, noting clicking, etc. deviated closure; muscle palpations, joint vibration analysis (JVA), and X-ray tomography.

Snoring is caused when the tongue partially blocks the airway. Obstructive sleep apnea (OSA) is caused when the tongue completely blocks the airway for 10 seconds or more, at least 35–40 times per night. Patients with class II division 1 skeletal malocclusions with retrognathic mandibles are prime candidates for snoring and OSA later in life. It is due to retruded tongue, occurring naturally with retruded mandible. With age, the patients gradually gain weight, increasing the fat in their necks and lessening the muscle tone, which reduces the size of the airway. Women with a neck size more than 16 inches and men with a neck size more than 17 inches are candidates for snoring and OSA.

With retractive technique for correction of class II division 1 skeletal patients, the maxillary teeth are subsequently retracted, which may predispose the patient to snoring and sleep apnea later in life. Before treatment, the mandible and tongue are in a retruded position. With the retraction of maxillary teeth, the tongue and the mandible are prevented from obtaining their normal forward position. The treatment of choice would be to bring the lower jaw forward with a functional jaw orthopedic appliance. With functional appliances, the tongue comes forward and opens the airway, which prevents snoring and sleep apnea. Continuous positive air pressure (CPAP) device, which forces air up the nose all night using an air compressor is recommended in mild to moderate cases of OSAS.

Counterpoint

Gianelly favors that the treatment should be started in late mixed dentition period. It is a better time for intervention due to following reasons:

- E space, if not lost by caries or premature loss of teeth, can be used to relieve mild crowding by maintaining it. Space maintenance can be done by using lingual holding arch, TPA, bent-in stop loops in arch wires, etc. Mild crowding can be resolved in many patients in mixed dentition stage by preserving and using the leeway space, especially the E-space.

What is E-space: The combined mesiodistal width of deciduous canine and first molar are essentially the same as that of permanent canine and first premolar, thus the space gain actually, is due to difference in size of E and second premolar, which is the "E" space.

"E" space can be maintained by starting treatment in late mixed dentition stage. However, a passive lingual arch may be needed to preserve the arch length, if a deciduous canine is lost prematurely. Otherwise, the incisors can tip lingually under lip pressure and lead to loss of arch length.

- Patients can be treated by non-extraction method, if space discrepancy is mild to moderate. Space can be gained by expansion, stripping, maintaining E-space, etc.
- There is no need of subjecting the patient to treatment for a prolonged time or in two phases. The treatment can usually be completed in a single phase.
- The time and cost of treatment will be lesser.
- Patient does not lose the interest in the treatment.
- Since this is the time of growth spurt, PHV, etc. the maximum advantages of ensuing growth can be obtained during treatment, e.g. with FJO, etc.

One-phase Versus two-phase Treatment

1. Patient remains cooperative because the total treatment time (calendar time) is less; there are less hospital visits; and 2–3 procedures can be done at the same time. The functional appliance (fixed/removable) can be given along with fixed orthodontic appliance, thus skeletal and dental correction go side by side.
2. Patients needing mandibular growth modulation for treatment of skeletal class II relation can be treated successfully in a one-phase therapy, by starting treatment in the late mixed dentition, as it parallels the active growth spurt.
3. But habit control, the use of passive appliances such as space maintainers and minor alignment of incisors for esthetic or trauma reasons, is not considered part of conventional two-phase treatment.
4. Patients with crossbites and a mandibular shift and patients with class III malocclusions should be given early treatment, as they can benefit from immediate resolution of the problem.

Early Treatment of Class II Malocclusion

Substantial evidence supports the theory that early growth modification therapy can lead to an improvement, if not complete correction, of the class II malocclusion.

Class II malocclusions: If treatment is started in late mixed dentition stage, then class II can be treated successfully in one phase, the treatment time lasts for 2–3 years. There are a number of procedures used to correct these problems. For example, distal movement of the maxillary molars to convert the class II malocclusion to a class I spacing problem.

Class II malocclusions due to mandibular retrognathism are treated by using functional appliances, with the intent to stimulate mandibular growth. The treatment should be started in late mixed dentition as the advantages of growth can best be taken at this stage. After postadolescent growth phase, fixed Herbst appliance can be used to take advantage of remaining growth.

Conclusion

Early orthodontic treatment is effective and desirable in specific situations. In the treatment of patients with class II malocclusion, correction at an early or late stage is equally beneficial. The immediate effect that early treatment may have on a patient's self-esteem and susceptibility to dental trauma. Patients with class III malocclusion benefit significantly from early orthopedic treatment. However, such therapy may produce more favorable changes for older children (aged 11 and 12 years) and adolescents (aged 13 and 14 years) than previously thought.

Palatal expansion appears to be effective and stable at any time before late adolescence, a stage of development when ossification of the midpalatal suture begins. Consequently, the timing of expansion may be better determined by the specific needs of each patient. A functional shift resulting from a crossbite is optimally corrected early so that asymmetrical growth of the mandible can be reduced or even prevented. Expansion for the relief of crowding is best timed on the basis of the specific nature of the crowding.

Treatment of arch length discrepancies depends on the nature of the crowding. Natural arch development has the potential to correct early mild incisor crowding. Management of the leeway space will resolve a majority of cases of crowding. This approach is best accomplished in the transitional to late-transitional dentition. Severe crowding may warrant the extraction of permanent teeth. A serial extraction protocol may be desirable and the extraction sequence for such an approach begins in the early-transitional dentition, while the appliance phase occurs in the early-permanent dentition.

Starting of orthodontics treatment is a controversial issue in orthodontics. There are certain conditions which need earliest intervention so that growth and development can take place in a normal way. It gives a psychological boost to the patients with improved esthetics and functions. Craniofacial growth should be kept in mind during treatment. Certain cases need to be treated during late mixed dentition. The onus of recognising the conditions to be treated at the particular stage lies on the orthodontist and the best possible intervention should be given to eliminate or reduce the severity of the condition.

Further Readings

1. Clark WJ. The Twin Block technique. Part 1. Funct Orthod 1992;9(5):32–37.
2. Clark WJ. The twin block technique. A functional orthopedic appliance system. Am J Orthod Dentofacial Orthop 1988;93(1):1–18.
3. Dugoni: Comprehensive mixed dentition treatment. Volume 1995 Nov 560.
4. Gianelly A: One-phase versus two-phase treatment. Volume 1995 Nov (556–559)
5. Graber, Thomas M., Rokosi, Thomas, Petrovic, Alexandre G. Dentofacial Orthopedics with Functional Appliances. 2nd ed., Mosby, 484–485.
6. Larry White: Early orthodontic intervention. Volume 1998 Jan (24–28):
7. Viazis: Efficient orthodontic treatment timing.

41

Management of Class I Malocclusion

INTRODUCTION

Normal occlusion is considered to have Angle's class I molar relation, well-aligned arches, no spacing and rotations, normal overjet and overbite relation. Angle's class I malocclusion is the most prevalent malocclusion condition, followed by class II and class III in that order. Angle's class I molar relation is not a guarantee for a normal occlusion because the teeth should be well aligned, with normal overjet/overbite relation, and well-formed arches. There may be other conditions, like crowding, proclination, spacing, retroclination, rotation, bimaxillary protrusion; or malocclusion in the vertical plane, like open bite, deep bite; or in transverse plane, like crossbite. Presence of any such condition leads to malocclusion.

Dewey modified Angle's class I in five types based on the upper teeth as below:

- Type 1: Crowding of maxillary anterior teeth.
- Type 2: Spacing in maxillary anterior teeth.
- Type 3: Crossbite of maxillary anterior teeth.
- Type 4: Crossbite of maxillary posterior teeth.
- Type 5: Loss of molar relationship due to early loss of primary tooth.

Ackermann and Proffit classified the malocclusion in the three planes of space. For simplification, the Angle's class I conditions can be divided in sagittal, transverse and vertical dimensions.

a. In **sagittal plane**:
   - Increased overjet
   - Proclination of the teeth
   - Bimaxillary proclination of anteriors
   - Retroclination of teeth
   - Anterior crossbite (discussed in Chapter 43 on Management of Crossbite)
   - Space maintenance and space regaining (discussed in Chapter 22 on Methods of Gaining Space)

b. In **transverse plane**:
   - Buccal crossbites (discussed in Chapter 43 on Management of Crossbite)
   - Narrow maxillary arch (discussed in Chapter 43 on Management of Crossbite)
   - Midline shift
   - Flaring of buccal teeth (discussed in Chapter 43 on Management of Crossbite)

c. In **vertical plane**:
   - Deep bite (discussed in Chapter 44 on Management of Open Bite)
   - Open bite (discussed in Chapter 44 on Management of Open Bite)
   - Vertical growth pattern
   - Extruded or intruded tooth or teeth

d. Miscellaneous:
   - Crowding
   - Spacing
   - Habits: lip trap, thumb sucking, tongue thrusting, etc. (discussed in Chapter 47 on Oral Habits)
   - Rotation
   - Maxillary frenum and lingual frenum problems

- Ankylosed teeth
- Unerupted teeth
- Supernumerary or missing teeth, etc.

Diagnosis and treatment planning: A proper examinations and diagnosis is done so that a proper treatment plan can be made. Before treatment of any condition, the underlying etiology should be considered and "remove the cause" philosophy should be followed. In the following pages, we will discuss different conditions associated with an Angle's class I molars (Figs 41.1a to v).

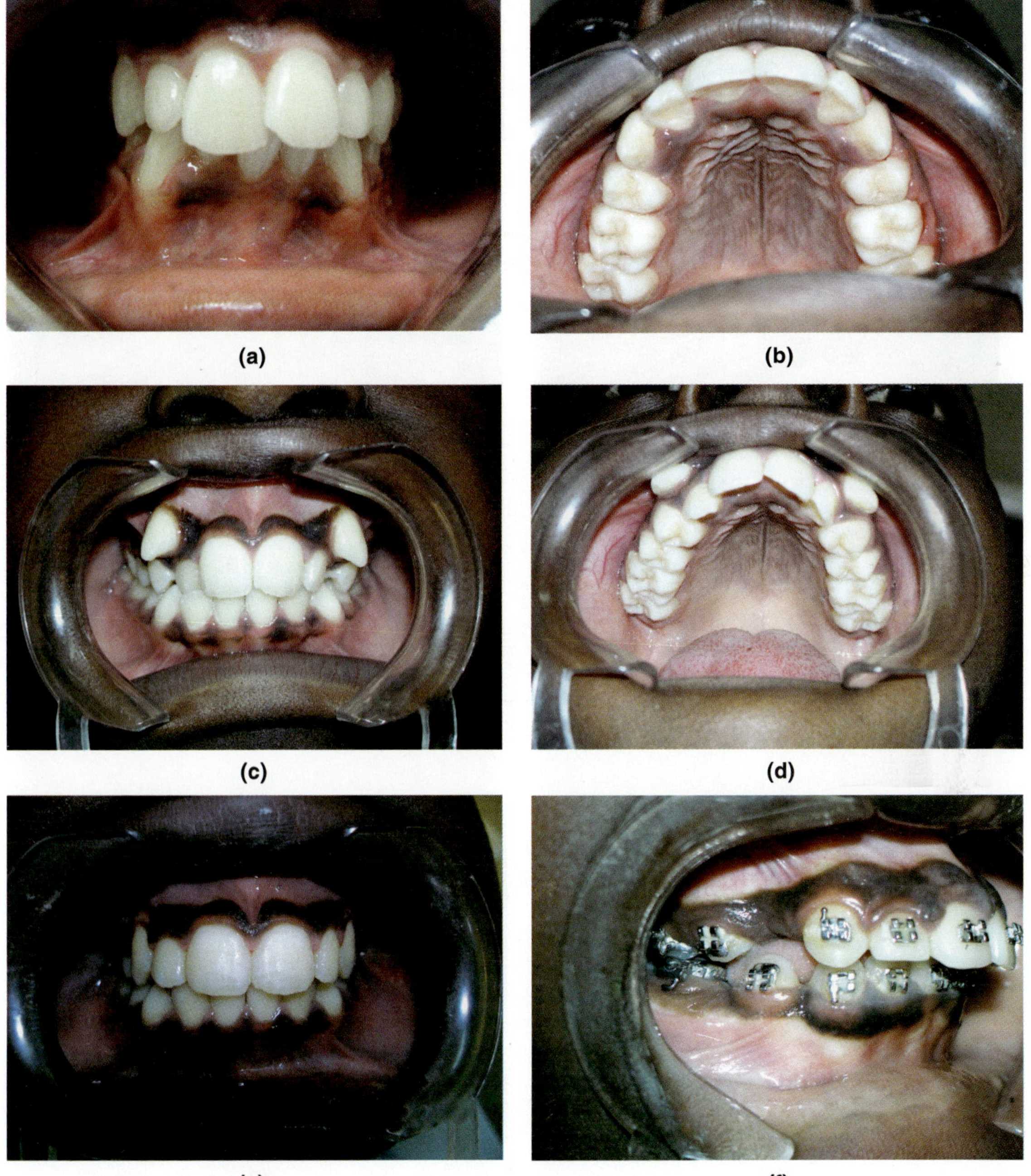

(a) (b) (c) (d) (e) (f)

Figs 41.1a to f:

(Contd.)

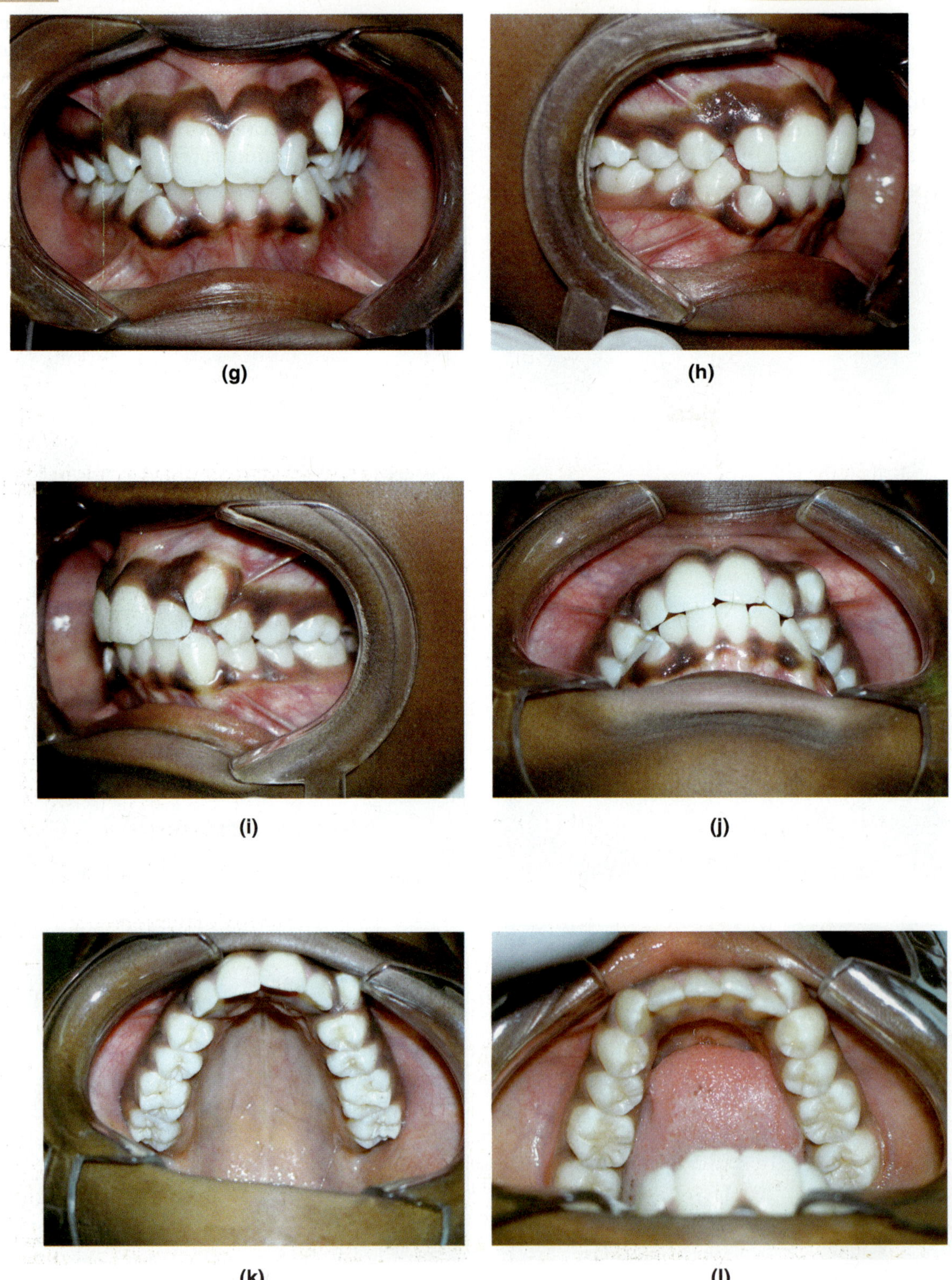

(g) (h)

(i) (j)

(k) (l)

Figs 41.1g to l:

(Contd.)

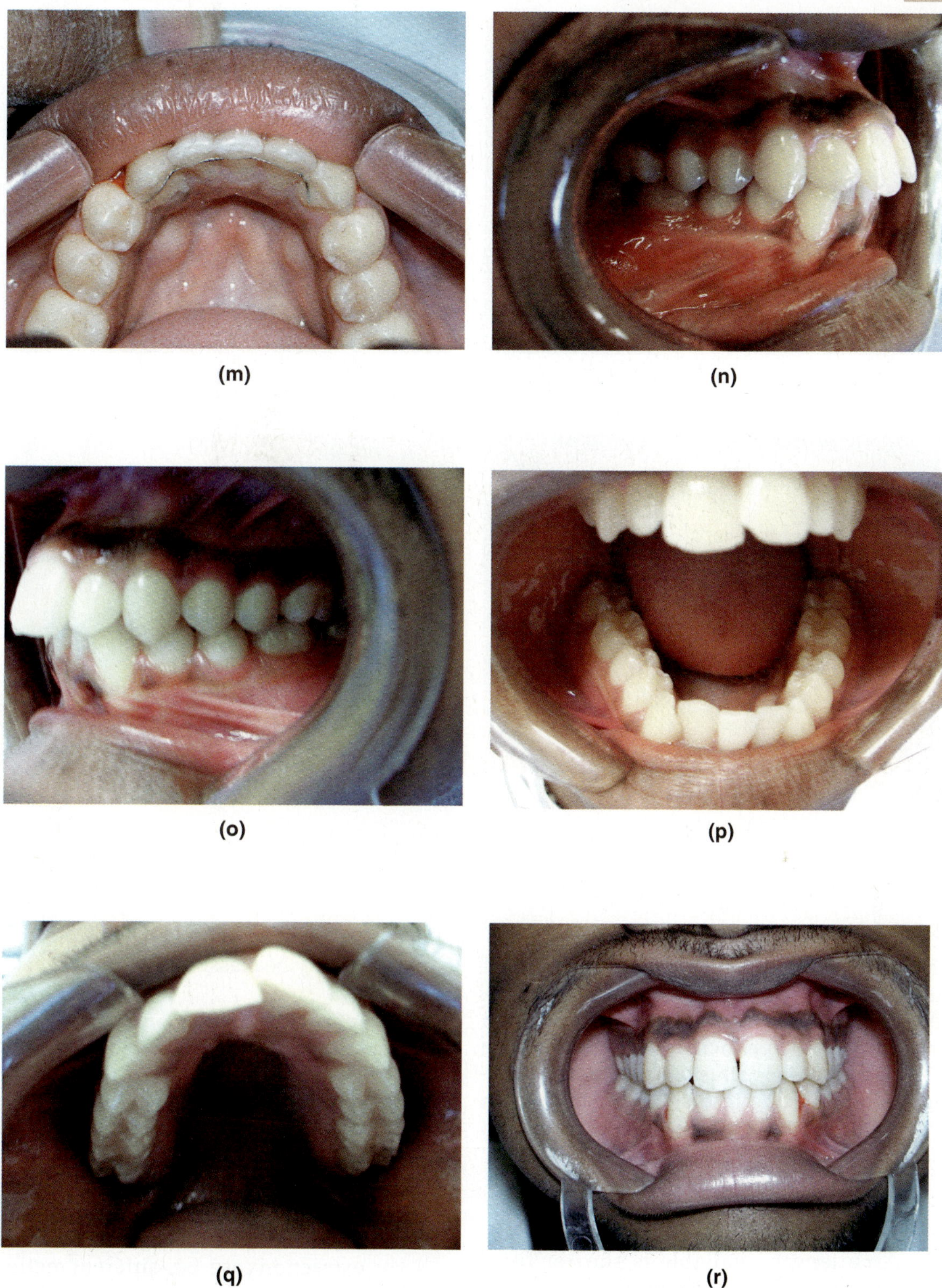
(m) (n)
(o) (p)
(q) (r)

Figs 41.1m to r:

(Contd.)

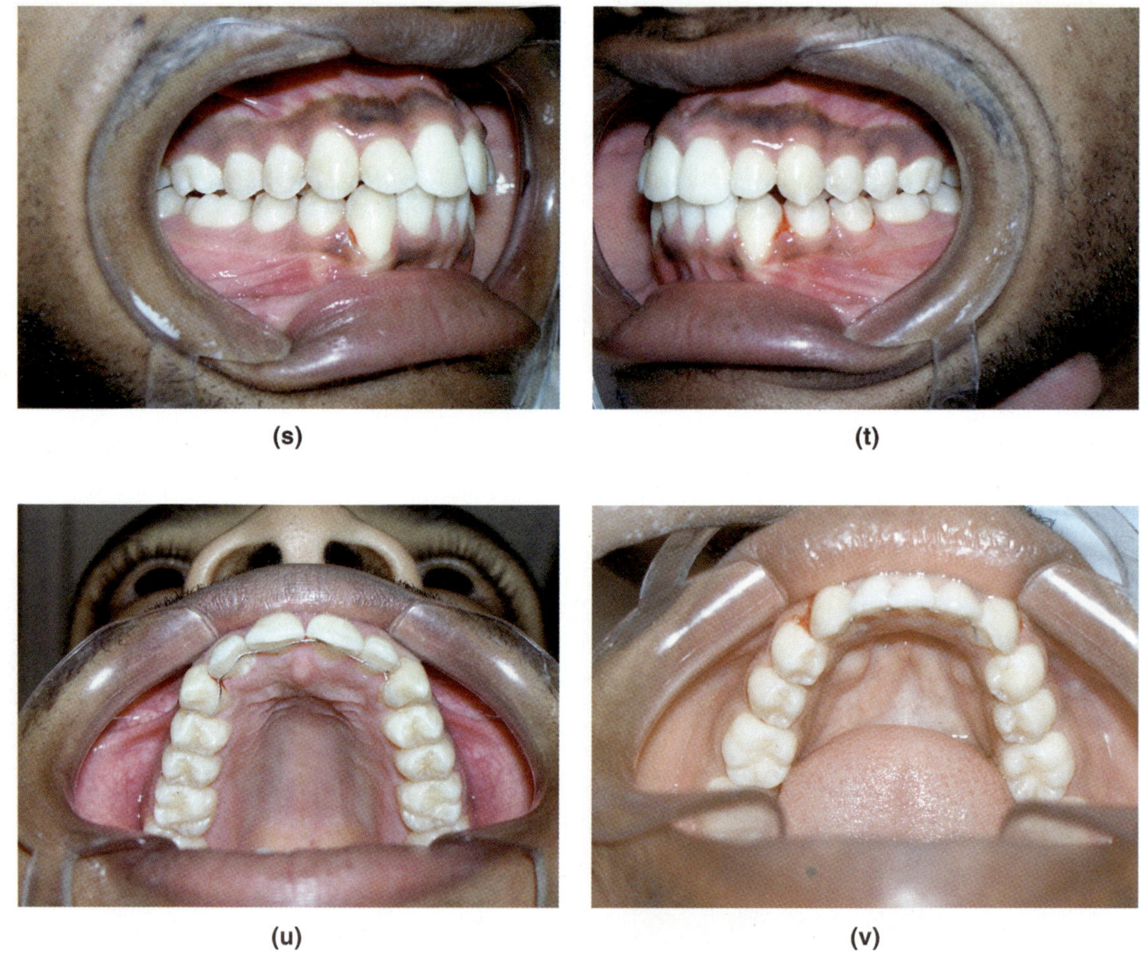

(s) (t)

(u) (v)

Figs 41.1s to v:

CROWDING

Crowding is the most common problem of malocclusion. The patients coming to orthodontic clinic cite it as one of their main complaints. Lower incisor crowding is the most common malocclusion condition. Crowding is mainly due to discrepancy between total tooth material (TTM) and arch length available (ALA) (i.e. TSALD). It can be due to:

a. Total tooth material is more in a normal arch length
b. Arch length available is shorter for a normal total tooth material
c. A combination of both.

Types of Crowding

Crowding may be classified in different types as follows:

A. **Depending on the amount of space deficiency:** Crowding can be first-degree crowding (mild crowding); second-degree crowding (moderate crowding); and third-degree crowding (severe crowding).

According to Proffit,

1. If TSALD is less than 5 mm: This is mild crowding and it is a non-extraction case. So, different methods of space gaining can be applied to treat the case.

2. If TSALD is more than 5 mm but less than 9 mm: This is moderate crowding and it is a borderline case. Other factors like growth pattern, nasolabial angle, growth completion, etc. should be considered for extraction planning.
3. If TSALD is more than 9 mm: This is severe crowding and is definite case of extraction (Figs 41.2 and 41.3).

B. According to etiology of crowding: It can be primary crowding; secondary crowding; and tertiary crowding.

a. **Primary crowding:** It is hereditary crowding, and is determined genetically. It occurs due to disproportion in tooth size and jaw bases.

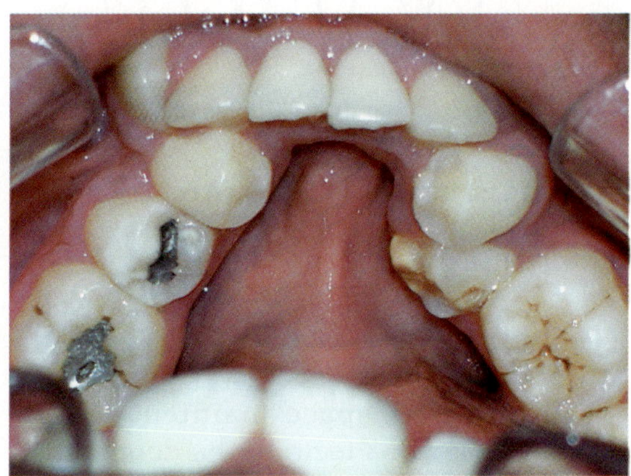

Fig. 41.2: Severe primary crowding in lower arch and narrow dental arch.

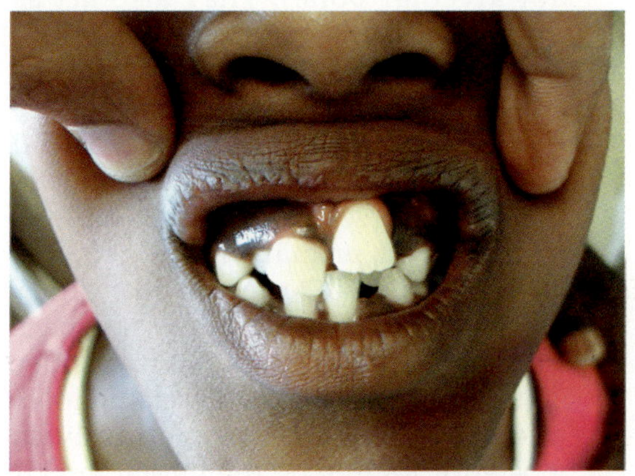

Fig. 41.3: Severe crowding in upper arch.

b. **Secondary crowding:** It is an acquired crowding which occurs due to mesial drift of posterior permanent teeth due to premature loss of primary teeth in buccal segments and leading loss of arch length, and thus deviated eruption or impaction of teeth.

c. **Tertiary crowding:** It occurs due to natural phenomenon, esp in the lower incisors region. It occurs during the late growth of jaws at around 18–25 years age, especially the terminal AP growth of mandible (which finishes later than the AP growth of maxilla). It thrusts the mandible forward and upward, lingual to the upper incisors. It leads to either spacing in upper teeth or crowding in lower incisors due to their lingual shifting. A small force from erupting mandibular third molars was also considered to be a factor in this crowding.

C. According to the inclination of teeth to their apical bases: Crowding can be coronal crowding and apical crowding. Apical crowding is the crowding of roots in the bone. It is due to the mesial inclination of long axes of roots of teeth, reducing the inter-radicular bone. Coronal crowding is the irregularity of crowns of teeth, which may be due to abnormal axial inclinations and also lack of space (Fig. 41.4).

D. According to location of crowding: It can be anterior crowding; mid-segment crowding; and posterior crowding.

Etiology of Crowding

There are many causes of development of crowding as follows:

1. **Heredity:** It is one of the main causes of any type of malocclusion. Certain conditions transmit from parents to children. Matching malocclusion conditions can be seen in MZ twins, e.g.

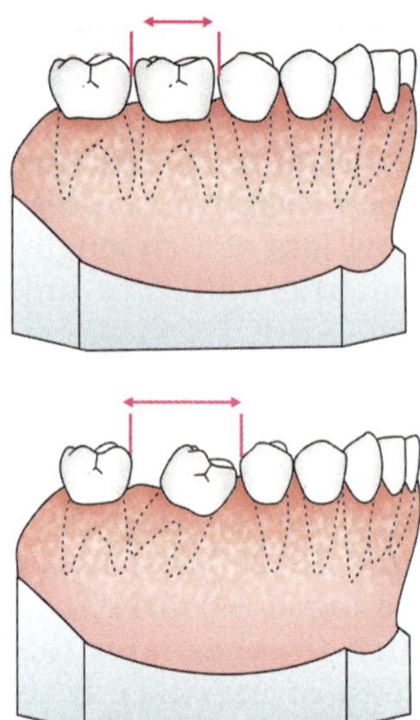

Fig. 41.4: Tilted buccal tooth occupies more space in dental arch, so correcting the axial inclination helps to gain space in the arch for other teeth.

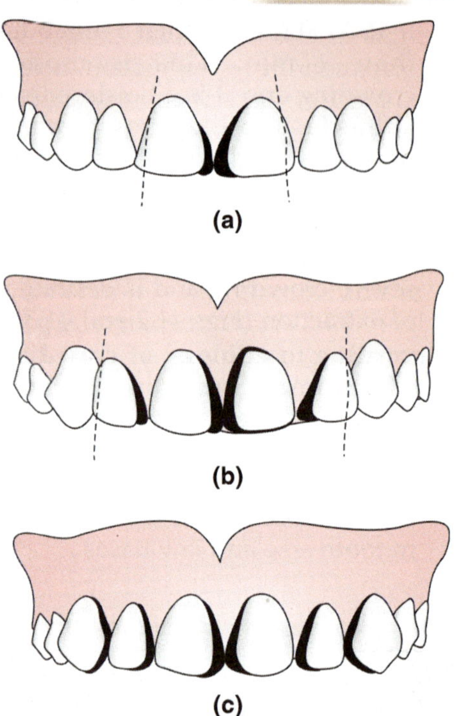

Figs 41.5a to c: Abnormally shaped incisors should be reshaped for better alignment and contact relation of teeth. Slicing also helps to get some spaces for correction of crowding.

crowding, spacing, congenitally missing tooth, etc.

2. **TSALD:** It may be due to increased TTM or decreased ALA or combination of both. Generalized increase in MD size of teeth on a normal sized dental arch will lead to crowding. It may also be due to small dental arch not able to accommodate the normal-sized tooth material.
3. **Abnormal size or shape of teeth:** For example, macrodontia, micrognathia or combination leads to crowding. It is mainly genetically controlled (Figs 41.5a to c).
4. **Presence of supernumerary teeth:** Extra tooth in the dental arch uses the space needed for normal alignment and thus leads to crowding, ectopic eruption or impaction of the tooth.
5. **Prolonged retention of primary tooth:** Primary tooth should get exfoliated timely or should be extracted timely to provide space for the permanent tooth. But if primary tooth remains in place, the succedaneous tooth gets either deflected in another location or gets impacted in the jaws.
6. **Premature loss of primary tooth:** Primary teeth have a very important function of space maintenance for succedaneous teeth in the dental arch. They also help in increase in dentoalveolar height of the jaws due to their eruption (teeth act as functional matrix for alveolar bone). They also act as stimulus for the permanent teeth to erupt. They should be retained in the mouth as long as possible, so as to keep space for permanent teeth and should follow the normal pattern and timing of exfoliation (see chronology tables). However, if primary tooth gets lost prematurely due to factors like caries, trauma, pulpitis, etc. then that space should be maintained with proper appliances. If space is not maintained, the space loss occurs especially in posterior region, by the mesial migration of the tooth distal to the space.

Most of the space loss occurs within first 6 months of extraction. It leads to space deficiency for the successor leading to crowding, e.g. if second primary molar is lost prematurely, the permanent first molar shifts in the space, and thus the space needed for second premolar is deficient. Second premolar may get impacted or deflected in eruption path erupting in abnormal locations.

7. **Caries of primary teeth:** Proximal caries of the primary tooth leads to space loss, because the adjacent tooth shifts in that defect. It is especially important for primary secondary molars which contribute to the total leeway space. Proximal caries should be adequately restored to maintain this space.
8. **Abnormal pressure habits:** They lead to disturbance in the force equilibrium around the dental arches. Lower lip trap is one of the causes leading to lingual tilting of lower incisors and their crowding (Figs 41.6a and b).
9. **Improper growth of jaws:** If the jaw bases do not grow to full potential, and especially in transverse dimensions, it leads to decreased space in arches and thus crowding.
10. **Racial factors:** Some races especially Caucasians are prone to crowding, while negroid have broader jaws and less crowding.
11. **Evolutionary trends:** Due to shift in dietary habits toward softer foods, the stimulus to growth of jaws is less as compared to the aborigines. It leads to impaction of third molars; development of crowding, and congenitally missing teeth, e.g. third molars, second premolars, etc.

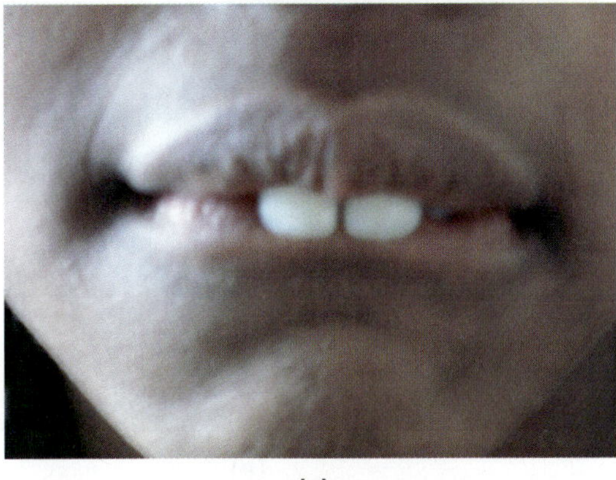

(a)

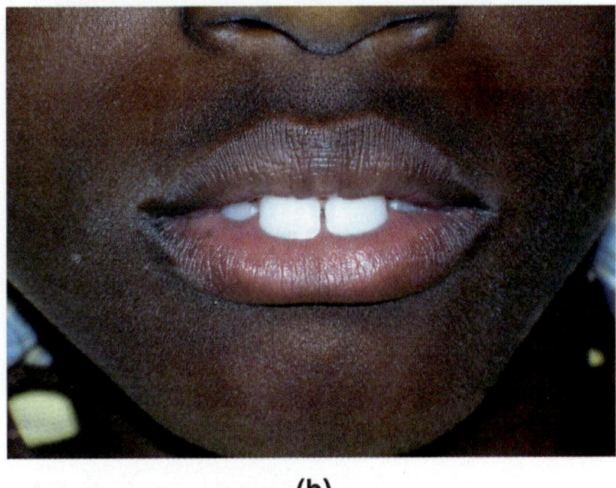

(b)

Figs 41.6a and b: Lower lip trap behind the upper incisors, which leads to constant labially directed pressure on them.

Diagnosis

A proper diagnosis is required for the treatment planning. The history, clinical examination, cast analysis and radiological analysis are performed. Clinical analysis is done to ascertain the causes of crowding, and the extent of crowding in the dental arches; shape and width of dental arches; abnormal habits, etc. Cast analysis is done to quantify the crowding and discrepancy. Various methods can be reviewed in the chapter of cast analysis. The radiographs help to locate any pathology, extra tooth, etc. in the jaws.

Treatment (Figs 41.7 to 41.10)

Treatment of crowding is based on the diagnosis. Following steps may be needed to correct the crowding.

1. **Space requirement and gaining:** Space is needed in the arches to treat the crowding. As a general rule, 1 mm space

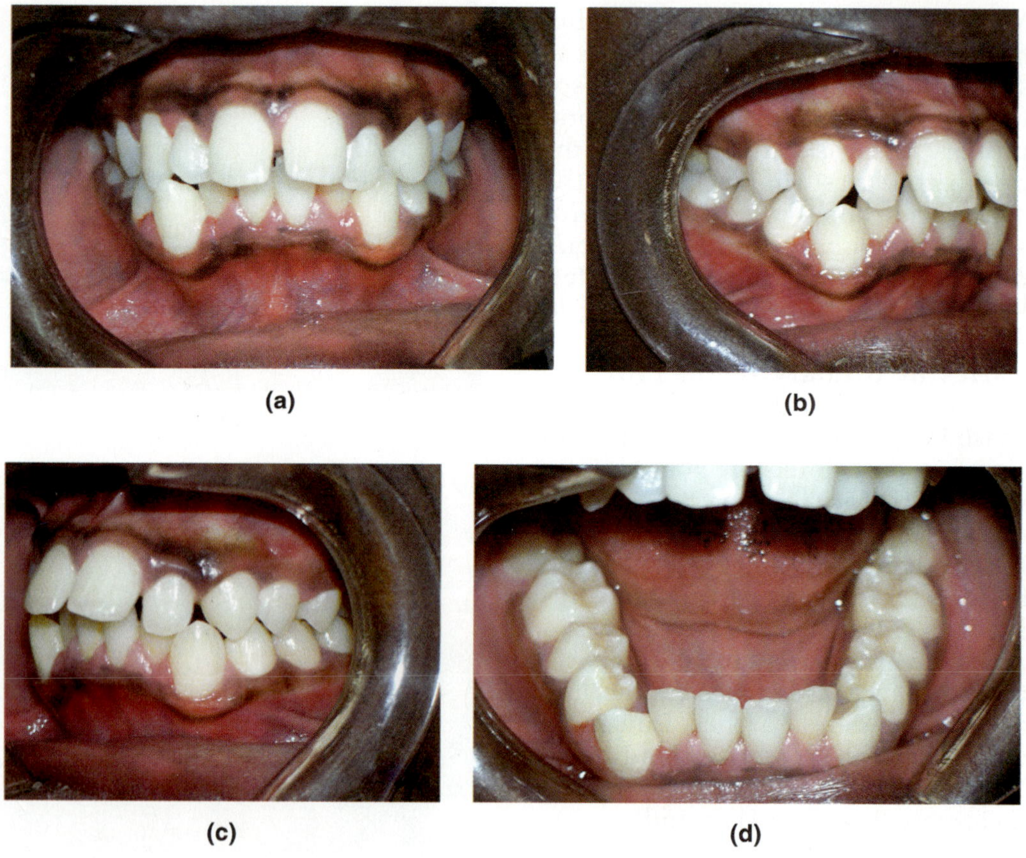

Figs 41.7a to d: CASE 1: Pre-Rx intraoral views.

is needed for every mm of crowding. The amount of crowding is calculated by model analysis. Methods to gain the needed space are determined based on the amount of space needed. It can be done by expansion, stripping or extraction of certain teeth. Extractions are needed in borderline and severe crowding cases, which need moderate or maximum anchorage respectively. The extractions should be decided after proper diagnosis. Some cases need only single lower incisor extractions the criteria of selection of such cases has been described below. Some cases having minimal crowding need to be treated with stripping or expansion. Details of methods of space gaining are described somewhere else in this book.

2. **Removable appliances:** Treatment can be done by removable or fixed appliance depending on the need. Removable appliances are used for treatment of minor crowding and for tipping purpose only. Springs, canine retractors, expansion screw, etc. can be used for tooth movements. Since the tooth cannot be controlled in all the 3D, the results achieved are not good.
3. **Fixed appliances:** They control the teeth in all the three planes of space, and provide best treatment results. Multi-loop archwires and soft flexible NiTi wires, etc. are very effective in resolving the crowding as they apply light continuous forces for alignment. Fixed expansion appliance help in gaining space by expansion, molar distalization, derotation, etc.

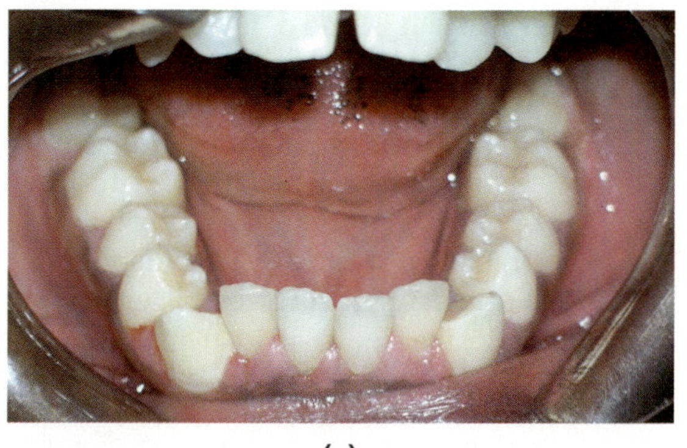

(a)

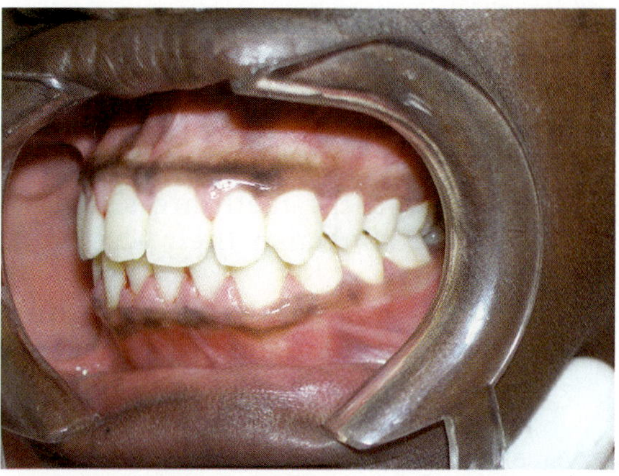

(b)

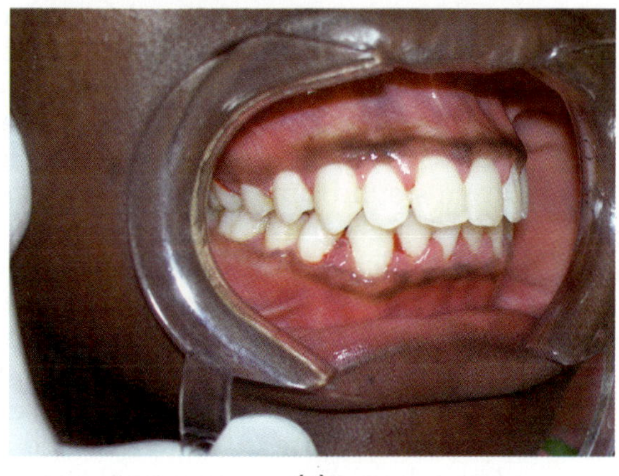

(c)

Figs 41.8a to c: CASE 1: Post-Rx intraoral views.

4. **Retention:** It is an important phase to stabilize the results. Retention is decided according to the initial malocclusion. Cases treated with non-extraction modality need prolonged retention. Details of retention can be studied in the relevant chapter.

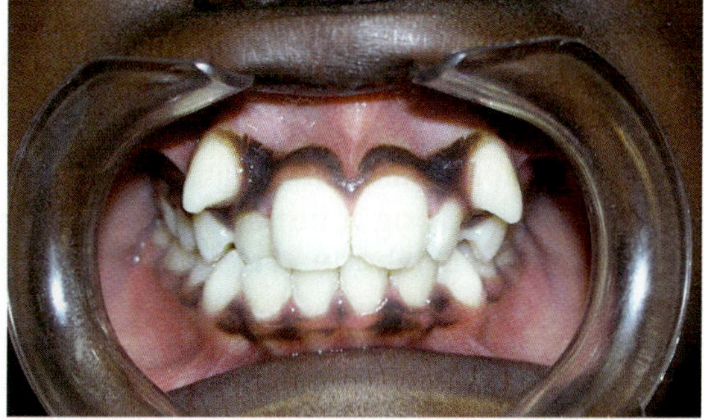

Fig. 41.9: CASE 2: Pre-Rx intraoral view with labially-blocked canines.

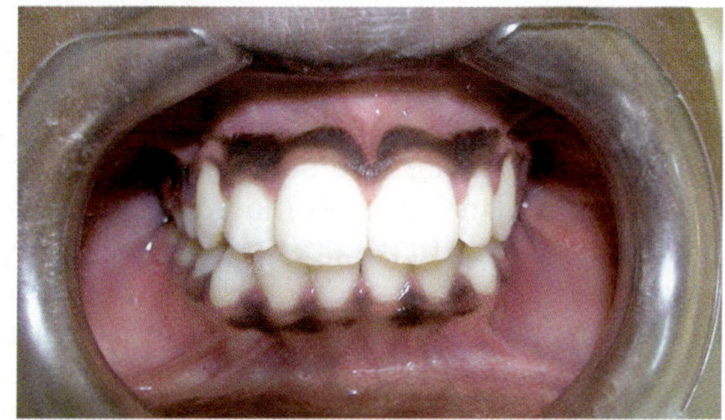

Fig. 41.10: CASE 2: Post-Rx intraoral view.

Single lower incisor extraction: Certain cases with following features can be treated with extraction of only one lower incisor:

- Class I molar relationship, with good buccal interdigitation.
- Moderately crowded lower incisors, where approx 5–6 mm space is needed. In such cases, extraction of one incisor is better than doing reproximation and making the teeth prone to caries. Severe crowding needs premolar extractions, while mild crowding can be treated without extractions.
- Mild or no crowding in upper anterior teeth, which can be corrected by interproximal reduction alone.
- The patients having acceptable soft-tissue profile, because there will be minimal change in upper arch.

- Minimal to moderate overbite and overjet, which can be treated by single lower incisor extraction. The lower anteriors just need an alignment and correction of axial inclinations.
- Patients having minimal growth potential having above criteria should be selected. In lower arch, after 9 years of age, minimal width increase is expected. In growing patients, first the nonextraction therapy with expansion should be considered before incisor extraction.

MANAGEMENT OF SPACING (Figs. 41.11a to h)

Spacing is a condition when there is absence of proximal contacts between certain teeth. Generalized spacing is seen in permanent dentition in some cases. It may cause various problems like esthetic, speech, loss of saliva during speaking, etc. Spacing in deciduous dentition is a natural phenomenon and is necessary as it develops due to growth of jaws and provides spaces for permanent teeth to erupt in good alignment. Mostly, the spacing is seen in anterior region of permanent dentition. Spacing in deciduous dentition is a normal and essential feature for proper development of permanent dentition. But in permanent dentition, spacing is an abnormal feature, and is unesthetic.

Types

It may be generalized or localized. Generalized means the spacing is present in the larger segment of dental arches; while localized means that spacing is localized to some area of dental arch.

Generalized spacing is due to causes, like heredity; large tongue size; larger dental arches; generalized smaller size of teeth.

Localized spacing is due to causes, like frenum, supernumerary tooth, abnormal shape of a tooth; habits, etc.

Etiology

It can be due to many causes.

1. **Heredity:** It is one of the main causes of spacing in dental arches. It controls the size of teeth and the jaws.
2. **TSALD:** Tooth size, shape, and number may be responsible for reduction in total tooth material. Discrepancy in teeth size and the jaw size also leads to the spacing. It may be due to either small size teeth in a normal jaw or normal sized teeth in bigger jaw or both. So microdontia, macrognathia, oligodontia, i.e. smaller number of teeth, etc. leads to generalized spacings.
3. **Larger dental arches:** Spacing also appears, if dental arch bases are larger than normal in size.
4. **Abnormal tooth form:** It also leads to spacing, e.g. peg laterals. In oligodontia condition, the teeth are smaller in number and also their shapes are abnormal.
5. **Deleterious oral habits** (thumb sucking and tongue thrusting) create spacing in anterior region due to abnormal forces on teeth and their shifting.
6. **Macroglossia:** Larger tongue size leads to generalized spacing by pushing dental arch outwards, and by overdevelopment of basal bones. It causes expansion of the dental arches to accommodate itself in the dental arches. It can be seen in amyloidosis, Down's syndrome, hypothyroidism, etc.
7. **Pathological conditions:** Unerupted supernumerary teeth, periapical pathology, cysts or tumors also lead to localized spacing.
8. **Abnormal frenum attachment:** Maxillary labial frenum is found attached at a lower level near the marginal gingiva orincisal papilla region in many patients leading to development of midline spacing.
9. **Congenital conditions:** In some congenital conditions, e.g. Down's syndrome; spacing is present in dental arches.

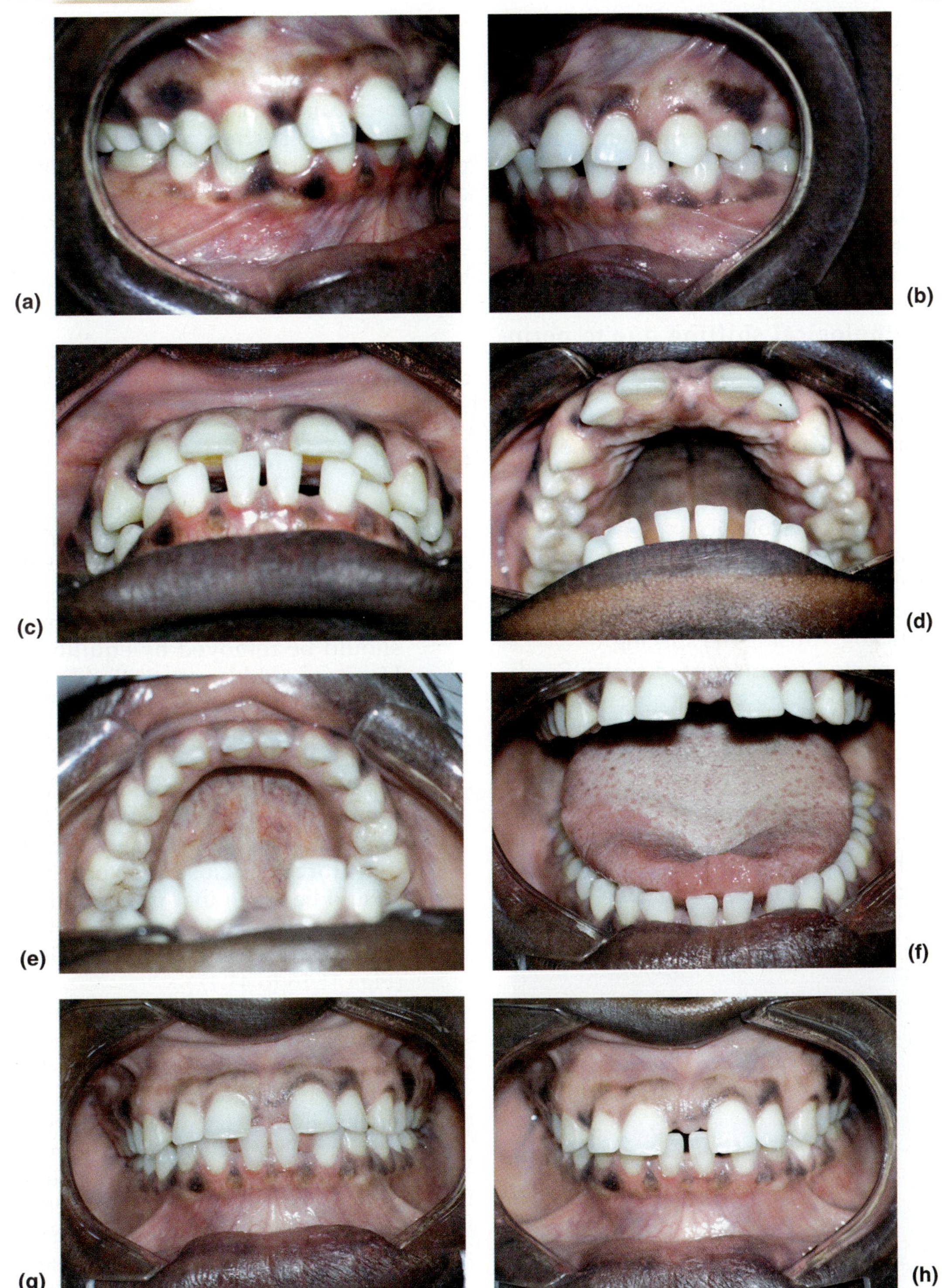

Figs 41.11a to h: Intraoral photos showing that larger sized tongue leads to creation of spacings, anterior teeth proclination, and wider arches.

10. **Abnormal growth patterns:** Fibrous dysplasia, hypertrophy, etc. lead to pathological shifting of teeth in the jaws and creation of spacing.
11. **Premature loss of permanent teeth:** It leads to formation of secondary spacings, but the side effects of premature loss, i.e. drifting of adjacent teeth and breaking of proximal contacts leads to appearance of spacing in the dental arches.
12. **Pathological shifting due to periodontal diseases:** In adult patients, the periodontal disease leads to shifting of especially anterior teeth leading to spacing. Due to periodontitis, the bone support of the teeth is decreased and the normal forces falling on the teeth become physiologically abnormal and lead to shifting of teeth. Even abnormal relation of incisors leads to trauma from occlusion TFO and leads to their shifting, causing the spacing.
13. **Impacted or unerupted teeth:** Sometimes, some tooth is not able to erupt in the dental arch due to some underlying reason, e.g. fibrous gingiva, abnormal path of eruption leading to impaction, delayed loss of primary tooth, etc. thus some space may be present in that area where the impacted/unerupted tooth was bound to erupt (Fig. 4.12).

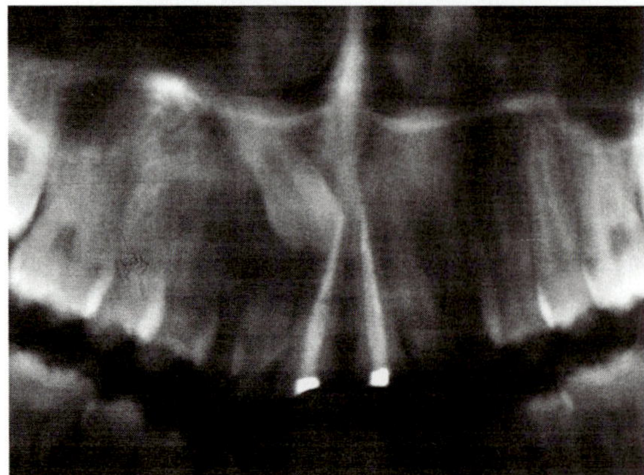

Fig. 41.12: Canine impaction and mesial migration; retained primary canine tooth.

Treatment (Figs 41.13 to 41.16): A proper examination and diagnosis is helpful in proper treatment planning. Model analysis is done to calculate excess space. Radiographic examination is carried out to find out any pathology or supernumerary teeth. Cause is determined and appropriate steps should be taken to remove etiology, if possible. For example, abnormal habit should be controlled; any pathology should be eliminated; supernumerary tooth is extracted, etc.

Appliances: Space can be closed by the use of removable appliance (labial bow, spring, etc.) or fixed appliance (with elastic chains or elastic threads, etc.). Removal of the cause is the first step for treatment.

a. **Removal of the cause:** Pathologies and supernumerary teeth should be removed. The periodontal condition should be treated by thorough prophylaxis and maintenance, and the TFO should be removed by equilibration. Habits should be controlled by appliances and counseling.
b. **Removable appliances:** They can be used if tipping movement is required esp if the anterior teeth have flared and can be retracted by tipping. A Hawley appliance can be effectively used with light forces to close the spaces. Care should be taken that upper and lower teeth should not strike during and after the treatment for effective closure (Figs 41.16 to 41.17).
c. **Fixed appliance:** They are used to control teeth in 3D. Brackets are placed on teeth and spaces can be closed with active ligature wires, elastomeric chains, thread, etc. to apply reciprocal or controlled forces as the need may be. If the tongue is of normal size, then spaces can be closed by retraction of anterior teeth. But if tongue is larger in size, then if spaces are closed by anterior teeth retraction, they encroach on the tongue space and thus relapse may occur. In such case, the spaces are closed by bringing the buccal teeth

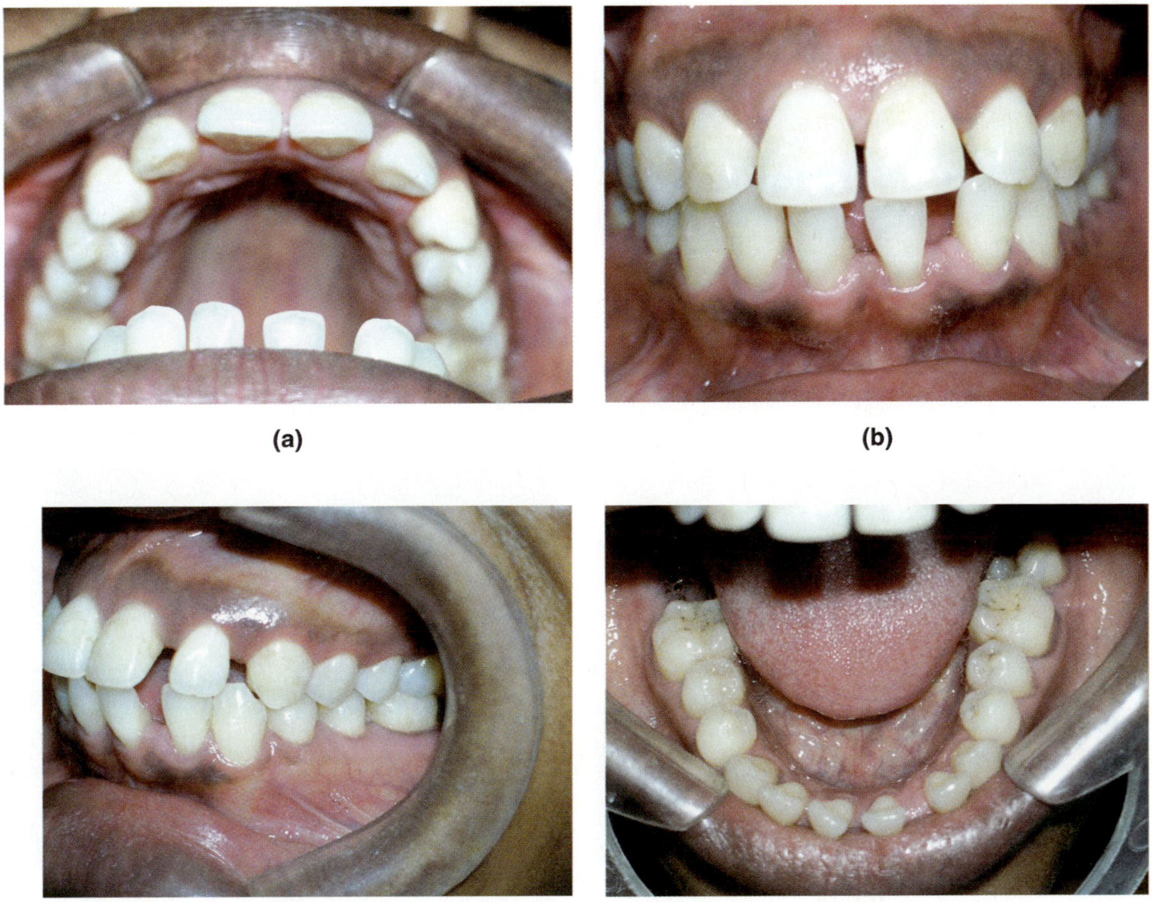

(a) (b)

(c) (d)

Figs 41.13a to d: Pre-Rx intraoral views showing upper and lower spaces.

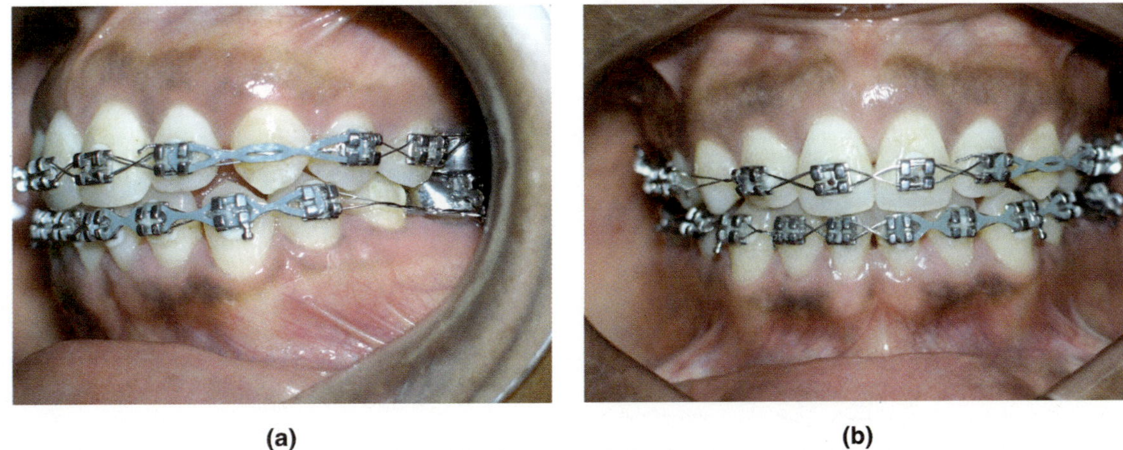

(a) (b)

Figs 41.14a and b: Fixed appliance to close the spaces.

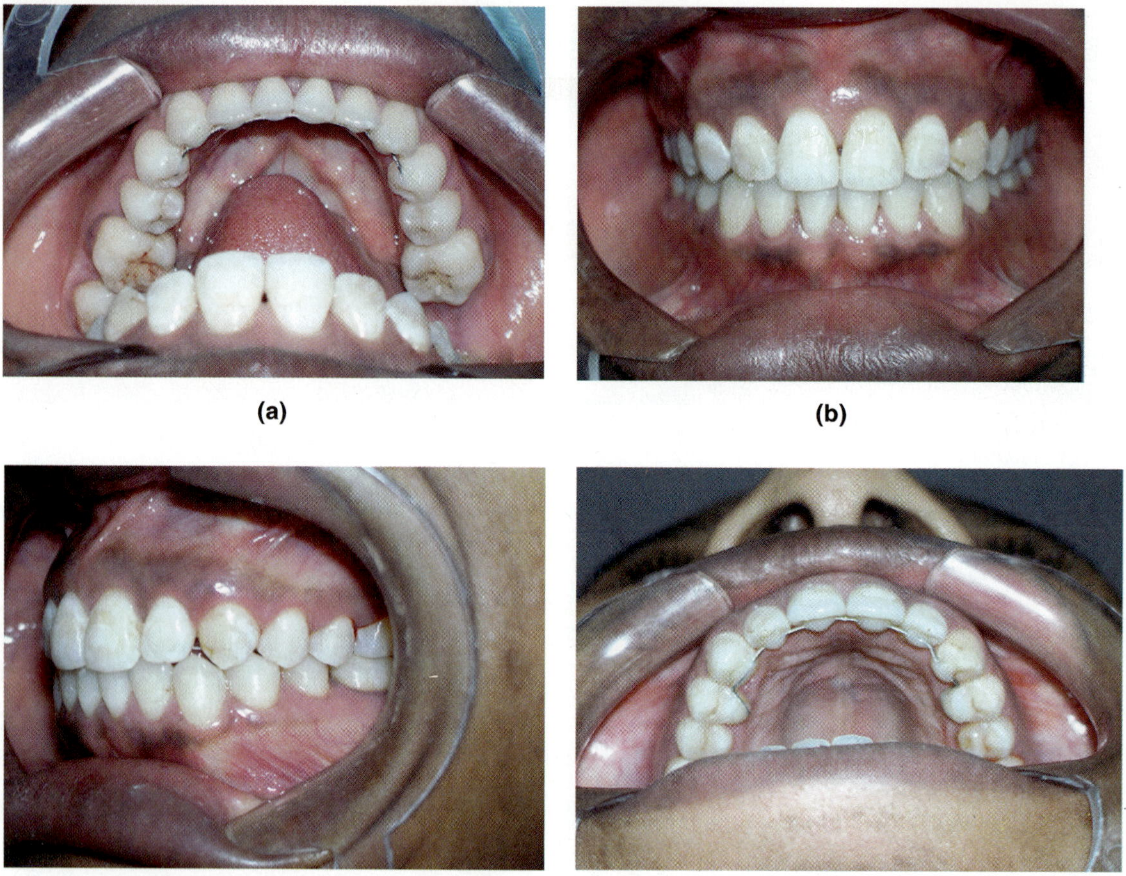

(a) (b)

(c) (d)

Figs 41.15a to d: Post-Rx views with upper and lower fixed retainers.

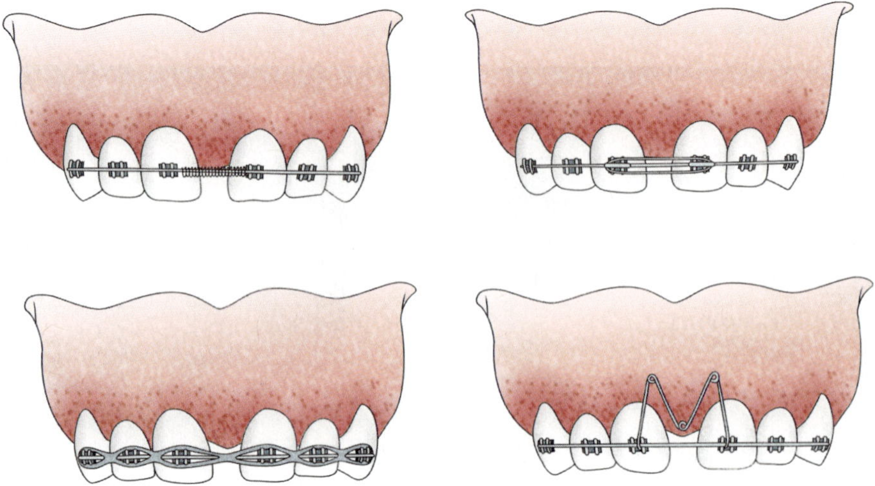

Fig. 41.16: Treatment of midline diastema by various means, e.g. active closed coil springs; elastic; e-chain; M-spring in that order.

forward, maintaining the anterior teeth in the position of best muscular equilibrium. More treatment time taken in this situation, since posterior teeth are moved mesially. Closure of generalized spacing needs prolonged retention.

d. If the space is in incisor region, and teeth are proclined needing simple tipping, then a Hawley appliance with active labial bow can be used to retract incisors and close the spaces.

e. **Midline space** can be closed by using a removable appliance with finger spring. If it is due to maxillary frenum, then **frenectomy** is done after closure of the space. It is followed by a prolonged fixed retainer.

f. **Habit control:** Abnormal habit control can remove abnormal pressure on the teeth, and the resultant spaces either get closed by normal muscular pressure or can be closed by active labial bow.

g. **Generalized spacing due to larger tongue size**; larger basal bone or smaller sized teeth is generally closed by using fixed orthodontic appliances, as they need bodily movement of teeth, and proper occlusal settling.

h. **Localized spacing** due to abnormal shape of tooth, e.g. peg lateral needs composite build up or jacket crowns.

i. **Space due to generalized microdontia:** Treatment is by fixed appliance and closing the space by bringing teeth together or by the use of jacket crowns on the teeth.

j. **Oligodontia:** Spaces due to this problem needs prostheses, after creating axial alignment of the teeth. If space loss has taken place due to migration of adjacent teeth, then space regaining is done before placing the prosthesis.

k. **Treatment of impacted or unerupted tooth:** With the help of wires, such teeth can be brought in dental arches.

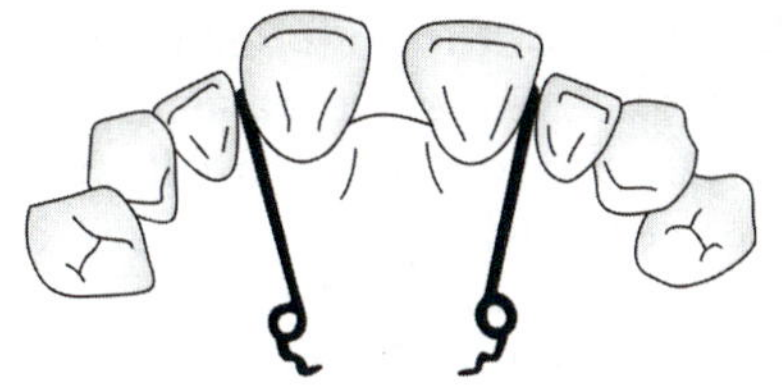

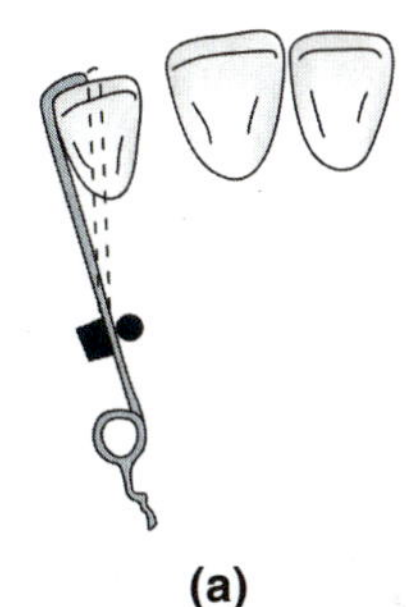

(a)

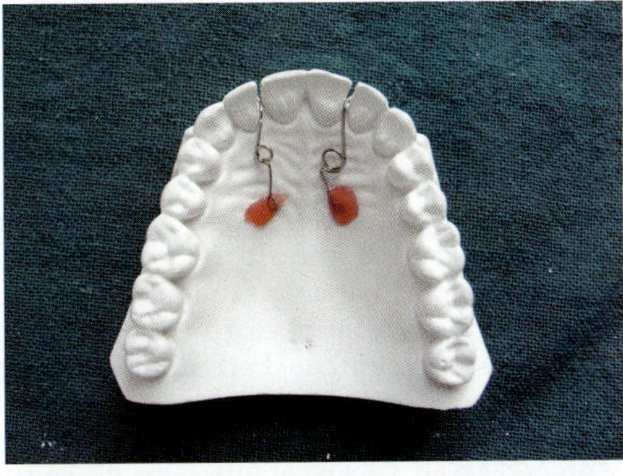

(b)

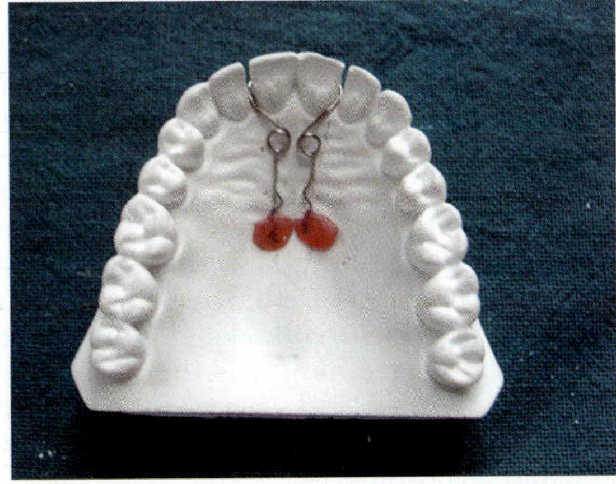

(c)

Figs 41.17a to c: Finger springs for mesial movement of central incisors.

l. **Surgery of tongue:** Partial glossectomy may be needed in cases of large-sized tongue to retain the results. Underlying causes leading to large size of tongue are also addressed as much as possible.

m. **Prosthesis and crowns:** Small-sized teeth, e.g. microdontia, or peg-shaped teeth, need fixed PFM crowns to maintain a normal MD width. Missing teeth need replacement with RPD/ FPD/implant, etc. after gaining the lost space with orthodontics, and uprighting the roots in the bone. Sometimes the spaces are very large, and it is not possible to orthodontically close all the spaces. In such situation, the spaces are closed in anterior segment, while that space gets moved in the buccal segment. There it can be left as such as it is not that unesthetic or prosthesis can be placed there.

Retention: After space closure, removable or fixed retainers can be placed for prolonged period. Habits should be kept under control. Tongue exercises should be continued if tongue thrusting habit was diagnosed. Partial glossectomy can be performed in cases of larger size of the tongue. Periodontal diseases should be kept under control.

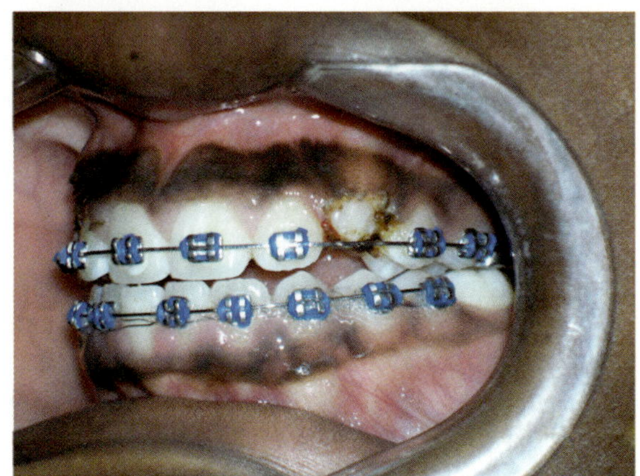

Fig. 41.18: Open bite in 23 region due to unerupted canine.

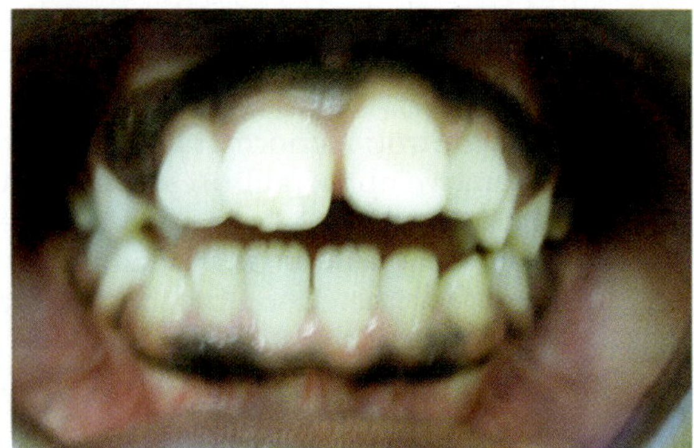

Fig. 41.19: Anterior open bite—pre-Rx.

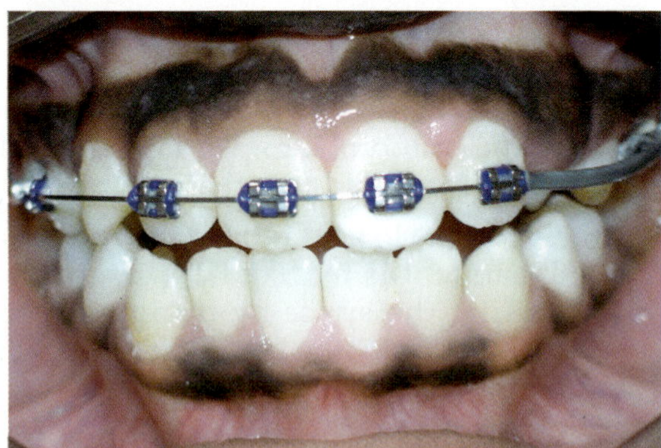

Fig. 41.20: Post-Rx after correction of anterior open bite.

MANAGEMENT OF OPEN BITE (Figs 41.18 to 41.20)

Definition

Clinically, the *dental open bite* is defined as the lack of vertical overlap between the maxillary and mandibular teeth when in occlusion. However, *skeletal open bite* is due to vertical growth pattern of the jaws, where there is an increased SN-MP angle well beyond the normal values of 32°. Dental open bite may or may not be present with skeletal open bite. The anterior face height is increased, the mandible shows a clockwise rotation pattern, convex profile, etc. It may also be called as long face syndrome.

Types

It may be classified in various types:

1. Depending on the location: It may be anterior open bite or posterior open bite.
2. Depending on the components involved: It may be skeletal or dental or skeletodental.

3. Combination, e.g. skeletal anterior open bite.
4. It may be localized, segmental or generalized.

Etiology

1. Heredity: It is one of the main causes of especially skeletal open bite as it influences the growth of jaws. Inherited factors, such as tongue size and abnormal growth pattern of jaws, lead to open bite.
2. Racial pattern: Some races are more prone to open bite, e.g. Africans.
3. Congenital and endocrinal disorder: For example, hypothyroidism, Down's syndrome, etc. which increase the tongue size also lead to open bite development.
4. Growth pattern: Vertical growth pattern leads to clockwise rotation of mandible leading to skeletal open bite.
5. Retention of infantile swallowing pattern: Improper transition in swallowing pattern form infancy to childhood and esp the tooth together swallow leads to development of anterior open bite which is well defined. Tooth apart swallow has poorly defined open bite.
6. Abnormal habit: Anterior or posterior tongue thrusting does not allow proper eruption of teeth. Thumb sucking habit also leads to open bite. Mouth breathing also disturbs the muscular balance and affects growth.
7. Trauma: Trauma and fracture to jaws and loss of tissues also may lead to open bite in certain cases. Condylar fractures in children lead to improper mandibular growth due to ankylosis leads to open bite.
8. Congenital abnormalities: Abnormal growth of tissues in some congenital conditions may cause open bite.

Clinical features: Open bite is generally perceived as lack of vertical overlap of upper and lower teeth. The teeth may be well aligned or may show crowding depending on TSALD. Tongue thrusting is seen during swallowing in the open bite. It may be presumed as a cause of open bite. But, it is also possible that the tongue thrusting can be secondary to the open bite.

In anterior dental open bite, proclined anterior teeth, narrow maxillary arch may be present due to habits (e.g. thumb sucking, mouth breathing). In posterior open bite, there is interocclusal gap between upper and lower teeth on occlusion, and tongue generally interposes between them. It does not allow proper eruption of teeth to come in occlusion. Open bite may also extend in both anterior and lateral regions.

Posterior open bite: It is usually due to infra eruption of posterior teeth; which may be due to lateral tongue posture/thrust; due to impacted or ankylosed posterior teeth, etc.

Skeletal open bite is generally associated with vertical growth pattern, the increased lower anterior facial height and decreased PFH, steep mandible (increased FMA), excessive maxillary incisor and gingival exposure, counter clockwise rotation of maxilla and clockwise rotation of mandible, or a combination, vertical maxillary excess, etc. Lips are generally found to be incompetent. This is also called as long face syndrome.

Treatment: Treatment of open bite depends on many factors. Etiologic factors should be considered during treatment, e.g. abnormal habits; abnormal growth pattern, etc. The mild forms can be treated with appliances, while moderate to severe forms need surgical treatment. Earlier the treatment, better and more stable the results. Prolonged retention protocol is needed after treatment.

1. Habits, such as thumb sucking, mouth breathing and tongue thrusting, should be controlled. It can be done by habit breaking appliances; tongue exercise; myofunctional therapy (used in mixed dentition stage) e.g. FR IV; modified activator, etc. Persistence of habit leads to relapse of open bite. A fixed retainer and a habit breaking appliance should be recommended.

2. Fixed orthodontic mechanotherapy: The archwires with extrusive loops in incisal region can be used. Elastics in box fashion or triangular fashions are also used for extrusion of upper and lower anteriors. Mild cases can be treated with this method. In another method proposed by Kalra, RCS NiTi wires are ligated in upper and lower arches, and heavy up-down (intermaxillary) elastics are used in canine regions. These elastics help to transfer the intrusive forces of RCS NiTi wires from anterior region to the posteriors, leading to their intrusion also.
3. Use of posterior bite plates has also been suggested which open the occlusion beyond free way space, thus applying intrusive forces on molars. But, it needs patient cooperation (Figs 41.21a to c).
4. Chin cap and high-pull headgear can also be used to apply intrusive forces on the molars, but they need patient cooperation.
5. Implant supported intrusion of posterior teeth: Microimplants and plates have been used successfully for buccal intrusion; along with some anterior extrusion by wires/elastics; and closure of open bite by autorotation of mandible.
6. Surgical correction: Severe skeletal problems, if growth of jaws has been completed, are treated with orthognathic surgical intervention along with the orthodontic therapy.
7. **Treatment of posterior open bite:** For control of habits, the lateral tongue spikes are given. Also the extrusion of posteriors can be done by fixed appliance therapy using loops, and extrusion elastics. In case of impacted or ankylosed teeth, the prosthetic intervention required.

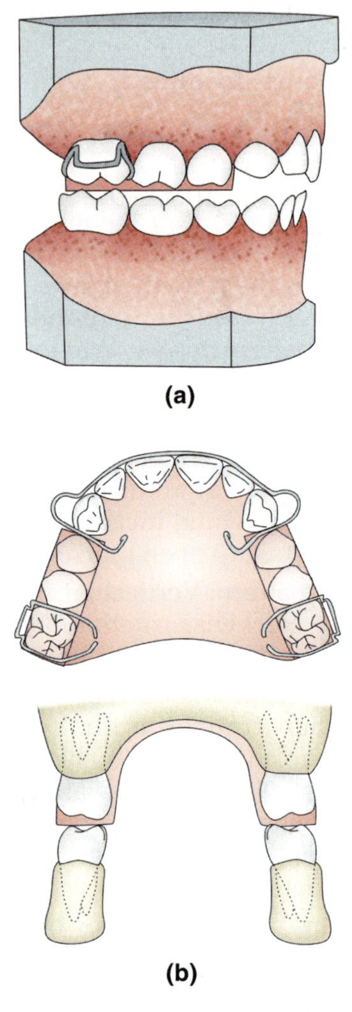

(a)

(b)

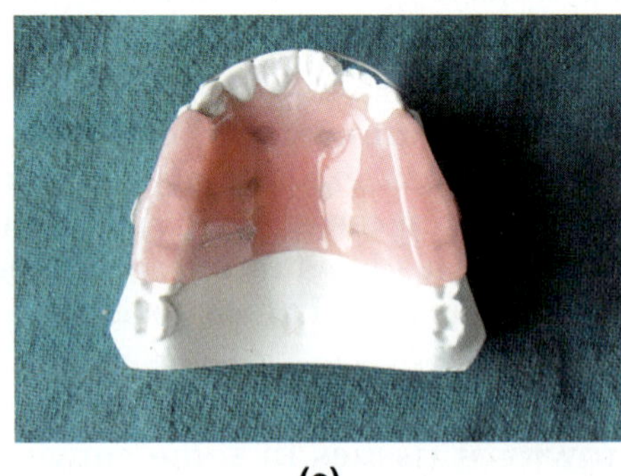

(c)

Figs 41.21a to c: Posterior bite plate appliance, which is used to raise the bite in anterior region to provide uninterfered movement of teeth in anterior crossbite. It is also used for reinforcing anchorage, and for applying intrusive force on buccal teeth to achieve open bite reduction.

TREATMENT OF PROCLINATION AND INCREASED OVERJET

Proclination is the labial inclination of tooth/ teeth. It can exist with Angle's class I molar relation. It can be present in upper or lower or both arches. It can be present as a normal or increased overjet. It can be of different types:

a. Proclination of a single tooth
b. Proclination of two central incisors
c. Proclination of all incisors
d. Proclination of upper anterior segment
e. Bimaxillary proclination
f. **Deck biss pattern:** The lateral incisors are labially inclined while centrals are either normal or retroclined.
g. Bimaxillary proclination with generalized spacing.

These can be present with or without spaces between the teeth. Presence or absence of spaces is a factor in determining the treatment plan.

Causes of Proclination

It may be due to some of the following factors:

- **Heredity:** It is one of the main factors leading to proclination.
- **Increased tooth material in upper arch:** Increased TTM in upper arch leads to either crowding or proclination of one or more teeth; or proclination of all anterior teeth such that they are well aligned.
- **Habits:** Deleterious habits, like tongue thrust, thumb sucking or lip trap, can lead to proclination of teeth.
- **Prognathism of premaxilla:** It also leads to anterior positioning of upper teeth.
- **Bimaxillary proclination:** It is the condition in which upper and lower incisors are labially inclined with respect to their apical bases, but most of the time they maintain a normal overjet.
- **Pathological migration:** In adults with periodontal diseases, the incisors start migrating generally in labial direction, leading to proclination.

Treatment

A proper diagnosis is essential to find out the underlying problem so that a proper treatment plan can be made. It depends on the factors, like growth status and pattern, presence of spaces; amount of TSALD; habits; soft tissue balance, etc.

Some of the treatment can be done as follows:

1. Habits if present should be controlled before treatment can be commenced.
2. Proclination of a single incisor can be treated with a removable Hawley's appliance with an active labial bow. A proper space should be present in the arch for its correction. It is easily possible in spaced area, otherwise space can be created either by expansion of the arch or by stripping (Fig. 41.22).
3. If the upper incisors are proclined and spaces are present between them, due to some habit, like lip trap or tongue thrust, then habit breaking appliance with active labial bow can be used to retract the incisors. Such teeth need only tipping for the treatment.
4. If upper anterior segment is proclined with no spaces between them, then upper first premolars are extracted to create space in which the anteriors are retracted with the help of fixed appliance (Figs 41.23 and 41.24).
5. Bimaxillary proclination generally needs fixed appliance in both arches with the removal of all first premolars.

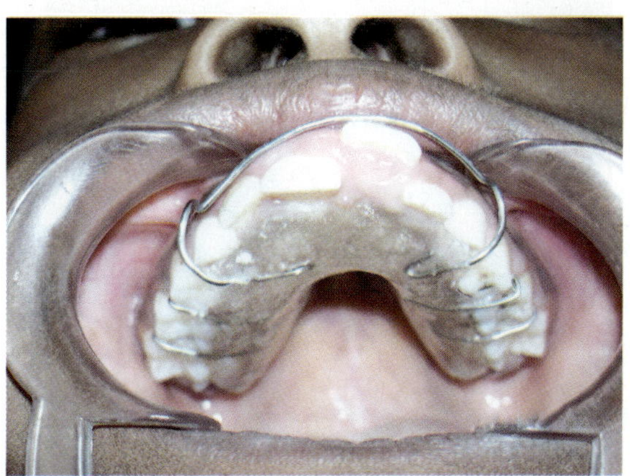

Fig. 41.22: Removable appliance with labial bow for palatal movement of labially-displaced central incisor.

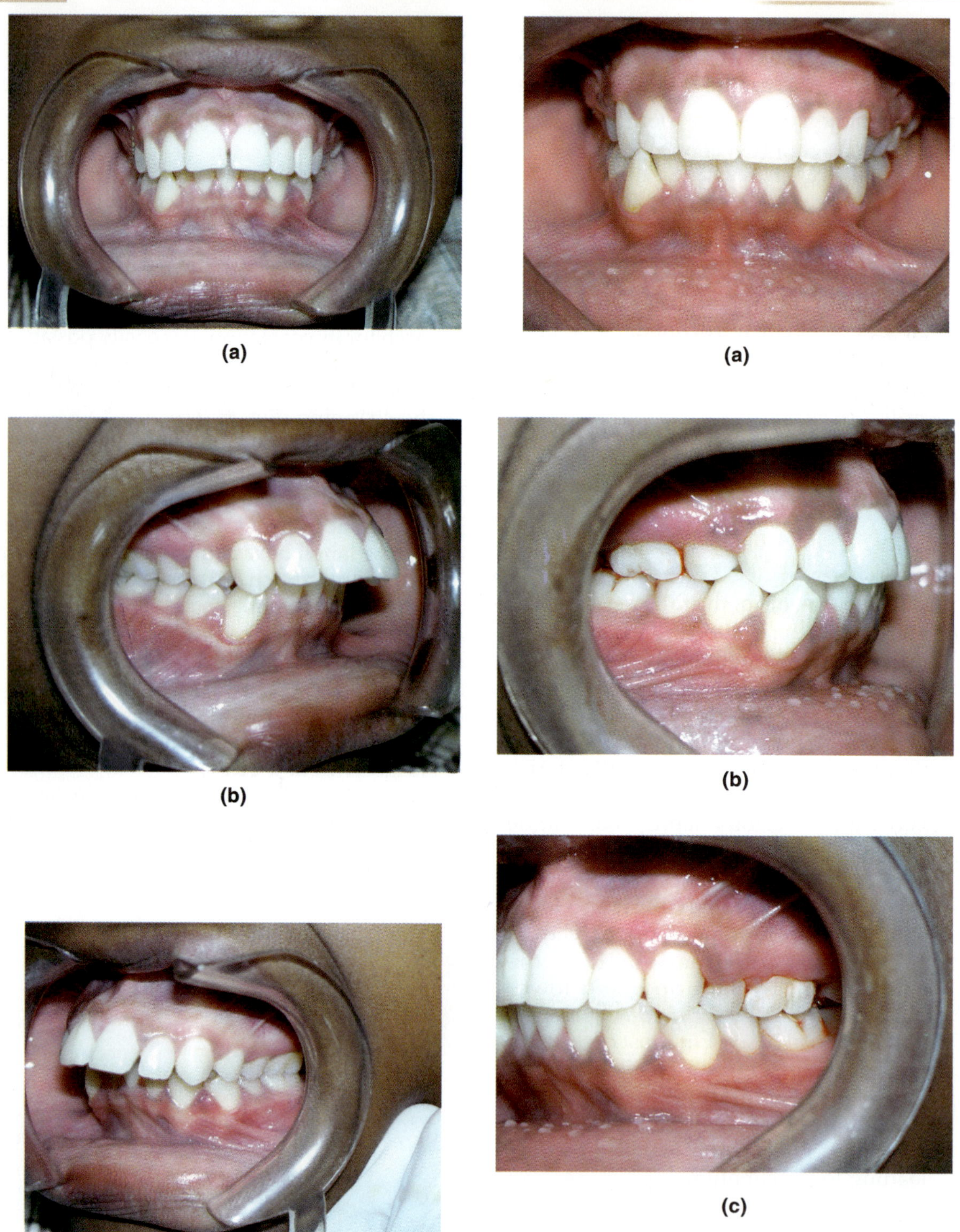

(a) (b) (c)

Figs 41.23a to c: Angle's class II division 1 with a very high overjet value.

(a) (b) (c)

Figs 41.24a to c: Post-Rx after first premolar extractions in upper arch and retraction of anteriors with maximum anchorage. Patient did not opt for lower treatment.

6. Deck biss pattern is treated by aligning the lateral incisors in the dental arch. The space can be created by stripping the anterior teeth.
7. Pathological migration due to periodontal disease leading to proclination is treated first by controlling the PD disease, and then using light forces either by removable or by fixed appliance.
8. Bimaxillary proclination with generalized spacing: This condition is generally seen in cases of larger tongue size, or a positive TSALD. It is treated by fixed appliances where the spaces are consolidated and are used for retraction of teeth to reduce the proclination.

Retention: A retention plan is important since these conditions are prone to relapse. Removable retainers can be used for at least 1 year in certain cases treated with extraction. Cases treated with non-extraction generally need fixed retainer. Also cases due to large tongue size or abnormal habits need to be retained with fixed retainers or prolonged removable retention plan.

RETROCLINATION OF TEETH

It means that the teeth are lingually inclined on their apical base. It may be limited to one or more teeth.

1. In deck biss pattern: Generally, upper central incisors are lingually inclined. Sometimes, lateral incisors can also be found retroclined. This condition is generally due to heredity factors or by hyperactive circumoral muscles. They may be treated with the help of removable appliance with Z-spring or using the fixed appliance. It needs a rigid prolonged retention appliance.
2. Lower incisors can be found retroclined if there is lip trap, which applies lingual force on them. The habit of lip trap or hyperactive lower lip needs to be treated, which can be done with lip bumper, oral screen, etc. The lower teeth can be proclined with the help of tongue forces or by using a removable appliance incorporating T-spring or paddle spring; or by using fixed appliances. A normal retention protocol can be followed afterwards.
3. Lower incisors also get retroclined during serial extraction procedures (a side effect of serial extraction), when primary canines are removed. The lower lip force gets directed on lower incisors causing their retroclination and extrusion. It leads to creation of deep bite; and loss of some space in canine region. They need the fixed appliance treatment for correction when all the permanent teeth have erupted.

MANAGEMENT OF MIDLINE DIASTEMA

Midline diastema is the space present in the midline between central incisors. It may be present in both upper and lower arches. But most of the time it is seen in upper arch.

Etiology: Many factors can lead to creation of midline diastema (Figs 41.25 and 41.26).

a. Heredity
b. Racial factor
c. Low attachment of maxillary labial frenum
d. Transient malocclusion
e. Supernumerary tooth, mesiodens: They do not allow the approximation of incisors.
f. Midline pathologies
g. Small sized tooth, TSALD
h. Large size arches
i. Habits: For example, tongue thrusting habit; finger-sucking habit, etc.
j. Proclined front teeth
k. During RME stage.

Heredity: It is one of the common causes of any malocclusion. Heredity controls the tooth size, shape, dental arch size and shape, facial shape, growth pattern, number of teeth, etc. Midline diastema is frequently seen in the child of a parent who is having midline diastema. It may be due to large size of frenum, jaw or small size of teeth, etc.

Racial predisposition: Midline spacing has racial predilection also. African people have more incidence of midline spacing.

Developmental stage of the occlusion/ transient malocclusion: Physiological/ developmental spacing is generally seen in the primary dentition which is due to jaw growth. Spacing in early mixed dentition is seen as transient/incipient condition which is self-correcting during normal course of the eruption.

Spacing in upper incisors is seen during ugly-duckling stage at 8–10 years age, when the permanent maxillary canines are trying to erupt. Canines during eruption apply physiologic forces especially on roots of lateral incisors, and push the roots of upper 4 incisors towards midline (root convergence), while the crowns of incisors get flared distally, thus creating spaces among incisors. It is because the buds of upper canine lie very high near the nasal floor, and the canines are the last succedaneous teeth to erupt in oral cavity. By the time, they start their eruption, the roots of lateral incisors are already near completion. This condition gets itself corrected with the eruption of crown of canine, when the pressure gets transferred on the crowns of canines. During ugly-duckling stage, the clinician should not tempt to treat it, since it may lead to root resorption of lateral incisors and deflected path of eruption of the canine. Parents should be advised to wait till canine eruption. However, this condition is not seen in lower arch.

Abnormal attachment of the maxillary labial frenum: Generally, during the gum pad stage, the upper labial frenum is attached to the incisive papilla and onto the alveolar crest. With the eruption of upper central incisors and dentoalveolar growth in that region, the frenum moves more gingivally, and comes to lie on labial side in attached gingival region, leaving the incisive papillary area. Any spacing developing in midline region occurs due to physiological growth of the upper jaw.

But sometimes, the frenum does not regress gingivally to the full, and thus prevents the

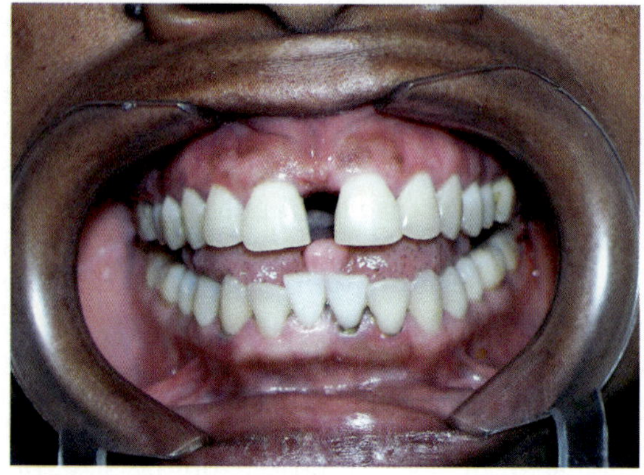

(a)

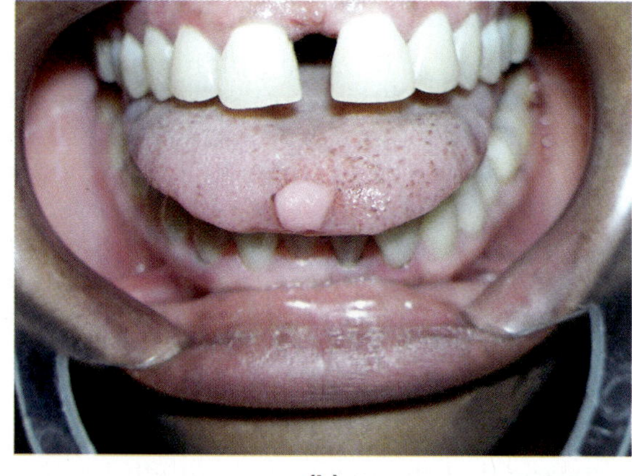

(b)

Figs 41.25a and b: Midline diastema leading to abnormal adaptive growth on the tip of tongue.

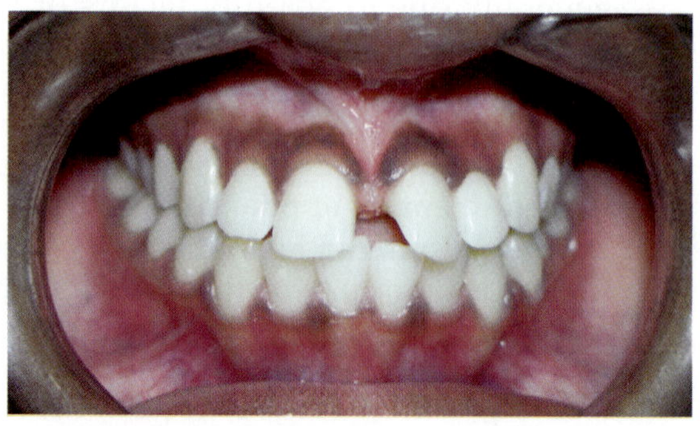

Fig. 41.26: Midline diastema, rotated 21, and low lying maxillary frenum.

approximation of the central incisors. This frenum mostly has elastic fibres with little or no muscular fibres. In many cases, the midline gingival papilla is seen hanging between permanent central incisors. The frenum needs frenectomy after the space closure and a permanent retention.

Tooth size–arch length discrepancy: Midline space can also appear, if the MD width of central incisors is less than normal. A generalized spacing is seen among incisors if MD width is less in a normally wide dental arch. Sometimes the MD width of teeth is normal but the arch width is more. Space can also be seen if lateral incisors are peg-shaped. Extraction of tooth with resultant drifting can also cause spacing.

Supernumerary teeth: Midline supernumerary teeth especially mesiodens, midline odontomes, midline cysts and other pathologies do not allow proper eruption of teeth and deflect them from their normal eruption path. It leads to spaces in midline.

Tongue thrust and finger-sucking habits: Pressure habits cause abnormal forces on the dentition, and disturb the pressure equilibrium around the dental arches. Habits generally lead to proclination of upper incisors and the generalized spacing in upper incisors.

During RME: Sometimes, the midline spacing is seen during certain therapeutic measures. When RME is done, the midpalatal suture opens up thus creating the midline space between central incisors, it is a prognostic sign for undergoing RME. With passage of time, the space gets closed due to contraction of midline transpalatal fibres.

Proclined incisors: Due to proclination, the teeth are arranged along a larger arch form, thus some spaces appear in incisal region.

Midline pathologies: For example, supernumerary tooth, cysts, etc. do not allow the central incisors to approximate.

Diagnosis: A proper history, clinical examination, and radiological examination are done to ascertain the cause and nature of midline diastema.

Blanch test: If frenum is abnormal attached, then a pull and blanch test is done to assess it. If during pulling, the palatal tissue around incisive papilla is seen whitish due to pressure. Also a movement of free gingival margin can be seen during the pull.

IOPA X-ray: In an IOPA X-ray, the notching of interdental alveolar crest in midline can be seen.

Radiographs, e.g. IOPA, occlusal view and OPG help in determining the midline pathology.

TSALD is calculated by model analysis and cephalometric analysis.

Treatment of Midline Diastema

1. **Removal of the causes:** Cause should be removed as a first step. Any supernumerary tooth should be removed, midline pathology removed surgically, abnormal habits should be controlled, etc.
2. **Active treatment:** Choice of the appliances needed for active treatment is made. The options are listed and the objectives of treatment and required steps/procedures are explained to the patient. Active treatment can be given by removal or fixed appliances (Fig. 41.27).

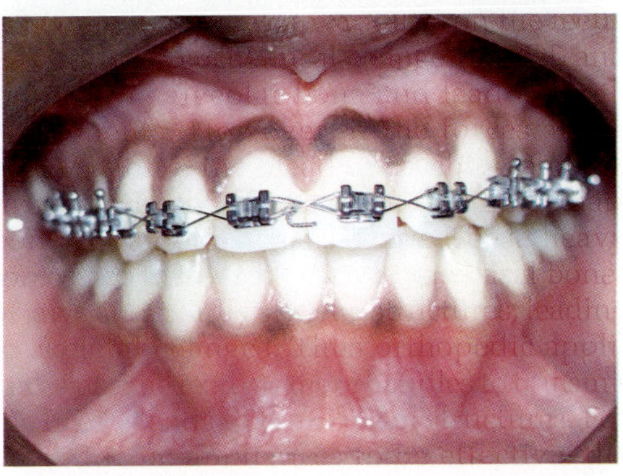

Fig. 41.27: During Rx: closed diastema and corrected rotation.

a. **Removable appliances:** A maxillary appliance with finger springs on central incisors to move them mesially can be used if tipping is needed. A split labial bow can also be used. These springs are activated by 2–3 mm at each activation. Removable appliance causes tipping movement of the teeth. If sufficient overjet is there, then the upper incisors can be tipped lingually which helps in closure of diastema.

b. **Fixed appliance** (Figs 41.28a and b): The brackets are placed in upper arch and the arch is aligned. Then, a hard wire is placed and the active force to close the space is applied by means of elastomeric chain, elastic, elastic thread, etc. Closed coil spring can also be stretched between the two central incisors to apply closing force. M-spring can also be activated and ligated on two central incisors.

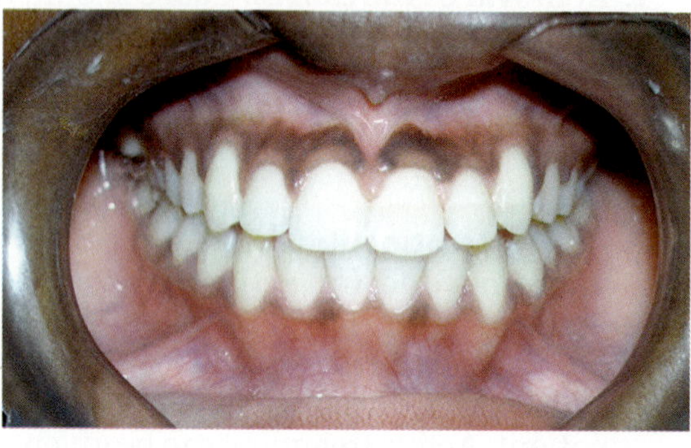

(a)

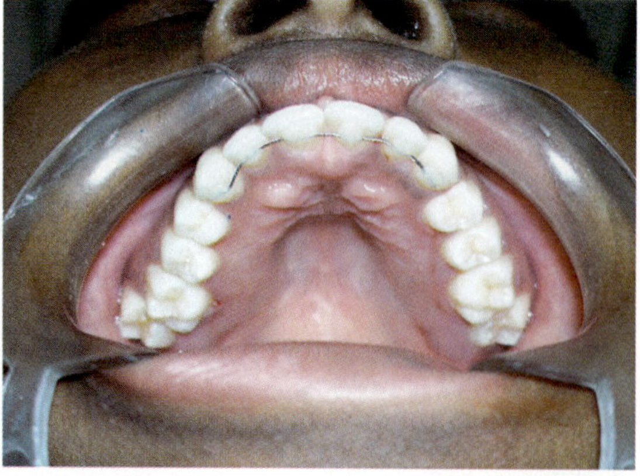

(b)

Figs 41.28a and b: Post-Rx and fixed palatal retainer.

3. **Retention phase:** It is very important phase, since the closed midline diastema has a tendency to relapse rapidly. Prolonged or permanent retention is planned by using lingual fixed retainers. The removable appliances can also be used but there are always a tendency of relapse since the patient cooperation cannot be ascertained. In some cases, a combination lingual retainer and an active labial retainer is given.
4. **Surgical removal of the frenum, Wanton's clipping** (Fig. 41.29): If the cause of the diastema is maxillary labial frenum, it should be removed surgically along with the fibres crossing the midline to the alveolar crest and palatal gingival. According to Proffit, the surgery should be done only after space closure, since the scar tissue formed helps in retaining the results. If surgery is done before space closure, the elastic fibres in scar tissue lead to relapse. It is due to the fact that during active closure, the scar tissue gets compressed, which being elastic, rebounds when the active force is removed, thus leading to relapse.
5. **Cosmetic build-up of teeth:** Composite restoration can be done after space closure on the teeth with smaller MD dimensions. In some cases, especially the

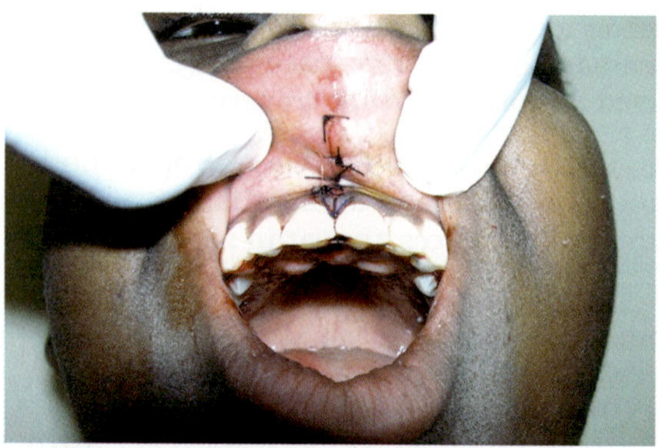

Fig. 41.29: Frenectomy.

adult cases (where orthodontics cannot be done), the gradual composite build up of the mesial surfaces of central incisors can be done to reduce the midline space, while the distal surfaces are gradually reduced to achieve natural contouring. Since in adult patients, the pulp chambers are small, the chances of pulpitis and sensitivity are less due to enamel removal. But if space is very large, then this method cannot give good results, and a first phase of orthodontics may be required to equally distribute the spaces before composite contouring is needed.

6. **Jacket crowns:** Since composite restorations are not life-long, the best method to achieve to permanent results in some cases are equal distribution of the spaces among the incisors according to the proportions of front teeth and then giving the permanent porcelain or PFM crowns. They are also used in teeth having generalized smaller size with generalized spacing. They also act as permanent retention besides fulfilling esthetic needs. They are also needed when 1 or more teeth are missing and if teeth have abnormal shape, e.g. peg laterals. Acrylic crowns can also be given but they lose their color with time and need to be replaced.

ROTATIONS

It is the deviation of tooth position around its long axis. Any tooth in the dental arch can be found rotated. It is of two types, i.e.

1. Mesiolingual rotation or the distobuccal rotation
2. Mesiobuccal or distolingual rotation

Space problems with rotations: Rotated anterior teeth occupy less space in the dental arch due to their triangular shape, i.e. less bucco-lingual dimension as compared to their MD width. So during their derotation/correction, they need space for alignment. of crown shape wheelers.

The rotated posterior teeth occupy more space. The trapezoidal shape of their crown has their maximum MD width less than the hypotenuse of the crown trapezoid. When they are derotated for correction, the space is gained in the dental arch (Fig. 41.30).

Upper molars rotate around their palatal root in the mesiolingual direction, when they migrate mesially in the extraction space or when they are moved mesially under orthodontic forces. Lower molars rotate mesiolingually around the mesial root.

Degree of rotation: Rotation can be mild, moderate or severe, depending on the angle of rotation of the tooth around the long axis.

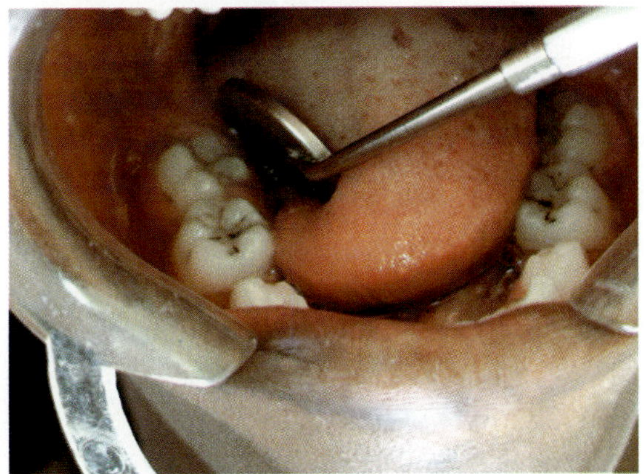

Fig. 41.30: Rotated molar occupies more space in dental arch.

Management of Rotations

Mechanics of treatment: Couple is needed to derotate the tooth. A couple is a set of two equal forces acting at a distance on the tooth in opposite direction. These forces generate a moment of force on the tooth and help in rotating the tooth along the long axis.

Treatment of rotation:

1. **Space management:** To derotate the anterior teeth, space is needed in the dental arch. For derotation of anterior tooth, the required space should be created before correction. The correction of rotations should be started in the initial stages of treatment since it needs long term retention after correction. The method to gain the space is decided to achieve the required space.

2. **Removable appliance:** Mild rotation of upper incisors can be treated with Z-spring and labial bow in the appliance. One force is provided by the Z-spring, while labial bow provides a reactionary force or the restricting effect. But removable appliances depend on patient cooperation and take a long time for treatment.
3. **Fixed appliances** (Figs 41.31 to 41.33): It is the best method for treatment of rotation, as it applies continuous force couple; and does not depend on patient cooperation. It can be used for treatment of multiple rotations simultaneously. A force couple is obtained with the help of flexible arch wires on labial side and the elastic thread or E-chain or springs or elastics from the lingual side. For incisors, the wider twin brackets help in producing the couple with flexible wires and may not need lingual force. Correction of rotated posterior teeth is difficult, needs more time, needs couple force from lingual side, due to their size, shape and number of roots, and bone morphology. Anterior teeth need less time for correction. The brackets are

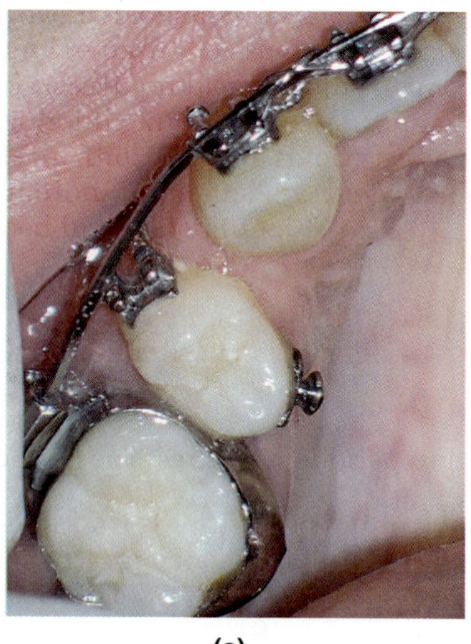

(a)

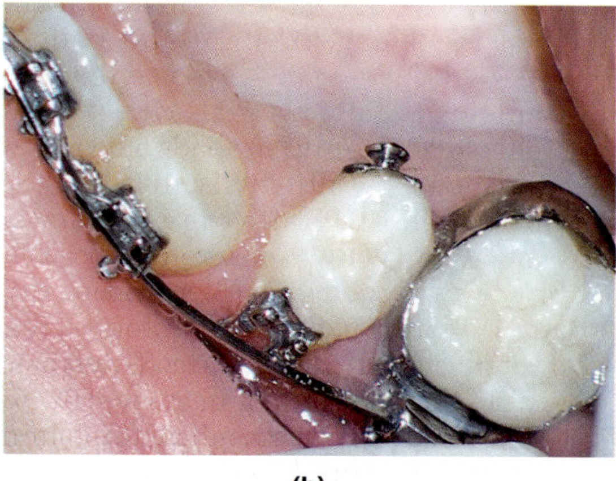

(b)

Figs 41.31a and b: Rotated premolar. A lingual button has been placed on palatal surface to apply rotational force.

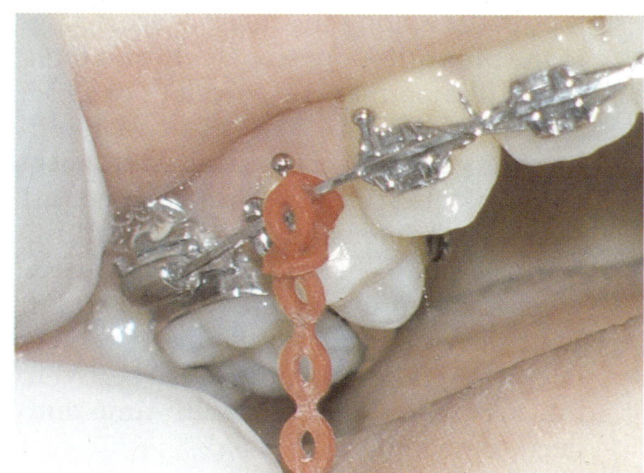

Fig. 41.32: E-chain wired around main archwire to be attached at lingual button.

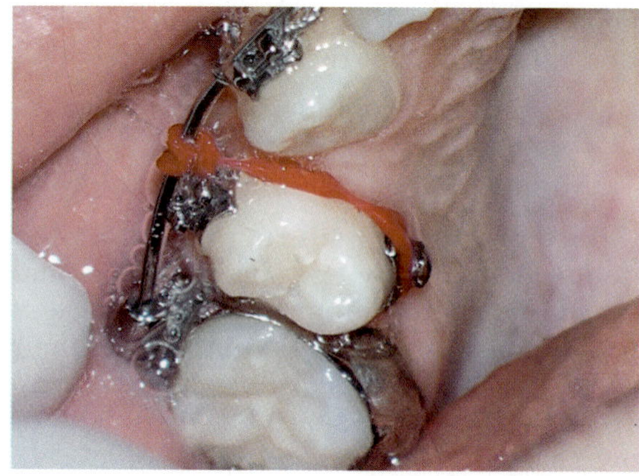

Fig. 41.33: E-chain attached at lingual button for rotation correction.

placed on the teeth and then mechanics are applied. Anchorage requirements should be decided and applied before starting the treatment. There are many methods for derotation.

a. **Rotation wedges:** Mild rotations can be treated by putting rotation wedges in between the tooth and the arch wire.
b. **Flexible wires:** For example, NiTi, multilooped arch wires, etc. are easily ligated due to their flexibility, they apply consistent force to derotate the mild to moderate rotations.
c. **Elastic threads:** Elastomeric chains, etc. are engaged on a lingual attachment and wrapped around the tooth in the direction of desired correction and then ligated to the main arch wire.
d. **Couple of forces:** Correction of severe rotation or rotated posterior tooth and canines generally needs a couple of forces. If two adjacent teeth are rotated in opposite directions, then lingual E-chain attached on these two teeth acts to derotate them by reciprocal movements.
e. **Derotation springs:** These are used with brackets having vertical slots (e.g. Beggs bracket) and their active arm is placed on the side of the tooth to be derotated to apply a pressing force on that surface, while the retentive arm is tucked to the main arch wire.
f. **Active transpalatal arches:** TPA can be effectively used to derotate the molars, without the need of brackets, etc. Before cementing, the TPA is activated in the required direction of derotation, so that it applies the force on the teeth. It can be used for correction of unilateral or bilateral molar rotations. For an optimum correction, it is necessary to insert the TPA in the passive state to determine its neutral position, and then it is activated by giving first-order bends at the arch ends. Normal position of upper first molar can be determined by passing a line through DB and ML cusps which should pass through maxillary canine in a normally placed tooth.
g. **Bends in the archwires:** Offset bends can be placed in the archwire in incisal regions to derotate the tooth.
h. **Offsetting the bracket or band position:** The bracket can be placed more on the side of rotated surface of the tooth rather than putting in the centre of the tooth. It automatically creates an offset and thus archwire can be further activated.
i. **Fixed Palatal expansion appliances:** Fixed palatal expansion appliance can be used to derotate the upper first molars, e.g. NPE; quad helix, etc.

Retention: Rotation after correction has high potential of relapse. It is due to the stretch of the supra-alveolar gingival, trans-septal fibers and periodontal fibres. The periodontal fibres (which are in PDL space, are small sized) take less time to adapt and do not lead to relapse. But, the supracrestal and the trans-septal gingival fibres (attached on two adjacent teeth crossing the interdenal septum crest, are long, have more elastic components) take a long time to readapt to new position due their more elastic component. Long-term retention is required because transseptal gingival fibers which get extended/stretched during correction, readapt very slowly to the new position. It generally requires more than 232 days.

Fixed retainer: A prolonged or permanent fixed lingual retainer should be given to the patient. At least one tooth should be involved on either side of corrected tooth in fixed retainer.

Pericision: It is also called **circumferential supracrestal fibrotomy** (CSF) as advocated by Edwards. It is the incising of the stretched supracrestal and the trans-septal gingival fibres. It is done under local anesthesia by a BP knife through the gingival sulcus. The knife is rotated all around the tooth till the alveolar crest of bone, thus cutting the fibres. An adequate time is given for them to reorganize before debonding. After that, new fibers get adapted to new position of the tooth. A fixed retainer is still placed but the duration of retainer can be reduced.

TREATMENT OF EXTRUDED OR INTRUDED TEETH

Extrusion of tooth is bodily shifting of the tooth along its long axis out of alveolar socket. Intrusion is opposite to extrusion. In both cases, the level of the incisal edge or occlusal surface is different than the adjacent teeth. Extrusion of incisor/s leads to increase in bite depth, while intrusion leads to decreased bite depth in that area. On the opposite hand, extrusion of posterior tooth leads to opening of bite/shallow bite, while intrusion can lead to deepening of bite.

Treatment of an extruded tooth: An extruded tooth as compared to adjacent teeth needs to be intruded to align the incisal/occlusal surfaces. Since intrusion is a difficult and slow process, lighter forces are needed. Also, the anchorage issue should be managed since there are extrusive forces on the adjacent teeth, leading to their extrusion, because extrusion is an easy movement. It especially happens when we want to intrude canines which are stronger and longer teeth, they lead to extrusion of adjacent teeth. Incisors can be easily intruded by maintaining anchorage, and using local intrusive loop in the main arch wire on the culprit tooth.

Intrusion of posterior teeth is difficult due to their size and bone morphology. It helps in closing the openbite, because 1 mm intrusion of molar can help to deepen the bite by 2–3 mm. Many appliances, e.g. head gear, posterior bite plates, composite blob bonding on the occlusal surface; elastics crossing over the occlusal surface which are supported by modified TPA and buccal side hooks, etc. have been used for intrusion of posterior teeth with variable success. Microimplants are the current method to help in intrusion. Segmental surgery can also be done in the localized area for intruding the teeth.

Treatment of an intruded tooth: A tooth may be found away from the occlusal plane level which needs to be brought towards occlusion. Intruded tooth may be due to trauma, ankylosis, habits, incomplete eruption, etc. (Fig. 41.34). Their treatment is done by pulling them towards OP, i.e. by their extrusion. Fixed appliances are best suited for this movement. Extrusion is an easy movement, and does not put pressure on the anchor teeth. But if the tooth is ankylosed, then adjacent teeth get intruded rather than the culprit tooth extruded. Ankylosed tooth needs surgical tearing of the tooth from the bone and then repositioned in normal position and retained there. Controlling the abnormal habits also removes the pressure from the teeth leading to their normal eruption. A tooth having closed apex intruded due to trauma can be extruded with lighter forces with fixed appliance. But a tooth with open apices which gets intruded due to trauma is given time to erupt naturally.

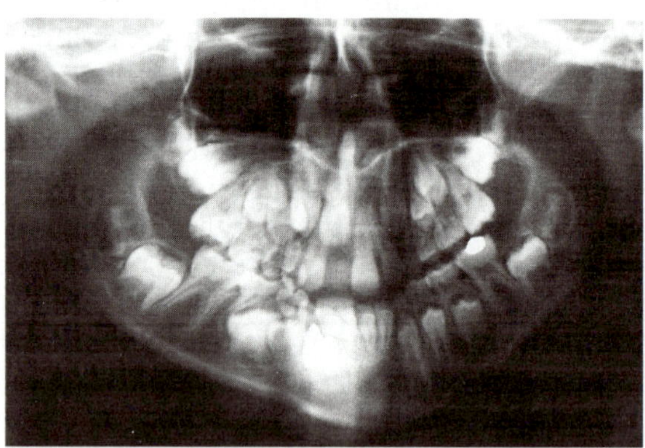

Fig. 41.34: An intruded upper central incisor due to trauma.

Conclusion

Class I malocclusion is easy to treat as it needs the correction of localized conditions. Various methods have been discussed above to correct varying colors of malalignment. Clinician has to decide best possible solution for the problem depending on the cause of the problem and anatomic features of the patient.

42

Deep Bite

INTRODUCTION

Vertical overlap of lower incisors by the upper incisors is called the overbite. Overbite can vary as normal overbite; edge to edge bite; open bite; and deep bite. Deep bite malocclusion is considered in the vertical plane. Deep bite is excessive vertical overlapping of mandibular anterior teeth by maxillary anterior teeth in centric occlusion. The normal value of overbite is 2–3 mm. However, in orthodontics, it is studied as the percentage overlap of lower incisors by the upper incisors. If the overlap is more than the normal range, it is termed as deep bite. Deep bite malocclusion is a common finding in many patients.

Importance of Normal Bite

A normal overbite is very important for the health of dental tissues, TMJs, and stomatognathic system. It is important for proper incisal guidance (IG). Incisal guidance is in consonance with the condylar guidance CG, i.e. condyle slides along the slope of condylar fossa during protrusion of mandible, which parallels the IG. If IG and CG do not match, it leads to abnormal forces on anterior teeth and TMJ especially the articular disc in TMJ along the slope of condylar fossa. To match IG and CG, the overbite should be corrected to normal values.

Deep Bite in Deciduous Dentition

There is a natural deep bite in primary dentition due to more upright position of upper and lower incisors on the jaw bases (interincisal angle is approx. 170°). When the permanent teeth start to erupt, the **natural bite opening** occurs due to eruption of molars. It occurs at the ages of 6, 12 and 18 years of age. When permanent molars are erupting, the soft tissue overlying them gets swollen and touches each other. It leads to a proprioceptive sensation, due to which patient avoids biting. It creates occlusal gap and leads to supraeruption of teeth anterior to molars, thus leading to bite opening. That is why the permanent molars are also called natural bite openers. Some bite opening effect is also occurs because upper and lower permanent incisors erupt in slightly labially proclined position (interincisal angle is approx. 131°) in a wider arch circumference, as compared to primary teeth.

Classification of Deep Bite (Figs 42.1 to 42.4)

A. **According to the tissues involved**, the deep bite is classified as: Dental deep bite and skeletal deep bite.
B. **According to bite depth:** Complete deep bite and partial deep bite.
C. **According to trauma caused:** Deep traumatic bite.
D. **According to Hotz and Muhlemann:** True deep bite and pseudo-deep bite.
E. **Cephalometric classification of deep bite:** It can be of two types:
   a. **Dentoalveolar deep bite:** It may be due to supraeruption of incisors or infraocclusion of buccal teeth.
   b. **Skeletal deep bite:** It may be due to horizontal growth pattern or retro-inclination of maxillary base, i.e. a clockwise rotation of maxilla.

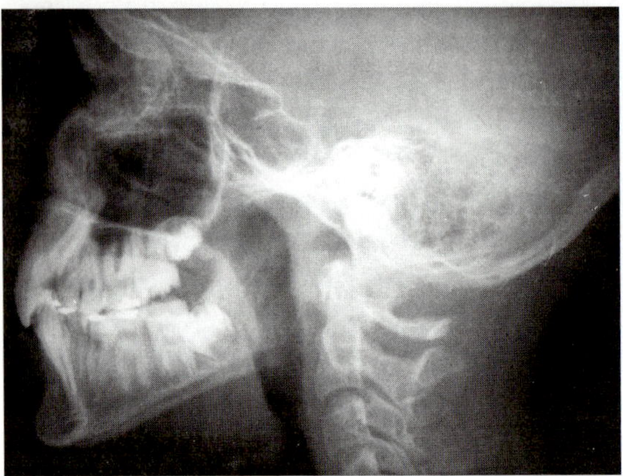

Fig. 42.1: Cephalogram showing deep bite. Note the incisal edges of upper and lower incisors approaching the CEJs of opposing teeth.

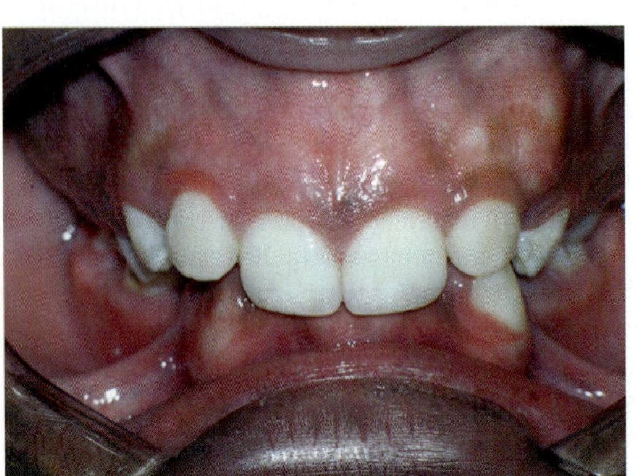

Fig. 42.2: Severe deep bite (>100 %). Upper incisal edges have crossed past the free gingival margins of lower incisors. It generally occurs due to supraeruption of teeth and has genetic component.

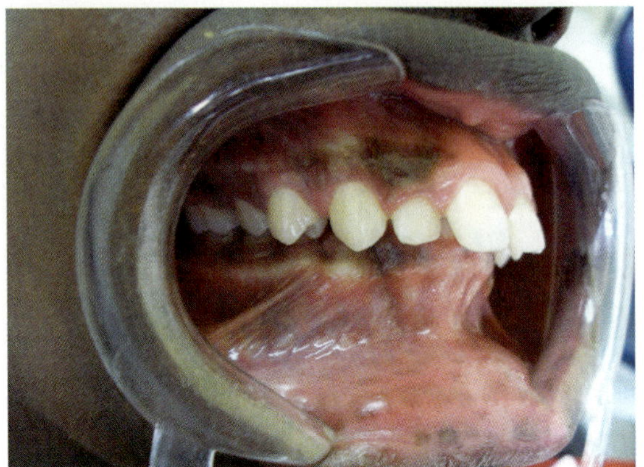

Fig. 42.3: Severe deep bite with lower incisors occluding in palatal mucosa. Also note scissors bite in premolar region.

Definitions

Dental deep bite: It is the increased overlap of anterior teeth, without any underlying skeletal component.

Skeletal deep bite: It is overclosure of the jaws. It may or may not be associated with dental deep bite. It is seen in horizontal growth pattern cases, which have short face height; reduced angles between the horizontal cephalometric planes, i.e. SN, FHP, PP, OP, and MP planes. The dentoalveolar height in the posterior region is reduced. It occurs due to U and F mandibular rotation during growth, which literally pushes it in the maxilla. Maxilla may also rotate D and F in some cases, contributing to the deep bite.

Partial deep bite: It is the partial overlap of lower incisors by the upper incisors. The incisal edges of upper incisors lie above the level of lower marginal gingiva, but still the overlap is more than normal bite.

Complete deep bite: It is the total overlap of lower incisors by the upper incisors. The incisal edges of upper incisors lie at or below the level of lower marginal gingiva.

True deep bite: It is due to infraocclusion of molars, and has large freeway space. It can be successfully treated with supraeruption/ extrusion of molars, especially with functional appliances and cervical headgear, and still an adequate freeway space can be maintained. Its treatment by molar extrusion is successful during active growth stage as the vertical growth of ramus compensates the vertical dentoalveolar growth.

Pseudo-deep bite: It is due to over-eruption of incisors. The molars have erupted fully and there is normal or small free way space. It is treated with intrusion of incisors. It cannot be treated with functional appliances causing molar extrusion, as it will affect the rest position, encroach/decrease the freeway space, strain the muscles and leads to relapse.

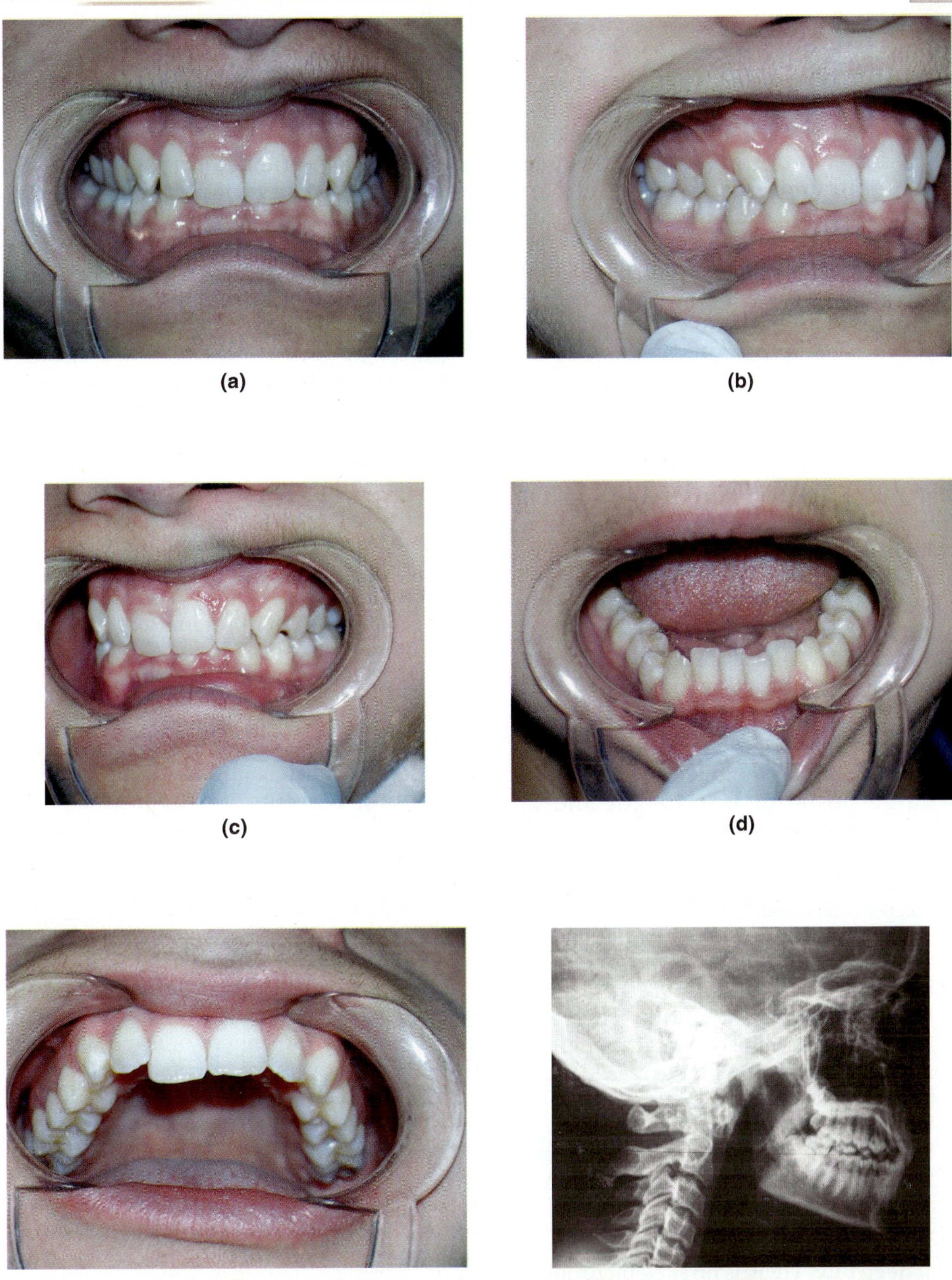

(a) (b) (c) (d) (e) (f)

Figs 42.4a to f: Pre-Rx intraoral views of deep bite and lower incisal crowding.

Closed bite (complete overbite): It is defined as a condition when lower incisors are completely overlapped by the upper anterior teeth.

Deep traumatic bite: It is the condition when the lower teeth contact the palatal tissue causing the trauma, or the upper incisors contact the labial gingival tissue in mandibular area, and the mandibular teeth are completely overlapped by maxillary anterior teeth in centric occlusion.

Generally, in orthodontics, the bite depth is considered as a percentage of overlap of lower teeth by the upper teeth, e.g. 100% deep bite, 50% bite depth, etc.

Clinical Features of Skeletal Deep Bite

Skeletal deep bite: It is generally of genetic origin, and is due to horizontal growth of mandible, where there is upward and forward rotation of mandible. It can also be due to D and F, i.e. clockwise rotation of maxilla during growth or a combination of both the jaw bases. Its severe form is also called short face syndrome, (SFS). Generally, some of the following features are seen in such cases.

a. Horizontal growth pattern of face
b. Small anterior face height
c. Large posterior face height and an increased Jarabak ratio
d. Increased ramal height
e. Decreased mandibular plane angle
f. Decreased/closed gonial angle
g. Prominent chin, and gonial angle region
h. The mandibular plane and the body is flat
i. Increased height of ramus
j. Some parallelism of basal and other horizontal planes, with decreased angulation between them.
k. Increased freeway space
l. Squarish face, prominent jaw angle and line.

Clinical Features of Dental Deep Bite

Dental deep bite: There is no skeletal problem in such cases, only dental tissues are affected which cause deep bite. It is the increased overlapping of lower teeth by upper teeth. It may be due to either supraeruption of incisors or infraocclusion of buccal teeth or a combination of both.

Deep bite due to supraeruption of anterior teeth may be contributed by both upper and lower teeth. The curve of Spee is increased. It may or may not be associated with increased overjet, e.g. in Angle's class II division 1, the overjet is increased, while in Angle's class II division 2, the overjet is decreased or almost zero. The lower teeth supraerupt when their incisal edges lie posterior to the cinguli of upper incisors, thus not getting an incisal stop. The upper incisors supraerupt in class II division 2 due to strong lips and circumoral musculature.

Deep bite due to infraeruption of molars is associated with horizontal growth pattern. It may also be caused by lateral tongue thrust or premature loss of posterior teeth. Also the deep bite may be caused by a combination of both, i.e. supraeruption of incisors and infraeruption of molars.

Deep bite due to over-eruption of incisors: Normally, the incisal edges of lower incisors lie just below the cingulum area (according to British society incisal classification), thus preventing eruption of upper and lower incisors. The incisors erupt more than the normal in deep bite if the incisors do not have proper incisal stops. It occurs in cases with increased overjet, e.g. in class II division 1; class I type 2 malocclusion. But an extreme deep bite is seen in class II division 2 cases also where overjet is minimal. It occurs due to hyperactive upper lip which leads to lingual and downward movement of upper incisors. This lingual movement of upper incisors may lead to lingual movement and uprighting of lower incisors, leading to deepening of bite.

Deep bite due to uprighting of lower incisors occurs during serial extraction procedure when lower primary canines are removed. The lower lip pressure leads to uprighting of lower incisors.

Deep bite due to infraocclusion of molars: It also leads to deep bite. It may occur if the tongue comes in interocclusal area, preventing eruption of bucccal teeth. Premature loss of posterior teeth leads to deep bite due to mesial migration of distal teeth. During this condition, partially erupted molars and large freeway space is present. Strong masticatory muscles are also responsible for infraeruption of molars as they apply heavy forces on the buccal segment. This condition is seen in horizontal growth pattern cases.

Etiology

Deep bite malocclusion is a common finding in many patients. The causes are:

Genetics: Heredity is one of the most important cause leading to deep bite; especially skeletal type, e.g. class II division 2 cases, horizontal growth pattern, etc.

Growth pattern: Horizontal growth patients have deep bite; this is skeletal deep bite. The mandible rotates upward and forward thus thrusting it in the maxilla and leading to deep bite.

Dental deep bite is generally seen when the teeth in the opposing arch do not keep the teeth to supraerupt, e.g. in Angle's class II cases, the incisal stops are lost, leading to supraeruption of the incisors.

Muscular forces: Especially in Angle's class II division 2 cases, the lower lip and the upper lip muscles have more activity leading to retroclination of incisors and thus deep bite. This is also supported by horizontal growth in these cases, thrusting the mandible in the anterior and upward direction.

Lower lip habit causes lingual pressure on lower anterior leading to their lingual inclination, supraeruption and deep bite. Hyperactive lower lip during lip trap also leads to lingual inclination and uprighting of lower incisors. Lip trap also leads to labial proclination of upper incisors. Hyperactive upper lip applying lingual forces on upper incisors lead to their extrusion and hence deep bite.

Deep bite caused during serial extractions: When the mandibular primary canines are removed, the lip forces cause the lingual tipping and uprighting of lower incisors, thus causing an increase in bite depth.

Diagnosis: A proper history, clinical examination especially extraoral examination, and cephalometric examination of the patient help to reach proper diagnosis. Examination of the dental casts also gives idea of dentoalveolar heights in especially molar region as the crown height of these teeth is found to be shorter. Cephalometric analysis helps to identify the skeletal and dental components which are at fault, and also the growth pattern of the face. It helps to devise a proper treatment plan. The status of development of cervical vertebrae helps to find out the growth status of the patient (Fig. 42.5).

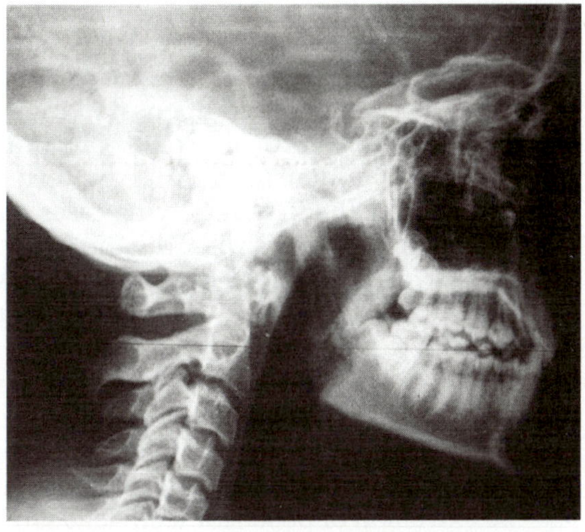

Fig. 42.5: Pre-Rx cephalogram showing deep bite.

MANAGEMENT OF DEEP BITE

Factors

Main factors to be considered during treatment are:

1. **Gummy smile:** If the patient exhibits gummy smile which may be due to short upper lip or over-eruption of the teeth, then intrusion of incisors should be done to reduce the deep bite. But, deep bite with normal lip relation to maxillary

incisors is to be treated with extrusion of posterior teeth. Deep bite having upper lip with normal length and more gingival exposure during smile is to be treated with incisor intrusion.

2. **Upper incisor exposure** during smile is also a factor to decide the intrusion. Normal exposure during full smile is that the lower border of upper lip lies at the gingival margin of upper teeth and the upper border of lower lip lies at the junction of incisor and middle third of upper incisors. If the incisal exposure is more, then intrusion of incisors is considered.
3. **Skeletal deep bite** (i.e. with reduced AFH and excessive horizontal growth). Such cases require extrusion of posterior teeth, which causes downward and backward rotation of mandible, leading to bite opening.
4. **Growth status** should also be considered. In a growing person, the extrusion of posterior teeth gets compensated by the simultaneous vertical growth of ramus and a stable neuromuscular pattern is established. But in nongrowing cases, the extrusion of molars disturbs the neuromuscular balance of the pterygomasseteric sling by stretching it, and thus leading to relapse.
5. **Growth pattern and vertical facial relationship:** Horizontal growth pattern leads to development of skeletal deep bite with decrease in anterior face height. So extrusion of posterior teeth leads to D and B rotation of mandible, leading to increase of anterior face height. A 1 mm extrusion of molar leads to approx. 3 mm opening in anterior region. Extrusion of posterior teeth, however, is beneficial in a growing case, as it can get compensated with increase of ramal height with growth and gets stable results.
6. **Muscular pattern:** In horizontal growth, the masticatory muscles are stronger and apply more forces, leading to deep bite. If treated with extrusion of molars, these muscles get stretched giving an intrusive force on molars, leading to relapse. Extrusion of molars can be done in growing patients where the increased dentoalveolar height is compensated by increased vertical growth of ramus. But in no-growing cases, extrusion of molars leads to stretching of muscles and hence relapse. Such cases need to be retained by prolonged, fixed and dynamic retention.
7. **Increased freeway space:** If IOG is more than 2–4 mm in premolar region, it indicates that the posterior teeth are infraoccluded. It may allow extrusion of posterior teeth, thus maintaining a normal freeway space. For stability of results, this dentoalveolar growth should be in consonance with the vertical growth of ramus. The normal freeway space should not be encroached by over-eruption of posterior teeth. It leads to stretching and activation of muscles leading to relapse. In such cases, incisor intrusion is recommended.

Treatment (Figs 42.6a to e)

A proper diagnosis and a treatment plan is considered to determine the mechanics. The treatment of deep bite is called as bite opening. The "**bite before jet**" philosophy is followed during the treatment of malocclusion. Opening the bite to edge to edge level (concept of over-treatment) helps in retraction of anterior teeth without binding by the lower teeth. If an attempt to reduce the overjet is done before opening the bite, then the crowns of upper incisors strike/interfered by lower incisors, producing a labial root torquing effect on upper incisors. It makes their roots prominent.

It depends on the diagnosis, and growth status of patient. Deep bite can be corrected either by intrusion of anterior teeth, extrusion of posterior teeth or a combination of both. Bite opening can mainly be done by (Fig. 42.7):

- **Absolute intrusion**, i.e. by intrusion of upper and lower incisors. It is also called as true bite opening.

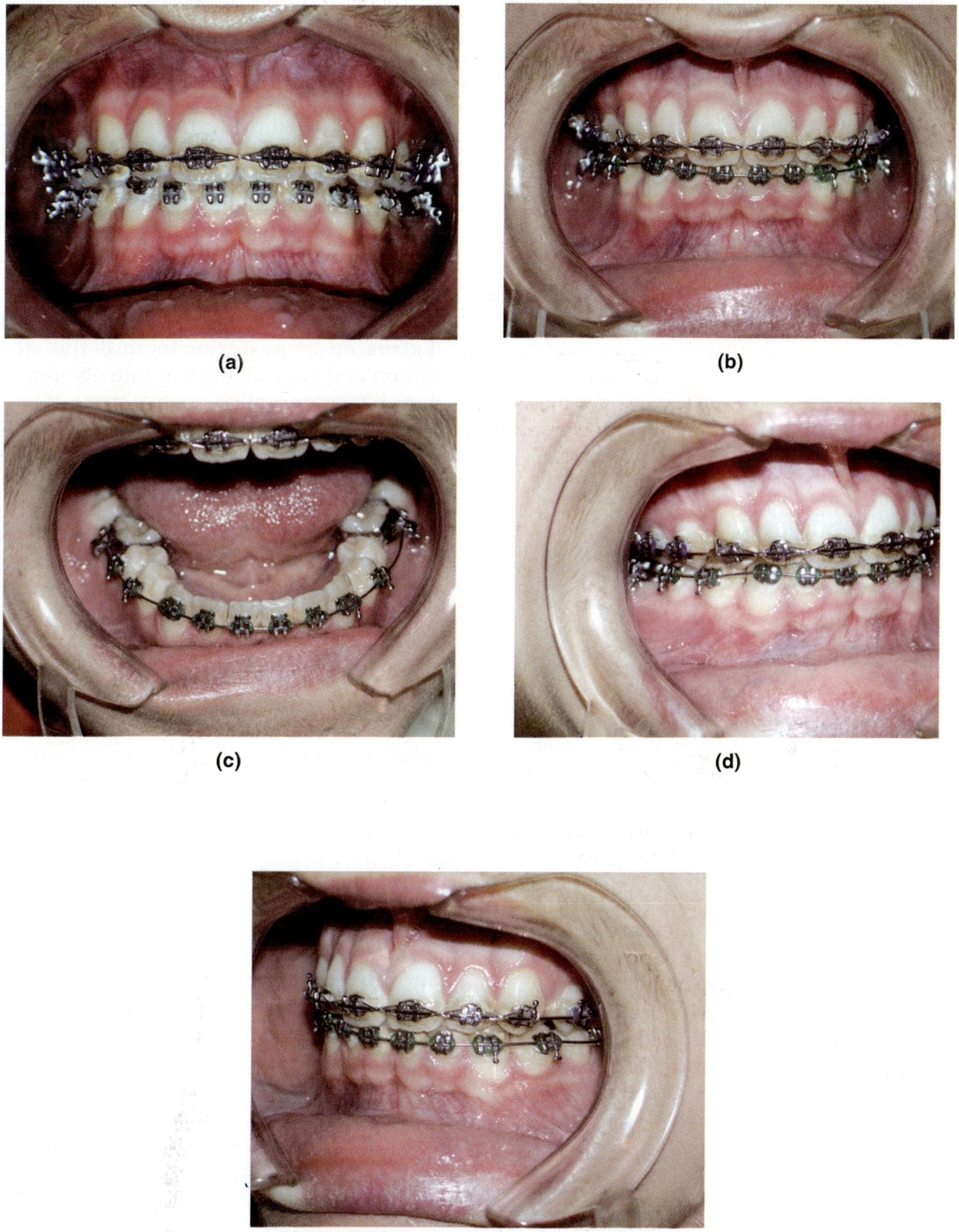

(a)

(b)

(c)

(d)

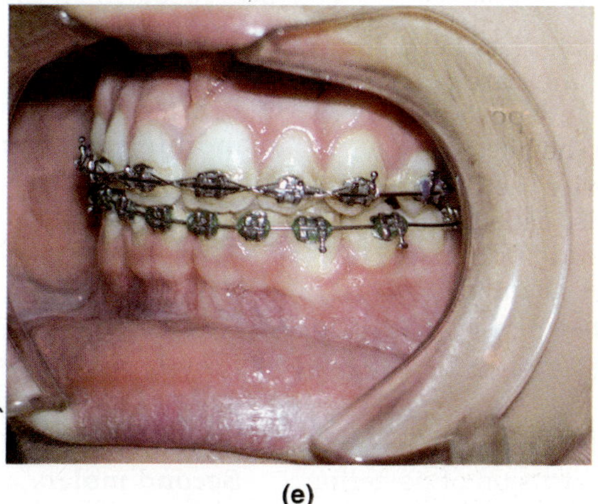

(e)

Figs 42.6a to e: Intra-Rx views of improvement of bite.

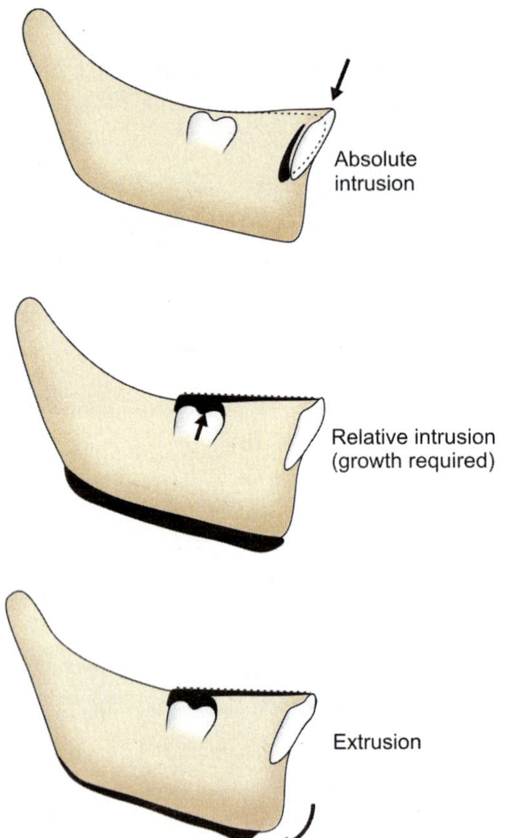

Fig. 42.7: Different modalities of treatment of deep bite: by absolute intrusion of incisors using orthodontic mechanics; by relative intrusion of teeth where growth is needed to rotate the mandible D, and the molars erupt further; and by extrusion of molars which leads to D and B mandibular rotation. *(Redrawn from Proffit and Fields for academic purpose only).*

- **Relative intrusion** of incisors, i.e. keeping the incisors where they are, while the mandible growth and posterior teeth erupt, thus opening the bite.
- **Extrusion of posterior teeth** and/or by distal tipping. It is also called as apparent bite opening, or pseudo intrusion. Here, the mandible rotates D and B.
- **Proclination of incisors:** It also leads to apparent bite opening
- **Combination**

The difference between the relative intrusion of incisors and the extrusion of posterior teeth is whether vertical growth of ramus compensates for increase in molar height. The mandibular plane angle is maintained in relative intrusion, while it increases as the mandible rotates downward and backward due to extrusion.

Forces required for intrusion: Light forces should be used for intrusion in the range of 15 gm per tooth. It is because all the forces get concentrated in the small apical area of the PDL. Since pressure is force per unit area (P = F/A), more force leads to increased pressure and hence compressing/necrosing the PDL in apical region.

Extrusion of posterior teeth is the most common and easy method of bite opening. It is done by incorporating reverse curve of Spee in the arch wires. With removable and functional appliance, it can be achieved by incorporating anterior bite plane in the appliances and creating gap between the occlusal surfaces of the posterior teeth, leaving them free to erupt. Cervical headgear appliance is used in the cases having horizontal growth pattern, with reduced posterior dentoalveolar heights. It helps to extrude the molars thus opening the bite.

Indications

Growth pattern: It is successful in the patients having normal to **horizontal growth pattern**. The patient is having the skeletal deep bite. Such patients have a low MP angle, Low FMA; decreased LFH, etc. With the extrusion of posterior teeth, the mandible moves downward and backward.

Profile: This downward and backward mandible movement is helpful in patients having a straight to concave profile, but it deteriorates the convex profile, further increasing the convexity.

Patient is in growing age: When the patient is growing, the increase in the dentoalveolar height is compensated/balanced by the simultaneous growth of ramus, thus leading to stability of the results.

Second molars are also included in fixed appliances during extrusion of molars in the horizontal growth pattern cases, especially in low angle and deep bite cases. Inclusion of second molars provides a lever for extrusion of premolars and assists incisor intrusion. The posterior the extrusion, more is the effective bite opening anteriorly. For every 1 mm extrusion posteriorly, a 3 mm anterior bite opening effect occurs.

Methods for bite opening: A number of options are available for treatment of the deep bite. Bite opening can be broadly done with following appliances:

- Removable appliances
- Myofunctional appliance
- Fixed orthodontic appliance
- Headgears
- Microimplants and miniplates
- Orthognathic surgery.

1. **Anterior bite plane** (Figs 42.8 to 42.10): It is a maxillary removable appliance having a flat bite plane in anterior region extending from canine to canine region. The lower anteriors are in even contact with this plane which creates an interocclusal gap in posterior region, thus helping the extrusion of posterior teeth by supraeruption. This occlusal gap should be limited to 3–4 mm only and when the supraeruption of buccal teeth has occurred in this gap, it is again

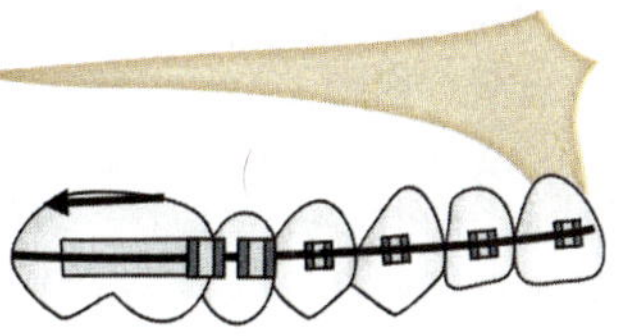

Fig. 42.8: Anterior bite plate with gap in molar region so that lower teeth are free to supraerupt to treat deep bite.

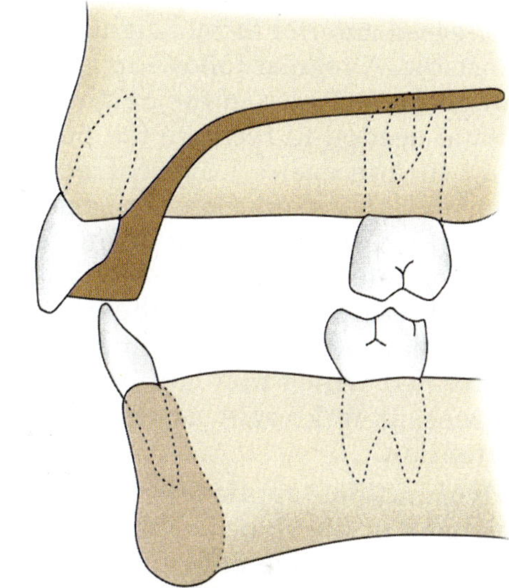

Fig. 42.9: Anterior bite plate helps to create gap in buccal region and thus the teeth are free to erupt in that space to treat deep bite.

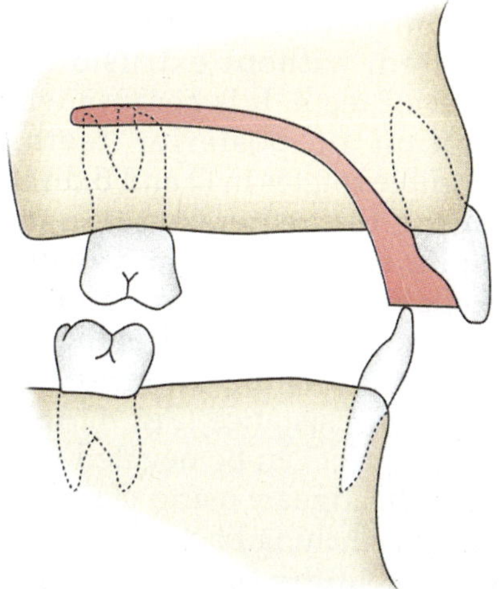

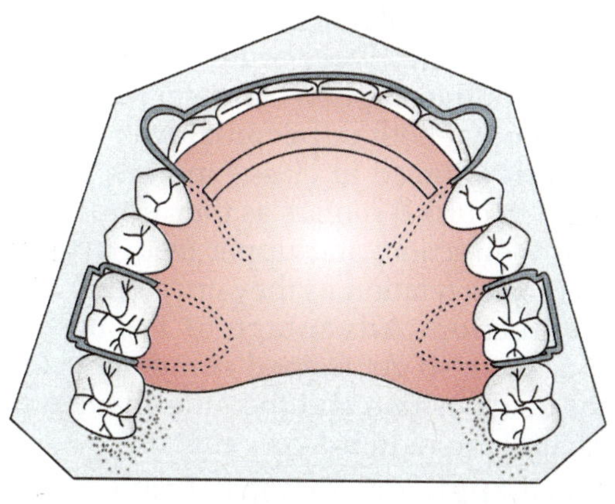

Fig. 42.10: Anterior bite plane and its mechanism. Interocclusal gap is created in buccal region when lower incisors touch on the bite plane, thus the lower buccal teeth are free to erupt in that space.

created by increasing the height of bite plane. If more gap is created initially, then the tongue may enter that gap and prevent the bite opening by preventing eruption of teeth. This appliance is suitable in patients having horizontal growth pattern. If given in vertical growth pattern cases, the molar supraeruption leads to downward and backward mandibular rotation, leading to worsening of facial profile and the increased anterior facial height which is unstable. A regular follow-up is done to judge the increase in the height of bite plane needed to recreate the posterior gap till the desired overcorrection is achieved. The same plate can be used for retention in a passive form for an appropriate time period, since with the increase in the facial height with extrusion of molars, the muscles get activated which may apply relapsing forces. It is known as the **dynamic retention**.

2. **Myofunctional appliances:** FR; activator, bionator or twin block appliances can be used during active growth period which help in correction of interjaw skeletal relationship also. These are mainly recommended in horizontal or normal growing cases, in which extrusion of posterior teeth can be useful. Posterior extrusion gets compensated with increased ramal height. The interocclusal acrylic is selectively removed to create space for the eruption of buccal teeth. The eruption of both upper and lower buccal teeth is allowed in class I molars; lower teeth in class II molars as they erupt in U and F direction; and upper teeth in class III molars relation as they erupt in D and F direction. Advantage of FA is that muscles also get trained simultaneously for new position and then the chances of relapse are reduced very much.
3. **Fixed appliance therapy:** Fixed orthodontic appliances including brackets and molar tubes are placed on the teeth. The arch wires are modified in various forms, like utility arch and its modifications; archwires with anchor bends; archwires with reverse curve of Spee, etc. In these cases, the extrusion of posterior teeth can be prevented by the use of TPA or the lingual holding arch, which also prevent the undesired rotations of molars.
   a. **Reverse curve of Spee archwires** (Figs 42.11 to 42.14): Preformed SS or NiTi archwires with RCS are available. It can also be incorporated in the upper archwire and a reverse curve of Spee in the lower archwire if the archwires are made on chair side. When they are placed, they apply intrusive forces on incisors and reciprocal extrusive forces on buccal teeth. If upper incisal exposure at rest below the upper lip is small, then deep bite is corrected by intrusion of lower incisors only.
   b. **Anchor bends** (Fig. 42.15) can also be incorporated in upper and lower archwires 2–3 mm mesial to molar tubes. On ligation, the wires apply extrusive forces on posterior teeth and the reciprocal intrusive forces on the anterior teeth. This protocol is helpful in patients having normal to horizontal growth pattern.

      But in vertical growing cases, the true intrusion of anterior teeth is required, without extrusion of the posterior teeth. It is because with the eruption of posterior teeth, the mandible rotates in D and B direction, leading to further increase in face height, and increase in convexity of profile. These wires also cause flaring of incisors due to their point of force application being anterior to their centre of resistance (Fig. 42.16). This flaring effect can be negated with the use of headgear; using class II or III elastics; cinching back the wires, etc.
   c. **Ricketts' utility intrusion arch:** It is a 2 × 4 appliance made of Elgiloy wire. The molars act as anchorage for incisor

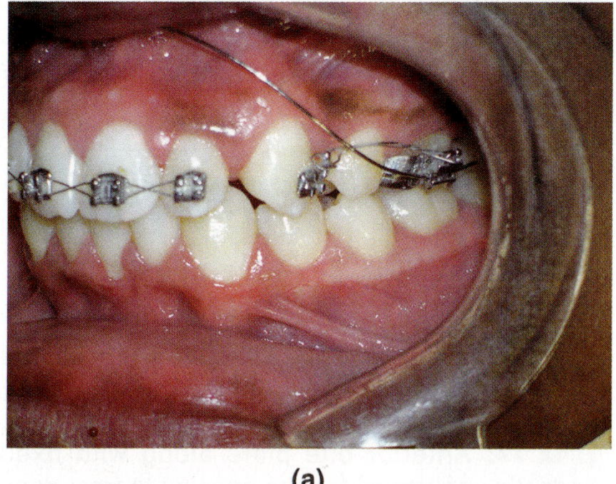

(a)

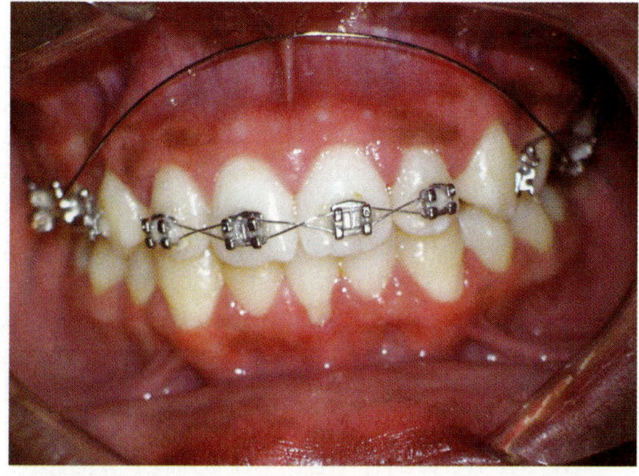

(b)

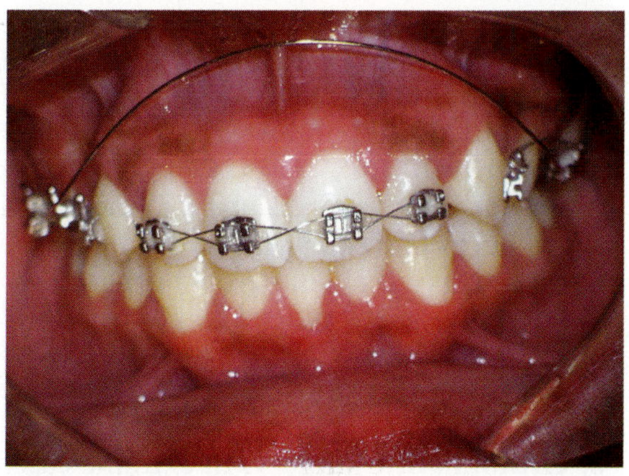

(c)

Figs 42.11a to c: Curve of Spee incorporated in the archwire, which helps in correction of deep bite, by applying extrusive force on molars and intrusive force on incisors. See the position of archwire deep in the labial vestibule.

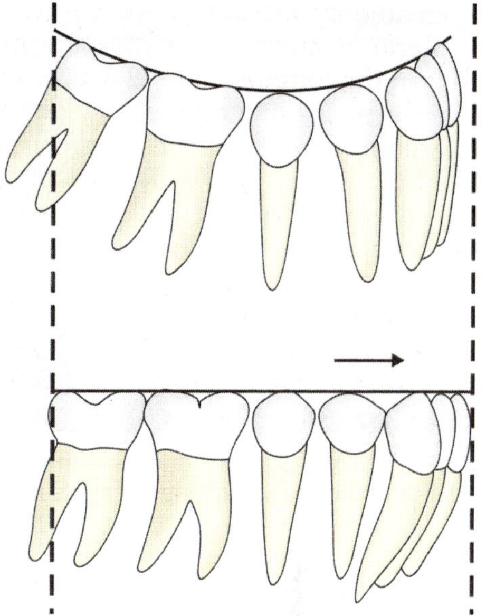

Fig. 42.12: Curve of Spee in the lower arch. To achieve a flat curve of Spee, it needs some space in the arch. Note that after flattening the curve, the lower incisors have moved forward.

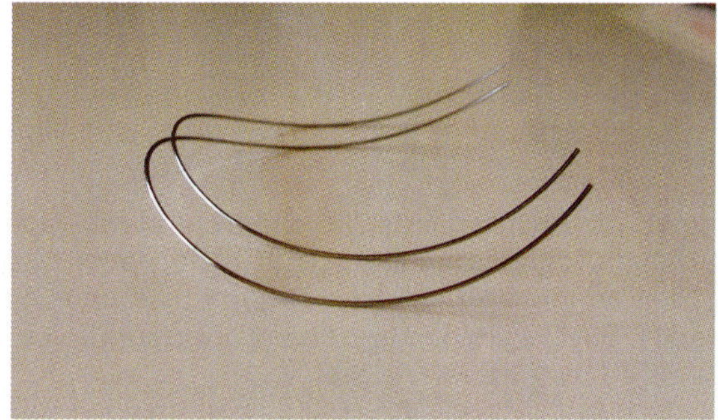

Fig. 42.13: RCS prefabricated NiTi wires.

intrusion. Light forces are used in the range of 50 gm, i.e. to apply approx 15 gm per tooth (Fig. 42.17).

d. The other variations have been proposed, e.g. Burston's intrusion arch, Connecticut intrusion arch, K-SIR wire, CNA intrusion arch, etc.

4. **Headgear appliances:** If maxillary incisor intrusion is required, **high-pull headgear is used.** The intrusive forces in U and B force direction are applied on the hooks attached on the upper arch

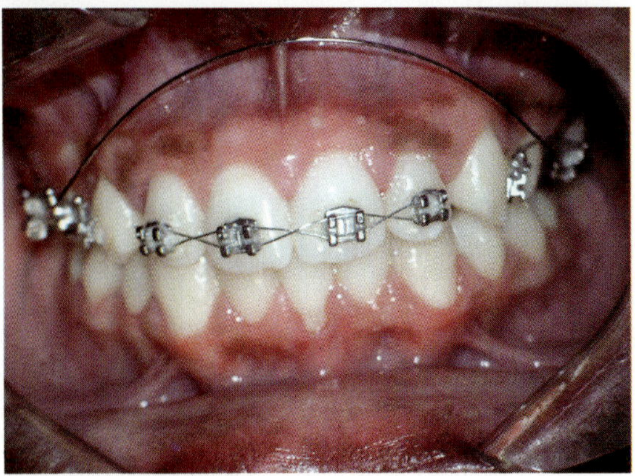

Fig. 42.14: RCS NiTi wires in place. See the position of wire in the vestibule, which helps to apply intrusion forces.

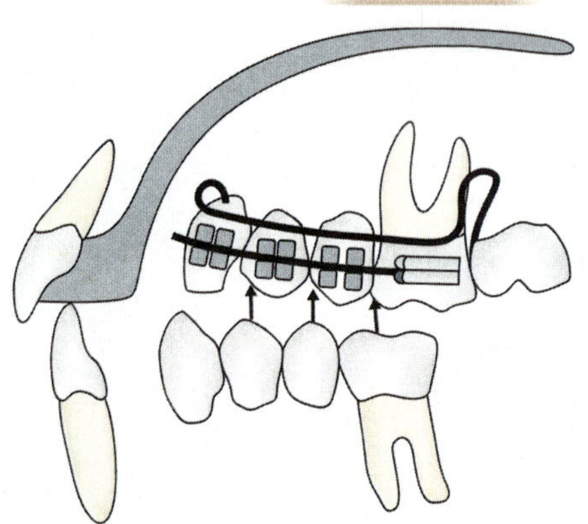

Fig. 42.17: Anterior bite plate along with fixed orthodontic appliances for bite opening to treat deep bites.

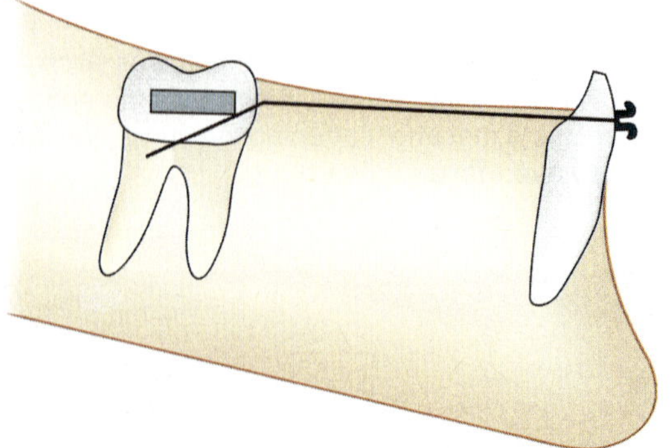

Fig. 42.15: Anchor bend in the wire helps in extrusion of molars, obtains anchorage at molar, and also applies an intrusive force on incisors thus opening the bite. But this also leads to flaring of incisors unless controlled by a backward force.

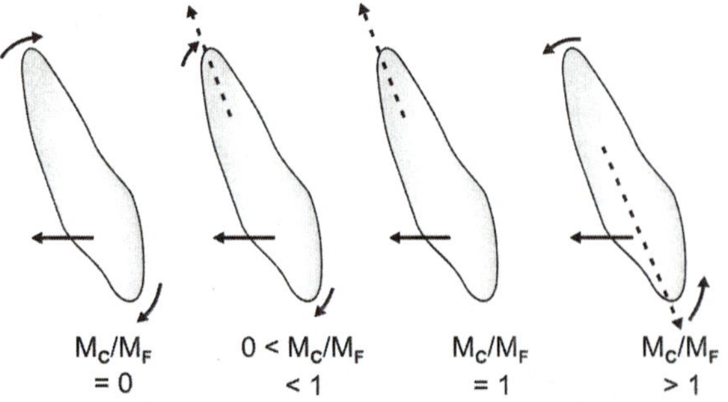

Fig. 42.16: Anchor bend given in molar region applies an intrusive effect on incisors, while a distal tipping and extrusive effect on the molar. A moment is also created at incisors leading to their flaring unless controlled by a reciprocal force.

wire between lateral incisors and canines. These forces help in achieving true intrusion, without any extrusive effects on the molars. However, patient's cooperation is a factor to succeed. It is an indicated method for patients having vertical growth pattern and with increased anterior face heights. In horizontal growth cases where molar extrusion is needed, then a cervical headgear is used to apply a D and B pull on upper molars or an upward pull on lower molars. Since it has a backward force component also, this may lead to distalization or distal tipping of molars. It may be beneficial for treatment of class II relation in upper arch; and treatment of class III relation in lower arch.

5. **Microimplants** (Figs 42.18a and b): Incisor intrusion can also be done with the help of microimplants/miniplates as they provide absolute anchorage. Two miniscrews are placed distal to lateral incisors. The intrusive force is limited to 15 gm per incisors and 30 gm per canine tooth.
6. **Orthognathic surgery:** In extreme cases where growth has ceased, cases having short facial height, called short face syndrome SFS, surgery has to be done. Generally, Le Fort I osteotomy with disimpaction/downward movement of maxilla is done. An autogenous graft is

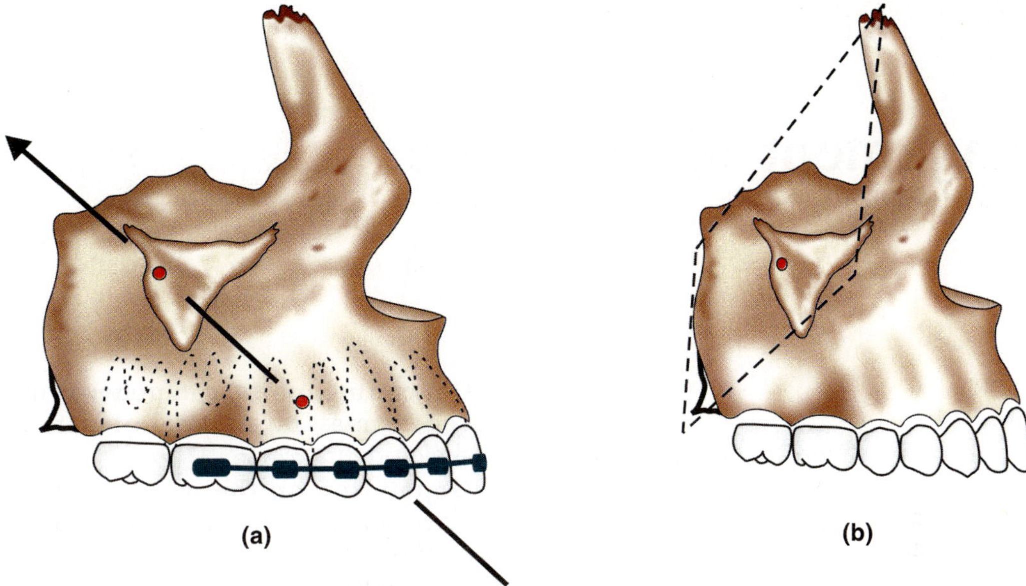

Figs 42.18a and b: Cres of maxilla in zygomatic region, and Cres of maxillary dentition in premolars root regions by red dot. For true intrusion of maxilla and maxillary dentition, the force should pass through their Cres, otherwise moments will be generated leading to rotations of these entities.

placed above the maxilla and is fixed with rigid fixation. However, it has been seen that this procedure activates the pterygomaxillary sling and thus applies an upward pressure on the maxilla and graft. It may lead to relapse. Long face syndrome having deep bite is treated with Le Fort I osteotomy with upward movement of maxilla.

Retention: It is very important phase. The condition treated by extrusion of posterior teeth may relapse fast. So a removable Hawley's appliance incorporating anterior bite plate touching passively to lower anterior teeth is used for retention. It is also called as dynamic retention (Nanda). Cases treated with incisor intrusion are retained with fixed lingual retainers. Since some amount of relapse is inevitable, so the **over-correction** should be achieved. Bite opening should be done till edge-to-edge bite status before debonding and then retention should be planned. Since the growth of maxilla and mandible continues to late adolescent and adult period, the retention appliance should be continued to avoid any after-effects of late growth.

43

Management of Crossbite

INTRODUCTION

Normal relation of upper and lower teeth is that "the buccal / labial surfaces of upper teeth lie buccal / labial to (the buccal / labial surfaces of) the lower teeth in centric occlusion". In posterior region, the palatal cusps of upper teeth lie in the central fossa of lower teeth. It is the condition of positive overjet.

In crossbite, the abovesaid relationship of upper and lower teeth is reversed, i.e. the buccal / labial surfaces of upper teeth lie lingual to (the buccal / labial surfaces of) the lower teeth in centric occlusion". In posterior region, the buccal cusps of upper teeth lie in the central fossa of lower teeth. In anterior region, the labial surface of upper tooth / teeth lie lingual to lingual surface of lower tooth. It is a condition of negative overjet. Literally speaking, there is crossing of bite by the tooth / teeth.

It may be seen in both the sagittal and the transverse planes. If it involves the anterior teeth, then the malrelationship is in the sagittal plane (one or more anterior teeth abnormally placed facially or lingually with reference to the opposing tooth or teeth); while posterior teeth are malrelated in the transverse plane.

Classification of Crossbite (Figs 43.1 to 43.7)

a. **Depending on the region involved**, it may be anterior crossbite or posterior crossbite.
b. **Depending on the sides** involved, it may be unilateral or bilateral
c. **Depending on the components** involved, it may be skeletal or dental or skeletodental.
d. **Depending on the number of teeth** involved, it may be single or multiple or segmental.
e. **Depending on the occlusal shift** during closure, it may be functional or non-functional.
f. **Depending on the jaw involved:** It may be maxillary or mandibular. Here, the clinician has to judge which jaw segment

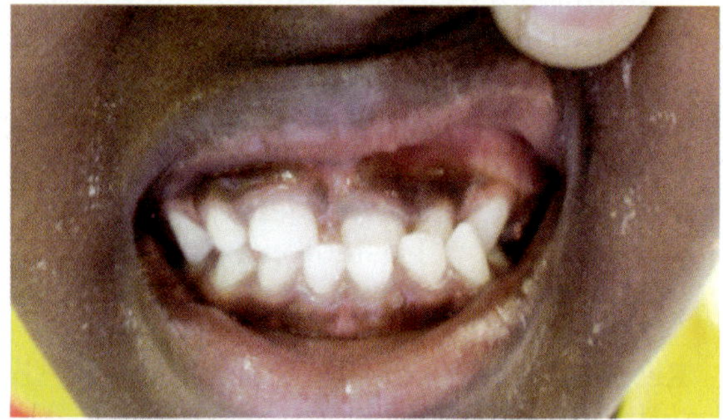

Fig. 43.1: Anterior segmental crossbite.

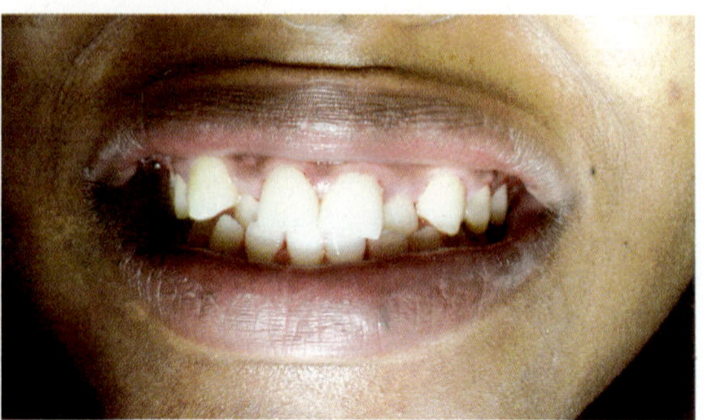

Fig. 43.2: Upper lateral incisors in crossbite.

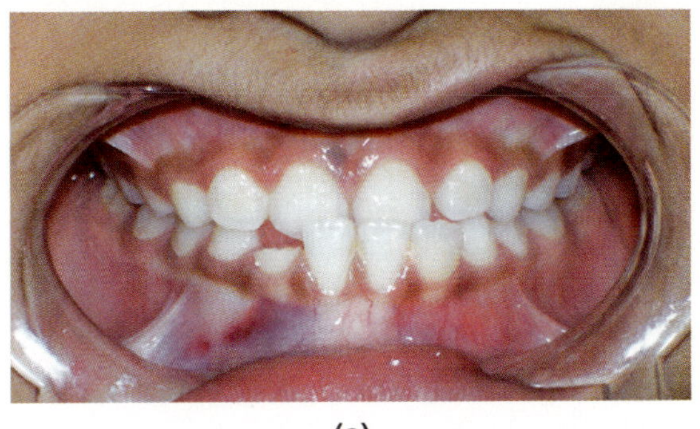

(a)

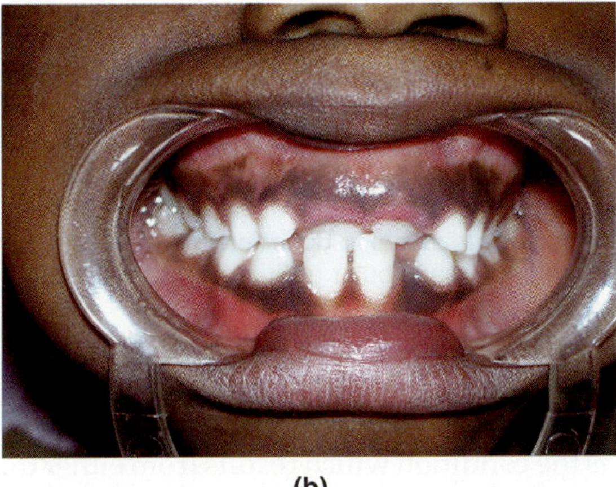

(b)

Figs 43.3a and b: Upper centrals in crossbite.

is at fault leading to crossbite. It is found in buccal region. They are of following types:

1. If the upper arch is narrow, but mandibular arch is normal width, then it is maxillary crossbite. Here, the buccal surfaces of upper teeth lie lingual to (the buccal/labial surfaces of) the lower teeth in centric occlusion. In posterior region, the buccal cusps of upper teeth lie in the central fossa of lower teeth. Sometimes, the buccal cusp can cross completely to the lingual side of lower tooth. It is called **maxillary dental palatal scissor bite**.
2. If upper arch is wide with normal mandibular arch, the crossbite is maxillary. It generally leads to scissors bite where buccal surface of lower tooth lies palatal to palatal

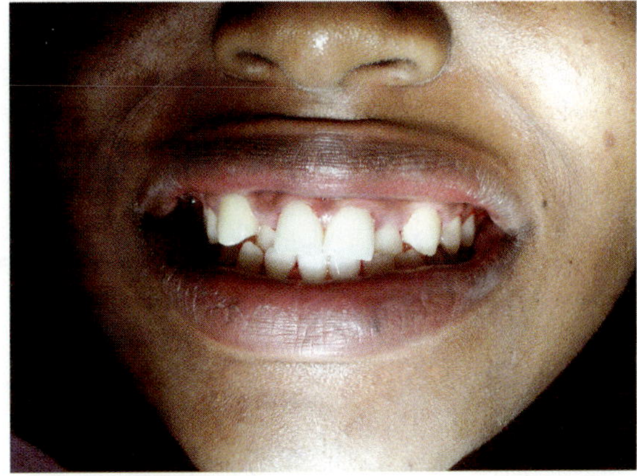

Fig. 43.4: Individual tooth crossbite.

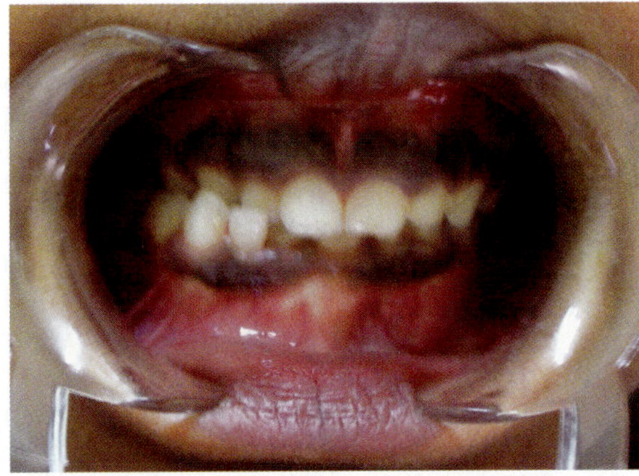

Fig. 43.5: Unilateral anterior and buccal crossbite.

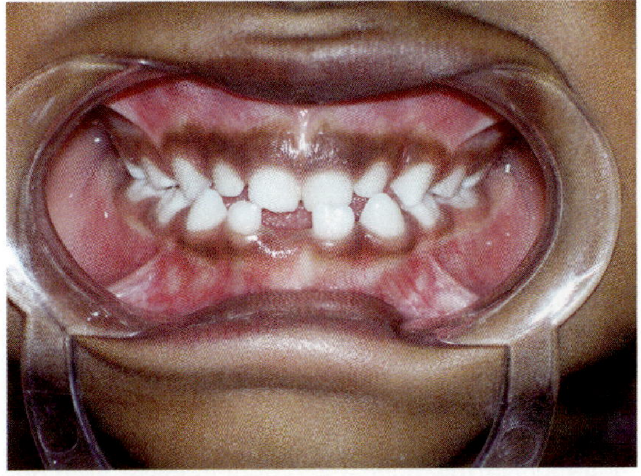

Fig. 43.6: Anterior segmental crossbite in deciduous dentition period.

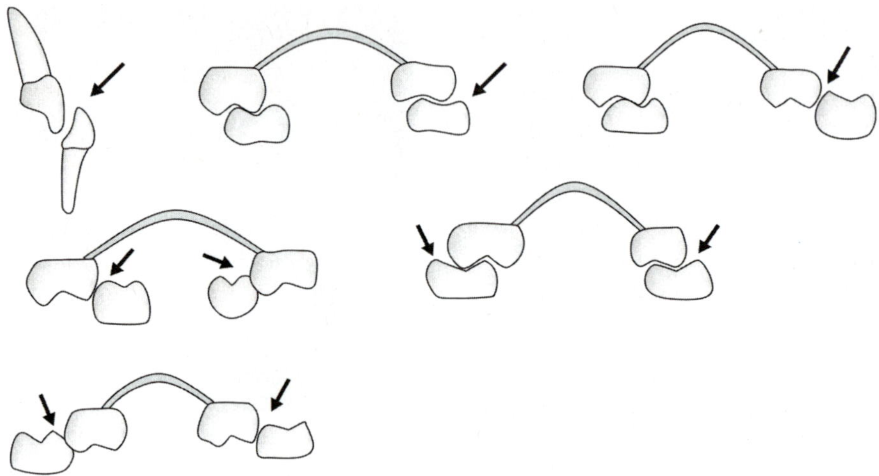

Fig. 43.7: Figures showing different types of crossbites:
- Anterior crossbite
- Buccal crossbite on one side
- Unilateral scissor bite due to lower molar occluding buccal to upper molar
- Bilateral scissor bite/telescopic bite due to narrow mandibular arch
- Bilateral crossbite due to narrow upper arch
- Bilateral scissor bite/telescopic bite due to narrow maxillary arch.

surface of upper tooth. It may be seen with full segment on one side, called **maxillary segmental buccal scissor bite** (Fig. 43.8).

3. If upper arch is normal, but lower arch is narrow, then it may lead to a scissor bite condition. If lower arch is wider, then the severity may vary from crossbite to scissor bite.

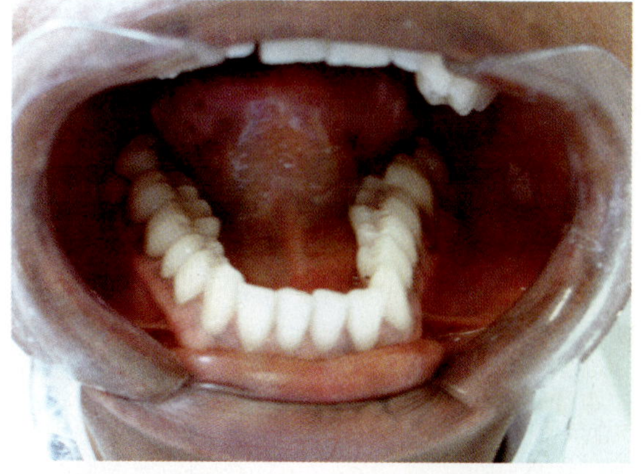

Fig. 43.8: Narrow buccal segment in lower arch due to unilateral complete scissors bite relation with upper teeth.

Anterior Crossbite

It is the condition which results from either the lingual relation of upper anterior teeth to lower anterior teeth or the labial relation of lower anterior teeth to upper anterior teeth. It is a very common findings in permanent teeth especially during the developing stages of dentition. It may also be seen in the primary dentition. It may be involving single tooth or a segment of the dental arch. Its presence should alert the clinician especially during the development of dentition, and it requires early treatment as soon as it is diagnosed. If crossbite of primary dentition is left untreated, then the permanent teeth also erupt in crossbite relation, because of the natural lingual positioning of the tooth buds. It has been shown in literature that with expansion of primary dentition, the permanent tooth buds also move with them and then erupt in normal relation.

Posterior Crossbite

It is seen in transverse dimension. It is the abnormal transverse relation of posterior teeth and occurs due to lack of coordination of width of upper and lower dental arches. Normally, the buccal surfaces of upper teeth lie buccal to buccal surface of lower teeth. In crossbite, the buccal surfaces loose this normal relation. Here, instead of mandibular buccal cusps occluding in the central fossa of upper teeth, they occlude buccal to upper buccal cusps. The upper buccal cusps are seen occluding in central fossa of lower teeth. Generally, clinically it is seen as unilateral in centric occlusion, but when examined in rest position, it is found to be bilateral. It is because during closure, there is a lateral functional shift of mandible for maximum intercuspation. It mostly occurs due to narrow width of upper dental arch (Figs 43.8 to 43.11).

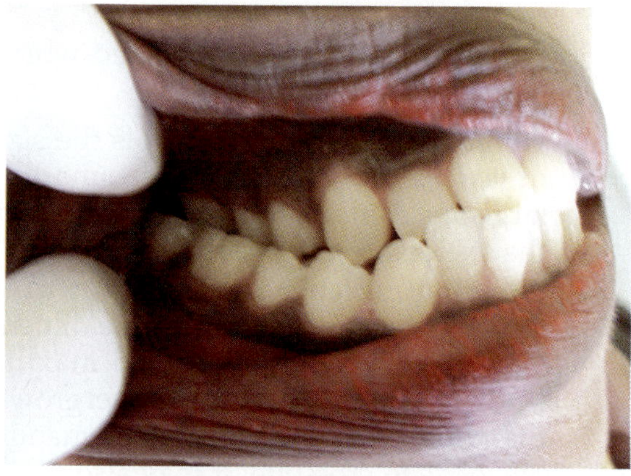

Fig. 43.9: Buccal segmental crossbite due to narrow maxilla and wider mandibular arch.

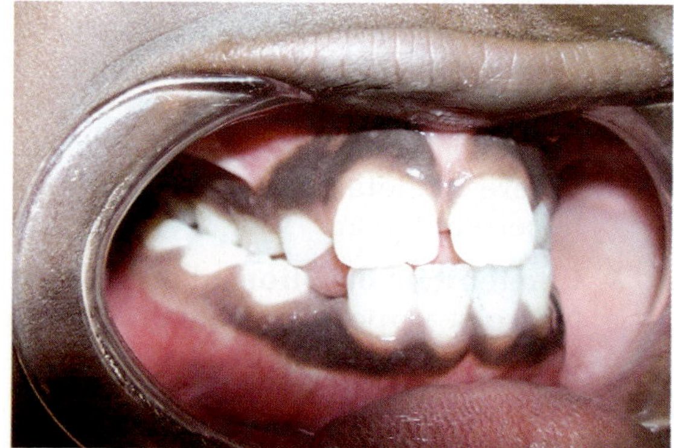

Fig. 43.10: Buccal segmental crossbite due to narrow maxilla. It can be treated by maxillary expansion.

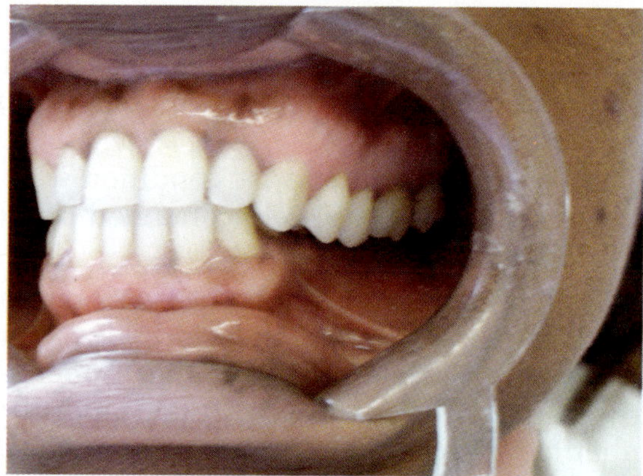

Fig. 43.11: Buccal segmental scissors bite due to narrow mandibular arch.

Its extent can vary depending on the width of arches as follows:

1. It can also be unilateral or bilateral.
2. **Edge-to-edge bite:** The tips of buccal cusps of upper and lower teeth come to lie in the same plane, rather than in a positive buccal overjet relation. It may occur due to either the mildly constricted upper arch or increased palatal crown torque of upper buccal teeth (Fig. 43.12).
3. **Scissors bite:** It is a condition where there is no intercuspation of cusp to fossa of the teeth. Either the upper teeth lie entirely buccal to lower teeth, when it is called as **buccal non-occlusion**; or the lower teeth lie buccal to upper teeth, when it is called **lingual non-occlusion** (Fig. 43.10).

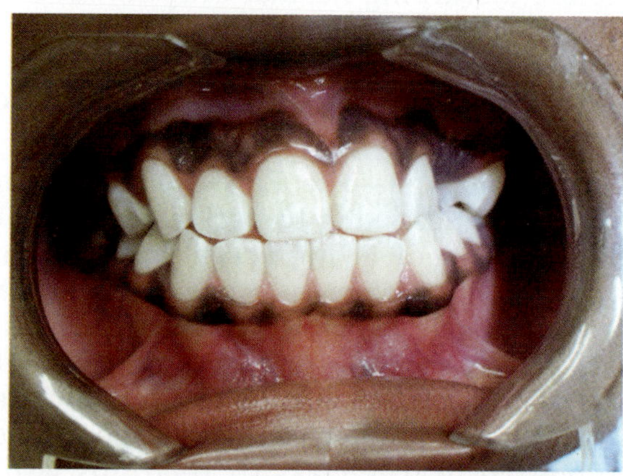

Fig. 43.12: Edge-to-edge bite in incisal region.

4. **Brodie bite:** A bilateral scissor bite with maxillary arch wide, with lower arch telescoping/contained in the upper arch.
5. **Telescopic bite:** It is the condition when one arch is completely contained in the other arch.

Skeletal crossbite: As the name suggests, it is due to discrepancy of the width of skeletal bases; and it may be due to either upper or lower or both jaw bases. It is generally inherited or occurs due to some congenital/developmental/syndromal/traumatic conditions, e.g. CLP. It can also be seen in extreme cases of mouth breathing or thumb sucking habit. It may be present in either anterior or posterior region. It may be unilateral or bilateral also. In unilateral cases, a facial asymmetry is also seen, while in bilateral cases, face is generally symmetrical.

In anterior region, it is due to either maxillary hypoplasia or mandibular prognathism or combination, i.e. due to either due to retarded growth of maxilla or increased growth of mandible or a combination of both.

Skeletal posterior crossbite is due to constricted maxillary arch. In some cases, it can be seen due to wider mandibular arch.

Dental crossbite: It is usually a localized condition and involves only the malposition of teeth without involving the skeletal bases. It may be single or segmental, may be unilateral or bilateral. It develops due to some local factors disturbing normal eruption of the teeth, e.g. prolonged retention of primary tooth; premature loss of primary tooth alongwith extreme space loss leading to ectopic eruption of successor tooth (Fig. 43.13).

Functional crossbite: Presence of occlusal pre-maturities leads to deflected path of closure of mandible during centric occlusion. It may occur either in lateral or anterior direction. Any prematurity in anterior region esp incisors leads a forward path of mandibular closure leading to **Pseudo-class III relation**. If not treated at early age, it gets converted to true class III relations with ensuing growth. Any prematurity in buccal region forces mandible to shift in lateral path of closure for attaining centric occlusion (Figs 14a and b).

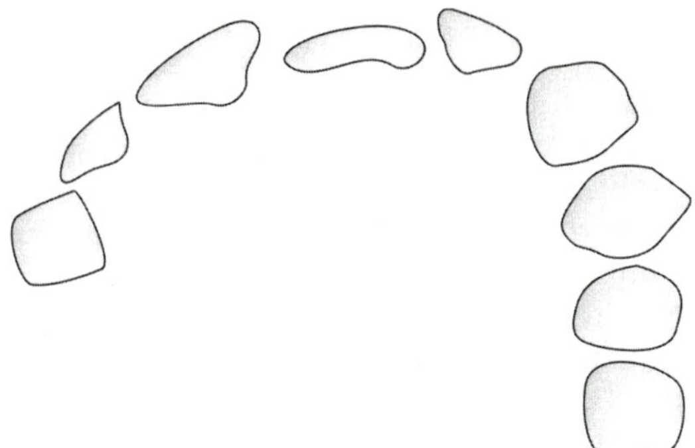

Fig. 43.13: Position of upper incisor which is in crossbite, as seen from top of the dental arch.

Etiology of Crossbite

Various causes have been implicated which can be summarized as below:

1. **Hereditary:** Heredity controls the size of jaw bases, which may be small or large or a combination. It mainly causes the skeletal type of defect.
2. **Growth problems:** Deficient growth of maxilla in anterior or transverse dimension or backward positioned maxilla leads to crossbite. Also the overgrown mandible or forward positioned mandible leads to crossbite. It may also occur due to a combination of above entities. When mandible is overgrown, it surpasses maxilla leading to anterior crossbite. Also, its wider posterior portion comes in relation with narrow middle part of upper arch leading to a posterior crossbite also. It is seen in moderate to severe skeletal class III cases, e.g. hyperpituitarism.
3. **Congenital conditions:** For example, Narrow upper arch (may also be associated with cleft palate).
4. **Trauma:** Fractures of maxilla and/or mandible and their malunion can lead to crossbite. Trauma to primary/secondary growth areas of maxilla or

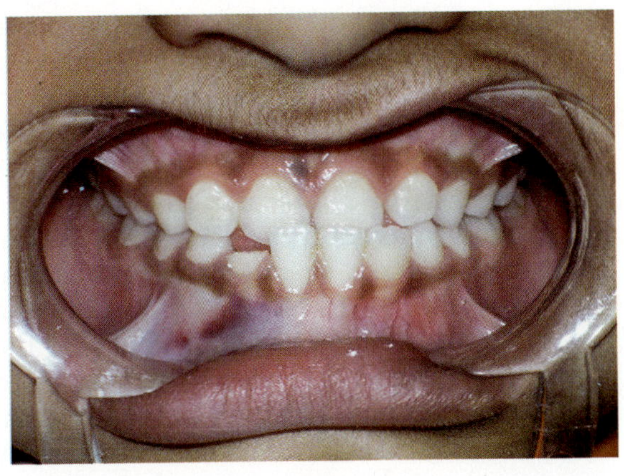

(a)

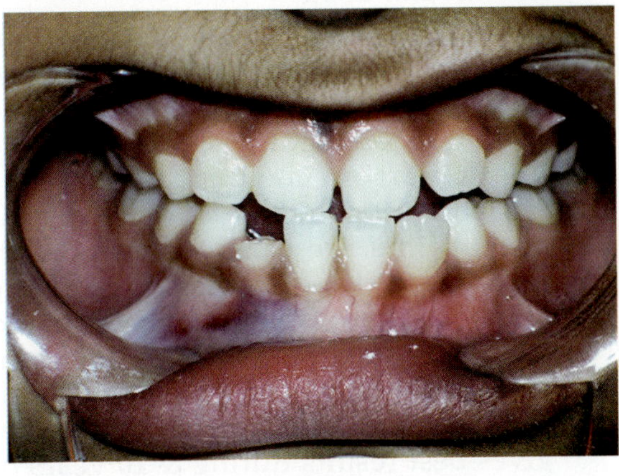

(b)

Figs 43.14a and b: Anterior crossbite due to anterior mandibular shift during occlusion due to premature contact in incisal region. It is a pseudo-class III condition. Note edge-to-edge bite with prematurities in incisal region when mandible is manipulated to close at first contact.

mandible may lead to abnormal growth of jaw bases. If condylar growth is impaired (e.g. by trauma, infections, arthritis, etc.), the mandible remains deficient while maxilla keeps on growing. Thus broader posterior part of maxilla occludes with narrow deficient anterior/middle section of mandible leading to buccal skeletal crossbite condition, e.g. as seen in Pierre Robin anomalad.

5. **Habits:** Thumb sucking habit leads to narrowing of maxilla and increased palatal depth due to disturbed buccinator mechanism, and thus leads to development of posterior crossbite. A prolonged presence of thumb during active growth period prevents natural descent of palatal shelves and thus the palatal depth is increased, while the nasal passage remains small and narrow. Mouth breathing habit also leads to such effects of narrow and deep maxillary/palatal region. In mouth breathing, the child keeps the mouth open with tongue positioned downwards to provide space for air-exchange. It leads to disturbed buccinator mechanism and thus narrow maxillary arch and wider mandibular arch may occur.
6. **Local causes:** For example, Over retained deciduous tooth/roots leads to lingual eruption of the successor teeth, since the tooth buds of permanent teeth lie lingual to primary teeth. It may be seen in upper incisor region, and upper and lower buccal regions.
7. **Early loss of primary teeth:** It leads to space loss to varying extent, thus not giving enough space for permanent tooth and it may erupt in dental crossbite.
8. **Prolonged retention of primary tooth:** When the primary tooth does not exfoliate before eruption of permanent tooth, then the successor erupts lingual to it because naturally they develop lingual to their corresponding primary tooth bud esp in anterior region.
9. **Arch length–tooth material discrepancy:** If there is not enough space for permanent teeth, they generally erupt lingual to the primary teeth in crossbite situation.
10. **Presence of supernumerary tooth; pathology, etc:** These may deflect the erupting tooth in abnormal position toward crossbite.

11. **Thickened fibrous gingiva:** It may also cause deflected eruption of tooth.

Diagnosis: A proper diagnosis is required to plan the proper treatment. Factors, like etiology, growth status of the patient, age, cooperation, etc. are also to be considered. The steps involved and records required during diagnostic process are:

- Case history and examination
- Study models
- Radiograph
- Photographs

Treatment

Any form of crossbite whether single or multiple or skeletal, etc. should be treated as soon as possible when it is first examined. This is the condition which requires an **early intervention**. A developing crossbite due to lingually erupting anterior tooth, if left untreated, leads to interference with the anterior growth of maxilla and thus maxillary hypoplasia may occur. Sometimes, all the upper incisors are locked lingual to lower incisors. If this condition is left untreated, it leads to restricted growth of maxilla, alongwith the un-interrupted manibular growth. Thus it develops in skeletal class III condition later on which is difficult to treat. Following factors should be kept in mind for treatment planning of crossbites.

a. **Remove the etiology:** The causative factors should be found and removed, e.g. prolonged retention of primary tooth; presence of supernumerary tooth; habits; thickened fibrous gingiva, etc.

b. **Role of ruling out the functional shift during centric occlusion:** Generally the posterior crossbite presents itself as unilateral type. It is because while examining the patient, the centric occlusion is considered, which leads to lateral functional shift of mandible to either side giving an impression of unilateral crossbite. So to diagnose such condition, the patient is also examined in rest position, and the relation of upper to lower jaws is studied. Patient is asked to close slowly till the first occlusal contact and then in centric occlusion while noting the functional shift. Thus a diagnosis of bilateral crossbite due to narrow maxilla or wider mandible can be established. The treatment of bilateral crossbite is different as compared to a true unilateral crossbite. Generally, the true unilateral crossbite is due to asymmetry of face or other skeletal problems. Also, the chances of narrow upper arch are more than wider mandibular arch.

c. **Role of age and growth status of the patient:** Age of the patient helps to determine the growth status of the patient. A bilateral posterior crossbite due to narrow maxilla can be better treated during the growth of maxilla, as at that time, we can achieve skeletal changes. With increasing age, the midpalatal suture gets interdigitated and ossified, so the attempts of expansion lead to dental effects and less stability of the results. Generally, expansion gives best results during 8–10 years of age, as during this age, the jaws are achieving the transverse growth.

Similarly, the developing anterior crossbite should be treated at an earliest, otherwise the growing mandible overshoots and maxilla may not grow to its full potential, leading to skeletal problems. Milder form can be easily treated with the help of removable appliance having Z-spring or E-screw. Skeletal defect requires the use of chin cup and/ or reverse face mask for growth control. The effects of the orthopaedic appliances are better during the growth stage only, giving skeletal effects. The reverse face mask treatment yields better results if started during 8–9 years of age. Since the mandible keeps on growing till at least 16 years of age, the maintenance with the chin cup is required till that time to keep the growth of mandible in control.

However, if the cause of the problem is genetic, then the genetic potential of growth of mandible or maxilla cannot be fully controlled, and in such cases, orthognathic surgery is required after the growth ceases, after 18 years of age, to establish normal skeletal interjaw relationship.

d. **Creation of space before attempting correction:** Proper amount of space equal to or more than the mesio-distal size of the tooth to be corrected should be created in the arch area before attempting the correction of tooth. If space is not there, the tooth will not come in line and attempts will fail. The space can be gained by various means, e.g. expansion, stripping, molar distalisation, extractions or correction of buccal rotations.

Treatment of Single Tooth Anterior Crossbite

It is the most common form of crossbite. It is easy to treat if diagnosed early. Later treatment may require some complex steps. For planning treatment, following general steps can be followed, viz.

- Determine the etiology
- Manage the space required for correction
- Select the appliance.

There are various methods to correct the anterior tooth crossbite, depending on the degree of development.

A. **Tongue blade therapy** (Fig. 43.15): It is a simple appliance and is use to correct the developing anterior crossbite of single incisor tooth during the eruption stages. The wooden or plastic tongue blade is used for 1–2 hours for about 2 weeks. It is positioned on the lingual side of the upper incisor and on the incisal edges of the lower incisors, and a labial force is applied to shift the tooth labially. There should be sufficient space for the tooth to be treated. But this is a crude method and requires extreme patient and parental cooperation. It can only be used with a tooth which is erupting and just developing in crossbite.

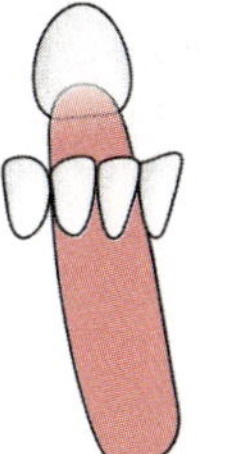

Fig. 43.15: Tongue blade therapy to treat anterior crossbite of upper incisor during its stage of eruption.

B. **Enamel equilibration:** Premature contacts in primary dentition lead to functional shift. The teeth can be grinded to remove the areas of premature contacts to prevent functional shifts and thus preventing development of crossbite and abnormal forces on TMJ.

C. **Lower anterior inclined plane:** It is also known as **Catalan's appliance**. This is a simple appliance made of acrylic and can be used to treat a single tooth anterior crossbite, where the upper tooth is in crossbite with normal lower incisors. It may be removable type or cemented / fixed type, and is **made on lower teeth** (Figs 43.16 and 43.17).

   a. **Removable type:** The lingual plate of the removable type is extended till the molars of both the sides. The anterior part of acrylic is made at an incline of 45°, and the lingual surface of the culprit upper incisor slides on it. The posterior teeth may be left out of occlusion or a posterior bite plate (PBP) may be incorporated in the appliance to prevent the supra-eruption of posterior teeth. But the height of PBP should be such that it should not contact upper teeth otherwise no force will be applied on the culprit tooth during closure of mouth. The forces of occlusion during closure are transferred on the upper tooth

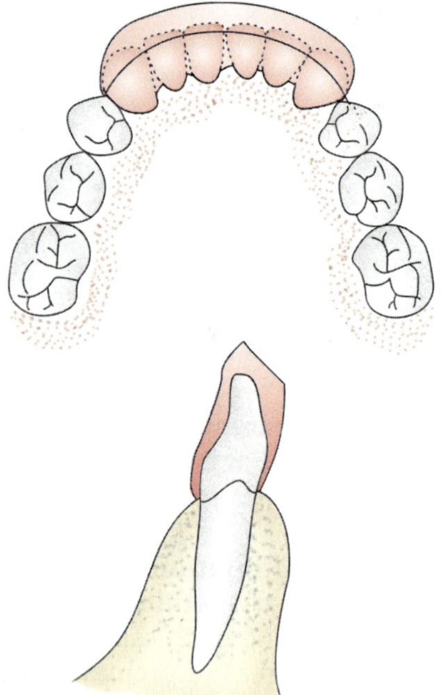

Fig. 43.16: Catalan's/(L) inclined plane appliance.

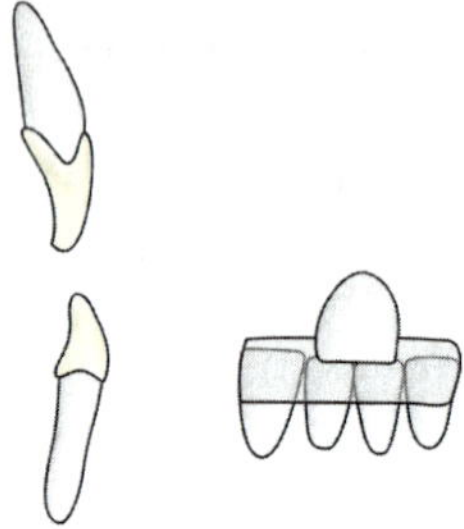

Fig. 43.17: Catalan's appliance

which starts moving labially out of crossbite position. It also requires patient's cooperation.

b. **The cemented/fixed type of appliance** can be made with acrylic, such that it covers at least 3–4 lower incisors teeth, is at an incline of 45 degrees, and the lingual surface of upper incisor resting on it. It is cemented in place with GIC cement. However, it should be in place for only 2–3 weeks, till the culprit tooth generally comes out of crossbite. Keeping it in place for extended time may lead to supraeruption of buccal teeth which may not be desirable in many situations. Once the crossbite is corrected, the appliance is discontinued as the corrected position is self-retentive.

c. In maxillary arch on the culprit tooth, different types of appliances can be fabricated to give an inclined plane effect, e.g. cast incline; inclined crown; banded incline, etc. but they are complex to make and need special laboratory support.

Advantages

- Easy to fabricate.
- Rapid correction
- Lack of soreness of teeth doing movement
- Rarity of relapse

Disadvantages

1. Limitations on diet
2. Temporary speech defect
3. Tendency for anterior open bite (if kept too long).
4. Appliance may loosen because of strong occlusal forces.

D. **Removable appliance with double cantilever spring (Z-spring)** (Fig. 43.13): This is one of the most common removable appliance used to treat single tooth crossbite or a group of teeth in crossbite, (usually the two teeth). It is more effective for the treatment of incisors only due to its lighter forces and delicacy. It is fabricated in the upper arch. The usual Hawley's appliance with Z-springs fabricated with 0.5 mm wires, and acrylic is extended on the occlusal surfaces of the posterior teeth (PBP) for disoccluding the anterior region. It also helps in prevention of supraeruption of posterior teeth. A proper space in the arch should be available before the culprit tooth can be brought in line. The spring is activated 2–3 mm each time to apply lighter forces. It generally takes 3–4 months for correction. After correction, the appliance is discontinued as the treated crossbite of incisors is self-retentive due to overbite. But if there is no overbite, then the same appliance can be modified by removing the posterior bite plane acrylic to serve as retainer.

E. **Removable appliance with expansion screw opening in sagittal direction** (Figs 43.18 and 43.19): If all the 4 incisors are in crossbite, this appliance can be used. The posterior bite acrylic is incorporated in the appliance to disocclude anteriorly to allow correction. The cuts are placed in the plate in a V-shape fashion extending from lateral incisor to other side. The E-screw is activated by one-fourth turn every second day, till the correction is achieved. It generally takes 3–4 months for correction. In this way, the arch is expanded in the anterior region mainly by tipping of teeth, which is also known as arch augmentation. Then the appliance can be modified as retainer if required depending on the bite depth.

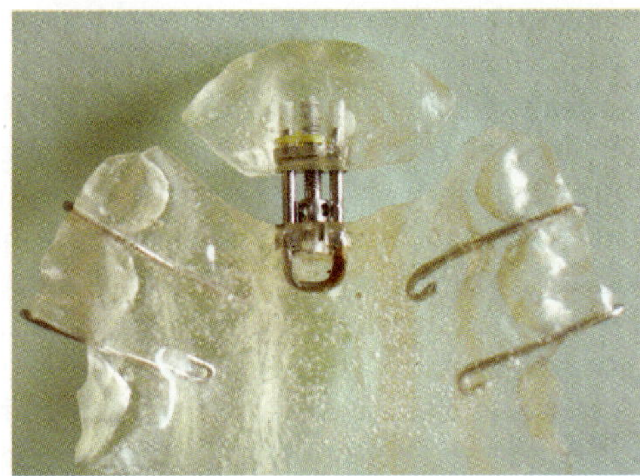

Fig. 43.18: Expansion appliance incorporating for anterior expansion of the arch.

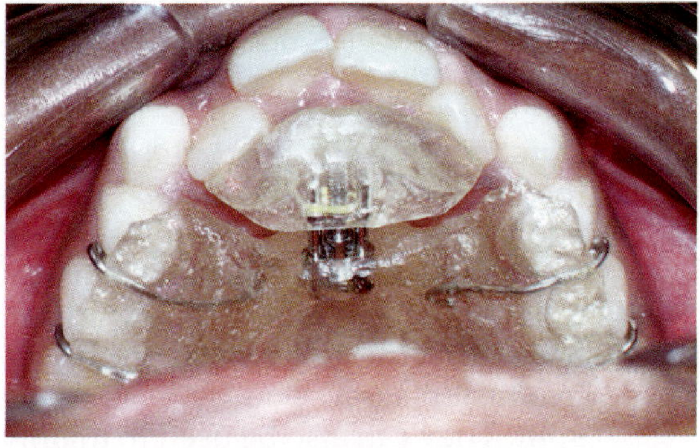

Fig. 43.19: Appliance in place.

F. **Fixed appliance:** Fixed orthodontic mechanotherapy or brackets can be used to treat the anterior crossbite involving single or multiple teeth. Since they are not dependant on patient's cooperation, it is a better and fast, but costly method. Proper space is gained in the arches, e.g. by expansion, stripping, or extraction before attempting the correction. The brackets are placed on all the teeth. Along with, a removable posterior bite plate or anterior bite plate appliance should be given to the patient to open the bite and to avoid brackets failure, but it will need patient's cooperation. Alternatively, a **composite block/button** can be bonded on occlusal surface of posterior teeth especially first or second molars to open the bite in anterior region. It is useful especially for the treatment of dental (segmental) anterior crossbite.

G. **Treatment of skeletal anterior crossbite:** Treatment of skeletal condition is most important otherwise it may lead to development of a permanent skeletal defect which requires surgical intervention later in life. It should be treated best during the growth period to achieve maximum skeletal changes. The condition is assessed properly with the help of diagnostic aids to determine the components of problem. The skeletal crossbite in anterior region may be due to underdeveloped maxilla or overdeveloped mandible or combination of both. It is mostly genetic. Also, the growth status of patient is assessed. Depending on the condition, the treatment options are:

- Protraction face mask or reverse headgear (if maxilla is retropositioned)

- Use of chin cap with high-pull headgear (if mandible is overgrown)
- A combination of both appliances.

H. Orthognathic surgery: After the active growth period has passed, the only treatment option for severe cases is orthognathic surgery. It is generally done after 18 years of age. Depending on the condition, the treatment options are:
   - If maxilla is retropositioned: Le Fort I osteotomy with forward repositioning.
   - If mandible is overgrown: BSSO with set back or segmental ostectomy with set back and/or genioplasty.
   - A combination of both

Treatment of Posterior Crossbite

(Figs 43.20a to e)

Posterior crossbite should be treated to avoid any growth discrepancy in transverse plane. It may be dental/skeletal; unilateral/bilateral; segmental; single/multiple.

A. Treatment of single tooth crossbite (Figs 43.21 to 43.23): If proper space is available for the tooth to be moved, then the **crossbite elastics** can be used. They produce reciprocal forces, thus moving both the teeth in opposite directions, so it is recommended, if both the teeth are at fault. But, if tooth in one arch is at fault, while in other arch is normal, then an anchorage unit is created in normal arch by involving more teeth, against which the cross-elastic can be applied to move the faulty tooth in line. Result also depends on the patient cooperation for changing the elastics. These elastics are given for approx. 6 weeks since a prolonged use can extrude the teeth. Once the crossbite is corrected, it is self-retentive due to occlusal interdigitation.

Removable appliance having Z-springs or a small expansion screw are not much effective in treatment of single tooth crossbite in posterior region due to larger size of the teeth. In all cases of posterior crossbite, the occlusion should be relieved for uninterrupted movements to occur. It is done by incorporating anterior bite plate in the appliances (Figs 43.24a to c).

Fixed appliances, e.g. TPA or Nance palatal arch can be made to provide anchorage in upper arch (Fig. 43.25), to which hooks may be placed at strategic locations to receive elastics, which will apply force on the culprit tooth. This applies palatal force on the tooth so it is used to correct those teeth which are buccally displaced to crossbite situation. A constricted TPA can also be used for treatment of such a tooth (Figs 43.26 and 43.27).

Transverse elastics can be placed from one side to other side in buccal region to bring the buccally-displaced tooth towards palatal position, but these elastics pass over the tongue, thus uncomfortable to patients and thus may not be used properly (Fig. 43.28).

B. Treatment of segmental unilateral or bilateral crossbite: Expansion appliances, removable or fixed, (e.g. removable or fixed Coffin spring, removable split appliance with expansion screw, etc.) can be used for treatment of segmental/unilateral or bilateral crossbite due to narrow maxillary arch. It primarily leads to dentoalveolar expansion. The expansion can be slow or rapid maxillary expansion (discussed separately in chapter on expansion).

   a. Removable appliances: Split acrylic appliances with expansion screw can be used for expansion of upper arch. They are helpful when the constriction is mild to moderate, and they lead to dentoalveolar expansion and they tip the teeth buccally. They can be used for symmetric/bilateral or asymmetric/unilateral expansion by modifying the placement of the expansion screw and by placing the split. They can also be used to mainly expand only intercanine region when

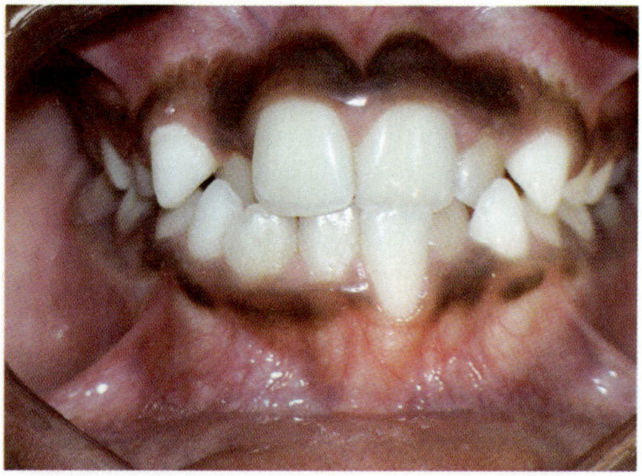

(a)

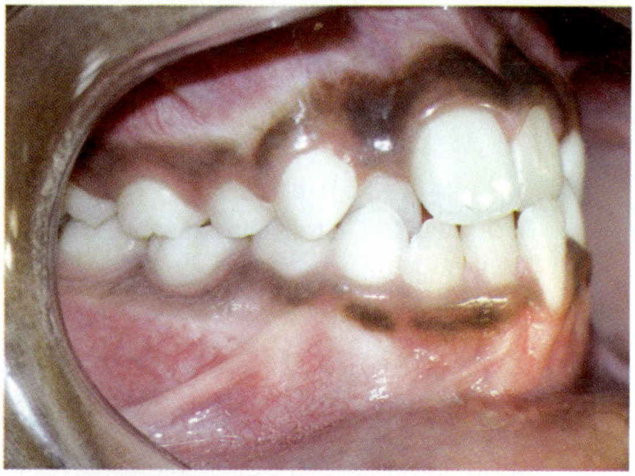

(b)

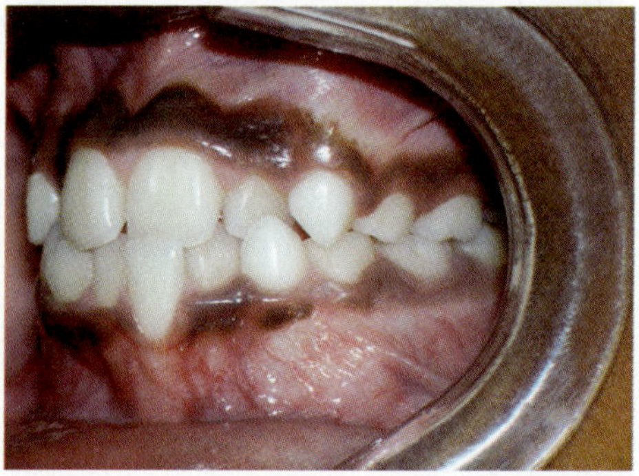

(c)

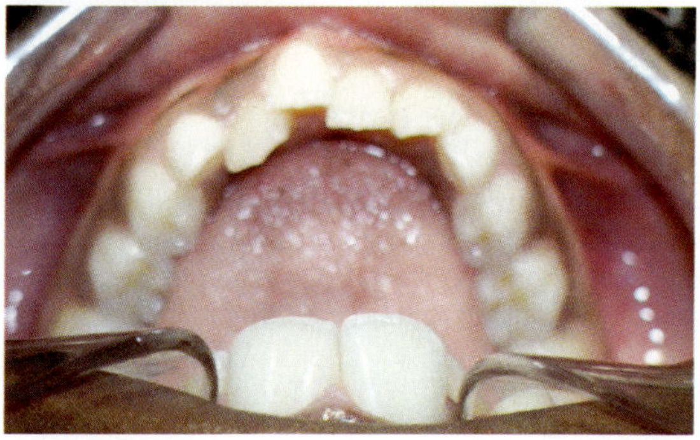

(d)

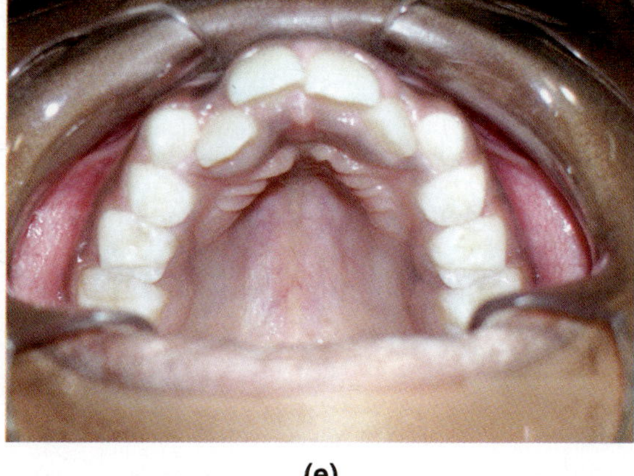

(e)

Figs 43.20a to e: Pre-Rx intraoral views of the occlusion and crossbite.

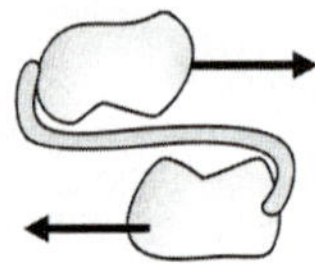

Fig. 43.21: Crossbite elastic

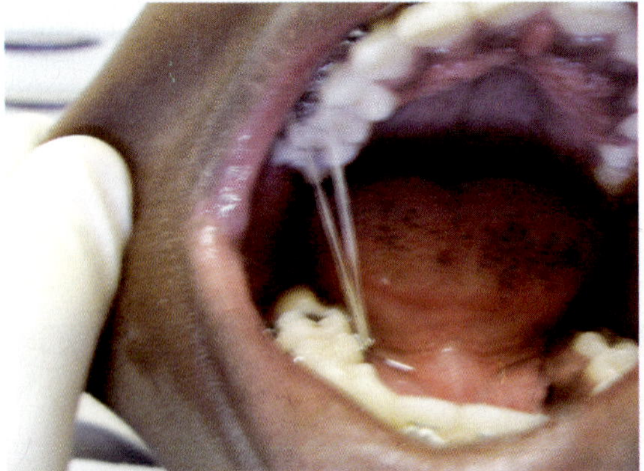

Fig. 43.22: Crossbite elastics can be used for treatment but need patient cooperation. They are good for single tooth in crossbite, but segmental crossbite is difficult to treat with them.

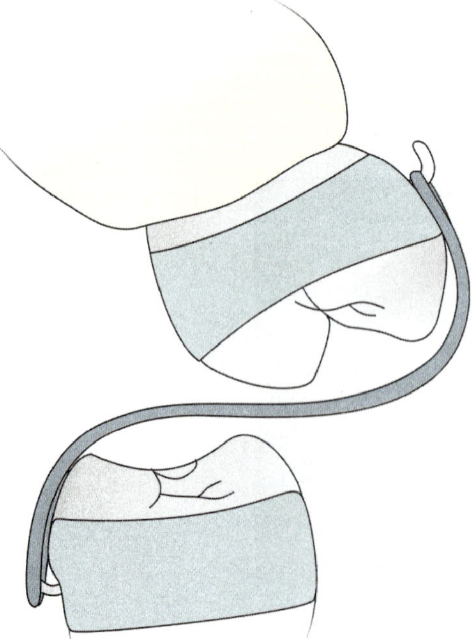

Fig. 43.23: Crossbite elastics to treat molar crossbite.

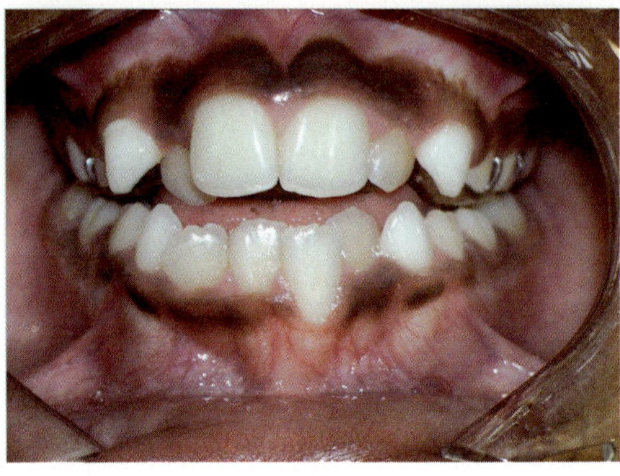

(a)

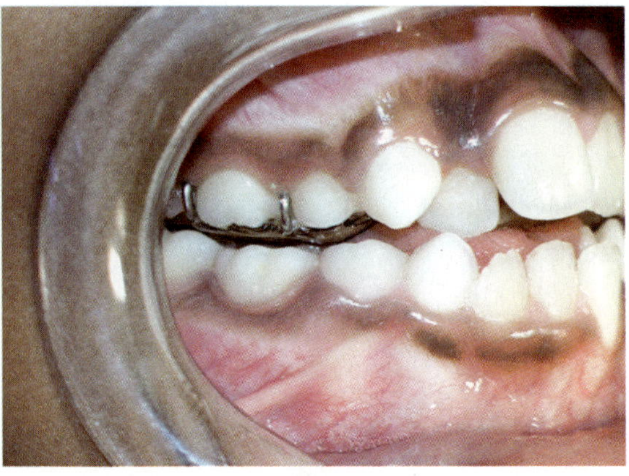

(b)

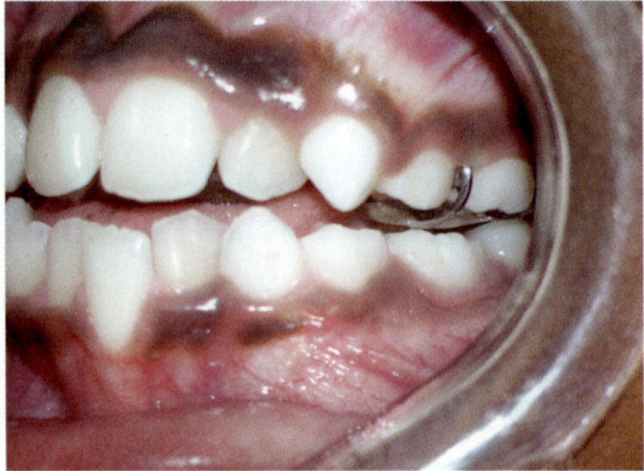

(c)

Figs 43.24a to c: Posterior bite plate helps to open the occlusion out of crossbite, so that there is unhindered movement of teeth.

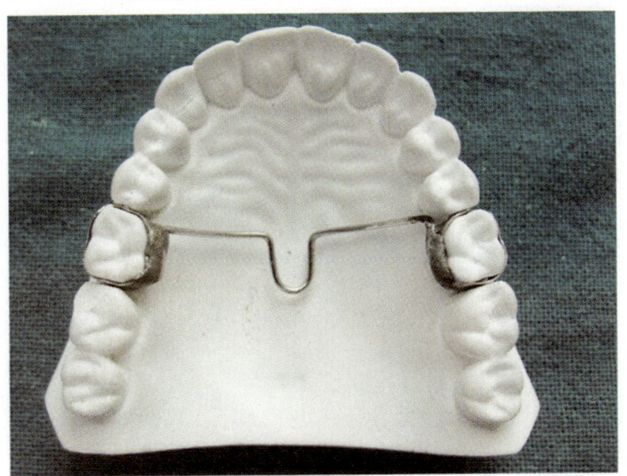

Fig. 43.25: Transpalatal arch: It can be used for expansion of molars, anchorage augmentation, space maintainer, etc.

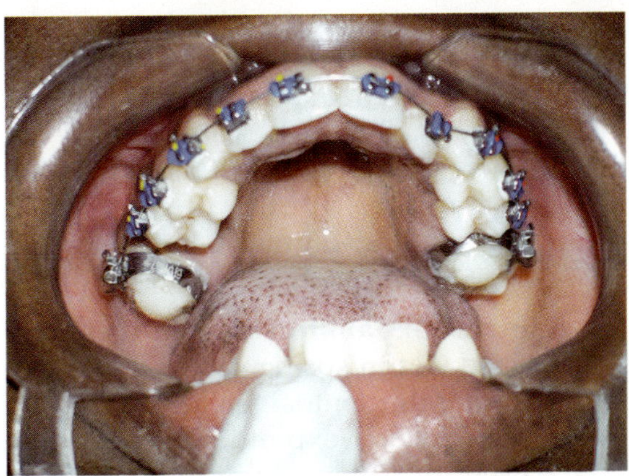

Fig. 43.27: Composite block fixed on upper first molars to help raise the bite in anterior region during correction of anterior crossbite.

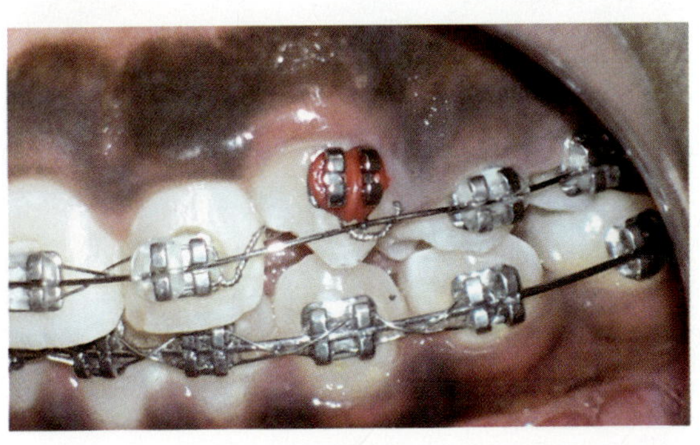

(a)

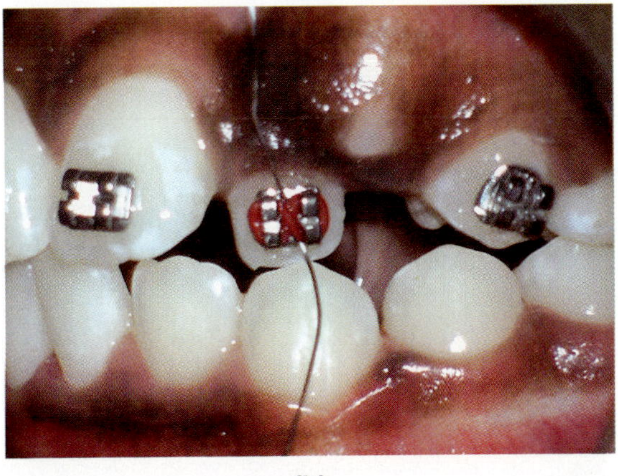

(b)

Figs 43.26a and b: Ligation of displaced teeth with the help of ligature wire which is activating the ligature ring applies a light force.

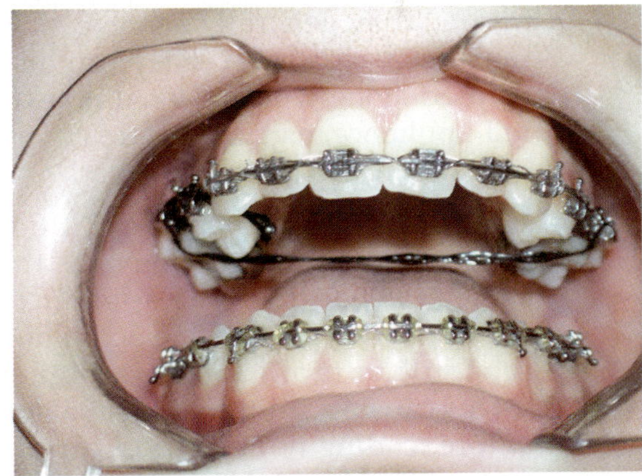

Fig. 43.28: Transpalatal E-chain to bring molars palatally, but it leads to tongue irritation.

the posterior end of the cut in the plate is restricted with a heavy wire spring which does not allow the opening of the posterior part of the plate, and all the force is directed to the anterior part of the arch.

b. **Unilateral crossbite** due to asymmetrical maxillary arch can be treated with a removable appliance with asymmetrically split expansion acrylic plate. The smaller part acts as active part while the bigger part acts as anchorage unit. During the treatment of unilateral crossbite, the occlusion should be relieved for uninterrupted movements to occur on the affected side, but on the unaffected side, the posterior bite plate is incorporated so that it uniformally touches the lower teeth. There it acts to prevent the extrusions and buccal tipping of unaffected teeth and also gives a better anchorage effect under the occlusal forces.

c. **Fixed expansion appliances**, e.g. fixed Coffin spring, Quad helix (primarily for dentoalveolar expansion), NiTi palatal expanders, etc. can be used for expansion of maxilla in the patients. Patient cooperation is not a factor, and they achieve rapid results as compared to removable appliance due to their continuous force and action. They generally achieve slow maxillary expansion. They can also be used along with the fixed bracketed appliance, e.g. during treatment of CLP (Figs 43.29 to 43.32).

d. **Rapid maxillary expansion:** RME is used primarily for achieving the skeletal expansion. The appliances are of fixed type, and the activation schedule is rapid to attain higher forces causing splitting of mipalatal suture leading to expansion. Appliances like Hyrex, Haas, banded or bonded splint type appliances are used for rapid maxillary expansion. They are very effective during active growth phase and also in patients who are nearing the end of their active growth. It can also be used

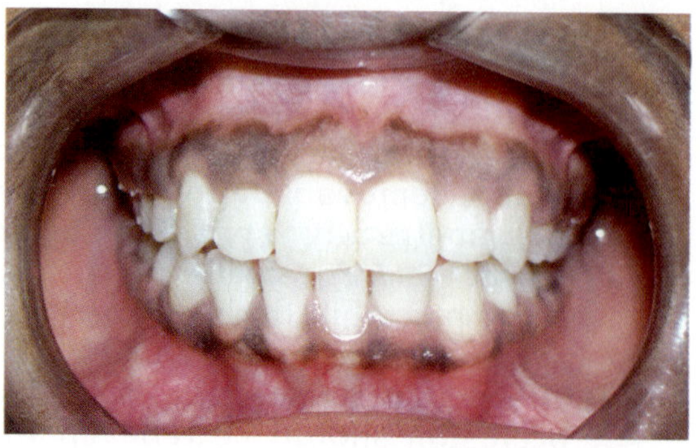

Fig. 43.29: Lateral incisor in crossbite.

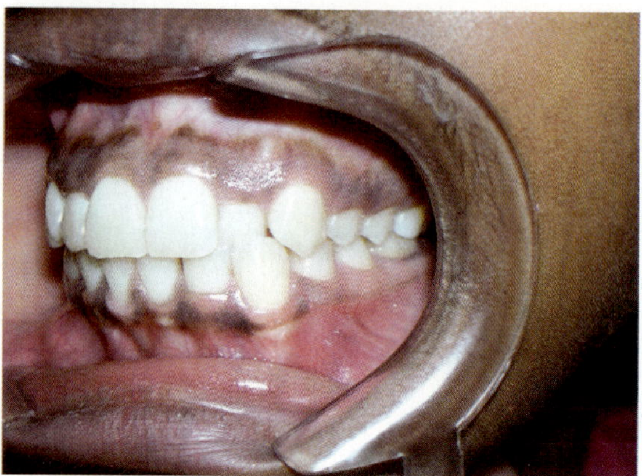

Fig. 43.30: Pretreatment view.

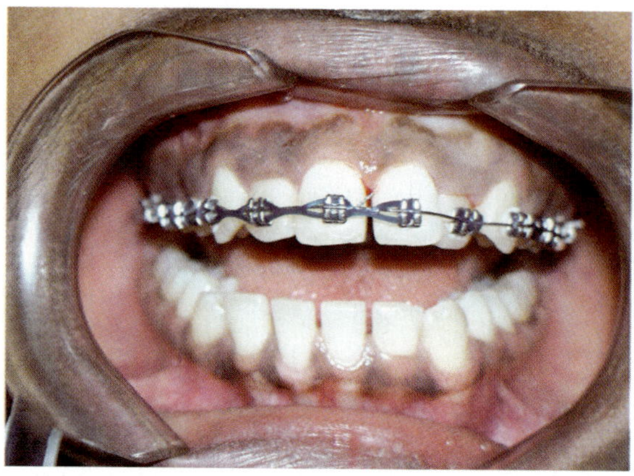

(a)

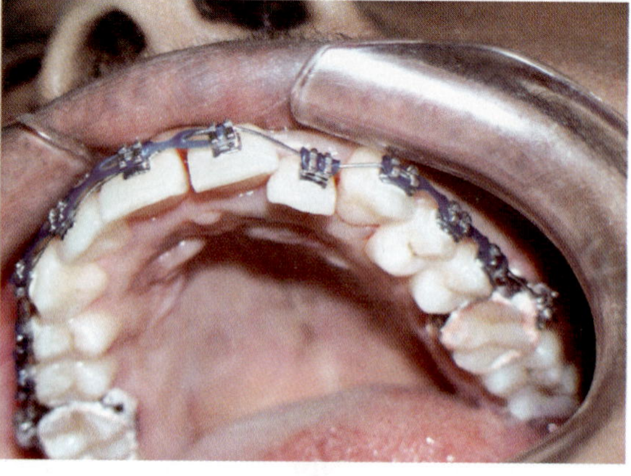

(b)

Fig. 43.31a and b: After placement of braces and slicing.

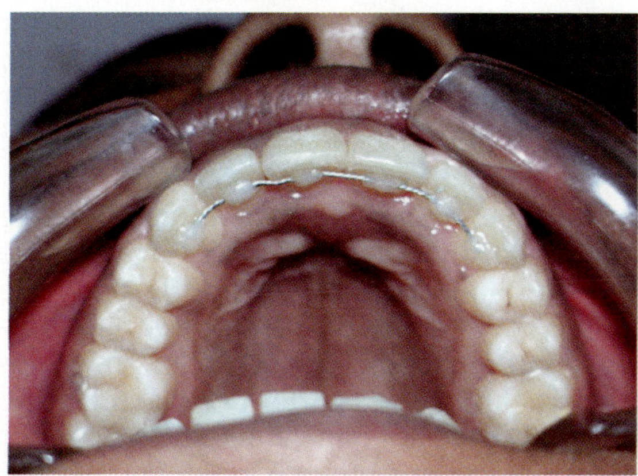

Fig. 43.32: Fixed retainer after correction of crossbite.

when maxillary constriction is severe. RME is also done before or along with maxillary protraction with reverse headgear.

e. **Fixed orthodontic appliance:** Expanded heavy archwires can be used for correction of narrow maxillary arches. Heavy wires are used for this purpose, since the lighter wires cannot apply sufficient forces to overcome the cheek muscle's forces. But, it can be successfully used for mild to moderate cases. **Jockey arch** (18 gauge SS hard wire expanded and ligated at molars tubes only) is used for 2–3 weeks for a rapid result, but the patient should be carefully monitored during this period.

f. **SARPE/SARME:** It is the surgically assisted rapid palatal/maxillary expansion. In adult patients with narrow maxillary arch and/or crossbite, the chances of correction with normal expansion are very less. It is due to the fact that the mid-palatal suture gets much inter-digitated and the growth of maxilla has already finished. So to achieve expansion, the palate is split surgically and rapid expansion is instituted to correct the narrow maxilla.

g. **Treatment of over-expanded upper or lower arches:** Wider lower arch causing buccal crossbite is difficult to treat. Constricted heavy archwires can be used with fixed bracketed appliances to move the teeth lingually. It can be supported by heavy transverse elastics extending from buccal of left to buccal of right side of lower arch, crossing the occlusal plane but these elastics are very uncomfortable to patients, since they interfere with function and position of tongue. However, the treatment of such a condition is very difficult, and may need surgical intervention, with variable results, torquing problems, and questionable retention of results. Same problems can be faced in upper arch. Rigid fixed appliance with bands on multiple teeth, incorporating fully opened E-screw can be placed on upper teeth. This opened screw is then closed according to a decided scheduled, which helps to bring the teeth towards each other. But it can be used only if there is bilateral widening of the arch, as it will use a reciprocal anchorage.

h. **Microimplants or palatal implants:** They can be adapted for deciding the mechanics for correction of different types of crossbites, but details are out of scope.

Correction of crossbite in primary dentition:

1. **Expansion of dental arch:** Expansion can help in correction of posterior crossbite due to narrow upper arch. It has been reported that permanent tooth buds also move during expansion with the primary teeth and thus later on erupt in normal relation. Thus problem of developing crossbite in future is taken care of.

2. **Planas direct tracks (PDTs):** They are the inclined planes made of composite materials to correct the crossbite in

deciduous dentition. They were introduced by Prof. Pedro Planas of Spain in 1994. It is used for early prevention of anterior or posterior crossbite. PDTs are used in deciduous dentition only, as they cover the occlusal surfaces of primary molars, resulting in a flat posterior occlusion until the molars are exfoliated.

Fabrication: It can be placed directly in patient's mouth as a chairside procedure but is very cumbersome. Best way is to fabricate them in laboratory by an indirect technique and then bond on the child's teeth. A wax bite registration is taken in an edge-to-edge incisor relationship, i.e. open occlusion position. The casts are mounted on articulator. The tracks are formed from self-curing acrylic or POP or wax, first on the lower cast. For a posterior crossbite, the inclined plane is contoured from lingual to buccal on lower primary molars on the crossbite side only. On this plane, the palatal surface of PDTs of upper teeth slide moving them buccally out of crossbite under the forces of occlusion. For anterior crossbite, the inclined plane is contoured from distal to mesial on the lower deciduous molars on both sides. These help to transfer the occlusal forces in an anterior direction on the upper teeth.

Mechanism of action: PDTs prevent deflection of jaws during occlusion, and thus help to locate both condyles concentrically in the glenoid fossae. PDTs help in repositioning the mandible, and prevent morphological and positional asymmetries in young children and allow a more symmetrical craniofacial development.

The tracks should cover the entire occlusal surfaces of each molar, and are extended to about the middle third of buccal and lingual surfaces for optimum retention. After finishing and contouring the lower tracks, they are covered with vaseline or transparent tape to separate it while fabricating the upper track, so that the acrylic of both tracks does not join. Both upper and lower casts are articulated, and the upper track is built by copying the inclination of lower tracks. The height is adjusted so that the all the posterior teeth touch the tracks evenly and comfortably, and there is no dental contact in anterior region. It allows the mandible to be repositioned in centric occlusion.

Bonding: An acetate transfer tray is made for each arch. The deciduous molars are etched with 37% orthophosphoric acid. The acetate tray is filled with light-cured composite in the areas of tracks. Incisor region is used as the reference point for setting the transfer trays. The composite resin is cured for at least 40 seconds on each molar surface and thus gets directly bonded to molars. Tracks should be placed in both arches at the same appointment. The occlusion is adjusted after removing the transfer trays.

Advantages

1. They are fixed appliances, so patient cooperation factor is eliminated.
2. They are easy to fabricate in lab and have faster action. They take advantage of pliable bone of the child for early readaptation of skeletal tissues in normal relation.
3. PDTs can be used to correct either posterior or anterior crossbite in the deciduous dentition, regardless of the severity of the malocclusion.
4. A higher rate of success is expected in young patients, as a skeletal discrepancy has not yet been established.
5. By reducing or eliminating the problem, the second phase of treatment, if necessary, will be simpler and shorter, as it prevents development of permanent asymmetries during prepubertal growth.

Retention

This is an important phase of treatment to keep the teeth in their corrected positions. Anterior crossbite are self-retentive after correction due to a positive overjet, unless there is anterior open bite, where it will need proper retainers. Buccal crossbites, if not severe, i.e. if limited to single tooth or small segment, are also self-retentive due to proper interdigitation of upper and lower teeth. But severe posterior crossbites treated with RME or SARPE, etc. need prolonged retention for maturation of bone and adaptation of soft tissues to the new positions of the teeth and dental arches. The fixed expansion appliance; TPA, Nance arch; the expanded archwires, etc. are left in oral cavity for a prolonged period. The E-screw in RME appliance after achieving over-expansion are blocked with acrylic to prevent the tendency of reversed movement of screw during retention period. Otherwise, new fixed retentive appliance extending from first molars to canine regions can be fabricated and cemented, e.g. TPA with extended arms till canines. Details can be found in the Chapter 55 on Retention and Relapse.

Conclusion

Treatment of crossbite is very important since it causes restriction in normal growth of jaw bases. It should be treated as soon as possible. A variety of appliances are available depending on the condition, and least complex appliance should be chosen for treatment for better cooperation of patient. Anterior crossbites after treatment are self retentive. A proper retention should be given to the patient after buccal crossbite treatment, with a regular follow-up.

44

Management of Open Bite

INTRODUCTION

A vertical overlap of upper and lower teeth is called as overbite. Normal values in anterior region are 2–3 mm. In posterior teeth, the buccal cusps of upper teeth overlap the buccal cusps of lower teeth. Vertical overlap / dental bite depth in the anterior region can vary as normal bite; deep bite; deep traumatic bite; edge to edge bite; open bite.

Definition

Open bite is the condition where there is a lack of vertical overlap between upper and lower teeth. This condition is expressed in the vertical plane of the space.

Classification of Open Bite (Figs 44.1 to 44.4)

a. According to the region:
   1. Anterior open bite
   2. Posterior open bite
   3. Combined anterior and posterior open bite
b. According to the side:
   1. Unilateral
   2. Bilateral
c. According to the involvement of tissues:
   1. Skeletal
   2. Dental
   3. Skeletodental
d. According to severity:
   1. Mild
   2. Moderate
   3. Severe.

Etiology of anterior open bite: It is a multifactorial condition. Following are some of the causative factors for anterior open bite.

1. **Heredity:** Genetics is one of the important causes of any malocclusion, and is a major factor for open bite. Children of parents having open bite generally have open bite condition.

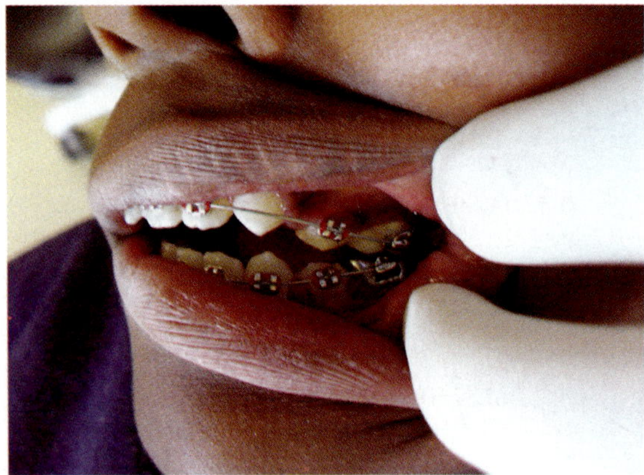

Fig. 44.1: Severe open bite involving anterior and posterior segments on both sides.

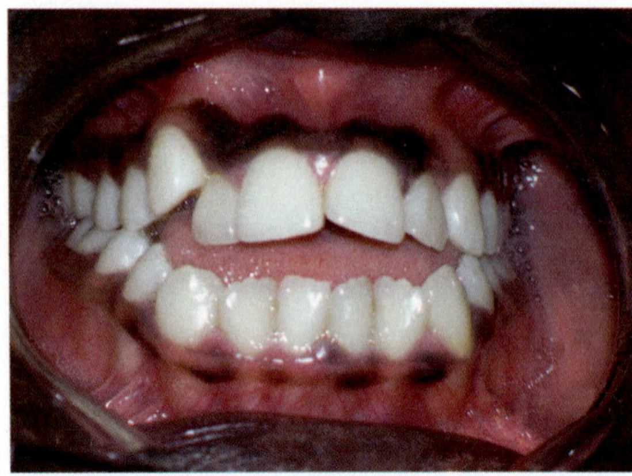

Fig. 44.2: Anterior open bite.

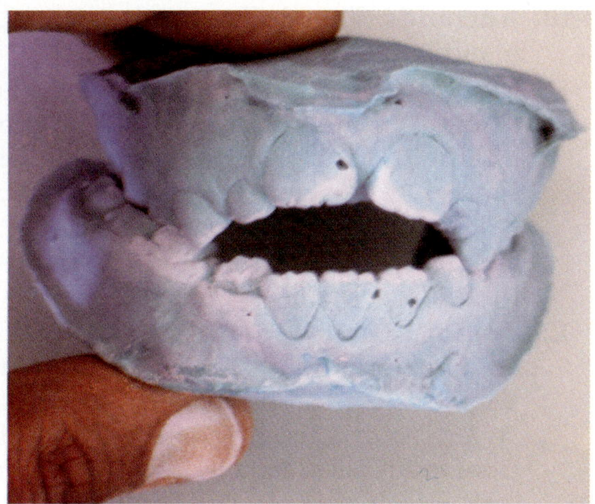

Fig. 44.3: Anterior open bite in mixed dentition due to persistent thumb sucking habit.

2. **Racial difference:** African people have more incidence of open bite as compared to Caucasians.
3. **Congenital:** Certain congenital conditions, e.g. Down's syndrome, have open bite.
4. **Abnormal growth pattern:** Excessive vertical growth of maxilla leads to increased facial height and D and B mandibular rotation. Vertical growth pattern of face leads to development of the skeletal open bite. D and B growth of mandible, with lack of ramal vertical growth also leads to skeletal open bite.
5. **Habits:** Abnormal pressure habits, e.g. prolonged thumb sucking; tongue thrusting, etc. interfere with the eruption of anterior teeth and lead to open bite. Persistent habits, e.g. prolonged thumb sucking or finger sucking habit leads to development of anterior open bite in incisor region. Initially, it represents as dental condition, but if left unchecked, it gets converted in skeletal open bite also. Its nature and severity depends on the position of the digits, frequency and intensity of sucking.

Mechanism of developing the open bite with digit sucking: When thumb is placed in the mouth, it causes the

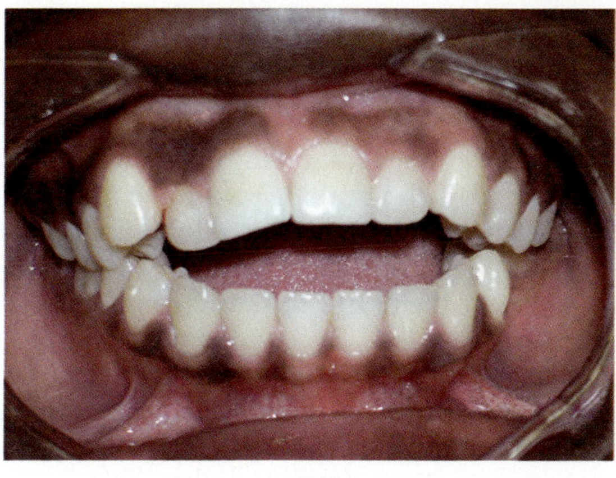

(a)

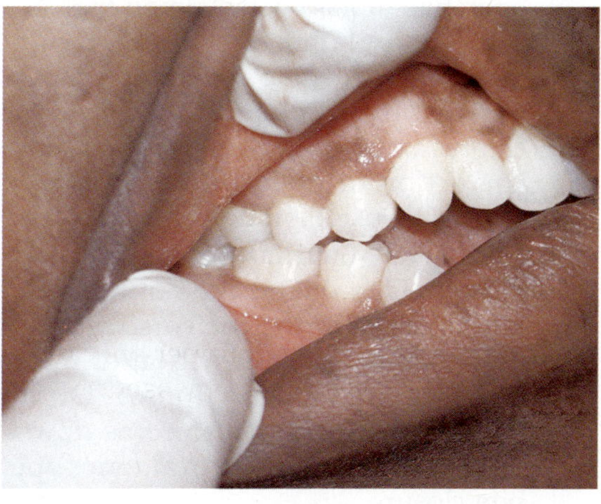

(b)

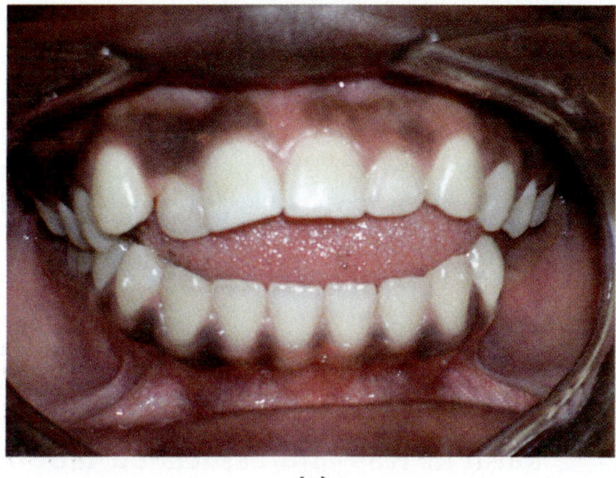

(c)

Figs 44.4a to c: Severe anterior open bite having associated anterior tongue thrust and a skeletal component.

mandible to go D and B. The interocclusal gap is created between posterior teeth, in which the buccal teeth are free to supraerupt, thus increasing the dentoalveolar height. The abnormal forces falling on incisors have intrusive effect. It also causes labial flaring of upper incisors, and lingual inclination of lower teeth and thus increased overjet may be seen. Buccinator mechanism is disturbed, as the tongue pushed down due to thumb, while the cheek muscles are hyperactivated. It leads to constriction of upper arch.

6. **Tongue thrusting** also causes anterior open bite. It has been claimed that they are inter-related in that the tongue thrust may develop due to presence of anterior open bite and vice versa. It creates a vicious cycle. It is claimed that correction of open bite may correct tongue thrust habit and vice versa.
7. **Excessive proclination of incisors:** It also leads to dental type of open bite and spacing in the incisors. It can be easily treated by retraction of upper and lower incisors by tipping. During tipping, the incisors also come down/ extruded and thus help in anterior open bite closure.
8. **Ankylosis** of one or more teeth may lead to presence of open bite in that area, e.g. due to trauma, upper incisor may get ankylosed. In deciduous dentition, sometimes a primary molar gets ankylosed due to infection and leads to submerged tooth. The adjacent teeth keep on erupting while ankylosed tooth remains there.
9. **Mouth breathing habit:** It leads to D and B rotation of mandible, supraeruption of posterior teeth, and thus skeletal open bite. The dental open bite may also be present. Obstruction of nasal airway and associated mouth breathing also leads to development of skeletal open bite. Due to mouth breathing, the mandible goes D and B, with supraeruption of posterior teeth.
10. **Adenoids:** They influence the airway, mandibular, and tongue postures.
11. **Macroglossia:** Large tongue size leads to development of open bite as the tongue tends to fill the interocclusal space. Large tongue size due to genetic factors or congenital conditions, e.g. Down's syndrome, amyloidosis, hypothyroidism, etc. lead to openbite.
12. **Trauma:** Trauma to jaws, condyles, etc. and their abnormal union, ankylosis of TMJ, etc. lead to improper growth of jaws. Trauma leading to intrusion of front teeth also leads to localised open bite, which needs correction by orthodontically extruding the intruded tooth.
13. **Retained infantile swallow:** Prolonged retention of infantile swallowing pattern, leads to complex tongue thrust which leads to open bite.

Diagnosis and Treatment Planning

A proper diagnosis is important to prepare a treatment plan to manage the cases of open bite. Treatment of open bite is quite difficult as compared to many other conditions and thereafter the retention is quite perplexing, needing a different combination of the retainers. Diagnosis should involve the identification of its causative factors, since removal of the cause is very important for its treatment and retention. If factors are not removed, they lead to fast relapse of the condition. There are many factors causing open bite as discussed above, e.g. heredity, abnormal growth, environmental and local, traumatic, congenital, abnormal muscular activity, habits, etc.

Diagnosis: Diagnosis involves the history of patient and family, trauma, habits, clinical examination, cephalometric examination, OPG, etc. A thorough clinical examination evaluating the dental occlusion, the functions of tongue and lips, history of habits and genetic history are important for the diagnosis and treatment plan (Figs 44.5 to 44.7). Cephalometric analysis can be helpful to find

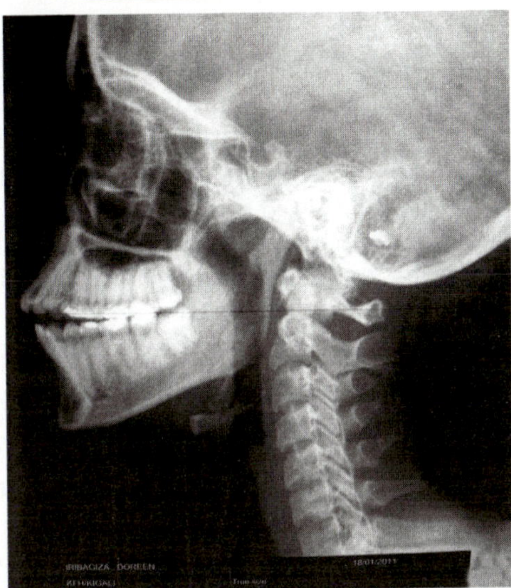

Fig. 44.5: Cephalogram showing anterior open bite.

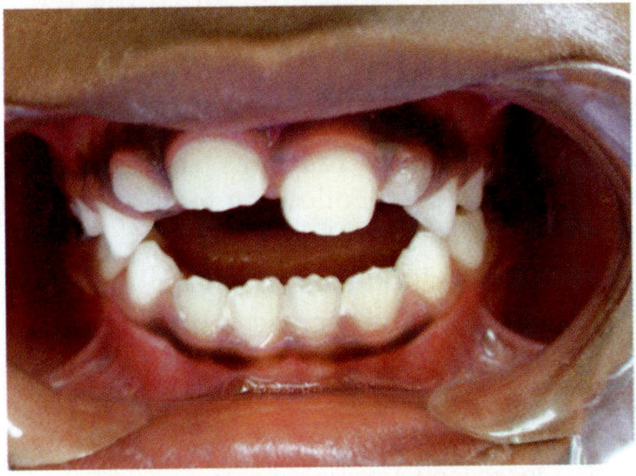

Fig. 44.6: Severe anterior open bite.

out the skeletal relations of jaw bases, and dentoalveolar heights to decide the mechanotherapy. Treatment planning and treatment depend on various factors, e.g. growth pattern, growth status, soft tissue morphology, abnormal habits, patient cooperation, TSALD, amount of open bite, etc.

Growth pattern: Vertical growth pattern leads to increased face height, D and B mandibular rotation, long face syndrome, thus leading to skeletal open bite. Various features are increased AFH, divergent horizontal cephalometrics planes; incompetent lips; narrow dental arch; proclined incisors; increased gonial angle, increased antegonial

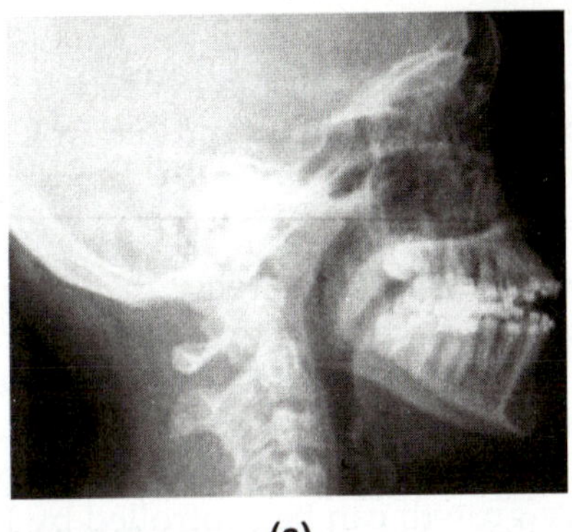

(a)

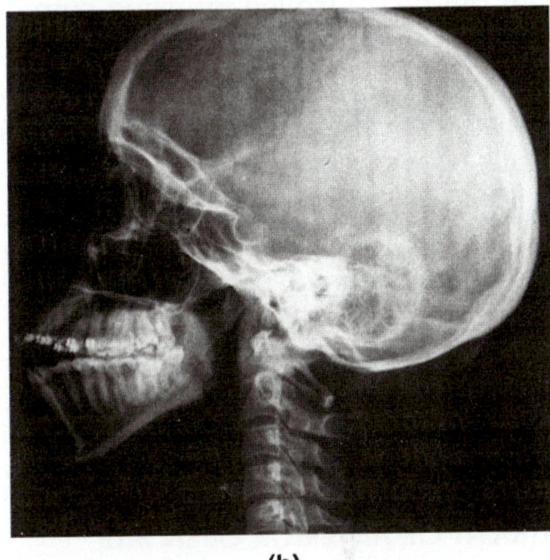

(b)

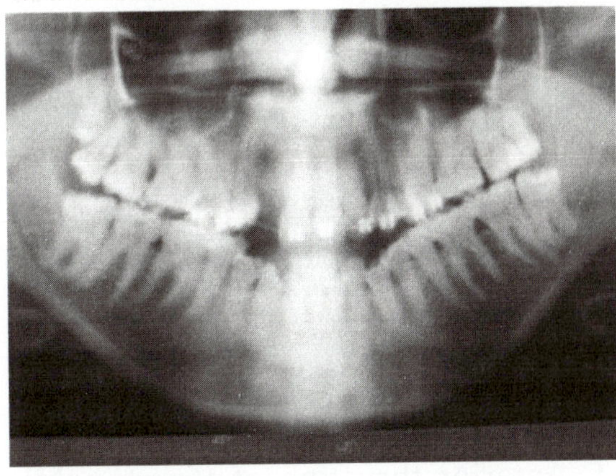

(c)

Figs 44.7a to c: Lateral cephalogram and OPG of a patient having open bite. A vertical growth pattern, downward and backward mandibular rotation; and long face are typical features.

notching; decreased ramal and mandibular length, etc. Molar intrusion is needed in such cases to autorotate the mandible in U and F direction. It can be done by headgear or implants.

Growth status: In actively growing child with abnormal vertical growth pattern, the growth can be redirected or controlled for advantage of the patient. Maxilla and mandible grow downward more in vertical growth. Maxillary growth can be controlled by HPHG with force in U and B direction. Mandibular growth can be controlled by using chin cup with HPHG or vertical-pull headgear.

Abnormal habits: If abnormal habit is not controlled, then the abnormal forces applied by habits lead to relapse of the condition.

TSALD: Generally, in vertical growth pattern, the arches are narrow and shorter dental arches, leading to crowding of teeth. In such cases, extraction of teeth is needed to resolve the crowding. Also, the closure of extraction space by mesial movement of molars leads to closure of anterior open bite because the point of lever moves anteriorly.

TREATMENT OF ANTERIOR OPEN BITE

Definition

It is a condition where there is lack of vertical overlap between upper and lower anterior teeth. It may vary from mild to severe form.

Problems with Anterior Open Bite

a. Unesthetic
b. Inability of incising the food from incisors
c. Speech problems because tongue cannot get proper lip seal and dental contact.
d. Escape of air while speaking
e. Escape of saliva
f. Anterior thrusting of tongue while swallowing
g. Psychological effects.

Classification: Open bites can be classified as either a skeletal open bite or a dental open bite or a skeletodental open bite.

Dental open bite is a condition where there is lack of vertical overlap of teeth. A dental open bite is characterized by normal facial proportions with or without a history of parafunctional habits. A dental open bite has a better prognosis than a skeletal open bite.

A skeletal open bite is usually characterized by abnormal vertical facial growth, vertical maxillary excess, excessive eruption of posterior teeth, downward and backward rotation of the mandible, and normal or excessive eruption of anterior teeth. There may be or may not be a vertical overlap of the teeth, but there is increased vertical distance between the jaw bases.

But, most of the time, it is a combination of skeletal and dental components. In skeletal open bite, there may or may not be the presence of dental open bite, since the teeth achieve compensatory positions during development. It can be properly diagnosed by cephalometric analysis.

Cephalometric features of skeletal anterior open bite: Following features can be found in such a case.

1. Increased total anterior facial height
2. There may be decreased upper anterior face height and increased lower anterior face height
3. Decreased posterior facial height
4. Decreased Jarabak's ratio
5. Steep angles, i.e. increased SN-MP, PP-MP, OP-MP, etc. angles. And divergent horizontal planes.
6. Vertical growth pattern, i.e. increased Y-axis angle
7. Small ramus and mandibular body; and D and B mandibular rotation.
8. There may be vertical maxillary excess in some cases
9. Upper lip may be short
10. More maxillary incisor exposure may be there
11. Increased anterior and decreased posterior dentoalveolar heights.
12. Long and narrow face/dolichofacial features/dolichocephalic pattern

13. Steep anterior cranial base. Since maxilla is attached to ACB, the maxilla is also moved anteriorly in U and F with ACB, while the posterior part of maxilla comes D and F. It leads to D and B mandibular rotation, leading to skeletal open bite.

Features of dental open bite: Dental open bites do not have any skeletal problem. Following features may be seen.

1. Lack of overlap between upper and lower anteriors.
2. There may be increased overjet due to proclined upper incisors.
3. Upper arch may be narrow.
4. Anterior tongue thrust during swallowing is seen
5. Lips may be short and incompetent.

Treatment of anterior open bite: Correction of skeletal open bite is one of the most difficult problems in orthodontics especially if it involves skeletal component. After correction, its retention creates a problem, since it has got a high relapse potential. In severe cases, the orthodontic treatment alone may be insufficient and need orthognathic surgery.

Following options are available for the treatment of anterior open bite depending on the need of the case, the growth status of patient, severity of the case, etc.

- True anterior extrusion, e.g. by extrusive archwires, box elastics
- Relative anterior extrusion and retroclination of anterior teeth, e.g. by tipping of anterior teeth
- Posterior intrusion with U and F mandibular autorotation, e.g. by HPHG, Magnts, implants, etc.
- Orthognathic surgery.

Following methods are used to treat this condition.

A. **Removal of the cause:** Abnormal habits leading to AOB should be controlled as early as possible, since if not intercepted, the severity of the condition increases. Habit breaking appliances, removable or fixed, are used to intercept the habits. As the habit gets controlled, the teeth start taking their normal position with continued normal eruption.

B. **Tongue exercises:** If anterior tongue thrust is present, the patient is advised to do tongue exercises so as to keep the tongue from coming in between the incisors during swallowing. With active mechanotherapy, the patient is given habit breaking appliance and advised to do the tongue exercises. If there is persistent imbalance between the activity of tongue and orofacial muscles, the treatment of open bite often fails.

C. **Removable appliance** for treatment of excessive proclination of incisors: Due to tongue thrust habit, the incisors get proclined, spaces appear between them, and open bite is there. It can be treated by using Hawley's removable appliance for retraction of upper and lower incisors by tipping. During tipping, the incisors also come down/extruded and thus help in anterior open bite closure. Habit breaking cribs and exercises should be included during treatment (Fig. 44.8).

D. **Removable appliance with posterior bite plate:** PBP appliance in lower arch is given to patient which applies a constant intrusive force on upper teeth

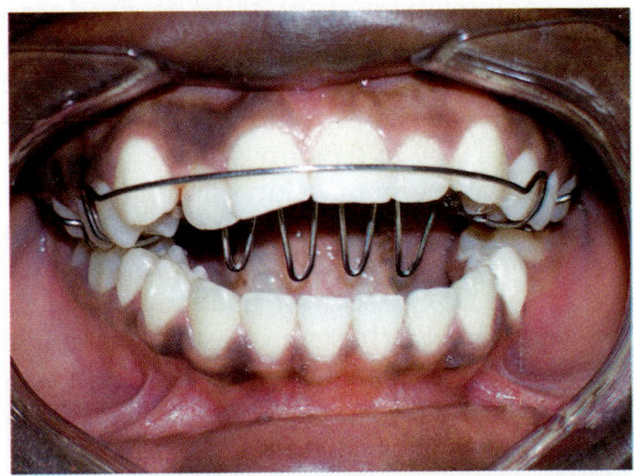

Fig. 44.8: Tongue thrust preventing appliance in place. A good control over the habit can be helpful during orthodontic treatment and surgical intervention. A continued habit leads to relapse.

leading to some improvement in open bite. If it does not lead to true intrusion, at least it prevents the further eruption of posterior teeth with growth, thus preventing increasing the severity of condition. But the success depends on patient cooperation. The composite bite blocks can be bonded on the occlusal surfaces of the molars for this effect which do not involve the patient cooperation. These composite blocks should be of different color (blue color) so that their removal is easy later on.

E. **Removable appliance in lower arch with spring-loaded bite blocks:** This appliance has been designed by Umal Doshi 2010 AJO, which applies a spring-initiated intrusive force on the posterior segment and helps in improvement of open bite.

F. **Myofunctional therapy:** Mild cases of skeletal open bites can be treated during growth periods using modified myofunctional appliances. These FAs have high occlusal bite blocks in posterior region, which apply intrusive forces on the teeth, and also prevent eruption of these teeth, e.g. vertical activator; Stockfisch kinetor, FR-IV appliance; modified bionator or twin block, etc.

G. **Orthodontic mechanotherapy by incisor extrusion:** Mild to moderate cases of open bite, with mild skeletal component, can be treated by extrusion of incisors with orthodontic appliances. The 2 × 4 extrusion arch is placed in incisal segment, taking anchorage from molars. To prevent abnormal movement of the molars, the TPA and LHA can be used. Box elastics are used to extrude the incisors. But in severe cases of open bite, extrusion of incisors may lead to excessive incisal exposure, imbalanced position and loss of supporting bone.

H. **Extraction therapy:** Open bite can be closed by extraction of posterior teeth during mechanotherapy. The more posterior the tooth is extracted, better are the chances of open bite closure, e.g. second premolars or first molars are removed and the remaining teeth are mesialised. It leads to removal of premature contact in the far posterior region, brings the level of fulcrum more anteriorly and helps in U and F autorotation of mandible.

I. **Orthodontic mechanotherapy by molar intrusion** (Figs 44.9 to 4.11): It is a better method to close the open bite especially in vertical growth pattern cases or increased dentoalveolar height cases, but molar intrusion is difficult to achieve. It needs a lot of patient cooperation to use extraoral appliances and elastics. Some methods used for posterior intrusion are:

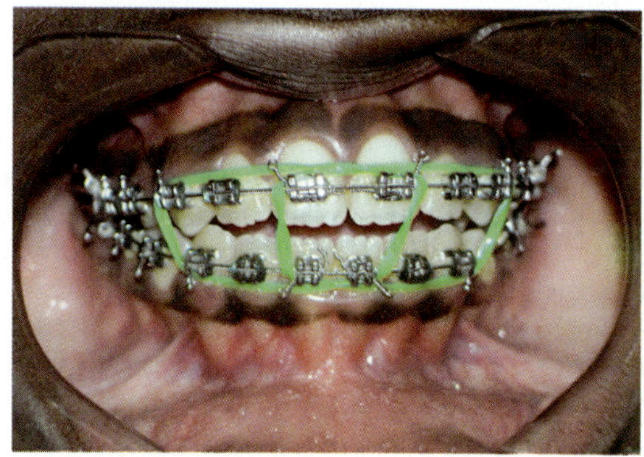

(a)

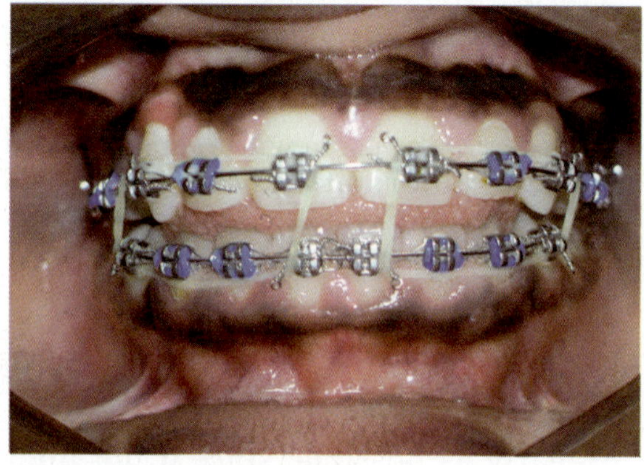

(b)

Figs 44.9a and b: Anterior box elastics can be helpful, if open bite is mild.

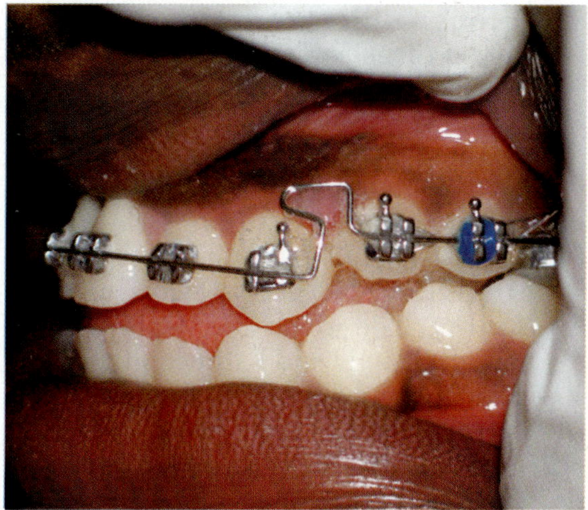

Fig. 44.10: Extrusive loops in the archwires can help to extrude the incisors to correct milder forms of open bite. But, they lead to steps formation in canine—first premolar region, i.e. in the area of loop's location.

a. **High-pull headgear or vertical-pull headgear with chin cup:** HPHG with U and B force on the upper molars is applied for their intrusion, which helps in U and F autorotation of mandible. Vertical-pull HG with chin cup also helps to apply intrusive forces on upper buccal teeth to close the open bite. It also helps to prevent abnormal maxillary growth. But, this therapy is successful if started in mixed dentition period. Vertical growth of mandible leads to its D and B rotation. A vertical-pull chin cup appliance is used which applies intrusive forces on upper teeth, prevents further eruption, redirects the abnormal growth and helps in U and F bending of mandible with growth. These orthopaedic appliances are useful during active period of growth and with proper patient cooperation.

b. **Removable appliance** for intrusion of posterior teeth by using elastics which are extended from buccal to palatal side of the molars pressing on its occlusal surface. It can be used to intrude individual tooth. Appliance with posterior occlusal coverage alongwith HPHG helps to apply intrusive forces on the whole buccal segment.

c. **Anterior vertical corrector, i.e. TPA with an acrylic button:** TPA is made on first molars and kept away from the palatal tissues by 2–3 mm. An acrylic button is made on the TPA. The pressure of tongue applies intrusive forces on the first molars, besides preventing their eruption.

d. **Using modified TPA (M-TPA):** This has been designed by Goyal and Goyal (cyberjournal of orthodontics). The E-chains engaging hooks are soldered on the buccal and palatal sides of the TPA, which are extended in the region of extruded teeth. E-chains are attached from these hooks from buccal to palatal side crossing over the occlusal surface of the tooth to be intruded. On the occlusal surface of the tooth to be intruded,

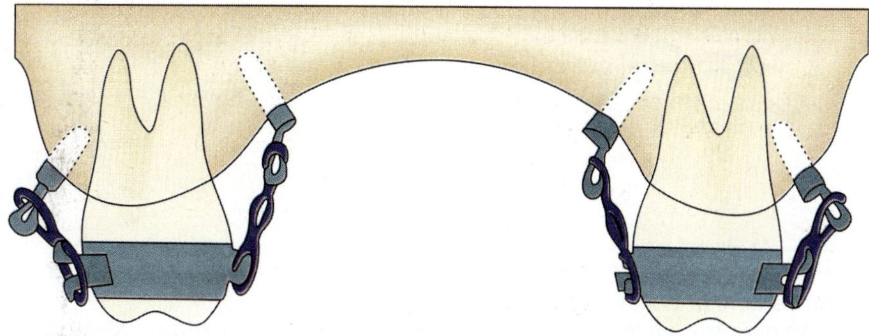

Fig. 44.11: Buccal and palatal implants to apply intrusive forces on the molars to treat anterior open bite.

the lingual button can be bonded to prevent slippage of E-chain in the contact area. It can be used to intrude more teeth simultaneously and does not need patient cooperation.

e. Using **reverse curve of Spee NiTi** wires in upper and lower arches and using heavy intermaxillary elastics in canine region or box elastics. The intrusive force in anterior region is cancelled by the elastics. The resultant force becomes intrusive on the molars.

f. **Using microimplants or zygomatic anchorage:** This is one of best methods providing the absolute anchorage and eliminating patient cooperation. The implants are placed in the buccal and palatal areas and intrusive forces are applied to the molars. Miniplates of L-shape can be placed in zygomatic buttress region to apply intrusive forces on the arch wire ligated in the teeth. There is no requirement of HPHG or removable appliance.

g. **Magnets:** Bite-blocks with repelling magnets can be placed on upper and lower posterior teeth for their intrusion (Fig. 44.12).

J. **Orthognathic surgical corrections:** Severe cases and cases beyond active growth, which cannot be properly treated with orthodontics need surgical treatment. Surgery is done only after the active growth has ceased. Choice of the surgery depends on the patient condition. Generally, it is done by **Le Fort I osteotomy with superior repositioning.** The mandible is allowed to autorotate in U and F direction. It helps in closure of open bite, decreases the profile convexity, decreases anterior face height, etc. It may need **advancement genioplasty** after re-evaluation of the results.

K. **Surgical osteotomy** in posterior segment followed by intrusion with the help of zygomatic anchorage (Fig. 44.13).

L. **Surgery of ankylosed tooth:** An ankylosed tooth does not move with orthodontics. In such cases, a segmental alveolar osteotomy is done and the segment is brought down in the normal level of other adjacent teeth to treat the open bite.

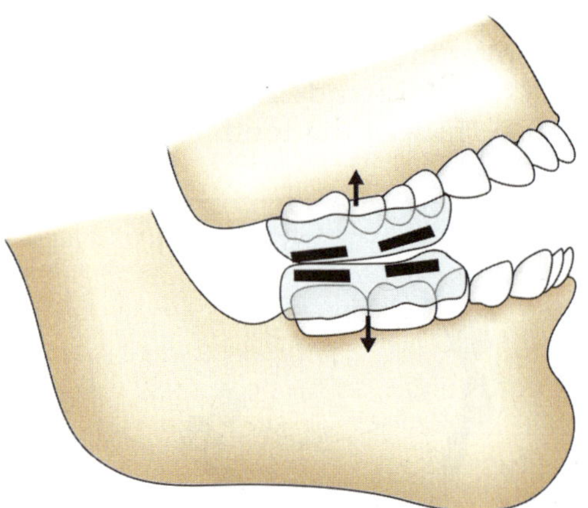

Fig. 44.12: Fixed posterior bite plates with magnets in repulsive mode to apply intrusive forces on molars to treat anterior open bite.

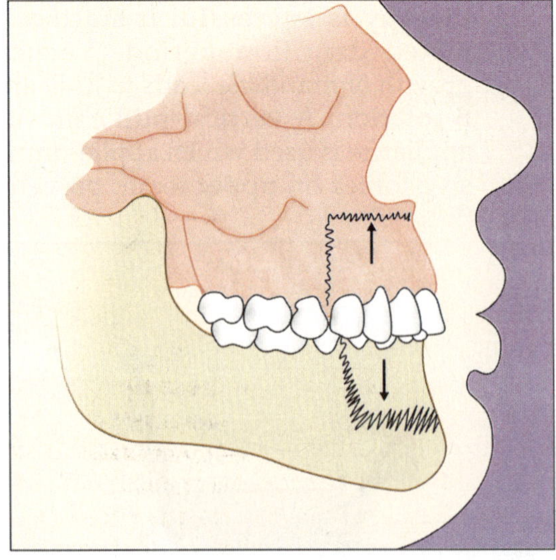

Fig. 44.13: Bimaxillary dentoalveolar anterior segmental surgery to treat anterior open bite.

M. **Invisalign** can also be used for treatment of open bite.

N. **Muscle exercise:** Clenching of muscles provides intrusive forces on molars and can help in open bite closure.

O. **Second molar extraction:** It helps to remove the wedge effect and thus closure of open bite by autorotation of mandible.

POSTERIOR OPEN BITE

It is a condition which is characterized by a lack of contact or overlap in posterior region during centric occlusion. It generally involves a segment of posterior teeth.

Causes

It is caused by following factors:

a. **Lateral tongue thrusting** habit, which leads to mechanical interference in the eruption of the posterior teeth.
b. **Ankylosed tooth:** Due to trauma or infection of tooth, which is not able to erupt.
c. **Ankylosed primary tooth:** It does not exfoliate and does not erupt and thus alveolar bone remains deficient, and it becomes submerged.
d. **Supernumerary tooth** in the area of erupting tooth does not let it erupt.
e. Disturbance of eruption mechanism of teeth due to some disorders.
f. **Congenital conditions** leading to impaction of multiple teeth.
g. **Growth problems.**

Treatment

Treatment of posterior open bite is important for proper mastication. Following methods are used:

1. Removal of cause: Abnormal position of tongue or digit sucking habit has to be controlled to avoid the interference in the normal eruption of teeth. Habit breaking appliance with cribs in posterior region can be given.
2. Extrusion of infraerupted teeth: It can be done by using intermaxillary elastics or extrusive loops in the arch wire.
3. Ankylosed permanent teeth which are infraoccluded are treated with jacket crowns.
4. Ankylosed primary teeth should be removed to pave way for eruption of successor tooth. The space should be maintained with proper methods.
5. Surgical: Localized segmental osteotomy can be done and the segment is brought to normal occlusal plane level and stabilized.

COMBINED ANTERIOR AND POSTERIOR OPEN BITE

Such conditions extend from posterior to anterior region, frequently having contact in the last erupted molar region, generally second molars. The patient is not able to chew and speak properly. It is generally a skeletal problem.

Treatment

Mild to moderate cases having normal growth pattern can be treated by camouflage with fixed appliance therapy. Extrusive force with the help of box elastics and extrusive loops can be used. In vertical growth pattern, extrusion method is not preferred. Extraction in posterior region with space closure by mesialization of molars is done to close the anterior open bite. In severe cases, surgical intervention with Le Fort I osteotomy is done. The maxilla is pushed upwards in the posterior region, thus mandible autorotates U and F.

Retention protocol: Retention is a very important phase after the correction of open bite. Open bite is one of the most difficult condition to retain, as the relapse is very fast. Also if etiology is not removed like persistence of abnormal habits, then the relapse is inevitable.

A prolonged retention protocol is followed. Mild to moderate open bite case treated with orthodontic extrusion of anterior teeth, needs a fixed 3–3 retainer in mandible and a removable Hawley's retainer in maxillary arch is given. Cribs can be incorporate in appliance to check the abnormal habit. Buccal bonded retainer can also be placed to augment the lingual anchorage.

A tongue crib and a passive posterior bite plane can be incorporated in the appliance. Posterior bite plane has an intrusive effect on the posterior teeth. HPHG for part time wear is also recommended. A regular follow-up is necessary to intervene timely.

45

Treatment of Class II Malocclusion

INTRODUCTION

Angle defined class II malocclusion as "the relation of upper and lower permanent first molars where the MB cusp of upper first molar lies mesial to MB groove of lower first molar". According to his classification, the malocclusion results due to distal relation of mandible to maxilla, (since he considered the maxilla as a stable entity), and hence it is also called as distocclusion. But, Angle's classification is merely a dental classification in sagittal dimension, and it does not consider the skeletal malrelationship. The class II malocclusion is mostly a skeletodental problem, with the dental compensations present due to abnormal relation of upper and lower jaws.

Classification of Class II Malocclusion

Class II malocclusions generally have either a dental, skeletal, and/or functional components.

A. According to **Angle's system** of classification: It is of two types divided according to certain peculiar features.

1. **Division 1:** In these cases, the overjet is increased.
2. **Division 2:** Here overbite is increased (which may vary from mild to more thatn 100% depth); overjet is decreased, and maxillary incisors erupt in a lingually inclined pattern. It also shows different variations as given below.
3. **Subdivision:** It is the unilateral class II relation, i.e. when molar relation on one side is class I and the other side is class II. Unilateral cases are classified as a "subdivision" of the affected side.

Class II division 2 can be of following types depending on the severity:

1. Type A: Central incisors are retroclined, and their distal margins are overlapped by lateral incisors.
2. Type B: Upper central and lateral incisors are retroclined, and the canines overlap them.
3. Type C: Central and lateral incisors, and canines are retroclined.

B. Skeletal classification: Ackermann-Proffit classification of malocclusion describes any condition in the three planes of space.

In **sagittal dimension:** Most of the skeletal class II problems are seen due to discrepancy in intermaxillary AP jaw relationship. These can be:

1. **Maxillary prognathism** (with normal mandible). It may be of following varieties:
   a. It may be normal sized maxilla which is placed forward; or
   b. A normal positioned maxilla which is overgrown; or
   c. An overgrown maxilla placed forwards than its normal position. It is the most severe form.
2. **Mandibular retrognathism** (with normal maxilla). It may be of following varieties (Fig. 45.1):
   a. It may be normal-sized mandible which is placed backward (due to posterior position of glenoid fossa); or

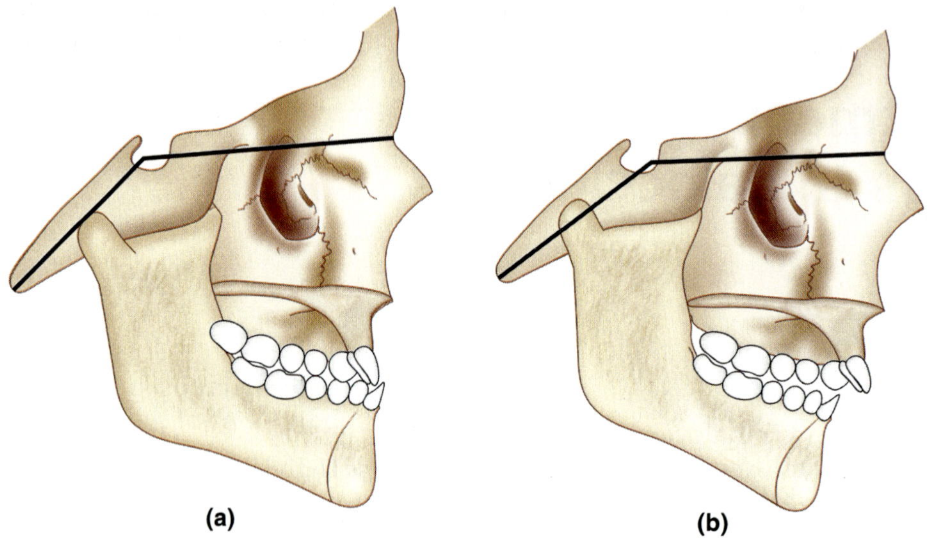

Figs 45.1a and b: Position of glenoid fossa in the middle cranial base also affects the position of mandible, thus creating skeletal imbalance of upper and lower jaw bases. Its anterior position leads to mandibular pognathism and thus skeletal class III, while the posterior position leads to mandibular retrognathism and thus skeletal class II.

   b. A small sized mandible which is at a normal position in space (mandibular length is less);
   c. A deficient mandible placed backwards. It is the most severe form.
3. **Combination** of any of the above.

In vertical dimension: There may be difference in facial height due to different growth pattern of the face, i.e.

a. Increased anterior face height, i.e. long face. It is due to vertical growth pattern. Maxillary height is also increased, which leads to D and B rotation of mandible, convex profile, etc. Thus, there are sagittal and vertical problems.
b. Normal face height: the growth pattern is normal, the height of maxilla and mandible is in normal range. Class II is due to sagittal problem.
c. Decreased face height, i.e. short face. It occurs due to horizontal growth pattern. The bite is deep. Maxillary and mandibular lengths are more. Muscles are stronger. Class II condition is due to sagittal discrepancy in jaw relation.

In transverse direction: The dental arches may be narrow or normal or wide. Generally in class II division 1, the dental arches are narrow, and it is generally associated with dolichocephalic, dolichofacial and vertical growth patterns.

In class II division 2, the upper arch is generally normal to wider in size, and it is generally associated with mesocephalic, mesofacial and horizontal growth patterns. The lower arch is normal or narrow. The mandible is retropositioned (although having normal length) due to it either contained in the upper arch and/or due to stronger soft tissues.

Combination: Any variation of skeletal class II can be a combination of discrepancy in these planes, which leads to increased severity of the condition.

Incidence of Class II Malocclusion

Incidence of class I malocclusion is the maximum (60–70%), while class II (20–30%) are lesser, and class III (5–10%) are least. But class II cases are seen maximum in the orthodontic clinics for treatment due to its esthetic implications. Also, the class II division 2 cases are less frequent than either class I or class II division 1, but slightly more frequent than class III.

Etiology: Development of malocclusion is a multifactorial. Factors such as heredity, environment and functional factors play role. Broadly, they can be divided in three types.

1. Prenatal factors
2. Natal factors
3. Postnatal factors

Prenatal Factors

1. **Heredity:** Jaw size and position is under genetic control. Parents with disproportional size and position of jaw may transmit it to their offsprings in different combination. It may lead to skeletal malposition. Abnormal axial inclination of maxillary central incisors is genetically determined. There is variation in morphology of maxillary central incisors; and a difference in the crown-root angulation also exists in some class II division 2 cases. Also, the crowns of the upper incisors are thinner labiolingually when compared with incisors in other malocclusions.
2. **Teratogens:** Certain chemicals, drugs, etc. taken during pregnancy affect the growth of bones of body, e.g. alcohol, smoking , certain drugs, etc. act as teratogens.
3. **Irradiation:** Exposure to irradiation during fetal life leads to developmental problems, e.g. it is a myth in some parts of world, that during pregnancy, if the mother gets exposed to solar eclipse, there are chances of development of CLP or other bony abnormality. It is esp due to fact that during eclipse, the dose of dangerous radiations, like UV and infrared rays reaching the earth increases.
4. **Fetal posture during IU life:** If abnormal posture leads to application of abnormal pressure on the mandible, it may lead to deficient growth of mandible, e.g. due to less amniotic fluid and thus intrauterine space, the chin may get pressed against the chest leading to deficient mandibular growth. It may lead to asymmetric development also. Pierre Robin anomalad is due to this problem.

Natal Factors

Trauma during birth: While passing through narrow birth canal may lead to trauma to the craniofacial region.

Forcep delivery: During difficult births, the head of fetus is held with forceps in the TMJ region to pull it out of the birth canal. This may lead to injury to TMJ/condylar region.

Congenital syndromes: Some congenital conditions also have deficient mandibular growth.

Postnatal Factors/Environmental Factors

Environment plays an important role in the development of certain types of malocclusion. It disturbs the normal development of dentofacial region. They are:

- **Trauma:** Many children may get trauma/fracture of the condylar region due to falling while playing, etc. which may lead to fibrous or bony ankylosis. It leads to deficient mandibular growth.
- **Infectious condition:** For example, rheumatoid arthritis in childhood may affect TMJ and thus mandibular growth.
- **Irradiation therapy:** Children with tumors of craniofacial region undergoing radiation therapy get their condylar area (active cartilage) affected by irradiation.
- **Muscles dysfunction:** The muscles affect jaw growth since the musculature is an important part of the soft tissue functional matrix. Growth of soft tissues helps in growth of the jaws. If a part of muscles or soft tissue is deficient, which may occur due to infection, trauma, some unknown causes, or due to birth injury, etc. then growth of bone in relation to that muscle is affected. If

injury to the motor nerve occurs, the muscle atrophies and thus the function stimulus to the bone is lost. It results in underdevelopment of that part of the face.

- **Abnormal habits:** Habits apply inadvertent forces on facial structures, e.g. thumb sucking leads to shifting of tongue D and B in the mouth; a D and B pressure on the mandible and thus deficient growth of mandible. A persistent finger habit displaces the maxilla and maxillary dentition anteriorly upward and forward, leading to the development of a class II molar relationship. The palatal plane gets oriented upward and forward, which leads to slight mesialisation/anterior positioning of maxillary arch, contributing to the class II relation. Habits also lead to contraction of upper arch due to increased activity of buccinators, effects of which are mainly concentrated in the region of modiolus, i.e. the upper canine region. A constricted upper arch, since it is narrow in anterior region, leads to locking of mandible, does not allow the mandible to come forward in due course of time, and thus the mandible remains retrognathic.

- In patients with an excessive overjet, the lower lip may become trapped behind the maxillary incisors, causing abnormal contraction of mentalis and other perioral muscles leading the maxillary incisors to further tip labially.

- **Abnormal muscles contraction:** For example, torticollis; scars of burns; fibrosis after injuries, etc. especially of submandibular region, apply abnormal D and B pressure on mandible and do not let it grow normally.

- **Milwaukee braces:** This is an orthopaedic appliance which is worn in the neck region and is supported by mandible and chest. It is used to treat scoliosis. It applies abnormal growth restricting forces on mandible.
- **Certain infections,** like acute tonsillitis, nasal polyps, etc., lead to mouth breathing habit and thus to D and B rotation of mandible, contributing to skeletal class II pattern.
- **Premature loss** of maxillary primary second molars: Early loss of maxillary second deciduous molars in a patient with an otherwise class I occlusion results in mesial migration, rotation and tipping of maxillary first molars, and the creation of a class II molar relation. Preventive measures can be taken in such situations to avoid development of class II.
- **Space loss due to proximal caries lesions in upper teeth:** Especially if maxillary primary second molars having distal caries, then the permanent first molar shifts mesially, leading to class II molar relation.

General Clinical Features of a Class II Division 1 Case (Figs 45.2 to 45.4)

Following are some clinical features.

1. Relation of first permanent molars is Angle's class II which may vary from half cusp to the full cusp.
2. Increased overjet due to proclination of upper incisors (Figs 45.2 and 45.3).
3. Bite depth may vary from deep to open bite. Generally, deep bite develops due to eruption of lower incisors, since there is no incisal stop.
4. The palatal gingival may be traumatised in extreme deep bite cases
5. Spacing in upper incisors may/may not be present
6. Deep curve of spee in the lower arch, which is due to overeruption of lower incisors
7. Upper arch narrow, generally due to disturbed circumoral muscles equilibrium
8. Convex profile

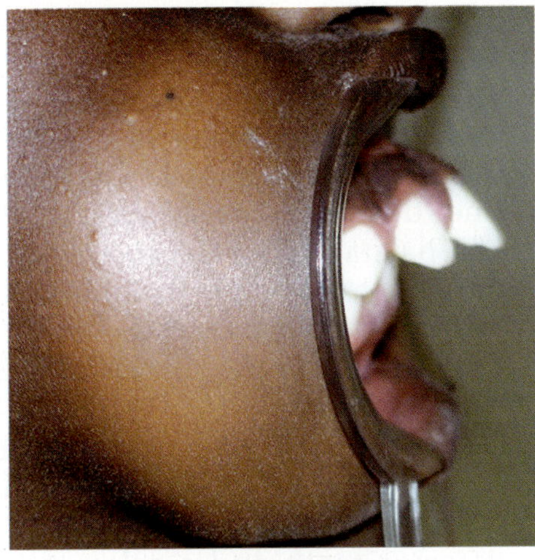

(a)

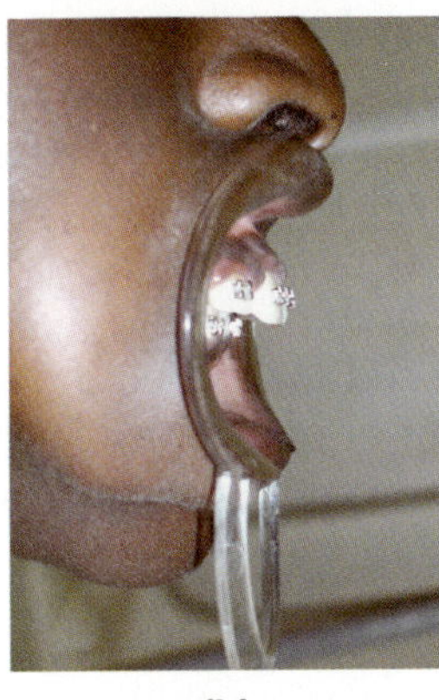

(b)

Figs 45.2a and b: Increased overjet.

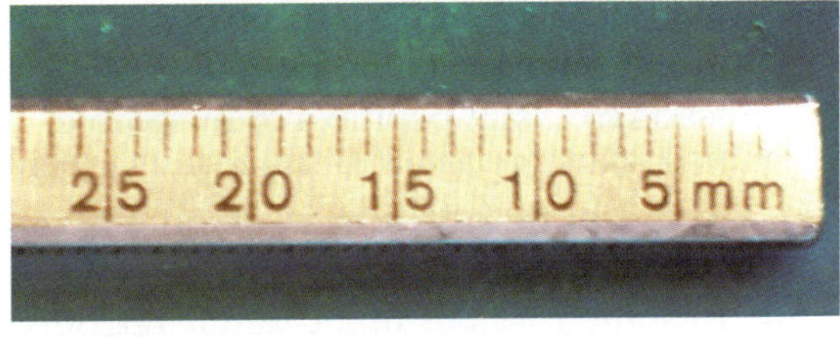

(a)

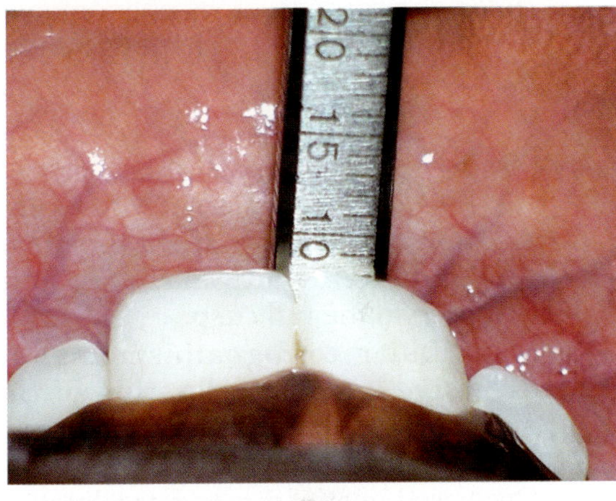

(b)

Figs 45.3a and b: A graduated handle of mirror can be used to measure overjet directly in the mouth.

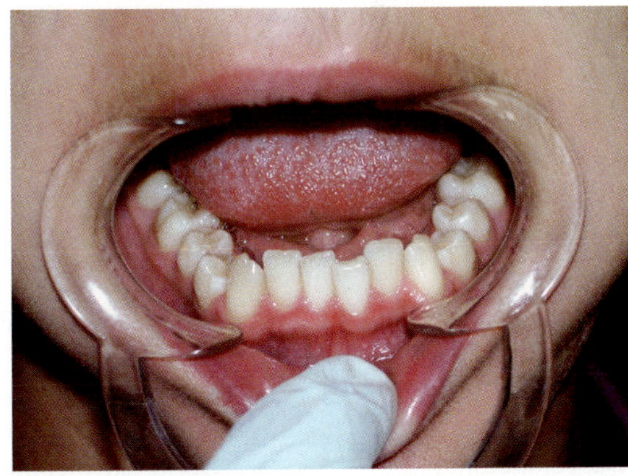

Fig. 45.4: Lower anterior crowding and a deep, concave curve of Spee.

9. Increased facial height, with D and B rotation of mandible, and posterior divergent facial pattern.
10. Lips incompetent, with upper lip short and hypotonic, and lower lip in lip trap relation with upper incisors. It may lead to further increase in overjet. Proper maintenance of lip seal is essential to maintain teeth in their normal corrected position.
11. Abnormal muscles activity: Buccinators mechanism is disturbed, leading to narrow upper arch, which may lead to buccal crossbite. Hyperactive mentalis is seen which may lead to lip trap and further increase of overjet and spacings among the upper incisors; while it causes lower incisors tilt lingually and crowded position.
12. Tongue position is downward and backward. Downward position of tongue disturbs the balance in posterior

region, leading to contraction of upper arch. Backward position of tongue leads to distal position of mandible.

13. Pharyngeal airway size is less and hyoid bone position is distal as compared to normal.
14. In some cases of mandibular retrognathism, the lower incisors are also proclined as a compensatory phenomenon to reduce the overjet. It happens under the tongue forces.

General Characteristics of Class II Division 2 Maloclusion (Table 45.1)

a. Relation of first permanent molars is Angle's class II which may vary from half cusp to the full cusp.
b. Mandibular retrognathism due to excessive lingual inclination of the maxillary central incisors and posterior functional shift.
c. Decreased overjet due to retroclination of upper central incisors. Central incisors are overlapped on distolabial by lateral incisors. In some cases, both the central and the lateral incisors are lingually inclined and the canines overlap the lateral incisors on the labial.
d. There is deep overbite. It develops due to linguoversion of upper incisors and the overeruption of lower incisors, since there is no incisal stop.
e. The palatal gingival and lower labial gingival may be traumatized in extreme deep bite cases.
f. Crowding of upper and lower incisors may be present.
g. Deep curve of Spee in the lower arch
h. An inverted maxillary occlusal plane is often seen due to supraocclusion of the anterior teeth and a relative infraocclusion of the posterior segments.
i. Upper arch is normal or wider.
j. Pleasant profile straight to mild convex profile. They are sometimes called as Hollywood faces.
k. Broad square face, with broad upper dental arch.
l. Decreased facial height, with U and F rotation of mandible.
m. Lips competent, with lower lip in lip curl relation.

Table 45.1: Difference between division 1 and division 2

Features	*Division 1*	*Division 2*
Overjet	Increased	Decreased
Overbite	Varies	Increased
Upper incisors	Proclined	Retroclined, variable
Lower incisors	Proclined, normal, retroclined	Generally retroclined
Arch width	Narrow	Wide
Growth pattern	Vertical/normal	Horizontal/normal
Face height	Increased/normal	Decreased/normal
Lip competency	Generally incompetent	Competent
Lower lip trap	Generally present	Absent
Lip curl	Absent	Present
Mentolabial sulcus	Shallow	Deep
Upper lip	Hypotonic	Normotonic
Masticatory muscles	Weaker	Stronger
Functional shift	Absent	Posterior functional shift on closure
Face width	Narrow and long	Wide and short; square type
Labial gingival trauma	Absent	Generally present
Freeway space	Decreased	Increased

n. Deep mentolabial sulcus is present due to prominent soft tissue chin and curling of lower lip.
o. Abnormal muscles activity: Generally, there is no abnormal muscle activity as is in class II division 1 cases. But some patients may have stronger mandibular muscles, which prevent proper eruption of teeth and thus lead to deep bite, and provide strong anchorage also.

Cephalometric Characteristics of the Class II Division 1 Malocclusion

According to Fisk, there may be six possible morphological variations in dentofacial complex:

- The maxilla and teeth are anteriorly placed in relation to cranium;
- Maxillary teeth are anteriorly placed (proclined), while maxilla is normally positioned;
- Mandible is of normal size, but posteriorly positioned;
- The mandible is underdeveloped;
- The mandibular teeth are posteriorly placed on a normal positioned mandible; and
- Various combinations of the above relationships.

Class II cases with anteroposterior skeletal discrepancies between the maxilla and mandible are characterized by a large ANB angle and Wits appraisal. The anteroposterior skeletal discrepancies may also be accompanied by a vertical and transverse discrepancy.

Cephalometric Characteristics of the Class II Division 2 Malocclusion

Posterior cranial base is larger in division 2 as compared to division 1 cases.

Mandible in a division 2 case has relatively more acute gonial, mandibular plane, palatal plane, occlusal plane angles, horizontal growth pattern, skeletal deep bite, etc.

Anterior face height is shorter especially the lower anterior face height due to horizontal growth pattern in which mandible rotates U and F which also leads to an excessive overbite.

Perioral Functional Characteristics of Class II Malocclusions

A. Abnormal muscular patterns are generally associated with class II malocclusions. In class II division 1, the increased overjet may lead to incompetency of lips and the lower lip trap behind the maxillary incisors, thus maintaining or accentuating the overjet. During swallowing, an abnormal mentalis muscle and buccinator activity, and the compensatory tongue function and position, could cause constriction of maxillary arch, protrusion and spacing of the maxillary incisors, and abnormal inclination of the mandibular incisors.
B. In class II division 2 cases, the orbicularis oris and mentalis muscles are often well developed and active. Lips are competent. The lingual inclination of maxillary incisors accentuates the appearance of lower "lip curl" which is associated with the vertical overclosure. Due to overclosure, the mandible is positioned U and F, thus thrusting the lower lip against the upper lip, causing the lip curl. The reduced vertical height also accentuates the chin prominence.
C. Class II division 2 cases have a larger freeway space.
D. In some class II division 2 cases, the path of closure is influenced by the lingually inclined maxillary incisors, resulting in a posterior shift on closure. The condyles are displaced posteriorly and superiorly in the articular fossa. The presence of such a "**posterior functional shift**" in some cases is favorable for the correction of the class II relationship. Such cases show a partial correction of the malocclusion

after labial repositioning of the maxillary incisors, as the mandible gets unlocked and moves forward to a normal centric relation position. But it is not a consistent finding in class II division 2 cases.

Relation of Growth and Treatment: Growth Patterns of Maxilla and Mandible

General concepts: The maxillary complex is usually displaced in a downward and forward direction. According to the functional matrix theory, bones adapt to the functional demands of various craniofacial components. Sutural and nasal septum growths are therefore passive processes and are secondary growth sites, which adapt to functional demands of various vital systems including respiration and mastication.

Mandible is translated in a downward and forward direction with growth. The growth of mandible usually exceeds that of maxilla due to cephalocaudal gradient of growth and so the bony face becomes less convex with age. Mandible is able to rotate either forward or backward depending on the growth pattern. Forward mandibular rotation is favorable for correction of class II malocclusions, while backward rotation is not favorable. Therefore, the direction and magnitude of growth, the type of mandibular rotation, patient cooperation and skill of the clinician determine the prognosis for treatment of a class II malocclusion.

If no Treatment is Given?

A distal step in deciduous dentition mostly converts in class II molar relationship in permanent dentition. Once the class II molar relationship is established, it does not self-correct although mandibular growth may occur at a faster rate and for a longer time than that of the maxilla. It is due to the functional locking of inclined planes of mandibular with maxillary teeth. So, this growth differential itself cannot correct the dental malocclusion. Facial profiles of untreated patients remain the same whereas those of treated patients show a tendency for the profile to improve. Untreated class II malocclusions with a retrognathic face maintain the class II dental relationship even if growth improves the skeletal mandibular retrusion.

TREATMENT CONSIDERATIONS

Diagnosis

A proper clinical examination, study cast and radiographic analysis, growth status analyses are done to diagnose the condition. Due to large variation in the class II cases, the clinician should thoroughly evaluate the occlusal relationships, anteroposterior, transverse and vertical skeletal discrepancies, the soft tissue morphology, and the presence of any abnormal function in each patient. The severity of condition depends on these combinations and hence the treatment is decided according to the relationship and size of jaw bases; growth status; and dental relationship. During treatment planning, the growth status of the patient plays a very important role. Different combinations of treatment may be needed depending on the underlying problem, especially a growing patient can be treated either with the functional appliance or dentofacial orthopedics/ headgear or a combination of both. An accurate diagnosis and estimation of growth are very important to reach a treatment plan. Broadly, for treatment planning, class II cases can be divided as follow. Treatment of class II can be broadly divided in following **three categories**.

1. Growth modulation
2. Camouflage treatment
3. Surgical treatment

Timing of treatment: Timing of treatment is very important for achieving good and stable results. Correction of skeletal problem can best be done during periods of active growth. According to the **early treatment concept**, the correction of skeletal class II malocclusions discrepancies is as effective in the preadolescent years as during adolescence, while other orthodontists believe that treatment should be postponed to coincide with the adolescent "growth spurt."

A **biphasic/two-stage treatment approach** has been suggested. In first stage, early correction of skeletal discrepancy taking advantage of active growth; correcting incisor flaring, arch expansion, correcting the molar relationship, and crossbite (if present) followed by a period of retention. In the second stage after the eruption of the permanent dentition, the fixed appliance is used for detailing the dentition.

Sexual dimorphism: Timings of growth spurts in females is 2 years earlier than the males. So growth modulation in females should be started earlier than the boys.

A. **In growing cases**:
   a. **Maxillary prognathism:** They are treated by head gear therapy, to restrict/redirect maxillary growth.
   b. **Mandibular retrognathism:** They are treated by functional appliances to enhance mandibular growth. Implant supported class II elastics can also be used to bring mandible forward.
   c. **Combination:** They are treated by a combination of headgear-FA therapy, e.g. headgear-activator therapy of Teuscher, etc.

B. **In non-growing cases:** Camouflage treatment is given in mild to moderate cases.
   a. **Dental class II:** It can vary from half cusp to full cusp molar relation. Variations can present, e.g. crowding of teeth, proclination of incisors, overjet, etc. which help in deciding the treatment plan and extraction decision. Orthodontic treatment with the extraction of some teeth to create spaces and retraction of teeth to better positions. Upper molar distalization can be done in some cases having mild crowding in upper arch.
   b. **Skeletal class II due to maxillary prognathism:** If severe, then orthognathic surgery is done, e.g. Le Fort I with maxillary set back. In some cases, anterior maxillary osteotomy with set-back can be done. If there is **vertical excess**, then maxilla is displaced upwards and backwards. If there is **vertical deficiency**, then maxilla is displaced downwards and backwards.
   c. **Mandibular retrognathism:** In severe cases, mandibular advancement is done by either segmental osteotomy or BSSO. Genioplasty may be required in some cases. If vertical excess, then AFH anterior facial height can be reduced by removing a chunk of bone in the chin region and bringing chin upwards and forwards. Distraction osteogenesis can be done in mandible to increase the length.

Treatment Objectives of Class II Division 1 (Figs 45.5 to 45.7)

Main objectives of orthodontic treatment are to improve function, esthetics, stability and health of the tissues. Specific objectives for treatment of class II div 1 cases are:

a. Reduction of overjet, reduction of overbite
b. Normalising inter-jaw relation
c. Correction of molar relation to proper intercuspation, e.g. either full class I or full class II.
d. Correction of crowding
e. Normalising the muscular function to help in stability of the results.
f. Improvement of arch width and treatment of crossbite, if any.

Factors to be considered in treating the maxilla: There are five possibilities for the treatment of the maxilla in a class II malocclusion depending on the case:

1. Inhibiting the forward and downward growth of maxilla
2. Inhibiting the forward movement of maxillary teeth
3. Distalization of maxillary denture

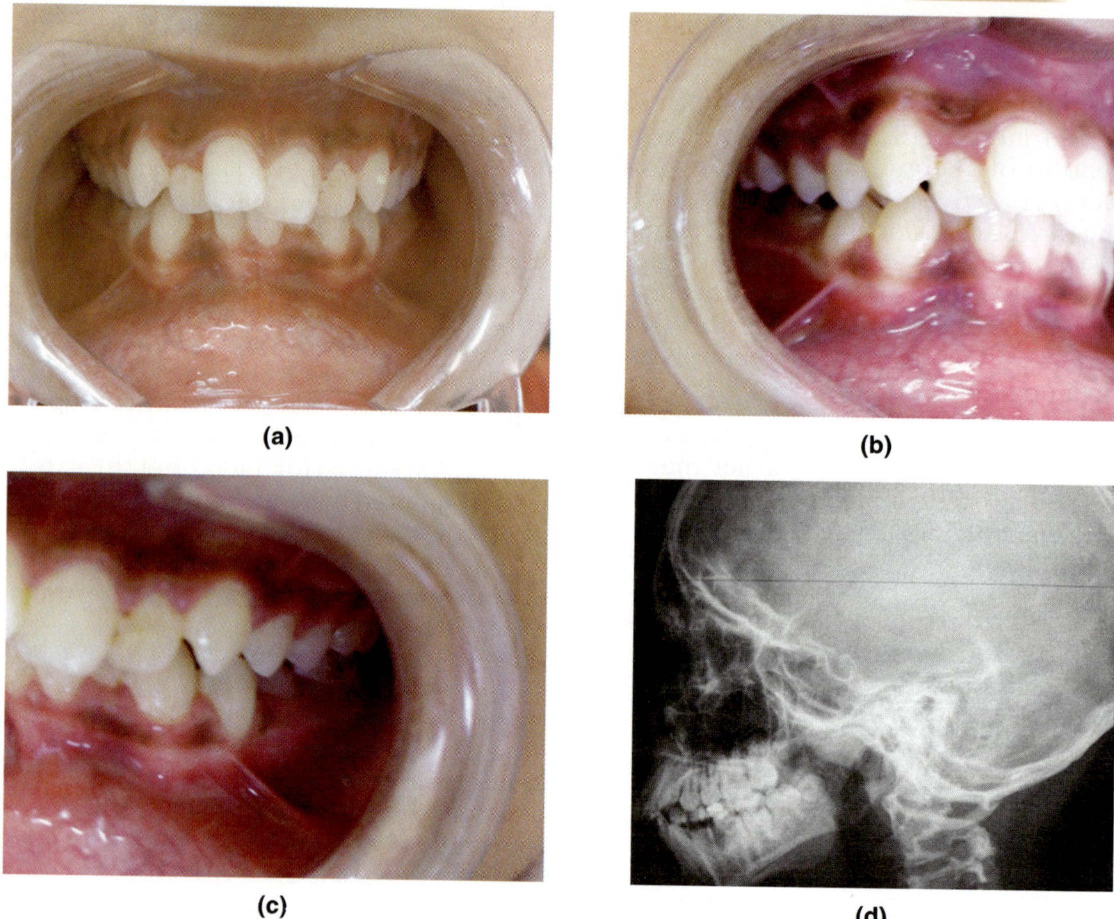

(a) (b) (c) (d)

Figs 45.5a and b: Pre-Rx intraoral photos and the lateral cephalogram.

4. Influencing the eruption pattern of maxillary teeth
5. Camouflage treatment by differential tooth movement using fixed appliances.

Factors to be considered in treating the mandible: Following five possibilities can help in the correction of a class II malocclusion:

1. Stimulating the horizontal growth of the mandible
2. Anterior repositioning of the mandibular body
3. Influencing the eruption pattern of the mandibular teeth
4. Moving the mandibular denture forward on its skeletal base
5. Creating space by selective extractions to allow for the desired tooth movements with fixed appliances.

Maxillary growth modulation by extra-oral orthopedic appliance: In a growing patient especially during mid-mixed dentition period, head gear is used to control abnormal growth of maxilla in D and F direction. It helps to restrict the maxillary growth, while at the same time, the mandible growth catches up. It also helps in restricting the further eruption of the maxillary dentition in D and F direction.

Mandibular growth modulation: During growth phase, the mandible can be repositioned anteriorly with a functional appliance. It helps to achieve skeletal as well as dental effects.

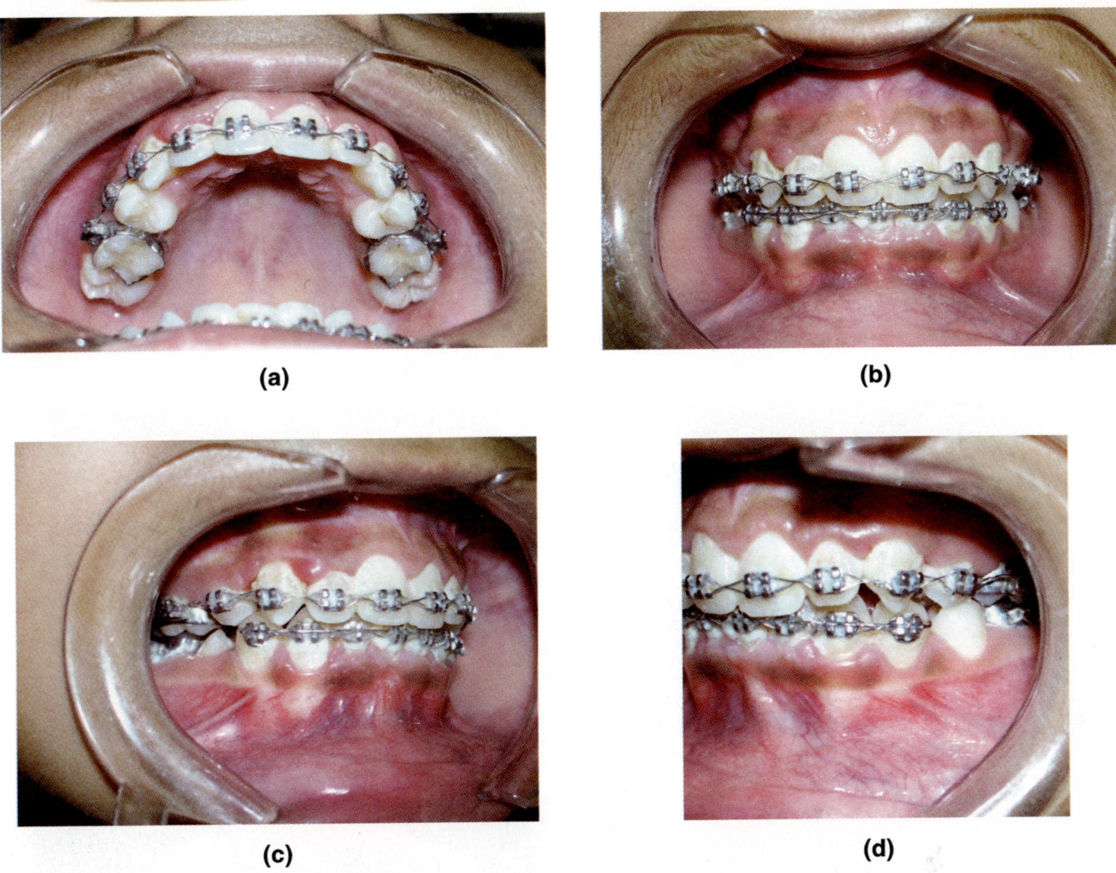

(a) (b) (c) (d)

Figs 45.6a and d: During treatment photos.

Combination, i.e. comprehensive orthopedic approach: If there is severe class II due to presence of both maxillary prognathism and mandibular retrognathism, then combined headgear-activator treatment is given.

In non-growing patients, camouflage treatment is given. Skeletal effects are minimal, but esthetics can be improved with orthodontic treatment. Following variations can be there depending on the case.

a. If lower dental arch is normally aligned, and overjet is increased, then the maxillary first premolars are removed and the anteriors are retracted in the space to reduce the overjet. The molars are maintained in class II relation, and class I canine relations are achieved. It helps to achieve better esthetics, lip competency, decreases the proneness of trauma to upper incisors, and helps in raising self-esteem of the child. It can be done by using either removable or the fixed appliances. But better results are achieved by fixed appliances only because of better control of teeth in 3D.
b. In mild crowding cases and mild proclined incisors cases in upper arch, the upper molars can be distalised to gain space. This process is, however, more effective before the eruption of second molars. But the treatment time and mechanics are increased.
c. If there is crowding in both arches, and lower incisors are also proclined, and increased COS leading to deep bite is there, then all first premolars or upper first with lower second premolars are

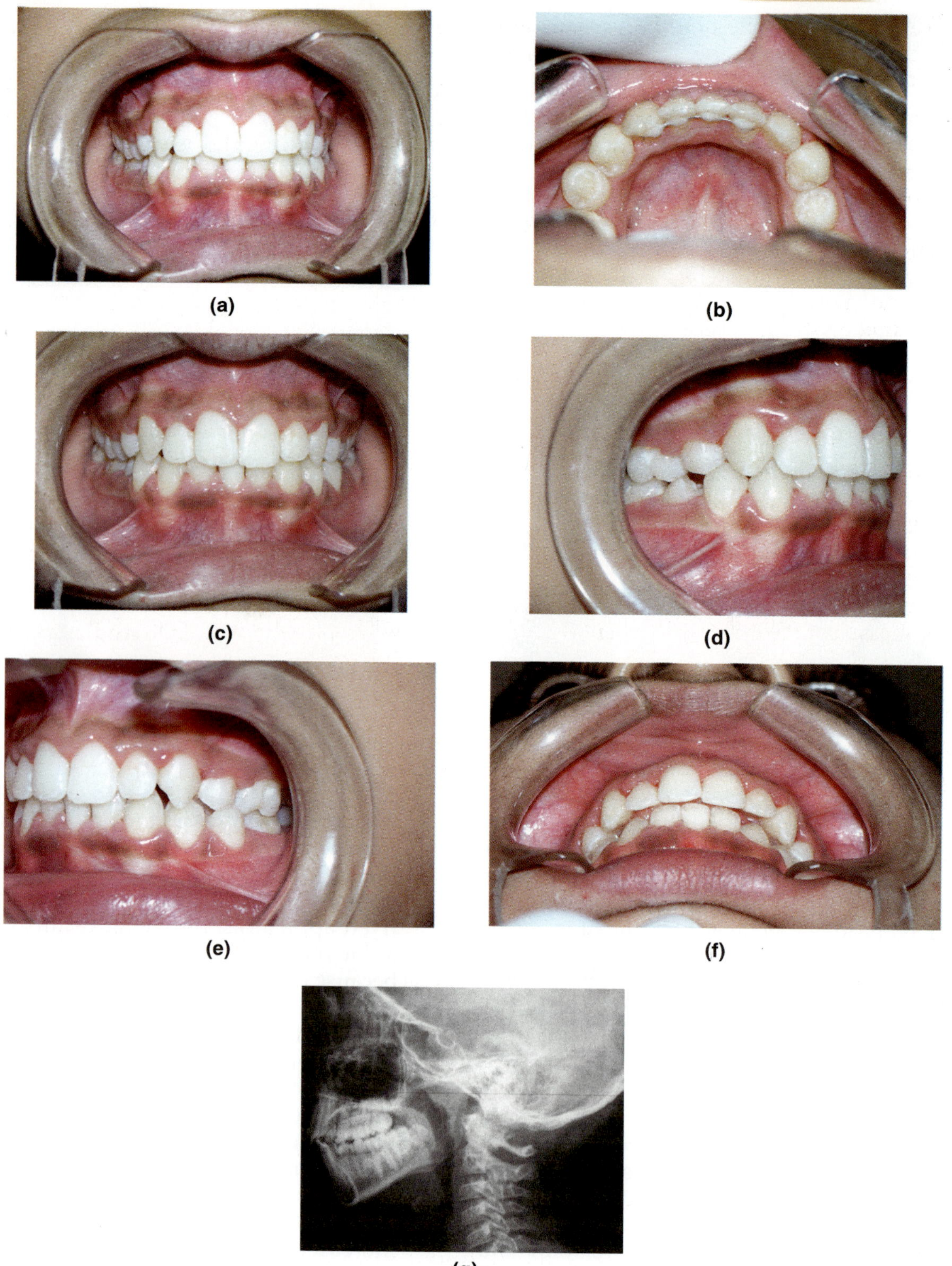

(a) (b) (c) (d) (e) (f) (g)

Figs 45.7a and b: Post-Rx intraoral photos and the lateral cephalogram.

removed and the dental positions are improved, achieving class I molar and canine relations.

Camouflage treatment in mandibular arch: In non-growing cases, the mandibular teeth can be moved in a mesial direction by moving the whole mandibular denture forward along its skeletal base using a functional appliance or with the use of class II elastics to achieve purely dental effects. It can be done with or without extractions, depending on the amount of crowding, deep bite, unstable molar relation, proclination of incisors, etc. The proclination of the mandibular incisors, extrusions of the molars, etc. can be achieved with the use of elastics.

Surgical intervention in maxilla: Severe cases of maxillary prognathism which cannot be treated by simple orthodontics, are treated by orthognathic surgery after the active growth phase is over. It may be anterior segmental with setback or Le Fort I with set back, etc. as per the case requirement.

Surgical intervention in mandible: In severe cases, the surgical option is viable after the active growth of mandible has passed. It is done at around 18 years of age. Various options are available as per the case requirement and choice of the surgeon, e.g. BSSO, segmental advancement; genioplasty with advancement, etc.

Treatment Considerations in Class II Division 2 Malocclusions

In general, class II division 2 malocclusions are easier to correct during the growth period than in adulthood, especially when favourable growth occurs during treatment.

Treatment objectives of class II division 2:

a. Correction of incisor inclination and angulation
b. Correction of overjet and overbite
c. Flattening of curve of Spee
d. Relief of gingival trauma
e. Treatment of crowding, etc.
f. Correction of molar relations

A number of factors need to be considered for these patients.

1. Correction of axial inclination of maxillary incisors. It can be done by 2 approaches, i.e. palatal root torquing of incisors and labial tipping of crowns of incisors. Excessive lingual inclination of maxillary incisors generally locks the mandible and lead to a functional mandibular retrusion. Mandible can be freed either by tipping the maxillary central incisors labially or by placing an anterior bite plate to disarticulate the anterior teeth and allowing the mandible to assume a position dictated by the musculature.

2. Correction of deep bite and exaggerated curve of Spee: To level the dental arches orthodontically, one must either extrude the molars and premolars or intrude the anterior teeth. It can be done by intrusion of upper incisors, or extrusion of lower posterior teeth or a combination of both. Bite plates, arch wires with exaggerated COS and anchor bends, intrusion arches, etc. are used for this purpose.

3. Extraction versus non-extraction. Treatment of class II division 2 malocclusions with a low mandibular plane angle and deep overbite are best managed with a nonextraction approach to avoid retraction of incisors and further labial movement of roots, and protraction of the molars; these movements tend to further deepen the overbite. Due to horizontal growth pattern, the mandibular body is horizontal, the muscles are strong, the trabecular pattern of bone is almost perpendicular to long axis of teeth. In such cases, the mesial movement of buccal teeth to close the spaces is very difficult. Any attempt to close the extraction spaces leads to overretraction of incisors and torque loss.

Even the patient's profile does not allow extraction because these patients have relatively retrusive lips, but prominent chin and nose. Extraction of premolars followed by incisor retraction will further retrude the lips. It worsens the profile and results in an unacceptable "edentulous look."

Before considering the extraction of premolars, there is need to evaluate several factors including the prominence of the nose and chin, nasolabial angle, presence of a functional mandibular retrusion, growth potential and headgear cooperation, extent of tooth size-arch length discrepancy, and the periodontal condition of lower anterior teeth. As a rule, in borderline crowded class II division 2 cases, it is best to start the treatment with a non-extraction approach. It has been seen that the relieving of anterior crowding, flaring of upper incisors unlocks the mandible, which can be redirected forward with the help of class II elastics.

Timing of treatment: Treatment of class II division 2 malocclusion should be initiated in the late mixed dentition. During active growth periods, the functional appliances can be used to correct the skeletal relationship. The incisors are proclined so that overjet is created just like in class II division 1, and then FA can be given to bring mandible forwards. During late growth period, fixed functional appliances should be used to take full advantage of remaining growth.

Retention: Cases with severe skeletal class II discrepancies should be retained with continued use of extraoral forces during the

Summary

Condition	*During growth*	*After growth*
Maxillary prognathism	Headgear class II elastics	Le Fort I with setback; anterior osteotomy with setback
Mandibular retrognathism	Functional appliances;	BSSO with advancement; genioplasty
Combination of above	Combined HG – FA treatment	Combined
Long face		Le Fort I maxillary surgery with upward positioning / impaction; allowing autorotation of mandible; reassess the case for mandibular surgery/genioplasty
Short face		Le Fort I maxillary surgery with downward positioning/ disimpaction; allowing D and B rotation of mandible; reassess the case for mandibular surgery/ genioplasty
Mild crowding in upper arch		Molar distalization
Increased overjet, with well-aligned lower arch		Upper premolar extraction
Upper and lower incisal crowding, proclination		All first premolar extraction
Upper crowding, increased overjet, with mild lower crowding and normally inclined lower anteriors		Upper first and lower second premolar extraction
Class II division 2	Alignment of teeth and FA Rx.	Nonextraction, alignment of teeth and class II elastics

remaining growth period to maintain the maxillary dental and skeletal correction, since the growth can only be restricted or redirected but cannot be completely stopped. It helps to minimize the forward rebound of maxilla due to continuing growth that may occur when the headgear is discontinued. In class II division 2 cases, the retention appliances should be left for a longer period, to allow for the musculature to adapt better. A Hawley retainer with an anterior bite plate should be used (dynamic retention), especially in patients with pre-treatment excessive overbite. Cases treated with fixed appliance with or without extraction need Hawley's appliance, fixed retainer or a combination.

Conclusion

Class II malocclusion is one of the common conditions needing orthodontic treatment. There are various types of this condition which need proper diagnosis and individualised treatment plan. A common treatment plan cannot be applied to every patient. During early treatment, the growth of the patient can be advantageous to achieve better skeletal and dental results. Later on, camouflage treatment is done to achieve improvement of dental condition, soft tissues, profile improvement, etc. In some severe cases having underlying skeletal discrepancy, the orthognathic surgery has to be combined with orthodontic treatment to achieve acceptable results.

46

Treatment of Class III Malocclusion

INTRODUCTION

Angle defined class III malocclusion as the condition in which "the MB cusp of upper first permanent molar lies distal to MB groove of lower first permanent molar". The degree of this relationship can vary from half cusp to full cusp or more. It is also called **mesiocclusion**, because the mandibular molar occludes more mesially than in class I. It is a condition in which the mandibular arch is mesial to maxillary arch. Since Angle's classification is based on dental relationship only and does not consider skeletal relationship, there are many variations in class III condition. Incidence of class III malocclusion is 5–10%. It is more often found in Chinese, Japanese and Koreans.

Classification of Class III Malocclusion

A. Dental and skeletal class III malocclusion
B. Pseudo and true class III malocclusion
C. Skeletal class III malocclusion can be due to
   a. Maxillary hypoplasia/retrognathism
   b. Mandibular excess/prognathism
   c. Combination of both.

Dental class III: According to Angle, the MB cusp of upper first permanent molar lies distal to MB groove of lower first permanent molar.

Skeletal class III: It is due to discrepancy in the relation of upper and lower jaw bases, where mandible is related mesially/anteriorly to maxilla as compared to normal class I relation.

Pseudo-class III: Here, the mandible shows a forward path of closure due to prematurities in incisal region, and assumes a class III molar and skeletal relation with maxilla. When examined asking the patient to stop at first point of contact during slow closure, the exact relation of molars and skeletal bases can be accurately examined. In early stages of development, it is class I/normal relation.

True class III: There is no anterior path of closure, but the relation of molars or skeletal bases is class III.

Clinical Features of Class III (Figs 46.1 and 46.2)

1. A class III molar relationship
2. Class III canine relations
3. Incisors can be in a normal overjet; edge-to-edge bite; or crossbite relation.
4. Upper arch is generally short and narrow, which may contribute to anterior and/or posterior crossbite.
5. Lower arch is long and wide. It contributes to posterior crossbite relation, because the wider posterior part of lower arch comes to lie in relation to narrow middle segment of upper arch.
6. Concave profile, and chin prominence
7. There may be crowding in upper arch. Lower arch may show crowding if incisors are in normal overjet relation. The lower incisors in such cases are lingually tilted and thus occupy less arch space and hence get crowded.
8. Lower incisors may not be crowded if they lie in anterior crossbite relation, as then they occupy larger arch space. In

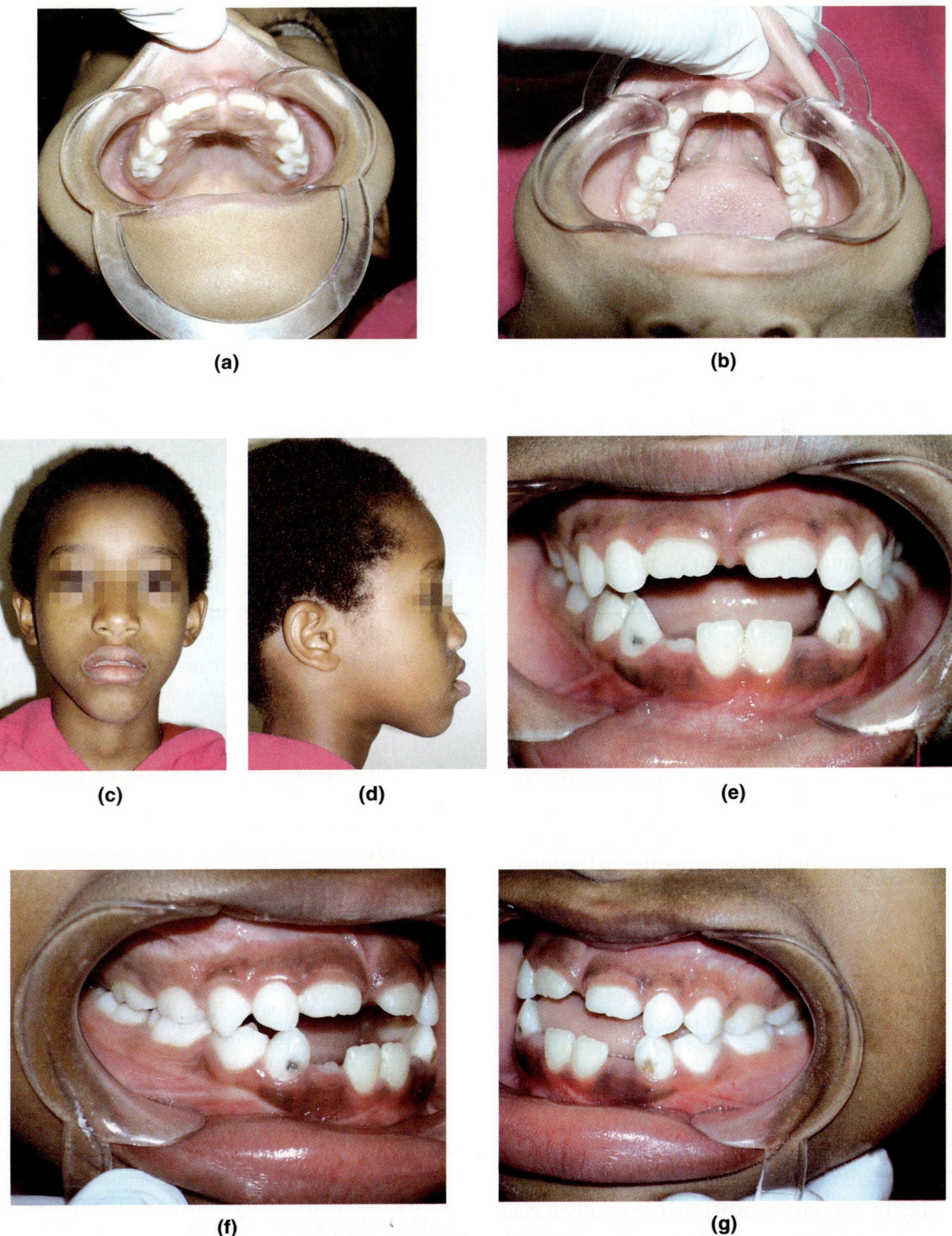

Figs 46.1a to g: Skeletal class III in mixed dentition period due to maxillary deficiency, anterior open bite, concave profile and anterior crossbite relation, obscured by anterior open bite.

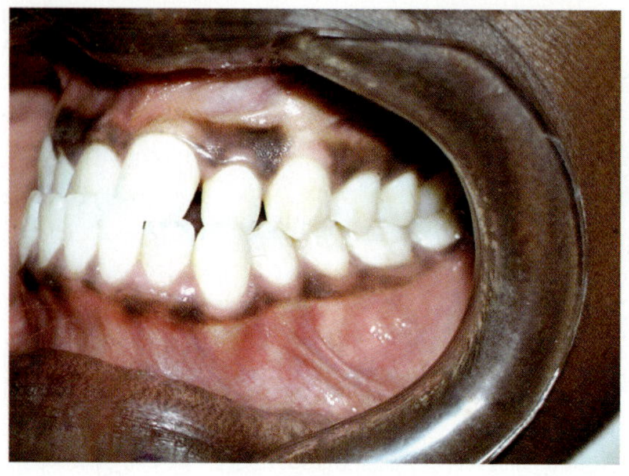

(a)

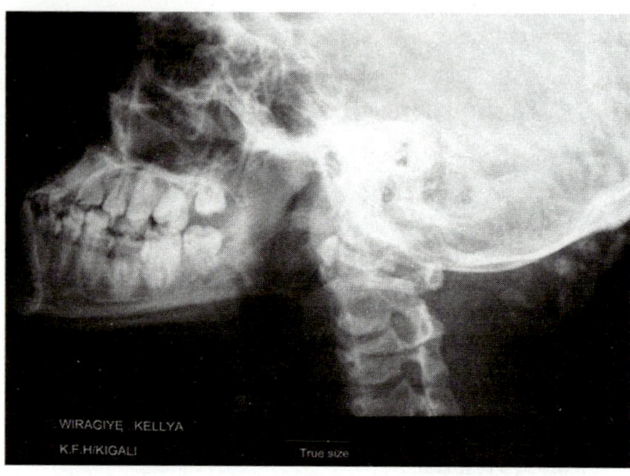

(b)

Figs 46.2a and b: Anterior crossbite, skeletal class III relation, and class III molar and canine relations, due to mandibular prognathism.

such a case, the lower incisors are well aligned under the moulding action of lower lip (if upper incisal arch is also aligned).

9. If mandible is large or maxilla is small, with an increased negative overjet, the lower incisors get lingually tilted under lower lip force in a compensatory position to come closer to upper incisors, in an attempt to reduce the negative overjet. Crowding may also appear.
10. Anterior open bite is seen in vertical growth cases. It has a racial predilection and genetic effect also.
11. **Pseudo-class III:** This is a condition where due to prematurities in the incisor region, the mandible has a forward path of closure and thus closes in a forward position/anterior crossbite relation during the centric occlusion. It should be treated as early as possible during the early age. If it is left unattended, then the mandible may overgrow maxilla and become a true skeletal class III relation. A proper overbite and overjet should be achieved as they provide an anterior stop to excessive abnormal mandibular growth.
12. In **primary dentition:** Generally a class III relation is rare in primary dentition stage. It is because the mandible growth lags behind that of maxillary growth in initial years (cephalocaudal gradient of growth). In primary dentition, the mandible growth is less. From a dental point of view, a **mesial step** may be present in some children which is an indication of future class III relation. These kids should be regularly monitored and timely interceptive treatment should be given to prevent development or increasing the severity of this condition.
13. In children during **mixed dentition:** The mesial step relation of primary second molars generally always leads to development of class III molar relation of permanent teeth during transition of dentition. It is aided by more E-space and leeway space in lower arch and more growth of mandible (as there is cephalocaudal gradient of growth) as compared to maxilla. Mixed dentition period is the right time of interceptive treatment in these patients to control and redirect the abnormal growth.

Skeletal feature of class III: A class III problem is generally found to be associated with skeletal problem. Skeletal class III occurs mostly due to heredity. Different components of skeletal class III are (Fig. 46.2):

a. **Maxillary retrognathism/deficiency:** Maxilla may be normal in size but is placed backwards due to abnormal relation of anterior and middle cranial bases (increased saddle angle). Or it may be deficient due to deficient maxillary growth.

b. **Mandibular prognathism/overgrowth:** Mandible is placed forward due to decreased saddle angle leading to mandibular prognathism, or its length has increased due to an abnormal increased growth.
c. **Combination of above:** These are most severe cases as the both jaws are involved.

Etiology

1. True class III cases with skeletal problem are genetic.
2. Pseudo-class III is due to incisal prematurities. But if it is not treated at an earliest, it gets converted in true skeletal problem with continued/unchecked growth of mandible.
3. Class III molar relation is also seen, if there is premature loss of teeth mesial to lower first permanent molars and their resultant mesial drifting. These are dental class III malocclusion as defined by Angle's classification.
4. Deficient growth of maxilla
5. Growth problem of cranial bases
6. Hormonal problem, e.g. hyperpituitarism, where mandible growth is excessive
7. Congenital conditions, e.g. Crouzon syndrome, CLP, anchondroplasia, etc.
8. Cleft palate and lip cases, where maxillary growth is generally deficient. If untreated, then mandibular growth overshoots causing mandibular prognathism also.
9. Improper surgically treated CLP where the damage to premaxilla; scarring on upper lip providing a restricting effect on maxillary growth, etc. lead to skeletal class III.

Diagnosis: Diagnosis is done by taking proper history, clinical examination, cephalometrics radiological examination, etc. The dental, skeletal, true or pseudo-class III conditions should be properly diagnosed so as to plan an appropriate treatment. Growth status of the patient is important to be considered as it influences the treatment planning and should be properly evaluated. Growth pattern of the patient also affects the treatment mechanics and direction of applied forces.

Growth of the Maxilla and Mandible

Endochondral growth of the cranial base (due to synchondroses) pushes the maxilla forward leading to its passive displacement. Also, the active growth in maxillary sutures is responsible for its growth. As maxilla is translated downward and forward, bone is added at the sutures and in tuberosity area posteriorly. Surface remodeling removes bone from its anterior surfaces. For this reason, the amount of forward movement of anterior surfaces is less than the amount of displacement. In roof of the mouth, bone is added, while bone is resorbed from nasal floor by surface remodeling. So the total downward movement of palatal vault is greater than the amount of displacement. The jaw bones follow the growth spurts at different ages when the amount of growth increases. The active growth spurt is the best time to intercept the problem. Understanding of the growth sequence of maxilla and mandible is important for treatment planning by dentofacial orthopedic means.

Growth of maxilla in sagittal plane: In the first years of life, the maxilla is displaced bodily under the influence of the growth of frontal lobe of brain which pushes frontal bone forward, and hence maxilla which is attached to frontal bone; growth of cartilages in cranial base; nasal capsule and median septal cartilage.

From age 4–10 years, maxilla moves forward with anterior cortex of frontal bone, pressure from nasal cartilage and median septal cartilage. Forces from facial soft tissues, tongue pressure on palatal vault and occlusal forces on upper arch also contribute to the growth of maxilla in anterolateral dimension due to activity in circummaxillary sutures. At 11–12 years, growth of maxilla occurs by remodeling of external cortices.

Vertical growth: During first few years of life, maxilla moves down by the growth of eyeball upto 3–4 years of age, and soft tissue forces from the lower parts. Later on, it occurs by downward movement of palatal vault; floor of sinuses; and alveolar growth.

Transverse plane: Upto 4–5 years, transverse growth of maxilla occurs by development of nasal capsule and pterygoid plates. Activity in midpalatal suture also leads to increased width. After 7–10 years of age, maxillary width increases by growth of maxillary sinus and displacement of their lateral walls. It is also aided by pressure of tongue and masticatory forces transmitted to upper teeth.

Mandibular growth occurs by both endochondral proliferation at condyle and remodeling of bone surfaces. Mandible is translated downward and forward by the growth of muscles and other adjacent soft tissues, and the addition of new bone occurs at condyles in response to these soft tissue changes. The maxilla and mandible grow in all three planes of space, in the following sequence: width, length, and then height. In both sexes, growth in vertical height of the face continues longer than growth in length, with the late vertical growth occurring primarily in the mandible.

Treatment of Class III Malocclusion

Rationale of treatment: Class III malocclusion should be diagnosed and treated as early as possible due to following reasons.

a. Early detection of the developing conditions helps to intercept and restrict the abnormal growth of the jaw bases and hence reduces the severity of the condition.
b. It helps to provide more favorable environment for the future growth of jaws.
c. To provide good facial esthetics
d. To provide a psychological advantage to patient
e. To improve occlusal function
f. To achieve good soft tissue balance; to modify soft tissue functional matrix for normalizing future growth.
g. Maxillary deficiency may present as anterior cross bite. It further leads to deficient growth of maxilla as it is locked anteriorly by mandible and hence does not grow to its full potential.
h. When mandible is overgrown, then there is no anterior stop for its growth (which is generally provided by maxilla), hence its continued growth leads to increased severity of the condition.
i. Pseudo-class III condition due to incisor prematurity, if not treated timely, may convert to a true skeletal problem due to continued unchecked growth of mandible.

Treatment during Active Growth Period

As discussed above, the class III condition is generally a skeletal problem which may represent as maxillary deficiency; mandibular excess; or a combination of both. An early diagnosis and treatment helps to prevent increased severity of the condition due to ensuing growth. These skeletal problems require interceptive procedures during growth phase, to intercept abnormal growth with the help of dentofacial orthopedic procedures. The best time to start the treatment of such problems is around 8–9 years age, because this time maxilla is growing actively in transverse and sagittal directions due to the starting prepubertal growth spurts. Timely treatment helps to achieve skeletal effects. Following appliances are used depending on the condition:

a. For mild maxillary deficiency, growth modification can be done with myofunctional appliances, like FR 3; reverse activator or bionator; class III twin block, etc.

b. For treatment of moderate maxillary deficiency, growth modification can be done with dentofacial orthopedic appliances, e.g. reverse face mask to protract the maxilla in D and F direction. Since maxillary width is also less, so RME appliance is also used to expand the maxilla. A phase of RME before initiating face mask therapy is beneficial since it helps to activate the circum-maxillary sutures system and thus the pull by face mask on maxilla is prompted. Details can be studied in Chapter 30 on Dentofacial Orthopedics.

c. For controlling overgrowing mandible, chin cup with HPHG is used for growth redirection, with the forces directed in U & B direction. It should be kept in mind that high forces for 12–16 hours per day for approx 1 year or till the condition is controlled are to be used. Also, since mandible keeps on growing till 18 years of age, this condition needs active retention phase with night time use of chin cup appliance till the active mandibular growth ceases. Otherwise it may lead to relapse. Details can be studied in Chapter 30 on Dentofacial Orthopedics.

d. **Vesco Protraction Units for rapid skeletal protraction of the maxilla and midface:** Vesco Protraction Units are a set of lip-pad attachments and molar tubes, which are passed through the rectangular base arch wire in maxillary fixed appliance. These maxillary lip pads relieve restrictive forces of upper lip on anterior maxilla. The elastic are attached from these pads to the reverse face mask to apply a pulling force on the maxillary arch. Also, these reverse-pull elastics create a labial root torque transmitted to maxillary incisors which prevents their proclination during maxillary protraction.

Vesco Protraction Unit includes a pair of an acrylic labial pad, a wire framework and a 0.018" × 0.025" buccal tube. It is used with stainless steel rectangular archwire in the upper fixed appliance (0.016" × 0.022" for 0.018" slot and 0.018" × 0.025" for 0.022" slot brackets). The buccal tubes allow easy positioning along the arch wire and excellent stability after crimping (Fig. 46.3).

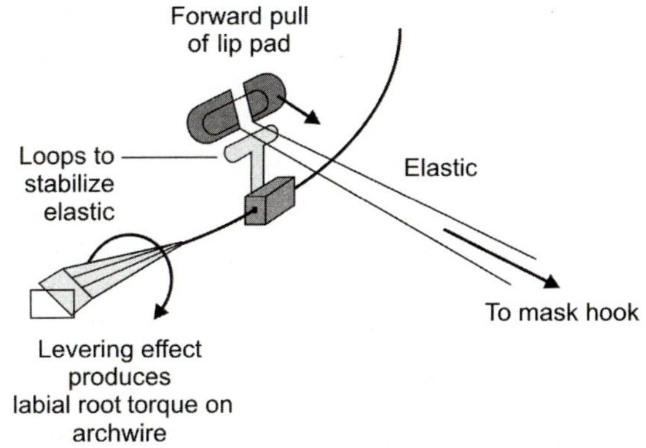

Fig. 46.3: Vesco Protraction Units *(Courtesy: Internet for academic purpose).*

Advantages

- Incisors torque control is automatically activated when the face mask elastic are placed on Vesco Protraction Unit.
- Lip pads shield lip musculature against maxillary arch.
- Maxillary protraction from anterior segment prevents molar extrusion.
- It can also be used to align dental midlines or to open space for cuspids, etc.
- It can be used to provide maxillary protraction and fixed orthodontic treatment/finishing with one appliance.

e. **Modified tandem appliance (MTA)** described by Klempner in 2003 for class III patients with mild skeletal midfacial deficiencies can be used for better patient cooperation.

Appliance design: The MTA has three components, one fixed and two removable. The upper appliance is a fixed maxillary expander, with or without palatal acrylic, or a

Nance appliance, which is placed with bands on permanent first molars. Buccal arms are soldered to be used for elastic traction. The lower appliance is a well retained removable acrylic plate with posterior occlusal coverage. The headgear tubes are embedded in the area of lower first molars to receive inner arm of 0.045" facebow, while the outer arms of face bow are bent in the form of hooks to attach traction elastics.

Lower midline expansion screw can be used in some cases. Heavy orthopedic elastics (400 g per side) are placed from the soldered buccal hooks in upper arch to the facebow which applies the protraction force to the maxilla for 14–16 hours per day.

Treatment of crossbite: Treatment of crossbite in both anterior and posterior segments is important for coordination of upper and lower arches, and for occlusal settling. Details of treatment can be studied in the Chapter 43 dedicated to crossbite, with a brief discussion here.

Mild anterior crossbite can be treated with upper Hawley appliance with Z-spring or expansion screw opening in anterior direction to bring incisors out of crossbite. Posterior bite plane is incorporated in the appliance to open the occlusion in anterior region so that the movement is not restricted by lower incisors.

Mild posterior crossbite is treated with transverse expansion. It can be done by fixed appliances, like NiTi palatal expander, quad helix, RME, etc. or by removable split plate type expansion appliance.

Pseudo-class III treatment: In such cases, there are incisal premature contacts which lead to forward path of closure of mandible during centric occlusion. In mild cases, the prematurities may be removed by grinding. A maxillary appliance with Z-spring and posterior bite plate helps to push upper incisors labially and brings them out of crossbite. It helps in proper closure of mandible, and provides a positive anterior stop to abnormal growth of mandible.

Fixed orthodontic appliance (Figs 46.4 to 46.7): It is used in patients with mild class III problems with anterior crossbite having dental compensation; mild pseudo-class III relation; and uncooperative patients. The composite stops or posterior bite plane can be placed on molars to open the occlusion anteriorly. The expanded and extended arch

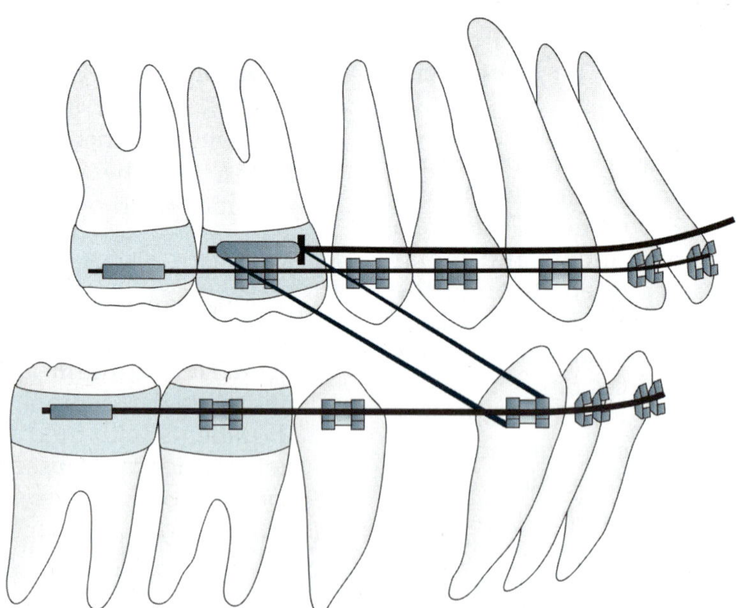

Fig. 46.4: Class III elastics to move the lower anteriors posteriorly.

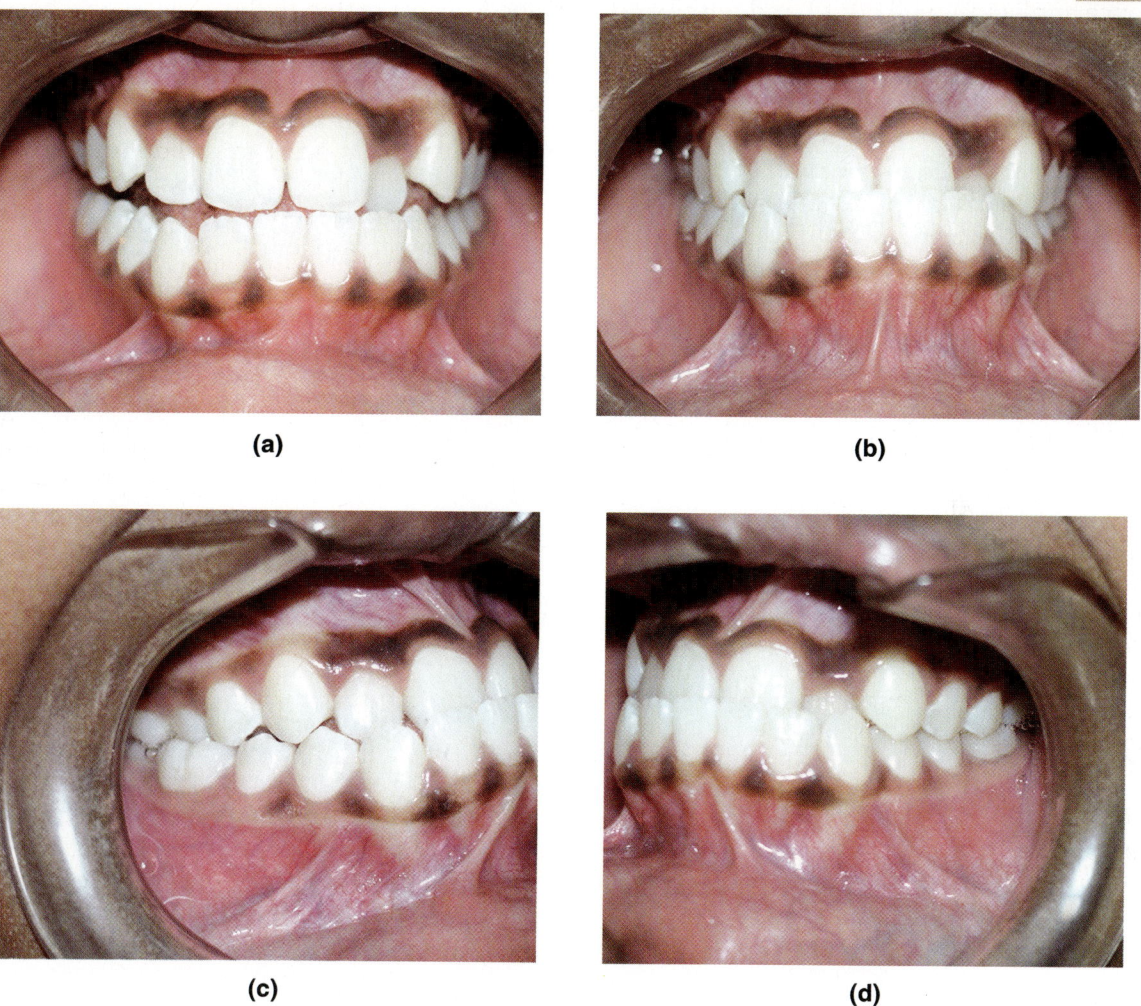

(a) (b) (c) (d)

igs 46.5a to d: Pre-Rx intraoral photos. She has a mild maxillary deficiency. See anterior crossbite due to
›rward path of closure.

ʼires are used to move the upper incisors
ıbially. Proper use of class III elastics can help
ı reciprocal movements of upper and lower
ːeth (Fig. 46.4).

ʼecision for Requirement of Extractions

ʼamouflage treatment: In mild cases of
‹eletal discrepancy having class III maloc-
.usion, generally fixed appliance is used to
rovide camouflage treatment. The lower first
remolars are removed and the lower
ıteriors are retracted to treat the crossbite
ɔndition. If there is crowding in upper arch also, then either first or the second premolars can be removed. Class III elastics are used to protract the upper teeth and retract the lower teeth. But if the retraction of lower teeth leads to relative chin prominence, then genioplasty can be considered.

Surgical treatment: However, if surgery is needed, then the extraction choice is different. Surgery is done in severe cases of skeletal discrepancy. Such cases generally have compensatory incisal positions. The upper incisors are proclined while lower incisors are retroclined under the force of tongue and

(a)

(b)

(c)

(d)

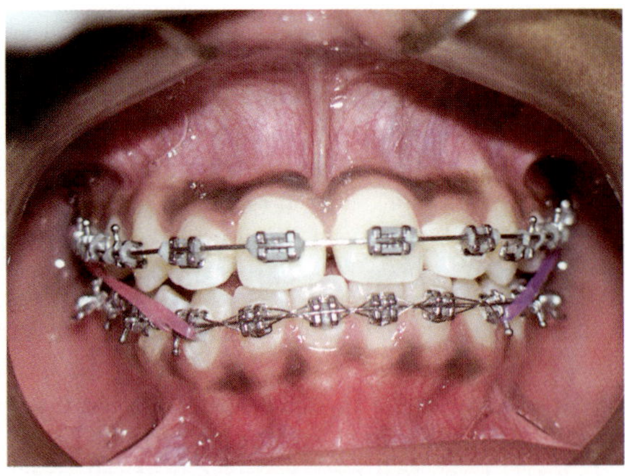

(e)

Figs 46.6a to e: During treatment photos. Class III elastics are used to achieve normal incisal relation.

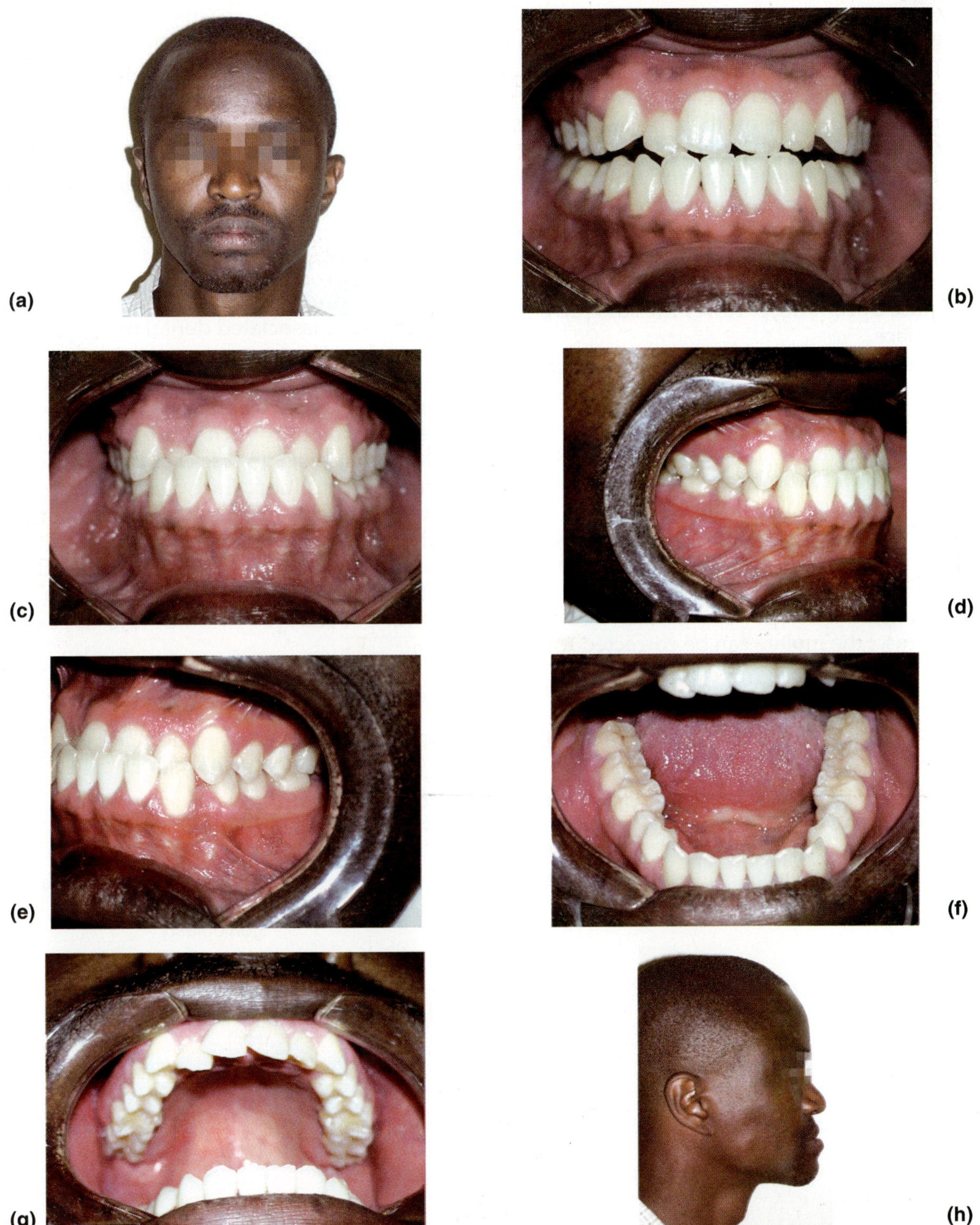

Figs 46.7a to h: Photos showing a case of skeletal class III due to mandibular prognathism, luckily the discrepancy is not very big. It can be treated by camouflage treatment by flaring the upper incisors to correct the anterior crossbite.

lower lip. It is a natural attempt to bring upper and lower incisors toward each other in a stable relationship and to reduce the extent of negative overjet. In such case, there is need to upright the incisors on their respective basal bones. When this is done, the actual skeletal discrepancy and extent of anterior cross bite becomes evident, showing the exact severity of the condition. To upright the upper incisors, upper first premolars are removed, while lower arch may not need extractions because uprighting of lower incisors provides the space.

Treatment of class III after growth phase: Surgery is needed to treat moderate to severe skeletal discrepancy.

a. For treating maxillary deficiency, the Le Fort I osteotomy with maxillary advancement is done.
b. For treating mandibular excess, mandibular set back is done either by BSSO or by segmental setback after removal of first premolars. In former case, the molars can be corrected to class I relation, while in later case, the molars are maintained in class III relation.
c. Genioplasty may be needed in some cases to provide chin contouring and to reduce chin prominence.
d. If there is combination of skeletal problems of both jaws, then both jaws surgery is done.

Conclusion

Class III condition is mainly a skeletal problem with associated dental malpositions, which arise due to compensatory changes. Interception of a developing class III problem during active growth phase helps to achieve skeletal correction with dentofacial orthopedic appliances; and prevents the increase in severity of condition. Early interception also helps to improve psychological status of the child. Once the growth period is missed, then only options available is either camouflage treatment in mild cases, or orthognathic surgical procedures in moderate to severe cases.

Summary

Condition	*Treatment during growth period*	*Surgery after growth completion*
Maxillary hypoplasia or retrognathism	Myofunctional appliances; reverse face mask, etc. appliances	Le Fort surgery with advancement
Mandibular prognathism	Chin cup with HPHG	BSSO with mandibular set back; with/without genioplasty
Combination	Combination of above appliances	Bimaxillary surgeries
Mild dental class III	Camouflage treatment with removable or fixed appliances; class III elastics	
Pseudo-class III	Relieve prematurities; relieve anterior crossbite;	
Maxillary arch constriction	RME; SME; expanded archwires	

47

Oral Habits

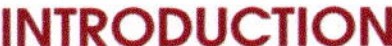

INTRODUCTION

Growth and development of dentocraniofacial complex depends on the strong interaction of various factors and tissues. Genetics, diet and drugs, hormones, pressure and balance of soft tissues, etc. have been found to affect the growth and development. Oral habits have a definite effect on the development of occlusion. During the period of growth, children have a tendency to acquire certain habits which may be temporary or permanent, and may be harmful to the occlusal development. So, the knowledge of diagnosing and treating a habit is important for every clinician so as to avoid or intercept the developing malocclusion or for proper timely referral to the specialist.

Definition

Habit has been defined as the tendency or an act, which has become relatively fixed, a repeated performance and is consistent and easy to perform by the patient.

In other words, a habit is defined as an – "autonomic response to a situation acquired normally as the result of repetition and learning, strictly applicable only to motor responses".

Patient may develop habits initially as a conscious act, which if left unchecked, may develop in semiconscious or unconscious acts. The treatment of habits in younger age is easier, but as the age increases, the neuromuscular patterns become matured and it becomes difficult or almost impossible to retrain or break those neuromuscular patterns.

Effects of habits on dentofacial complex is mainly determined by a combination of three factors, i.e. intensity, duration and frequency. It is mainly the pressure which is exerted by the tissues under the influence of habit which leads to maldevelopment. Klein in 1952 classified the pressure as follows.

CLASSIFICATION OF PRESSURE: KLEIN 1952

I. Intentional Pressure (Planned Pressures)

A. Orthodontic treatment appliances
B. Myofunctional therapy
C. Intentional head deformation (in some races)
D. Giraffe-necks of the Padaung women
E. Chinese custom of foot binding (to keep feet small size)
F. Reshaping horns of cattle.

II. Unintentional Pressure (Abnormal Pressure Habits)

A. Intrinsic Pressure Habits (within the Mouth)

1. Thumb sucking
2. Finger sucking
3. Tongue sucking
4. Lip sucking
5. Cheek sucking
6. Blanket sucking
7. Nail biting
8. Lip biting
9. Tongue biting
10. Tongue thrusting

11. Macroglossia, overgrowth of the tongue
12. Incorrect swallowing, anesthesia throat
13. Mouth breathing.

B. Extraneous (Extrinsic) Abnormal Pressure Habits (Face)

1. Chin propping
2. Face leaning on hand
3. Abnormal pillowing, positions, leaning on forearm or hand
4. Habitually sleeping on right side of face may cause the nose to turn leftward or vice versa; a deflected septum may also result from this sleeping habit.

C. Functional Pressures

1. Bowlegged cowboy (sprung legs)
2. Warping bones of the foot by wearing shoes that do not fit properly
3. Narrowing the external auditory meatus on one side by sleeping on that side of the head more than on the other
4. Flattening of an infant's head by laying infant habitually in one position for prolonged periods. To avoid it, the position of baby should be changed infants frequently.
5. Flattened Indian skulls, base of skull mushroomed over spinal column caused by carrying heavy loads on their heads throughout their lifetime.
6. Malocclusion frequently developed in musicians (playing flute, trumpet, etc.) from pressure exerted on their teeth or face.
7. Kyphosis or round shoulders common among dentists, school children, tailors, cobblers, carpenters, and laborers, caused by occupational pressures/positions.
8. A bent and sometimes notched breastbone of chickens and turkeys that roost in trees from the pressure exerted
9. Spinal curvature can result from abnormal sleeping positions and postural irregularities.

"Anesthesia throat" (from Klein, 1952): "Anesthesia throat" is a term coined by Stenson to describe a throat with no sensory nerve supply and is immune to sensation. The individual has no normal impulse to swallow. There is no gagging sensation on touching the uvula, soft palate, velum, or any other trigger point in throat. In order to swallow, the patient must seize the tongue between the anterior teeth and, by a series of muscular contortions involving even the face, perform the act of deglutition.

Various habits: In orthodontics, we generally see and treat some of the following pressure habits for correction of malocclusion.

- Thumb sucking and digit sucking
- Tongue thrusting
- Lip sucking
- Bruxism
- Lip biting, cheek biting and nail biting
- Mouth breathing
- Abnormal swallowing habits
- Speech defects
- Pshychogenic habits.

All these habits are functional aberrations which disturb the normal balance of circumoral tissues, and produce abnormal forces on surrounding tissues. These forces are capable of bringing about a permanent deformity in the developing musculoskeletal unit. Deformity developed by a habit depends upon the triad of factors, viz. **intensity, duration and frequency**.

Classification of habits:

Habits can be classified as:

1. Useful/harmful; By William James, 1923
2. Empty/meaningful; by Earnest Klien (1971)
3. Pressure/nonpressure/biting
4. Compulsive/non-compulsive; by Finn and Sim (1975)
   - **Useful habits:** These are those acts which are considered essential for normal function, e.g. proper tongue positioning, swallowing, etc.

- **Harmful habits:** They have a deleterious effect on the dentofacial structures, e.g. tongue thrusting, thumb sucking, etc.
- **Unintentional/empty habits** (meaningless habit, which has no need for support); these habits are not associated with any psychological problems.
- **Intentional/meaningful habits:** These habits have a definite psychological connection.
- **Pressure habits:** These are those sucking habits which apply pressure on the teeth and supporting tissues thus leading to malocclusion, e.g. tongue thrusting, thumb sucking, etc.
- **Non-pressure habits:** Habits which do not apply direct forces on the teeth and supporting tissues, e.g. mouth breathing.
- **Biting habits:** Habits like nail biting or lip biting.
- **Masochistic habits:** These habits lead to tissue damage as incurred by the patient himself, e.g. scraping of gingival tissues with nails or pins, hair pulling, etc.
- **Compulsive habits:** They are the deep rooted habits which the child does when he feels that his security is in danger or when he feels unsafe. The anxiety level of child is high and it may have a psychological connection.
- **Non-compulsive habits:** These are those habits which are easily learned and dropped as the child matures. No abnormal response results from attempt to restrain this habit.

According to cause of the habit:

- **Physiological habits**—those required for normal physiologic function e.g. nasal breathing, suckling during infancy.
- **Pathological habits**—those that are pursued due to varied reasons, e.g. mouth breathing due to DNS.

According to origin of the habit:

- **Retained habits:** These are carried over from childhood to adulthood.
- **Cultivated habits:** Those that are cultivated during socioactive life of an individual.

According to awareness to the habit:

- **Unconscious habits:** They are sustained by unconscious behavior, simple attenuation of sensory feedback mechanism and in cessation.
- **Conscious habits:** They involve choice or need, making the treatment difficult and complex.

Classification by Kingsley (1956)

1. Functional: Mouth breathing
2. Muscular: Tongue thrusting, cheek or lip biting
3. Combined muscular: Digit sucking
4. Postural: Chin propping.

Etiology

Various causes have been proposed for abnormal habits:

1. **Anatomical:** For example, posture of tongue. Infantile swallow occurs due to large tongue in small oral cavity coupled with anterior open bite in the gum pads region.
2. **Mechanical interferences:** If permanent incisors are erupted forward with increased overjet and lip incompetency, then while swallowing to achieve the vacuum, the child may thrust his tongue forward to make a seal with upper lip. Also, the mouth breathing may result due to incompetent lips and loss of lip seal.
3. **Pathological:** Pathologies also lead to development of abnormal habits as they interfere with normal functions, e.g. tonsillitis, DNS, hypertrophy of inferior nasal turbinates, etc. interfere with normal breathing and lead to mouth breathing. Increased size of adenoids pushes the tongue forward and downward, thus disturbing the normal balance.
4. Emotional
5. Imitation
6. Random behavior.

In the following section, we have described some of the habits in detail.

THUMB AND DIGIT SUCKING

It is defined as the placement of thumb or digits in the oral cavity in varying positions or depth. It is one of the most common habits seen in children. However, it has also been seen in the intrauterine life for some children. Till, 3½ to 4 years of age, it is considered normal, as there is a change in swallowing and eating patterns of the child. Sucking reflex is seen in oral stage of development and disappears during 1–3.5 years. But if it persists, after that age, it is a cause of concern as it may lead to maldevelopment. According to Moyers, repeated and forceful sucking of thumb is associated with strong buccal and lip contractions, causing abnormal pressures on the teeth and bones.

Two forms of digit sucking habits have been described as nutritive form and non-nutritive form.

Psychology of non-nutritive sucking: A number of theories have been described to explain the development of the digit sucking.

1. **Psychoanalytical theory of psychosexual development** (by Sigmund Freud): It is also called Freudian theory. According to this theory, a child passes through various stages of psychological development during early life. Here, oral and anal phases are seen in the first 3 years of life. The oral cavity acts like an oro-erotic zone. The child has a tendency to place his fingers or any object he holds to put in the mouth. Prevention of such an act may result in emotional insecurity, and may lead the child to acquire any other habit.
2. **Learning theory:** According to Palermo, 1956, the sucking is merely a learned pattern with no underlying cause or psychological connections.
3. **Oral drive theory:** Sears and Wise 1960 proposed that prolonged suckling may lead to thumb sucking.
4. **Benjamin's rooting reflex theory:** 1962 According to this concept, the rooting or placing reflexes in infants lead to development of thumb sucking habits. Rooting reflex is the movement of head of the infant towards an object touching his cheeks. Like during feeding, the mother touches her breast to the cheek of child who then moves to suckle the milk. This reflex generally persists up to 7–8 months of age.
5. **Oral gratification theory:** Sheldon 1932.
6. **Psychological aspects:** Sucking habit has also been linked to the psychological insecurity in children who are deprived of the parental love and care.

Phases of Development

Phase I: This is normal and clinically non-significant sucking. It is generally seen in first 3 years of life and considered normal. It itself terminates during that period.

Phase II: If the habit persists beyond 3 years of age, it is considered as clinically significant sucking habit. This phase extends from 3–6½ years of age. If not controlled, it leads to abnormal development of occlusion and growth. It may be an indication of great anxiety of the child. Treatment should be started to disrupt the habit.

Phase III: It is the phase of intractable sucking. The habit may have a psychological connection, and a psychologist should be consulted during this phase. Persistence of habit leads to maldevelopment, the longer the habit, more are the problems, and it becomes more difficult to control the habit with increasing age. So, "the earlier the better" should be the motto to control the habit.

Classification of thumb sucking (by Subtleny, et al, 1973): It is depending on the length of thumb insertion in the oral cavity.

1. Group I: Thumb inserted above the first joint and occupies large area of hard palate vault pressing against palatal mucosa and alveolar tissue. Lower incisors press out the thumb.

2. Group II: Thumb extended up to the first joint or just anterior to it. No palatal contact; there is contact only with maxillary and mandibular anteriors.
3. Group III: Thumb as in Group I, but without contact with mandibular incisors.
4. Group IV: Thumb did not progress appreciably into mouth. Lower incisors made contact approximately at level of thumb nail.

Effects of digit sucking: Severity of malocclusion depends on the trident of factors, i.e. duration, frequency and intensity of factors. The effects of digit sucking depend on the level of insertion of the digit, the force of sucking; the length of habit; and the direction of forces. The main effects appear due to disturbance in the balance of intraoral and extraoral forces, due to disturbance of **buccinator mechanism**, i.e. loss of equilibrium of tongue and circumoral forces (Figs 47.1 to 47.3).

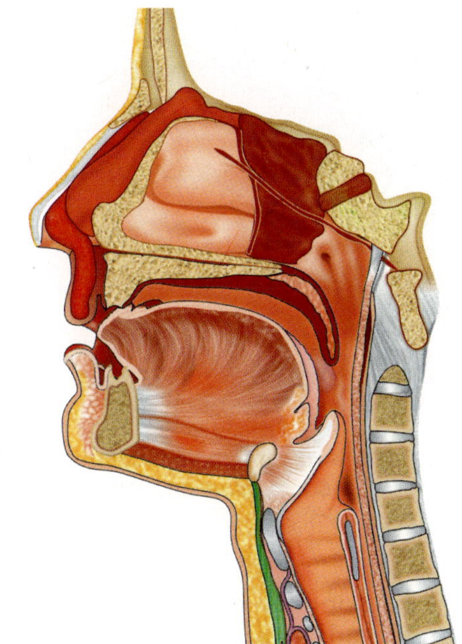

Fig. 47.1: Normal anatomical features of oral cavity.

With the thumb in the mouth, it pushes the tongue downwards and lips are pursed around the thumb. The cheek muscles and modiolus get hyperactivated, applying abnormal force on the buccal surfaces of teeth. Since there is no opposing force of tongue, the buccal forces lead to narrowing of the upper arch. Forces of thumb apply protrusive forces on upper incisors causing their flaring and increase in overjet (Figs 47.4a and b).

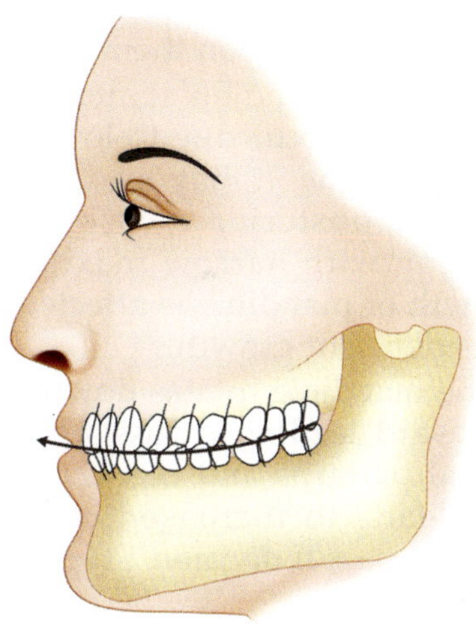

Fig. 47.2: Normal arrangement of teeth with a mild curve of Spee.

1. On maxilla: Proclination of incisors and premaxilla occurs due to anteriorly directed forces of thumb sucking and loss of inhibiting forces of upper lip. When thumb is placed in mouth, the tongue is shifted lower in the oral cavity. Narrowing of maxillary arch and decreased width of palate occurs as the forces of cheeks become more active and the counteracting forces of tongue from palatal side are lost.

   The thumb is placed in between the upper and lower arches, it creates gap in posterior region leading to supra-eruption of posterior teeth, which leads to an increased clockwise rotation of mandible. It also leads to a vertical growth pattern, long face and convex profile.

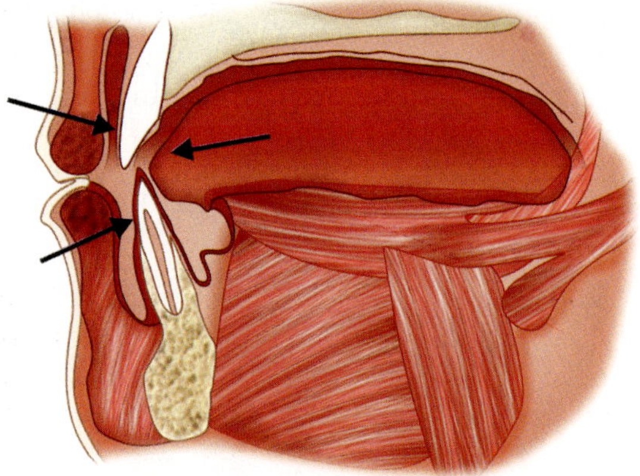

Fig. 47.3: Lips and tongue musculatures are in equilibrium in a normal situation, with teeth in well balanced, arch form.

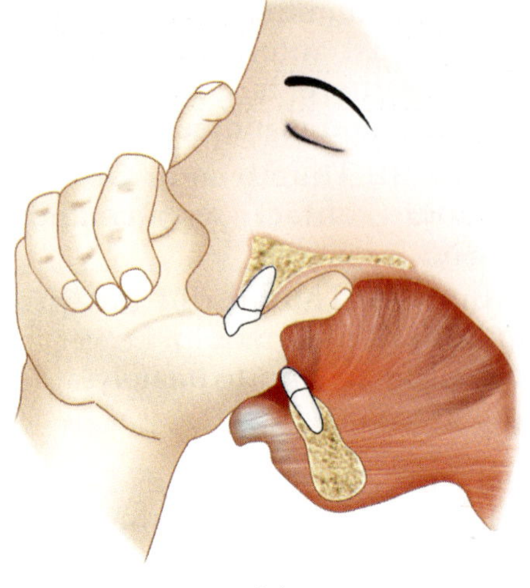

(a)

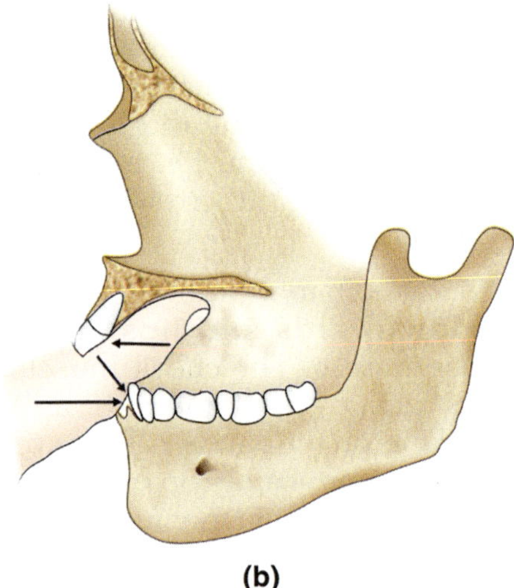

(b)

Figs 47.4a and b: Position of thumb during thumb-sucking habit. Note that the thumb applies forward pressure on upper incisors and anterior palatal region, while a lingual and intrusive pressure is applied on lower incisal region. It leads to increased overjet, anterior open bite, and maxillary proclination.

Anterior open bite develops since the upper and lower incisors are inhibited by the intervening thumb. If thumb is placed in the posterior region, the open bite may develop there.

2. On mandible: Retroclination of lower incisors occurs as the forces of thumb are directed lingually on them.

   Increased mandibular inter molar arch width may occur due to lowered position of tongue. It may lead to development of posterior crossbite in conjunction with narrow maxillary arch. Growth of mandible is affected leading to its deficient growth.

   The mandible rotates downward and backward, leading to class II skeletal and dental patterns and convex profile. It also leads to increased overjet, and Angle's class II division 1 type of malocclusion.
3. On interarch relationship: Decreased interincisal angle, increased overjet, posterior cross bite, anterior open bite, high palatal vault, unilateral or bilateral class II molars can be seen.
4. On lip: It leads to increased lip incompetence, hypotonic upper lip, and hypertonic lower lip/mentalis muscle due to its tendency to make a seal during the sucking. Hypertonic lower lip also leads to increased pressure from lingual side on upper incisors further causing their flaring.
5. On tongue: Tongue thrust may also develop to make the lip seal during sucking and due to developed anterior open bite or increased overjet. Upper lip

to tongue rest position gets disturbed. Lower tongue position occurs in the oral cavity due to thumb position which may lead to wider lower dental arch. It may / may not cause flaring of lower incisors also depending on tongue and thumb habit.

Diagnosis

History obtained from parents regarding feeding habits, emotional status of child, frequency and duration and time of sucking, etc. clinical examination of child and occlusion; examination of thumb or finger to see the presence of callus or thickened skin on them, observation of lips and facial soft tissues, etc. should be done.

Treatment

Habits should be treated as soon as possible to avoid abnormal development. There are three approaches which can be followed for habit treatment which are:

- **Reward approach:** The children are motivated to shun the habit, and they are promised to get some reward in return.
- **Reminder approach:** This involves the tying of the tape on the digits, applying some bitter substances; making elbow joint immovable by tying hard wooden stick on the arm; putting the gloves on hand, etc.
- **Appliance approach:** Certain removable or fixed appliances can be used for breaking the habits. They can be punishment appliance if they are sharp and cause some soft tissue trauma.

Psychological approach: Since the habit develops in children lacking parental care and love, the parents are advised to take care of the child. They are also advised to divert the attention of the child. Since the cooperation is very essential, the child should also be motivated to break the habit.

Dunlop has suggested his **beta hypothesis** to control the habit. It states that the best way to control the habit is by its conscious purposeful repetition. The child is asked to suck his thumb in front of the mirror and observe the changes occurring to his face. It is very effective if the child is asked to do the same when he is involved in an enjoyable activity, like playing or watching his favorite TV program, etc.

Mechanical aids/reminder therapy: They act as **reminders** (but not as punishing appliances) which are used when a child wants to quit the habit, but is not able to quit it as the habit has entered his subconscious level. Certain appliances, removable or fixed, can be used to control the habit. Other aids, like adhesive tapes, bandages, distasteful liquids, etc., can also be used as reminder.

Removable appliances: These appliances are modified Hawley's appliances, which have cribs made of heavy hard SS wires, located in the palatal rugae area which is the most common site of thumb placement. Modifications can be introduced in the appliance in the form of sharp acrylic ridge in this area in place of cribs. They help to break the sucking seal during the habit, so the child does not enjoy the sucking and slowly leaves the habit.

Fixed appliances: Children who do not cooperate with removable appliances, they should be treated with fixed appliance. It can be Hayrakes, rakes, fixed cribs, etc. which are soldered on the base wire which is then soldered to the bands on permanent first molars and cemented in place. But, due to a longer span of such an appliance supported by bands on permanent first molars, it gets frequently loosened, and can be easily removed or damaged by the strong forces of sucking. An uncooperative child may also pull it out. For better retention, a **4-band appliance** involving permanent first molars and first premolars/primary first molars or canines can be used to give extra support and resistance to dislodgement. If the narrow upper arch is present, then the cribs or rakes can be introduced with expansion appliances, e.g. Quad helix with cribs; expansion appliance with cribs or rakes, etc. Fixed appliances like quad helix and its modification with cribs, maxillary lingual arch with palatal crib, etc. can also help in controlling the habits, and they can also be used in conjunction with braces.

Triple loop corrector TLC, as designed by Viazis, has been an effective appliance, as the wire is bent in circular loops rather than vertical cribs. So the wire maintains its rigidity in TLC and is not distorted easily, still maintaining its function.

Corrective therapy: When a child is not cooperative to stop the habit, the corrective, **punishing appliances** are used. They are generally the appliances having sharp ends like tongue spikes, tongue guard, spurs/rake made of hard s.s heavy gauge wires. When a child sucks the digit, he gets hurt by the sharp ends of the wires. They can be inserted in removable appliances but generally are soldered to make fixed appliance to control uncooperative child.

Chemical approach: Some bitter or foul smelling chemicals can be applied on thumb or digit. When the child inserts it in the mouth, he may not enjoy the habit, e.g. quinine, red pepper, asafetida, etc. may be used.

TONGUE THRUSTING HABIT (Fig. 47.5)

Definition: According to Proffit, it can be defined as the placement of tongue tip forward between incisors during swallowing.

During the normal act of swallowing, the tip of the tongue contacts the cervical-lingual area of upper incisors and rugae area of the palate. But, in certain patients, they are not able to achieve this position, rather the tongue slides beyond the incisors' edges forward, between upper and lower incisors. It is called as **anterior tongue thrust**. It may lead to development of anterior open bite, spaces between teeth, flaring of teeth, bimaxillary proclination, etc. Tongue thrust has been said to cause anterior open bite. It may develop secondary to the anterior open bite. In certain cases, the lateral border of tongue comes in between the occlusal surfaces of upper and lower teeth, leading to posterior open bite. It is called as **posterior/lateral tongue thrust**.

Swallowing is a natural phenomenon, which develops in stages to maturity from infancy to childhood. When a child is born, he shows infantile swallowing pattern. It passes through a transition phase, and development of adult swallowing pattern ensues.

Infantile swallow is characterized by placement of tongue between the lips by bringing it forward to make the seal, active contractions of musculature of lips, and there is little activity of posterior tongue or pharyngeal musculature. The mandible is stabilized by the muscles supplied by 7th cranial nerve. Suckling consists of small nibbling movements of lips, which is a reflex

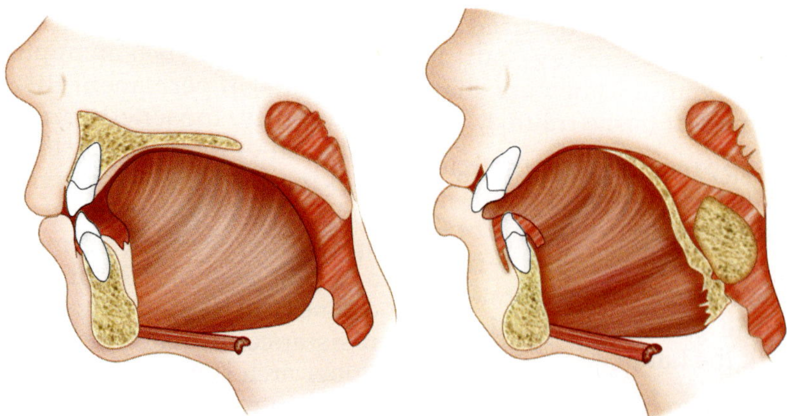

Fig. 47.5: First figure showing normal tongue position with its tip resting in rugae area, and the normal incisal relationship. Second figure shows that the tongue slips between incisors during anterior tongue thrusting.

action in infants. When the milk is squirted into mouth, it is necessary for the infant to groove the tongue and allow the milk to flow posterior into the pharynx and esophagus. The tongue must be placed in contact with lower lip, so that the milk is deposited on tongue. The suckling reflex and infantile swallow disappears during first year of life, with a transition to adult swallowing pattern.

Adult swallowing pattern is characterized by cessation of lip activity, placement of tongue tip against palate and behind upper incisors, while the posterior teeth come into occlusion during swallowing. The mandible is stabilized by muscles supplied by 5th cranial nerve.

Etiology

According to Fletcher, following factors may lead to development of tongue thrust.

1. Genetic factors: Certain anatomic or neuromuscular patterns can cause this habit, e.g. Down's syndrome,
2. Learned behavior: It can be acquired as a habit. Certain factors may lead to the learned behavior, e.g. prolonged thumb sucking, improper bottle feeding, chronic tonsillar and upper respiratory tract infections; anterior open bite, etc.
3. Maturational factors: With the eruption of posterior primary teeth, the infantile swallowing pattern gradually matures in adult pattern. But, in some children, this gets delayed or they cannot learn the normal adult pattern, which may be due to presence of some predisposing factors. So, this normal infantile pattern gets developed as abnormal habit in the adults.
4. Mechanical restriction: The tongue is forced to lie in a forward position leading to tongue thrusting by certain factors, e.g. enlarged adenoids, narrow dental arches, macroglossia or increased size of tongue, etc.
5. Neurological disturbances: Some neurological disorders affecting the orofacial structures can also lead to tongue thrust, e.g. motor disability, etc.
6. Psychogenic factors: Psychogenic factors, e.g. anxiety, stress, fear of separation or neglect from parent or teachers, etc. may also cause the development of certain habits, e.g. thumb sucking, tongue thrusting, etc. Also, some patients who are forced to shun the digit sucking habit may start tongue thrust.
7. Systemic causes leading to increased size of tongue, e.g. amyloidosis, hypothyroidism, Down's syndrome, etc.

Classification

Types of Tongue Thrust

1. Physiologic: This comprises of the normal tongue thrust swallow of infancy
2. Habitual: The tongue thrust swallow is present as a habit even after the correction of the malocclusion.
3. Functional: When the tongue thrust mechanism is an adaptive behavior developed to achieve an oral seal, it can be grouped as functional.
4. Anatomic: Persons having enlarged tongue can have an anterior tongue posture.
   - By Backlund,1963: Anterior tongue thrust, posterior tongue thrust
   - By Pickett's,1966: Adaptive; transitory; habitual
   - By Moyers, 1970: Simple tongue thrust; complex tongue thrust; retained infantile swallow

Simple tongue thrust: It is characterized by the presence of proper intercuspation/ occlusion of teeth during swallowing, (so it is also called as **teeth-together swallow**), there is presence of well-defined anterior open bite so the tongue protrudes in the gap to make an anterior lip seal. There is contraction of muscles of lips, mentalis and mandibular elevator muscles. A history of digit sucking causing anterior open bite is generally found. It may diminish with age and has a good treatment prognosis. Speech problems, like sibilant distortions and lisping, may also be present. The teeth are generally proclined and spacing is present. The simple tongue thrust is characterized by a normal tooth contact during the swallowing act. They exhibit good intercuspation of posterior teeth in contrast to complex tongue thrust.

Complex tongue thrust: It is also called as **tooth-apart swallow**. Here, the posterior intercuspation is absent during swallowing, and there is diffuse open bite. It is severe form of tongue thrust, where there is no contact between teeth. The tongue fills the spaces between teeth during swallowing. The tongue thrusts between anterior and posterior teeth. There is abnormal contraction of muscles supplied by the seventh cranial nerve, like lips, facial and mentalis muscles. However, the muscles of fifth nerves, i.e. mandibular elevators are not activated, which otherwise should support the mandible in normal swallowing. These features are characteristic of **retained infantile swallow**. It does not diminish with age and has got poor prognosis. It is usually associated with chronic nasorespiratory distress, mouth breathing, tonsillitis, and pharyngitis.

Pain and lessening of space in the throat precipitate a new forward tongue posture and swallowing reflex. Because maintenance of airway patency is a more primitive and demanding reflex than the mature swallow, the later is conditioned to the necessity for mouth breathing. The jaws are thus held apart during swallow in order that the tongue can remain in a protruded position.

Differences between simple and complex tongue thrust are described in Table 47.1.

Lateral tongue thrust (posterior tongue thrust): In some patients, the tongue thrusting is seen in the premolar-molar region, and the lateral open bite is frequently seen. It may be unilateral or bilateral.

Classification by James Braner and Holt

- Type I (non-deforming)
- Type II (deforming anterior tongue thrust)
    - Subgroup 1: anterior open bite
    - Subgroup 2: anterior proclination
    - Subgroup 3: posterior crossbite

Table 47.1: Differences between simple and complex tongue thrust

S. No	*Simple tongue thrust*	*Complex tongue thrust*
1.	It displays the contraction of lips, mentalis and mandibular elevators.	It displays the contraction of lips, mentalis, and facial muscles. But contraction of mandibular elevators is not seen.
2.	Teeth come in contact during swallowing	Teeth do not come in contact during swallow.
3.	Open bite is well defined with definite beginning and ending.	Open bite is diffuse, ill defined.
4.	Mandible is stabilized by muscles of mastication	Mandible is stabilized by muscles of lips and cheeks (facial muscles)
5.	Proper, secure, posterior occlusal fit is present except anterior open bite	No proper posterior occlusal fit.
6.	Usually will have a previous history of thumb sucking.	Usually will have history of tonsillitis, chronic airway disease or airway obstruction.
7.	Treatment is simple with less relapse tendency.	Treatment is difficult with more relapse tendency.
8.	Occlusal equilibration may be needed.	Occlusal equilibration is mandatory.
9.	Tonsils may not be so inflamed	Tonsils are found to be very much inflamed
10.	It tends to diminish with age	It does not diminish with age
11.	Prognosis is good	Prognosis is poor

Type III (deforming lateral tongue thrust)

- Subgroup 1: posterior open bite
- Subgroup 2: posterior crossbite
- Subgroup 3: deep over bite

Type IV (deforming anterior and lateral tongue thrust)

- Subgroup 1: anterior and posterior open bite
- Subgroup 2: proclination of anterior teeth
- Subgroup 3: posterior crossbite

The non-deforming tongue thrust implies that the interdigitation of teeth and the facial profile is within acceptable limits, while deforming tongue thrust means that there is dentoalveolar defect created by the habit. The subgroups have been created depending on the effect caused by the habit.

Clinical Features

Habit leads to disturbance of the balancing forces leading to development of abnormal forces on certain tissues. It causes the development of malocclusion. Following features can be seen:

1. Open bite—anterior and posterior
2. Proclination of the anterior teeth
3. Protrusion of anterior segments of both arches with spaces between teeth.
4. Narrow maxillary arch which may cause posterior crossbite.
5. Lips incompetence, and convex profile, hyperactive muscles, etc.

Management of simple tongue thrust: Management of this habit involves interception of habit, followed by the treatment of the malocclusion. However, both the phases can be done simultaneously. Since anterior open bite has been found as a cause of this habit, treatment of open bite should eliminate the habit. **Retraining exercises** should be advised to the patient. However, during treatment, the tongue should be prevented to shift in the open bite with the help of appliances.

Interception of habit: It can be done with the help of appliances; retraining exercises, etc.

Appliances (Figs 47.6 to 47.12): Various habit breaking appliances having cribs or rakes can be used. They can be removable or fixed type of appliances. Various modifications can also be done in the removable appliances used, e.g. using a rotating bead in wire; using an acrylic bead in the anterior area; roughening the anterior area for tactile sensations of tongue, etc. Posterior tongue cribs are used in case of posterior tongue thrust habit.

Mechanotherapy: Different types of fixed and removable appliances (cribs or rakes) can be used to treat this habit. These appliances prevent the tongue coming forward during swallowing. The appliance also helps to develop conditional reflex and guides the tongue so that the dorsum of tongue approximates the palatal vault and the tip of the tongue contacts the palatal rugae during deglutition. As a result, the tongue spreads laterally leading to expansion of maxillary buccal portion thereby preventing the narrowing of the arch.

Removable appliance therapy: Modified Hawley's appliance with cribs or rakes or spikes is used. The crib serves as a reminder. The spikes should be bent such that it does not irritate lower anteriors or anterior lingual alveoli. Open bite gets corrected naturally when the teeth erupt themselves when tongue stops coming in between them. It may also be corrected to some extent by activating the labial bow, which reduces proclination of upper teeth. The acrylic should be trimmed along the gingival marginal area on lingual surfaces of maxillary anteriors so that incisors can move palatally (Figs 47.9, 47.10 and 47.12).

Habit breaking appliance with a bead in rugae area: Tongue tip keeps its position at the bead thus acquiring a new position. Such an appliance can also be modified by creating a depression/rough area in rugae area where the tongue can be fixed during swallowing.

Fixed habit breaking appliance: First permanent molars are banded and a 0.040 inch stainless steel "U"-shaped wire is adapted from one molar to the opposite

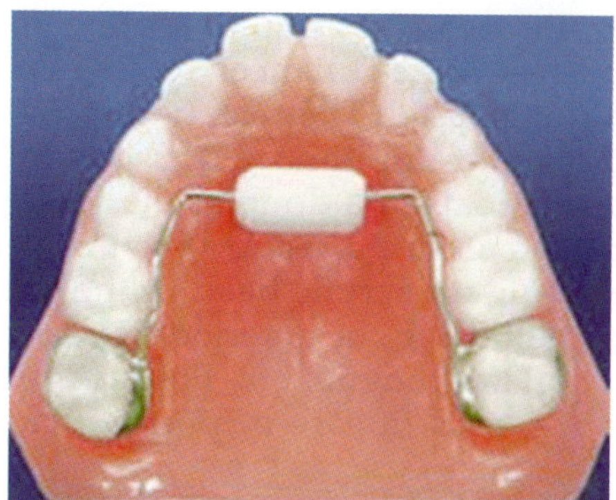

Fig. 47.6: Fixed habit—breaking appliance for tongue thrust with a roller in rugae area for proper tongue positioning *(Courtesy: Internet)*.

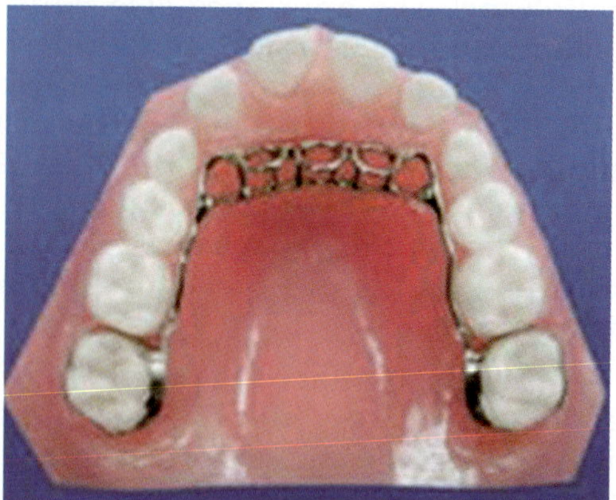

Fig. 47.7: Fixed habit—breaking appliance for tongue thrust with cribs in rugae area for proper tongue positioning and preventing anterior tongue trust *(Courtesy: Internet)*.

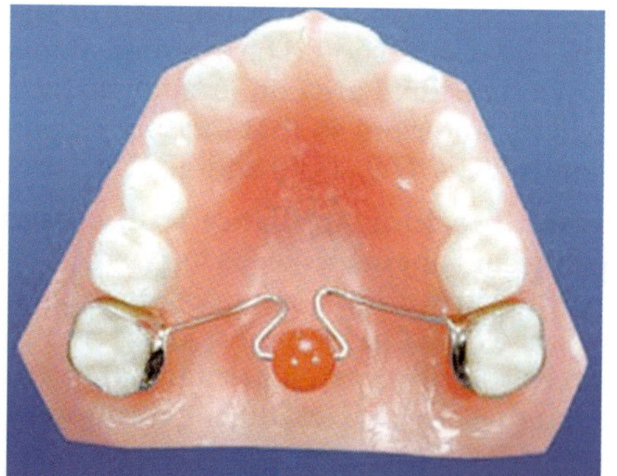

Fig. 47.8: Fixed habit—breaking appliance for tongue thrust with a roller in posterior palatal area for tongue positioning exercise *(Courtesy: Internet)*.

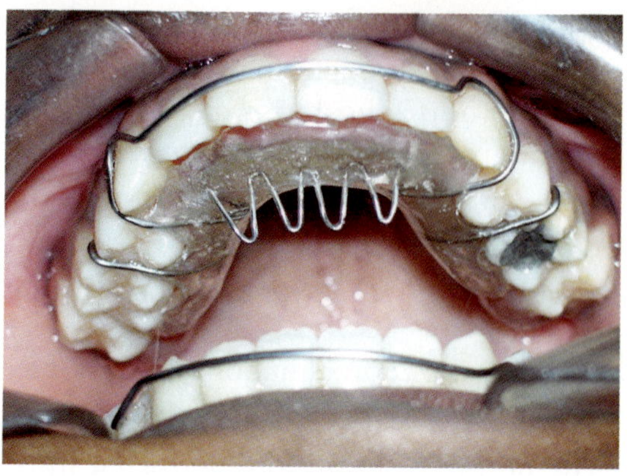

(a)

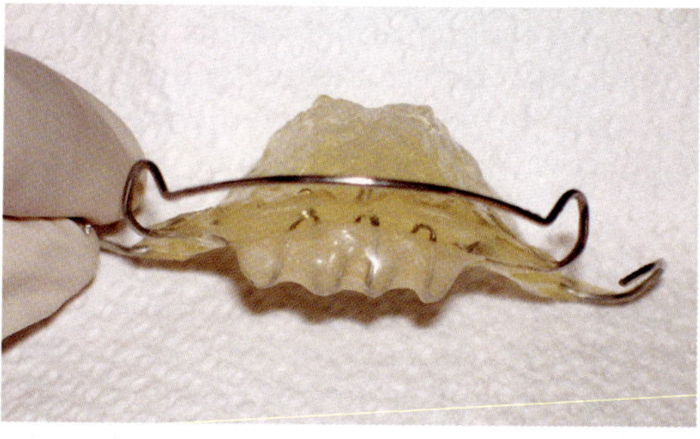

(b)

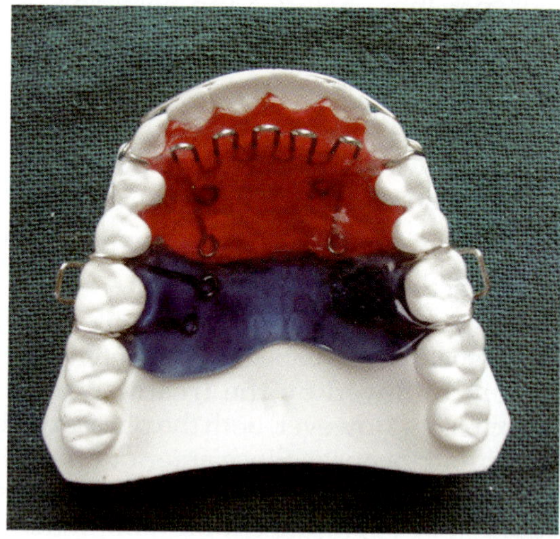

(c)

Figs 47.9a to c: A modified Hawley's appliance with tongue cribs for tongue thrust habit breaking. Sometimes, the cribs' edges irritate the tongue, so the composite material can be bonded in cribs to block the sharp wires.

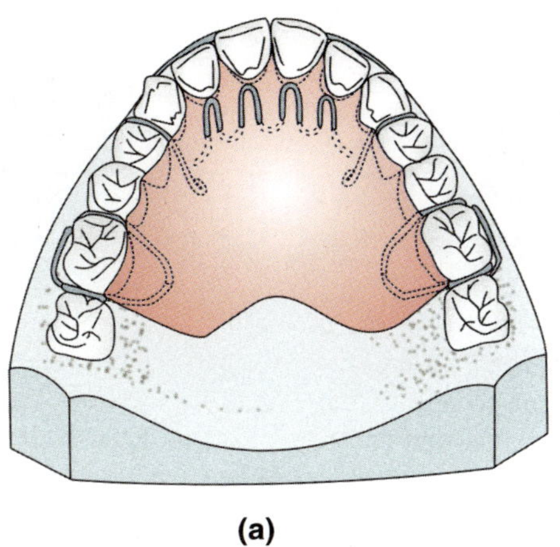

(a)

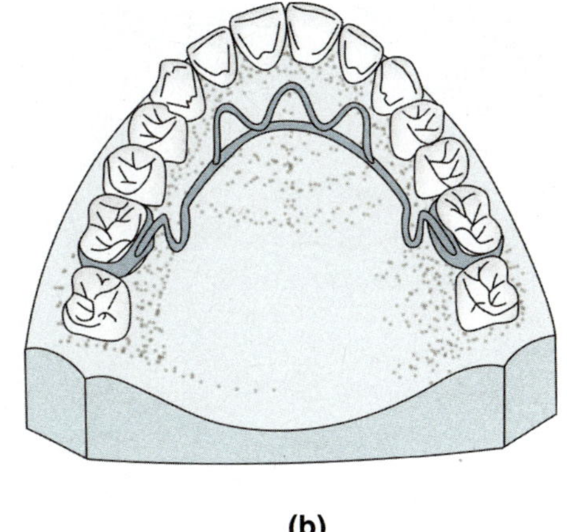

(b)

Figs 47.10a and b: Habit breaking cribs appliances: Removable appliance; fixed appliance.

molar. Cribs are formed and soldered to the base wire. These appliances create a new neuromuscular behavior for the tongue and lips. The cribs can be fabricated with expansion appliances, like quadhelix and expansion screw, if the arch is constricted.

Oral screen: It can be used to control abnormal muscle habits like tongue thrusting; and uses the muscular force for the correction of developing malocclusion. It is mostly used to intercept mouth breathing, tongue thrusting, lip biting and cheek biting. They also correct mild proclination of anterior teeth.

Modified oral screen with cribs: It helps in preventing tongue thrust, mouth breathing, helps in expansion, etc. It was designed by Kraus.

Blue grass appliance: It has been designed by Haskelt and Mink. The bands are placed on permanent first molars, with a hard SS 0.9–1.0 mm wire adapted. This wire is passed through a three-side beveled Teflon roller of 5/8 inch long, ¼ inch diameter. This roller rests in the palatal rugae region, where the tongue tip lies. Thus a new position of tongue develops.

Various muscle retraining exercises: Muscle training using elastics have been used to eliminate it. Details are presented in Chapter 48 on Role of Muscles Exercises in Orthodontics.

Myofunctional exercises: Educate the patient about normal swallowing by asking

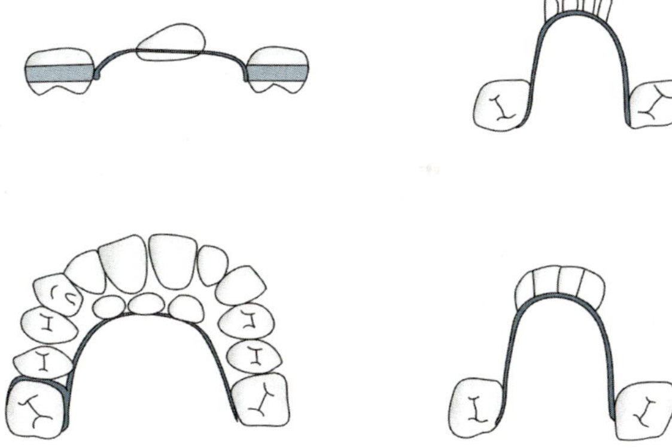

Fig. 47.11: Fixed appliance for habit breaking:

- Fixed appliance with acrylic button or a rotating bead in the wire placed in the rugae area
- Fixed appliance with cribs
- Triple loop corrector, TLC (Viazis)
- Appliance with cribs, having spaces between cribs blocked either with molten solder material or light cure composite, to avoid tongue irritation

the patient to keep the tongue tip in the rugae are on the hard palate. Various muscle exercise of the tongue can help in training it to adapt to the new swallowing pattern.

Appliances to guide the correct positioning of tongue: Once the patient is familiar with the new tongue position, an appliance is given for training the correct positioning of the tongue.

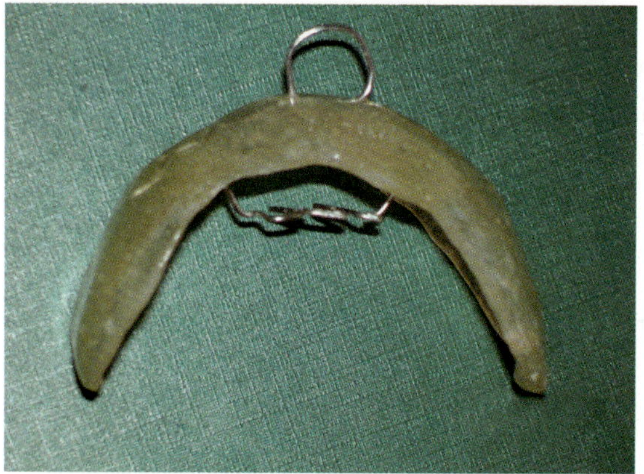

Fig. 47.12: Modification of oral/vestibular screen which includes the tongue cribs for habit-breaking and a ring on labial side.

Preorthodontic trainer/tongue trainer: This appliance aids in the correct positioning of tongue with the help of tongue tags. The tongue guards prevent the tongue thrusting when in place. It can also used to correct mouth breathing habit (Figs 47.13a to c).

MOUTH BREATHING

It is the condition in which the patient breaths through the mouth more than the nose. During physical exertion, most of the people also breathe through mouth, but that cannot be called as a mouth breathing habit. But there are certain pathological conditions which cause the person to breathe through mouth. This habit leads to altered posture of head, tongue and jaws, which disturbs the craniofacial balance leading to malocclusion. Sassouni has defined mouth breathing as habitual respiration through the mouth instead of nose.

Classification

It can be of three types, i.e. obstructive, habitual, and anatomic, as given by Sim and Finn.

1. **Obstructive:** Complete or partial obstruction of nasal passage leads to increased resistance to normal nasal airflow. Some causes leading to nasal obstruction are: nasal polyps, DNS, chronic inflammation and/or allergic reactions of nasal mucosa, localized tumors, adenoids, enlarged turbinates, etc. The obstructions can lead to total or partial blockage.

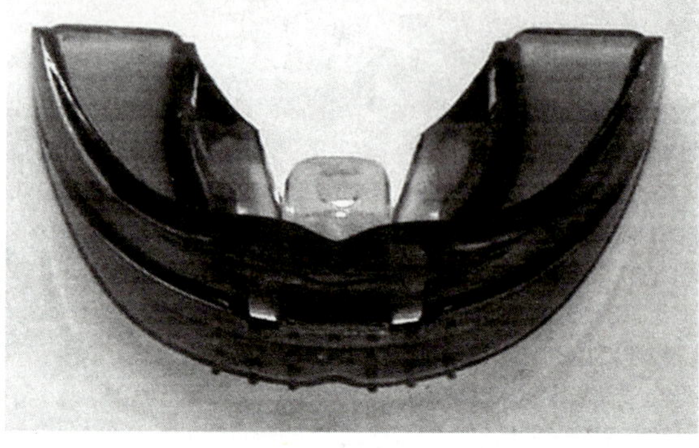

(a)

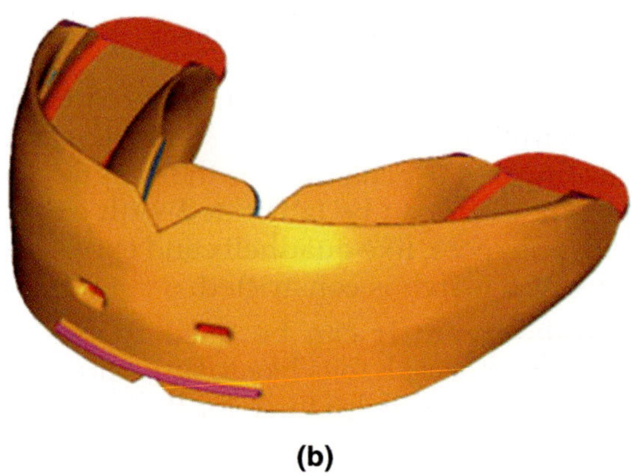

(b)

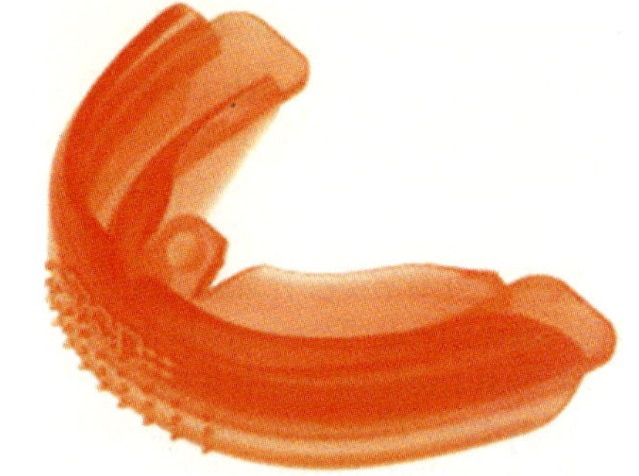

(c)

Figs 47.13a to c: Prefabricated appliances for interceptive Rx like habit-breaking, skeletal class II correction, e.g. T4M appliance *(Courtesy: Internet)*.

Etiology of nasal obstruction:

1. Enlarged turbinates
2. Hypertrophy of pharyngeal lymphoid tissue/adenoids
3. Intranasal defects (e.g. DNS, subluxation of septum, thickness of septum, bony spurs, polyps)
4. Allergic rhinitis.

2. **Habitual:** The patient keeps on breathing through the mouth even if nasal passage is normal or after the removal of obstruction. Here, it is a deep rooted habit, being performed unconsciously.
3. **Anatomic:** In such patients, the lip morphology does not permit complete closure of the mouth, e.g. patient having short upper lip.
4. **Postural:** In certain children, the mouth breathing is postural and may be due to the racial features and craniofacial anatomy, e.g. in certain African children, they keep the mouth/lips open, with an anterior open bite and mouth breathing.

Clinical features in mouth breathing: An uncontrolled habit leads to development of features typical of **long face syndrome**, LFS. They are also called as **classic adenoid facies**. They are:

- Long and narrow face
- Vertical facial and growth patterns
- Convex profile
- Incompetent lips
- Narrow and flat nose and narrow nasal passages
- Underdeveloped nasal bridge
- Short and hypotonic upper lip
- Increased posterior dentoalveolar height
- Narrow upper arch and may be posterior cross bite
- Proclined upper incisors with increased overjet
- An expressionless or blank face
- Anterior marginal gingivitis due to drying of gingival tissues
- Dry lips
- Dryness of mouth may lead to increased caries
- Anterior open bite may be seen.

How the mouth breathing leads to malocclusion: During mouth breathing, the mandible drops downward and backward, tongue is placed downward and forward, and tipping back of the head occurs to allow more space for oral respiration. These changes lead to disturbances in the balance of orofacial muscles especially the buccinator mechanism gets disturbed. The forces from buccal side increase relatively because opposing forces from lingual side get decreased due to its downward positioning. It leads to constriction of upper arch and posterior crossbite.

Hypotonicity of upper lip (moulding action of upper lip on incisors is lost) leads to proclination of upper incisors and increased overjet, etc. When mandible drops downward and backward, the interocclusal space increases, in which the posterior teeth are free to erupt, leading to vertical face and growth, convex profile, etc. Lower incisors are free to erupt and may touch the palatal tissues.

Distal relation of mandible to maxilla occurs due to down and back rotation of mandible. It leads to skeletal class II relation and convex profile.

Diagnosis of mouth breathing: History: Chronic allergic rhinitis, nasal discharge, stiffness, sore throat, repeated attacks of cold, etc. can give idea of the habit.

Clinical examination: Various clinical features are noted. Certain tests to diagnose mouth breathing can be done, e.g. mirror test, double side mirror test, cotton wisp test, water in mouth test, etc.

Diagnostic tests:

1. **Rhinomanometry** is the study of nasal air flow and nasal resistance by using special equipment.
2. Mirror test
3. Cotton/Massler's butterfly test
4. Water test

Mirror test: A one-sided mirror is placed facing the nostril. If it fogs, it implies that patient is a nasal-breather.

Double-sided mirror test: A double side mirror is placed near the nostril. The mirror which gets fogged during respiration implies the type of breathing.

Cotton/Massler's butterfly test, i.e. cotton wisp test: A wisp of cotton is placed near the nostrils. Its movement during inhaling and exhaling shows that patient is a nasal breather, otherwise not.

Water-in-mouth test: the patient is asked to full the water in mouth and to hold it for 1–2 minutes. A nasal breather has no difficulty in holding the water while the mouth breather can't hold water for long.

Cephalometrics: It helps to find the presence and size of adenoids, and size of pharyngeal space, position of tongue, hyoid bone, skeletal and dental features, etc.

Management: Treatment of mouth breathing is important so that a normal growth of dentofacial complex can be achieved. After establishing the causes, a proper treatment is given to the patient (Fig. 47.14).

1. **ENT referral and management:** To treat any nasal or pharyngeal obstruction, rhinitis, etc.
2. **Interception of habit:** It is done by using appliances, e.g. oral screen, taping the lips to attain lip seal. The appliances are given only if there is no nasal obstruction. A modified oral screen having holes in the anterior region is given to the patient, so that he does not face problem while breathing through both nose and mouth. These holes are gradually sealed off as the patient gets used to breathing mainly from nose.
3. **Myofunctional therapy:** It helps to bring the mandible forward so that the pharyngeal space can be increased, thus decreasing resistance to air flow.
4. **RME:** It helps to increase the width of arch, increase the size of nasal passage, decreasing the nasal resistance, etc.
5. **Muscle exercises:** To achieve lip seal, etc. e.g. holding water in mouth; holding a piece of paper between lips; inflating the balloon; flute-blowing, etc. to increase the tonicity of lips.

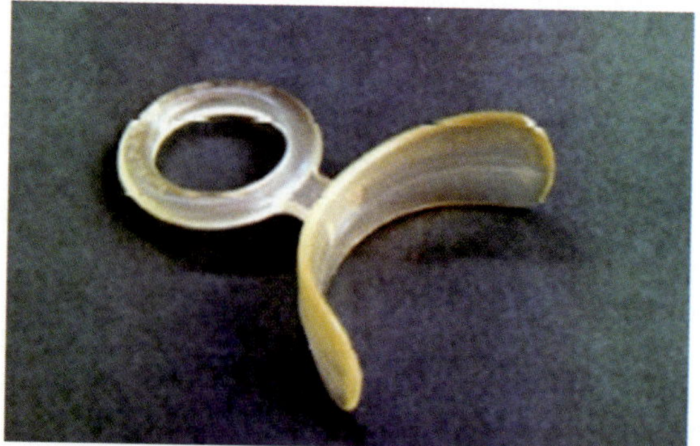

Fig. 47.14: Prefabricated vestibular screen *(Courtesy: Internet)*

BRUXISM

It is the non-functional contact of teeth which may include clenching, grinding, and tapping of teeth. It mainly refers to nocturnal, subconscious activity but can occur in day time also (bruxomania). It is a conscious activity when parafunctional activities are included in it.

Etiology according to Nadler:

1. Psychological and emotional stress factors have been attributed as the most common causes.
2. Local factors (e.g. faulty restorations, calculus, pericoronitis, periodontitis, functionally incorrect occlusions, malocclusions), as they lead to tactile stimulation/irritation.
3. Systemic factors [e.g. nutritional deficiencies, intestinal parasite infections, GI disturbances, hyperthyroidism, pubertal growth, increased negative pressures in the tympanic cavities from intermittent allergic edema of the mucosa of Eustachian tubes (chronic middle ear disturbances may promote reflex action to the jaws by stimulating the trigeminal nucleus)], CNS disturbances, etc.
4. Occupational factors

Sign and symptoms:

1. Tooth mobility
2. Dull percussion sounds
3. Soreness to biting stresses

4. Nonfunctional pattern of occlusal wear
5. Increased senstivity from excessive abrasion of enamel.
6. Atypical facets
7. Muscular facial pain
8. Muscle tenderness or fatigue on rising in the morning
9. Tenderness of jaw to palpation
10. Compensatory hypertrophy of muscles
11. Muscular incoordination
12. Locking of jaws
13. Difficulty in opening of mouth for a long time.
14. Order of muscle senstivity: lateral pterygoid, medial pterygoid, masseter
15. Pain, clicking restricted jaw movements, jaw deviation in TMJ.

Management:

1. Determine the underlying cause and eliminate it
2. Muscular deprogramming using bite guards, etc.
3. Psychotherapy
4. Drugs like vapocoolants (ethyl chloride) for pain in the TMJ, LA injections in TMJ for muscle relaxing, tranquilizers and sedatives
5. Occlusal adjustments
6. Electrogalvanic stimulation for muscle relaxation.
7. Tens
8. Acupressure
9. Others—oral exercises, desensitizing agents, occlusal correction, counseling on nutrition, supplements for nutritional deficiencies.

Nocturnal bruxism can be effectively reduced with occlusal appliance therapy, i.e. bite/night guards, e.g. muscle relaxation appliance is used to treat muscle hyperactivity. It is fabricated for maxillary or mandibular arch and provides an occlusal relationship in which the condyles are in the most musculoskeletaly stable position and the teeth are evenly contacting. It helps in muscle-deprogramming. Night guard appliances can be of soft or hard material.

LIP Sucking (Figs 47.15 and 47.16)

This is the habit in which the child sucks his lip/s. In many cases, it may be a compensatory activity resulting from an excessive overjet and the relative difficulty of closing the lips properly during deglutition. So, the child places his lower lip behind the upper incisors to make a seal with tongue. This in turn starts a negative feedback cycle, leading to further increase in overjet. The hyperactive lower lip causes an increased labial pressure on upper incisors, and an increased lingual pressure on lower incisors, thus increasing overjet.

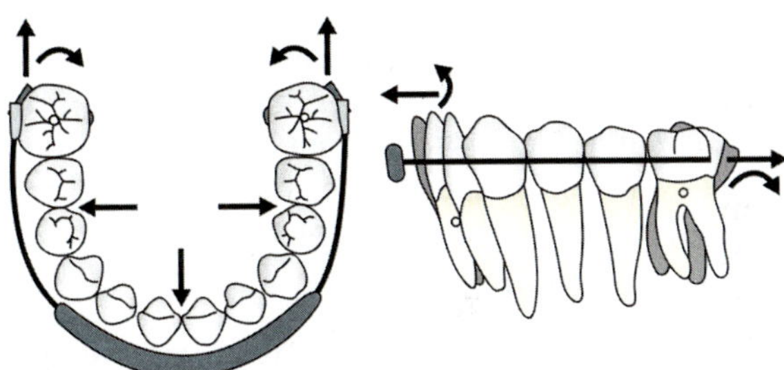

Fig. 47.15: Lip bumper: Used for treatment of hyperactive lower lip and lip trap/lip sucking habits. The lower arch expands under the tongue forces, as shown by the arrows. Lower molars also get uprighted distally with the forces of lower lip.

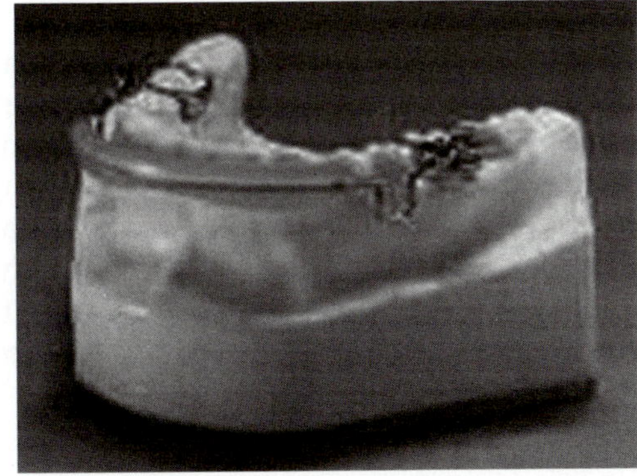

Fig. 47.16: Prefabricated fixed lip bumper for controlling lip sucking habit *(Courtesy: Internet).*

Following features are seen:

1. Retruded teeth according to the lip which is sucked
2. Vermillion border becomes hypertrophic and redundant during rest.

3. Reddening below the vermilion border
4. Flaccid lip
5. Mentolabial suclus is accentuated
6. Chronic herpes with areas of irritation and cracking of lip.

Lip wetting: It is a minor habit of repeated wetting of lip/s by tongue. It rarely leads to any dentoalveolar problems, but the lips get cracked, reddened, may become sore and infected.

Lip biting: It is also a minor habit, seen in many people even in adults. It generally involves lower lip which is placed between the incisal edges of teeth and a part of mucosa is bitten. It may exert pressure on lingual surfaces of upper incisors in certain cases, leading to features like increased overjet due to proclined upper and retroclined lower incisors; cracking of lips; hypertrophy of lip, etc.

Management:

1. Appliances: Such lip habits are treated with lip bumpers, or oral screen. They help to keep the lips away from teeth, and improve the axial inclination of teeth due to forward unrestricted action of tongue.
2. Lip over lip exercises
3. Playing bass instruments.

Cheek biting: It is the habit of sucking and biting the buccal mucosa between the occlusal surfaces of upper and lower teeth. It may affect both the sides. Biting the cheeks, if not unchecked may contribute to ulceration, pain, discomfort, or malignancy. Generally, a white line is seen along the occlusal plane in the buccal mucosa which is called as **linea alba**.

Etiology:

1. Buccoversion of erupting molars
2. Stress
3. Flabby cheeks
4. Atrophy of muscles in paralysis.

Treatment:

1. Identify and remove the causes, e.g. sharp edges of tooth or restoration; edge—on bite of cusps of molars;
2. Occlusal grinding, e.g. buccal reduction of lower molars
3. Analgesics and local anesthetic ointments
4. Appliance therapy, e.g. cribs, oral screens, to keep the buccal mucosa away from the occlusion.

Conclusion

Normal growth and development of dentofacial complex occurs in the presence of an equilibrium of forces of surrounding soft tissues. Abnormal habits apply the pressures and disturb this equilibrium and thus affect the development of dentofacial complex. If not controlled, the effects on the dentofacial complex become permanent. Habits should be diagnosed and controlled as early as possible to reverse these changes. Interceptive modalities deal with the control of habits, alongwith establishment of the normal balance of the forces, which in turn direct the normal development. Various appliances and muscle training exercises are advised to the patients to establish a normal neuromuscular pattern.

VIVA VOCE QUESTIONS

1. **What are the three main factors of a habit, which lead to its effect on the dentofacial complex during development?**

   The three factors or the trident of the factors is = frequency, duration and intensity of habit.

2. **Up to what age, the digit sucking may be considered as normal habit?**

   Up to 3½ to 4 yrs age, it can be considered as normal habit.

3. **What is the difference b/w simple tongue thrust and complex tongue thrust?**

   Teeth come in full ICP during swallowing in simple tongue thrust; but there is gap b/w the teeth in complex TT, in which 7th n ms contract and no temporalis m contraction occurs.

4. **What are the adenoid facies?**

   It occurs due to chronic mouth breathing habit. The face is long and narrow; blank face; dry lips and gingiva; short and flaccid upper lip and narrow upper arch.

5. **What is lip trap?** (Fig. 47.17)

   When there is increased overjet, the lower lip falls behind the lingual surfaces of upper incisors and on the labial surfaces of lower incisors. With continuous function due to swallowing, etc., the lower lip keeps pressing the incisors in opposite directions and also prevent proper forward growth of the mandible. It contributes in the development of forward growth of the mandible. It contributes in the development of class II skeletodental relation. With the help of the myofunctional appliances, we can treat this condition, e.g. lip bumper, etc.

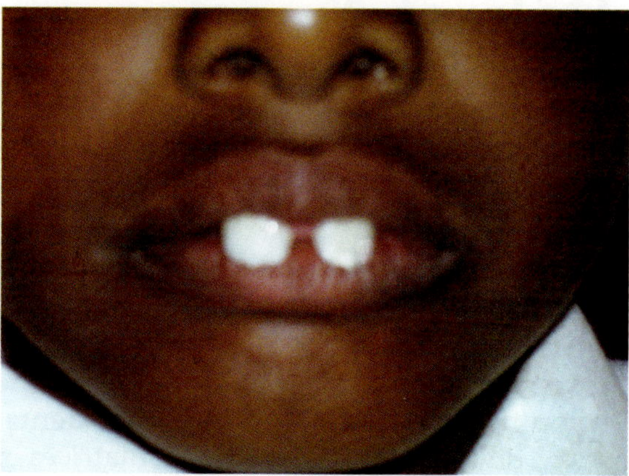

Fig. 47.17: Lip trap.

48

Role of Muscles Exercises in Orthodontics

INTRODUCTION

Soft tissues play an important role in the development and growth of face and dental arches. They work as the functional matrices of growth of the associated skeletal tissues. Circumoral, masticatory, hyoid group, tongue muscles, periodontium and other surrounding soft tissues have important influence during the development of size and form of jaws and dental arches. The dental arch is molded in its form under the influence of equilibrium of forces of buccinator mechanism. The muscles surrounding the dental arches, i.e. orbicularis oris, tongue and buccinators muscles guide the teeth during eruption and help to attain the shape of dental arches, which develop in the "neutral zone". There exists equilibrium of forces between them, as shown by Profit, with a slight difference that the force of tongue is slightly more than the outer forces. This force is balanced by the eruptive forces of the teeth. The functional matrix concept of growth also emphasizes that the soft tissues are the primary driving force for the growth of craniofacial complex. Any disturbance of this equilibrium leads to disturbance in proper development of dentition. Certain habits apply abnormal forces on the skeletodental structures and lead to abnormal development. The effects of habits are described below.

Definition

According to Thompson 1927, a habit is a fixed practice produced by constant repetition of an act. With each repetition, it becomes less conscious and then later on, it settles in the subconscious mind of an individual". Certain habits are useful as they are part of normal function and play an important role in craniofacial growth and occlusal physiology, as they serve as stimuli for the normal growth; e.g. normal action of lips, tongue and mastication. Abnormal habits interfere with normal facial growth, and must be differentiated from the normal habits. If the abnormal muscles pattern is not corrected or controlled, then it also leads to failure of orthodontic correction. So for long term stability of orthodontic treatment, such perverted abnormal patterns should be controlled.

Various reflexes develop during intrauterine life. By 14th week of intrauterine life, there is stimulation of lips which causes the tongue to move. At about the same time, stimulation of upper lip leads to mouth closure and even deglutition. Gag reflex develops by about 18½ weeks. Sucking and swallowing develops by 32 weeks. Many times the fetus can be seen as sucking his thumb or finger during ultrasound.

Negative Oral Habits

Harmful sucking or chewing habits develop because the respective functions could not be completely fulfilled and matured at the appropriate age. Therefore, to eliminate any negative habit, all functions should be exercised as they are mutually dependent. After that, it is beneficial to focus on those functions which did not mature properly. So, more sucking exercises are assigned to the patient who sucks a finger or a pacifier. Exercises for mastication are given to patients with chewing habits (e.g. bruxing, finger nail biting, and so on). But always all the functions are exercised together at the time of exercises, so that all muscles are activated naturally. Thus a **neurological memory** is established or re-established with exercises to attain a normal pattern. Since the functions/reflexes get established and stronger with increasing age. So, sooner the treatment is provided to correct the function, the better. It will be easier and stronger for the fixation of new pattern in the CNS. With delay, it becomes more difficult to restore a normal function of chewing and swallowing, as has been advised by Moyers. Also, no orthodontic correction can be adequately maintained unless optimal occlusion obtained at the end of treatment harmonizes with the patient's musculature (Moyers). Certain forces act on the bony and dental structures during the developmental stages and help to shape them. There are certain antagonistic forces which are continuously acting on the masticatory apparatus as described below.

1. Lips on outside and tongue from inside in the anterior dental region.
2. On the buccal region, the cheeks on outside and the tongue from inside.
3. On the eruption of teeth, certain muscles, e.g. tongue, buccinators, and masticatory muscles.
4. Action of lateral pterygoid muscle in anterior movement is opposed by the posterior one third of temporalis, suprahyoid group, digastric and muscles of neck.
5. Action of lateral pterygoid muscle of one side for the lateral movement is opposed by lateral pterygoid muscle of the opposite side.

Breitner in 1942 described the **concept of functional equilibrium** that a balance should exist between the tongue forces from within the dental arches and compensating action of the lips and cheek musculature.

Buccinator Mechanism

The teeth and supporting structures are constantly under the influence of musculature. Any abnormal muscle function leads to development of malocclusions. The dental arches are surrounded by a sheath of muscles which is formed by the orbicularis oris muscle in the lips, which join the buccinator muscles around the corner of the mouth. Buccinator muscles run posteriorly to insert into the pterygomandibular raphe just behind the dentition. There they intermingle with fibers of superior constrictor muscle which arises at pharyngeal tubercle of the occipital bone. At the corners of mouth / lips, there is a junction of 8 muscles which is called modiolus. It lies in the region of canines, thus having a direct effect on the maxillary canine region. When modiolus becomes active, it applies more pressure in the intercanine region of maxilla, leading to a constriction of arch in canine region. It happens when the child sucks the thumb or fingers, when he activates the entire orbicularis oris and the muscles attached at the corners of the mouth. The tongue shifts down and comes to lie below the thumb/ finger. It applies strong constrictive forces in the canine region and leads to narrowing of intercanine width and the dental arches. The buccinator mechanism is opposed/balanced by the tongue. Balance between these muscle forces is very important for development of shape and width of dental arches. Any deviation in these reflexes or mechanism leads to malocclusion. If the tongue force becomes less, the imbalance leads to increased forces by the buccal muscles. It leads to constriction of dental arches. If tongue has a thrusting effect or is larger than normal size, then it leads to development of open bite, spaces between teeth, wider arches, etc.

Thumb sucking habit: When the thumb is placed in the mouth, it leads to shifting the tongue downward, thus increasing the net inward force of cheek muscles. The buccinator muscles become more active. It leads to maxillary protrusion, as it may lead to an increased pressure from buccinator muscles activating pterygomandibular raphe just behind the dentition and forcing the maxillary teeth forward. It also leads to narrowing of the upper arch. An open bite may develop, because the intervening digit hampers the eruption of front teeth. It also leads to a gap creation between posterior teeth which are then free to over-erupt. A developed open bite leads to development of the tongue thrust to attain an anterior oral seal, which is called as "compensatory tongue thrusting". Nasal floor fails to drop vertically to its expected position during growth because the thumb prevents its natural descent, leading to a narrow nasal floor and high palatal vault. Upper lip becomes hypotonic and lower lip becomes hyperactive, since the tongue tries to make a seal with lower lip. It leads to creation of overjet by retroclining the lower teeth, while the upper teeth get proclined.

Mentalis hyperactivity: A marked mentalis muscle contraction compresses the lower lip inward on swallowing, to make a seal lingual to upper anteriors. It leads to flattening of lower anterior arch and crowding; flaring and spacing of upper incisors, and increased overjet. If not controlled, it becomes a vicious circle. The mentalis becomes hyperactive, upper lip hypoactive, lip incompetence, and a deficient chin. Correction of overjet by upper anterior retraction, and the lip bumper can help in treating this habit. Lip bumper helps in obtaining proper lip seal and lip competency by keeping lower lip away from the lower anteriors and shifting it closer to the upper lip. It also decreases the overjet by labial flaring of lower incisors under the tongue pressure.

Tongue thrust habit: Subtenly and Subtenly (1962), Proffit and Mason (1975) have described that in patients having a tongue thrust habit, there is a contraction of circumoral muscles, the mandible is supported by contraction of facial muscles rather than by masticatory muscles, and the tongue protrudes between the incisors to make the seal with the lips during swallowing. Facial grimace, puckering of mentalis muscle, and/or pursing of the lips is observed during swallowing.

Muscular effects of the mouth breathing habit: When a patient does mouth breathing, the mouth is opened beyond normal opening, mandible goes D and B, the tongue drops down and forward in the oral cavity, and lips are separated. The upper lip is hypotonic. It leads to loss of molding action of upper lip on incisors resulting in proclination and spacing of maxillary anteriors. Also, the upper lip loses its tonicity, remains short and incompetent. The lower lip gets everted. Downward positioning of tongue leads to disturbed equilibrium of buccinators mechanism, leading to constriction of upper arch, and narrow maxilla. Respiratory needs act as functional matrix and a primary determinant of posture of jaws, tongue and head. A disturbance could alter the equilibrium of pressures on the jaws and teeth, influencing jaw growth and tooth position. In order to breathe through the mouth, it is necessary to lower the mandible and tongue, and extend the head. Since functional matrix of respiratory system of nasal area is not functioning properly, it leads to underdeveloped nose and nasal bridge, and high palatal vault. An increased interocclusal gap allows supra-eruption of teeth and hence increased facial height. Mandible gets rotated in a clockwise (D and B) direction.

Role of muscle exercises or muscle retraining: Any imbalance in the equilibrium of forces leads to abnormal shaping of dental arches and abnormal relation of jaw bases, e.g. abnormal oral habits. The growth pattern of the patient is also affected which further leads to deterioration of muscular balance. If this abnormal muscular pattern is not controlled by retraining the involved muscles at an early age, the pattern becomes fixed in the neuro-muscular circuits, and then it becomes difficult to establish the new pattern as the age advances. Habits being causative factors, need to be addressed during treatment for successful and stable results. Along with, the involved muscles need to be retrained to develop normal patterns. Some of the exercises have been discussed below.

Exercises for circumoral/lip muscles: Some patients have small upper lip thus the lips are incompetent and hypotonic. Also, some may have lip biting habits. If the soft tissue growth is still continuing, then the timely lip exercises can give good results, leading to improvement in tonicity and length. Following exercises can be taught to the patient:

1. Upper lip can be stretched towards the lower lip to attain a lip seal, especially if upper lip is small or hypotonic.
2. The patient can be asked to hold a piece of paper between the lips.
3. They can be asked to over-stretch the upper lip and then the lower lip is extended above the upper lip to cover it and hold it for count upto 10. This exercise can be repeated many times per day.
4. To inflate the balloons is also a good exercise involving lips and cheeks.
5. Patients can improve by playing flute.
6. Patient can be asked to hold water in mouth for 10 sec and then repeat the exercise. He can also be told to pump the water back and forth behind the lips to stretch them.
7. Patient can be asked to stretch the lip toward the chin.
8. Massaging the upper lip in downward direction can also help in stretch.
9. Button pull exercise: A big button of approx 1½ inch diameter with a strong thread through it is used. It is placed behind the lips in the vestibule and held by the lips. The thread is used to pull it outward, while the lips restrain it from being pulled outside.
10. Tug of war exercises: It uses 2 buttons in the same fashion as above, one button is inside and other is outside for pulling.
11. Oral screen with a lip loop: Oral screen used for treatment of mouth breathing problem also has a loop at incisal level. The patient is advised to pull his upper lip towards the ring, and the lower lip tries to catch the upper lip.

Exercises for Tongue

Tongue is a very strong and important muscle in oral cavity. It helps in speech, mastication, swallowing, etc. It also helps in molding the dental arches in proper shape, by maintaining equilibrium of forces with extraoral muscles of cheeks and lips. Many habits disturb this equilibrium, e.g. tongue thrust, thumb sucking and mouth breathing habits. Some of tongue exercises can be used as given below:

a. **Positioning of tongue and swallow exercises:** The patient is asked to position the tip of tongue in the rugae area of palate. The teeth are lightly brought in occlusion. Lips should be kept lightly touched without any strain or kept apart. The patient is instructed to swallow keeping the tip of tongue fixed in rugae area, and not letting it to slip forwards in between the teeth. He can be advised to use a sip of water or juice each time he swallows. This exercise is to be repeated for 10–15 minutes, 3–4 times daily for many months.

b. **4S exercises:** This includes identifying the spot, salivating, squeezing the spot and swallowing. First step is spotting exercise. Spot should be the rest position of tongue. Next is the salivating exercise. Place the tongue on the spot. It results in salivation. It should be followed by squeezing the tongue vigorously with the teeth closed against the spot. 'Squeeze' is done by squeezing followed by relaxing. This is third step. This should be followed by fourth step of swallowing. The patient should practice the new swallowing pattern at least 40 times a day. Citric acid tablet can be is used for this exercise. Ask the patient to hold the tablet using the tongue tip against the palate as long as possible. Initially the patient can hold for only a few seconds, gradually the duration can be extended. It helps to develop the new neuromuscular pattern.

c. **One-elastic swallow:** A small elastic is placed on the tongue tip and patient is asked to hold the elastic in rugae area and swallow without ingesting it.

d. **Two-elastic swallow:** One elastic is kept at tip of tongue and other at dorsum of tongue. Patient is asked to swallow, maintaining the elastics in place.
e. **Hold pull exercise:** The patient is asked to keep the tip and mid of tongue against the palate and then he is asked to open the mouth gradually. It also helps to stretch the lingual frenum, besides training the tongue.

Exercise for lip biting: Patient is asked to keep his one lip over the other lip to avoid bringing the lip between the teeth.

Exercise for Mouth Breathing

1. If there is no pathology in the nasal passage, the patient is advised to breathe through the nose gradually increasing the frequency.
2. He may be asked to do breathing exercise by closing one nostril at a time and breathing through the other nostril, and vice versa, e.g. Anulom vilom yogic exercise.
3. He may be advised to breathe heavily deliberately through nose while keeping his mouth and lips closed.
4. He is advised to hold water in the mouth and then breathe through the nose.

Muscles exercises for treatment of TMD, excessive mouth opening; subluxation: Patient is advised to do resistance exercises to strengthen the muscles around the condyles. The palm is placed below the chin to apply an upward pressure while the patient tries to open the mouth against resistance. Another exercise is that the fingers are placed on the lower incisors to apply a downward pressure, while the patient tries to close the mouth.

Muscles exercises for masseter muscle: To strengthen the masseter, the patient is asked to clench the teeth and count upto 10. It should be repeated for some duration of time. Alternatively he may be asked to chew the gum for some duration.

Myofunctional appliances as muscle exercisers: Oral gymnastics was the term introduced by Frankel. He said that the skeletal malrelation is due to abnormal muscular patterns of the orofacial muscles. He introduced the Frankel appliances which are loose fitting appliances in the oral cavity. To retain them in position, the patient has to keep his orofacial/masticatory muscles active, thus achieving a new retrained pattern. This helps to guide the growth of jaws in a normal direction. With myofunctional appliances, mainly the lateral pterygoid muscle achieves a new pattern to keep condyle in a forward position. Along with it, other masticatory muscles, like temporalis, tongue, etc. also get readapted. Bionator has a capacity to retrain the tongue muscles during treatment by caressing the dorsum of tongue by Coffin spring and stimulating it to achieve a more D and F positioning during skeletal class II treatment. Activator also stretches and activates the masticatory muscles to achieve a new pattern.

Myofunctional Orofacial Therapy: Padovan Method of Neurofunctional Reorganization

Padovan method has been developed as a treatment approach in which all functions of orofacial region are considered, e.g. respiration, speech, mastication, breathing, swallowing, etc. This method can be applied to any patient, with any kind of pathology and at any age. In Padovan method, all the muscles related to functions are exercised in each therapeutic session. These functions are not isolated but are interdependent on the same muscles and the same nerve impulses. So, if one function gets altered, the others are also affected. Conversely, proper functioning of one group also helps the other ones. Patient's own reflexes are used to establish adequate function.

Some exercises of the method: There are some simple materials used in the Padovan training which are easily available, e.g. party blowers, pacifiers, flexible rubber tubing of different sizes, spatulas, catheters, orthodontic elastics, drinking straws, a small massage vibrator and wooden whistles.

Respiration: The entire respiratory tract of patient is taken into account, from the diaphragm up to the nose and mouth. The patient leans back comfortably in a chair and is asked to speak vowels one by one. Clinician applies gentle pressures on the region of diaphragm. This light pressure interrupts the sound and stimulates the vocal folds. The diaphragm and vocal folds are addressed simultaneously. Blower is used to increase the lung capacity. Exercises to re-establish nasal airflow are done with the blower in nostrils. The patient is asked to close the lips, to occlude one nostril with finger and insert the blower into other nostril. Then he blows through the nose to unfurl the blower and keep it inflated as long as possible. When the blower deflates it is immediately removed, and the patient automatically breathes deeply through the open nostril. The exercise is repeated a varying number of times, depending on the patient.

Sucking: A special orthodontic pacifier is used to stimulate sucking, as it will not deform the dental arches. These exercises involve all facial muscles and those supporting the head. To have an efficient suction, it must be continuous and rhythmic. Muscle tonus is improved through the rhythm of alternating contraction and relaxation. The exercises are performed along with rhythmical poems, so that the rhythm gets incorporated into the patient's movement patterns. The pacifier may be slightly pulled out to make the suction more vigorous.

Mastication: Surgical rubber tubing is used for the exercise of masticatory muscles. It is placed transversely in the mouth between the molars of both sides. The patient is asked to chew first bilaterally; and then unilaterally with the bent tubing inserted between the molars on one side, then on the other, and then on the anterior teeth. The tube ends, during mastication, pinch the tongue slightly, providing a beneficial stimulus.

Deglutition: EMG studies have confirmed that the activities of various muscles, i.e. superior constrictors, buccinators and orbicularis oris ms are interrelated. They perform as a unit during swallowing, blowing, chewing, coughing, etc. The buccinator and orbicularis oris play a definite role in starting the swallowing by producing a peristaltic-like wave of contraction originating in oral cavity and tongue, which then passes through the pharynx and esophagus. Activity of superior constrictor begins before the simultaneous contraction of buccinators and orbicularis oris has ceased. Swallowing exercises help to stimulate the muscles of suprahyoid, infrahyoid and the posterior tongue regions. During deglutition, the supra- and infra-hyoid muscles elevate the hyoid.

For swallowing exercise, the water is injected in patient's mouth, and the tongue is held and pushed with a tongue depressor. Patient is advised to gargle quickly, to move the water into position where it will trigger the swallow reflex, and then to swallow. The exercise is repeated many times during the session. After this procedure, the patient himself becomes capable of positioning the tongue back without tongue depressor. Then, correct positioning of tongue tip (on the rugae area and incisal papilla) is exercised, which helps to establish the process of normal deglutition.

Certain other exercises can be helpful to stimulate and strengthen the buccofacial musculature. One of them is very helpful to improve proprioception of tongue as well as its propulsion and retraction. An orthodontic elastic is placed around the tongue. The patient retracts the tongue, sliding the elastic forward until it comes off. It can be repeated few times every day.

Conclusion

Since the normal functioning of soft tissues is important for the dentofacial growth, all the attempts should be made by the clinicians to normalize the functions. Abnormal habits disturb the balance of the forces leading to abnormal development causing malocclusion. Habits can be easily controlled at an early age, thus reducing the severity of malocclusion and even normalizing the functions and growth. With increasing age, the correction of habit becomes difficult and a prolonged treatment is needed. It also needs a prolonged retention period to maintain the orthodontic correction. Muscles retraining methods are very important during treatment of habits, as they help in achieving a normal function of associated muscles and thus normalizing the development and growth of dentofacial complex. These exercises play a crucial role during habit-treatment and should be regularly advised and reinforced to the patients.

49

Adenoids and Orthodontics

INTRODUCTION

Adenoids are lymphatic tissues embedded in the posterior wall of nasopharynx. They are known as pharyngeal tonsils, and are part of the Waldeyer's ring. The group of lymphoid tissue encircling the pharynx is known as Waldeyer's ring. It includes: adenoids/ pharyngeal tonsils, lateral pharyngeal tonsils, lateral pharyngeal bands, faucial/palatine tonsils, and lingual tonsils.

Enlarged tonsils and adenoids have been implicated in abnormal growth of dentofacial tissues by affecting the patency of upper respiratory tract. Blockade caused by them leads to mouth breathing and the open mouth posture. Although they are commonly implicated as the cause for dentofacial abnormalities by orthodontists, but the decision for tonsillectomy and/or adenoidectomy remains on ENT specialist who considers other factors before any surgical intervention.

Immunologic Aspects of Tonsils and Adenoids

Tonsils and adenoids, because of their strategic locations, constitute the primary sites of initial exposure to inhaled or ingested antigens. Nasopharyngeal mucosa, tonsils, and adenoids are replete with immunocompetent tissue. Tonsillar lymphoid tissues may also be involved in the development of human immune system, like thymus. Newborn infants do not have antibodies in their bodies except IgG at birth acquired through mother. After birth, the bacterial colonization of oral cavity and exposure to other antigens occurs, so the immune system begins to mature rapidly. During the early years of life, all available immunocompetent lymphoid tissue is required for optimal development of immunoglobulins. Waldeyer's ring also contributes to stimulate the immunologic response.

Basic Facial Growth and Development

Postnatal facial growth is influenced by genetic and environmental factors. Most facial growth and development occurs during the two growth peaks seen in childhood. The basic facial growth and development is dependent on interrelation of multiple functional matrices. According to studies, by the age of four, 60% of the craniofacial skeleton has reached its adult size, and by 12 years age, 90% of facial growth has already occurred. By age seven, majority of the growth of maxilla is complete, and by age nine, the majority of the growth of mandible is complete. The growth of nasomaxillary complex, NMC, is dependent on the growth of anterior cranial fossae upto 6 years of age, and after that the growth occurs mainly by growth of nasal cartilage, surface remodeling and adaptive changes. The abnormal growth of adenoid tissues affects the growth of NMC.

Natural Growth of Lymphoid Tissues

According to Scammon's theory, there is a rapid growth of lymphoid tissues during infancy and early childhood, and a continued but slower increase during late childhood and prepuberty. It may be due to the requirement of the body, which needs immunocompetent cells during initial years of life to fight form the pathogenic assault. Growth of lymphoid tissues reaches upto 200% growth, peaking before adolescence and then gradually declines thereafter to adult values.

Bacteria may play a role in adenoid hyperplasia. Specifically, pathogens, like *Haemophilus influenzae* and *Staphylococcus aureus*, have been associated with lymphoid tissue hyperplasia. The adenoid lymphoid structures are lined with ciliated respiratory-type epithelium which is normally distributed throughout the upper and posterior nasopharynx walls. During the presence of disease, there is an increase in dendritic cells in the crypts, and extrafollicular areas, and a decrease in surface epithelium dendritic cells.

There is also some suggestion that adenoids and hypertrophic tonsils are a consequence of a thyroid hormone deficiency. This hormone deficiency acts as a catalyst for activating the organism's defense mechanisms which include hypertrophy of lymphoid tissue.

Growth of the Pharynx and its Physiologic Implications

The pharynx can be anatomically divided into two parts: upper (the nasopharynx) and lower (the oropharynx). Normally, the nasopharynx enlarges to accommodate the growing adenoids maintaining a patent nasopharyngeal airway. Any imbalance between this increase in the size of nasopharyngeal airway and the concomitant growth of adenoids may result in reduced patency and nasopharyngeal obstruction. The main growth direction of pharynx is vertical. The hard palate grows downward due to remodelling, and the growth contribution of spheno-occipital synchondrosis, SOS, is also in upward and forward direction. Growth in SOS takes place till maturity and parallels sexually determined growth of the skeleton (in boys until 18 years of age or later, in girls until about 13 years of age). The nasopharynx's ultimate patency, however, depends on the growth and relative size of soft tissues lining the skeletal boundaries.

Growth of oropharynx is related with vertebrae also. The cervical vertebrae also grow in height (atlas 31%, other cervical vertebrae a mean of 41%). This process continues until adulthood and shows two periods of accelerated growth (between 5 and 7 years and between 12 and 15 years of age). Also, height of each vertebra lower in the neck or farther down the spinal column grows bigger (cephalocaudal gradient of growth), and an increase in thickness of intervertebral disks also contributes to the total length gain of the cervical column. The vertical growth behavior of hyoid bone closely parallels that of the vertebral bodies. During growth, hyoid maintains a relatively stable superoinferior position between C3 and C4, and it descends together with the mandible and the vertebrae.

Pharynx and the Somatotypes

Size and shape of pharynx also varies with shape of the head, which can be dolichocephalic, normocephalic, or brachycephalic. The relation of face, head and the dental arches has been discussed in the chapter of diagnosis. Dolichocephalic form is oval, horizontally long and relatively narrow and is associated with a narrow and long face and dental arches (leptoprosopic). The brachycephalic head form is horizontally shorter and broader, and associated with a short and broad face and dental arches (euryprosopic). Nasopharyngeal depth (the distance of PNS to the posterior pharyngeal wall) is significantly shorter in long face syndrome, LFS, than in the short face syndrome (SFS). Dolichocephalic persons have longer necks than persons with euryprosopic features. The hyoid bone is also displaced more closely to the cervical spine in LFS. An increased mandibular plane angle and the U & B rotation of cervical spine against the cranial base helps to restore the pharyngeal space at the level of the base of tongue.

Euryprosopy is characterized by lesser vertical increase in vertebrae and by a forward only movement of hyoid bone, whereas in vertical growth pattern, cervical vertical growth is considerable and is associated with a concomitant downward movement of hyoid bone under the influence of infrahyoid muscles. The latter may be an explanation for higher occurrence of dental crowding in persons with LFS. Concomitant with the lowering of hyoid, the tongue also falls back leading to a disturbance in the buccolingual muscular equilibrium, thus a decrease in lingual support for dental arches, and thus leading to narrow arch form in anterior region.

The Effect of Adenoids on Dentofacial Morphology

Grossly enlarged tonsils and adenoids are among the reported causes of mouth breathing. Two physiologic factors have received particular attention with regard to their possible relation to craniofacial development, namely, (1) the adequacy of the nasopharyngeal airway and (2) the postural relations of the head and the cervical column. Development of nose and nasal bridge is affected in mouth breathing, the bridge being flatter as compared to normal patients. The nasal breathing function acts as a functional matrix for the growth of nasal passage. They lead to disturbed development of occlusion and craniofacial growth as discussed below.

Effects on Maxilla and Mandible

Dentofacial changes associated with nasal airway blockage were described by CV Tomes in 1872 as **adenoid facies**. He reported that children, who were mouth breathers, often had narrow V-shaped dental arches. It is due to that the mouth breathers keep their mouth open, their lips apart and the tongue position low. It leads to an imbalance between the tongue pressure, and the cheek muscles (buccinator mechanism), resulting in cheek muscles compressing the dental arches thus narrowing them. These simultaneous actions have been termed the **compressor theory**. Simultaneously, the lower jaw drops D and B, with increased interocclusal gap, in which the posterior teeth are free to erupt. It leads to increased dentoalveolar and facial height, convex profile, long and narrow face; D and B rotation of mandible; decreased posterior face height, etc. occurs. These features are found in patients having long face syndrome LFS.

Positioning of the tongue also plays an important role in mandibular development. The tongue gets displaced downward which can lead to a retrognathic mandible; and an interposed tongue can lead to open bite.

Airway obstruction, and thus the imbalance of lingual, palatal and buccal pressures produce alterations in the maxilla. Maxillary narrowing occurs which may lead to cross bite. In sagittal direction, it may produce maxillary retrusion. Vertical height of the maxilla also increases; the palatal plane may be found tipped up in the anterior part, while tipped down in posterior part, contributing to Angle's class II molar relation by bringing the molars mesially.

Respiratory Pattern and Dentofacial Form

Mouth breathers often have narrow, V-shaped dental arches however it may be an inherited feature and should be evaluated properly. Adenoid obstruction appears to be most common among children who have long faces and small nasopharynx, while larger nasopharyngeal cavities are in SFS. Mouth breathing has been incriminated in dentofacial deformities as supported by experiments in which nasal obstructions were created in growing monkeys. Moss's functional matrix theory in orofacial growth supports this idea, since due to nasal obstruction, the nasal passage and soft tissues are not able to act as proper functional matrix and thus growth of related part (nasopharynx, nasal cavity, nostrils, nasal bridge, nasal tip, etc.) is affected. Facial structures are modified by postural alterations in soft tissue that produce changes in the equilibrium of pressure exerted on teeth and the facial bones.

UPPER AIRWAY OBSTRUCTION AND MOUTH BREATHING

Mouth breathing is usually defined as "habitual respiration through the mouth instead of the nose." During normal nasal respiration, the nose filters, warms and humidifies the air to prepare it for entry into lungs. This nasal airway also provides a degree of nasal resistance to assist the movements of diaphragm and intercostals muscles by creating a negative intrathoracic pressure. According to blood gas studies, mouth breathers have 20% higher partial pressure of carbon dioxide and 20% lower partial pressures of oxygen in the blood. Contributing factors in the obstruction of upper airways include: anatomical airway constriction, developmental anomalies, macroglossia, DNS, enlarged tonsils and adenoids, nasal polyps and allergic rhinitis.

Adenoid Evaluation

Adenoid size is assessed relative to the dimensions of nasopharynx. Adenoids are best assessed clinically by direct nasopharyngoscopy, and by lateral view of nasopharynx in extended neck position. Lateral cephalograms have also been used for assessing nasopharyngeal and adenoid size by the orthodontists. It has been found that there is a significant relationship between the size of adenoids measured on lateral cephalograms and as assessed clinically; and the greater the size of adenoids, as measured on lateral cephalograms, the less the nasal airflow. But these radiographs reflect the nasopharynx in only two dimensions. Grossly enlarged tonsils can create an obstruction in oropharyngeal space posterior to tongue leading to its forward protrusion to maintain an adequate oropharyngeal space for respiration. A protrusive tongue may also occur due to other factors causing nasorespiratory obstruction to maintain a patent oral airway, e.g. macroglossia. Degree of airway obstruction is expressed in terms of **nasal resistance**. Watson, Warren, and Fischer showed that the incidence of clinically observable mouth breathing was greater among subjects with a nasal resistance above 4.5 cm. water per liter per second. But it may vary according to age of the patient. Nasopharyngeal space and the size of adenoids have been evaluated using different methods of assessment, e.g. Determination of the roentgenographic adenoid/nasopharyngeal ratio (from a lateral cephalometric X-ray); flexible optic endoscopes; acoustic rhinometry; direct measurements during surgery. Direct measurements are considered to be the most accurate because space can be assessed in three dimensions. A lateral cephalometic radiograph is an added valuable diagnostic tool for the orthodontist in the evaluation of children with upper airway obstructions. Direct measurement of the adequacy of the nasopharyngeal airway can be performed by rhinomanometry.

Treatment of Nasal Obstruction

Use of nasal sprays (e.g. mometasone, fluticasone), nasal decongestants (xylometazoline), and anti-allergic medications (loratidine, cetrizine) are given in initial phases in patients having allergic rhinitis, etc. to control the inflammation of soft tissues lining in nasal passage.

Adenoidectomy with or without tonsillectomy is indicated if hypertrophied adenoids (and tonsils) are the cause of upper airway obstruction.

Powered-shaver adenoidectomy: Adenoidectomy coupled with endoscopic visualization will assist in achieving adequate removal of adenoids particularly high in the nasopharnx. Use of the powered-shaver technique allows for better clearance of obstructive adenoids. The end result is more reliable restoration of nasal patency. Septal surgery is rarely indicated in the child, but may be considered in the presence of a marked nasal septal deflection with impaction. Conservative septal surgery in growing patients will not have an adverse effect in dentofacial growth.

Maxillary expansion (RME or SME) can be done to expand the upper dental arch. It also helps to widen the nasal cavity, and decreases the nasal resistance.

Cryosurgery or electrosurgery is also a viable option for certain patients with rhinitis.

Bipolar radiofrequency ablation is another technique for treatment of allergic rhinitis, and can be performed under local anesthetic.

Inferior turbinectomy is required in hypertrophy of turbinates, thus blocking the nasal passage.

Surgical intervention should be done after judicious evaluation of certain factors because

1. The removal of tonsils and adenoids during the growth period may compromise subsequent local nasopharyngeal immunologic responses and overall immunity to infections in the respiratory tract, since (a) tonsils and adenoids are located strategically at sites of initial antigen exposure and (b) tonsils are possibly involved in the development and maintenance of the immune system.
2. There is a lack of scientific evidence of actual health benefits resulting from tonsillectomy and/or adenoidectomy.

Conclusion

Adenoids have been considered as important cause of abnormal growth of face and development of malocclusion. By the age of 12 years, almost 90% of facial growth has already occurred so most formation and/or deformation has already occurred, if there lies any uncontrolled causative factor. Thus to prevent any abnormal growth, early interceptive measures must be initiated as soon as possible. A multidisciplinary approach should be followed for management of young patients with increased nasal airway resistance, which includes physicians, dentists, allergists, otorhinolaryngologists, and orthodontists. After diagnosis, a comprehensive risk benefit analysis regarding early intervention must be considered. Thus, a universal goal of intervention is the promotion of proper nasal respiration throughout a child's early years of facial growth.

50

Obstructive Sleep Apnea Syndrome

INTRODUCTION

Obstructive sleep apnea (OSA) is characterized by repeated episodes of airway obstruction for more than 10 seconds during sleep, resulting in pauses in breathing. It is the condition of recurrent episodes of cessation of respiratory airflow during sleep due to collapse of upper airway (UA) at the pharyngeal level. It is usually associated with reduction in blood oxygen saturation. A reduce airflow and increased resistance to nasal breathing may cause narrowing of upper jaw. Deviated nasal septum deviations, swelling of turbinates, allergic nasal congestion, etc. cause a reduction of total airflow. Because this condition is affected by jaws and related structures, dentists play an important role in diagnosing and treating such patients. Correlations exist between obstructive sleep apnea syndrome (OSAS), malocclusion and maxillofacial malrelationship.

Obstructive sleep apnea syndrome (OSAS) can affect children also due to various causes affecting the nasal breathing, leading to disturbed sleep and thus lead to negative consequences. It can affect growth, development and behavior. One of the main causes of childhood OSA is enlargement of the tonsil tissues and, in most cases, their removal serves as an ultimate treatment of OSA. **Risk factors** for development of OSA in children include a family history of snoring or OSA, obesity, physical abnormalities, cerebral palsy, muscular dystrophy, Down's syndrome, mouth breathing and any condition that may lead to a narrowing of the upper airway.

Causes of OSAS

1. Anatomic abnormality leading to narrowing or obstruction of the airway, e.g. deviated nasal septum, swollen turbinates, chronic allergic rhinitis, narrowing of the nasal passage, etc.
2. Gross facial deformity can contribute to anatomic factors leading to OSAS. Cephalometric radiography showed that these patients have smaller retropositioned mandible and maxilla, narrower posterior airway spaces, larger tongues and soft palates, inferiorly positioned hyoid bones, etc.
3. Obesity.

Symptoms of OSA include snoring, pauses in breathing while asleep, restless sleep, bizarre sleeping positions, paradoxical chest movements, cyanosis, bedwetting, hyperactivity, stunted growth and disruptive behavior in school. OSAS results in oxygen desaturation and arousal from sleep. The reduced blood oxygen saturation may give rise to hypertension, cardiac arrhythmia, nocturnal angina, and myocardial ischemia. The impaired sleep quality leads to excessive daytime sleepiness, deterioration of memory and judgment, altered personality, and reduced concentration.

Effect on dentofacial structures: Abnormal dentofacial morphologies, e.g. retrognathia, long face, mandibular deficiency, bimaxillary retrusion, steep occlusal plane, increased mandibular plane angle, and a more caudally positioned hyoid bone, and inferior positioning of hyoid bone are found in patients with OSAS. Also, reduced cranial base length and angle, large ANB angle, steep mandibular plane, elongated maxillary and mandibular teeth, narrowing of upper airway, long and large soft palate, and large tongue have also been reported. Most of these symptoms are also present in patient with mouth breathing habit. Sites of obstruction and narrowing of upper airway differ in patients with OSAS. The retropalatal (posterior to the soft palate) and retroglossal (posterior to the base of tongue) regions are commonly affected sites, and multiple sites of obstruction and narrowing are not rare.

Prevalence: The prevalence of OSAS in the middle-aged population (30–60 years) is less than the elderly people. It is more common in males (4%) than females (2%).

Clinical manifestations: They are related to cyclic obstruction of upper airway, disturbed sleep, and respiratory and cardiovascular consequences due to disturbed breathing. OSAS patients show episodes of gasping, choking or periods of apnea, with repeated arousals through the night. Patient feels sleepy in daytime which is a key feature of OSAS. Snoring, mild to extremely loud, is also present. Patients also have a feeling of tiredness despite full sleep, fatigue, morning headaches, and symptoms of depression. OSAS may lead to cardiovascular problems, like systemic hypertension, cardiac arrhythmias, myocardial infarction, etc. and the respiratory problems, like pulmonary hypertension, cor-pulmonale, chronic carbon dioxide retention, etc. So OSAS can be a potentially life-threatening condition; and it needs both proper diagnosis and appropriate treatment.

Diagnosis: A proper history is taken by asking some questions, e.g.

- Do you have difficulty staying awake when inactive (e.g. while reading, watching television or driving)?
- Do you snore while sleeping?
- Do you pause in your breathing while you are sleeping, as observed by your family member or partner?
- Is there a decrease in work performance; concentration, memory or mood?

Polysomnography: It is main method of diagnosis and assessing the potential success of treatment. Parameters, like the apnea index, the hypopnea index, the respiratory disturbance index (RDI) and the lowest oxyhemoglobin saturation, are noted.

- Apnea is the cessation in air flow for 10 seconds or more, and the apnea index is the number of apneic episodes occurring per hour.
- Hypopnea is a 50% reduction in tidal volume for more than 10 seconds, and the hypopnea index is the number of hypopneic episodes per hour.
- The RDI is the number of apneic and hypopneic episodes per hour of sleep.
- The lowest oxyhemoglobin saturation is measured by pulse oximetry.
- OSAS is diagnosed if RDI reaches a threshold level, typically 5 or 10. OSAS becomes clinically significant when the RDI is greater than 20 and oxygen desaturation fall to a level below 80–85%.

Management: OSAS can be managed by nonsurgical or surgical methods. Etiological factors should be removed first during treatment. The severity of the patient's condition and diagnostic features must direct the treatment plan. Treatment of OSA in children depends largely on the underlying cause of the problem and may include one of the following.

Nonsurgical Management

1. Obesity is a risk factor for OSAS, so reduction in body weight is advised.
2. **Continuous positive airway pressure (CPAP):** The most common nonsurgical treatment for OSA is continuous positive airway pressure therapy. This treatment involves wearing a mask overnight that exerts pressure on the upper airway to prevent collapse. Continuous positive airway pressure is often considered as a

treatment for children whose OSA symptoms are not relieved after adenotonsillectomy. CPAP was first described in 1981, and is the gold standard for its treatment. But, patient cooperation is low due to dislodgement of appliance during sleep, physical discomfort, drying of nasal and oral mucosa, etc.

3. **Oral appliances for mandibular advancement** are used for treatment of OSAS (Figs 50.1a and b). They bring the tongue forward, thus removing interference from airway, and have been found better than CPAP from patient's cooperation point of view. Various types of appliances have been designed for OSAS treatment. The basic idea is to keep the mandible and associated tissues in a forward position so that they do not fall back to obstruct the airway and interrupting normal breathing patterns. Thus they act by preventing airway obstruction and allowing the patient to breathe easily and continuously. The purpose of oral appliance is to reposition the lower jaw, tongue, soft palate, and hyoid bone into a certain position, to keep the airway open with stabilization of the tongue and jaw, or to provide artificial muscle tone to prevent collapse and resulting airway blockage. They may be made from acrylic, elastomeric materials, or silicone, or thermoplastic materials which remain soft at mouth temperature for comfort to patient; can be preformed or custom made; can be adjustable for incremental advancement of mandible; can be modified to keep tongue forward, etc. The appliance may have clasps also for better retention on the teeth. Few of the appliances are mentioned below briefly.
   - **Mandibular advancement appliances** (MAA) are modified functional appliances. Treatment with MAA is recommended especially for patients for whom improvement of sleep hygiene and removal of etiological factors are not possible. It can also be used in moderate to severe degrees of OSAS where the patients refuse nasal continuous positive airway pressure (nCPAP) therapy. The appliance brings the mandible and adjacent soft tissues in protrusion/forward during

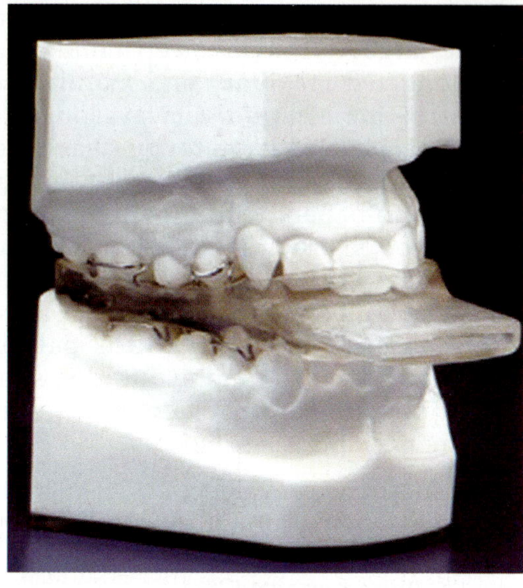

(a)

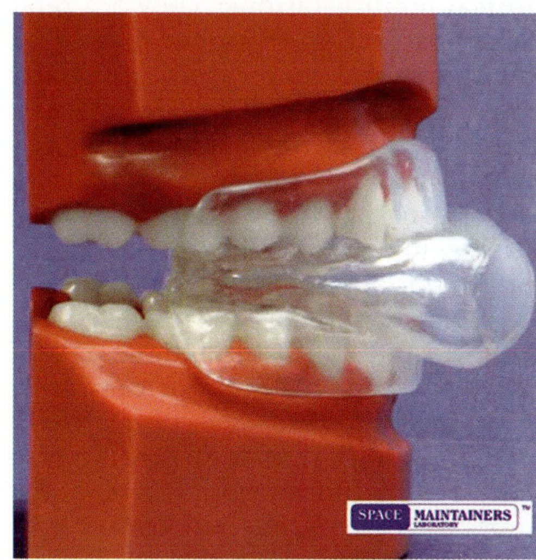

(b)

Figs 50.1a and b: Appliances for Rx of OSAS: The anterior/incisal extension in the appliances is for keeping the tongue in forward position so that it does not fall in pharynx during sleep *(Courtesy: Internet)*.

sleep. It helps in increasing the pharyngeal space, in particular the area of oro- and hypopharynx and prevents their nocturnal collapse.

- **Herbst telescopic appliance:** It is an adjustable appliance and can be extended incrementally by adding sleeves. It is comfortable to the patient as it allows various mandibular movements, speech, etc.
- **Tongue retaining device:** It is a custom made device made of flexible polyvinyl material. A tongue bulb is created in the front part to keep the tongue in a forward position by creating a negative pressure.

4. **Diet and medications:** For obese children, weight loss and maintaining a healthy diet might prove to be the ultimate treatment for their OSA. Antibiotic medication has been used as a short-term treatment for snoring and obstruction, particularly when these problems are not persistent.
5. **Medications:** For example, protriptyline, a tricyclic antidepressant, leads to symptomatic improvement of OSAS and may reduce the degree of oxygen desaturation, but its anticholinergic side effects limit its use.

Surgical Management

1. **Tracheostomy** is done for normal breathing as it bypasses the upper airway.
2. **Adenotonsillectomy:** Enlarged tonsils and adenoids can be removed to remove blockage form the airway and to normalise the breathing.
3. **Uvulopalatopharyngoplasty** (UPPP) involves removal of tissues coming in the airway, e.g. shortening the soft palate, removing the uvula, and lateral and posterior pharyngeal wall mucosa from the oral pharynx. But postoperative lateral cephalograms of patients of UPPP show that the soft palate gets shortened but its thickness increases, resulting in a narrow nasopharyngeal airway. Risks associated with UPPP are risk of hemorrhage, postoperative pain, velopharyngeal insufficiency and nasophyarngeal stenosis. There are currently two commonly performed laser procedures for snoring and mild sleep apnea: laser-assisted uvulopalatoplasty (LAUP) and laser assisted uvulopalatopharyngoplasty (LA-UPPP).
4. **Orthognathic surgery** to treat OSAS with mandibular advancement leads to correction of symptoms of OSAS. Advancement of the maxilla, may also be required, the treatment plan depends on cephalometric analysis. The advantage of orthognathic surgery is that patient cooperation is not a factor. Depending on the type of OSAS patient classification, different orthognathic procedures may be recommended. The most prevalent procedures are either mandibular advancement (MA) or maxillomandibular advancement (MMA).

Conclusion

OSAS is a common condition which may lead to significant morbidity and mortality. It also affects the children and thus their sleep and development, behaviour, school performance, etc. In adults, it may lead to cardiovascular and respiratory problems, behaviour problems, affecting their work performance, etc. The dental doctors should be aware of signs and symptoms of OSAS, so that diagnosis can be confirmed, and proper treatment and referrals may be done. Treatments should be directed to the specific causes of the condition. The treatment may involve non-surgical and surgical methods. CPAP and mandibular advancement appliances are the main methods of OSAS treatment. Surgery may be needed in patients who are non-cooperative and/or do not improve from non-surgical methods.

51

Space Management in Orthodontics

INTRODUCTION

One of the main roles of an orthodontist is the efficient management of spaces in dental arches to minimize extractions of teeth during orthodontic treatment. Space needs arise in situations, like crowding of teeth, proclination of teeth, loss of space with tooth impaction, etc. Various methods have been described to create the space in the arches to correct the malocclusion. Space management is an important procedure used in preventive and the interceptive phases of orthodontics. Preventive procedures aim at preventing the space loss in the dental arches, e.g. by restoration of proximal caries, fixing the space maintainers, etc. Interceptive procedures are used to control the developing condition so that its severity does not increase. Any loss of space may be gained by using space regainer appliances.

During growth, the physiological spaces also develop in the arches, which help to accommodate bigger permanent teeth in place of smaller primary teeth. A balance or surplus space in the arches helps in proper alignment of successors, while a deficiency of space leads to crowding. In some cases, this natural space can be efficiently utilized to correct the mild cases of crowding, e.g. by using E-space especially in lower arch, mild crowding can be resolved (Figs 51.1 to 51.3).

Rationale of Space Management

Space management is a broad concept which involves the orthodontic planning in consonance with the space availability and space need. Most of the problems in orthodontics are due to space deficiency, thus space is needed to correct the malocclusion. It involves the use of available space, maintaining the space and preventing its loss; and/or regaining the lost space. In some cases, there is excessive space, which needs to managed keeping in view the size of teeth, soft tissues esp tongue and lips, retention planning, possibility of prosthodontic intervention, etc. Broadly, space management can be divided as follows.

I. **Using the natural spaces:** Utilize the space present in the normal developing dentition, e.g. primary/developmental spaces, i.e. physiological spaces, primate spaces, and leeway space.

II. **Space maintenance:** Maintain the space after loss of a tooth. Space due to loss of a primary tooth should be managed with a space maintainer; while space due to loss of a permanent tooth is managed with prosthesis or by orthodontics as the case demands.

III. **Space regaining:** Loss of space occurs due to proximal shifting of adjacent teeth if it is not managed properly after loss of teeth. In certain cases, the lost space has to be regained to correct the position of other teeth to receive a proper prosthesis or for correction of malocclusion. It can be done by space regaining appliances, expansions screws, finger springs (Cetlin appliance), molar distalization, molar uprighting, active lingual arch, etc. It will avoid future crowding and allow the normal eruption of developing permanent teeth.

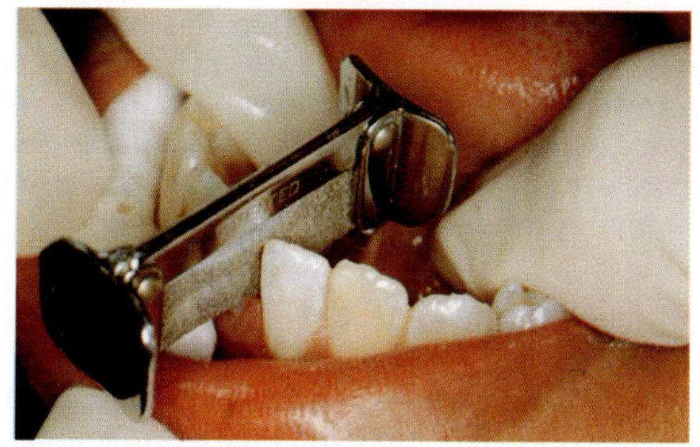

Fig. 51.1: Metallic strip holder for slicing the teeth for space creation *(Courtesy: Internet)*.

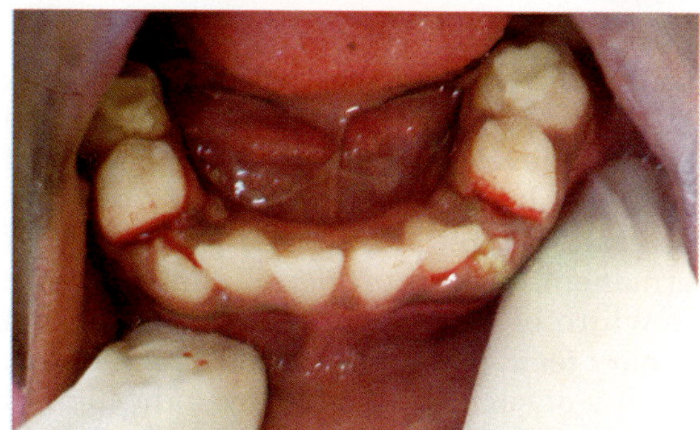

Fig. 51.3: Judicious slicing of the contact areas of primary teeth to create space for erupting permanent tooth. In this case, mesial surface of primary molar has been sliced to make some space for erupting canine.

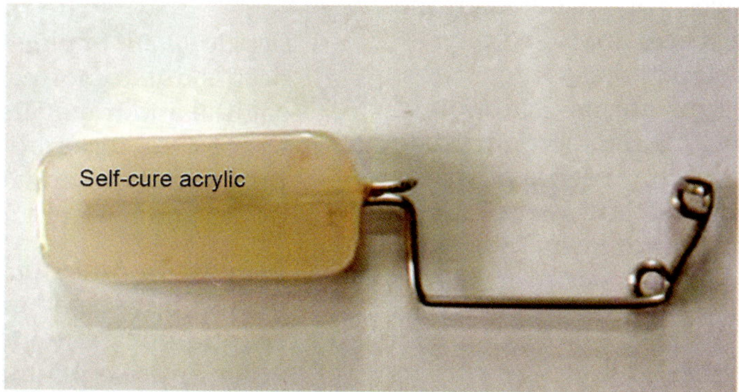

(a)

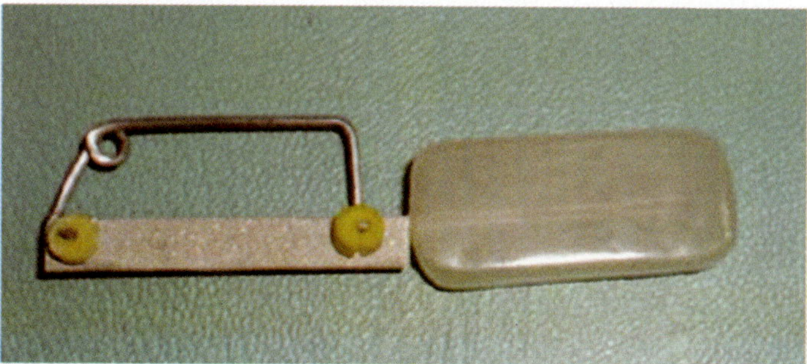

(b)

Figs 51.2a and b: Custom made strip-holders *(Courtesy: Internet)*.

IV. **Management of excess space:** Excess space in the dental arches can be due either to the small sized teeth; or broader arches or a combination of both. Broader arches are generally seen in horizontal growth cases, comparatively larger than normal tongue size, excessive growth of jaws, etc.

Need to Maintain the Space

Primary teeth are the best space maintainers for the proper eruption of successors in normally developing arches. Maintenance of space left by the loss of primary teeth is necessary to keep the space for eruption of permanent teeth in proper alignment. Since the width of permanent teeth is more than primary teeth (except the second premolars), any loss of such space is a sure indication of crowding and disturbance of occlusion in permanent dentition.

DEVELOPMENT OF DENTITION

During normal growth and development of arches and jaws in sagittal and transverse dimensions, the spaces appear between the primary teeth. These spaces are called physiological spaces or developmental spaces. These spaces are important for normal eruption of permanent teeth which help to accommodate the larger permanent teeth. Absence of spaces is an indication that crowding will occur in permanent dentition. It is evident in Table 51.1.

Table 51.1: Crowding in permanent teeth

Class	*In deciduous teeth*	*Chances of crowding in permanent teeth*
I	Crowded	10 in 10
II	No spaces	7 in 10
III	< 3 mm spacing	5 in 10
IV	3–6 mm spacing	2 in 10
V	> 6 mm spacing	None

Primate spaces: These spaces are seen mesial to maxillary canine and distal to mandibular canine. These physiological spaces are also called simian spaces or anthropoid spaces. These spaces help in achieving the relation of of upper and lower canines.

Incisal liability: It is the difference in the combined MD sizes of primary and permanent incisors; it is 7.6 mm in upper and 6.0 mm in lower arch. It is overcome by utilization of physiological interdental spacing, incisors erupting labially, and increase in intercanine width with growth **(Warren Mayne's principles).** In a normally developing dentition, this is overcome by following sources (Table 51.2):

1. ***Development of physiological spacing*:** It occurs due to normal growth of jaws in sagittal and transverse dimensions, thus spaces get created in the arches. It provides approximately 4 mm space in upper and 3 mm in lower arch.
2. ***Increase in intercanine width*:** It occurs during transverse growth of jaws, and eruption of permanent canines. It provides approx. 4.5 mm space in maxilla and 3 mm space in mandible. It occurs more in males than in females (M > F); more in upper arch than the lower arch (U > L); and for longer time in upper arch than the lower arch (U > L). Thus the girls have greater liability to incisors' crowding. It increases upto 12 years in females, and upto 16 years in males in maxilla. In mandible, it increases upto 9 years age in both males and females.

Table 51.2: Incisal liability

Method	*Maxilla*	*Mandible*
Interdental spacing	0–10 mm Average: 4 mm	0–6 mm Average: 3 mm
Increase in intercanine width	4.4 mm	3 mm
Incisor position	2.2 mm	1.3 mm

3. **Labial positioning and eruption of permanent incisors:** Although the permanent incisors develop on lingual side of the primary teeth, but they erupt in more labially inclined position and erupt labial to the primary incisors. It may be due to forward growth of jaws and a push factor from tongue. It helps to compensate approx. 1–2 mm space. It is more in upper arch than the lower arch.
4. During eruption, the mandibular lateral incisors apply a distal-push force on the primary canines and push them in the primate space. It leads to create approx. 1 mm space for alignment of incisors. But this phenomenon is not seen in upper arch, because the primate space is present distal to lateral incisors which is utilised by the erupting permanent lateral incisor.

Leeway space of Nance: Combined mesiodistal width of primary canine, first and second molars (CDE) is larger than the combined mesiodistal width of permanent canine, first and second premolars (345). This difference in mesiodistal widths of CDE and 345 is the leeway space of Nance. This is 1.7 mm as either side of lower arch, totally it amounts to 3.4 mm in the lower arch, whereas it is only 0.9 mm per side of upper arch, amounting 1.8 mm in upper arch.

Importance of leeway space: In normally developing jaws and dental arches, the upper and lower primary second molars related in a flush terminal plane. It is because the MD size of lower molar is more than the upper molar. Thus the permanent first molars erupt in end-on relation. When the lower primary second molars are lost, the permanent first molars shift mesially to achieve Angle's class I molar relation. It is allowed by the leeway space. Since leeway space in lower arch is more than upper arch, the lower molars shift mesially more than the upper molar.

Leeway space can be conserved by interceptive orthodontic means and then used for alignment of erupting permanent teeth in mild crowding cases. The half-cusp class II or flush terminal/end-on relation of permanent molars is corrected by distalizing maxillary first molars to achieve class I molars.

Ugly-duckling stage: It has been described by Braodbent. It is a self-correcting condition seen in maxillary incisor region at around 8–9 years of age, during eruption of permanent maxillary canines. As the permanent canines erupt, they displace the roots of incisors mesially, leading to root crowding; development of spaces between crowns and distal divergence of crowns of incisors. This stage usually resolves naturally when permanent canines erupt in dental arches, thus relieving the pressure from the distal sides of lateral incisors roots and transferring it to the crowns, thus pushing them mesially and roots distally in a better axial inclination. This stage should not be disturbed to close the developing spaces with any orthodontic mechanics, otherwise it will push roots of lateral incisors against the canines, thus leading to root resorption and the displacement of the path of eruption of the canines.

SPACE ANALYSIS

Space analysis is the comparison between the amount of space available in the dental arches for alignment of teeth and amount of space required to align them properly. The analysis can be done either on dental casts or by a computer method after appropriate digitization of arches and tooth dimensions. A comparison of space available with the space needed can represent one of the three situation, i.e.

1. A deficiency of space: Which will lead to crowding
2. Correct amount of space: Lead to normal alignment of teeth
3. Excess space: Will result in spaces between the teeth.

Spacing Problems in Primary Dentition

In primary dentition, especially around the age of 5 and 6 years, some spaces are present in the anterior segment of dental arches. These are the physiological spaces which develop due to growth of jaws, and are necessary for proper alignment of permanent incisors. Absence of these spaces indicates high probability of crowding. Also, the leeway space as discussed above are important for permanent dental alignment and should be preserved. Certain situations can cause due to premature loss of primary teeth, e.g. traumatic avulsion, gross caries, infection, etc. where the teeth are not salvageable. The space left by the primary teeth should be preserved as discussed below.

1. **Loss of primary incisors:** In the incisal region, the physiological spaces are present and there are no adjacent dental contacts, so an early loss of a primary incisor generally does not lead to any space loss. As there are no dental contacts, the occlusal forces in mesial direction are not transmitted to adjoining teeth and thus shifting does not occur. Also, the anterior component of masticatory forces does not go toward the incisal region around the curve of dental arches. So, space maintenance is not necessary in incisal region. But it needs a prosthetic management for esthetics for psychological benefit, and as an aid in speech. It may also help to prevent development of tongue thrust habit.

2. **Loss of primary canine:** Permanent incisors shift laterally into the space left by the premature loss of a primary canine, creating a midline deviation and dental asymmetry. Space maintenance is not needed here during primary dentition, but it is desirable to intercept during eruption of permanent incisors. To prevent shifting of permanent incisors laterally, a symmetrical/ balanced extraction of other side of canine may be needed. However, premature extraction or loss of canines has been noted as a negative factor for proper increase in intercanine width and transverse jaw growth. It may also lead to uprighting of lower incisors, and deepening of bite as seen during serial extraction.

3. **Loss of primary first molar:** Space of first primary molar may be lost due to movements of adjacent teeth in certain situations. It may be more crucial in closed dentitions. Thus, space maintenance should be considered in this region.

4. **Loss of primary second molar:** Primary second molars preserve the spaces for second premolars, and also their distal root guides the erupting permanent first molar into position. It is a very crucial area of dental arches because any space loss in this region leads to loss of leeway space and deficiency of space for permanent teeth. Premature loss of primary second molar needs a space maintainer to preserve the space and to guide the eruption of permanent first molar in proper position (distal shoe appliance). Primary second molars are the best natural space maintainers and all efforts should be done to preserve them.

Problems in Early Mixed Dentition

Many situations may be seen during MDP, and the clinician has to act according to the situation. Main objective is to prevent loss of any space or to regain the lost space so that the permanent teeth are able to erupt in normal position. The dental arches should be evaluated for developmental and primate spaces and an evaluation of the growth pattern of face and jaws should be done. Some of the situations of space problems have been described by Proffit can be discussed as follows.

Situation I: Missing Primary Teeth with Adequate Space

In cases with is no loss of space, the space maintenance is done if there is expected a delay of 6 months or more for the eruption of permanent tooth. Unilateral space is best managed by unilateral fixed appliance, e.g. band and loop SM, band and bar SM, etc.

Space due to bilateral loss of molars is best managed with TPA or LHA. In mixed dentition, unilateral loss of an anterior tooth needs the balancing extraction of contralateral tooth to prevent the midline change so that the arch symmetry is maintained. If contralateral canine is extracted, then a lingual arch space maintainer is still needed to prevent lingual movement of incisors.

Situation 2: Localized Space Loss (3 mm or less)

Space regaining appliances are needed. Up to 3 mm of space may be regained by tipping the molar distally. It may be done by using simple appliances, e.g. Cetlins' removable appliance; Gerber space regainer; etc.

Situation 3: Generalized Moderate Crowding (4–7 mm)

It is a borderline type of problem which may need treatment by non-extraction or extraction method, depending on the soft tissues, and growth pattern of the patient. Depending on the magnitude of discrepancy, and presence of crowding in incisors region, 2 treatment possibilities are there for treatment during early MDP. Either reduce the MD size of primary canine to gain some space for alignment of incisors, or expand the arch to gain space, including mild distal tipping of molars, some proclination of incisors, and widening arch in premolar region.

Severe Space Problems

If space discrepancy is more, then the extraction of some permanent teeth is needed to align the remaining teeth following the guidance of eruption.

Serial Extraction

It is an interceptive procedure followed during the mid-mixed dentition period when severe crowding is anticipated. It involves planned and sequential extraction of certain primary and permanent teeth in an orderly sequence to provide space and guide the erupting permanent teeth in favorable positions.

SPACE MAINTENANCE

Space maintenance can be defined as the preservation of spaces left due to premature loss of primary teeth. Primary teeth act to stimulate the alveolar bone during mastication and help in growth of alveolar bone and stimulating the dental eruption. Primary teeth are the best natural SM for the succedaneous teeth. They help in avoiding crowding and allow normal eruption of developing permanent teeth. A ***space maintainer*** (SM) is an appliance which maintains the MD width of the space left by lost primary tooth or teeth, and sometimes helps in restoring function depending on the design used. It is a passive appliance since it applies no force on the abutment teeth.

Principles in designing of a space maintainer: Certain factors should be kept in mind while making an SM appliance.

1. Anchorage: Abutment teeth must be strong to withstand the occlusal forces, and should be having proper root length and bone support.
2. Passivity: It should be passive that is should not apply any abnormal force on the abutment tooth so that it remains stable.
3. Simplicity: The design must be simple so that it allows easy manipulations by the clinicians and should be tolerated by patient.
4. Interference: It should not interfere with the erupting permanent teeth, occlusion and surrounding tissues.

Planning for Space Maintenance

Factors considered during planning for space maintainers are as follows:

1. **Number of teeth lost:** It is a major factor to plan the design of the SM. SM should be sturdy while in use. Loss of a single tooth needs SM which can be supported at one end, i.e. cantilever type, e.g. band

and loop type which is the most commonly used SM. But an longer span of space needs an SM which should be supported at both ends and should be made of thicker wire. Design of SM depends on the number or position of the teeth lost. Loss of a single posterior tooth needs unilateral SM. A bilateral loss of teeth needs either 2 unilateral SMs or one bilateral SM, e.g. LHA / TPA, etc. Span of extraction space also affects the design of SM. If 2 or more teeth are lost on one side of dental arch, then a functional type and sturdy SM is required. An RPD may be used as SM in such cases and in bilateral multiple loss of teeth. In the anterior region, a fixed SM cannot be placed as it will not have the artificial tooth. So an RPD is to be placed to satisfy the esthetic demands and for speech functions.

2. **Time elapsed since tooth loss:** Most of the loss of space occurs during first 6 months after extraction, because of the softness of bone and also the refilling of extraction socket take time. The appliance should be inserted immediately after extraction or as soon as possible, if more than 3–4 months time is expected for eruption of the successor tooth. It is always better to fabricate the appliance before the extraction and then insert it on the day of extraction.
3. **Amount of bone covering the unerupted tooth:** A long-standing extraction socket becomes calcified and bone thickness is increased. It takes more time for its resorption and thus delays eruption. The more the thickness of bone occlusal to the tooth, the more time will be required. For 1 mm movement of the tooth during normal eruption, approx. 3–4 months time is needed. If the amount of bone covering the permanent tooth in that area is more than 1 mm, then SM should be given. Approximately 3–4 months time is needed for a tooth to move 1 mm in the bone during eruption. If the bone is destroyed by infections, etc. then the eruption is accelerated since there remains no need to resorb the bone while eruption.
4. **Dental age of patient:** The chronological age of the patient is not important as the dental developmental age. It helps to determine the time of eruption of succedaneous tooth. Permanent teeth erupt in oral cavity when the root is approx. two-thirds to three-fourths of its normal size. So if the tooth is at or near to this stage, the space maintainer may not be needed. IOPA view of that area provide the best information regarding root development, level of crown near the alveolar bone, quality of bone, etc. Early loss of tooth delays the eruption of permanent tooth, since the bone above it becomes calcified and more resistant to resorption comes into play. The root development may continue but apically only, not giving enough thrust for bone resorption and eruption. In such case, the surgical removal of the bone to uncover the tooth should be attempted, along with space maintainer.
5. **Sequence of tooth eruption:** Sequence of dental eruption and the status of adjacent teeth also influence closure of the space and thus the choice of SM. A proper check is done of the position of other teeth in the jaw near the site of space created by tooth loss, e.g. in case of premature loss of primary second molar, if the permanent second molar is ahead of eruption of second premolar, then it may push the permanent first molar mesially leading to space loss for second premolar. Such cases need sturdy SM and regular follow up.
6. **Amount of root development:** If the root length of the tooth is less than two-thirds, the SM should be given. The tooth generally erupts in oral cavity when the root length is two-thirds to three-fourths completed.
7. **Congenital absence of tooth:** It also influences the choice of SM. Some teeth may be congenitally absent in the dental arches. In such cases, clinician has to decide whether the space is to be

retained for future prosthesis or for relief of crowding during orthodontic treatment or it can be allowed to be closed by drifting of the teeth in the space.

8. **Delayed eruption of secondary teeth:** In such cases, space maintainer is must to avoid space loss.
9. **Level of support of the abutment teeth:** For fixed SM, the abutments should be strong to support the appliance till the permanent tooth erupts. So the level of root resorption of primary tooth to be used as abutment should be evaluated by IOPA view. If the root is less than half or tooth has mobility, it should not be used as abutment, and some other design should be planned for SM.

Prerequisites of Space Maintainers

1. They must be simple to fabricate, comfortable, painless, durable and should not be costly.
2. They should maintain the mesiodistal dimension of the space.
3. They should be functional and prevent overeruption of opposing teeth.
4. They should be simple and strong enough to withstand functional forces.
5. They should not cause stresses on abutment teeth.
6. They must permit maintenance of oral hygiene.
7. They must not restrict the normal growth and development which takes place during transition from primary to permanent dentition.
8. They should not interfere with normal functions, like mastication, speech and deglutition.
9. They should not interfere with the normal eruption of the successor tooth in that space.

Essential Steps to Make a Space Maintainer

1. Proper examination
2. Collection of diagnostic records
3. Analysis of tooth development stages
4. Analysis of tooth size
5. Analysis of space available
6. Prediction of growth and future occlusal relationship.

Classification of space maintainers: SMs have been variously classified. Generally, the design depends on the clinical requirement and may vary from case to case. Hicthcock classified the SMs in very simple terms as follows:

1. Removable or fixed or semi-fixed.
2. With bands or without bands
3. Functional or non-functional
4. Unilateral or bilateral
5. Active or passive
6. Certain combination of above.

SMs can be fixed at both ends or may be of cantilever type, e.g. distal extension SM.

SM can be made of acrylic as RPD or Complete denture.

Removable Space Maintainer

It is the appliance that can be removed and reinserted by the patient. It is made of acrylic, with/without a tooth as a replacement. It can be functional or non-functional type. Functional type has a tooth, it can help in chewing, speech and esthetic functions. Non-functional type may be having an acrylic extension in the space or it may have two clasps in the space holding the adjacent teeth from shifting.

Advantages of Removable SM

- It is easy to clean and so oral hygiene can be better maintained.
- Functional types help in restoring the functions of chewing, speaking and esthetics especially in anterior area, and help in maintaining the vertical dimension.
- It stimulates tissues in edentulous area and accelerates the eruption of teeth beneath them.
- It applies minimal stress on the adjacent teeth.

- It is easy to fabricate, involves less chair-side time and are cheaper.
- It is less traumatic as band fabrication is not required.
- It does not interfere with growth. If needed for a longer time, then it can be easily refabricated so as to allow growth to take place normally.
- Acrylic can be adjusted easily to provide space for erupting permanent tooth by trimming it.
- Routine oral health check up is easier as it can be removed.

Disadvantages

- It requires patient cooperation for proper use.
- It may be lost or broken.
- It is a bulky appliance, which encroaches on the space of tongue, so the patient has initial difficulty in adjustment to the appliance.
- It may restrict lateral growth of the jaws if clasps are used esp in canine regions. So a regular replacement is needed in consonance with the ensuing growth.
- It may cause irritation to underlying soft tissues as it creates the niches for accumulation of debris.
- If not cleaned properly, it may lead to bad breath and bad taste.

Indications

- It is mostly required in anterior region to maintain the esthetics.
- If a fixed SM cannot be supported by a mobile tooth, then it is used.
- It can be modified for use in the cleft patient to help in obturation of palatal defect.
- In incompletely erupted permanent teeth, the bands fabrication is not possible, then it can be used.
- It can be modified to act as guiding plane for erupting teeth by judicious trimming.
- If multiple primary teeth have been extracted then it should be used to maintain the function, in the form of RPD or CD.

Contraindications

- It should not be used in uncooperative patients, since they will not use it.
- It should not be used in patients having allergy to acrylics.
- It should not be used in epileptic patients.
- It should not be used in very small children.

Some Commonly Used Removable Space Maintainers

Acrylic removable partial denture (Figs 51.4 and 51.5): It is used in patients having multiple extractions, since there are not enough teeth to support the fixed SM. The impression is taken, and teeth are fitted in the extraction spaces on the acrylic base. Advantage of this appliance is that it can be readily adjusted to make space for the erupting teeth. It restores masticatory, esthetic and speech functions, and maintains VD also. The clasps can be fabricated on remaining deciduous teeth for retention.

Full or complete dentures: It is used when the child looses all his primary teeth due to rampant caries, if they cannot be restored. The advantages are it restores masticatory

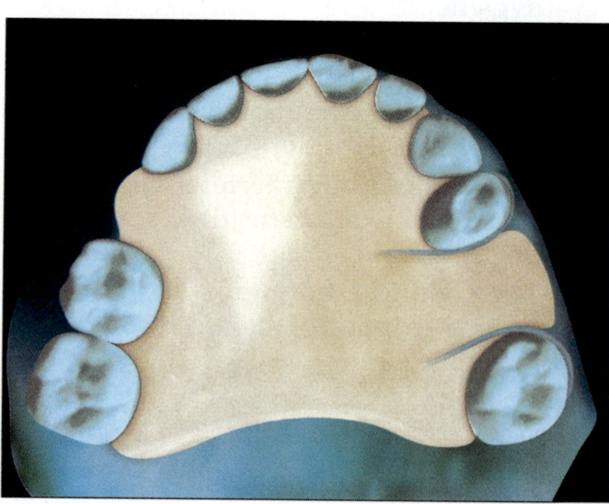

Fig. 51.4: A removable, functional space maintainer with acrylic pads.

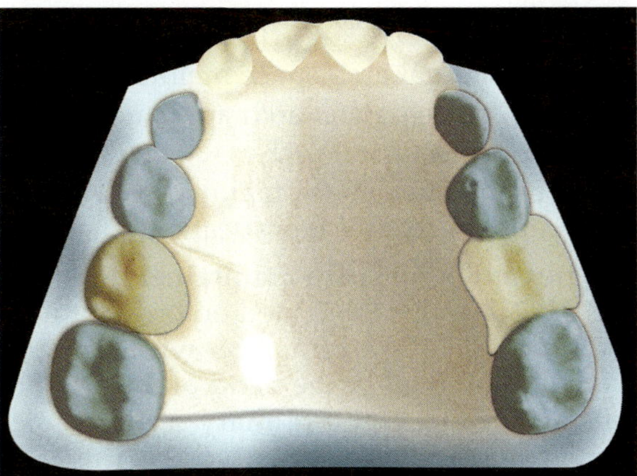

Fig. 51.5: A removable, functional space maintainer with acrylic teeth. Anterior teeth give esthetic advantage also.

functions, stimulates the tissue for enhancing teeth eruption, maintains esthetics and function, and helps first permanent molars to erupt into their correct positions by guidance through the distal border of the denture. It can also be readily adjusted by grinding to give space for the erupting permanent teeth. However, the denture should be changed frequently usually within 3–6 months, so as not to interfere with the growth of the jaws.

Removable distal shoe space maintainer: An acrylic denture with an acrylic distal shoe extension can be used to guide first permanent molar into the position when deciduous second molar is lost shortly before first permanent molars. It should not be used if there is more time remaining for the eruption of first permanent molar. It can be prepared and placed immediately. The deciduous second molar tooth to be extracted is cut away from stone model and a depression is made into the stone model at the position of distal surface of the deciduous second molar socket, which allows the formation of an acrylic extension. This acrylic will extend into the extraction socket after removal of primary tooth and help in guiding the erupting first permanent molar. The extension should be adjusted and then subsequently removed after the eruption of permanent tooth, maintaining a light contact with the mesial surface of first permanent molar to prevent its mesial tilting in the extraction space. Otherwise, it can be replaced with a fixed type of SM. Main disadvantage is that it needs patient cooperation, and may be uncomfortable and painful to place in the tissues every time.

Fixed Space Maintainers (Figs 51.6a and b)

These appliances are fixed to the abutment teeth either by banding or bonding, and cannot be removed by the patients.

Advantages

- Patient cooperation is not needed as it cannot be removed by the patient.
- It does not restrict or interfere with the lateral growth of the jaws.

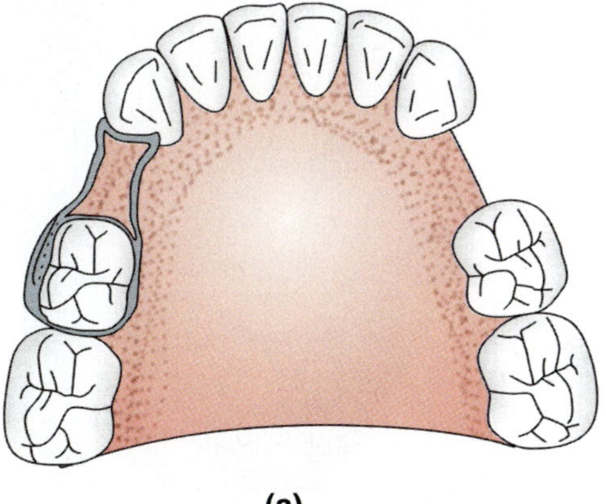

(a)

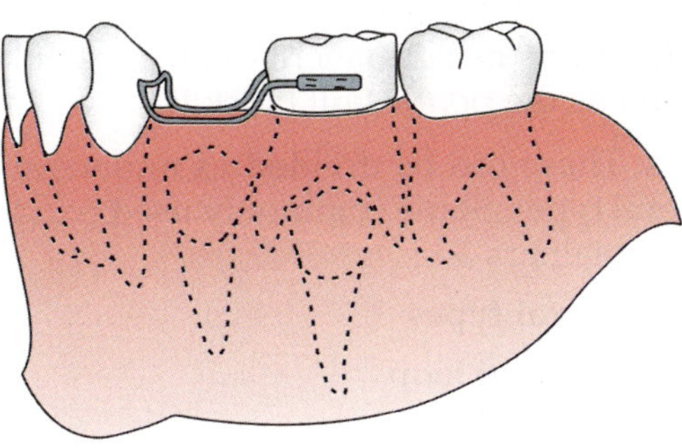

(b)

Figs 51.6a and b: Band and loop type of fixed space maintainer appliances.

- It can be made of functional type to help in restoration of masticatory function if pontic is placed.
- It does not interfere in maintenance of oral hygiene, since the deposits are less as compared to removable ones.
- It does not encroach on tongue space so patient can easily get used to its presence in the oral cavity.
- Permanent successor are free to erupt through the appliance, as provision of proper space is given during fabrication.

Disadvantages

- Maintenance of oral hygiene around the abutments is difficult since it can't be removed.
- It needs special lab work, instruments for fabrication and is costly.
- Fabrication of bands on abutment teeth is traumatic to the patient.
- It is smaller in size, so there is chance that the small child may accidently swallow it if it gets loosened.
- Plaque build-up may cause decalcification under or around the bands.
- Supraeruption of opposing tooth may occur if pontic is not used, i.e. in non-functional types.
- If pontic is used, it will interfere with active eruption of permanent tooth. It needs regular grinding on the tissue-side to make space for erupting tooth. It needs removal and recementing of the appliance. If the patient fails to report for follow-up, the permanent tooth does not erupt as the pontic will block it.

Types: These can be divided as unilateral or bilateral types. Some commonly used fixed space maintainers are:

I. Unilateral types:
   - Band and loop
   - Band and bar
   - Crown and loop
   - Crown and bar
   - Buccally bonded wire (Goyal S).

II. Bilateral types:
   - Lingual arch space maintainers
   - Nance palatal arch appliance
   - Transpalatal arch

III. Distal shoe space maintainer, Willet's appliance, and modification.

Band and loop space maintainer (Figs 51.6 and 51.7): Band is fabricated on the abutment tooth and a loop of hard SS wire is made which is soldered to the band on buccal and palatal surfaces, e.g. if primary second molar is lost, a band is fabricated on the first permanent molar. A hard SS wire of 0.9 mm or more size is fabricated in the form of loop, extending from buccal surface of band to its lingual surface. The loop touches the distal surface of the tooth mesial to the extraction space. Loop is gingivally bent and contoured along the alveolar contour to avoid any irritation to the buccal or lingual tissues. The loop should be wide enough not to interfere with the buccal or lingual surface of the erupting tooth. So it will not need the frequent removal of the appliance for adjustments to allow the eruption of the permanent tooth. It is cemented with fluoride containing cements, e.g. GIC, or resin modified cements.

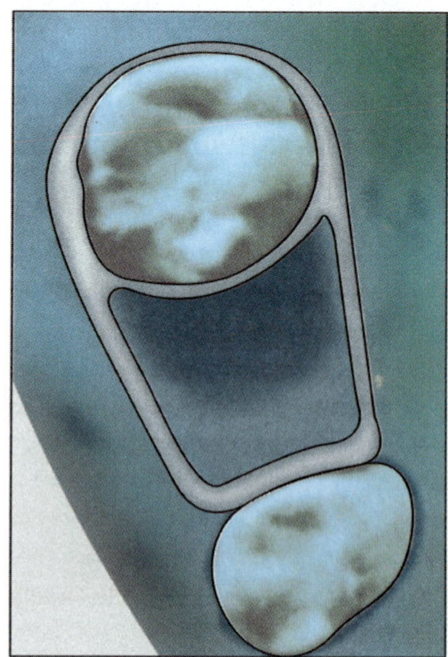

Fig. 51.7: A unilateral, fixed space maintainer: band and loop type.

Indication:

- It is used for single tooth space. If there is loss of a tooth in different quadrants, then it can be used in each quadrant individually.
- It should be used when span of space is short, i.e. for a single tooth space. It will not be stable and stronger if space is larger.
- The abutment tooth should be firm and strong.
- Regular follow-up is required to adjust if it is causing any interference in eruption of the tooth. It should be removed as soon as the tooth erupts to almost half of its crown. Since after that the tooth itself is capable of maintaining the space (Figs 51.8 and 51.9).

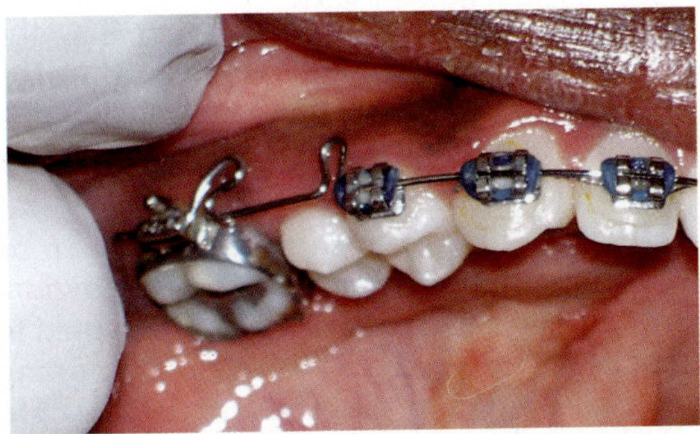

Fig. 51.8: Loops can be incorporated in the base archwires to prevent space loss for the erupting tooth. Loops prevent the shifting of adjoining teeth in the space.

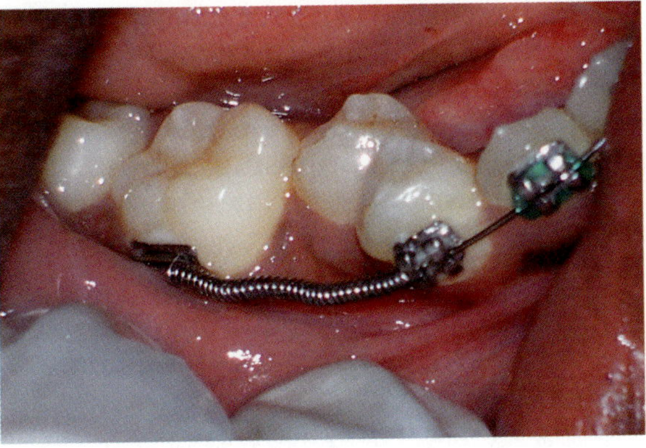

Fig. 51.9: Active open coil spring to create space for lingually blocked premolar.

- Since it is a non-functional type, there are chances of supraeruption of the opposing tooth, so a proper care is to be taken if it is a permanent tooth.

Crown and loop appliance: It is a variation of band and loop type. The crown if present or is to be placed on a primary abutment tooth adjacent to the extraction space can be used instead of the band. The loop is fabricated in the same way as described above and is soldered to the crown on a primary tooth. Then it can be cemented on the abutment tooth.

Band and bar, and crown and bar (Figs 51.10a and b): Bands or crowns are fabricated on the two proximal teeth adjacent to the extraction space. A piece of a hard SS

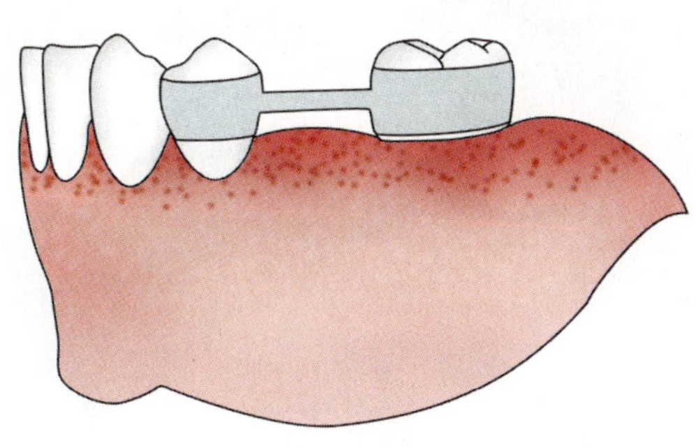

(a)

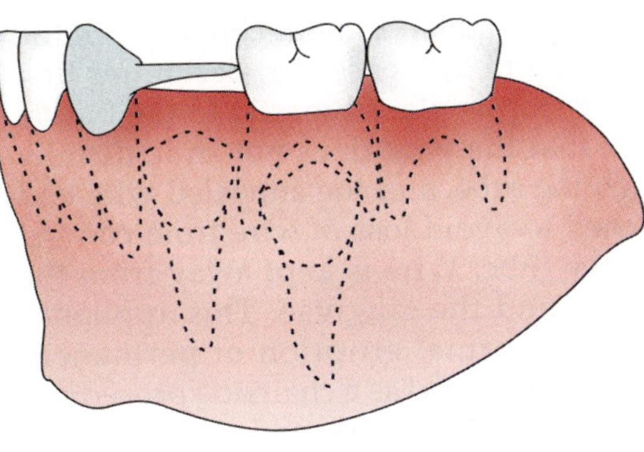

(b)

Figs 51.10: Band and bar type of fixed space maintainer in the first figure; the second figure is crown and bar type of fixed space maintainer.

wire or bar of size 0.9 mm or more is soldered on both the bands on proximal surfaces of bands just above the HOC near the occlusal level. It helps in preventing the supra-eruption of the opposing tooth. Once succedaneous tooth penetrates the soft tissue, bar should be cut-off.

Indication: When a tooth is prematurely lost in posterior segment and opposing tooth has to be prevented from supraeruption.

It should be used only for short spaces, i.e. for single extraction space only.

Bonding of wire in proximal pits: The cavities are formed in the proximal pits of the teeth adjacent to the space and a hard wire is placed there with the help of composite resin. The resin should be trimmed out of occlusion. But this method leads to loss of normal enamel, especially if it uses a permanent tooth for abutment. Thus, this design is not considered much.

Bonded space maintainer: It was suggested by Coican (JCO 1992). For example, if primary second molar is lost at early age, and a band-loop space maintainer is contraindicated if the permanent first molar is partially erupted. A removable appliance is also not suitable in cases with lack of patient co-operation, less retentive capability, short clinical crowns, and in very young patients.

Design: A buccal tube is bonded on the buccal surface of erupting first molar and a full-size rectangular wire segment is placed equal to the size of the space to be maintained. This wire is adapted in light contact with the tooth mesial to the space, e.g. deciduous first molar. A stop is placed mesial to the buccal tube so that the wire does not slide distally through the tube, and the annealed wire end is cinched to avoid loss of wire from coming out of the tube. Wire is kept away from the occlusion and the gingivae. This appliance allows the normal eruption of permanent molar, can be placed as a chairside procedure, needs no laboratory work, and also maintains the space. It does not interfere with the erupting tooth in the space also. The wire can be easily removed, adjusted or replaced to adapt to the changes in the area due to occlusal forces or the loss of the mesial deciduous molar.

Chairside space maintainer (Fig. 51.11): This is also a modified space maintainer as suggested by Goyal. Here, a segment of full size rectangular wire is bonded on the buccal surfaces of teeth adjacent to space with the help of composite resin. It can be used in upper and lower arches. This wire is kept out of occlusion in the lower arch to prevent breakage. It can be used on both sides in case of bilateral loss of tooth as individual appliances. It does not create a problem of oral hygiene as no bands are needed. It does not interfere with the erupting tooth as it lies on the buccal side of the space. It can be easily removed when the tooth has sufficiently erupted. It can be easily placed as a chair side procedure. It does not involve any cost, as the wire segments are easily available in the clinics. It does not need any laboratory work. No banding is needed so it does not cause any trauma to soft tissues.

Dentapreg strip: Dentapreg strip can be used to maintain the space in incisor region. An adequate sized piece is cut and adapted to the space. It is then fixed with regular bonding material to say in place. The strip is also light cured to polymerise it to gain the strength. Later on, the strip and the bonding material is finished adequately.

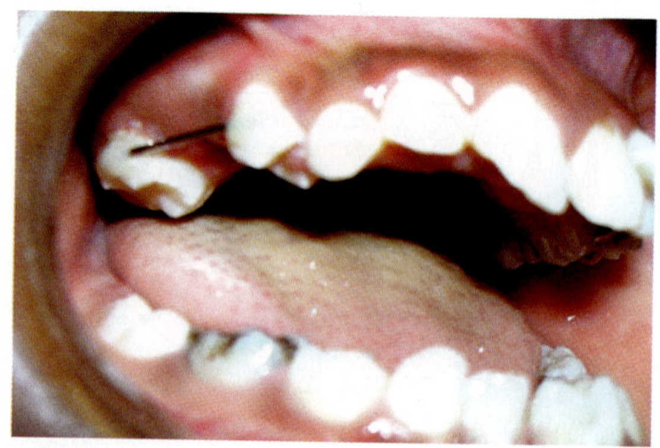

Fig. 51.11: A simple, chairside space maintainer by bonding the piece of wire on buccal surfaces of teeth adjacent to extraction space.

Bilateral Appliances (Figs 51.12 to 51.14a and b)

Lingual holding arch as a space maintainer: LHA is a bilateral type of SM and is used in lower arch.

Indications: It is used in cases of bilateral loss of primary teeth. Its modified form with U-loops can also be used for gaining some lost space by activating the U-loops. It can also be used to augment the anchorage if the patient is in need of fixed orthodontic appliance.

Fabrication: Bands are fabricated on both first permanent molars and transferred on the working cast. A hard stainless steel wire of 0.9 mm or more size is adapted from lingual surface of band on one side, passing forward touching the lingual surfaces of other primary teeth and also contacting lingual surfaces of mandibular incisors, to the band of the other side. If it is to be made active, then a U-loop can be incorporated just mesial to the band on both sides. The wire is soldered to the bands, finished and cemented.

Transpalatal arch: This is a bilateral type of SM, used in maxillary arch. The bands are fabricated on the teeth just distal to the extraction spaces, e.g. permanent first molars. A hard stainless steel wire of 0.036" diameter/ 0.9 mm or more size is adapted from lingual surface of band on one side to the band of the other side, crossing the palate transversally. The wire is kept at least 2–3 mm away from the palatal tissues to avoid irritation. If it is to be made active, then a U-loop can be incorporated in the centre of the wire, which may open either mesially or distally. The wire is soldered to the bands, finished and cemented. It is generally used when primary second molars are removed and thus made on first permanent molars. It can help in expanding, derotating and distally tipping the molars by activating the U-loop. It can be used to augment the anchorage, if fixed orthodontics is to be done for the patient. However, since it does not have an anterior stop, some mesial movement of the anchor teeth is noted.

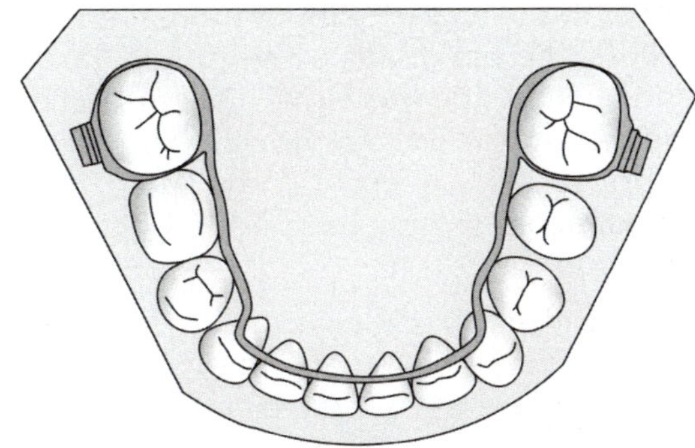

Fig. 51.12: Bilateral space maintainers: lingual holding arch. It also helps to maintain leeway space which then can be used for resolving mild crowding.

Nance's arch holding appliance: It is modified form of TPA and is used as bilateral SM. The bands are fabricated on both the teeth just distal to the extraction space. A hard stainless steel wire of 0.036" diameter/0.9 mm

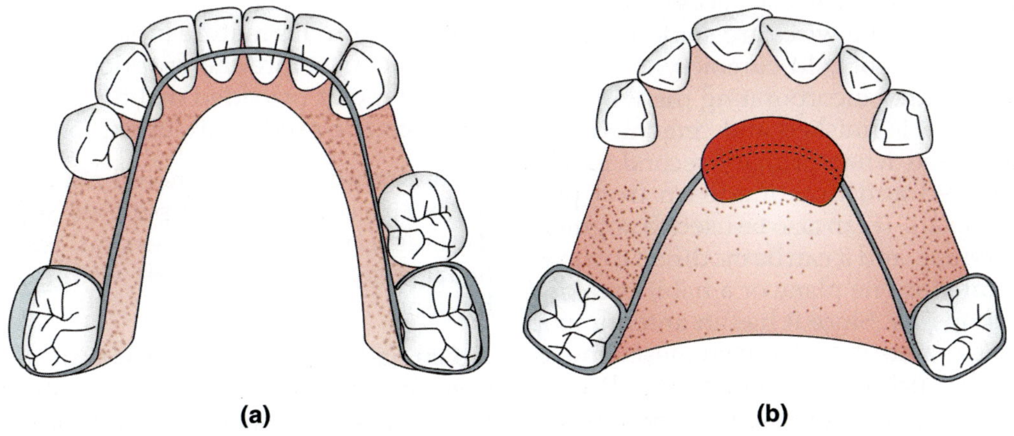

Figs 51.13a and b: Bilateral space maintainers: lingual holding arch; Nance's palatal arch.

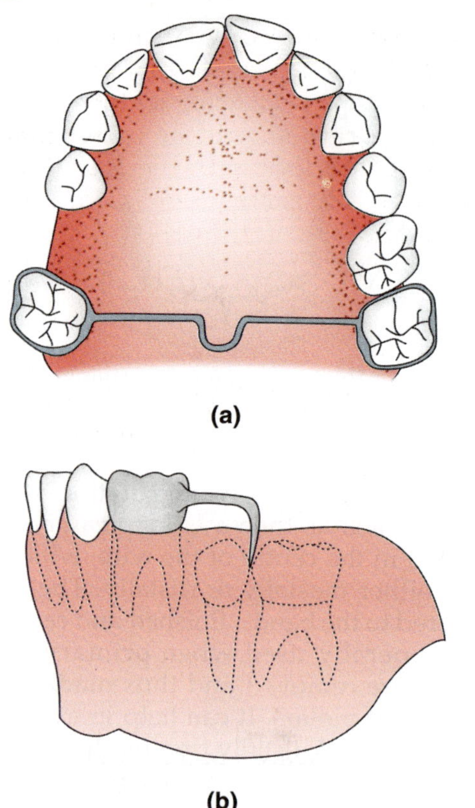

Figs 51.14a and b: (a) A fixed space maintainer: the transpalatal arch (TPA); (b) figure shows a distal shoe appliance, to guide erupting permanent first molar in lower arch.

or more size is adapted from the palatal surface of band on one side to the band of the other side, passing through rugae area. Alternatively, 2 segments of wires can be adapted from the palatal surfaces of bands till the rugae area. The wires are soldered to the bands. A button of cold-cure acrylic is made in the rugae area incorporating the wire/s in it, and then it is finished and cemented. It is generally used when primary second molars are removed and thus made on first permanent molars. It can also be used to augment the anchorage, and it can be modified to incorporate anterior bite plane or a habit-breaking crib or loop in it. Since it has an anterior stop in the rugae area, it can prevent mesial movement of the anchor teeth better than TPA.

There are chances of food impaction below the acrylic button, which can cause tissue inflammation, so it needs a good oral hygiene schedule and session of frequent removal-cleaning-recementing.

Also, since the span of wire is longer, it is not that sturdy as TPA, and can be easily distorted or removed by the un-cooperative patient. So in such cases, – 2 bands can be made on both sides and then wires can be fabricated to be soldered on these bands which are incorporated in the acrylic.

Distal shoe space maintainer (Fig. 51.14b): (**Willet's appliance**, intra-alveolar guidance appliance): It is a unilateral type of SM. It is used when there is premature loss of primary second molar before the eruption of permanent first molar. It is best to plan the distal shoe at the time of extraction of primary second molar, since it can be place immediately after its extraction and then another surgery will not be needed to make a place in the alveolar and gingival tissues to receive the vertical arm of the appliance. Vertical arm helps to guide the eruption path of permanent first molar to normal position. Its placement should be confirmed with IOPA view that it is in contact with the mesial surface of first molar, below the height of contour. If permanent first molar is not guided, it may tilt in the space resulting in space loss and impacted second premolar, and will need extensive orthodontic treatment later on. It may be made with the bands or the metal crown on the abutment tooth to which the guide wire assembly is soldered.

Indication: Premature loss of a second primary molar before the eruption of first permanent molar provided that the primary first molar can be used as abutment tooth.

Contraindication: It should not be used in medically compromised patients, e.g. blood dyscrasia, immunosuppression, congenital heart diseases and patient with poor oral hygiene.

Garcia-Godoy appliance: It is an appliance used for space maintenance in cases of early loss of primary second molars before the eruption of permanent first molars. It is like a distal shoe appliance and also helps to guide the erupting permanent first molar in position. It consists of a 0.036" stainless steel wire extending distally from buccal and lingual surfaces of the deciduous first molar. A groove is made in the cast in the approximate area of mesial surface of erupting first molar, where wire is adapted, and later on the appliance is inserted under local anesthesia. One U-loop on each side extends across the edentulous span, submerging subgingivally, and one small loop on each side contacts the mesial surface of permanent first molar. It is also suggested that the contralateral first or second deciduous molar could be used as an abutment tooth, by involving in a lingual holding arch.

Its advantages over the distal-shoe type are that its construction and insertion are simple; it is adjustable and can be activated to regain small amounts of space or to correct mesial tipping of the molar.

Modified Willet's appliance by Dhindsa and Pandit (JISPPD Sept 2008): It is used in case of bilateral loss of primary second molars before eruption of permanent first molars. Bands are made on lower first deciduous molars on both sides. Deciduous canine can also be banded and involved in the appliance for increasing the anchorage and stability of appliance. Cuts are placed in the cast at approximate location of mesial surfaces of erupting first molars. The wire components are made of a single piece of 20 gauze SS wire. Anteriorly, the wire component is shaped as a lingual holding arch extending bilaterally, and posteriorly the wire is bent in the shape of a modified Willet's appliance bilaterally. The wire is soldered on bands on both the buccal and lingual sides for better strength. Proper clearance is created to prevent any interference in the path of eruption of permanent mandibular incisors. The appliance is cemented in place under local anesthesia and is regularly followed up with IOPAs for the status of erupting first molars.

Disadvantages of this appliance are that it is non-functional, difficult fabrication, cannot be used in un-cooperative patients, and since it has a long span, it is not that sturdy and stable, and can get loose frequently.

However, care should be taken that it should not interfere with the eruption of mandibular permanent incisors which generally erupt lingual to the primary teeth. In such cases, the appliance needs a prior removal and should be replaced with the unilateral type. Even after eruption of permanent first molars, the space has to be maintained by the new appliances which may be of uni-/bilateral types, depending on the situation of permanent incisors.

SPACE REGAINERS (Fig. 51.15)

Space regainers are the interceptive appliances which are used to regain the lost space which was left by the premature loss of primary tooth. Thus, they are active in nature, applying orthodontic forces in the physiological range and affecting the tooth movement to gain the spaces. Some of the designs have been discussed in the chapter of interceptive orthodontics.

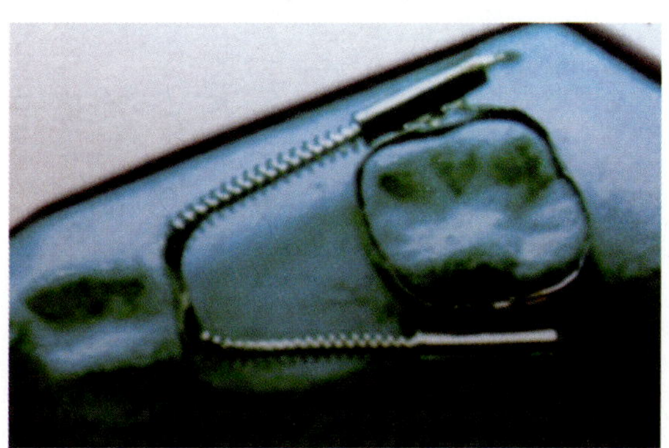

Fig. 51.15: A fixed space regainer with open coil spring *(Adapted from Internet)*.

Conclusion

Space is the very crucial factor during orthodontic treatment. A sufficient space is needed in the dental arches for proper alignment, leveling and correction of the teeth. Nature has its own growth mechanism to provide space for permanent teeth, but in many cases, it remains deficient.

Primary teeth are the best natural SMs and all the efforts should be done to maintain them as long as possible in the oral cavity. They help to stimulate alveolar growth, and eruption of permanent teeth and also maintain space for them.

The space maintainers are important part of orthodontics to prevent any loss of space after premature loss of primary teeth. Any lost space increases the complexity of orthodontic mechanics and timings. So, preventive efforts should be done at an earliest to preserve the spaces in the dental arches.

In some cases, the space gets lost either partially or fully due to lack of awareness. In such cases, some of the space can be regained with the help of orthodontic appliances to be used for correction of malocclusion. But in many cases where complete space has been lost, the permanent tooth in that area may become impacted or ectopically erupted and mostly needs to be sacrificed. To prevent the extractions of permanent teeth, all the effort should be done to maintain or regain the spaces.

52

Evidence-Based Orthodontics

INTRODUCTION

The contemporary view on clinical care of patients is the evidence-based care, which integrates the accrued scientific evidence in clinical practice, to improve clinical care based on informed decision making. According to American Dental Association (ADA), the "Evidence-based dentistry" can be considered as "an approach to oral health care that requires the careful integration of systematic assessments of clinically relevant scientific evidences, relating to the patient's oral and medical condition and history, with the dentist's clinical expertise and the patient's treatment needs and preferences".

Evidence-based treatment concept has been adopted by almost all medical fields, and orthodontics is one of them. In orthodontics, the concept of evidence based orthodontics, EBO was introduced in 1990s. Systematic reviews have been conducted on various topics of orthodontics. It helps to find out how effective and efficient is the particular treatment modality being used in orthodontics to provide the best possible treatment to our patients. The decision of continued use of these treatment method or choosing another method has been left to clinicians because further studies based on sound principles, e.g. randomized clinical trials, are required, and till they prove the superiority of one method over the another method.

Process of Evidence Based Care

Following steps are taken to find the evidence on a particular question.

1. **Need for the evidence:** Evidence is required to evaluate the efficiency and the efficacy of the Rx being provided to the patient.
2. **Formulation of a question,** i.e. any query you want to evaluate from the available literature. For example, should we provide early treatment to a patient or not, having Angle's class II division 1 condition? Formulation of a question is done by the PICO Process, which means
   - **P** – Patient problem
   - **I** – Intervention
   - **C** – Comparison
   - **O** – Outcomes.

   The PICO forms the foundation for the search terms to be used during the search.
3. **Search of the evidence:** Clinical evidences are required to prepare the answer for the question fabricated. It should be kept in mind during searching the literature that not all the publications in the literature are appropriate for consideration in evidence based decision making (EBDM) process, because there is a hierarchy of evidences based on their relevance and validity.

The EBD model paradigm for clinical decision making has **three hierarchical levels**, of which only levels 2 and 3 are significant and truly evidence based.

Level 1 is the lowest level which is based on information gained by practitioner's clinical experience. It contains case reports, opinions, and consensus of experts in the field. It has a strong bias-factor.

Level 2 is information obtained from the clinician's experience which is gained by a review of selected published articles and research. It has cross-sectional studies, cross over studies, cohort studies, where the bias factor is not string but still exists.

The highest level of evidence is **Level 3**, which consists of a systematic review of articles by meta-analysis, RCTs and non-RCTs published in literature. A goal of Level 3 literature search is to select the best studies, which are randomized controlled trials (RCTs).

Sources of evidence: There are following sources of evidence.

1. **Primary sources:** These are original research publications that have not been filtered or synthesized, e.g. Systematic Reviews, Meta-Analysis, Evidence-Based Article Reviews and Clinical Practice Guidelines and Protocols.
2. **Secondary sources:** These are synthesized publications of primary literature, e.g. Cochrane Library, which provide the best evidence.

All treatment modalities are evaluated from two perspectives:

- **Effectiveness:** How well it works or how successful it is in overcoming patient's problem.
- **Efficiency:** How much benefit the patient receives relative to the cost, time and risks of treatment. Efficient treatment produces large benefits with minimal cost and risk.

4. **Appraisal of evidence:** Evidences are gathered from the literature and are selected and analyzed based on certain pre-set guidelines. These guidelines help to see whether the methods used in studies were appropriate and were rigorously conducted. International evidence-based groups have developed guidelines that help the user through a structured series of yes/no questions to determine the validity of the research. Many guidelines such as consolidation standards of reporting trials (CONSORT), quality of reporting of meta-analyses (QUOROM), critical appraisal skill program (CASP) and meta-analysis of observational studies in epidemiology (MOOSE) have been established to help in EBDM process. The scientific evidence along with experience and judgment, patient preferences/consent and clinical patient circumstances complete the EBDM process. This is also called as "**the interactive model of orthodontic treatment**".

RANDOMIZED CONTROLLED STUDIES IN ORTHODONTICS

Randomized controlled trial (RCT) has become the standard experimental tool for evaluation of any medical treatment, and same principals have been applied in dentistry also. During the research, the process of randomly assigning the subjects to different study groups is the best method, as it helps to ensure the comparability of the treatments and ensures that different treatment groups are "statistically equivalent".

According to Meinert, RCT is that clinical trial which involves at least one test treatment and one control treatment. There is concurrent enrollment and follow-up of the test and control-treated groups. Also, the treatments to be administered are selected by a random process, such that neither the patients nor the persons responsible for their selection or treatment can influence the assignments, and the assignments remain unknown to the patients and clinical staff, until the patients have been determined to be eligible for enrollment into the trial.

Ismail and Bader have described a three-tiered model of evidence based dentistry (EBD). At the lowest level:

- Model 1: An experimental, biased model based on the opinions of a clinician or an educator.
- Model 2: A combination of one's experience in addition to a search for the best clinical and scientific studies Limitations. Model 2 are that all relevant researches are not identified by an exhaustive and systematic review, so the biased conclusions can result.

- Model 3: It has got the highest level of evidence. A systematic review and evaluation of all evidence is taken.

Clinical study: It is "any systematic study in human subjects undertaken to verify the safety and performance of a specific device under normal conditions of use". A clinical study should make a clear distinction from other (non-clinical) studies, and include all possible study designs that meet the following criteria:

- It represents a research activity in humans and not an in vitro, ex vivo, or laboratory study.
- Enrolled participants are alive, at least at the beginning of their follow-up period.
- There is a question of clinical relevance with regard to a disease or health condition.
- At least has been, direct contact with the participants to collect data about a clinical characteristics or condition.
- Clinical trials are designed to answer a specific question about a treatment, usually the safety and efficacy of the treatment.

CURRENT SCIENTIFIC EVIDENCES IN ORTHODONTICS

There are myriad of clinical situations and queries in the field of orthodontics which need the knowledge of current scientific evidence to provide best clinical care to patients. Most of the evidence has been generated by systematic reviews of available literature on many clinical situations. So the researchers have found the strong need of RCTs to be conducted on the problems seen by clinicians to find the best method of treatment, which will take many years to generate. Till that time, we have to depend on the results of the systematic reviews published in the literature on many of the clinical problems, combined with the personal judgement and experience of the clinicians. In the following paragraphs, we describe some of the current scientific evidences generated by systematic reviews and by available RCTs in orthodontics.

1. Factors Affecting Duration of Orthodontic Treatment

In a systematic review to explore the factors affecting the duration of orthodontic therapy, following conclusions regarding the duration of orthodontic treatment: (1) extraction treatment takes more time than non-extraction therapy; (2) age does not have a role in treatment duration provided the patients are in permanent dentition; (3) in Class II division 1 malocclusions, the earlier the orthodontic treatment begins the longer its duration; (4) combined orthodontic-surgical treatment duration is variable and is operator sensitive; (6) various other factors, e.g. the technique used, the skill and number of operators involved, patients' cooperation level, and the severity of the initial malocclusion, all seem to play a role; and (7) impacted maxillary canines appear to prolong treatment. Also there is a need for more conclusive research.

2. Early Treatment

It is one of the most important topics of discussions among orthodontists in past decades, and has changed the paradigm of treatment. There are several conditions which need special attention as early as possible to avoid the increased severity of the problem with growth and development. Multiple modalities have been devised by clinicians to treat such problems, but their efficacy has to be tested with controlled studies. In some of the systematic reviews and RCTs, following results have been found.

A. Chintakanon (2000) found that the treatment with twin-block showed no evidence of any increase in mandibular protrusion after treatment.
B. Popovich (2003) in a systematic review on Herbst's appliance found no conclusive evidence on the effect of Herbst appliance on TMJ morphology and condylar position changes.
C. **O'Brien et al** (2003) in an RCT found no differences in skeletal and dental changes achieved between the **Herbst or twin-block** appliances.

D. Kalha (2004) in a summary trial found that changes in skeletal relation were not clinically significant with twin block.

E. Huang (2006) found that F. As do not permanently influence mandibular growth.

F. Cozza (2006) in a systematic review on effect of FAs in enhancing mandibular growth found that Herbst appliance was more efficient than twin block appliance, at pubertal peak of skeletal growth. However, the final occlusal result and skeletal discrepancy were better for girls than for boys. Because of the high cooperation rates of patients using it, the Herbst appliance could be the appliance of choice for treating adolescents with class II division 1 malocclusion.

G. Rubin has said that there is still no consensus on whether we can influence the growth of mandible.

H. **Orthodontic treatment for prominent upper front teeth in children:** In a systematic review, it was found that providing early orthodontic treatment for correction of prominent upper front teeth is no more effective than providing one phase of orthodontic treatment at an early adolescence age of the patient.

I. Tulloch et al (2004) stated that the optimal timing for treatment of a class II malocclusion remains controversial and that the decision for early treatment should be based on individual indications for each child.

These statements list is not exhaustive, and there are multiple evidences which have not been covered here. According to above results, it can be stated that the functional appliances do not have much clinical effect on the skeletal changes in mandible; there is no consensus which appliance is better than other; and whether the early treatment is better than late treatment.

3. Soft Tissue Changes with FAs

In a new paradigm, there is more consideration of soft tissues than the hard tissues during diagnosis and results evaluation. The soft tissues changes achieved with fixed orthodontic appliances and/or functional appliances have been widely published. Various systematic studies have been published some of which have been discussed.

- Flores Mir (2006) found that soft tissue changes with twin block in C2D1 malocclusion were not clinically significant, with no changes in AP position of lip, soft tissue menton or facial convexity.
- Flores Mir (2006) found that soft tissue changes with fixed FAs in C2D1 malocclusion were not clinically significant, with only a secondary level of evidence. Soft tissue changes were similar b/w growing and non-growing patients.
- Ren (2007) and Flores-Mir, Major (2006) have found that there is significant controversy regarding soft tissue changes achieved with activator and bionator Rx. Soft tissue changes which were reported as being statistically significant were of questionable clinical significance.
- **Proffit** compared 1-phase to 2-phase Rx of class II cases, he observed that: There is no difference in the quality of occlusion between these 2 groups. Early treatment did not reduce chances of extractions later on. Also, the early Rx did not reduce the eventual need for orthognathic surgery. It can be concluded that preadolescent Rx for most Class II malocclusion is no more effective than the later Rx and is less efficient.

4. The Effect of Functional Appliances on Skeletal Pattern

Mills (1991) reviewed effects of Andresen and Fränkel appliances, analyzed from cephalometric radiographs. Generally, no appreciable maxillary advancement restriction was there in either group (although a slight relative reduction in SNA was seen). There is a slight mean increase in mandibular growth, mainly in a vertical direction. In another review by Aelbers, Dermaut (1997, 2006), the orthopedic effect of functional appliances, such as activators and Herbst appliances, and the orthopedic effect of extraoral traction appliances, were assessed. Only Herbst therapy was able to change mandibular growth to a clinically significant extent.

In a nut-shell, it can be said that there is no benefit of subjecting the patients to prolonged treatment of two phases.

The literature has also suggested the reason why the functional appliances are not effective and efficient for early Rx of the patients. Recent growth theories have suggested that the growth is dependant on genetic make-up of patient, it is not so superficial what was considered initially, and its roots are lying deep in micromolecules of the cells, so the evidences to the efficacy of FAs is questionable.

5. Maxillary Protraction

Skeletal and dental effects of maxillary protraction in patients with Angle class III malocclusion. Jäger et al reviewed the literature with meta-analysis to find the treatment effects of maxillary protraction in patients with Angle class III in which 12 studies cephalometric measurements were selected for further analysis. Maxillary protraction was shown to have a significant treatment effect.

The effectiveness of protraction face mask therapy: In a meta-analysis done by Kim et al to examine the effectiveness of maxillary protraction with orthopedic appliances in class III patients, it was found that more skeletal effect and less dental change are produced in the expansion appliance group. Greater treatment changes in younger group are achieved. Results indicate that protraction face mask is effective in growing patients, but has lesser effects in patients older than 10 years of age, and that protraction in combination with an initial period of expansion may provide more significant skeletal effects.

6. Slow and Rapid Maxillary Expansion

Expansion is generally used to widen the maxilla, maxillary arch to treat the crossbite, and to loosen the circummaxillary sutures during maxillary protrusion with reverse head gear.

- Gianelley commented that RME in non-posterior crossbite cases gives 3–4 mm of space for incisor alignment, but has no effect on mandibular arch perimeter. So the E-space should be maintained esp. in mandibular arch. It can be concluded that any added benefit of RME non-posterior crossbite cases is "challenging to define".
- Yijin Ren in 2005 found the same results of maxillary expansion in adolescents and young adults. Significantly less indirect mandibular molar and cuspid expansion was attained in young adults compared with adolescents. More transverse dental arch changes were found after puberty than before, but the difference may not be clinically significant.
- **Lagravère, Major, Flores-Mir** (2005) in a systematic review (SR) found only a lower level of evidence for skeletal and dental changes with fixed slow maxillary expansion treatment . So there exists limited evidence regarding SME treatments.
- **Lagravere, Major, Flores-Mir** (2005) in **another SR** found that long-term transverse skeletal change is approximately 25% of the total dental expansion for prepubertal adolescents. Better long-term transverse changes are expected in less skeletally mature patients.
- **Lagravère, Major, Flores-Mir** (2006), in an SR for dental and skeletal changes following surgically assisted rapid maxillary expansion found that the

results should be considered with caution because only a secondary level of evidence was found.

- Meta-analysis of immediate changes with RME found that the greatest changes from RME were dental and skeletal changes in transverse plane, while only few vertical and anteroposterior immediate changes were statistically significant, though they probably are not clinically important.
- Dental and skeletal changes after surgically assisted rapid maxillary expansion (SARME) were studied. It was found that expansion was greater at molars and diminished progressively to anterior part of dental arch in all the evaluation periods. Vertical and sagittal skeletal changes were nil or not clinically significant. The nasal portion of maxillary complex showed an increase in dimensions thereby improving nasal patency. An overall dental relapse of 0.5–1 mm was reported after 1 year of orthodontic treatment. The conclusions should be considered with caution because only a secondary level of evidence was found.

Long-term dental arch changes after rapid maxillary expansion treatment in a systematic review found that similar maxillary molar and canine expansion could be found in adolescents and young adults. But in young adults, significantly less indirect mandibular molar and cuspid expansion could be attained as compared to adolescents. Also, a significant overall gain in maxillary and mandibular arch perimeter was found in adolescents. Also, although more transverse dental arch changes were found after puberty as compared to before, but these differences were not clinically significant. **Long-term skeletal changes with rapid maxillary expansion were evaluated with a systematic review** in transverse, anteroposterior and vertical planes in clinical trials by cephalometric analysis. It was found that the transverse skeletal maxillary increase is approximately 25% of the total dental expansion for prepubertal adolescents. Better long-term transverse changes are expected with RME in less skeletally mature patients. RME appears not to produce clinically significant anteroposterior or vertical changes in the position of the maxilla and mandible. It was concluded that the conclusions from this systematic review should be considered with caution because only a secondary level of evidence was found. Long-term randomized clinical trials are needed.

Skeletal and dental changes with fixed slow maxillary expansion treatment were evaluated in a systematic review. The authors found only a lower level of evidence. Therefore, they could make no strong conclusions on dental or skeletal changes that occurred after SME treatment. Clinicians need to rely on their clinical experience, experts' opinions and the presented limited evidence concerning SME treatments.

It can be seen that controversy still exists for SME/RME's efficacy. The conclusions from these systematic reviews should be considered with caution because only a secondary level of evidence exists. Long-term randomized clinical trials are needed for finding best evidences.

Orthodontic treatment for posterior crossbites: The evidence from the trials reported by Lindner (1989); Thilander (1984) suggests that removal of premature contacts on baby teeth is effective in preventing posterior crossbite from being progressing in mixed and permanent teeth. When grinding alone is not effective, an upper removable expansion appliance can be used which will decrease the risk of posterior crossbite from being continued in permanent dentition.

Orthodontic treatment of posterior crossbites (Harrison, Ashby, 2000): The aim of this review was to evaluate orthodontic treatments used to expand the maxillary dentition and correct posterior crossbites. Five RCTs and eight CCTs were included in the study. Occlusal grinding in primary dentition with/without an upper removable expansion appliance in mixed dentition for those children who did not respond to grinding, was shown to be effective in preventing a posterior crossbite in primary dentition from progressing in mixed and permanent dentitions.

But there was no evidence of difference in the treatment effects (molar and canine expansion) of appliances, e.g. banded versus bonded and two point versus four point rapid maxillary expansion, banded versus bonded slow maxillary expansion, transpalatal arch with/without buccal root torque, or upper removable expansion appliance versus quad-helix.

It can be concluded that removal of premature contacts of baby teeth is effective in preventing a posterior crossbite from being perpetuated to mixed and permanent dentition. It can be combined with upper removable expansion plate to expand upper arch to decrease the risk of posterior crossbite from being progressed to permanent dentition. But other effects were inconclusive and thus strong recommendations for using these appliances cannot be made in clinical practice, and experience of the clinicians has to be used.

Effects of RME on nasal airway cross-sectional area and volume measured by acoustic rhinometry were evaluated which suggest that some increases in nasal dimensions were noted which are small and should not be used as clinically significant indication for therapeutic maxillary expansion.

7. Orthodontic Tooth Movement

Medication effects on the rate of orthodontic tooth movement: a systematic review. There are many OTC and prescription medications which can affect the rate of OTM. Eicosanoids resulted in increased tooth movement, whereas their blocking led to a decrease. Nonsteroidal anti-inflammatory drugs (NSAIDs) decreased tooth movement, but non-NSAID analgesics, such as paracetamol (acetaminophen), had no effect. Corticosteroid hormones, parathyroid hormone, and thyroxin increase tooth movement. Estrogens probably reduce tooth movement, although no direct evidence is available. Vitamin D_3 stimulates tooth movement, and dietary calcium seemed to reduce it. Bisphosphonates had a strong inhibitory effect. It can be concluded that medications might have an important influence on rate of tooth movement, and information on their consumption is essential to adequately discuss treatment planning with patients.

In a systematic review to find the different intervention modalities to control pain during fixed orthodontic appliance therapy, it was found that there was no difference in pain control between ibuprofen, acetaminophen, and aspirin. Some analgesics, e.g. tenoxicam and valdecoxib had relatively lower visual analog scale (VAS) scores in pain perception. Low-level laser therapy (LLLT) has also bben found to be an effective approach for pain relief. Thus the analgesics remain the main treatment modality to reduce orthodontic pain despite their side effects. Some long-acting nonsteroidal anti-inflammatory drugs (NSAIDs) and cyclo-oxygenase enzyme (COX-2) inhibitors are recommended for their comparatively less side effects. Other approaches, like LLLT, have also been under research.

Optimum force magnitude for orthodontic tooth movement: In a systematic literature review, regarding the optimal force or range of forces for orthodontic tooth movement, over 400 articles both on human and animal experiments were found. Data from human research on the efficiency of forces was very limited. Systematic review of current literature found no evidence about the optimal force level in orthodontics. It can be concluded that well-controlled clinical studies are required to find the relation between applied force and rate of tooth movement.

Esthetic considerations: Traditionally, flat profiles were preferred which was achieved by extraction of 4 premolars and retraction of anterior teeth to maximum. But it was found to lead to aging effect, especially in patients with thin lips. Now, evidences say that somewhat convex profile is preferred, and the pendulum has swung towards the non-extraction treatment.

8. Retention and Stability

There has been a long quest on finding the best methods and duration for retention, and numerous articles have been published. Julian O'Neill (2007) in a systematic review showed that evidence-based conclusions are few. Chung How Kau (2006) showed there are insufficient research data on which to base our clinical practice on retention at present. Littlewood, Millett, et al (2006) described that there is weak, unreliable evidence that teeth settle quicker with a Hawley retainer than with a clear overlay retainer after 3 months. There is currently insufficient evidence on which to base the clinical practice of orthodontic retention. This is mostly because of inferior study design. There is a great need for well-designed prospective studies; sufficient sample sizes; and sample selection according to type of malocclusion, age and growth pattern.

Retention procedures for stabilizing tooth position after treatment with orthodontic braces by Littlewood et al (2006). Retention is the phase of orthodontic treatment to keep teeth in corrected positions after treatment with braces. Without a phase of retention, there is tendency for the teeth to return to their initial position (relapse). To prevent relapse almost every patient who has orthodontic treatment will require some type of retention. This review was done to evaluate the effectiveness of different retention strategies. Five trials compared different interventions: circumferential supracrestal fiberotomy (CSF) combined with full-time removable retainer versus a full-time removable retainer alone; CSF combined with a nights-only removable retainer versus a nights-only removable retainer alone; removable Hawley retainer versus a clear overlay retainer; multistrand wire MSW retainer versus a ribbon-reinforced resin bonded retainer; and three types of fixed retainers versus a removable retainer. There was weak, unreliable evidence that teeth settle quicker with a Hawley retainer than with a clear overlay retainer after 3 months. The quality of trial reports was generally poor. Thus presently there is currently insufficient evidence on which to base the clinical practice of orthodontic retention. Thus high quality RCTs are needed for further elaboration of results.

Stability: Bondemark, et al (2007) in a systematic review found that changes in the dental positions occur post-treatment. Following changes were found:

- There was reduction in post-Rx arch length and intercanine width of mandible.
- Crowding of lower incisors was found to increase.
- Angle's class II division 1 treatment with Herbst appliances normalized dentition and occlusion and relapse occurred but could not be predicted at individual level.
- Regarding the stability of treated cross-bite, insufficient scientific evidence was found.
- Stability of class III problem using RME with face mask has not been supported with conclusive scientific evidence.
- Regarding the stability of open bite after treatment, no evidence base conclusion was found.

Overall, regarding the long-term stability, no evidence based conclusion could be found. Long-term stability after orthodontic treatment remains inconclusive. Thereby, there is an urgent need for high quality randomised controlled trials in this crucial area of orthodontic practice.

9. TMD

TMD has always given shivers to orthodontist, as there has been legal cases filed against clinicians by the patients who could not get relief from TMD or got TMD during/after orthodontic treatment, thus implicating the clinicians. But, Rinchuse and McMinn 2006 in a systematic review of TMD literature found that

- Traditional orthodontic treatment does not increase TMD. Orthodontic treatment has no relation with TMD. Joint hypermobility does not have a clear relation with TMD.
- CT scan is not recommended for routine diagnosis of TM disc displacement.
- EMG biofeedback treatment is effective in TMD. Use of occlusal splints may be beneficial in TMD. Occlusal adjustment is not recommended for Rx or prevention of TMD.

TMD in relation to malocclusion and orthodontic treatment: It has been found that TMD is not correlated to any specific type of malocclusion. Also, there is no evidence to support any association of orthodontic treatment causing TMD. Thus, there is still a need for longitudinal studies. In another meta-analysis, the relation between traditional orthodontic treatment, including the specific type of appliance used and whether extractions were performed, and the prevalence of temporomandibular disorders (TMD) did not find any association that traditional orthodontic treatment increased the prevalence of TMD.

10. Role of Fluorides in Orthodontics

Decalcification, i.e. development of WSLs is a significant problem during fixed orthodontic treatment. Topical fluorides can reduce or eliminate the problem, but the relative effectiveness of different treatments or combinations of topical fluoride preparations is unknown.

In a systematic review to evaluate the effectiveness of fluoride and to compare all modes of fluoride delivery in preventing white spot lesion (WSL) demineralization during orthodontic treatment, it has been found that some evidence exist that use of daily NaF mouthrinse and GIC for bonding brackets reduces the occurrence and severity of WSL during orthodontic treatment. However, more high quality, clinical research is required to find different modes of delivering fluoride to the orthodontic patient.

Use of topical fluorides in addition to fluoride toothpaste reduced the incidence of decalcification in patients with both fluoridated and non-fluoridated water supplies. Different preparations and formats appear to decrease decalcification, but there was no evidence that any one method was superior. There was some evidence that the potency of fluoride preparations might be important.

Use of fluoride-containing orthodontic adhesives and decalcification: According to current literature, it is impossible to recommend the use of fluoride-containing orthodontic adhesives during fixed orthodontic treatment. But there is evidence to suggest that GIC is more effective than composite resin in preventing white spot formation, but the evidence is weak. Further research is required to determine the effectiveness of various fluoride-containing orthodontic adhesives.

Adhesives for fixed orthodontic brackets and bands: Various bracket adhesives have been evaluated, but it is difficult to draw any conclusions from the current systematic review regarding the best material, and thus improved future research is needed involving orthodontic adhesives. Similarly, for determining the adhesives for fixed orthodontic bands, the systematic review found insufficient quality evidence with regard to the most effective adhesive for attaching orthodontic bands to molar teeth. Thus, further RCTs are required.

11. Root Resorption

Root resorption has been found to occur in many cases and is associated with multiple factors. It can also be found in patients who are not undergoing orthodontic treatment. Constantinou in a systematic review found that RR can occur in individuals whether they undergo orthodontic treatment or not. During orthodontic treatment, frequency and severity of RR may increase, which in turn is affected by many factors. RR also undergoes certain degree of repair. Whether age, time, and OTM can increase RR remains controversial.

Root resorption associated with orthodontic tooth movement: a systematic review: In an another systematic review, it was found that comprehensive orthodontic treatment causes increased incidence and severity of root resorption, and heavy forces might be particularly harmful. There is not effect of archwire sequencing, bracket prescription, and self-ligation on the root resorption. Previous trauma and tooth morphology are unlikely causative factors. There is some evidence that a 2 to 3-month rest period during treatment decreases total root resorption. In conclusion, the results have been inconclusive in clinical management of root resorption, but evidence supports the use of light forces, especially with incisor intrusion.

In a meta-analysis performed on the treatment-related factors of external apical root resorption, it was found that the total distance the apex had moved and the time it took are also the treatment-related causes of root resorption.

12. Miniscrews in Orthodontic Treatment

Review and analysis of published clinical trials on the effects related to patient, screw, surgery, and loading on the stability of miniscrews was conducted. Miniscrews were found to have success rates sufficient for orthodontic treatment. There were different placement protocols. It is recommended to avoid screws with less that 8 mm length and 1.2 mm diameter. Immediate or early loading up to 200 cN was adequate, with no significant influence on screw stability.

Critical factors for the success of orthodontic mini-implants: a systematic review: Mini-implants are effective as anchorage, and their success depends on proper initial mechanical stability and loading quality and quantity.

A systematic review on use of mini-implants as anchorage in orthodontics: Miniscrews have biologic damage, inflammation, and pain and discomfort as some common adverse effects. Mini-implants can also be used as TADs, but research in this field is still in its infancy. There is lack of clarity and poor methodology of most studies and thus the interpretation of findings is poor by. Thus future studies are needed to clarify lots of issues related with TADs.

Survival and failure rates of orthodontic temporary anchorage devices: a systematic review: Palatal implants and miniplates provide reliable absolute orthodontic anchorage based on available evidence. But reliability regarding the use of multiple miniscrews to provide adequate anchorage in certain situations is questionable. Some cases needing variable force vectors or need of the roots to be moved past the anchors, there the, palatal implants or miniplates should be the TADs of choice.

Reinforcement of anchorage during orthodontic treatment with implants or other surgical methods: Anchorage refers to the control of unwanted tooth movement. It is conventionally provided either by intraoral anchor sites, e.g. the teeth and palate, or from outside the mouth (headgear). Orthodontic implants which are surgically inserted intraorally in the bone are increasingly being used as alternatives for anchorage reinforcement in orthodontics.

A systematic review to evaluate the effectiveness of surgical methods for preventing unwanted tooth movement compared with conventional anchorage reinforcement techniques was done which found limited evidence in favour of osseointegrated palatal implants as acceptable means of reinforcing anchorage. Thus, this is a dynamic area of orthodontic practice needing high quality, randomized controlled trials.

Systematic review of the experimental use of temporary skeletal anchorage devices in orthodontics: Experimental literature was reviewed to determine functional and morphological tissue reactions around orthodontically loaded temporary skeletal anchorage devices. Healing times ranged from 0 to

12 weeks, and the amount of force varied from 25 to 500 gm. Implant stability was generally achieved without severe side effects. Direct bone-screw contact was reported to be 10% to 58%, and osseointegration increased with loading time. Also, no significant difference in bone-screw contact was found between loaded and unloaded screw implants, or between tension and pressure sides of loaded implants. Future well controlled research based on standardized protocols to test specific hypotheses is needed.

Implant vs screw loading protocols in orthodontics: Systematic review for loading protocols for implants and screws found that a minimum waiting period of 2 months is needed for implants before applying orthodontic forces, while loading protocols for screws involve immediate loading or a waiting period of 2 weeks to apply forces. Success rates for implants were on average higher than for screws.

Another systematic review found two main anchorage situations: anchorage of molars during space closure after premolar extractions and anchorage loss in the incisor or premolar region (or both) during molar distalization. But the scientific evidence was too weak to evaluate anchorage efficiency during space closure due to contradictory results and the vast heterogeneity in study methods. Controlled RCTs with sufficient sample sizes are needed to determine the most effective anchorage system in the respective anchorage situation.

13. Maxillary Molar Distalization with Noncompliance Intramaxillary Appliances in Class II Malocclusion

Antonarakis and Kiliaridis in a systematic review evaluated quantitatively the dental effects of fixed molar distalisation appliances in individuals with class II malocclusion. Prospective or retrospective clinical studies matching inclusion criteria were considered. It was found that maxillary first molars showed distal crown movement and tipping greater than mesial crown movement and tipping of incisors and premolars. Incisors and premolars showed extrusion, but molars showed intrusion or extrusion, depending on the study and type of appliance used. Palatally acting appliances produced lesser distal tipping movement, as well as smaller incisor and premolar mesial tipping movements, as compared to buccally acting appliances. Friction-free appliances, e.g. pendulum, produced a large amount of mesiodistal movement and tipping, if no therapeutic uprighting activation was applied. In conclusion, the intramaxillary fixed molar distalization appliances act by distalizing molars with a concomitant and unavoidable loss of anchorage, as revealed by incisor and premolar mesial movement. Palatal acting appliances showed less tipping. Friction-free palatal acting appliances appear to produce better molar distalizing effects.

14. Early Orthodontic Treatment of Skeletal Open-bite Malocclusion

Cozza et al (2006) conducted a systematic review of the literature to assess the scientific evidence on the actual outcome of early treatments of open-bite malocclusions. It was found that no RCTs of early treatment of anterior open bite were performed. Most of the studies had serious problems of small sample size, bias and confounding variables, lack of method error analysis, blinding in measurements, etc. Thus, the quality level of studies was not sufficient enough to draw any evidence-based conclusions.

15. Orthodontic Therapy and Gingival Recession

Movement of incisors out of the alveolar process may be associated with a higher tendency for developing gingival recessions. A systematic review was done to assess the effects of changes in incisor inclination due to orthodontic treatment and the occurrence of gingival recession. A low level of evidence from the included studies for the amount of gingival recession was found, thus the results should be considered with caution. It needs further RCTs including clinical examination of hygiene and gingival conditions before, during and after treatment are needed to find such effects.

16. Prevalence of Nickel Hypersensitivity in Orthodontic Patients

In a meta-analysis, it was found that orthodontic treatment is not associated with an increase in the prevalence of nickel hypersensitivity unless subjects have a history of cutaneous piercing. There is need of high-validity studies to find strong evidence to further support these results.

17. Self-ligating Brackets

In a systematic review on frictional resistance in self-ligating brackets and conventionally ligated brackets, it was found that compared with conventional brackets, self-ligating brackets produce lower friction with small round archwires in the absence of tipping and/or torque in an ideally aligned arch. But, sufficient evidence regarding friction with large rectangular wires was not found; in the presence of tipping and/or torque; and in arches having considerable malocclusion. It has been concluded that at this stage there is insufficient high-quality evidence to support the use of self-ligating fixed orthodontic appliances over conventional appliance systems or vice versa.

Systematic review of self-ligating brackets: It was found that the shortened chair time and slightly less incisor proclination appear to be the only significant advantages of self-ligating systems over conventional systems supported by the current evidence. Despite claims about the advantages of self-ligating brackets, evidence is generally lacking.

18. Invisalign

The treatment effects of Invisalign orthodontic aligners: Lagravère, Flores-Mir (2005) conducted a systematic review of literature to determine the treatment effects of Invisalign orthodontic system (Align Technology). The authors reviewed clinical trials that assessed treatment effects in non-growing patients treated only with Invisalign. It was found that the studies were inadequately designed and only a lower level of evidence (level II) was found. Thus, no strong conclusions could be made regarding the treatment effects of Invisalign appliances. Future prospective RCTs are required to find Invisalign's treatment effects. Presently, the clinicians will have to rely on their clinical experience, experts' opinions and limited published evidence for using Invisalign appliances.

19. Incisor Intrusion

True incisor intrusion attained during orthodontic treatment: Flores-Mir et al (2005) in a meta-analysis quantified the amount of true incisor intrusion attained during orthodontic treatment. The goal was to identify clinical trials that assessed true incisor intrusion through cephalometric analysis and factored out craniofacial growth when required. Only 4 articles could be selected based on inclusion criteria which showed that true incisor intrusion is achievable in both arches, but the clinical significance of the magnitude of true intrusion as the sole treatment option is questionable in severe deepbite. In nongrowing patients, the segmented arch technique can produce 1.5 mm of incisor intrusion in the maxillary arch and 1.9 mm in the mandibular arch.

Conclusion

EBDM has become the recent tool in the medical science to use the best available evidence to treat the patients. It has also been incorporated in dental and orthodontic fields. The vast literature of orthodontics is being searched through systematic reviews and meta-analysis to find the best available method/s for treating the particular problems. These reviews have been widely published in leading journals and Cochrane data base. Based on the findings of these systematic reviews and meta-analysis, it has been concluded that the literature on most of the orthodontic procedures cannot provide strong scientific evidence on which the treatment planning can be based, and thus there is strong need to conduct further research based on strong methods like RCTs, etc. Some of the conclusions drawn from EBDM process in orthodontics can be summarised as below.

- There are no strong evidences to recommend the particular methods of treatment for the problems. There are brewing controversies in orthodontics for different methods of treatment, their efficacy and efficiency and long term results.
- It is mostly because of inherent problems with inferior study designs and retrospective data. There is a strong need for well-designed prospective studies with sufficient sample sizes and sample selection criteria should be well defined.
- There is need to integrate the accrued scientific evidences into clinical orthodontic practice.
- Research should be based on the need of practice. Practice should guide the research to find out the lacunae in the information available. Practice should be demanding what kind of research should be conducted for what has not been covered by the research. Currently, the research and the practice go independently, while the need of the hour is that both should go hand-in-hand.

53

Self-Correcting Anomalies

INTRODUCTION

Anomaly is defined as a deviation from the normal. Self-correcting anomalies are the conditions which are seen during the different stages of developing dentition, extending from gum pads stage to the permanent dentition and get corrected on their own without any dental treatment.

These conditions are developmental, which appear to be abnormal at that stage but are perfectly normal and in fact, a natural requirement for normal development. They should be recognized and should not be disturbed. Wait and watch for their natural disappearance, and if parents of the child are very much concerned, then refer the patient to a specialist. They are part of developing dentition and should not be considered as developmental or pathological abnormality.

Incipient Malocclusion

During normal development of dentition, there are certain clinical features which point towards the developing malocclusion in future. Some of the main features are lack of interdental spacing in primary dentition, crowding in permanent incisors in MDP and premature loss of primary canines esp mandibular due to the eruption of lateral incisors which cause root resorption of canines if arch length is deficient in the mandibular arch. Self-correcting anomalies can be discussed based on the different periods of dentition development.

A. Predentate Period

It is the period from birth to the eruption of first deciduous tooth in the oral cavity. During this stage, following SCA problems can be seen.

1. **Retrognathic mandible/skeletal class II pattern:** At birth, the mandible is seen retrognathic in relation to maxilla, and thus a convex profile is seen. It is due to cephalocaudal gradient of facial growth, so maxilla is more developed at birth as compared to mandible. Self-correction occurs when this retrognathic condition normally gets improved and corrected in postnatal life by rapid mandibular growth and its forward displacement to establish orthognathic or skeletal class 1 maxillomandibular relationship. This yet again conforms to the cephalocaudal gradient of growth pattern, where mandible grows more than maxilla with age. But an inadequate mandibular growth results in skeletal class II, while the overgrowth of mandible produces skeletal class III relation.

2. **Anterior open bite:** It is seen in the anterior region when upper and lower gum pads occlude. Upper pad is wider and longer than mandibular gum pad. On occlusion, they touch only in the future first molar region, and thus a space exists between them in the anterior region. This is considered normal and helps in suckling. *Correction:* It corrects with the eruption of primary incisors.

3. **Infantile swallowing pattern:** During the period before eruption of incisors, the tongue lies between the gum pads. It helps in holding the nipple during suckling in close apposition with lips. Contraction of facial muscles helps to stabilize the mandible during suckling, while the mandibular elevators show minimal activity. *Clinical implication:* During suckling, the mandible comes forwards, the tongue makes seal with upper lip to squirt the milk. Milk flows directly to the pharynx by an automatic peristaltic movement of tongue. *Correction:* With the eruption of deciduous teeth, many changes occur in the functioning of orofacial musculature. Tongue assumes a retracted position with eruption of incisors, open bite gets closed, and it also marks the learning of process of incising and mastication. Mature swallow begins as soon as the posterior occlusion is established when primary molars erupt. Gradually, the fifth cranial nerve muscles assume the role of mandibular stabilization during swallow. If the transition of infantile to mature swallow does not occur with eruption of teeth then it leads to tongue thrust.
4. **Anterior tongue thrust:** At birth, the tongue size is almost equal to adult size, while the oral cavity size is not. Also, there is open bite when the gum pads occlude. Thus, the child has a tendency to keep the tongue between the gum pads, and tongue comes between pads on swallowing. It gets corrected by natural growth of jaws and dentition.

B. Deciduous Dentition

It refers to the period from the eruption of first deciduous incisor till the eruption of first permanent molar.

1. **Anterior deep bite** (Fig. 53.1): Deep bite may occur in initial stages of development. It is accentuated by fact that the deciduous incisors are more upright than their successors. *Correction:*

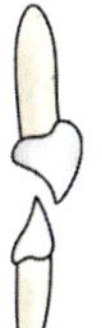

Fig. 53.1: Upright primary incisors contributing to deep bite in primary dentition.

It is corrected by eruption of deciduous molars; attrition of primary incisors; and downward movement of mandible due to growth.

2. **Flush terminal plane:** Mesiodistal relationship between the distal surfaces of upper and lower deciduous second molars is called the terminal plane. A normal feature of the deciduous dentition is a flush terminal plane where their distal surfaces are in the same vertical plane. It is because the MD size of lower second molar is larger than that of upper; and also the growth difference between upper and lower jaws. *Correction:* It gets corrected mesial shifting of permanent lower first molars in the leeway space; and by more mandibular growth as compared to maxillary growth (Fig. 53.2).

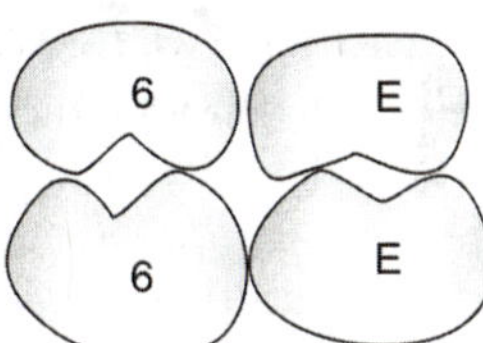

Fig. 53.2: When primary second molars are in flush terminal plane, then permanent first molars erupt in end-on relation.

3. **Spacing** (Fig. 53.3): Spaces are found in between the primary teeth and are required for proper eruption of larger sized permanent successors. These spaces are of two types: primate spaces and physiologic/developmental spaces. They appear due to continuing transverse growth of jaws. *Correction:* These spaces are naturally required for normal alignment of permanent teeth. If they are

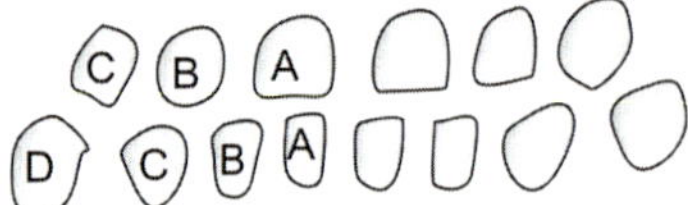

Fig. 53.3: Primary/physiological spacing in the anterior segments of primary arches which help to accommodate the wider permanent teeth.

not present, then there are chances of crowding in the permanent dentition.

4. **Retrognathic mandible and convex profile:** It is due to the growth differential where still the maxilla is larger than mandible.
5. **Attrition of teeth:** Attrition of teeth is seen during this stage, which is normal. The attrition leads to flattening of the cusps and also removes the overbite. It is important to keep the mandible free from interdigitation so that it can move forward with the ensuing growth.

C. Mixed Dentition

It is the most crucial stage and must be watched carefully. The interception of malocclusion can be done during this stage. Many SCA are seen in MDP.

1. **End-on relation:** The erupting permanent first molars are generally seen in end-on relationship where their mesial surfaces are in the same plane (at 6–7 years of age). It is due to flush terminal plane relation of deciduous upper and lower second molars. Correction occurs when the lower first molars move forward more than the upper molars (by 3 to 5 mm). It occurs by utilization of E-space, physiologic spaces and leeway space in lower arch and by differential forward growth of mandible.
2. **Mandibular anterior crowding:** Some crowding of lower incisors is seen with eruption of permanent incisors (at 6–8 years of age), because permanent incisors are wider than deciduous teeth. This difference is called incisal liability. Generally, upto 2 mm of crowding gets corrected itself. *Correction:* It occurs by increase in intercanine width with growth, by utilization of interdental spaces, and by tongue pressure which has a moulding action on incisal segment, and may also cause their mild labial shifting.
3. **Ugly-duckling stage:** It is seen in maxillary incisor region between 8 and 9 years of age, especially when the permanent canines start their journey of eruption. As the permanent canines erupt, they displace the roots of lateral incisors mesially. This results in transmitting of the force on to the roots of the central incisor which also gets displaced mesially. It leads to a resultant distal divergence of crowns of incisors which causes spacing between incisors. If any mechanical attempt is done to close the spaces between the incisors, the roots of lateral incisors will move distally, thus coming in contact with canines. It may lead to root resorption of lateral incisors. That is why, the condition should not be disturbed, and should be allowed to resolve naturally. *Correction:* It usually gets corrected when the canines erupt intraorally and the pressure is transferred from the roots to the crowns of incisors, thus leading to mesial movement of crowns.
4. **Anterior deep bite:** During normal development, the deep bite is seen in anterior region. It is more than the normal as seen in permanent dentition. *Correction:* It gets self-corrected by proprioceptive response when the first permanent molars erupt leading to swelling of overlying mucosal tissues. A premature contact of the pad of tissues leads to pain response and the child tends to keep the jaws apart, in which space the teeth are free to supraerupt, thus reducing deep bite. This is called natural bite opening, and it also occurs with eruption of permanent second and third molars also. Permanent molars can thus be called as natural bite openers. It also gets improved with vertical growth of jaws.

5. **Retrognathic mandible and convex profile:** It is present during MDP also, which is due to growth differential where still the maxilla is larger than mandible, although the degree of convexity is less as compared to the primary dentition period, because the mandibular growth in forward direction starts catching up during middle to late MDP.
6. **Attrition of teeth:** Attrition of teeth is also present during this stage, which is normal. The attrition leads to flattening of the posterior cusps, and helps to free the mandible from occlusal interdigitation so that it can move forward with the ensuing growth.

D. Permanent Dentition

In a normally developing early permanent dentition, increased overjet and overbite may be present. It gets corrected by differential growth of mandible, and by natural bite opening with the eruption of all permanent molars respectively.

Conclusion

The clinician should be watchful of certain developmental conditions seen at different stages of development of dentition, which are normal for that stage. These conditions should not be disturbed by mechanical means, and should be allowed to correct naturally.

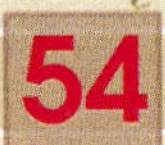

Cleft Lip and Palate

INTRODUCTION

Cleft of lip and palate is the most common congenital anomalies of face; and the second most common congenital anomalies of the body after club foot. It represents clinically as a defect in the continuity of upper lip and/or the palate. It may or may not be associated some syndrome and is present in varying degrees of severity. It is associated with multiple problems, e.g. esthetics, psychological, socioeconomic, malocclusion, improper growth of maxilla and mandible, difficulty in speech, mastication, swallowing, etc.

Incidence: Its incidence varies in different races and ethnic groups. It varies as 1 : 600 to 1: 2000 in live births in different races. It is found least in Negroids and most in Mongoloids. It may vary as isolated cleft lip or cleft palate or combination, to varying degrees. Cleft lip is more common in males and cleft palate is more common in females. Unilateral clefts are more common than bilateral condition. Left side is involved more than right side of the face.

Prenatal Development (Figs 54.1a to e)

Face is derived from fusion of 5 embryonic processes, i.e. the frontonasal process FNP, 2 maxillary processes and 2 mandibular processes (derived from the mandibular arch, the first branchial arch). Mandibular arch gives rise to maxillary process on each side. When nasal pits are formed, the fronto-nasal process gets divided into medial nasal process and 2 lateral nasal processes. Maxilla and palate are formed by the maxillary process, medial and lateral nasal processes. FNP descends and forms nose, and premaxilla.

During 3–4 week IU life, the neural crest cells proliferate and form five facial primordia, i.e. the frontonasal prominence, two maxillary prominences, and two mandibular prominences. Frontonasal prominence forms the forehead and nose. Maxillary processes form the lateral stomodeum (primitive mouth), while the mandibular process form the caudal part of the stomodeum. The neural crest cells within these prominences differentiate into skeletal and connective tissue of the face, bone, cartilage, fibrous connective tissue, and all dental tissues except enamel. Medial and lateral nasal processes develop on either side of frontonasal prominence.

Development of Lips

The lower lip and jaw are formed from mandibular process. Upper lip is derived from the fusion of the medial nasal and maxillary processes. The mesodermal base of its lateral part is formed by maxillary process. Its overlying skin is derived from the ectoderm of maxillary process. Mesodermal basis of median part, i.e. philtrum is formed by frontonasal process. The overlying skin forms from the ectoderm of maxillary process. Hence the skin of entire upper lip is formed by maxillary process.

During the fourth week, the medial ends of the mandibular prominences merge to form the mandible, lower lip, and lower cheek region. During 6th and 7th week, rapid proliferation of maxillary process results in the fusion of medial nasal prominences

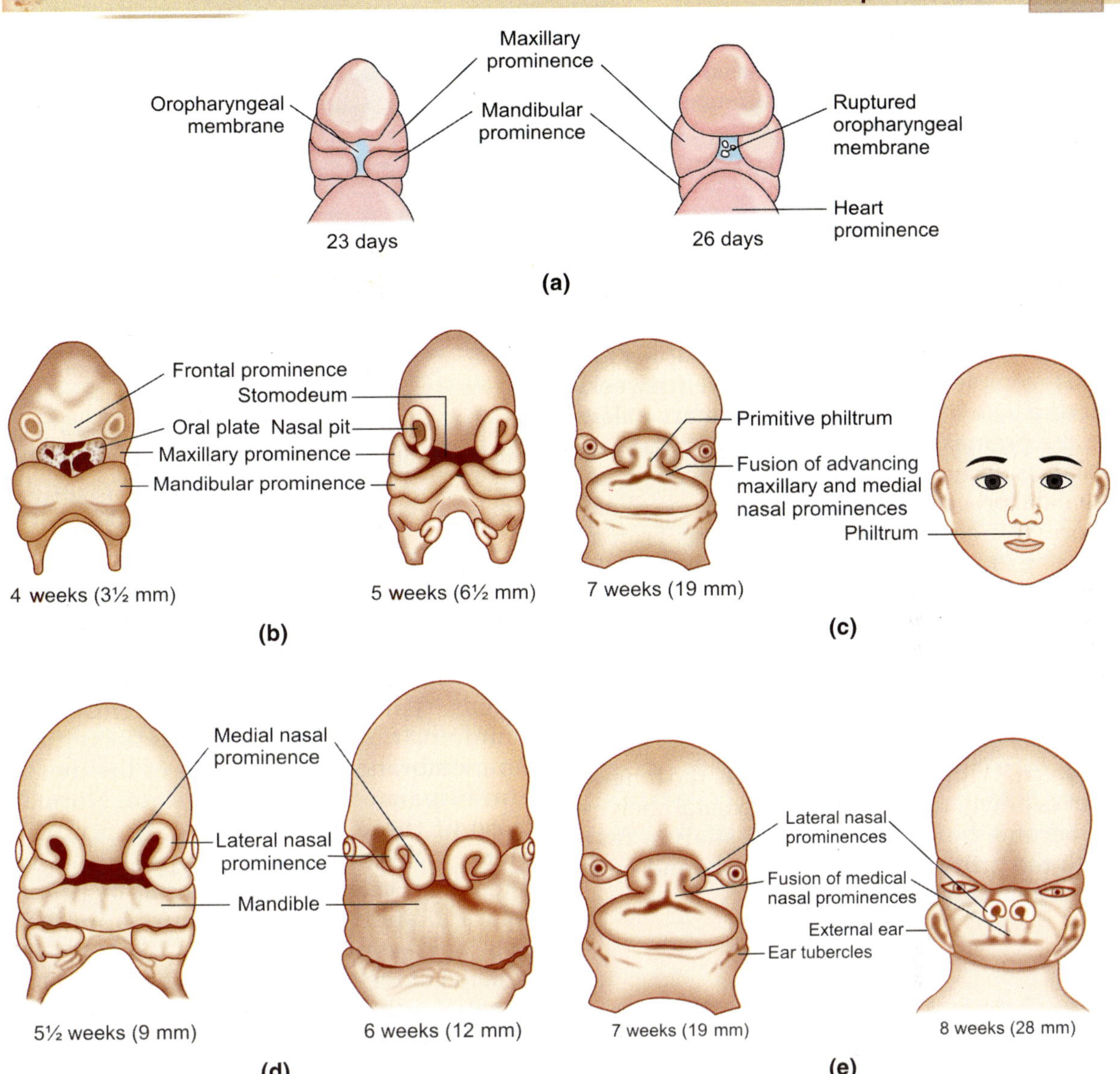

Figs 54.1a to e: Different stages of embryonic development of facial parts.

merging with each other and the lateral nasal prominences to form the lateral nose and cheek regions. Maxillary processes grow forward and medially below the lateral nasal processes, and continue to grow medially fusing with medial nasal processes, and then growing over them to meet in the midline. The face is fully formed by the eighth week. These processes consist of an epithelial surface with a mesenchymal core. It is believed that epithelial fusion is followed by mesenchymal penetration of the fused processes. Failure of these processes may cause a cleft lip. The upper lip is formed during this period by the lateral movement of the maxillary prominences and medially by the fused medial nasal prominences. Thus, the upper lip is formed by the fusion of maxillary processes. The premaxilla, the primary palate in front of the incisive foramen and the alveolus between the canines is formed from frontonasal process.

Clefts of lip are the result of the failure of the lateral nasal and median nasal processes, part of the frontonasal prominence, and the maxillary prominence to merge. Unilateral clefts occur when the maxillary prominence on the affected side fails to unite with the merged medial nasal prominences.

Development of Palate (Figs 54.2 and 54.3)

Palate development begins during the fifth week of gestation, after fusion of the upper lip, and is complete at the end of the twelfth week. Hard palate has two parts, i.e. primary palate or the premaxilla and the secondary palate. Palate is derived from the three processes, i.e. 2 palatal processes which arise from maxillary process; and the frontonasal process. Frontonasal process forms the primitive palate (premaxilla). Development of the secondary palate begins during the sixth week with the movement of palatal shelves toward the midline. Palatal shelves grow out from the inner aspect of the maxillary processes. At first they grow vertically as the tongue lies in between. With the growth of neck, the tongue moves down, thus helping the palatal shelves to become horizontal. Palatal shelves fuse with the primary palate anteriorly and with each other more posteriorly.

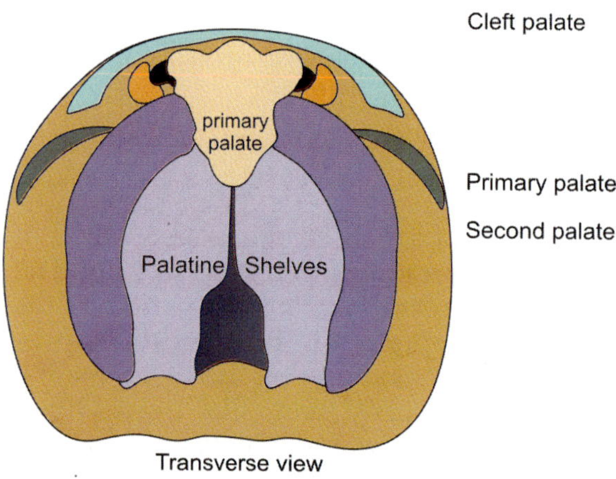

Fig. 54.2: Development of palate, and different embryonic palatal processes.

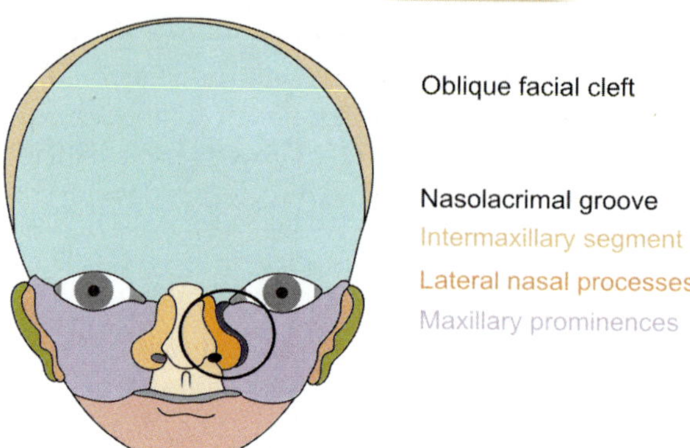

Fig. 54.3: Different embryonic facial processes, and formation of oblique facial cleft.

At 8–9 weeks of IU life, the palatal shelves start fusing. The fusion starts in the middle area first and then progresses anteriorly and posteriorly. Also, the palatal processes fuse with free lower edge of nasal septum which is derived from the posterior part of fronto-nasal process. This fusion helps to close the communication of oral and nasal cavities. Intramembranous ossification of the mesoderm of palate forms hard palate. Normal fusion of these processes during primary palate formation forms upper lip and premaxilla. Secondary palate forms by fusion of palatal shelves which occurs approx 2 weeks after primary palate.

Fusion of the palatal shelves is a process of epithelial adhesion and fusion followed by epithelial seam disintegration and mesenchymal in-growth. There is programmed cell death of the medial edges that thins the epithelium and allows the tissue from each side to join in the midline. Fusion of the hard palate is completed by the tenth week. Development of the soft palate and uvula is completed in the twelfth week. Thus the palate is formed from the palatal processes of the maxillary processes.

Anomalies of Face

Development of clefts occurs due to disturbance during fusion of the embryonic processes. The type and extent of clefting is dependent on the stage of embryonic development and age. Cleft lip occurs due to non-fusion of medial nasal process and the maxillary process. Midline cleft of upper lip occurs from the clefting of lower part of the fronto-nasal process. Midline cleft of lower lip occurs due to non fusion of mandibular process of one side with that of the other side. Cleft of lip and palate can be present together. An isolated cleft palate occurs if the developmental disturbance occurs after complete formation of lip has occurred. The degree of clefting in palate depends at the time when the developmental disturbance occurs. It may vary from a complete cleft to partial cleft to only a notch in its posterior extent or sometimes only a bifid uvula. Oblique facial cleft arises due to non fusion of the maxillary process and the lateral nasal process. Microstomia is small oral opening which occurs due to too much fusion of maxillary and mandibular processes. Lateral facial cleft arises due to unilateral non-fusion of maxillary and the mandibular processes. Incomplete fusion of maxillary and mandibular processes leads to wide mouth, or macrostomia.

Causes of cleft lip and palate (Fig. 54.4): Various theories have been proposed to explain the development of this congenital anomaly. Some of them has been discussed briefly.

a. **Theory of fusion of processes:** According to this theory, during embryonic development, separate processes fuse to form the face. Different processes grow toward the midline, epithelium and ectodermal layers disintegrate and endoderm and the mesoderm of the opposite side fuse. Any interference in this process may result in a cleft palate or cleft lip.
b. **Theory of mesodermal migration:** According to this theory, cleft palate occurs due to failure of epithelial membrane on the palatine shelves to disintegrate upon their approximation. Mesoderm grows and migrates to form different embryonic processes in head and neck region, which move towards each other in an ordered fashion due to mesodermal growth and migration. If mesodermal migration is interfered, then it may lead to clefting.
c. **Failure of palatal shelves to fuse:** The palatal processes which arise from maxillary process first grow vertically and then horizontally to fuse in midline

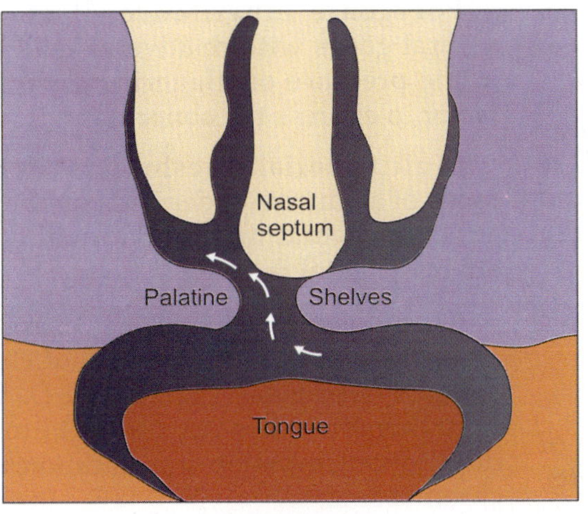

Fig. 54.4: Development of cleft palate, and oronasal communication.

to form palate. Factors which lead to failure of palatal shelves to elevate are:

- Failure of the head to elevate and become erect at around the 7th–9th weeks.
- Failure of tongue to descend downwards, thus causing a mechanical interference to fusion of the palatine shelves.
- Deficiency of oxygen
- Shift of blood supply of face during the 6th week. Most of the midface is supplied by the stapedial artery which is the branch of the internal carotid artery. At around the 7th week, stapedial artery severs from the internal carotid and its terminal branches join the external carotid artery. Delay in this vital step can lead to cleft palate.

Predisposing Factors

- Maternal and paternal age: Increased age of father and mother increases the chances of clefting.
- Racial differences: Clefts are more in some races as compared to other races. It is least in Negroids and most in Mongoloids, Japanese and Chinese.
- Socioeconomic status and nutritional status are also interlinked. Poor nutrition of expecting mother also may be predisposing factor for CLP development.

Etiological factors: A multifactorial etiolgy has been considered for this anomaly. It is mainly believed to occur due to genetic and environmental causes. Causes can be broadly classified as:

- Genetics
- Teratogens
- Nutritional factors

Heredity: It is one of the main causes of CLP. If one or both parents are having clefts, the chances of their offspring having clefts increase. Even if the parents are not having cleft, but grandparents were having cleft, then also chances of clefting are more. If both the parents are unaffected, and if they have an affected child, their next offspring has a risk developing CL/P. If there is an affected relative, then risk of CL/P is increased. If both parents are affected a probability of offspring developing the analomy is 60%.

Inheritance of CL and CP in twins: In monozygotic twins, there is approx 40% concordance of CL and CP; while in the dizygotic twins, there is 5% concordance of CL and CP.

Genes: Several genes have been associated with development of cleft lip and palate, e.g. MSH homeobox homolog-1 (Msx1), transforming growth factor-β3 (TGF-β3), T-box transcription factor-22 gene (TBX22), poliovirus receptor like-1 (PVRL1), interferon regulatory factor-6 (IRF6), etc. Transforming growth factor alpha (TGFA), transforming growth factor beta 3 (TGFB3), and MSX1are genes have been identified as having a major role in the development of CL/CP. AP2 is another gene identified through having a role in the development of CL/CP.

Monogenic inheritance: A single gene is considered as the cause of CLP. There is equal distribution among autosomal dominant and recessive disorders, e.g. Van der Woude's syndrome, X-linked submucous clefts.

Polygenic inheritance: It means that several genes with relatively small effect act in the presence of triggering environmental factor to express the abnormality.

Multifactorial/threshold model: Occurrence of an anomaly depends on the additive effect of several minor abnormal genes and environmental factors.

Chromosomal anomalies: Chromosomal abnormalities account for 18% of clefts-associated syndromes, e.g. trisomy-D. Chromosomal abnormalities may occur due to deletion; duplication; inversion; translocation, etc. of the chromosome/s.

Environmental causes: They affect during especially first trimester which is the time of maximum tissue differentiation.

Teratogens: They are the substances like drugs, medications, etc. which disturb the normal developmental process, e.g. phenytoin, alcohol, thalidomide, aminopterin, trimethadione, corticosteroids, smoking, rubella viral infection, toxoplasmosis during the first trimester, valium, methtrexate, retinoids, hyperthermia; maternal obesity and diabetes mellitus, etc.

Drugs: Taking vasoactive drugs by expecting mothers, e.g. pseudoephedrine, aspirin, ibuprofen, amphetamine, cocaine, or ecstasy, cigarette smoking, alcohol, corticosteroids, have been associated with higher risk for oral clefts. Anticonvulsant medications, such as phenobarbital, trimethadione, valproate, and dilantin, also increase incidence of cleft lip and/or cleft palate. Isotretinoin (Accutane) has been identified as potential causative factors for oral clefts. An association between maternal intake of sulfasalazine, naproxen, and glucocortisoids during the first trimester has been suggested. Aminopterin (a cancer drug) has also been linked to the development of oral clefts.

Nutritional deficiencies: Deficiency of B_6, B_{12}, (riboflavin) and reduced levels of folic acid also predispose to developmental defects. Deficiency of folic acid interferes with the neural crest cells migration and thus deficiency of the tissues.

Blood groups: Blood group AB and O show significantly increased frequency with CL and CP patients.

Distorted growth patterns: This may be due to hypervitaminosis A.

Rupture of the palatal plates: Small epithelial islands trapped along the line of closure may cause the post-closure opening.

Distortion or malpositioning of facial processes: This may be caused by excessive or prolonged compression of face against the chest.

Radiations: Abnormal exposure to radiations during the first trimester period, which is the time of extreme cellular differentiation and migration, produces somatic or genetic defects.

Syndromes: Many syndromes have been found to be associated with some form of cleft palate, e.g. Kabuki syndrome, Van der Woude syndrome, Treacher Collins syndrome, Stickler syndrome, DiGeorge syndrome, Opitz syndrome, etc.

Minor symptoms as prodromal symptoms: Some features may also be associated with clefts, and they have been considered as microclefts of face, e.g.

- Lip pits: midline/corners of mouth
- Malformed ear/pinna
- Malformed teeth
- Missing teeth
- Malformed and asymmetric alar base
- Asymmetrical nostrils

CLASSIFICATION OF CLEFT LIP AND PALATE (Fig. 54.5)

Many classifications have been proposed by various authors to classify CL/P cases for ease of learning and treatment planning. Few of them are:

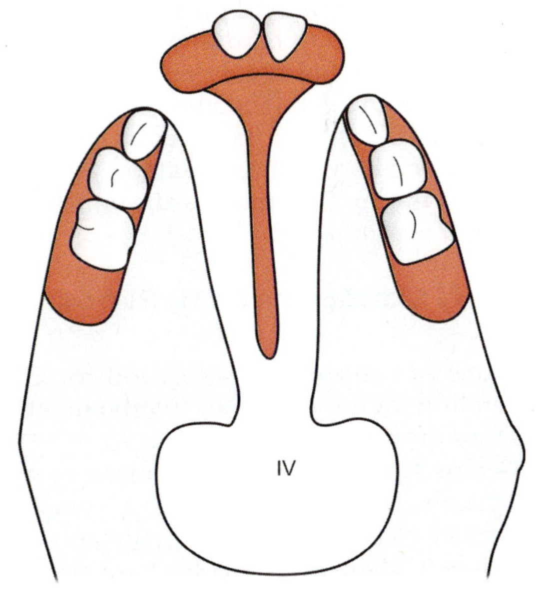

Fig. 54.5: Different types of cleft lip and cleft palate.

A. Most Simple Classification of Clefts of Lip and Palate

a. CL, cleft lip only: Unilateral or bilateral
b. CLA, cleft lip and alveolus: unilateral or bilateral
c. CP, cleft palate only: Cleft of hard palate/cleft of soft palate/cleft of hard and soft palate/bifid uvula.
d. CLP, cleft lip and palate: Unilateral/bilateral
e. Submucosal clefts.

B. Indian Classification of Cleft Lip and Palate by Balakrishnan (1975)

Group - I	Cleft Lip alone.
Group - Ia	Cleft lip and alveolar
Group - 2	Cleft Palate only.
Group - 3	Cleft lip and palate.

C. Davis and Ritchie Classification (1922)

It is based on the location of cleft relative to alveolar process. It has three groups:

Group I: Pre-alveolar clefts: These clefts involve only the lip, which may be unilateral/bilateral/medium. They do not involve the alveolar ridge.

Group II: These are the **postalveolar clefts**, which are limited to hard and soft palate to variable degree, not involving the lip. They may also be unilateral/bilateral/medium.

Group III: These are the **alveolar clefts**, i.e. complete clefts involving palate, alveolar ridge and the lip. They may also be unilateral/bilateral/medium.

D. Veau's Classification (1931) (Figs 54.6 to 54.9)

It is one of simplest classification for CLP depending on the degree of involvement. It has four groups.

Group 1: These clefts are limited to soft palate only, to varying degrees, e.g. complete soft palate cleft/partial/bifid uvula only.

Group 2: These clefts involve hard and soft palates extending upto incisive foramen, to variable degrees, e.g. partial hard palate cleft, etc. They are in the midline.

Group 3: These clefts are the complete unilateral clefts involving soft palate, hard palate, alveolar ridge and lip.

Group 4: They are the complete bilateral clefts involving soft palate, hard palate, alveolar ridge and lip.

E. Kernahan's Stripped 'Y' Classification (Figs 54.10a and b)

It is a symbolic classification, in the form of Y. Y is divided in 9 blocks, out of which 6 blocks are in the 2 forks of Y, while rest 3 blocks are

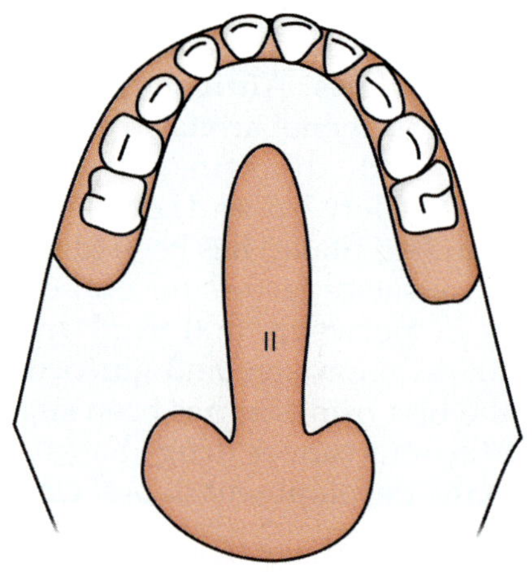

Fig. 54.6: Veau's classification of CLP: Group 2. Partial cleft of hard and soft palates.

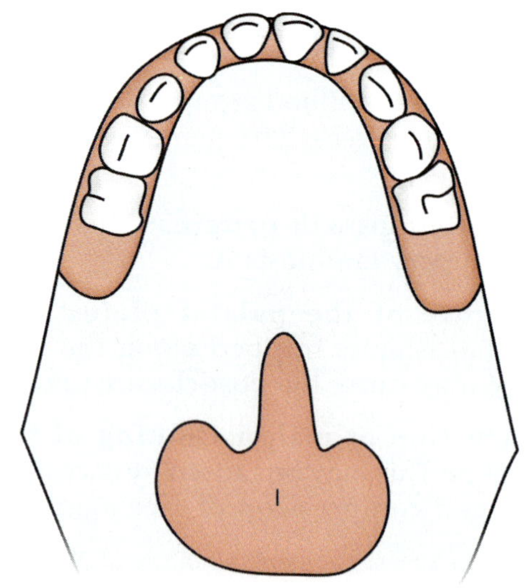

Fig. 54.7: Veau's classification of CLP: Group 1. Cleft of soft palate.

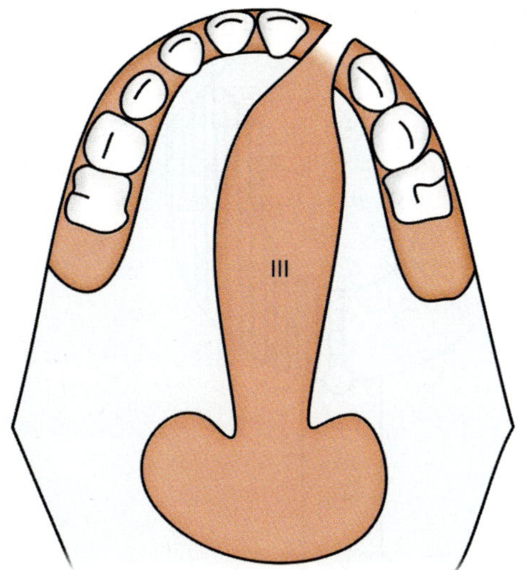

Fig. 54.8: Veau's classification of CLP: Group 3. Complete unilateral cleft of lip, alveolus, hard and soft palates.

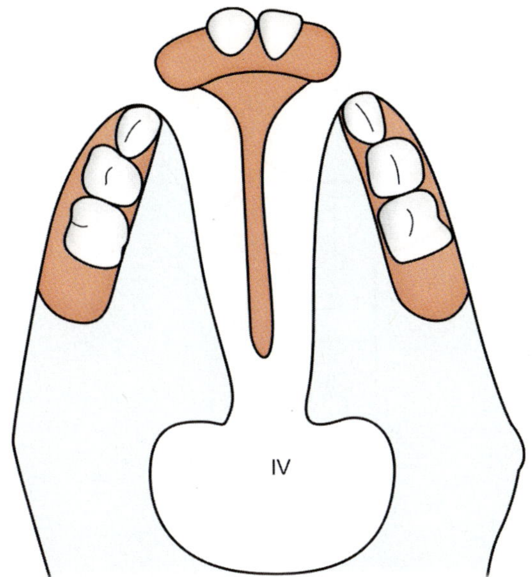

Fig. 54.9: Veau's classification of CLP: Group 4. Complete bilateral cleft of lip, alveolus, hard and soft palates.

in the vertical arm of the Y. they are numbered as 1–9.

Two forks of Y represent left and right sides of the lip, alveolus and the premaxillary part of hard palate. The vertical arm represents hard and soft palates.

- Lip: blocks 1 and 4.
- Alveolus: blocks 2 and 5.
- Hard palate anterior to incisive foramen: 3 and 6
- Hard palate posterior to incisive foramen: 7 and 8.
- Soft palate: 9.
- Boxes are shaded in those areas where the cleft has occurred.

It is a very simple and easy to learn classification.

F. Lahshal Classification (Figs 54.10a and b)

It was proposed by Otto Kreins (1987). It represents the areas affected by the cleft by their initial letters.

L – Lip (right)
A – Alveolus (right)
H – Hard palate (right)
S – Soft palate
H – Hard palate (left)
A – Alveolus (left)
L – Lip (left).

PROBLEMS ASSOCIATED WITH CLEFT LIP AND PALATE

A patient affected by CL/P is affected by a lot of problems. They can be broadly classified as follows.

- Feeding problems
- Speech and hearing problems
- Upper respiratory tract and middle ear infections
- Dental problems and malocclusion
- Growth problems: general body growth and facial growth
- Skeletal problems and facial deformity
- Esthetic problems
- Psychological problems.

Feeding problems: A child born with CL/P is not able to suckle and swallow properly. If there is cleft palate, generally there is naso-oral communication leading to nasal regurgitation of fluids. He is not able to make proper seal with lips, palate and tongue and thus suckling is difficult. The parents are

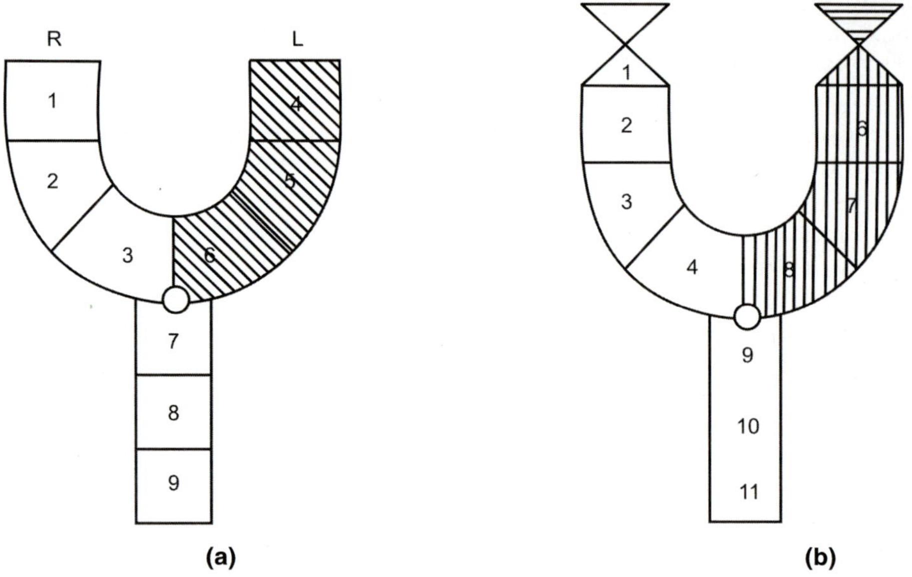

Figs 54.10a and b: Kernahan's classification system of CLP; modified classification.

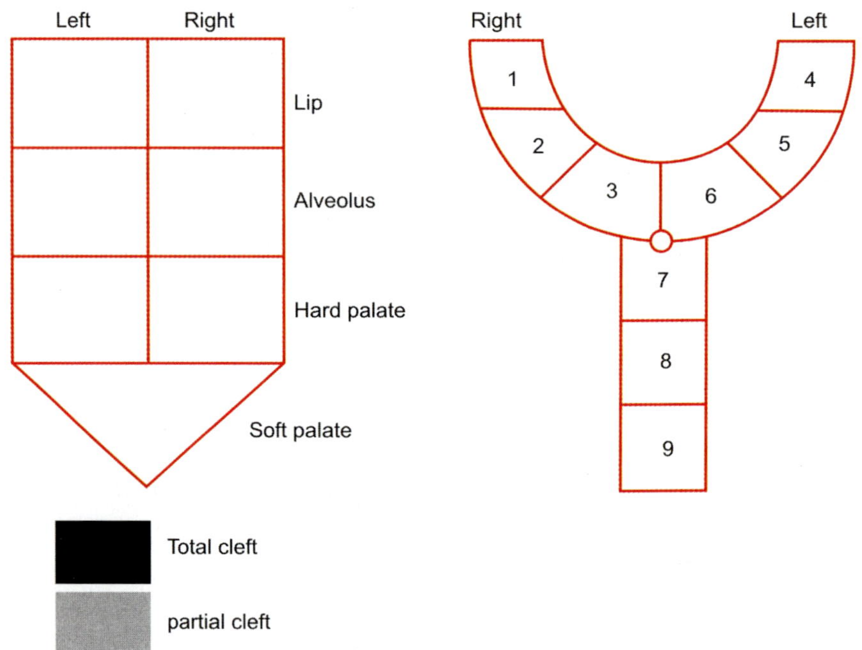

Fig. 54.11: Classification method of CLP: LAHSAL classification; Kernahan's classification.

trained to feed the child with spoon to put the milk directly in the oral cavity behind the cleft area or in the buccal vestibule of mouth. Special nipples have been designed to feeding through bottles, e.g. Nuk Sauger nipple. These nipples are flat, long and have a cross-cut opening which helps to deposit the milk more posteriorly and without much effort.

Speech development problems: The child is not able to properly articulate because proper air seal and escape routes are not formed and thus he is not able to learn speaking properly. Nasal twang and unclear sound is present in them.

Hearing problems: Due to oronasal communication in CLP/CP, the Eustachian tube gets affected and recurrent infections may lead to otitis media, i.e. middle ear infections, which may be chronic, suppurative or purulent, etc. and may lead to hearing problems if not attended properly.

Respiratory tract infections: Recurrent URTIs are very common in such cases due to oronasal communication, leading to infections of nasal cavity, maxillary sinus and upper respiratory tract. It may also lead to blockage of Eustachian tubes and otitis media.

Dental problems: Many dental problems are seen in these patients. The development of certain teeth may be affected during initiation, histodifferentiation and morphodifferentiation. Following dental problems can be seen.

- Congenitally missing teeth (commonly upper lateral incisor on the cleft side),
- Presence of natal teeth,
- Presence of supernumerary teeth
- Ectopically erupting teeth
- Impacted teeth esp maxillary canines
- Abnormal shaped (malformed) teeth
- Fused teeth
- Enamel hypoplasia
- Abnormal sized teeth: microdontia or macrodontia. Generally, teeth size is smaller in cleft patients.
- Mobile teeth due to weak periodontal support
- Spacing/crowding/rotations
- Teeth prone to caries.

Facial skeletal problems: Growth of maxilla is deficient leading to maxillary deficiency. Mandibular growth is almost normal, which may lead to skeletal class III defect. Width of maxilla is also decreased leading to buccal crossbite and functional shift. The maxilla may get locked by mandible in anterior crossbite and is not able to express itself properly. In case of bilateral cleft, initially, the premaxilla is protruded and thus a crossbite may not be seen. But after its repair, the scar tissue may restrict growth of maxilla and thus maxillary deficiency occurs. The alveolus on the cleft side gets deviated towards the midline leading to development of asymmetry of the dental arch and crossbite.

Transverse growth of maxilla is affected due to discontinuity of palatal halves. The nasal septal cartilage is also deviated in cleft palate. In cleft lip cases, there is no anterior molding effect on the maxilla, and hence asymmetry of maxilla develops. Normal mandibular growth leads to development of anterior crossbite and hence a skeletal class III relation is established.

Esthetic problems: Abnormal growth of jaws and malposition of teeth lead to esthetic problems. Nasal deviation occurs on the cleft side, nostrils are abnormally shaped which get widened and flattened on cleft side. Nasal bridge is flattened in some cases. Deficient maxillary growth leads to concavity of face profile.

Psychosocial problems: Multiple problems, e.g. hearing, speech, malocclusion, facial disfigurement, esthetic problems, etc. lead to psychosocial problems. The child faces problems in studies due to his inability to speak properly due to nasal twang, and social acceptance is low due to esthetics.

Velopharyngeal insufficiency: It is due to improper closing of velopharyngeal sphincter (soft palate muscle in the mouth) during speech, allowing air to escape through the nose instead of mouth. It leads to formation of

- Improper consonants such as "p", "b", "g", "t" and "d".
- Hypernasality and nasal air emission occurs.

Management

Management of CL/P cases needs a comprehensive management involving a dedicated team having following members.

- Orthodontist
- Plastic surgeon

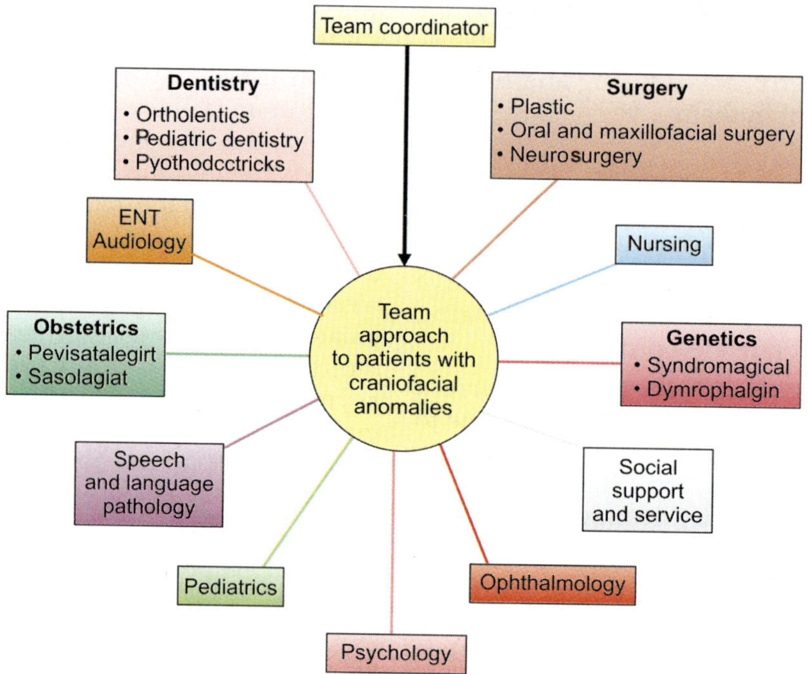

Fig. 54.12: Diagram depicting multi- and interdisciplinary approach to manage a case of CLP.

- ENT surgeon
- Oral/maxillofacial surgeon
- Dentist/pedodontist
- Pediatrician
- Psychologist
- Prosthodontist
- Speech pathologist
- Nurse
- Audiologist
- Genetic counseling
- Opthalmologist
- Neurologist
- Social worker

Interdisciplinary vs multidisciplinary approach: For the comprehensive management of a CLP patient, a team work is needed. The members of teams should meet regularly and discuss the treatment and progress of the cases. Cases should be regularly followed up till at least postpubertal age.

Interdisciplinary approach means the involved members interact with each other frequently during the entire treatment at a common platform, and share their views face to face.

Multidisciplinary approach (Fig. 54.12): Means the involved members do not interact with each other face to face during the treatment, but only give/write their opinions about the treatment without discussing the needs of the patient. Later approach is not fruitful, as without proper discussion, many aspects of the treatment and progress can be missed out.

Protocol for CLP cases: A proper protocol or clinical guideline should be established for the comprehensive management of CLP patients by the team. This protocol should be flexible and regularly updated based on latest knowledge and experiences of the team members. Here, a brief protocol is presented, based on which the treatment of CLP patient can be planned according to the age and stage the patient visits the health facility.

- **Feeding appliances**
- **Presurgical nasoalveolar molding, (PNAM)**
- **Presurgical orthopedics**
- Lip repair: at 3 months.
- Pediatric dental care: 6–8 months Onwards

- Palate repair: b/w 18–24 months/5–6 years or later
- Speech therapy: as soon as possible and continued/palate repair.
- Orthodontic intervention to treat premaxillary cross bite: at 4–5 years.
- Sulcus repair and columellar lengthening: at 5 years.
- Contd. Speech therapy and dental care: at regular intervals.
- Early ortho. Phase: 6–8 years.
- Alveolar bone graft : 9–11 years.
- Final ortho. Phase: till 14 years.
- Prostho. Rehab: after ortho.
- Surgical intervention, scar revisions, etc: adult age.
- Continuous FU: till early 20s age

The management of a CLP patient can be divided in **following stages**:

A. Neonatal period
B. Primary dentition period
C. Mixed dentition period
D. Permanent dentition period
E. Late permanent dentition period/adult hood
F. Retention period.

Neonatal period: A child born with CL/P has main problems of feeding and maintaining the airway. He is prone to infections of nose, ear and respiratory tract. In a child, the foremost importance lies to protect the airway. It can be done by proper feeding technique to avoid inhaling of food and resultant choking.

Feeding: Proper feed is important for the overall physical and mental growth of child. Breast feeding is not precluded for CLP cases. The breast feed is the best feed during first 6 months of life, as it provides immunity to child against many infections. Since a child with CL/P is not able to suckle due to lack of proper seal around the nipple, the parents are advised to spoon feed the child. The mother should extract the fresh breast milk in a bowl and feed the child. Alternatively, the bottle feeding with special nipples having large hole to allow easy flow of milk are used.

During feeding following simple guidelines should be followed:

1. The infant is held upright or at about 30–45° angle to decrease nasal regurgitation.
2. Place nipple to intact part of the palate.
3. Burp the infant frequently
4. Adjust the flow of the milk so that milk is delivered slowly in child's oral cavity.
5. If spoon feeding is done, the milk should be directed in the buccal vestibule from where it can easily flow down.
6. Holes in the nipple should not be too small or too large. It should be soft and easily squeezable.

Mead-Johnson cleft palate nurser: It is a soft, squeezable, plastic bottle that is easy to squeeze and has a large crosscut nipple. As the baby begins to suck, squeeze the bottle with a firm steady pressure to the count of "three," and then relax. Thus an intermittent flow of milk is provided. Pause every few seconds to allow the baby to take a breath. The person feeding the baby controls the amount of flow of milk.

Haberman feeder: It works well for babies who have only cleft palate. It has a one-way valve that keeps milk in the nipple. The milk is obtained by compressing the nipple against the roof of mouth, without need for suction. Most of the babies can obtain milk from this feeder by themselves, because no bottle squeezing is needed. This is a specially designed bottle system with a valve to help control the air the baby drinks and to prevent milk from going back into the bottle.

Pigeon nipple: It can be used with any bottle. It has a faster flow than Haberman or squeeze bottle, and works well for slightly older infants. It works by compression only. The nipple has a firm side that faces the roof of mouth and a softer side is on the tongue side. A small notch at the base of nipple serves as an air vent, which should be kept uppermost under the baby's nose while feeding for escape of air. A one-way valve is fitted into the nipple to keep milk in the nipple. The valve is placed with the flat side toward the tip of the nipple. It allows milk flow only when the baby begins to suck. The infant controls the flow of milk and no squeezing is needed.

NUK nipple: This nipple can be placed on regular bottles or on bottles with disposable bags. The hole can be made larger by making a criss-cross cut in the middle.

Syringes: These may be used in hospitals following cleft surgery and may also be used at home. Typically, a soft, rubber tube is attached on the end of the syringe, which is then placed in the infant's mouth.

Feeding obturator: Obturators were used to cover the cleft defect so that the milk, etc. does not enter the nasal cavity during suckling or feeding. It helps to obturate the defect and prevents the tongue from entering the defect and interfering with growth of palatal shelves. It helps in development of jaws and contributes to speech development. It has an acrylic palatal plate with wires coming out of oral cavity adapted parallel to the cheeks. Acrylic plates are made with wax spacers to provide space for naturally growing tissues, and are adjusted time to time to keep pace with changes and growth. It is retained in the position with the help of tape stuck to the cheeks of the child. It should be replaced regularly so as not to restrict the growth of jaws. Nowadays, they are used rarely, because the parents are trained to feed the child by spoon putting the milk in the buccal vestibule, so that the milk directly reaches the back of oral cavity for swallowing. Also, special nipples have been designed to be used for bottle feeding in such patients.

Infant orthopedics, (IO) (Fig. 54.13): It was initially advised by Burstone in 1950s. Forward displacement of pre-maxillary segment esp in BCLP makes lip repair more difficult, as it does not allow proper approximation of the tissues and needs stretching the tissues more to suture them over the displaced premaxilla. It, **IO,** is done to retract the premaxillary segment in the dental arch line to help in lip surgery. It can be done by various methods like:

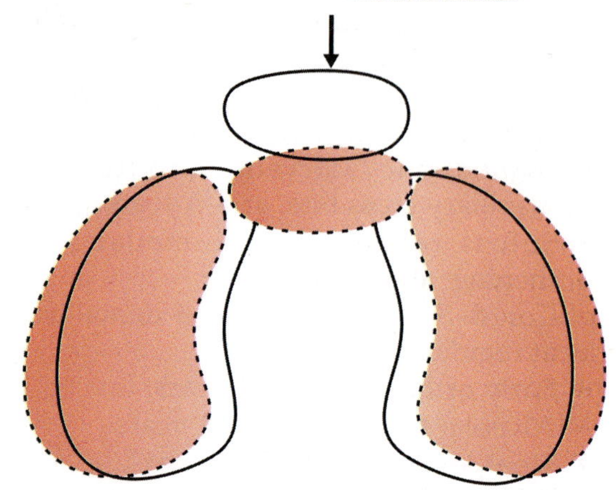

Fig. 54.13: Molding of premaxilla and alignment with other alveolar segments with the elastic strap before surgery.

Elastic strap: A light elastic strap is placed across the anterior segment that applies a contractile retraction force on pre-maxilla. Elastic band is taped on the sides of cheeks with micropore tape.

Latham appliance: It is a pin-retained fixed appliance which helps to retract the protruded premaxilla in line with lateral segments of maxillary arch, esp in BCLP cases, before the lip surgery and also expands the collapsed arch in BCLP cases. It has a special type of expansion screw, and a pin is inserted in the nasal septum. The E-chain is attached between this pin and a posterior point, which gets activated during expansion and thus applies a retraction force on premaxilla. It is placed surgically under anaesthesia.

Pre/postsurgical nasoalveolar molding (PNAM) (Grayson et al, 1999): It is a non-surgical method of reshaping the premaxilla, lip and nostrils before/after cleft lip surgery, reducing the severity of the cleft. Naso-alveolar moulding appliance (NAM) consists of an intraoral moulding plate and nasal stents which helps to mould the alveolar ridge, columella and nasal cartilages. It helps to reduce the deflection of maxillary and nasal segments to approximate them. The objective of PNAM is to reduce the severity of cleft deformity and thus enable the surgeon to achieve better repair of alveolus, lip and nose so that the surgery can be performed without applying much stress on the tissues. It actively molds and repositions the deformed nasal cartilages and alveolar processes and lengthens the deficient collumella. Use of NAM also reduces the need of surgical columella reconstruction. Resultant scar tissue is reduced after surgical correction. It is much helpful in BCLP cases where premaxilla is deflected outwards. The elastic strap helps to bring protruding premaxilla back in line with the lateral segments. The nares are shaped by inserting the acrylic hollow tube to help in adaptation of the cartilages. These tubes are changed frequently to allow the growth.

Procedure: Initial impression of the patient is obtained within the first week of birth with heavy-bodied silicone impression material, under a clinical setting that is prepared to handle airway emergency, if at all encountered. The infant is held upside down and the impression tray is inserted into the oral cavity. The infant is held in an inverted position to prevent the tongue from falling back and to allow fluids to drain out of the oral cavity. The cast is made in dental stone.

A 2–3 mm thick moulding plate is fabricated on the cast with hard, clear self-cure acrylic and is lined with a denture soft material. All the undercuts and the cleft space are blocked with wax. A retention button is fabricated and positioned anteriorly at an angle of 40° to the plate. In the unilateral cleft only one retention arm is used. The exact location of retention arm is determined at the chair side. It is positioned so as not to interfere with bringing the cleft lips together. The vertical position of the retention arm should be at the junction of upper and lower lips. The retention button adequately secures the moulding plate in the mouth with the help of orthodontic elastics and tapes. The appliance is secured extraorally to the cheeks by surgical tapes that have orthodontic elastic bands at one end. The elastic on the surgical tape is placed on the retention arm of the moulding plate and the tape is secured to the cheeks. The elastics (inner diameter 0.25 inch thick, heavy) should be stretched approximately two times their resting diameter for proper activation force of about 100 grams. Additional tapes may be necessary to secure the horizontal tape to the cheeks. Parents are instructed to keep the plate in the mouth full time and to remove it for daily cleaning.

The patient is seen weekly to adjust the moulding plate to bring the alveolar segments together, by selectively removing the hard acrylic and adding the soft denture base material to moulding plate. No more than 1 mm of modification of the moulding plate should be made at one visit.

The nasal stent component of NAM appliance is added when width of cleft alveolar gap is reduced to about 5 mm. The rationale for delaying the addition of the nasal stent is that as the alveolar gap is reduced, the base of the nose and lip segment alignment is also improved. The stent is made up of 0.36 inch, round stainless steel wire and takes the shape of a 'swan neck'. The stent is attached to labial flange of moulding plate, near the base of the retention arm. It extends forward and then curves backwards (in the form of a swan neck) entering 3–4 mm past the nostril aperture. It is shaped into a bilobed form resembling a kidney. The upper lobe enters the nose and gently lifts forward the dome until a moderate amount of tissue blanching is evident. The lower lobe of the stent lifts the nostril apex and defines the top of the columella. After adding the nasal stents, the non-surgical lengthening of the columella is done. A horizontal band of the denture material is added to join the left and right lower lobes of the nasal stent, spanning the base of the columella which sits at the nasolabial junction and defines this angle as the nasal tip continues to be lifted and projected forward. A tape is adhered to prolabium underneath the horizontal lip tape which stretches downward to engage the retention arm with elastics. This vertical pull provides a counter stretch to the upward force applied to the nasal tip by nasal stent. Taping downwards on the prolabium helps to lengthen the columella and vertically lengthens the often small prolabium. The horizontal lip tape is added after the prolabium tape is in place.

Surgical lip closure: It is done at around 10 to 12 weeks of age. At that time, the lip tissues have gained sufficient strength to maintain the suturing and are not friable. Lip surgery helps to create the continuity of lip; helps in feeding and suckling; and prevents pre-maxillary displacement. Before lip surgery, **Millard's "Rule of 10"** is followed, which has following criteria. The infant should be at least 10 weeks age; 10 lbs. weight; 10,000 WBC; and 10 gm% Hb.

Palate closure: The timing of palate closure is controversial. It can be done early at 18–24 months or as late as 9–12 years. Its objectives are to join the cleft palatal edges to achieve continuity; thereby preventing nasal regurgitation and to help in vacuum achievement during eating and speech; and to lengthen the soft palate, and help in speech development.

Early repair: If it is done at 18–24 months, it helps in development of normal speech. But it generally leads to maxillary underdevelopment and constriction. It is because the post surgical scar tissue created in mid-palatal region has elastic fibers, which does not let the transverse growth of maxilla express fully.

Late repair: Research has shown that palatal closure done at later age, i.e. at 9–12 years age has following advantages. The vomero-premaxillary suture is a significant growth site and affects maxillary growth. There is almost normal growth of maxilla if cleft is left unrepaired. It also reduces surgical morbidity and infections. During this time, the speech can be improved by placing obturators and speech therapy. Adult patients with unoperated clefts had normal growth of the middle third of the face (almost same as of non-cleft children).

Latest suggestion:

- Closure of soft palate first at the age of 12 months and wait for later hard palate closure. It helps in development of Speech.
- No growth retardation with early soft palate closure.
- Closure of hard palate: done at the age of 5–6 years or even later

Facial growth in un-operated child as compared to operated child: Growth of maxilla and mandible is near normal in unoperated child as compared to the operated child. So minimal surgical intervention should be done during major growth periods of the face of the child

Orthodontic Treatment

Orthodontic intervention starts at 7–8 years of age depending on the requirements. After initial treatment, there is a break until the patients are 12–14 years of age, with all permanent teeth erupted, when final orthodontic treatment is performed.

Aims of Orthodontic Treatment

Orthodontic treatment is done to achieve optimum alignment of teeth esp incisors to facilitate in lip and palate surgery. Expansion of constricted arch leads to exact expression of the cleft defect which helps to plan the alveolar bone graft and palatal surgery. It harmonizes the relationship of the dental arches, to create functional occlusion, and to prepare for alveolar bone graft. Orthodontic treatment is a prolonged procedure in CLP patients than the routine patients.

Special precautions should be taken during orthodontic treatment:

- Avoid overzealous tooth movement into the cleft sites
- Use lighter forces.
- Do not procline the upper anteriors into the tight scarred upper lip.
- Use permanent retention for expansion, rotations, etc

Phases in Management

Orthodontic treatment can be divided in following phases of dentition.

A. In deciduous dentition: During primary dentition, no major treatment is indicated except crossbite treatment; grinding of premature contacts, and extraction of unfavorable supernumerary teeth. Oral hygiene and dental caries treatment are done. Objectives of treatment during deciduous dentition are:

- Child conditioning for future treatment
- Equilibration of deciduous canines or other teeth to prevent mandibular shifts
- Speech therapy
- 3–6 monthly review
- Motivation of family
- Monitoring of caries status and oral hygiene
- Diet counseling

B. Mixed dentition phase: It is a very important phase regarding orthodontic treatment. The upper incisors are generally crowded, rotated, and deviated. The upper arch is narrow. There is maxillary retrusion due to restricted growth. The orthodontics procedures involved are:

a. **Growth modulation** and protraction of maxilla by reverse face mask. It helps to correct anterior cross bite, and helps in achieving proper skeletal relation of the jaw bases. This phase helps to prepare patient for bone grafting in the cleft area. The expansion helps to align the lateral segments and widens the cleft area. Thus it helps to reveal the exact size and nature of the defect. This is helpful for proper bone grafting.
b. **Expansion of upper arch** by quad helix, NPE, RME, etc. Expand collapsed segment to improve surgical access to the graft site.
c. Alignment of teeth, e.g. by using 2 × 4 appliance.
d. Correction of rotations, anterior and posterior cross bites, etc
e. Space management for proper dental eruption esp in lateral incisor-canine region.

Alignment of Incisor Teeth

Upper incisors are usually rotated and are in cross bite. They do not allow proper surgical closure of lip defect; may poke in the surgical site and open the wound. They are corrected by using partial fixed orthodontic appliance. It helps in proper lip surgery/scar revisions, etc. Early treatment of incisors helps to improve esthetics; improve oral hygiene; to allow secondary lip surgery; prior to lip repair in neglected cases. It can be done by using a 0 × 2 anterior sectional twin bracket appliance (0 × 2 **ASTBA**) as suggested by Utreja et al. It works on the principles of reciprocal anchorage. The 2 twin brackets are used only on 2 centrals incisors and a sectional wire is ligated (Fig. 00). A 2 × 4 appliance can also be used for alignment of upper 4 incisors.

Correction of Lateral/Transverse Dimension

There is narrowing of maxillary arch, due to medial deflection of the arch segment on cleft side, it needs correction prior to palatal surgery and bone grafting. It is best done by using a fixed expansion appliance, which are more efficient than removable appliances and patient cooperation is not required, e.g. by using Hyrax, NiTi palatal expander, Quad helix, etc. rapid maxillary expansion (RME) is done to achieve rapid skeletal changes. It opens up the cleft site and reveals the proper dimensions of the defect for a better alveolar bone grafting. Treatment of collapsed maxillary arch is required for the

- Prevention of lateral shifts of mandible
- Promotion of favorable inter-arch development
- Preparation for bone grafting and stabilisation
- To provide space for tongue
- It has a potential of stimulating immature bone which may enhance graft survival.

Maxillary protraction: It is indicated for the treatment of maxillary deficiency/retrusion; anterior crossbite; and to align maxilla in proper relation to mandible, so that future growth of maxilla may occur unrestricted by mandible. if the maxillary growth is not enhanced, then it may get locked by the mandible which is growing normally. Locking then leads to further restriction of sagittal and transverse growth of maxilla. Its favorable age is generally at around 8 years, when more skeletal changes can be achieved. In higher age groups, there are more dentoalveolar changes. It is done by using reverse face mask therapy. A session of RME before/alongwith face mask is favorable, as it activates the circum-maxillary sutures.

Face mask therapy for growth modulation of maxilla: It helps to treat the mild to moderate maxillary deficiency in the cleft patients. Orthopedic force of 350–500 gm per side over 10–12 hours/day for an average of 12–15 months is used. A disadvantage of this appliance is that patient cooperation is required. Also, the treatment is started at an early age, which may lead to patient burn-out. Different methods have been tried for this phase eliminating the factor of need of patient cooperation, e.g. implant-supported maxillary protraction; distraction osteogenesis; class III myofunctional appliances, etc.

Studies have shown that the stability of results by face mask is questionable because of two reasons. There is a counter-pressure of a tight lip due to postsurgical scarring on the maxilla which inhibits its growth; and there is scarring in pterygomaxillary region after extensive tissue mobilization for palatal closure, which also restricts and causes the relapse of the results.

Alveolar Bone Grafting

Autogenous cancellous bone graft is placed in the cleft defects which are obtained from iliac crest, tibia or febula, or rib. Its role is:

- To close the defect and to provide a medium for the tooth eruption especially maxillary canine. It is done at the time when the crown of canine is still covered with a thin shell of bone (9–11 years).
- To stabilize premaxilla in BCLP cases.
- To close oroantral fistulae and anterior clefts.
- To ensure better PD support for teeth.
- To aid in better speech.
- To build up piriform rim, support alar base to provide lip support

Alveolar bone grafting divided in two types:

a. **Primary alveolar bone grafting:** It is done at the time of lip closure at around 10–12 weeks. But it causes hinderance in maxillary growth.
b. **Secondary alveolar bone grafting:** It is done after lip closure at later stage. It helps in eruption of teeth through graft sites as it provides a medium for movement of teeth during eruption. For optimum age of bone grafting, there is primary vs secondary debate. Consensus favors secondary grafting. This is can be dived into three phases, i.e.
   - Early (2–5 years): Performed in primary dentition. Rationale is to allow eruption of the lateral incisor if present. But it can affect growth of midface.
   - Intermediate (6–15 years): Performed in late mixed dentition time to allow the eruption of the permanent canine in the graft. There is minimal interference in growth.
   - Late secondary alveolar bone grafting (adolescence to adulthood): Aids in replacement of missing teeth with implants.

Tissue engineering is one of the latest emerging concept for treating the cleft defect rather than grafts, e.g. BMP; PDGF, etc.

3. Early permanent dentition treatment: After the eruption of canines, and premolars, the comprehensive fixed orthodontic treatment is resumed for final correction of dental relations. Permanent rigid fixed retainer is given for stability of expansion and growth modulation until growth ceases. Prosthesis to replace missing teeth are given, which may be in the form of RPD, FPD or implant-supported teeth depending on the requirement and age of the patient.

Use of riding pontics: These are artificial acrylic tooth having a bracket bonded on the labial surface, and is ligated on the arch wire in the space of missing tooth. They are placed in case of missing tooth during fixed Rx. Riding pontics are like RPD in the wire; have esthetic value, and maintain space. Preferably

Standard or Reversed SWA/ PAE bracket is placed on the tooth. They are ligated when the rectangular arch wire is in place, so that they do not rotate around the wire during use. They have a positive psychosocial effect on the patient; and aid in lip support and speech. They are self-cleansing. However, it is best to close the space due to missing tooth by orthodontic movement to avoid future prosthesis or implant, etc. Orthodontic treatment is usually completed by 14–15 years of age. The results should be retained by rigid fixed retention esp of expansion and anterior correction. Removable prosthesis is given till the age of 18 years, after that permanent bridge, implants, etc. can be given.

Permanent dentition: If a patient has not achieved any treatment since birth and is seen at a late stage, say in permanent dentition, then the clinical feature of this stage are generally severe malocclusion, constricted upper arch; maxillary skeletal retrusion; anterior and posterior cross bite, deep bite due to overeruption of upper incisors, space deficiency, impacted and supernumerary teeth, etc.

Aims of the treatment in the permanent dentition:

- Correcting axial inclination of teeth.
- Improving the dentofacial relationship.
- Balancing the relationship between dental and skeletal components
- Establishing favorable maxillo-mandibular balance and proportion
- Establishing normal incisal and buccal occlusion.
- Establishing harmonious dental arches in both jaws.
- Correcting midlines.
- Avoiding prosthetic replacement of teeth when possible. Spaces are closed with orthodontics, so that future prosthesis and implants, etc. can be avoided.
- Establishing functional occlusion in centric relation.
- Establishing optimal lip contour and contact

Surgical intervention: In severe skeletal discrepancy, orthognathic surgery involving maxilla and/or mandible has to be done. Maxillary length can be increased by distraction osteogenesis. Orthognatic surgery is required in later years or in severe cases of skeletal discrepancy. It is done after the completion of facial growth. Usually maxillary advancement is required to correct maxillomandibular relation. But if mandible has grown more, then mandibular setback may also be required with maxillary advancement. Genioplasty may occasionally be required. Distraction osteogenesis has given good results in terms of stability of the results.

Relapse and retention in CLP: Relapse of expansion and maxillary protraction is very common in cleft cases. It is due to the surgical scars which have elastic fibers and are extremely unyielding. Since some relapse is almost certain, so overcorrection of the malocclusion is done. Long-term rigid fixed retention is essential especially for expansion; maxillary protraction; corrected rotations, etc., e.g. maxillary fixed appliance with soldered rigid lingual retainers for retention of expansion; bonded spiral wire for derotated incisors. Protraction face mask is continued as retainer till facial growth has ceased. In mandibular arch, a routine Hawley retention appliance is used, as there are no major orthodontic changes are required. Follow-up should be advised on a regular basis till at least 21 years of age. The original and post-treatment records should be reviewed at every visit. Strict monitoring of oral hygiene and caries control measures are instituted, with regular follow-up.

Conclusion

CLP patients need a dedicated team of careproviders and interdisciplinary approach is the most suitable for them. They need a long-term management plan, which may need to be modified according to the emerging needs of the patient and emerging new trends of the management.

VIVA VOCE QUESTIONS

1. **What are the various epidemiological features related to cleft of lip and palate in the human beings?**
   - The incidence in India is approx. 1:800 patients.
   - Incidence increases with increased mother's age.
   - Unilateral is more common than the bilateral CLP. (U>B)
   - CL is more common in males; CP in females.
   - CLP more in males than females (M > F)
   - CL is 3 times more on left side than on right. (L>R)
   - Isolated CP is more common in females.

2. **How do you classify the CLP conditions?**
   - Class I = Soft palate with possible notching of hard palate.
   - Class II = Soft and hard palate but no alveolar ridge.
   - Class III = Complete unilateral lip–jaw–palate cleft.
   - Class IV = Complete bilateral lip–jaw–palate cleft.

3. **How does the clefts of lip and /or the palate develop?**
   - CL = MNP–LNP not fused = during 6th wk. i.u.
   - CP = Palatal shelves not fused = during 8th wk. i.u.

4. **Which embryological processes are involved in the formation of palate, upper lip and the maxilla?**

   Palate is formed by palatal shelves which arise from maxillary process; and the frontonasal process (which forms premaxillary part)—(First pharyngeal arch).

   Upper lip and maxilla are formed by fusion of maxillary process with the medial and lateral nasal processes.

5. **What is "Millard's rule of 10" considered during lip repair?**

   It is 10 wks age, 10 lbs wt., 10 gm% Hb, 10,000 WBC count

6. **Why lip repair is essential at an early age?**

   It helps in suckling the milk by making a seal around nipple.

7. **Why palate repair is to be done at the age of 12–24 months?**

   It is the time of start of development of the speaking skill, i.e. child starts learning how to speak at around this age. A broken palate leads to failure in proper articulation of the words and a proper vacuum is not created for escape of air during speech.

8. **What are the disadvantages of an early repair of palate?**

   It leads to constriction of maxilla and improper growth of maxilla due to the scar formed by the surgery of palatal tissues.

9. **What is the recent concept of palatal repair?**

   It is proved that the surgery can be postponed till the completion of maxillary growth and the palatal defect can be filled by some obturator like device for proper sound development and to prevent nasal regurgitation of the food and liquids.

10. **Which is the proper age of primary alveolar grafting and why?**

    The proper age is during the eruption of permanent maxillary canines, i.e. approx. 10–11 yrs. It is because a sound bony medium is required for the eruption of any tooth. The canine erupts at around this age.

11. **Which is most common missing tooth in CLP cases?**

    Mostly the maxillary lateral incisor is missing, because the cleft generally passes in b/w lateral incisor and the canine thereby affecting its tooth bud.

SELF-ASSESSMENT QUESTIONS

1. What is Veau's classification of clefts?
2. What do you mean by Riding Pontics?
3. Why long-term retention is required after expansion in CLP patients?
4. What is the reason behind that all possible efforts should be done to save the incisors in bilateral CLP cases?
5. Which is the appliance fabricated to block the defect of CLP in un-operated cases?
6. Which of the problems develop in untreated CLP cases?
7. What are different speech defects in CLP cases?
8. Why middle ear infections are common in CLP cases?

55

Retention and Relapse

INTRODUCTION

Correction of malocclusion requires movement of teeth within the bone under the influence of forces within biological limits. Teeth thus moved by mechanical appliances have a tendency to return to their former positions. This phenomenon is called **relapse**. Thus, the process used to prevent relapse is called **retention**.

Thus retention can be defined as "holding the teeth in their post treatment esthetic and functional positions". Retention is a passive phase of treatment, after the active treatment phase with the mechanical appliances has been completed. Thus the retention plan is a part of main treatment plan of the patient, and is decided at the time of diagnosis and treatment planning. The duration of the retention phase should be included in the total duration of treatment and explained to the patient/parents at the beginning of treatment and an informed consent should be obtained. Studies have shown that relapse is inevitable, and some degree of relapse always takes place.

Causes of Relapse

Relapse of the treatment result is perplexing to all orthodontists because relapse is inevitable. There are many causes which have been implicated leading to relapse as mentioned below.

1. Persistence of etiological factor of the malocclusion. If the underlying etiology is not removed, the relapse generally occurs.
2. Stretching/compression/activation of the soft tissues around the neck of tooth. The transseptal fibers take maximum time to reorient and are the main cause of relapse especially after rotational correction, diastema closure, extraction space closure, etc. (Fig. 55.1).
3. The perioral soft tissues take longer to adapt to new position of teeth than the bone. Activation of circumoral and buccinator tissues during expansion to correct narrow jaws leas to rapid relapse if not retainer properly.
4. Differential jaw growth in growing individuals also leads to relapse, e.g. in class III skeletal pattern due to mandibular overgrowth; class II skeletal

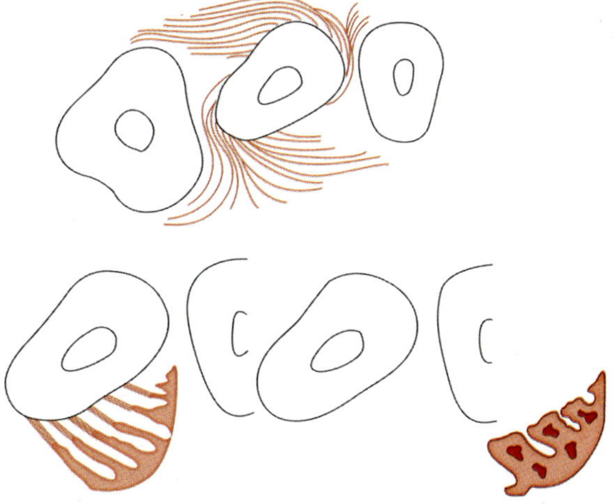

Fig. 55.1: Attachment of transseptal fibers on a rotated tooth, which get activated/stretched when rotation correction is done and leads to relapse unless properly retained *(Adapted from Graber and Vanarsdall for academic purpose)*.

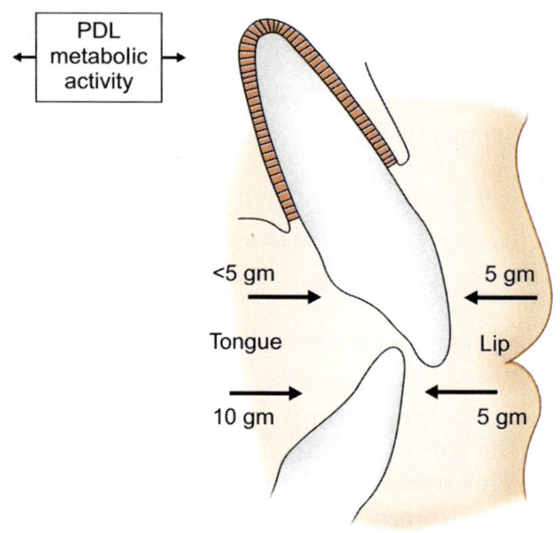

Fig. 55.2: Balance of forces to keep the dental arch in an equilibrium position *(Redrawn from Proffit for academic purpose).*

pattern due to maxillary overgrowth, etc.
5. Lack of normal cuspal interdigitation
6. Incorrect arch size and harmony
7. Incorrect axial inclinations
8. Improper contacts
9. Tooth size disharmony.

Definition: Moyers defined retention as "the holding the teeth after orthodontic treatment in the treated position for the period of time necessary for the maintenance of the results."

HISTORY OF RETENTION

Relapse has perplexed the clinicians for many decades, and after so much research, the scientists are still groping to find out the best way to prevent relapse. Relapse can occur due to many factors, and thus the modalities have been devised accordingly. Over the years, different philosophies or schools of thought have emerged, and present-day concepts generally combine many of these theories. Main theories which have been considered are as follows.

The occlusion school of thought: Kingsley stated, "The occlusion of the teeth is the most important factor in determining the stability in a new position." Many writers have considered that proper occlusion and interdigitation is of primary importance in retention.

The apical base school: Lundstrom suggested the apical base as one of the most important factors in the correction of malocclusion and maintenance of a correct occlusion. Any alteration in the original dimension of apical base is bound to relapse. McCauley suggested that intercanine width and intermolar width should be maintained as original.

The mandibular incisor school: According to Tweed, the mandibular incisors must be kept upright and over basal bone for better stability.

The musculature school: Roger proposed the necessity of establishing proper functional muscle balance. Since soft tissues guide the growth and development of facial growth and dental occlusion, any abnormal muscular activity will lead to loss of achieved results.

In view of above information, all these concepts are important during the treatment to achieve the stability of results, i.e. a proper occlusion should be achieved within the equilibrium of normal muscle balance, teeth should be properly related to their respective apical bases, and the relationships of these apical bases should be balanced to one another (Fig. 55.2).

Rationale of retention: According to Proffit, the muscular, gingival, periodontal and alveolar tissues are affected by orthodontic tooth movement and require time for reorganization after removal of active appliances. The thus activated soft tissues apply pressure which leads to a relapse tendency. The teeth come to occupy new position after the treatment which is an unstable position and needs time to achieve equilibrium. Disorganized gingival and PDL fibers lead to an increased susceptibility to tooth movement. Collagenous fibers take 4 to 6 months to reorganize structurally. Supracrestal elastic fibers of gingiva take up to 1 year to adapt to new position of the teeth. Rotational relapse is caused by the activated and stretched elastic gingival fibers. Remodeling of craniofacial skeletal and soft tissue structures continues into the adult life, leading to changes in dental alignment.

Why is retention necessary: Retention is needed because the balance of muscle forces of stomatognathic system has not been achieved. Reorganization of periodontal and gingival tissues is needed for stability. Also the occlusal balance has not been established. Occlusion changes related to growth also lead to relapse.

Twelve keys to stability: Gorman has described following keys for stability.

1. Whenever possible, allow lower incisors to align themselves either through serial extraction or use of lip bumper in early mixed dentition (Figs 55.3a to c)
2. Overcorrect lower rotation as early in treatment as possible
3. Reproximation of incisors early in Rx and again at retention enhances stability
4. Avoid increasing the intercanine width during active treatment.
5. Extract bicuspids where mand arch discrepancy is 4 mm or greater, except where facial esthetics dictates otherwise.
6. Recognize that more a tooth is moved, more likely it is to relapse, overcorrect accordingly
7. Upright lower incisors to atleast 90° whenever the profile permits
8. Create a flat occlusal plane during Rx and overcorrect the overbite.
9. Prescribe supracrestal fibrotomy for severely rotated teeth
10. Retain the lower arch until all growth is complete
11. Place retainers the same day appliance is remove
12. Recognize that compromise often necessary in the interest of facial esthetics and that sometimes lifetime retention is necessary.

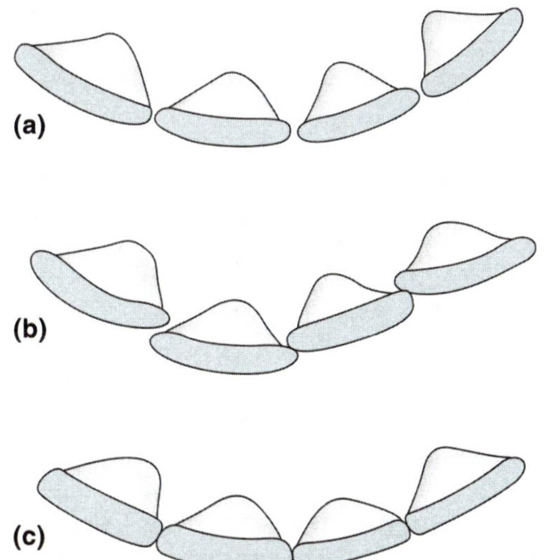

Figs 55.3a to c: Crowns of lower incisors in a well-aligned position. Figure (c) shows that wider incisors need to be slenderized for better and stable alignment *(Redrawn from Proffit for academic purpose).*

Basic Theorems

Riedel described 9 theorems in 1960 regarding the concept of relapse and retention. The 10th theorem has been added to it later on.

Theorem 1: Teeth that have been moved tend to return to their former positions. Experts do not agree on the reason for this tendency; they have suggested certain factors like musculature, apical base, trans-septal fibers, and bone morphology. Teeth should be held in their corrected positions for some time after treatment to prevent this tendency.

Theorem 2: Elimination of the factor/s causing malocclusion will prevent recurrence. Caused for certain conditions can be find out, while for others it may be obscure, so little can be done about their elimination. It is important that the causative factors for a given malocclusion be prevented from recurring, e.g. habits like tongue thrusting, thumb sucking, etc. Open bite may be secondary to mouth breathing resulting from nasopharynx obstruction due to anatomic blockage, allergic disease, or adenoid hyperplasia.

Theorem 3: Overcorrection should be done as a leeway factor to allow some amount of relapse so that the teeth settle down in normal positions, e.g. class II malocclusions overcorrected into an edge-to-edge incisor relationship, overcorrection of deep overbite and rotation correction, etc.

Theorem 4: Proper occlusion is a potent factor in holding teeth in their corrected positions. The occlusion usually referred to is the intercuspal position. Correct intercuspation is an essential factor in occlusal stabilization.

Theorem 5: Bone and adjacent tissues must be given time to reorganize around the newly positioned teeth. This is the rationale for use of retainers after active tooth movement. Histological evidences show that bone and tissues around the moved teeth get and considerable time is needed for complete reorganization to occur.

Theorem 6: Lower incisors are placed upright over basal bone to remain in good alignment. Proper angulation and placement of mandibular incisor should be attained. Stable results are obtained when the mandibular incisors are either upright or slightly retroclined over the basal bone.

Theorem 7: Corrections carried out during periods of growth are less likely to relapse. When treatment needs a control or redirection of growth (e.g. headgear or functional appliance therapy), treatment must be instituted during periods of active growth, which lead to long-term stability.

Theorem 8: The further teeth have been moved, the less likelihood of relapse. It is desirable to move teeth further during orthodontic treatment.

Theorem 9: Arch form, particularly the mandibular arch, cannot be permanently altered by appliance therapy. So the original arch form should be maintained during orthodontic treatment. Strang in 1946 described that the mandibular intercanine width is an accurate index to the muscular balance inherent to the individual and dictates the limits of the denture expansion in this area of treatment.

Theorem 10: Many treated malocclusions require permanent retaining devices. The type of retentive measures and the duration of their use allegedly are determined by many factors, e.g. the occlusion; age of the patient; cause of a particular malocclusion; health of tissues involved; size of the arches or arch harmony, muscular pressure, etc.

Summary of the concepts: Different authors have worked for retention and have suggested important principles like the following:

- Overcorrection of all malpositions should be attempted. Rotation should be corrected by overrotation in the opposite direction.
- Retention should depend on modification of structure and function of tissues.
- Intercanine and intermolar widths should be maintained as in the original malocclusion.
- Mandibular incisors should be maintained upright over basal bone.
- Slight movement is more difficult to retain than extensive movement.
- Attempt functional treatment (i.e., to achieve muscle balance).
- Functional adaptation of occlusion occurs with growth.
- Discrepancies in tooth sizes may cause problems in retention.
- Early treatment is more desirable than treatment at a later age.
- Use mild forces.

Raleigh Williams rules: Raleigh Williams proposed six keys of retention to achieve stable results in mandibular teeth (Figs 55.4 and 55.5).

1. Incisal edge of lower incisor should be placed on A-Pog line or 1 mm in front of it.
2. The lower incisor apices should be spread distally to the crowns. The apices of lateral incisors should be spread more than those of the central incisors.
3. All four lower incisor apices must be in the same labiolingual plane.

4. The apex of lower canine should be positioned distal to the crown.
5. The lower canine root apex must be positioned slightly buccal to the crown apex.
6. The lower incisors should be slenderized as needed after treatment.

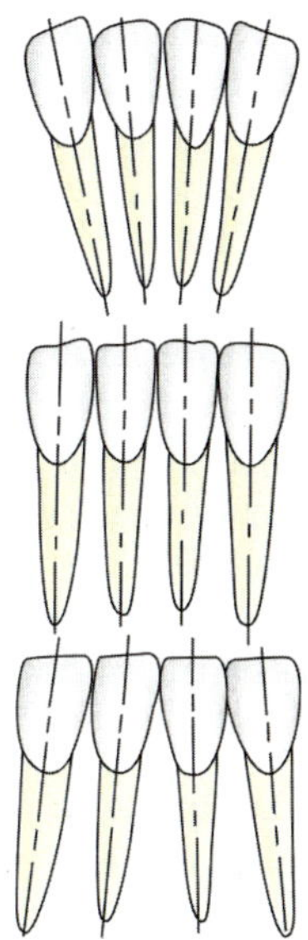

Fig. 55.4: Root position of lower incisors for stability according to **Raleigh Williams rules.**

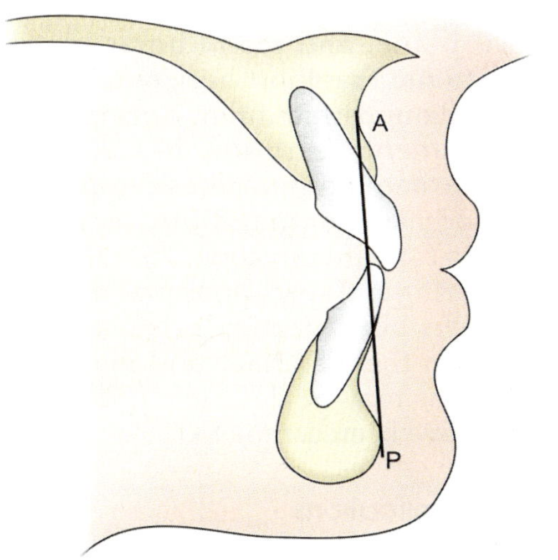

Fig. 55.5: Position of incisal edges of lower incisors should be 0–1 mm from A-Pog line according to **Raleigh Williams rules.**

Relationship of Third Molars

There are different arguments regarding the role of third molars in relapse after orthodontic treatment. Some authors have implicated third molars for pre- and post-treatment changes in mandibular teeth; while according to others, the third molars play very little role in long-term mandibular arch changes. The recommendation for mandibular third molar removal with the objective of alleviating or preventing mandibular incisor irregularity may not be justified. The long-term changes in the mandibular anterior alignment have been found to occur mainly due to postpubertal growth changes in mandible especially when it moves U and F with ensuing growth, leading to development of mandibular anterior crowding. It is called as **late mandibular growth**.

Growth Factors

Advantage of active growth is taken during the correction of many types of orthodontic problems, but it may also lead to relapse in treated orthodontic patients, e.g. during class II treatment with headgear, the normal downward and forward growth of maxillary alveolar process can be controlled, and it is possible that the growth of the maxilla itself may be retarded or redirected. The normal forward movement of maxillary molars gets restrained while the mandible continues in its course of growth, and a normal tooth relationship can be obtained. But, it generally happens by the distal tipping of maxillary buccal segments, which tend to upright themselves again, with the crowns moving in a mesial direction. If sufficient mandibular forward growth occurs, the occlusion may remain satisfactory, but if not then the relapse of class II relation occurs. Similarly, the forward translation of mandibular teeth on its base after the use of class II elastics or functional appliances is undesirable, because during relapse, the mandibular posterior teeth do not migrate distally, while the anterior teeth, during their attempt to upright to their former positions, break the contacts and become crowded.

Gender Differences

As we have studied during growth and development, there exist significant gender differences. Thus gender of the patient is an important consideration during treatment and retention planning. It has been found that the female skeletal and dental pattern gets matured earlier than boys, i.e. by 13 years; while in boys, it occurs after 15 years on the average. Treatment of skeletal class II malocclusion, particularly in girls, should be started earlier than boys, before the maturation of skeletal pattern.

Further implications of growth: Growth of the craniofacial complex is a complex phenomenon, and it keeps on occurring till late adult age, albeit at a very slow and imperceptible rate. During initial years, the rate of growth is more and it can be used to the advantages of the patients during orthodontic/orthopaedic/functional treatment. After treatment also, the growth plays a perplexing role for the orthodontist. It continues till late pubertal age and may cause the post-Rx relapse of certain conditions if not retained properly.

Maturation changes generally occur, esp in boys, in apical bases and alveolar processes. Facial structures literally emerge out from beneath the cranium in late adolescence (cephalocaudal gradient of growth), which helps to bring mandible forwards thus reducing the angle of convexity, and reducing angle ANB.

The amount and direction of mandibular growth is of great importance in correction and retention of corrected malocclusions. The mandible keeps on growing till approx 18 years of age, so a patient treated with chin cup to control excessive forward growth of mandible should be retained with night time use of chin cup till 18 years of age. If the skeletal class III due to mandibular prognathism is severe and needs mandibular orthognathic surgery, the surgery should be performed only after the growth has ceased. If the surgery is done before the cessation of active growth, then the continued growth may lead to recurrence of the skeletal class III condition again, because the pattern of growth remains unchanged.

Similarly, in case of maxillary prognathism treated with HPHG, the night time wear of HPHG is maintained till the maxillary growth is complete, i.e. till around 16 years of age.

Functional appliances can be used to play an important role during the retention period to assist in maintaining correction of skeletal components. These can be worn during sleep to prevent changes in maxillomandibular position that may take place through continued unharmonious growth.

The treated overbite in horizontal growth cases has a tendency to relapse due to continued U and F mandibular growth. To prevent it, the anterior bite plane is incorporated in the upper Hawley's retainer to create a minimal gap in interocclusal area, where the teeth continue to erupt in consonance to the ramal vertical growth.

Late mandibular growth: Mandible keeps on growing in U and F direction in late pubertal age. It leads to thrusting of mandible against the maxilla, which may lead to restriction of mandibular denture. It causes the force to be transferred to the lower incisors and thus resulting in their lingual uprighting and crowidng. It also leads to flattening of occlusal plane, and mandibular plane in relation to the Frankfort horizontal. Also, it has been demonstrated that during growth the permanent dentition has a natural tendency to become more recessive in relation to the body of the mandible, as it keeps growing in forward direction. The other effect may be flaring and space appearance in upper incisors. In boys particularly, continued retention in the maxillary and mandibular incisor areas may be desirable until growth changes have been completed.

Clinical Applications

Planning of retention: Generally, a full-time retainer is used for first 6 months. It is continued on a part-time basis for at least 12 months, to allow time for remodeling of gingival tissues. If significant growth remains, continued part-time until completion of growth.

Factors important in the planning of retention:

1. Original malocclusion and patient's growth pattern.
2. The type of treatment performed.
3. Type of retainer.
4. Duration of retention.

Duration of retention: As yet, there is no consensus how long the retention period should be. Clinicians generally advise the retainers according to their experience. Since removable retainers have the problem of patients' cooperation to be successful, the fixed retainers are generally preferred. Since the main function of retainers is to give time for the reorganisation of the tissues, many clinicians, after achieving the finishing stage of treatment, keep the fixed appliances in passive state for few more months. It gives the time for tissues organization, and thus period of retention is reduced, and the factor of patients cooperation is also minimised. The literature has shown that the some amount (upto 30%) of relapse is inevitable and is bound to occur. Theoretically and by experience, the duration of retention has been divided into following categories, depending on the malocclusion:

- No retention
- Limited or short term retention: for 3–6 months
- Medium term: 1–5 years
- Prolonged or permanent retention: in CLP cases, where prosthesis can be used as retainer.

1. No Retention

Minimal or no retention is needed in certain cases which are generally self-retentive post-treatment, e.g.

a. **Corrected crossbites**:

1. Anterior crossbite: This does not need retention when adequate overbite has been established.
2. Posterior crossbite: It is treated generally by expansion of arch, which leads to buccal flaring of crowns of posterior teeth. With proper torquing, the axial inclination of posterior teeth is normalised, and proper interdigitation of upper/lower teeth is achieved, which leads to stability. Also during treatment of posterior crossbites, the overcorrection should be done so that the teeth settle down in a stable normal relation during retention phase.

b. **Dentitions that have been treated by serial extraction:** Serial extraction is generally done in extreme crowding developing during mixed dentition period. An advantage of natural eruption potential of teeth and their physiological migration is taken, e.g.

1. **High canine/labially blocked out canine cases:** Such cases need extraction of first premolar/s to align them in the arches. After first premolar extraction, either the canines erupt themselves or they can be aligned with the help of fixed appliances. This condition does not relapse as canines will not be moving back apically.
2. **Cases needing extraction of one or more teeth,** e.g. subdivision types of malocclusion, or when the posterior teeth are in class II relationship and the anterior teeth are normal. Such cases need minimal retraction movements of anterior teeth even after extraction of first premolars. Most of the extraction space is used by mesialisation of posterior teeth to achieve proper interdigitation. This has minimal relapse tendency.

c. Conditions where the teeth have been separated to allow for **eruption of blocked out teeth** due to lack of some space, e.g. partially impacted mandibular second premolars and maxillary canines, which after coming in the dental arch become self retentive.

2. Moderate Retention

a. **Class I non-extraction cases**, having protrusion and spacing in anterior teeth. They are treated by space closure and retraction. Retention is needed to achieve the equilibrium in lip and tongue function.

b. **Class I or class II extraction cases** need retention to prevent relapse of overjet, and to prevent opening of the extraction spaces. Time is also needed to achieve balance of lip and tongue function. It is generally desirable to use a maxillary Hawley type of retainer until normal functional adaptation has occurred.

The time of retention appliance usage can be reduced as **the patient** adapts to new tooth positions, proceeding from full-time wearing of appliances to night time wear only, once or twice a week, and finally discontinuing all retention as tooth positions remain stable. Corrections of adult dentitions require longer retentive procedures. Time of retention depends directly on the patient's compliance and tissue reaction during retention. Lip exercises and tongue-training may be advantageous in these cases. Corrected deep overbites in either class I or class II malocclusions usually require retention in a vertical plane, as discussed below.

1. If **anterior teeth were intruded** to achieve overbite correction, an **anterior bite plate** is included on a maxillary retainer which should be worn continuously for at least few months, or during the active mandibular growth (it is called **dynamic retention** as described by Nanda). In deep overbite cases, overcorrection should be done so that during relapse, the overbite gets settled down at normal depth of 2–3 mm. It is essentially necessary in horizontal growth cases, where the mandible rotated U and F due to vertical ramal growth. It tends to push mandible inside the maxilla tending to increase the bite depth. In turn, it also creates a gap in molar region. So if an anterior bite plate is maintained, then the ABP will not let the mandible to go in maxilla while the interocclusal gap thus created will be covered by extrusion of buccal teeth, thus maintaining the corrected bite.
2. If overbite correction was achieved **by posterior extrusion**, leading to D and B mandibular rotation, and thus an increased anterior facial height, the vertical dimensions should be maintained until growth (i.e. mandibular ramal height) can catch up.

c. **Early correction of rotated teeth** to their normal positions especially before root completion. Stability of the correction of rotations can also be augmented by severing of trans-septal fibers (CSF).

d. Cases of **ectopic eruption of teeth** or supernumerary teeth require varying retention times, usually prolonged, and occasionally a fixed or permanent retentive device is needed. Supernumerary teeth are frequently found in maxillary anterior area, blocking the eruption of incisors. Upon their removal, the maxillary incisors often erupt slowly and incompletely, which are brought to a normal level through orthodontic therapy. In such cases, it is desirable to leave the appliance in a passive state for several months before giving retention because these teeth have a tendency to re-intrude when released due ot activated apical group of PDL fibers.

e. **Excessive spacing between maxillary incisors** (e.g. by habits, large tongue size, frenum, etc.) requires prolonged retention after space closure.

f. The corrected class II division 2 malocclusion requires extended retention to allow adaptation of surrounding musculature. These cases are generally treated on non- extraction basis, and may need an increase in mandibular intercanine width to relieve the crowding. It is maintained with prolonged retention.

3. Permanent or Semipermanent Retention

a. Cases in which expansion has been done, esp in mandibular arch, require either permanent or semipermanent retention.

b. Cases of considerable or generalized spacing require permanent retention after space closure, e.g. spacing due to larger tongue size; due to larger basal bone; etc.

c. Severe rotation (particularly in adults) or severe labiolingual malposition require permanent retention. At least 232 days are needed to retaine corrected rotation, and still there are chances of relapse. Circumferential fibrotomy, CSF is also recommended to augment the retention.
d. Maxillary midline diastema in otherwise normal occlusion, due to larger maxillary frenum, supernumerary tooth, tongue/lip sucking habit, e.c, requires permanent retention, particularly in adult dentitions.
e. Cleft lip/palate cases needing expansion, rotation correction, alignment, etc
f. Skeletal class III cases due to mandibular prognathism or maxillary retrognathism treated by denotfacial orhtodpedic appliances like chin cup. Kloehn headgear, etc. should be retained till active growth has ceased, i.e. 18 years of age.
g. Cases treated with myofunctional appliances also need prolonged retention esp in adult cases; and actively growing cases.

RETENTION APPLIANCES

Many types of appliances have been used for retention as described in literature, many of which have become obsolete after the new comfortable appliances have been designed by clinicians. They are passive in nature, do not apply any force on the teeth, and their main motive is to keep the teeth in new position and provide time for tissue reorganization. They can be classified as:

1. Removable
2. Fixed
3. Active retainers.

Removable Retainers

These include Hawley retainers, wrap around retainers and modifications. They can be modified for active tooth movement by activating the labial bow or by incorporating springs, hooks, cribs, etc. They are routinely worn full time for three to six months, part time for one year to 18 months, followed by continued wear twice a week. Disadvantages of these retainers include speech difficulties in the initial period of wear, poor esthetics and a marked dependence on the patient for continued compliance. These appliances can be removed and replaced by the patient, thus patient cooperation is necessary. **Hawley retainer** is one of the most frequently used appliances, and can be used in both the arches (Fig. 55.6). It is made of acrylic, contacting the lingual surfaces of teeth and the mucosa. The acrylic should be passively and completely in touch with the lingual surfaces of teeth to avoid any undesired movement of teeth. A labial bow of round, hard, stainless steel 0.8 to 1.2 mm wire is made to contact the labial surfaces of teeth. It can be made in the regions of 2–2, 3–3, 4–4, 5–5, 6–6, 7–7, depending on the requirement. Labial bow and retention clasps should not pass through extraction sites because it may lead to reopening of spaces.

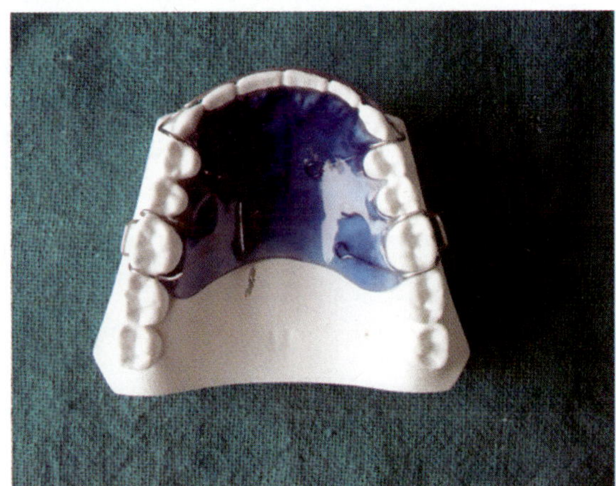

Fig. 55.6: An ideal Hawley's retainer.

Modifications of Hawley Retainer

A number of modifications have been designed by clinicians.

1. **Circumferential labial bow:** It is used so as not to pass through the occlusal embrasures to eliminate occlusal interference.

The labial bow is made to pass distal to last erupted molars. It can be activated for closure of minor spaces developing in anterior or extraction areas. Some hook type keeper wires can be wound around the main labial bow between lateral incisors and canines to enhance the stability of the labial wire. Acrylic should be extended distally to retain second molar position. Pontics can be included in the retainers to enhance esthetics and retain the edentulous area till permanent prosthesis can be placed.

2. **Beggs' appliance:** A labial bow is formed from 6–6, thus not passing through the extraction spaces.
3. **Hawley's appliances with cribs:** The cribs can be used in the appliance to prevent tongue thrusting, thumb sucking habits, and in cases of treated anterior open bite (Fig. 55.7).
4. **Removable wraparound retainers:** They are made of acrylic on both the labial and lingual surfaces of the teeth, with the wires like labial bow, retentive clasps, etc. They can be made from 3 to 3 or 6 to 6. They help to firmly hold each tooth into position. Another modification of **wraparound cantilever retainer** was suggested by Tremont 2003. It has a cantilever arm in the middle of first bicuspid soldered to labial bow. Bow adjusted by giving a slight bend in the cantilever arm.

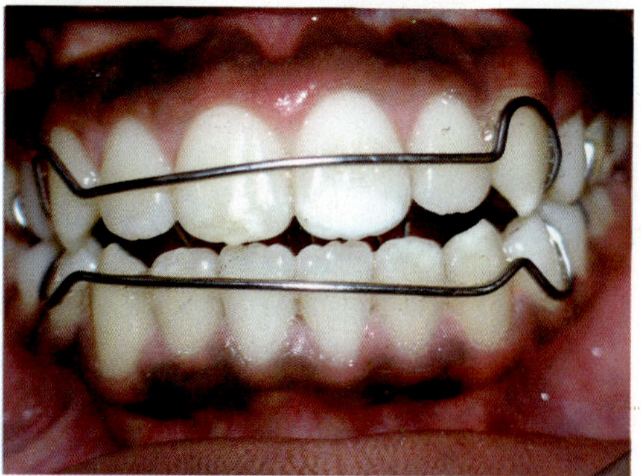

Fig. 55.7: Upper and lower Hawley's retainers. Note the cribs on upper appliance as this case was having anterior open bite.

Other Removable Retainers

Mandibular spring retainer can be used to include only the six anterior teeth. It helps to eliminate the difficulty of seating the appliance over buccal segment undercuts. Spring retainers combine the principles of Hawley-type retainers with those of the tooth positioners. A working model is required on which the teeth are sectioned and repositioned with wax in aligned positions. It is a sectional appliance using 0.028" (0.7 mm) stainless steel wire contoured to labial and lingual surfaces of the teeth, incorporating vertical loops, and passing distal to the canines. Acrylic is added on lingual and labial sides on the wire following the occlusal and gingival contours of the teeth. When inserted, the retainer springs to engage the malpositioned teeth and move these teeth into the alignment established on the working model. Due to the potential for dislodging, swallowing or aspirating the appliance, the design has been modified to include acrylic flanges extending lingually to the first molar and incorporates an occlusal rest. Spring aligners may also be used with interproximal reduction to correct lower mandibular crowding.

All wire retainer: The retainer is made of the hard sturdy wires and having no acrylic. Different components, e.g. C-clasps, Adams clasp, labial bows, etc. are soldered to each other. These retainers are very comfortable to patients; and easy to clean.

Removable vacuum formed retainers (Figs 55.8 to 55.17): Vacuum formed retainers (VFRs) are relatively inexpensive and can be quickly fabricated on the same day of appliance removal. They can be modified to produce minor tooth movements if required. For that purpose, the modification is done on the working model by creating pits/mounds of POP to create active/relief areas, and then the appliance is made. Full posterior occlusal coverage (including second molars if present)

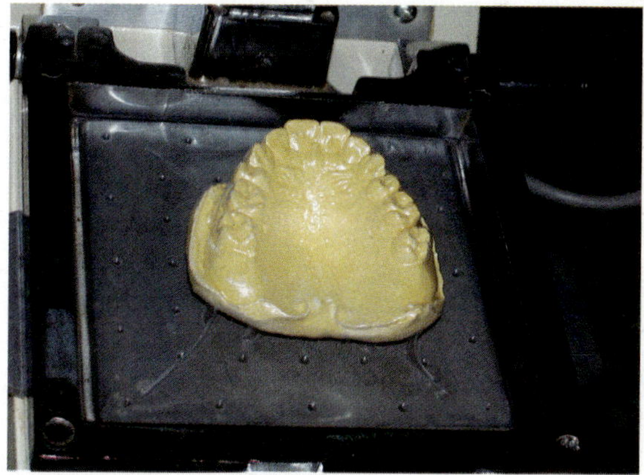

Fig. 55.8: Night guard appliance or vacuum-formed retainer on the maxillary cast.

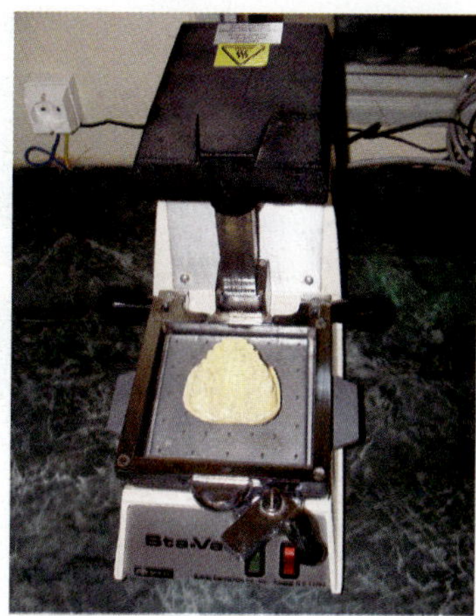

Fig. 55.9: Steps to form vacuum-formed retainer: maxillary cast on the Sta-Vac machine.

is advisable to reduce the risk of overeruption of these teeth during retention.

Invisible retainer by McNamara: It is used as an active retainer when some crowding reappears during post-treatment period. The irregular teeth are cut from the models and are repositioned with the wax. Retainer is made with 1 mm thick sheet of Biocryl in Biostar positive pressure thermal forming machine The distal half of the last molar should be covered to prevent extrusion of these teeth with full-time appliance wear. The facial and lingual surfaces are trimmed to approximate the gingival margins. Invisible retainers need trimming in the area of tissue impingement. If teeth have been reset in the invisible retainer, the patient should be told that the appliance will take a few hours to a few days to seat in place.

Kesling's tooth positioner: It was described by Kesling in 1945. It is made of thermoplastic material. It covers the occlusal surfaces also, occupies the interocclusal space, and covers clinical crowns and a small portion of gingiva. But the patient faces difficulty in speech and risk of TMJ problems.

Positioners: Positioners are elastomeric or rubber removable retainers which are either preformed or custom made. But preformed positioners may not be fitting properly due to variation in tooth size, shape, etc. and thus are not good for long term use. Custom-made

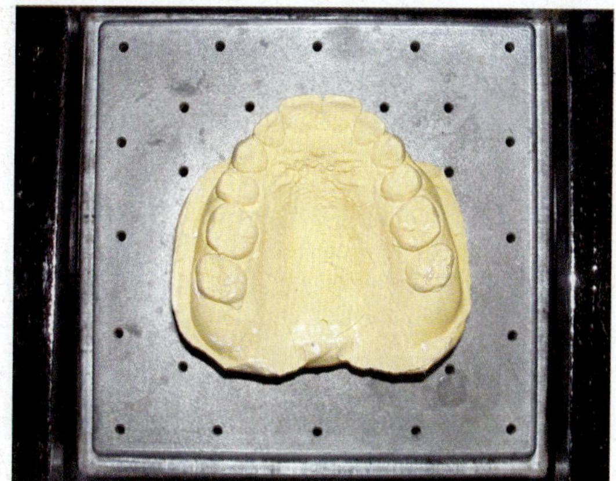

Fig. 55.10: Maxillary cast on the Sta-Vac machine base.

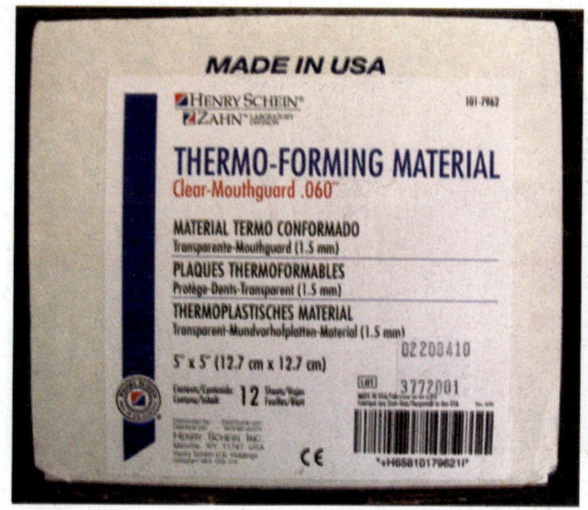

Fig. 55.11: Thermo-forming material used in making a night guard.

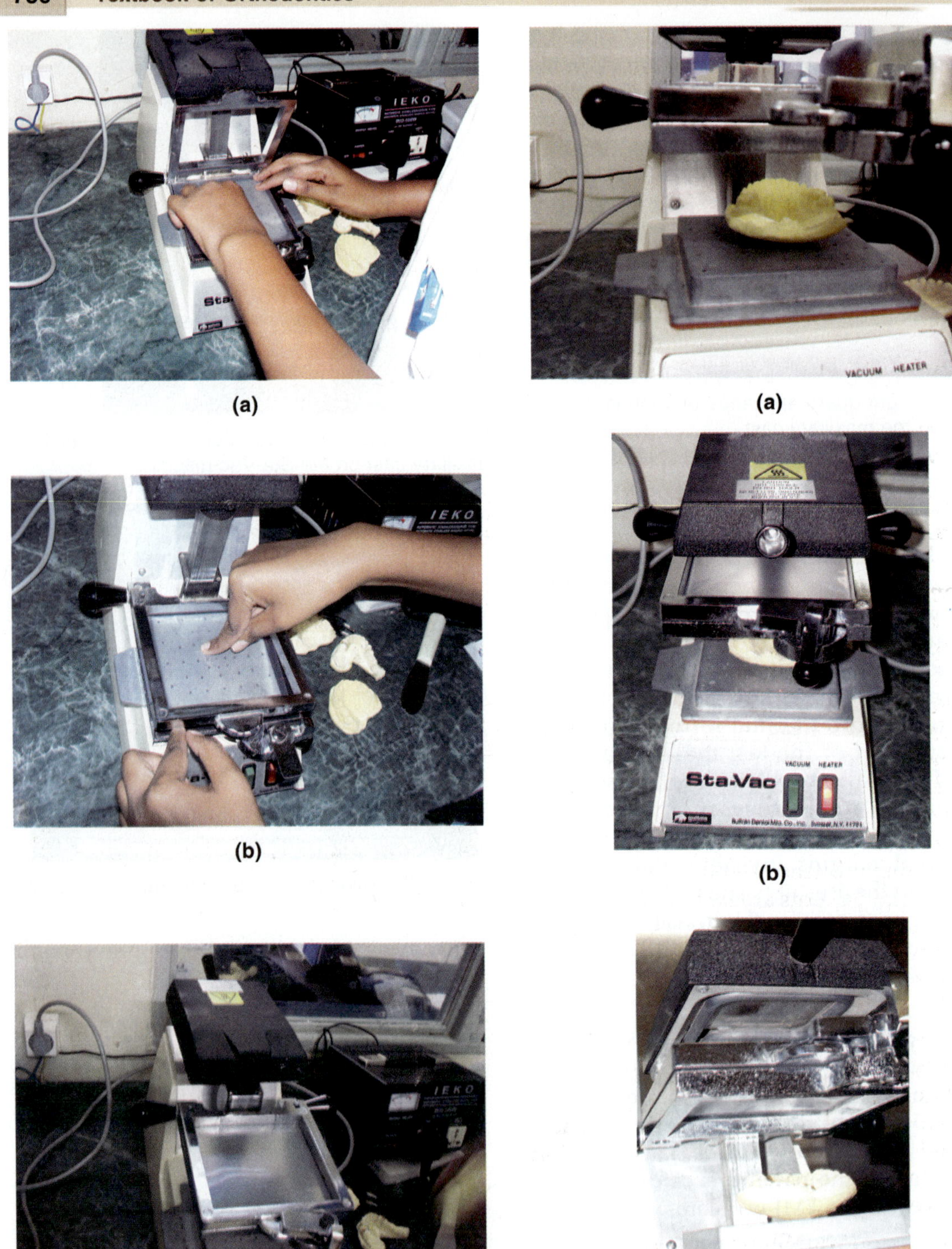

Figs 55.12a to c: Fixing the thermo-forming sheet in the Sta-Vac machine.

Figs 55.13a to c: Sheet holder raised to near the heating element, with maxillary cast in position on the base.

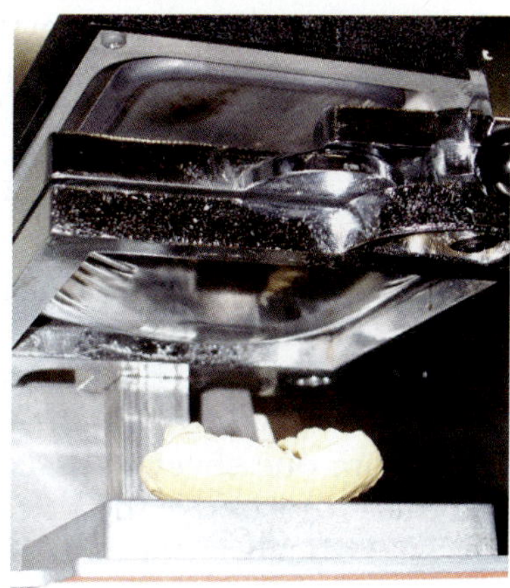

Fig. 55.14: Sheet starts softening under heat and starts moving down towards the cast. When it reaches near the cast, the heating is turned off and the vacuum switch is turned on, which leads to adaptation of sheet on the cast.

positioners are fabricated on the patient's models in the lab. These can also be used for minor corrections in tooth position and occlusal relationship. For such purpose, the teeth are sectioned from the models, realigned and waxed in an ideal configuration. The elastomeric or rubber material is then deposited around the teeth and the coronal portion of the gingiva. Positioners are worn full time for first two days, and for four hours daily plus during sleep after that. For the four hours of wear, patients are advised to repeat a cycle of biting and clenching for 20 seconds followed by a rest of 20 seconds. If this routine is followed, the desired tooth movements should have occurred in the first three weeks and the positioner becomes a passive rather than an active appliance. Disadvantages of this technique include the cost and delay in fabrication of appliance, the inability to hold rotational and overbite corrections, and the general lack of patient cooperation and acceptance.

Essix retainers: Sheridan, et al 1993 described Essix Retainers. They are made of clear, thermoplastic copolyester material, vacuum-formed, are thinner, but stronger, extended **cuspid-to-cuspid**. Advantages include: absolute stability of the anterior teeth; durability and ease of cleaning; low cost and easy fabrication; minimal bulk and thickness (.015"); esthetic.

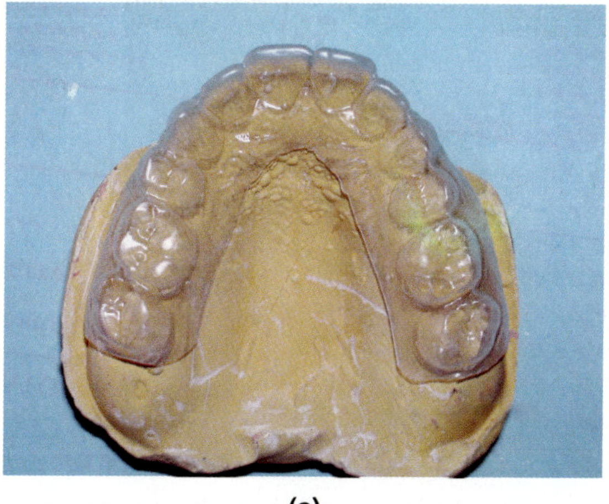

(a)

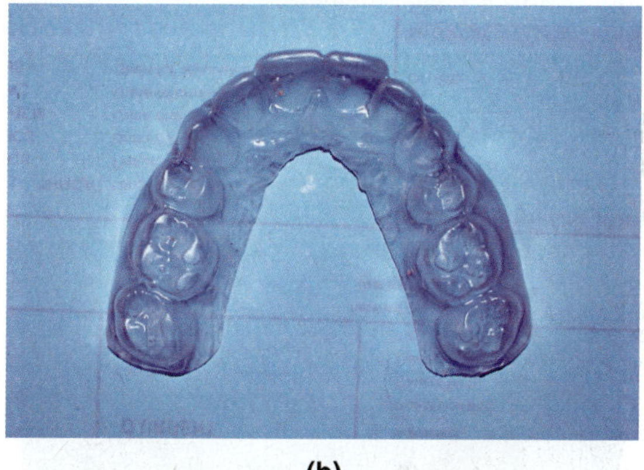

(b)

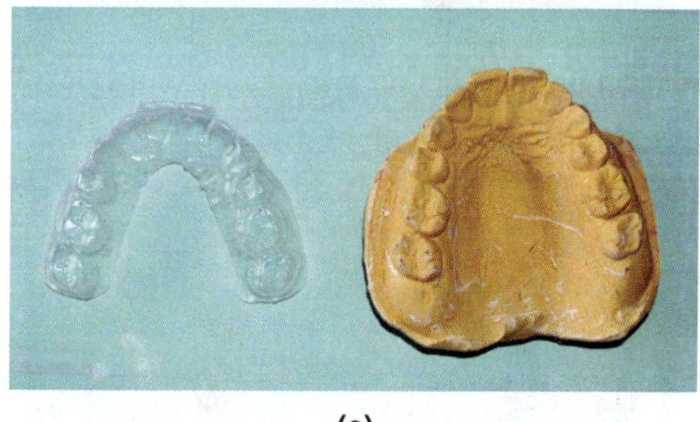

(c)

Figs 55.15a to c: Night guard/vacuum-formed retainer on the cast after cutting and shaping before delivering it to the patient.

Fabrication: Impressions of the arches are taken with alginate or vinyl polysiloxane, and

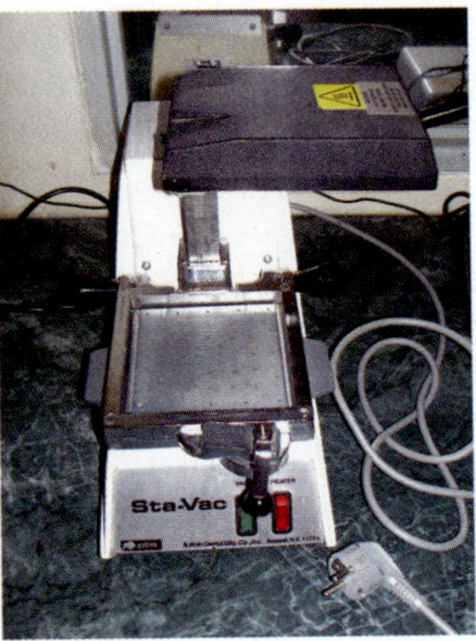

Fig. 55.16: Sta-Vac machine which is used to make night guard or Essix retainers.

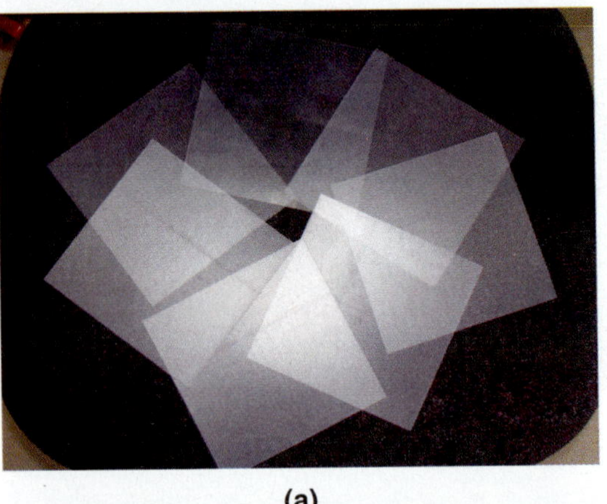

(a)

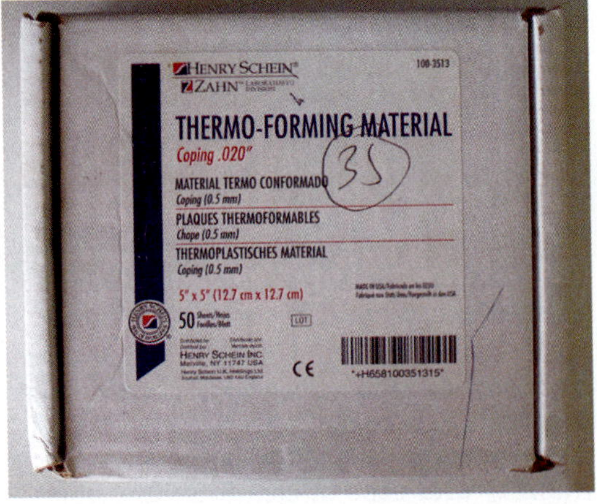

(b)

Figs 55.17a and b: Thermoform sheaths used to make night guard, these are available in different thicknesses.

cast is poured. A pressure-type thermoforming unit such as a Biostar is used for fabrication. Essix 0.75 mm (.030") thermoplastic copolyester sheet is used for fabrication of Essix retainers. **Copolyester**, unlike polycarbonates, does not require heat treatment before thermoforming. It is much stronger, clearer, and resistant to abrasion than acrylic sheet, and thus produces thinner yet sturdier appliances. Two or three retainers can be made from one sheet of Essix plastic. During the thermoforming, the thickness of the plastic is reduced from .030" to .015". Labial/lingual flanges of the retainer are extended 2–3 mm cervical to gingival margin. Essix thermoplastic copolyester retainers are a thinner, but stronger, cuspid-to-cuspid version of the full-arch, vacuum-formed devices. Advantages include that it can serve as a night guard against bruxism; alternative to spring retainers in correcting minor tooth movements; can be used to reduce occlusal forces from the opposing arch when moving posterior teeth. Due to their inherent flexibility, however, they cannot be used to retain cases in which arches have been expanded during orthodontic treatment.

Occlusal splint type retainer, RPDs; cast partial denture may also be used as removable retainers in certain cases.

Fixed Retainers

They are used to retain more rigidly to reduce the dependency on patient compliance. The wires used for such retainers should be flexible enough to allow physiologic tooth movement. they can be bonded or banded types. But banded retainers esp on 3–3 or 5–5 in extraction cases are unesthetic. They also lead to plaque retention and thus caries potential/enamel decalcification in the vicinity of bands increases. Bonded retainers are used to avoid the banding. They may also be effectively used to hold extraction spaces closed. Removable retainers may be fabricated to fit over bonded retainers to minimize potential relapse in the other planes of space and to maintain interarch relationships. Fixed retainers have been proposed to improve the long-term stability.

Indications of Bonded canine-to-canine retainer as described by Lee in 1981 and Zachrisson in 1983:

- After non-extraction treatment in mildly crowded cases
- After advancement/proclination of lower incisors during active treatment
- Planned alteration in the lower inter-canine width
- If expansion is done in lower arch
- Maintenance of lower incisor position during late mandibular growth.
- After correction of deep overbite
- Diastema closure maintenance
- Maintenance of extraction spaces for future pontic or implant.
- Keeping extraction spaces closed in adults
- Spaced anterior teeth
- Adult cases with potential post-orthodontic tooth migration; having PD disease
- Spacing reopening, after mandibular incisor extractions
- Severely rotated maxillary incisors.

Commonly used fixed retainers: Mostly 3–3 retainers are used, but can be extended distally as needed. Zachrisson introduced the mandibular bonded lingual 3–3 retainer as follows:

- First-generation mandibular bonded lingual 3–3 retainer was a plain round 0.032 to 0.036" blue Elgiloy wire with a loop at each end.
- Second generation was a twisted, 3-stranded 0.032-in wire.
- The third generation in 1995, was a plain round 0.030 to 0.032″ wire with both ends sandblasted with 50–90 μm aluminum oxide particles to increase the micromechanical retention.

Following have been described some of the fixed retainers, e.g. MSW retainers; resin fibreglass retainers; preformed 3–3 retainers with mesh pads at canines; twisting 3–4 strands of ligature wires (spiral wire retainers), Dentapreg retainers, Tru-tain retainers, etc.

Preformed 3–3 retainers with mesh pads at canines: Preformed 3–3 retainers made of rigid steel round wires with mesh pads at canines are available in different lengths. They are adapted on the patients' models in a passive state, and then bonded in place at canines with composites.

Twisted 3–4 strands of ligature wires (spiral wire retainers): 3–4 strands of 0.010" SS ligature wires (spiral wire retainers) are twisted by holding the two ends in Mathew's holders, or by twisting with the help of a slow–speed micromotor. The exact length of this wire is cut for 3–3 or 5–5 in case of extraction cases. The wire is stabilised with the help of floss, ligature wire, e-chain, elastics, etc. and then bonded. In lower arch, the wire is bonded on the mesial pits of premolars, while in upper arch, it is bonded on palatal surfaces of premolars.

Buccal retainer to prevent extraction space opening: A small segment of wire can be bonded on buccal surfaces of 3–5 in extraction cases to prevent space opening. The lingual or palatal retainer is placed 3–3 (Fig. 55.18).

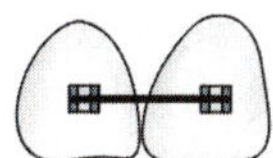

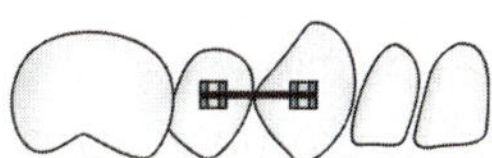

Fig. 55.18: Segmental fixed retainer at upper central incisors to prevent re-opening of midline diastema; while another figure shows fixed retainer at 3–5 region.

Bonded cuspid to cuspid retainers: These fixed retainers are made from 0.0195" or 0.0175" multistranded (MSW) stainless steel archwire. The wire is adapted passively on a working model to make the retainer by indirect technique. This wire is stabilised to lingual surfaces of the teeth using ligature wire, floss or a specially constructed jig, and is bonded in position using a light-cured composite resin. The retainer in the maxillary arch should not come in occlusion, otherwise it will break during use. The inherent flexibility of multi-strand archwire allows for physiologic tooth movement and prevents bond fracture due to occlusal forces. Disadvantages of this method retention are difficult hygiene maintenance especially gingival to retainers, the risk of decalcification and caries, and localized relapse if there is a partial debond of the retainer. A regular follow up every 3–4 months should be done.

Retainer for midline diastema: 1–1 palatal or labial retainer can be placed to prevent relapse, accompanied by frenectomy if needed. 1–1 Labial retainer can be used to augment palatal retainer in some cases to avoid reopening of midline diastema. In some cases, the palatal wire of 0.018 SS wire can be made with a loop in the midline region, which can be closed to keep the midline diastema closed actively. Alternatively, the meisal incisal edges of central incisors can be bonded with composite to keep the space closed.

Magnetic retainer: The use of magnets has also been reported to retain treated teeth. For example, in a case report by Springate and Sandler (1992), small, thin NdFeB magnets were bonded on the palatal surfaces of upper incisors in order to prevent re-opening of a diastema.

Rigid retainers: They are generally used in cases of CLP which have been treated with expansion. The molars are banded and the rigid SS wire of 0.9 mm size is bilaterally adapted to the palatal surfaces of teeth, and a section from molar to molar as transpalatal arch. The wire is soldered, and then the retainer is cemented in place.

Molar-to-molar mandibular retainer (Christie, 1985): It is lingual holding arch type of the appliance, and is extended between lower first molars. It allows natural/physiological settling of mandibular canines and molars. It is placed when the mandibular arch can be expanded or contracted. Even the corrected rotations can be retained by ligating the teeth to the lingual arch. Lower incisors can be advanced by activating it; can be retracted, intruded or extruded by ligating them to the lingual arch. It can be modified by adding spurs in incisor region to control tongue thrust habit. Second and third molar eruption can be facilitated by adding the auxiliary springs. Class II elastics can be used in retreatment.

Resin fiberglass bonded retainer: It was described by Michael Diamond in 1987. Problems faced with most bonded cuspid-to-cuspid retainers are holding the lingual arch in position during bonding, adapting the arch to contours of the teeth, and repairing a broken arch in the mouth. Retainers of glass fibers from woven fiberglass fabric can be made. A piece of fiberglass thread is measured between distal aspects of the canines, contacting the lingual surfaces of the incisors and cut, which is soaked in light-cured bonding resin. Make a second mixture of resin and restorative paste to the consistency of heavy cream, and incorporate a small amount of this paste into the fiberglass thread to increase its strength. This creamy paste is applied to the lingual surfaces of the teeth to be bonded. The resin-soaked fibers are placed to the teeth and positioned with an explorer, with adequate clearance of the gingival embrasures. The visible-light-curing unit is used to cure the retainer to the tooth surfaces. Paint a small amount of the creamy paste over the bonded junction on each tooth and cure. Advantages of this type are that it is rigid and impervious; tooth-colored, esthetic; comfortable; retainer sections can easily be recontoured, removed, or repaired in the mouth. Because no metal wires are used, additional material can be applied to the teeth or the fiberglass or both. The fiberglass material allows the retainer to be adjusted so as not to interfere with the functional contacts of the opposing teeth.

Dentapreg-fixed retainers: Dentapreg strips which are available commercially can be used for retention in anterior region. An adequate sized piece is cut and adapted in the region. It is then fixed with regular bonding material to say in place. The strip is also light cured to polymerise it to gain the strength. Later on, the strip and the bonding material is finished adequately.

Bondable multipurpose attachment (MPA) has been designed by Vashi and Vashi, 2010 which is useful for bonding lingual retainer wires. The MPA, shaped like the letter "P" in its profile view, which is only 0.4 mm thick at its base and 1 mm thick at the lumen. As it has a low profile, it is comfortable for the patient and versatile in many lingual and labial applications.

Bonding procedure: MPA is placed on the lingual surface of canines in the desired position with the lumen on the gingival side with normal bonding process. In the upper arch, the MPA should be placed at an appropriate height to avoid occluding with the lower canines. A twisted (MSW) wire is passed through the lumens of both MPAs. The wire is passively adapted to lingual surfaces of incisors. Excess wire is cut, leaving 2–3 mm extending from the distal end of each MPA and is bonded to the teeth with composite adhesive. The protruding distal ends of the retainer wire are bent gingivally, and more flowable adhesive is added to prevent the wire from sliding out the tubes and potentially causing relapse. The retainer can be extended to the premolars if necessary to prevent first-premolar extraction spaces from reopening. Advantages are that this method is quick and simple, as it does not require floss, ligature wires, or other stabilization to keep the retainer wire from moving during the bonding process. Attachments can easily be bonded at the desired heights, with vertical adjustments made to accommodate the patient's occlusion.

Chairtime is shorter, and bond failures are minimal compared to other techniques.

Short-span, low-profile bonded retainer: Proposed by Davis and Cooke. Many attachments, e.g. mesh pads, staples, composite, lengths of wire, and preformed rigid retainers with mesh pads at terminal ends, have been proposed for fixed retention devices. But these present problems especially when treating incisors with prominent marginal ridges and cingulae. Mesh pads are difficult to maintain plaque-free, and they can irritate the patient's tongue. Composite and wire may interfere with the occlusion. Precontoured wire sections are difficult to bond in the exact planned position. Preformed retainers rarely provide an ideal fit, and the rigid connecting wires do not permit physiological tooth movement during function. A simple short-span retainer can be custom-made from blank bracket bonding bases and multiflex wire. It has the advantages of close fit, low profile, smooth surfaces, and ease of cleansing. Its flexibility allows minor tooth movements and avoids bonding failures. Bracket bases are adapted to the palatal surfaces of the teeth on the model, taking into consideration the occlusion of the opposing teeth. A length of 0.018" spiral wire is tack welded and then soldered to the bases, and polished smooth. The retainer is stabilised with dental floss during bonding. It must be free of interference and closely adapted to the teeth, with no voids or flash around the bases or gingival margins. However, it should be used on only adjacent teeth, because longer lengths of connecting spiral wire become too flexible and difficult to control during bonding. If more than two teeth need to be retained, we suggest using additional two-unit retainers.

Direct-bonded lingual retainer: It has been described by Kenneth Lew, 1989. The major drawback with current designs is the difficulty of flossing between the retained teeth. This new design eliminates that difficulty. Before appliance removal, take an alginate impression. Passively adapt a length of 0.0195" spiral wire to the model so that the straight portion follows the middle or cervical third of the lingual surfaces and the "V" portions crosses the interdental papilla. 0.0195" spiral wire is used, instead of 0.015" wire advocated by some authors, to compensate for the increased flexibility introduced by the "V" loops. Use inlay wax to affix the wire to the model at several teeth. Construct hourglass-shaped stops from light-cured composite resin at two convenient points to act as reference landmark during positioning. Adapt the composite over the incisal edges to allow three-dimensional positioning. Melt the wax and remove the retainer from the model. Coat the etched enamel and under-surfaces of the resin stops with a thin film of unfilled light-cured composite resin. Cure the resin with a light source to secure the retainer. Bond the wire to the remaining teeth with composite resin. Remove the incisal portions of the hourglass stops with a rotary instrument to complete the retainer. The "V" loops in this design allow the patient to floss into the interproximal areas. The flexible wire and extended inter-adhesive spans permit the teeth to move within the periodontal space.

Modified bell-shape bonded lingual retainer (by Dr KFL, 1995): A bell-shape splint, contoured to the cingulum and interdental papilla, has been advocated to allow more gingival positioning, thus reducing bond failures from occlusal forces. Such a retainer is not rigid enough to keep the interdental space closed, so activate the bell-shape retainer in the "bell" area. A light force applied with a Weingart plier is enough to ensure a closing pressure that will maintain the treatment result. Double back the ends of the twisted wire to prevent the wire from sliding out from the composite resin. Also, check for any occlusal interferences before curing the resin.

Banded mandibular adjustable retainer (by Balenseifen, 1991): B-MAR combines fixed retainer's advantages—cooperation and hygiene; ability to adjust the appliance one to three months after insertion.

Active Retainers

They are active in nature and used to treat minor relapse of incisal crowding, e.g. removable spring retainers, vacuum formed retainers, Essix retainer, NiTi retainer; Osamu retainer, etc. as discussed below.

Removable spring retainer, vacuum-formed retainers, Essix retainer: They have been described in the section of removable retainers.

Osamu active retainer for correction of mild relapse: It was developed by Dr Osamu. It is a transparent removable appliance that can correct individual tooth positions during the retention phase. There are 2 superimposed layers. Inner layer is 1.5 mm ethylene vinyl acetate copolymer (Bioplast) adapted to the interproximal areas and covers the palatal and lingual aspects of the teeth. The outer layer is of 0.75 mm hard elastic polycarbonate, covers the occlusal aspects of the teeth and makes the retainer elastic and stable.

Active NiTi retainer: (byLliou, Huang 2001): The relapse of mandibular anterior crowding is very common. Several causes are associated with relapse, e.g. reorganization of the periodontal tissues, overexpansion of the arch, and changes due to mandibular growth. The best way to re-treat mandibular anterior crowding is using brackets and archwires. But, patients are often reluctant to wear braces again. Theoretically, the nickel-titanium (NiTi) archwire is an excellent alternative to use as a bonded lingual retainer or as an active appliance for solving relapse of mandibular anterior crowding without brackets. Bonding a segment of mandibular NiTi archwire lingually canine to canine to can be used to solve relapse of mandibular anterior crowding and to serve as a post-treatment bonded lingual retainer. Medium-force 0.018" NiTi mandibular arch wire is bonded with light-cured resin on the lingual surfaces of the canines at a position along the contact points of the mandibular anterior teeth.

Clinical procedures: NiTi archwire is first coordinated for the lingual curvature and arch form along the contact points of mandibular incisors on the dental cast obtained at completion of orthodontic treatment. NiTi archwire is then bent and adjusted for the intercanine width with a three-prong plier.

Both ends of the NiTi archwire were then cut to adjust the canine-to-canine arch perimeter and were microetched with sandblast before bonding. NiTi archwire is loosely ligated to the mandibular incisors with several .010-in ligature wires through the embrasures. NiTi archwire is oriented horizontally along the contact points, and either the right or the left end was first fitted and bonded onto the lingual surface of the canine on that side. The archwire is then tightly tied to fit each incisor, one by one, toward the other canine. Finally, the other end of the archwire was bonded to the opposite canine. Thus the bonding is only at canines. The ligature wires are left in situ to control the orthodontic tooth movement. The patients are seen once a month, and the ligature wires were retied, changed, or removed as needed. After completion of the retreatment, the ligature wires were removed and the NiTi archwires were left in situ for permanent retention.

Conclusion

Retention is a very important phase of orthodontic treatment. It should be included in the total treatment time and its importance should be explained to the patient. Retention period is for the reorganisation of tissues and achieving muscular equilibrium for stability of dentofacial structures in the new environment. Myriad of retention appliances have been described by clinicians. Relapse is inevitable so the best method of retention is the indefinite retention. But this is not possible clinically. Thus a prolonged retention is mostly advised. Also the retention depends on the nature and etiology of malocclusion. Evidence-based research has shown that there is a paucity of high quality evidence on which to base our clinical practice of orthodontic retention. There is an urgent need for high quality research in this field, which affects the vast majority of our orthodontic patients (Littlewood, 2006).

56

Risks in Orthodontic Treatment

INTRODUCTION

Orthodontic treatment can help to improve functions like mastication, speech and appearance, as well as overall health, comfort, and self-esteem of the patients. Like any medical or dental treatment, orthodontic treatment is also associated with some risks. These are seldom serious still the possibilities should be discussed with the patients/ parents and an informed consent should be obtained before proceeding with treatment. Some patients may be more at risk than others; they need to be identified early and managed appropriately to avoid adverse sequelae. The common complications of orthodontic treatment are given below.

Some possible **complications** related to orthodontic treatment are:

1. Enamel: Crowns decalcification; enamel wear; enamel fracture, white spot lesions; dental caries and decay
2. Bone: Crestal bone resorption, abnormal development
3. Chemical burn from etchant, thermal burns from overheating handpiece
4. Cross-infection: Operator to patient, patient to operator, patient to patient, any source to third parties
5. Face: Skin trauma from displaced headgear whisker, eye damage from displaced headgear whisker, bruising from headgear strap (uncommon)
6. Gastrointestinal tract/respiratory tract: Swallowing or aspiration of small parts
7. Growth: Unfavorable growth
8. Heart: Infective endocarditis
9. Allergy to orthodontic components: Nickel-induced allergy/sensitivity
10. Periodontal: Gingivitis, periodontitis, burns, recession, dark triangle
11. Psychological: Teasing, abnormal patients/parents behavior, ignorance from teachers
12. Pulp: Early closure of root apex, pulpitis; devitalization of the tooth
13. Resorption: Root resorption
14. Soft tissues: Direct trauma, mucosal ulceration due to appliances; trauma from headgear whisker, clumsy instrumentation, soft-tissue clefts, poor gingival contours
15. Temporomandibular joint: Temporomandibular dysfunction, condylar resorption
16. Treatment results: Unfavorable results, unable to maintain results, unable to complete treatment, failed treatment
17. Tooth staining
18. Relapse of orthodontic problems
19. Prolonged treatment time
20. Ankylosis.

Some of them are being discussed below.

Enamel Demineralization/Caries (Fig. 56.1)

Caries is a common risk in orthodontics and usually occurs on smooth surfaces around the brackets. It is due to improper oral hygiene; increased dental plaque; lowering of resting pH; and a rapid shift in bacterial flora. Subsurface demineralization is called **white spot lesion (WSL)**. Any WSLs present before

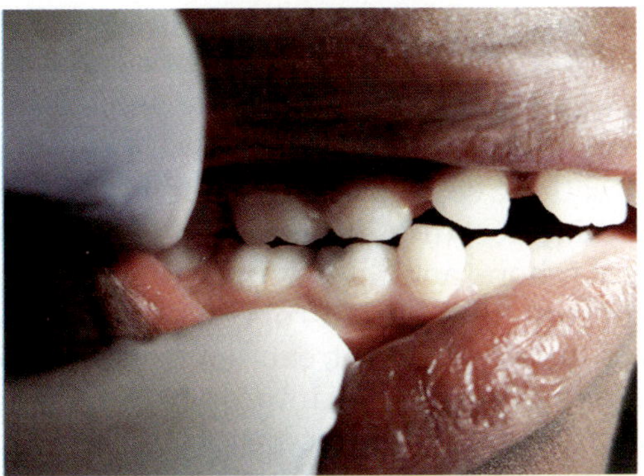

Fig. 56.1: White spot lesions and partially decalcified on buccal surfaces of lower teeth.

treatment should be recorded and treated. Remineralization and reversal of lesion is possible with proper fluoride treatment if the demineralized surface remains intact. Cavities need to be restored. Preventive measures should be reinforced at each visit, i.e. intensive oral hygiene and dietary education. With 0.05% sodium fluoride daily **mouth rinse** or 0.2% sodium fluoride weekly rinse or using **fluoridated tooth paste** daily, the occurrence of caries decreases (Figs 56.2a and b). In severe cases and as a last resort, early removal of the appliance may be required to prevent further damage. For more severe cases of staining, WSLs, e.c, an acid/ pumice **microabrasion** technique has been advocated, but should be performed at least 3 months after debonding to allow natural initial remineralization.

Physical Damages on Enamel

Enamel abrasion can occur due to contact with both metal and ceramic brackets. Hardness of ceramic is more than enamel, so ceramic brackets are more abrasive. The incisal edges of upper anterior teeth and buccal cusps of upper posterior teeth are frequently affected as they are in contact with faulty placed brackets. It is also common on upper canine tips during retraction, as the cusp tips hit lower canine brackets. Direct contact between orthodontic brackets and opposing teeth may also lead to dislodging of brackets. Careless use of an orthodontic band seater or band remover can also result in **enamel fracture**. **Debonding** of brackets may lead to enamel fracture in some cases esp with ceramic brackets. Extreme care should be taken when large restorations are present, since these can result in fracture of enamel and fillings while band removal. Care must always be taken during removal of brackets and residual bonding agents to minimize enamel fracture. Burs used to remove the remaining bonding material leads to scratches and removal of enamel. Very fine grit diamonds should be used followed by polishing. Any lesions of enamel erosion should be recorded before starting the treatment and appropriate dietary advice given to minimize further tooth substance loss. Patients with history of gastric acidity

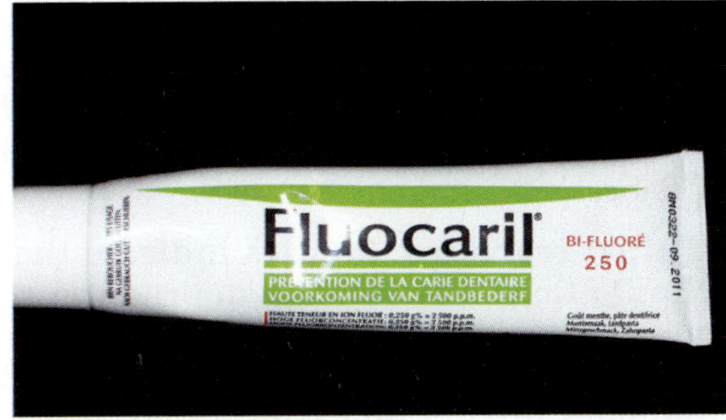

(a)

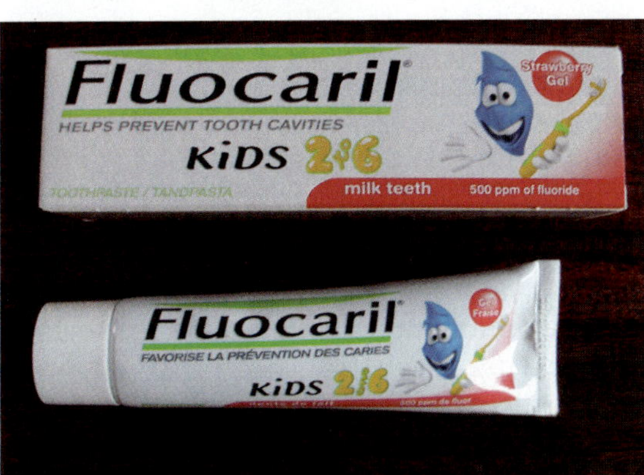

(b)

Figs 56.2a and b: Fluocaril, a fluoridated tooth paste, available commercially for different age groups with different fluoride concentration. It can be recommended to patients having active orthodontic treatment to prevent development of WSLs.

and regurgitation should be noted. Carbonated drinks, lemons and pure juices are the most common causes of erosion and should be avoided in patients with fixed appliances.

Pulpal reactions: Studies indicate that orthodontic forces cause a depression of oxygen utilization in pulp cells. It is more severe with application of greater and prolonged force. Light continuous forces produce mild and transient inflammatory response within the pulp, so some degree of pulpitis is always expected with orthodontic tooth movement, which is usually reversible or transient and has no long-term significance. But there may be increased pulpitis in previously traumatized teeth, so only light forces should be applied. Devitalisation can occur if heavy forces are applied. Removal of bonding material may also increase local temperature resulting in pulp damage. Temperatures of 46–50 C for 30 seconds lead to thrombosis and prevent pulpal circulation. So, water must be used as a coolant.

Dead teeth: A tooth may lose its vitality due to excessive forces, and can get discolored during orthodontic treatment. It may also be related to a previous injury.

Stability or relapse: According to studies, teeth move irrespective of whether or not they are orthodontically treated and also they move throughout life. The teeth positions can change adversely due to various causes like eruption of wisdom teeth, growth of soft tissues and their pressure, size of tongue and jaws, growth and/or maturational changes, mouth breathing and other oral habits. After the treatment, tooth and/or jaw position may change and may require additional treatment which depends on the nature of the problem. Relapse is inevitable after orthodontic treatment. It is due to tissue changes in gingival, periodontal and supporting bone during treatment, which needs time for re-organization after appliance removal. Also the teeth come to lie in new and unstable position after treatment, so they are easily affected by unbalanced soft tissue pressure. Continual growth of jaws and alveolar processes also affects orthodontic results. It generally takes 4 to 6 months for PDL and supporting bone to complete re-organization. During this time, the teeth have a stronger tendency to move and this effect diminishes gradually when the alveolar bone and the periodontium return to their normal pattern. Proper use of retainers helps to reduce post-treatment relapse. Most relapses occur due to improper use of retainers and inadequate monitoring. Therefore the long-term retention and monitoring is a must.

Gingivitis/gingival enlargement: Plaque retention increases with fixed appliances and plaque composition gets altered. There is an increase in periopathogenic anaerobic organisms and a reduction in facultative anaerobes around bands. **Gingival inflammation occurs in almost all patients after** fixed appliance placement due to problems with oral hygiene. Gingival hyperplasia, recession; alveolar crestal bone loss, are common sequelae of orthodontic procedures. Usually it is mild in nature and gets resolved after removal of the appliances, and does not lead to attachment loss. Bands induce more gingival inflammation than bonds, since they are more plaque retentive and their margins are often placed subgingivally. The interdental areas are affected more than facial areas, and posterior teeth more than anterior teeth. Adult patients are at higher risk of periodontal problems, and esp with preexisting periodontal loss. Treatment mechanics need to be modified in such patients having decreased alveolar support, and lighter forces are used. Patients with systemic diseases such as diabetes or epilepsy, poorly controlled diabetics and the patients on phenytoin drugs can cause gingival hyperplasia.

Oral hygiene should be maintained and the use of adjuncts such as electric toothbrushes, interproximal brushes, chlorhexidine mouthwashes, fluoride mouthwashes, and regular professional cleaning must be used. Bonding rather than bands on molars and premolars should be done. Compressed gingiva in extraction sites may produce a long-lasting epithelial tissue fold; esp on the buccal aspect of mandibular first premolar extraction sites. Plaque gets hardened to calculus which may interfere in space closure. Presence of plaque and calculus leads to rapid resorption of alveolar bone with orthodontic force.

Gingival recession: Gingival recession and loss of alveolar bone have been reported as a result of teeth moving in the presence of inflammation. Labial movement of mandibular incisors may also result in gingival recession.

Dark triangles: Dark triangles are unaesthetic open gingival embrasures which are more bothersome in the incisal region. It can be due to loss of attachment due to periodontal disease due to improper oral hygiene maintenance; and incisally positioned contact points and/or abnormally shaped teeth. Adequate oral hygiene should be maintained. Abnormally shaped tooth/contact area are treated by removing enamel at contact points and moving them apically so that the teeth can be moved closer together. However, proportional relationships of teeth should be maintained. Any pre-existing and expected black triangles should be noted and patient should be informed about the possibility of reshaping the teeth later to minimize the esthetic problem.

Profile changes: Unsatisfactory profile changes (e.g. flattening; dishing-in of face or increase in facial fullness) have been common complaints after treatment. Soft tissue changes also occur naturally with age, regardless of orthodontic intervention. Extraction of premolars and retraction of anteriors, without proper torque control of anterior segments; excessive expansion of dental arch in anterior-posterior direction, etc. leads to unusual changes in facial profile. Careful planning and proper communication with patients reduces the chances of complaints. Proper diagnosis should be done, and record of skeletal form, tooth position, and soft tissue form is done. A proper treatment planning and mechanics should be designed to avoid detrimental effect on profile.

Prolonged treatment time: Generally, the average treatment time is in the range of 18 to 24 months, but it may increase markedly in different situations and in non cooperative patients. Loose brackets, broken wires, not using the elastics and missed appointments, etc. are common causes of prolonged treatment.

Root resorption (Fig. 56.3): Some degree of external root resorption (approx. 2 mm) is inevitable during orthodontic treatment. Resorption may occur on apical and lateral surfaces of roots, but radiographs can only show apical resorption. In some cases, only microscopic surface changes may be present. Upper and lower incisors are affected more than other teeth. Excessive force and hyalinization of PDL results in excessive activity of cementoclasts and osteoclasts. The risk factors associated with severe resorption are application of excessive forces; longer duration of treatment; previously traumatized teeth; hormonal and hereditary component; shorter than average roots; teeth lacking vitality after RCT, increased overjet, pre-treatment trauma to maxillary incisors, torquing with rectangular wires, use of Class II elastics, systemic disorders such as hypothyroidism; familial risk; individual susceptibility to root resorption, etc. Treatment of ectopic canines, tooth intrusion, movement of root apices against cortical bone, increased age at the time of treatment increases the risk of resorption. All patients should therefore be warned and it is important to recognize specific risk factors. When resorption is observed during treatment, the forces should be removed and rest periods must be used. The root length

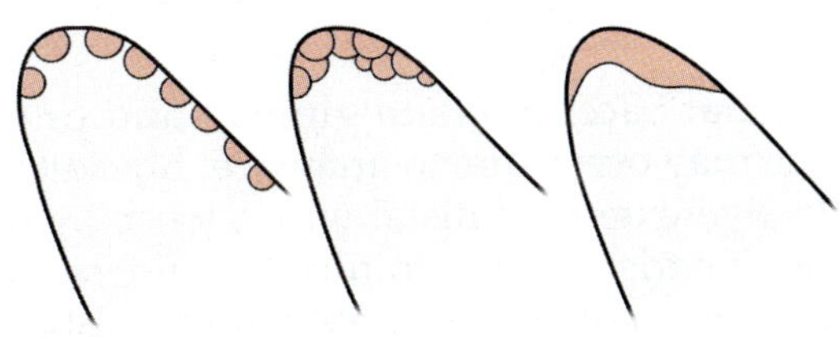

Fig. 56.3: Stages of apical root resorption which can be seen during orthodontic treatment.

should monitored with 6-monthly radiographs. In severe cases, treatment may have to be stopped to prevent further resorption. If not treated timely, it may lead to mobility, devitalisation and loss of such teeth.

Swallowing/inhalation of small parts: Orthodontic appliances are composed of various small parts like brackets, tubes, cleats, buttons, etc. which can be accidentally swallowed, or aspirated, and can irritate or damage the tissues. Small foreign bodies in alimentary canal do not present major problem because they pass through without any incidence, unless they get impacted or cause perforation. But aspiration of foreign body in airway leads to complications like spasm, breathing problem and accidental death. Precautions should be taken during placement of smaller sized orthodontic components, e.g. during cementing of molar bands, esp second molar, the band should be secured by dental floss passing through the molar tubes. If any object falls, the patient's face should be turned to the side so that the object comes towards the cheek, or the patients face should be turned down to allow object to fall out of the mouth.

A barrier of gauge piece can be placed towards oropharynx while working. Removable appliances esp lower, should be made of bigger size. The appliance should have good retention to avoid its accidental loosening. The safety hold distal end cutter should be used during intra-oral arch wire cutting and a cotton role should be placed distally while cutting to avoid insertion of wire part in the mucosa.

Loose appliances and discomfort: Gums, cheeks and lips may get lacerated by braces, loose or broken wires. It leads to ulceration and pain.

Trauma: Lacerations to gingiva and oral mucosa may occur due to archwire, brackets, bands, overextended distal wires, loose ligature wire ends, leading to ulceration. Use of dental wax over the brackets and rubber tubing on unsupported archwire may reduce trauma and discomfort. **Transpalatal arch/lingual arch** may cause trauma to the palate, lingual mucosa or tongue if adequate soft tissue clearance is not provided during their fabrication and placement. Extraoral appliances can cause both extra- and intra-oral injuries, e.g. injuries to cheek, eye, buccal mucosa, etc. **Headgear** can cause injury if it is displaced either during sleep or play. The inner arch of facebow is sharp and rich in oral microorganisms. A penetrating eye injury may cause damage and infection of the eye. **Samuels and Jones** classified headgear injuries as Accidental disengagement when playing; incorrect handling; disengagement by another child; and Disengagement while asleep. Headgears are now prepared with safety features which stop them from being accidentally displaced or recoiling back into the face or the eyes. They should not to be worn while playing and the headgear strap should always be removed before the facebow is disengaged. **Loops, utility arches** are often used during orthodontic treatment and are prone to tissue impingement causing ulceration or tissue hyperplasia around the loop and free ends. Sometimes, the loop may become completely embedded in hyperplastic tissue requiring surgical excision for removal.

Ankylosis: A tooth may become fused (ankylosed) to the bone and cannot be moved under orthodontic forces. It also happens due to some previous injury or due to genetic problems. An ankylosed tooth which needs to be moved needs alveolar surgery to be aligned. An ankylosed primary tooth needs to be removed.

Damage to teeth: The enamel edges of some teeth may get abraded if the teeth bite or grind against the brackets esp ceramic brackets. Premature contacts may also lead to loosening of the brackets, fracture of wings, etc. also.

Temporomandibular dysfunction: Some people are naturally susceptible to joint problems with or without orthodontic treatment. A lot of attention has been focused on the relationship between temporomandibular dysfunction (TMD) and orthodontic treatment. TMD is quite common in general population. However, current evidence says that there is no link of orthodontic treatment as a causative factor of TMDs. Pre-existing TMD should be recorded, and the patient should be advised that treatment will not improve this condition and also that some may experience increased symptoms. During or after orthodontic treatment, patients may experience pain or tenderness of jaw muscles and joints.TMD is managed with the standard approach to eliminate discomfort, occlusal disharmony and joint noises. Patient is also reassured. Other forms of standard treatment (e.g. soft diet, jaw exercises and analgesics) may also be required.

Infection control: Spread of infection should be prevented by adequate infection control procedures, like using gloves, masks, sterilized instruments, and clean working areas, are important. A detailed medical history of the patient must be taken to determine risk factors. Patients having cardiac problems are at risk of bacterial endocarditis, so proper care and an antibiotic cover should be given for invasive procedures such as during band placement/removal, scaling, extractions/surgery, separation, etc. Bonding attachments should be used rather than banding in such cases, which also reduces unwanted plaque in stagnant areas caused by bands. Chlorhexidine mouthwash should be used prior to any treatment to reduce bacterial population. Proper oral hygiene is essential to prevent gingival problems.

Allergy: Hypersensitivity reactions may occur to certain components like nickel, chromium, cobalt. Other allergens may also be released from bonding materials, cold curing acrylics, or latex elastics. Some patients may have some form of contact dermatitis with orthodontic appliances. **Nickel allergy:** Nickel is found in orthodontic wires, bands, brackets, etc. Females are more susceptible. Intraoral signs are highly variable and difficult to diagnose. They may be loss of taste or metallic taste, numbness, burning sensation, soreness at the side of the tongue, angular cheilitis and erythematous areas or severe gingivitis in the absence of plaque. Since such signs and symptoms are difficult to identify, nickel allergy in response to orthodontic appliances may be under-diagnosed. **Latex allergy** may occur due to contact with latex gloves, elastomeric ligatures or elastics. The commonest sites affected are the gingivae and tongue. Natural rubber latex sensitivity is associated with atopy, reflecting a predisposition to producing IgE antibodies. The main type of reaction to natural rubber latex (NRL) is allergic contact dermatitis. In latex sensitive patients, steel ligatures or self-ligating brackets may be used. However, now latex-free elastics and gloves are available.

Complications Related to Implants

Microimplants are excellent source of skeletal anchorage but they are not free from potential problems and soft tissue complications. Some of the problems associated with mini-screws are:

a. **Inadequate primary stability:** Poor stability of a mini-implant occurs if the cortex is thinner and the density of trabecular bone is low. It can also occur due to an over-drilled hole (more than the diameter of the miniscrew).
b. **Ulceration/trauma to soft tissue overlying the implant:** The implant head irritates the surrounding soft tissues leading to ulceration, pain, infection, etc. It should be covered with a layer of composite to avoid trauma and subsequent ulceration. Also, the implant should be placed in the immobile mucosa.
c. **Peri-implantitis:** Inflammation of gingival tissue and infection of surrounding tissues around the implant can occur if adequate oral hygiene is not maintained. The implant becomes lose and needs replacement. Patients should be instructed to maintain oral hygiene throughout treatment. 0.2% chlorhexidene mouthwash can also be prescribed.
d. **Delayed mobility:** A miniscrew can withstand is a force of 50–450 N. Delayed

mobility and failure of implant can occur due to overloading. Such screw should be removed and replaced.

e. **Screw fracture during removal:** Lateral forces during removal can cause fracture. If implant is left for a very long time, this also could lead to fracture on removal as a result of partial or full osseointegration.

Systemic diseases: General medical problems, e.g. cardiac diseases, blood dyscrasias, neurological, cancer, or endocrine disorders, can affect orthodontic treatment. The patient may be on medications which may affect the tooth movements. Any changes in the patient's health and updation of history should be monitored on a regular basis.

Treatment results: Due to multitude of factors, e.g. uncooperative patients; unexpected growth of jaws/soft tissues; skeletal disproportions; improper treatment planning; missing/extracted/grossly carious teeth; hereditary factors; shifting of the patients from one place to other; patients not coming regularly for follow ups; different treatment plans of clinicians attending the cases; getting orthodontic treatment from general dentists without sufficient orthodontic knowlege, etc. proper results may not be obtained; some cases may see unfavorable results; unable to maintain results, unable to complete treatment, etc.

Conclusion

Although not very common, but still the orthodontic treatment is associated with some risks and complications. Some of the risks are inevitable and reversible, while others are irreversible and may be iatrogenic. The most common are enamel lesions and gingival problems. Root resorption and devitalisation are mainly associated with application of heavy forces. Factors like late mandibular growth; soft tissue growth; heredity tendency, tendency of relapse, etc. should also be discussed. Possibility of risks should be discussed with the patients/parents and informed consent should be obtained.

57

Enamel Scars in Orthodontics

INTRODUCTION

One of the most common complications during the fixed orthodontic treatment is the formation of white opaque lesions or enamel demineralization around the attachments. The patients often complain of the loss of color on crown surface during and after the fixed treatment. It is generally due to improper oral hygiene during the treatment. Also, the improper bonding technique leaving excess bonding material around the brackets leads to the niches for bacterial growth, plaque, food and stains accumulation. The presence of white lesions at the end of orthodontic treatment is a major esthetic problem. To prevent such problems, proper preventive protocols must be followed.

Enamel decalcification occurs due to plaque accumulation and subsequent acid production, thus resulting in an alteration in the appearance of the enamel surface. Early lesions appear clinically as opaque, white spots due to loss of mineral in the surface and subsurface enamel. If mineral loss continues, then a frank cavity is formed. Clinically, formation of white spot lesions (WSL) around orthodontic attachments can occur within 4 weeks of start of the treatment. The labiogingival area of the lateral incisor is the most common site for white spot formation and the maxillary posterior segments are the least common site. It is usually more among males than females, which has been attributed in part to their poorer oral hygiene.

Etiology

Its development is just like caries development, where the co-existence of the four factors namely, bacterial plaque, fermentable carbohydrates, a susceptible tooth surface and a sufficient period of time are necessary for white opaque lesions to develop. WSL is the first step toward frank caries development.

Histopathology of the White Spot Lesion

Early enamel caries is seen clinically as a white spot lesion, which occurs due to an optical phenomenon owing to subsurface tissue loss

Four zones have been described in a carious lesion from dentin outwards. The first zone is called the **translucent zone,** where there is an absence of structural rod outlines and a tenfold increase in the amount of space compared to normal enamel. Progressing into the lesion, the next zone is the **dark or positive zone,** as seen in polarized light microscopy. There is further increase in the volume of spaces. Translucent zone results from preferential dissolution of structure at the rod periphery, which then proceeds to the cross-striations producing the dark zone. It has been shown that remineralization occurs in the dark zone. Finally, when the core of the enamel rods gets involved, it produces a zone of maximum tissue destruction which is termed the **body of the lesion**.

The outermost layer of enamel (i.e. above the lesion) remains relatively intact and appears radiopaque in radiographs known as **surface zone**. It is also **a zone of remineralization**. It is in approximation to saliva and hence has a tendency of remineralization, if surface is intact.

Pathogenesis

White opaque lesions on enamel surface occur basically due to subsurface demineralization resulting in porosity and changes in the optical properties of the enamel. The affected enamel may appear as chalky or may associate with erosion of the surface. This process is an interrupted process with episodes of repair and destruction depending on the oral environment, especially the fluctuations in plaque pH. Till the surface of the porous lesion remains intact, there is the possibility of arrest or even reversal of the lesion. This remineralization may occur spontaneously through the combined action of the salivary minerals and fluoride from the dentifrices, proper brushing to remove plaque, or through therapeutic intervention. But if pH of the plaque remains low for a prolonged period of time, the remineralization lags behind the demineralisation, resulting in cavity formation.

Salivary factors: Saliva acts as a buffer to neutralize the acidic pH of plaque on the teeth surfaces. It influences the dynamics of mineral loss and deposit at the enamel–plaque interface. The amount and the rate of demineralization and the likelihood of enamel remineralization is influenced by salivary factors, such as pH, rate of flow and buffer capacity. It also influences pH and microbial composition of plaque. Saliva also acts as a vehicle to deliver fluoride ions to the enamel and plaque. Tooth surfaces that are more exposed to carbohydrate with less exposure to saliva are common sites for demineralization. That is why the maxillary anterior teeth have highest incidence of demineralization during fixed orthodontics, while the lingual surface of the lower incisors is often the site of calculus formation, indicating mineralization where salivary flow is adequate due to opening of sublingual gland ducts. Thus, the presence of the sufficient amounts of saliva acts in preventing enamel demineralization.

Also, the salivary flow rate influences both caries risk and caries activity. Adequate flow of saliva helps in physical cleansing of carbohydrates from tooth surfaces, and thus preventing fermentation and acid production by bacteria. So it is an important factor for prevention and management of enamel demineralization, which is caused by acidic pH of plaque. It is countered by the alkaline pH and buffering capacity of saliva. The pH and buffering capacity of the saliva is maintained by the rate of salivary secretion. An intraoral environment with low pH favors colonization of the cariogenic bacteria, particularly *Streptococcus mutans*, whereas a high salivary pH maintains a higher buffering capacity and thus prevents caries.

Microbial factors: Initiation and progression of smooth surface caries is associated with *Streptococcus mutans*. After initiation of caries lesion, its progression is caused by *Lactobacillus*. Increased number of *Streptococcus mutans* and *Lactobacillus*, and new sites of plaque appearance on enamel around the orthodontic attachments is common in patients on fixed appliance. This is also influenced by the duration of the orthodontic treatment, the number of orthodontic attachments, and oral hygiene of the patient.

Oral hygiene: The orthodontic attachments make tooth cleaning more difficult leading to more plaque accumulation. They also restrict the self-cleansing action of the tongue, lips and cheek to remove food debris from the tooth surface. Therefore, accumulated food debris encourages growth of the cariogenic bacteria. Most growth sites are usually found on the gingival margin and on the edges of orthodontic bands. A study showed a five-fold increase in *Lactobacillus* count in patients undergoing active orthodontic treatment.

Diet: Frequency of carbohydrate ingestion has a significant influence on enamel demineralization. After ingestion of fermentable carbohydrate, acids are produced inside the plaque leading to fall of pH, which can by countered by salivary buffering. However, as the frequency of carbohydrate intake increases, the enamel surface may be exposed to more acid without intervening repair, resulting in a net loss of minerals over time.

Fixed orthodontic appliances: They create new plaque stagnation areas due to their irregular surfaces and also restrict self-cleansing action of the tongue, lips and cheek. The reduced access by saliva also encourages lowering of plaque pH. Plaque deposition is greater on resin bonding material than on enamel and also more on the gingival side of bonded brackets. The archwire ligation materials also cause plaque accumulation, bacterial colonization and enamel decalcification. The elastomeric rings attract greater number of cariogenic microorganisms than stainless steel ligature, which is due their more plaque retaining capacity. Studies have shown that the resting salivary flow increases during fixed orthodontic treatment, which helps in increase in salivary pH and buffering capacity and thus counteracts the demineralization tendency. This could be the reason why in some patients there are less white spots around orthodontic appliances despite moderate plaque accumulation.

Thus, before starting the fixed orthodontic treatment, an assessment of patient susceptibility to enamel demineralization must be made taking an account of factors like patient's oral hygiene procedures and cooperation; assessment of salivary flow rate, caries incidence over the past years, plaque scores, caries activity tests, dietary pattern and residence of fluoridated or non-fluoridated communities.

Prevention and Management

The enamel demineralization can be prevented by either eliminating plaque deposition by improving oral hygiene or by enhancing enamel resistance to acids by using topical fluoride. Fluoride inhibits the development of white spots and also reduces the size of white spots. Fluoride also enhances enamel remineralization due to flourapatite and calcium fluoride formation. For maximum caries inhibition, continuous presence of fluoride, even at low concentrations, in saliva and plaque is necessary. Proper oral hygiene maintenance, combined with daily use of topical fluoride, is found to significantly reduce enamel decalcification. Home use of topical fluoride agents needs patient co-operation. So, different non-compliant topical fluoride delivery measures can be used. Best is to use a fluoride-containing tooth paste, and patient is advised to brush the teeth at least 3 times per day.

Dietary Modification

Patient is advised to change dietary habits by avoiding carbohydrates, sticky foods, chocolates and biscuits, etc.

Mechanical plaque control: Since plaque is the primary cause of demineralization, thorough mechanical plaque control is very important. Proper method of tooth brushing during fixed orthodontic treatment is the most practical and acceptable method for plaque control. Standard tooth brush can be modified for use during fixed orthodontic treatment. Use of disclosing agents helps for self-monitoring of oral hygiene manouvers. Using power toothbrush or water irrigation with manual tooth brushing is a more effective method in reducing plaque accumulation than manual tooth brushing alone. Proximal surfaces of teeth are prone to enamel demineralization because of the difficulty in maintaining oral hygiene with archwires in place, so the dental flossing has proved helpful in interproximal cleaning. A floss threader can be used for threading the floss under the main archwire. A soft rubber inter-dental stimulator is also helpful in cleaning and massaging the interproximal areas.

Fluoride toothpaste: Regular use of fluoride toothpaste is a very common recommendation by the orthodontist, but it is shown to be inefficient in inhibiting white spot development. So, additional measures may be required.

Fluoride mouthrinse: Sodium fluoride mouthrinse can almost totally eliminate white spots if used throughout therapy and should be recommended to all orthodontic patients. Daily mouthrinse with sodium fluoride (.05% or 0.2%) and/or weekly with acidulated phosphate fluoride (1.2%) rinse have been found to reduce the incidence of enamel demineralization. After a systematic review, it has been recommended that the best method to prevent enamel demineralization during fixed orthodontic treatment is daily use of 0.05% sodium fluoride mouthrinse.

Fluoride gel: It has been found that use of Stannous fluoride gels (0.4%) during orthodontic treatment decreases enamel decalcification. Boyd has found that a 1100 ppm fluoride toothpaste alone or together with either a daily 0.05% sodium fluoride rinse or a 0.4% stannous fluoride gel applied twice daily by toothbrush provided additional protection against decalcification when compared to toothpaste alone, but neither was superior.

Fluoride varnish: Fluor Protector, a polyurethane varnish has 0.7% diflurosilane and it decreased white spot lesion formation under molar bands. Other studies have also found that fluoride varnishes are effective in preventing enamel demineralization. Thus the use of fluoride varnishes under orthodontic bands can be an effective way to prevent white spot formation. Recently, chlorohexidine varnish has also been suggested for reducing plaque accumulation and enamel decalcification.

Pit and fissure sealant: Frazier et al used light cured pit and fissure sealants on the labial enamel adjacent to orthodontic attachments and found it effective in preventing enamel demineralization without patient cooperation. But, the main problem with placing the sealants is that it is very technique sensitive, and also the mechanical and chemical discontinuities in the sealant layer may lead to enamel decalcification below the sealant.

Fluoride in bonding agents: Fluoride containing bonding agents have the potential for decreasing enamel decalcification. Fewer white spot lesions develop with the fluoride containing composites as compared to conventional bonding agents. Using glass ionomer cement and teh resin-modified glass ionomer cement for bonding brackets significantly reduced enamel demineralization around orthodontic brackets. It has been found that with the resin modified glass ionomer cements, the fluoride release is greater and also occurs over a prolonged period, as compared to the fluoride containing composites. The resin-modified glass ionomer cement alone and composite with added fluoride have almost equal cariostatic effects. The formation of white spot lesions can best be prevented by using resin-modified glass ionomer cement supplemented with topical fluorides. Thus the glass ionomer cement bonding agent, is more effective at preventing enamel demineralization and post-orthodontic white spot lesions than a conventional composite resin.

Fluoride in luting cement: Use of fluoride containing cements for banding has been advised by Kaswiner. Glass ionomer cement has fluoride-releasing property and can reduce enamel demineralization. Also the fluoride releasing cements like zinc polycarboxylate and resin modified glass ionomer cement lead to less enamel demineralization than the zinc phosphate cement. Glass ionomer cements decrease enamel decalcification when compared with zinc phosphate and zinc polyacrylate cements. Millett et al also found less enamel decalcification around orthodontic brackets with glass ionomer cement as compared to the composites, but the difference was not statistically significant.

Fluorides in elastomers: Elastic ligatures and power chains containing fluoride have also become available recently, and are effective in reducing plaque accumulation and enamel decalcification around the brackets. Joseph, Grobler and Rossouw found that release of fluoride from a fluoride containing elastic chain is high for the first week and decreased significantly after that and thus require a weekly-change for, for optimum fluoride release, which is against the laws of orthodontic forces/activation. Thus, these elastomeric ligatures had no significant anti-cariogenic benefits. It was also found that in the presence of fluoridated toothpaste and mouthrinse the fluoride release is also significantly more. Thus, fluoridated elastomers may imbibe fluoride from their environment.

Argon laser: The mechanism of action of the argon laser for the prevention of enamel decalcification is by altering the crystalline structure of the enamel. Blankenau, et al found an average of 29.1% reduction in the depth of enamel decalcification with argon laser. Other studies have also found significant reduction in lesion depth with it. So it can be considered as an effective method in reducing enamel decalcification during orthodontic treatment.

Microabrasion

If the WSLs/decalcification is limited to superficial layer of enamel, then enamel microabrasion can be used to eliminate the damaged tissue completely and conservatively, improving tooth appearance and the restoration is not needed. It is done with a compound (PREMA) having a mild concentration of 18% hydrochloric acid (HCl) and a fine-grit silicon carbide abrasive in a water-soluble gel, under the protection of rubber dam. A high torque-low rpm hand piece is used to rub this compound on the enamel surface. It leads to a uniform removal of an insignificant and undetectable amount of enamel (about 50–150 microns), and the decalcified tissue goes with it.

Microabrasion creates a smooth, polished "enamel glaze" layer by deposition and compacting of calcium and phosphate breakdown products which occur due to simultaneous erosive and abrasive action of microabrasion compound. In vitro polarized-light and SEM studies have shown this lustrous enamel glaze surface is more resistant to demineralization and colonization of *Streptococcus mutans*.

Air-powder Polishing

It can be an efficient and effective method for removal of stain and plaque. Air-powder polishing systems use air, water, and sodium bicarbonate to deliver a controlled stream that propels specially processed sodium bicarbonate particles to the tooth surface at 65 to 100 psi pressure. The particle size of the sodium bicarbonate is that which fits through a 200 mesh screen. This technique is time efficient and needs less physical exertion than polishing with a rubber cup and prophylaxis paste. In addition, no heat is generated with this type of system.

Also this does not damage either composite resin or zinc phosphate cement used to attach orthodontic brackets and bands when the spray is directed at a 90° angle to the bracket or band with the nozzle kept at a distance of 3 to 5 mm from the bracket or band. Handpiece should be positioned at 60° to gingiva for use on anterior teeth, 80° toward the gingiva for posterior teeth, whereas an angle of 90° has been recommended for occlusal surfaces. A constant circular motion should be used, with an exposure time of 30 to 60 seconds.

Fate of Enamel Scars

It has been found that demineralization ceases after the removal of fixed orthodontic appliances, which is due to removal of the overlying acid-producing plaque and improved accessibility to saliva, causing buffering action and recalcification of subsurface lesions and because of surface abrasion or from a reparative precipitation of mineral deposits. Fitzpatrick and Way had demonstrated that after acid etching the return to a normal enamel surface was due to a filling-in and not due to wearing away of the etched area. It has been suggested that polishing or abrasion of the dull and irregular enamel surface results in the exposure of the more tightly packed enamel crystals which give a harder and glossier clinical appearance.

It is important to enhance the remineralization by fluoride. So, routine fluoride mouthrinse serve a valuable purpose even after debonding. It has been suggested that lesions that develop in a highly fluoridated environment, during orthodontic treatment, may form a diffusion barrier against subsurface uptake of minerals from saliva, leaving the subsurface area hypomineralized. Such lesions do not disappear completely and remain as white spot after treatment. However, the appearance of white lesions can be improved by using hydrochloric acid-pumice microabrasion technique.

Conclusion

White spot lesions are one of the common complications of fixed orthodontic treatment. The orthodontist must minimize the risk of decalcification during orthodontic treatment. Thus the necessity for excellent oral hygiene practice must be explained. Patients must be advised a vigorous fluoride supplement using the mouthrinses to prevent enamel decalcification during and after fixed orthodontic treatment.

58

Lasers in Orthodontics

INTRODUCTION

'Laser' is an acronym for 'Light Amplification by Stimulated Emission of Radiation'. It is based on the Einstein's theory of stimulated emission of radiant energy. An active medium is stimulated to generate photons of energy, which are then released in a beam of specific wavelength unique to the active medium. In dental practice, laser is used as adjunctive tool for hard or soft tissue management procedures. Dental lasers produce light energy within a narrow frequency range.

Properties: Laser has two main properties:

1. **Monochromatic:** The energy emitted by lasers is of a single color.
2. **Coherence:** Laser light is coherent, i.e. each wavelength is of same size and shape. The photons are collimated into an intensely focussed energy beam. Dental tissues have a specific affinity to absorb laser energy of a specific wavelength. Wavelength of laser is the main determinant of the degree to which the laser energy is absorbed by the target tissue.

Basics of Laser Technology

Each laser releases a beam of light of a specific wavelength. Every target tissue has its own optical properties. These two factors determine laser–tissue interaction. Soft tissue lasers are diode laser, CO_2, neodymium-doped yttrium aluminum garnet (ND:YAG). For hard tissue, best choice is ER:YAG laser. The diode laser is the most suitable in orthodontics.

History: In 1960, Maiman, developed the first working laser device. In 1960, the first uranium laser was invented by IBM Laboratories. In 1961, Bell Laboratories invented the first helium-neon laser, while Robert Hall 1962 introduced the first semiconductor laser. Later on, Nd:YAG laser, CO_2 laser, argon laser in 1964, chemical laser in 1965 and metal vapor laser in 1966 were developed. In 1965, Goldman et al noticed painless surface crazing of the enamel. Subsequently, lasers were used for treatment of oral soft tissue lesions and periodontal procedures, tooth whitening, curing of composites, sulcular debridement, and removal of coronal pulp, RCT and for selective ablation of enamel caries. Use of lasers has seen an upsurge in orthodontic procedures, like bonding, debonding, craniofacial imaging, gingival contouring and prevention of enamel demineralization, etc.

Classifications of Lasers

Lasers can be variously classified, but a simplified classification is mentioned below. They are generally identified by the active medium which is used to generate the radiant energy.

According to the type of tissue on which laser is used:

a. **Hard tissue laser:** It is used to cut precisely into bone and teeth, to remove small amounts of tooth structure, to prepare teeth surfaces for bonding, and to repair certain dental restorations.
b. **Soft tissue lasers:** They penetrate soft tissue and seal blood vessels and nerve

endings. That is why no postoperative pain is felt and healing is faster.

Hard tissue laser equipment is costly, bulky and heavy. Soft laser instruments are cheap, light and handy and portable. Mostly, in dental practice, soft laser is used.

According to their mode of emission: They can be pulsed / fractioned / continuous.

According to their power: They can be high power / medium power / low power lasers

According to the emitting material: They can be gas laser / solid state laser / dye laser / semiconductor diode laser / ring laser.

According to their potential of causing biological hazard: It depends on the wattage emitted by the beams.

a. Class I: These lasers are found in laser caries detectors. Viewing these lasers with naked eye does not implicit any risk.
b. Class II: These lasers are found in laser pointers. There are risks in viewing light emissions, both to the naked eyes and when using magnification.
c. Class III: These are of three types, i.e. Class IIIa, IIIb and IIIr.

   Class IIIa lasers are non hazardous to an unprotected eye.

   Class IIIb lasers include 'soft' medical lasers, and laser measuring devices. These lasers can be hazardous to unprotected eyes if viewed directly or from reflected light. So the environmental controls, protective eyewear, and training in laser safety are required by personnel using these lasers.

   Class IIIr are include low-level medical devices and targeting lasers. The same safety measures as mentioned above are required.
d. Class IV: This class includes high-powered, surgical and other cutting lasers. All surgical lasers used in dentistry and in oral and maxillofacial surgery are included in this group. The protective measures are required. This group of lasers represents the greatest risk of damage, both to unprotected persons and target tissues.

Various Types of Lasers

Some of the common lasers used in dentistry are:

Argon laser: Argon lasers have an active medium of argon gas. It has two wavelengths, 488 nm (blue) and 514 nm (blue-green). They are poorly absorbed by dental hard tissues and water. The obvious advantage is that during soft tissues surgeries, there is no damage to tooth surface. Argon laser also illuminates the tooth and can be used for caries detection, the carious enamel appears of dark orange-red color.

Diode laser: Diode laser is a soft tissue laser. It is made of semiconductor crystals, which emit light when an electrical current passed through it. It is available in varying wavelength for dental use in the range of 800 to 980 nm. The semiconductor is made of either Al, Ga, Ar; or In, Ga, Ar. It is a soft tissue laser used for sulcular debridement and gingival surgeries. It is not well absorbed by dental hard tissues.

Nd:YAG laser: Its full name is yttrium-aluminum-garnet with neodymium, based on its composition. It is the first laser produced exclusively for dentistry. The available wavelength is 1,064 nm and is highly absorbed by water and pigmented tissues. It is absorbed slightly by dental hard tissues, thus allowing soft tissue surgery adjacent to the tooth to be safe without any effects on hard tissues. This laser is used in various periodontal procedures and cleaning of pigmented carious surface lesions. In orthodontics, it is used for debonding of brackets.

Ho:YAG laser: It has yttrium-aluminum-garnet with holmium as an active medium. The wavelength is 2120 nm. Its absorption by water is more than Nd:YAG but has little affinity for pigmented tissues. It is absorbed less by hard / tooth structure, thus the tissue surgery near the enamel, dentin or cementum is quite safe. The Ho:YAG laser is commonly used in TMJ surgery.

Er, Cr:YSGG and Er:YAG lasers: They have high wavelength range of 2790 nm and 2,940 nm, respectively. These are highly absorbed by water and hydroxyapatite and thus are ideal for caries removal and tooth preparation. Both lasers can ablate soft tissue readily because of its water content, but have limited hemostatic ability. They should be used with the water spray to avoid heat build up and pulpal damage. The advantage of these lasers is that a carious lesion in close proximity to the gingiva can be treated, and the soft tissue can be recontoured at the same time.

CO_2 laser: It is a gas-active medium laser and has a wavelength of 10,600 nm and is well absorbed by water. It is a rapid soft tissue remover and is useful in cutting dense fibrous tissue. It has the highest absorption in hydroxyapatite than any dental laser. It is useful in orthodontics for bracket debonding procedures.

Interaction with Biologic Tissues

Laser shows different types of interactions with the tissues as described below.

Photothermal interactions: Primary interaction of laser with the tissues is photothermal. When the tissue temperature reaches 100°C, the water of tissues boils and evaporates. It leads to soft tissue ablation. Beam size, power setting and the duration of exposure are the factors controlling the cutting efficiency of laser. In general, smaller the diameter of beam size, and greater the power density, the better is efficiency of laser to cut the tissues. Chromphores, e.g. Hb, melanin or other pigmented proteins are required to absorb the laser light which are present in soft tissues only. So the diode laser is not absorbed by hard tissue, ceramics, etc. And thus has no apparent effect on them.

Photochemical interactions: They include biostimulation, i.e. the stimulatory effects of laser on biochemical and molecular processes normally occurring in tissues, such as healing and repair.

Photomechanical interactions: Photomechanical interactions include photodisruption or photodissociation, i.e. the breaking of the structures apart by laser light and photoacoustic interactions which involve the removal of tissues with shock wave generation.

Photoelectrical interactions: Photoelectrical interactions include photoplasmolysis, i.e. the removal of tissues through the formation of electrically charged ions which exist in a semi-gaseous, high energy state.

Biological effects of laser: Lasers affect the biological response of the tissues by activation in ATP production; multiplication of collagen fibers; improvement of microcirculation; and increase in protein synthesis and DNA.

It thus helps in regulating the biological process; helps in regeneration of tissues; reestablishes equilibrium; and improves healing by better cellular reorganization.

Advantages

Laser has following advantages as compared to conventional surgical procedures:

- It provides painless, bloodless surgical field. There is increased coagulation of proteins in surgical field thus controlling the bleeding, leading to a dry field and thus better visualisation is there.
- It also helps in faster healing; lesser post-surgical swelling, edema, scarring, less pain.
- Increased patient acceptance.

Ideal average therapeutic dose is 4 joules/ cm^2 of energy; it should be directed perpendicular to the tissues. There should be maximum contact between tissue surface and tip of device. The therapeutic effect is not limited to the tip spot, but also includes the area of energy distribution.

Orthodontic Applications of Laser

Laser has found widespread use in dentistry in various procedures especially involving soft tissues. Some of the uses in dentistry are:

1. Cavity formation by hard tissue lasers.
2. Retraction and surgical removal of the soft tissues for better impression making after crown cutting.
3. Desensitizing the aphthous ulcers
4. Gingival contouring
5. Better soft tissue contouring around implants.
6. Gingivectomy and gingivoplasty; exposure of impacted teeth; removing the gingival interference from the eruption path of teeth
7. Root canal treatment
8. As a diagnostic tool, e.g. diagnosis of cuspal factures.

Laser has been used widely in the clinical orthodontics and the manufacturing of orthodontic components also. Laser can be used for following purposes in orthodontics.

1. **Laser etching of enamel for direct bonding:** Laser etching of enamel can be done with lasers to prepare for the direct bonding. Light energy acts as a thermal energy, which causes ablation of enamel surface. Etching occurs by direct vaporization and microexplosions of water entrapped in hydroxyapetite matrix of enamel. Experiments of shear bond strength testing have shown that the composite bonded to laser etched enamel would fail without fracturing the enamel, which indicates that the laser treatment does not make the enamel brittle. Also, the time required for laser etching is far less than the acid etching, laser etching takes 12 seconds. Laser etching is safe to pulp. Due to the extremely short pulse length of some nanoseconds and sudden removal, there is no sufficient heat conduction through the hard substance and thus there is no harmful increase in the temperature of the pulp.
2. **Polymerization of light-cure adhesive:** *Laser bonding:* Argon laser is used for light curing the orthodontic adhesives during bonding. After etching with 37% phosphoric acid for 15 seconds, the enamel surface is treated with the primer. The brackets are bonded with laser at a 10 sec exposure time per bracket. No enamel damage occurs by argon lasers at energy levels of 1.6 to 6 watts. It has been found that curing with argon laser produces bond strengths comparable to those achieved with 20 to 40 seconds of curing with a conventional high intensity light. Decreased curing time for bonding orthodontic appliance is an important for better efficiency during treatment. Camphorquinone is the photoinitiator present in visible-light-cured composite adhesives, which is highly sensitive to blue part of visible light at 470 nm. The argon laser is having single wavelength, enhances better bonding by achieving a more thorough curing in a less exposure time. Curing time of 10 seconds with argon laser is required. Studies to compare microleakage **after bonding by** using argon laser, halogen light and the plasma arc found that the microleakage is less in argon lasers bonded samples as compared to other curing methods. The bracket bond strength is increased with laser bonding as some studies have shown that the laser treated teeth may show increased bond strength.
3. **Laser debonding of ceramic brackets:** Enamel and bracket fractures and cracks are the common problems during debonding of ceramic brackets. Lasers can be used for debonding the ceramic brackets easily and safely. It occurs by degrading the bonding resins by thermal softening or photoablation of resin adhesive by the laser-induced heat transmitted through brackets to the resin. Studies found that no enamel and bracket damage occurred during debonding by lasers. The debonding of polycrystalline brackets occurs by thermal softening of the bonding resin resulting from heating of the bracket by laser energy. The hot bracket then

slides off the tooth. Ideal debonding time is 0.5 seconds. There is no adverse pulp reaction during this time. Pulp irritation increases only with increased lasing time.

4. **Management of impacted teeth:** Diode soft tissue laser is used to remove overlying tissues to provide access to the crown for placing an orthodontic attachment. Operculum on second molar often prevents banding of these teeth, so the clinician has to wait for its further eruption and thus it results in the increased treatment time. The diode laser can be used to remove the soft tissue and thus providing the place for placing the bracket or band.
5. **Gingival shaping and recontouring: Gingivoplasty/gingivectomy:** Gingival problems, like gingival margin discrepancies and improper zenith locations; hyperplasia, sharp interdental papillae and tapered gingival margins, gingival polyp/growth, etc. Adolescent patients generally have short clinical crowns due to incomplete eruption of teeth or asymmetric crown heights, and rolled margins due to improper oral hygiene. Gingival recontouring can be easily done with a diode laser. The diode laser does not cut hard tissues thus making it ideal for gingival contouring without risk of damage to the teeth. Other advantages of a diode laser are that it creates a bloodless field by coagulation of tissues, and thus better visibility and clear field; it helps in sterilization of surgical field; and it seals the tissues as it incises, thus creating a "**biological dressing**".
6. **Crown lengthening:** Crown lengthening by doing gingivectomy helps to enhance the aesthetics by improving tooth-to-tooth ratio; gingival contouring, matching the marginal gingival levels, etc.
7. **Frenectomy: Abnormally attached** frenal attachments can be relieved by using the soft tissue laser. It thus helps in removal of the causes of midline diastema, recession of marginal gingiva; relieving tongue tie and thus improving speech, etc.
8. **Prevention of enamel scars: Laser exposed enamel has better** resistance to acid attack. Research has shown that argon laser irradiation of enamel reduced the amount of demineralization by 30–50%. Combining laser irradiation with fluoride treatment could have a synergistic effect on acid resistance.
9. **Low-level laser treatment (LLLT) in reducing orthodontic post-adjustment pain:** Laser in the form of LLLT has been used to reduce pain in many clinical situations. In LLLT, a low energy output is used, so that the temperature of treated tissues is not increased above 36.5 C or normal body temperature. Biostimulatory effects of LLLT help in its anti-inflammatory and neuronal effects. According to Harris, LLLT stimulates the depressed neuronal and lymphocyte respiration. It helps in stabilization of membrane potential and release of neurotransmitters. Although LLLT is unable to provide immediate pain relief, it has a potential in reducing the intensity of pain with one or two applications. Orthodontic pain can be controlled by laser therapy, e.g. Nd:YAG, He:Ne, and CO_2 laser. Low-level CO_2 laser therapy can be used in reducing pain in patients with TMD problems. Analgesic action is due to that it prevents the formation of action potential in the peripheral nerves affecting the conduction of nervous stimuli. Also, there is an increase encephalin and endorphin synthesis in lab animals after single LLLT session. It helps in formation of microcirculation, improves tissue nutrition and peripheral nerve regeneration and tissue repair.

10. **Laser holography: Image scanning and reconstruction (holography):** A hologram is a recording of an interference pattern made by the interaction of two beams of light. It has been used to study the tooth positions on dental casts at different stages. Burstone and coworkers used pulsed laser hologram inferometry to study the dynamics of incisor extrusion. Holography is a wave front reconstruction technique in which low coherent beams converge to produce an interference pattern which is recorded in a film. The recorded three-dimentional (3D) image is called a hologram. 3D digital imaging of the craniofacial region can be done by laser holography techniques. Various applications of laser holography in orthodontics are: facial soft tissue analysis and digital models. Holograms are less prone to damage; a minimal storage space is required and is readily available chair side. Its disadvantages are that holograms are less convenient to some clinicians because of the inability to place holograms immediately next to the patient and to make detailed side to side comparisons. Some holograms may be somewhat harder to see in sufficient detail which makes them less informative.
11. **3D laser scanning:** Scanning can be used to record the dental casts, intraoral dental relation, tissues, facial morphology, etc. in the digital form, which can be used for storage, making virtual models, using them for CAD-CAM purpose; for making orthodontic appliances, and wires, invisalign, etc. Hand-held scanner in the form of a laser scanning wand is used in smoothly sweeping motion over an object to acquire three dimensional surfaces by gathering measurements in 3 coordinates. The details are fed directly in a computer and processed by a software to construct a 3D virtual model of the object.
12. **Laser spectroscopy:** It is used to analyze the surface structures of dental materials, e.g. it is used for evaluating the surface roughness of orthodontic wires, brackets, comparison of different materials, surface changes of orthodontic materials during use, etc.
13. **Measurement of pulpal blood flow during orthodontic treatment:** Orthodontic treatment causes a decrease in blood flow to the pulp. Pulpal blood flow decreases when continuous light tipping forces are applied. Nowadays, laser-Doppler flowmetry is a commonly used method to determine the pulpal blood flow.
14. **Laser-orthopedics:** Laser can be used in controlling the growth of facial structures. Light energy lasers might be applied to manipulate human facial growth to treat the problems of either overgrowth or undergrowth. Low energy laser at 650 nm is applied which affects the cartilaginous growth of condyles. Diode laser has also been tried in animals for controlling the excessive growth of the mandibular condyle and it was found that a laser is effective in regulating facial growth. It could be a substitute for current conventional methods such as a chin-cup in future.
15. **Treatment of dentinal hypersensitivity:** DH occurs due to exposed dentinal tubules. About 15,000–40,000 tubules/sq. mm are exposed. The hydrodynamic theory of Branstrom is most accepted theory explaining DH, i.e. there is movement of fluids in the tubules which exert pressure on odontoblasts and stimulate adjacent nerve fibers. Low-level laser therapy (LLLT) causes formation of reparative/tertiary dentin sealing the canaliculi and thus flow of fluid in tubules is eliminated. It also decreases the pain intensity due to maintenance of resting potential of nociceptors.

(Dose = 4J / cm^2 distributed at 4 points, i.e. 1 J / cm^2 at each point).

16. **Diagnosis of carious lesion:** Fluorescent laser diagnosis (Diagnodent) is a new method which detects lesion by measuring the quantity of fluorescent light irradiated from tooth demineralisation. Fluorescence occurs in organic part of tissues; larger the demineralized area, higher the values observed by equipment. 655 nm diode laser is used. When laser penetrates a tissue of heterogenous texture, e.g. demineralised dentin and enamel, the phenomenon of multiple refractions among its crystals takes place. Light diffuses as it falls upon demineralized tissue and it is absorbed by fluorophors in organic content. These fluorophors reemit laser light with longer wavelength. This phenomenon is called fluorescence. Laser can detect the carious lesion through fluorescence of carious dentin.

Uses of laser in manufacturing process of orthodontic materials:

1. **Laser welding:** Laser welding has the advantage of welding dissimilar metals while producing very low heat. It produces deep penetration welds with minimum heat effective zones. It is a non-contact process using a laser output of 2–10 kW into a very small area. The laser beam makes a 'keyhole' and the liquid steel solidifies behind the traversing beam, leaving a very narrow weld and heat-affected zone (HAZ). The weld is approximately 1 mm wide and the surrounding material is not distorted. Because the weld bead is small, there is usually no need for finishing or reworking and this reduces costs. Since there is no heat production, the metal does not become dead and thus does not lose its properties.

   Orthophaser: This is an argon laser welder, bigger than the conventional spot welder. All metals including titanium can be welded with it and it provides a strong weld.
2. **Laser welding of commercially available pure titanium:** Titanium is used in dentistry for crowns, bridges and partial denture framework. Titanium is a highly reactive metal and forms an oxide layer in contact with air giving a passivating effect to the surface, i.e. converting it into a passive state. Thus a proper solder or weld is not formed by conventional soldering / welding process, thereby debonding occurs from the parent metal. Laser welding in an argon gas atmosphere is done to join the titanium components. Its advantage is that the metal is subjected to very minimal heat and hence the welded joint has same pure titanium as the substrate components. The joint is stronger.

   Advantages of laser welding: The quality and strength of joint is very high. It can weld high alloy metals without difficulty. It can be used in open air. It involves minimal heat generation and has a narrow heat affected zone. It can weld dissimilar metals. It does not need any filler metals. The joint is clean and thus no secondary finishing is needed, thus reducing the cost. It is an extremely accurate process.

   Disadvantages of laser welding: The equipment is very costly. Rapid cooling rate may cause cracking in certain metals. High maintenance cost is involved with the equipment. Thus laser welding process can be incorporated in the manufacturing facilities with high turnover. **Fully automated laser welder** has been developed specifically for joining orthodontic brackets to their pads, customized weld spot sizes.
3. **Intraoral laser microwelding:** Neodymium laser equipment has been used for intraoral microwelding. It is safe intraorally and does no damage to dental tissues. It can be used for placement of space maintainers, orthodontic retainers, periodontal splints, hooks and

brackets to existing bands, wires and auxiliaries. It eliminates time consuming procedures like removal of whole arch wire, eliminates the need of laboratory steps for soldering/welding etc.

4. **Bracket mesh designing:** Laser has been applied during designing and manufacturing of orthodontic brackets also. Brackets with laser reinforced bases enable the force to be applied even closer to the crown. The laser structured base and mesh of brackets results in a better bond and thus less failure rate during the treatment.
5. **Laser markings:** Laser has been used to put non-erasable markings on the brackets in the form of numbering of tooth, arrow markings for proper direction and placement of bracket on the tooth. The advantages of laser markings on brackets are: for Easy identification of brackets; It cannot be abraded; It does not contain harmful coloring agents like regular markings.

Dental Laser Safety

Safety is an integral part of providing dental treatment with a laser instrument. There are three main factors to achievelaser safety, i.e.

a. The proper manufacturing and maintenance of the instrument
b. Proper handling and operation of device
c. Personal protection of the surgical team and patient.

Harmful effects of laser: Laser is also not free of harmful effects on the operator and patient, as some have been discussed below.

- **Pulpal damage:** Polymerizing the composite resins can increase intrapulpal temperature. The temperature increase should not exceed 55°C for proper uneventful recovery of pulp. Resin polymerization by argon laser is safer for pulp as the temperature is not increased much.
- **Eye damage:** Correct protective eyewear while using dental lasers is essential because it can damage various parts of unprotected eyes. It can cause ablation, scarring and distortion of vision, and retinal damage.
- **Skin risks:** Lasers can cause "skin burns" due to ablative interaction with chromophores.
- **Laser plume:** When non-calcified tissue is ablated, e.g. caries removal and soft tissue surgery, a complex chemical mixture of water vapor, carbon monoxide and dioxide, hydrocarbon gases and particulate organic material, bacterial and viral products, etc. is emitted, collectively termed a "laser plume". Plume inhalation can cause nausea, breathing difficulties and distant inoculation of bacteria.
- **Fire and explosion hazards:** Proper precautions like avoiding inflammable materials in the operating area. Protection of healthy tissue adjacent to the surgical site is required.

Conclusion

Laser is a very effective treatment modality both for hard tissue and soft tissue procedures in the field of dentistry. It can provide more comfortable, efficient and predictable outcomes in certain dental treatments. It has also made inroads in the clinics of orthodontists with its use in various applications in clinical, research as well as manufacturing processes pertinent to orthodontics. In future, with continued research, its use in orthodontics will make the life of clinicians and patients a lot easier, with its successful effects on growth of jaws, orthodontic movements, and pain control.

59

Magnets in Orthodontics

INTRODUCTION

In dental field, magnets were used initially for denture or maxillofacial prostheses retention. The magnets most commonly used were made of either aluminum-nickel-cobalt (AlNiCo) or platinum-cobalt (PtCo) alloys. In the 1970s and 1980s, rare earth magnets, i.e. samarium-cobalt (SmCo) and neodymium (NdFeB) magnets came in existence having improved properties. Use of magnets in orthodontics was introduced by Blechman and Smiley. First magnetic orthodontic brackets were designed by Kawata et al in 1977, made of iron-cobalt and chrome alloy, but were not used widely due to inferior properties. Later on, rare earth magnets were made which have better properties and produced sufficient tooth moving forces.

Biological Implications

Studies found the corrosion resistance of SmCo magnet similar to dental casting alloys and the magnet had virtually no toxic or other negative effects on the tissues. It was concluded that SmCo magnets could be safely used as a dental material after proper coating of magnets to seal them from oral environment to decrease their corrosive activity. Animal studies have shown that SmCo magnets have no adverse effects on blood cells; no change in dental pulp, periodontal and gingival tissues, buccal mucosa or alveolar bone.

Darendeliler et al., (1993) studied the effects of pulsed electromagnetic fields (PEMF) and static magnetic fields (SMF) on the rate and quality of hard tissue repair and found faster wound healing; increased amounts of bone formation and hard tissue density in the osteotomy sites. Another study on the rate of orthodontic upper incisor movement showed a significant increase in the rate of tooth movement for both PEMF and SMF. A reduced 'lag phase', and an increased organization and amount of new bone between the incisors was found.

Coulombs law: This law states that force between two magnetic poles is directly proportional to magnitude and inversely proportional to square of the distance between them.

Advantages of Magnets

1. They can be used for frictionless mechanics in attractive configuration.
2. They provide a predictable force level.
3. There is no force decay associated with the material structure and crystallographic make-up of the material, as in arch wires.
4. During the guided eruption of impacted teeth, there is reduced irritation of palatal mucosa.
5. There is more control over force application.
6. Requirement for patient cooperation is less.
7. Magnets apply light forces and thus there is decreased risk of external root resorption.

Disadvantages of Magnets

1. Decrease in force with increasing distance between magnets during repulsive mode.
2. Corrosive products may pose some toxicity or localised reactions.
3. Increased bulk of appliance with magnets.
4. Unpredictable forces in repulsive mode.
5. Expensive
6. Since there are less clinical studies, the use of magnets is still very limited in orthodontic clinics.

Types of Magnetic Materials

- Platinum-cobalt (Pt-co)
- Aluminum-nickel-cobalt (Al-Ni-Co)
- Ferrite
- Chromium-cobalt-iron
- Samarium-cobalt (Sm-Co)
- Neodymium-iron-boron

Clinical Application of Magnets

Magnets can be used for many purposes in orthodontics:

1. Tooth movements
2. Tooth intrusion
3. Expansion
4. Tooth impaction
5. Space closure
6. Molar distalization
7. Magnetic edgewise brackets
8. Functional appliances.
9. Retainers.

Tooth movement: Magnets provide relatively continuous and consistent force and lead to more rapid tooth movement, are less traumatic; and safe in oral environment. Blechman (1985) used magnets for intra- and intermaxillary force application and found them to be superior to intermaxillary elastics, as they provided a better control of force and required no patient cooperation.

Molar distalization: Repelling magnets can be used for distalization of maxillary molars, with a modified Nance appliance to augment the anchorage. The molars can be distalized at a rate of nearly 0.75–1 mm per month. Molar movement is faster when second molars are absent and it results in less anchorage loss. However, with distalization, the distance between the magnets increases and hence the repelling force decreases.

Space closure: Magnets can be used for space closure, e.g. magnets in attracting mode are used for median diastema closure. Similarly, the canines can be retracted using magnetic method, it helps to reduce the treatment time, no pain or discomfort, periodontal problems, root resorption, etc.

Root extrusion: Magnets have been used to extrude the roots/root eruption in case of traumatised tooth to increase the crown height and thus enabling a better accessibility for endodontics and prosthesis.

Eruption of impacted teeth: Magnets can be used for guided eruption of impacted canine and unerupted premolars. After surgical exposure of an impacted tooth, a magnet is bonded to the tooth surface and the mucosal flap is sutured in place, completely covering the tooth with its bonded magnet. Guided eruption of impacted tooth is achieved by placing a second intraoral magnet in a removable plate and placed in such a way as to attract the submucosal magnet.

Expansion: Vardimon et al. in 1987 used repulsive magnets for maxillary expansion. They devised two types of magnetic expansion device (MED), one is bonded type, and other is banded type, which applied around 250–500 grams of force. Tooth borne appliance and Tissue borne appliance configurations can be made.

Skeletal class II correction: Many appliances have been designed for skeletal class II correction. Vardimon et al. (1989) designed FOMA II, a functional orthopedic magnetic appliance. It has magnets in anterior part places in attractive mode and it protrudes the mandible as a result of attraction.

Magnetic activator device (MAD): Darendilier (1993) developed a series of magnetically active functional appliance of different varieties to be used in different conditions, e.g.

- MAD I s used to treat mandibular deviations.
- MAD II is used to correct class II malocclusions.
- MAD III is used to correct class III malocclusions.
- MAD IV is used to correct open bite malocclusions.

MAD II corrects skeletal and dental class II malocclusion by growth modification with minimal dental effects. Clark (1996) introduced magnetic twin block appliances which have samarium cobalt magnets embedded in inclined surfaces of the twin block in attractive mode.

Skeletal class III correction: A FOMA III appliance with two magnets in attractive force configuration placed in anterior region was designed by Vardimon et al. (1992) for the treatment of class III malocclusions. This activator has upper and lower plates having two pairs of attracting magnets placed in sagittal direction to pull the mandible distally and the maxilla mesially.

Correction of open bite: Active vertical corrector was the first appliance designed for open bite treatment, introduced by Dellinger in 1986. Samarium cobalt magnets were used in the repelling mode in the posterior region to cause intrusion of posterior teeth. This appliance was considered as an 'energized' bite block. It can be made as removable or fixed appliance. The MAD IV, was designed in 1989 for correction of open bites. It has a combination of posterior repulsive and anterior attractive magnets. It has an advantage of guiding the mandible to a midline centric position due to attractive forces. These anterior attractive magnets have anterior closing effect by extrusive action on anterior teeth, and they also accentuate and facilitate the anterior rotation of the mandible. Three types of MAD IV have been designed to be used in different types of open bite cases:

a. MAD IV-a is used in cases which need posterior intrusion and mandibular autorotation are required, i.e. gummy smile cases;
b. MAD IV-b is used where an additional extrusive effect is also needed in the anterior maxilla; and
c. MAD IV-c is used if only extrusion of anterior area of maxilla is needed.

Magnetic retainer: The use of magnets has also been reported to retain treated teeth. For example, in a case report by Springate and Sandler (1992), small, thin NdFeB magnets were bonded on the palatal surfaces of upper incisors in order to prevent re-opening of a diastema.

Conclusion

Magnets have been used in orthodontic and dentofacial orthopedics since last few years. Magnets have tendency of getting oxidized in oral cavity and formation of corrosive products, leading to deterioration of magnetic properties. It can be overcome by coating magnets. Also, the magnetic force between two magnets has a negative correlation with the square of the distance between them, and thus the force markedly increases in attraction and decreases in repulsion. Some advantages and disadvantages of magnets have been identified over traditional techniques. The advantages of magnets over traditional systems are the frictionless mechanics, especially when magnets are oriented in attractive configuration; predictable force levels, no force decay over time and lesser need of patient co-operation. Main disadvantages involved are due to size, i.e. an increased bulk of appliance. Also there is a limited three-dimensional control in repulsive magnets configuration. Magnets also require a coating to prevent corrosion and there may be possible side effects of corrosive products.

60

Soldering and Welding in Orthodontics

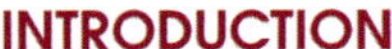

INTRODUCTION

The force is applied to the teeth with the help of various appliances which may be removable or fixed or combination. The appliances are retained intraorally with the help of various wire components. Some of the components of the appliances can be directly attached to the teeth, while others need to be supported by each other. It needs the attachment of the various metal parts to each other to make an assembly most useful for the situation.

The removable appliances need joining of certain clasps, hooks, labial bow to clasp, buccal tube to clasps, etc. to help in force application and for attachment of elastics, etc. The all-wire form of removable retainer which does not contain acrylic but only wire-components, all the wire components are joined together to form a single assembly.

In fixed appliances, the conventions fabrication of molar and other bands needs the joining of ends of band material strip together. The attachment of certain components, e.g. buccal tube/brackets, etc. need a mechanism of attachment of metal parts together.

Sometimes, hooks are required to be attached to arch wires for attaching the elastics. The heavy wires are used to attach on the bands to augment the anchorage. Nowadays, many of the prefabricated components are available in the market which are joined together with different forms of attachment processes, and have improved the clinical efficiency of the orthodontist by reducing his lab efforts.

Soldering and Welding

Most often, following two procedures are used by an orthodontist in his clinic to join the metal parts and make an assembly of appliances for various use in his patients.

1. Soldering
2. Welding.

Some of the common definitions are as below:

Soldering: Soldering is defined as the procedure of joining two metal parts by using an intervening filler metal at a temperature below the solidus temperature of the parts being joined and done at a temperature below 450°C. The molten solder flows between the two parts by capillary action.

Brazing: It is defined as the joining of two metals using a filler metal at a temperature below the solidus temperature of the metals being joined and at a temperature above 450°C. Thus, the difference between soldering and brazing is the difference between the liquidus temperature of filler metal.

Welding: It is defined as the joining of two or more metals without using an intervening filler/metal. It is done by applying heat/pressure or both to produce localized union across interface by fusion or diffusion.

Difference between soldering and welding/brazing is the possible absence of filler metal and partial fusion of parts being joined by welding.

Cast joining: It is the joining of two metal parts of FPD, by base metal alloys by using a molten alloy in between the interface region of the invested parts.

Required Features of a Dental Solder

1. It should possess equivalent strength as that of metal parts.
2. The corrosion resistance should be good.
3. Fusion temperature of solder should be 50–100°C less than the parts being joined so that excessive heat does not transfer to the parts, thus maintaining their properties of strength and elasticity.
4. It should be free flowing and should properly wet the metal parts being joined.
5. Color of solder should match the parts being joined.

Components of Soldered Joint

A soldered joint has the following components:

- Parent metal: These are the parts to be joined together.
- Solder metal: It is the filler metal used to join two or more parent metal parts.
- Flux
- Antiflux.

Solder

It is a filler material which has lower fusion temperature than the parts to be joined. Fusion temperature of the solder **should be 50–100°C less than** the parts to be joined. It should have the melting point in 28–56°C of solidus temperature of the metal units.

Types of Solder

Mostly, they are of two types, i.e. hard and soft.

Solders above 650 fine should not be used where considerable stress is involved.

In orthodontics, the MP of solder should be less than that of the SS wire, so gold solder cannot be used. Silver solder should be used to which Sn and In are added to decrease the fusion temperature and improve solderability. Cu increases the melting range. Ag narrows the melting range, more free flowing, greater adherence to the metals. Solder temperature is in the range of 620–665°C, and solidus–liquidus ranges of the solders should be small. Solder is **anodic to SS,** so it leads to corrosion.

Flux

Flux means "to flow". Flux helps to remove the oxide layer from the surfaces of metals being joined. The solder will flow and join that area only which have been deoxidized by the flux. It displaces gas layer and tarnish film, protects surface from oxidation.

Flux = borax + boric acid.

Borax = 55%, sodium perborate is better,

Boric acid = 35%—it decreases the fusion-point.

Silica = 10%, gives viscosity and toughness.

Flux contains **fluorides/KF** to **dissolve the passivating film** of chromium while soldering for better union.

Boric acid is more in conc. than in gold solders as it decreases the fusion temperature.

Types of Fluxes

Different types of fluxes used are:

1. Surface protection type: It prevents the formation of oxide layer on the metal surface. It covers the metal surface and prevents oxygen contact.
2. Reducing agent type: It reduces any oxide present and exposes the metal surface.
3. Solvent type: It dissolves the oxides and drives them away.

According to composition:

- Borax fluxes: Which contain sodium borate, sodium tetraborate; disodium tetraborate.
- Fluoride fluxes: Which has mainly potassium fluoride, KF 50–60%; + boric acid 25–35%; borax glass 6–8%; potassium carbonate 8–10%.

According to the pH: Fluxes can be of three types:

- Acidic flux: SiO_2
- Basic fluxes: CaO, $CaCO_3$, lime stone
- Neutral: e.g. fluorspar, CaF_2; Borax, $Na_2B_4O_2$

Most commonly, a superflux is used which contains borax glass 55% + boric acid 35% + silica 10%.

Antiflux: It is the material used to restrict the area of flow of flux during heating and melting of flux. It thus prevents over-flow of solder metal during soldering, i.e. confines the flow of solder. A low temperature of solder (than the metal parts being joined) is preferred to prevent carbide precipitation and thus weakening of the wire/metal parts. So, the silver solders are preferred for orthodontic purpose. The wettability of the metal parts by solder is also an important feature. The solder chosen should have a low contact angle so that it can wet a larger area and thus the joint formed is stronger. Graphite, rouge or lead pencil is used as antiflux. It is applied before applying the flux or solder.

Types of Soldering

- Soldering can be of two types, i.e. investment soldering and free hand soldering.
- Flame soldering (different flammable gases mixed with compressed air or oxygen)
- Post-soldering (porcelain furnace)
- Infrared soldering (IR).

Types of Welding

- Resistance welding (spot-welding)
- Plasma welding (torch)
- Laser welding (Nd:YAG laser machines)
- Single pulse tungsten inert gas welding (TIG).

Different Equipments Used

- Flame soldering torch
- Hydrosolder machine
- Electric solder
- Spot-welding machine
- Laser welding.

Investment soldering: Here the metal parts being joined are fixed in the investment material so that they are precisely placed. It is also used when the gap between the parts is more. It is used when precision of joint is needed, e.g. during repair of parts of cast partial denture and FPDs. Soldering investment is the same as quartz investment, also investment with low NSE is better than higher.

Free hand soldering: In orthodontics, mainly free hand soldering is used as precision of parts being joined is not needed that much. The parts being joined are stabilized with POP or clamps, etc. without investing them, and soldering is carried out with hand held microtorch or hydrosolder unit.

Steps in soldering:

- Cleaning of the ends of the parts: Irregular ends should be smoothened for better contact.
- Assembling and approximation of part ends with minimal gap in between: parts should be adequately assembled at proper position to produce adequate appliance.
- Flux application: Wet flux is placed in the areas to be joined, and it should be limited by antiflux.
- Flux heating and melting/diffusion.
- Heating and flow of solder: The reducing zone of the flame is used to prevent oxidation of the metals.
- Controlling the spread of heat to adjacent areas which is done by placing wet cotton near the area being heated, if possible.
- Cooling and quenching of parts: Wait for few seconds before quenching. Immediate quenching makes the area soft.
- Smoothening and finishing: The soldered area is lightly smoothened and polished to make is comfortable.

Solder joints: A proper solder joint should be used for maximum strength of the joint. Point contact is weakest. The wire end can be wrapped over the other part for increased area of contact. It provides best type of joint. Larger area of the joining by placing wire bends at ends and soldering them also increases the area of joint. Maximum strength is attained if soldered parts are cooled slowly for 5–7 min. and then quenched. Total bench cooling causes brittleness. **Gap** between the parts to be soldered should be = 0.13 mm/ 0.005". **Reducing zone** of the flame should be used. Color of the parts being joined should never exceed the dull-red during heating. If color becomes bright-red, it leads to dead softening of the wire parts, they become brittle and plastic. Use as little heat as possible, for the least possible time to avoid carbide precipitates, loss of strength, etc.

Uses of soldering in orthodontics:

1. It is used to join various clasps; labial bows, etc. to each other in the removable appliances.
2. It is used to make various appliances, e.g. space maintainers; TPA, LHA, expansion appliances, etc.
3. An all-wire removable appliance definitely needs soldering of various parts to be joined.
4. Soldering is used to join hooks to arch wires for attaching elastics, headgear hooks, etc.
5. After spot welding of molar tubes to the molar bands, the soldering is used to make the joint stronger to avoid of loss of tube during the treatment.
6. Solder can also be flown on the seam after band fabrication to make the seams smoother to avoid soft tissue irritation.
7. Soldering is used to join inner and outer bows of face bow during conventional chairside fabrication of the face bow.
8. Soldering is used to make the ball-end clasps to be used in removable appliances, e.g. twin block appliance, so make the ends smoother.

Welding

It is the process of joining two or more metal parts directly under pressure without using a filler material. Cold welding is done by pressure or hammering. Hot welding uses heat of adequate intensity to melt the metal parts being joined together. In orthodontics, mainly spot-welding is used, which generates the heat through electric current. The copper electrodes are used in spot welder, between which the metal parts to be joined are placed and held under pressure. Current is passed through them for a very short time to prevent change in physical properties of the materials being joined. The heat generated leads to softening of the metal parts and pressure leads to their squeezing together and joining. The size of the electrodes is important for the processes. A thin electrode is used for joining thick materials while a thick electrode is used to join thin materials. It is because the high heat generated has to be localized and used to join thick metal parts, while for joining thin parts, the heat generated has to be dissipated to avoid heat localization in the parts being welded.

Welding is used in orthodontics to fabricate bands; to attach the attachments to bands; to join hooks to wires and to join the wire parts together.

Principle of Spot-Welding

Heat and pressure are used during spot-welding process. Electric current (A/C; low volt, high amperage) is passed through the electrodes. The resistance offered by metal parts to be joined generates high temperature at electrodes. Thus the area of metals under the electrodes becomes plastic, which then get joined by the pressure being applied by the electrodes. The current should be passed for a very short period, i.e. 1/10th of a second. If current is passed for a longer duration, it may results in weld decay due to precipitation of carbides from the metal parts. This carbide joint has less corrosion resistance. To avoid this, the spot welders are fitted with a timer to control the passage of current.

Procedure of Spot-Welding

The electrodes should be free of carbide; they should be smooth and flat. They should be in total contact and perpendicular to its long axis. The timer of the welder is set to the required reading. The parts are placed between the electrodes and current is passed.

The pressure is maintained for few seconds to obtain the good joint. Spot welder is used in orthodontics. The weld spot is seen as **nugget** of the resolidified cast structure. Strength of weld joint decreases by increasing recrystallization of wrought structures. Weld joint is **susceptible to corrosion** due to chromium carbide precipitates and loss of passivation.

Uses of welding in orthodontics:

1. Band fabrication on teeth
2. To join hooks on archwires, e.g. TMA wires are weldable.
3. Fixing brackets, tubes, lingual sheaths on the bands.

Effects of soldering and welding: Heat used during soldering gets transferred to the adjoining metal parts thus reducing their strength. Also localized heat is produced during welding process which leads to formation of carbide precipitates which help in forming a weld of metal parts. This carbide makes the joint prone to corrosion and also decreases the strength of the joint. It may reduce corrosion resistance because of galvanic corrosion between metals. The high corrosion rates can influence the biocompatibility. Research has shown that there is superior biological quality of laser-welding over brazing. Traditional silver solder has been found to be toxic for osteoblast differentiation, fibroblast viability and keratinocyte growth.

Laser welding in orthodontics: To weld dental alloys, crystals of yttrium aluminum garnet (YAG) doped with neodymium (Nd) are mainly used to emit laser beams (Nd:YAG laser). The factors affecting the mechanical strength of laser welded joints are the wave length, peak pulse duration, power and pulse energy, output energy, pulse frequency, and spot diameter of laser-welding machine, and the type of metal used. It is widely used in orthodontic manufacturing process, e.g. the buccal tubes are laser-welded to the molar bands in preformed, prewelded molar bands. Laser welding is also used in laboratories to make appliances, like space maintainers, TPA and LHA, etc. Laser welding is also used to make various orthodontic appliances like Jones jig, face bows, myofunctional appliances, removable retainers, etc. An accurate fit and gap-free preparation of the parts to be joined is needed for successful welding. Parts must be prepared so that they lie flat against one another to join these parts directly to one another without using filler material. Laser welding should always be done under a protective argon atmosphere in order to prevent any oxidation of the weld. This is essential to give it the strength it requires. The welding spots must have a metallic lustre.

Benefits of laser welding: There is zero heat transmission to wire parts or molar bands reducing breakage. It is 260% stronger than soldering. Laser welding reduces bulkiness of appliances due very small weld joints, and offers a 96% alloy retention.

Tungsten inert gas (TIG) welding: It is an **arc welding** process. The welding heat is produced with a light bow between tungsten anode and metal. Laser and TIG welding can weld parent metals without use of a solder or any other metal. Therefore, the corrosion resistance may be increased because the same metal is used. Studies have shown that laser and TIG welding are solder-free alternatives for joining the metal parts. TIG welding needs less investment and is comparable with laser welding. However the laser technique is a sophisticated and simple method, but is expensive.

Heat treatment: It is the process of heating the wires to remove the residual stresses after cold working. A low-temperature heat treatment is done for orthodontic appliances made of stainless steel. The wire is passed over the flame and heated till its color changes to straw-color. Research has shown that heat treatment leads to changes in mechanical behavior, and in particular causes a marked increase in elastic strength. The increased elastic strength is the most significant effect of heat treatment. An elastically stronger working appliance is more likely to return to its original shape without any permanent deflection, and remains active to apply the force. It has been found that twenty minutes at 500°F; ten minutes at 750–820°F are adequate for heat treatment. The heat treatment should be done carefully not to heat the wire components to "red-hot", as it leads to dead softening status of the wire, which becomes weak and brittle and does not apply any force.

61

Computer Applications in Orthodontics

INTRODUCTION

Computers are widely used in every field of life, and have made deep inroads in medical field also. No aspect of medical / dental field is untouched with computers use. Orthodontics is no exception. Computers have become an important part of everyone's life. Computer uses in orthodontics are not entirely new. The history of computer applications for orthodontics can be traced back for decades. Basic parts of the desktop computers are the CPU, monitor, mouse, key board, UPS. But with constant innovation in computer field, the desktop is going to be in oblivion very soon. Now a days, the people are widely using laptops, i-pads, galaxy tabs, etc. for daily uses, even in the clinical settings.

Although, the basic function of all these gadgets is the same, the main difference is created by the software used for different purposes. Different software have been developed for record maintenance; appointment scheduling; growth prediction; diagnosis; cephalometric analysis; orthognathic surgical planning; soft and hard tissue changes to be expected by orthodontics and/ or surgery, CAD–CAM, appliance fabrication; invisalign appliances fabrication; automated formation of step wise appliances and wires; storage of diagnostic records, e.g. casts, photographs; video imaging, CT and MRI scans; patients education softwares, etc. which have found varied applications in different areas of orthodontics.

Below are briefly discussed some uses of computers in orthodontics.

1. **Medical information-processing systems:** Patient record management, e.g. photos, digital X-rays, like OPG, cephalograms, casts, e.g. holograms, etc. can be stored in the computers and can be retrieved with a click of mouse. It can be used for patient education, treatment progress analysis; orthodontic education, etc.
2. **Diagnosis and treatment planning** can be divided in two groups, i.e. for model analysis, and for cephalometic analysis. Also, the two-dimension and three-dimension (3D) techniques, and various surgical simulation techniques have been devised for these purposes. Analysis of data can be done to classify the severity of malocclusions.
3. **Patient records and treatment knowledge base**, i.e. a collection of orthodontic treatment cases can act as knowledge base and data and can help to provide a better justification on treatment planning based on past success or failure of treatment cases.
4. Three-dimensional e-model, i.e. e-cast, and digital patient records can be obtained and stored digitally, rather than physical models. It reduces the storage space needs to keep all patient records and dental models. Such models can be directly sent to labs through internet to be used to fabricate the appliances, arch wires, etc. Through computerized process in future, the wire-bending robots may produce the arch wires with precise angulations of wire needed by an orthodontist.

5. **Orthodontic practice management** include patients scheduling, appointment arrangement, patient charting or examination form handling, electronic patient recording and the use of electronic patient's identification cards. Software can be used to record the appointments, work done, their personal data, etc.
6. **Digital recording** applications are for recording and visualizing patient information in an electronic form. It can be done by using different devices, e.g. digital camera, three-dimensional measurement device, intraoral scanner or intraoral camera, digitizer and computerized tomography (CT) scanner.
7. **Forecast of growth** from serial cephalograms. The serial records of the patients are evaluated and analyzed over a prolonged period. The management information services can be integrated both nationally and internationally so that information from all sources can be recorded in a uniform manner. Thus the orthodontist can become a member of an oral health management team having all relevant information readily available.
8. **Digitizer** and **cephalographic analysis:** This instrument helps to record the landmarks from a cephalograms in a software which then calculates various angles and linear measurements for that particular patient. The obtained values are also compared with the norms of that particular ethnic group and can also be compared with other races to find out the differences. The data is sued for diagnosis of the conditions and can also be used for research purpose. **Dentofacial planner plus (DFP)** is a cephalometric program which helps in rapid and accurate analysis of a cephalogram to aid in treatment planning. Also, the photographic video image of patient's profile can be linked to digitised cephalogram. Manipulation of the tracing will show corresponding changes in the video image. It thus helps to simulate the orthodontic treatment or orthognathic surgery changes and thus is a valuable aid in treatment planning, communication with oral surgeon, discussion with patient/parents and patient education.
9. **Research purpose:** Various types of data recorded in the software systems can be subjected to comparison, statistical analysis, etc. which can be interpreted for various research analysis, e.g. treatment outcomes; growth prediction; changes in cast parameters; changes in hard and soft tissue parameters with treatment, etc. Serial cephalometrics, OPG, CT and MRI scan images can be superimposed to study the tissue changes with growth and treatment.
10. **Three-dimensional modeling for diagnosis and planning in orthognathic surgery:** This technique utilizes two stereo pairs of videocameras, a stereo pair at each side of the patient's face. It helps to capture the face in three dimensions and precise measurement of anatomic landmarks. It can be used to capture the facial image and a cephalogram almost simultaneously, allowing more accurate superimposition of soft and hard tissues. It facilitates development of surgical treatment plan. A computer program uses the data generated by this biostereometric measurement system to predict soft tissue changes following orthognathic surgery.
11. A computer vision technique can be used to record and process 3D images of the profile of dental impressions for automated diagnosis. This technique enables 3D image analysis for the detection of the interstices between the teeth. 3D imaging of dentition can be done by an intraoral scanner, which can be used for diagnosis and treatment.

12. The computerized technique can also help to predict approximate force values applied to each tooth. It can also be used to select the arch wire and to incorporate the amount of correction in arch wire needed for the treatment which allow the clinician to modify various simulated treatment until optimal treatment plan is found.
13. **Three-dimensional imaging in orthognathic surgery:** C3D is a relatively new 3D imaging system which captures 3D geometry of the face. Landmarks are identified on 3D facial models by a software-based facial analysis tool. This method is useful in studying facial soft tissue changes after orthognathic surgery and assessing facial soft tissue growth and development of the craniofacial complex.
14. **Case presentation and telemedicine:** It is a modern system of electronic face to face discussion between far-sitting doctors about the treatment of a case based on the records of patient. Remote medical examination and evaluation through the technology of telecommunication and Internet is known as telemedicine.
15. **Continuing medical education and conference presentations:** Computers are universally used to prepare the papers to be presented in conference and CME meetings for education and discussion purposes. Videos can be incorporated in the presentation. Also, live surgery and other procedures can be shown to the participants.

Conclusion

Uses of computer orthodontics are numerous. It is used for applications from simple databases for orthodontics practice to complex image processing techniques for efficient diagnosis. The computerized 3D dental model is an important method helpful for more accurate diagnosis, treatment planning and a better understanding of patient's treatment progress. It also helps in communication, telemedicine and education.

62

Sterilization and Disinfection in Orthodontics

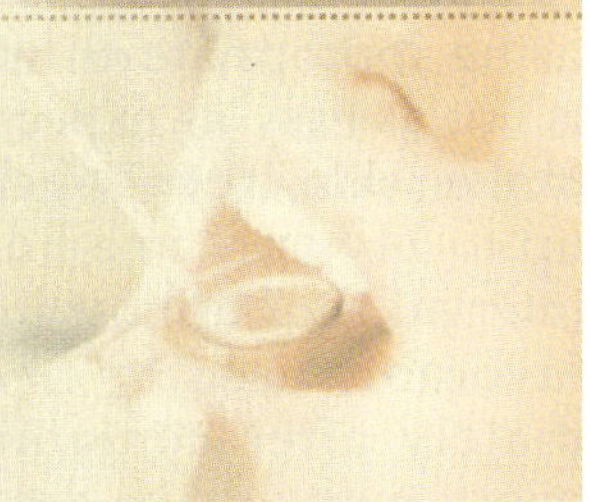

INTRODUCTION

On a daily basis, the practicing dentist and his personnel are at risk of being exposed to a wide range of patients with blood borne diseases such as HIV/AIDS, hepatitis B, hepatitis C, and airborne diseases, such as influenza and tuberculosis. Infection can be directly transmitted by oral fluids, blood, contaminated instruments and surfaces or via the respiratory system. To accomplish infection control accurately and to reduce the risk of cross-contamination, all patients have to be treated while practicing universal precautions, the latter including the imperative steps of disinfection and sterilization.

Cross-infection in Dentistry

Microorganisms are easily transferred between patients, dentists and dental staff in private offices. Infection involving these people is called cross-infection.

Hepatitis Viruses

Six types of hepatitis viruses are identified as A, B, C, D, E and G. Infection with hepatitis B virus (HBV) is most prevalent and occurs via the parenteral route. Contaminated blood and secretions are the main sources for transmission of infection. The incubation period for HBV is 45–160 days.

Hepatitis C Virus is transmitted by parenteral route. Incubation period is 15–150 days after viral contact.

Hepatitis D virus or delta agent: Hepatitis D virus needs HBV for existence, replication and infection. Therefore, HDV is found in individuals having either acute hepatitis B infection or are chronic hepatitis B carriers. Hepatitis G virus (HGV) is high in opiate users and in patients who receive dialysis and/or are hemophilic.

Herpes Simplex Virus

Herpes simplex virus (HSV), having two antigenic types, is responsible for oral or genital infections. HSV-1 is responsible for oral mucosal infections, whereas HSV-2 is responsible for genital herpetic lesions. HSV infections are generally asymptomatic. Antibodies are found in most of the adults. Avoiding direct contact with the ulcerated tissue is the most effective protection.

Epstein-Barr Virus

The first infection by Epstein-Barr virus (EBV) is generally asymptomatic. It may cause nonspecific illness during infancy. Viral diffusion and contamination occurs by the way of saliva and oropharyngeal secretions. EBV exists in lymphoid nodules primarily but also can be colonized on pharyngeal epithelial tissue where it can be hidden. Standard precautions are sufficient to prevent contamination from EBV.

Human Immunodeficiency Virus

Human immunodeficiency virus (HIV) is a member of Retroviridae. Virus attaches to its receptor on the surface of the CD4 lymphocyte. HIV can be contracted via the parenteral route, mucosal contact or contact with broken skin. HIV is a fairly weak virus that can be inactivated at 56°C for 10 minutes using appropriate disinfectants and its spread is not as easy as expected. If HIV penetrates broken skin, it can be held by the macrophages up to 24 hours in a human body. This time interval is of utmost importance and can be favorably used by health officials. Immediately after contamination, the area in question should be cleaned and washed with warm water and soap, and antiretroviral therapy is to be initiated within two hours following exposure for optimal effect.

Influenza Virus

Influenza virus causes flu, the most common epidemic worldwide. It is transmitted via body droplets. The incubation period for the illness varies between 1 and 4 days, but symptoms usually display after 2 days.

Vaccination

Dentists and dental staff are always recommended to be vaccinated against tuberculosis, rubella, diphtheria, tetanus and most importantly, against HBV (Deger, 2004). Hepatitis B vaccine consists of 3 injections. Five years after vaccination, immunity remains only in 7% of the individuals. Therefore, booster doses are required. Booster doses are given at 3–5-year intervals after vaccination.

Personnel Protective Equipment

Dental personnel should wear gloves during cleaning and touching contaminated instruments and surfaces. Hands should be washed after removal of gloves after each patient. Surgical masks, protective glasses, disposable gowns and plastic face masks should be worn during oral procedures that are likely to splash blood, saliva and oral fluids.

Protection of Hands and Skin

Gloves prevent blood and saliva-borne microorganisms entering from cuts, abrasions and wounds in hand. But, the hands and nails should be cleaned with appropriate skin antiseptics both before wearing and after removing gloves.

Protection of eyes: protective eye wear/goggles should be used to protect eyes. Plastic masks completely covering the face can also be used instead of glasses. Glutaraldehyde can be used for cleaning glasses.

Hand Instruments

The hand instruments must be sterilized by autoclaving. Chemical antiseptics are not the proposed methods of cleaning. Disposable parts are recommended to be changed after each use.

Removal of Sharp Instruments and Infectious Wastes

The patient's blood and saliva-contaminated sharp instruments are infected and necessary precautions should be taken for preventing injuries. To avoid cross-infection, use the disposable syringes. The needles should be destroyed by needle cutter machines. Sharps, e.g. blades, needles, RC files, etc. should be placed puncture-resistant boxes to be disposed off as per the disposal guidelines.

Sterilization and Disinfection Procedures in Orthodontics: Definitions

Sterilization: Sterilization destroys all forms of microorganisms including viruses and bacterial and mycotic spores.

Disinfection: Disinfection is the process of destroying or inhibiting most pathogenic microorganisms and inactivating some viruses, hence reducing microbial contamination to safety levels.

Antisepsis: Application of chemicals on living tissue to avoid infection.

Asepsis: It means an environment free of germs. That is the destruction of all disease-forming microorganisms in the working environment.

Presterilization cleaning: It involves debridement of all instruments contaminated with blood, saliva, etc. before their sterilization. It can be done by hand washing instruments with a solution of detergent and brushes. Recently, the ultrasonic baths have been recommended for this purpose. The instruments are dried of any moisture before packing them for sterilization.

Sterilization techniques/sterilization stages:

a. Cleaning
b. Packaging—loading
c. Sterilization
d. Unloading—registration
e. Storage—distribution

Sterilization and Disinfection of Orthodontic Instruments and Material

Prior to dry-heat sterilization, to prevent corrosion, orthodontic pliers should be dried with pressured air. Corrosion can also be prevented by oiling the joint surfaces with appropriate solutions. Autoclaving will negatively affect orthodontic instruments causing blunting and corrosion of their sharp cutting edges. Hence, soaking in 1% sodium nitrate or 2% glutaraldehyde can be recommended as an alternative. Unsaturated chemical vapor sterilization of pliers is appropriate to minimize corrosion, but this method requires a well ventilated area to eliminate noxious odors.

Autoclaving: Autoclaving is the most popular method of sterilization. The basic principle is that when the pressure inside a closed chamber increases, the boiling point of water also increases. Bacillus sterothermophilus is used for testing the efficiency of autoclaving. It is used for every kind of material or instrument which does not get damaged by heat, e.g. heat resistant plastics, dental hand pieces, dental instruments, cotton rolls, gauze, anesthetic syringes, glass slab, towel packs. It uses a pressure of 15 to 20 psi at a temperature of 121°C for 15–21 minutes or 3 minutes at 134°C is required for proper sterilization. However, steam vapor has detrimental effect on orthodontic pliers leading to rusting, blunting of tips of instruments, etc. Also, the tried-in molar bands should be autoclaved before reusing it.

Hot air oven is the most widely used method of sterilization by dry heat. A holding period of 160°C (320°F) for 1 hr or 190°C for 6–12 minutes called as *Rapid dry-Heat Sterilization*. It is an effective and safe method of sterilization for metal instruments, such as pliers and mirrors as it does not cause corrosion of carbon steel instruments and burs.

Glass bead sterilizer: It uses a metal cup filled with glass beads of 1.2–1.5 mm in diameter. Larger beads are not effective in transferring heat due to presence of large air spaces between beads which reduces the efficiency of sterilizer when operated at a temperature range of 218–240°C for 3–5 seconds for instruments, like root canal files. It can be used to sterilize orthodontic bands, pliers, etc. A longer sterilization time is needed for larger instrument. The recommended protocol for sterilization of bands or pliers is 220°C for 45 seconds.

Chemical immersion/cold sterilization: This method is recommended only for heat sensitive non-surgical instruments, alginate impressions, etc. 2% *glutaraldehyde* is the most popular high level disinfectants used in dentistry. It is very effective method of inactivation of bacterial spores. It is used as an as immersion solution for metallic instruments, face masks, heat sensitive plastic, cheek retractors, rubbers, and fiberoptics. The duration of sterilization is about 6–10 hrs at room temperature. It can be used for elastomeric materials also. Studies have shown that cold sterilization causes a pitting type of corrosion of orthodontic instruments as compared to surface corrosion caused by other methods.

Alcohol: Ethyl and isopropyl alcohols are most frequently used. Isopropyl alcohol is preferred to ethyl alcohol as it is a better fat solvent, more bactericidal and less volatile. It is active at a conc. of 50–70%. It denatures proteins and lipids and leads to cell membrane disintegration. It lacks sporicidal activity and also causes corrosion of metals.

Disinfection of orthodontic brackets: Chlorhexidine is an appropriate disinfectant to be used on metal or ceramic brackets.

Decontamination of orthodontic bands: Band selection for appropriate size requires several trials. Introrally tried/used band should be autoclaved for future use.

Sterilization of orthodontic wires: Autoclaving them for 18 minutes in 134°C is best method. No significant changes occur in the mechanical properties of wires that would affect their utilization.

Disinfection of elastomeric ligatures: The unused parts of elastomeric ligatures are generally sterilized via cold sterilization since they are not heat-resistant. Disinfection of these materials in a 2% glutaraldehyde solution for 10 minutes is recommended. Autoclaving at 121°C does not lead to permanent deformations or to increased shrinkage.

Bacterial contamination and disinfection of removable acrylic appliances: Disinfection methods of acrylic orthodontic appliances should inactivate pathogenic microorganisms immediately, without damaging the composition of the appliance. Chlorhexidine gluconate was found to be significantly more effective than cetilpyridinium chloridine.

Surface disinfection: Surfaces, e.g. air-water sprayers, aspirator heads, reflector arms, cuspidors, drawers, head rest and arms, etc. should be cleaned with sodium hypochlorite 1% or solutions including 70% alcohol are used for surface disinfection in orthodontic clinics.

Antibacterial agents in orthodontics: Chlorhexidine is an antimicrobial agent that is very efficient against *Streptococcus mutans*. 0.2% chlorhexidine solution significantly decreases *Streptococcus mutans* levels and bacterial levels in dental plaque and saliva.

Sterling Winthrop Research Institute has developed a topical antimicrobial agent Octenidine dihydrochloride. It is an antimicrobial effective against bacterial plaque formation

Conclusion

Although orthodontists usually do not work on tissues and treat infectious diseases, still chances of cross contamination exist. Proper sterilization techniques should be used in the orthodontic practice, providing full range sterilization. Diseases, like HIV/AIDS and hepatitis B and C, make it an absolute necessity to protect clinic staff and patients from cross-contamination, by using proper sterilization techniques.

63

Drugs and Orthodontics

INTRODUCTION

Orthodontic tooth movement is a biochemical process. Biochemical reactions occur in periodontal tissues, leading to bone resorption and deposition which help in change in tooth position when force is applied. The patients may experience pressure, pain, ulcer formation, gingival problems, etc. during orthodontic treatment needing medications. They might also be taking some medications for treatment of other diseases. Research has shown that rate of tooth movement is affected by certain drugs when applied locally or systemically. There are certain drugs which affect the rate of orthodontic tooth movement. Drugs and their effect in orthodontics can be discussed under following headings:

a. Drugs promoting the rate of OTM
b. Drugs suppressing OTM
c. Drugs for pain management
d. Drugs for TMD m/m
e. Drugs for prohylaxis in congenital heart problems, e.g. antibiotics, etc.
f. Drugs for saliva m/m
g. Anxiety m/m
h. Drugs for preventing white spot lesions
i. Drugs for prevention of gum problems
j. Drugs affecting gingiva, etc., e.g. cyclosporine
k. Multivitamins and calcium
l. Drugs used during cancer therapy
m. Effect of thyroid, parathyroid and steroid hormones

Biochemical Reactions in Tissues

Orthodontic forces lead to biochemical changes in the tissues. Eicosanoids are signalling molecules involved in inflammatory and immune responses, anaphylaxis, vasodilation and vasoconstriction, blood clotting, etc. Four families of eicosanoids, i.e. leukotrienes, thromboxanes, prostacyclins, and prostaglandins have been found. They all arise from arachidonic acid by the action of various enzymes. Cyclo-oxygenases (COX) helps in its conversion to thromboxanes, prostacyclins, and prostaglandins. Research has shown that therapeutic administration of eicosanoids resulted in increased tooth movement, whereas their blocking led to a decrease.

Leukotrienes: Leukotrienes are the only eicosanoids formed from arachidonic acid by the action of lipoxygenase, and not by COX. Leukotrienes play important role in inflammation, allergies, and diseases like asthma. Their effects can be counteracted by **Montelukast** and **Zafirlukast**, which block leukotriene receptors. It can also be done by a drug such as **Zileuton** which inhibits leukotriene synthesis by selective blocking of enzyme lipoxygenase. It can result in **inhibition of bone resorption**, but also in stimulation of bone deposition, thus influencing OTM. The effect of the selective inhibitor of leukotriene synthesis AA861 on OTM in a rat model led to a significant **decrease in rate of OTM**. Findings suggest that drugs like zileuton, montelukast, and zafirlukast might also decrease the rate of OTM.

Thromboxanes: Thromboxanes are vasoconstrictors and facilitate platelet aggregation. They increase in oral cavity in inflammatory conditions. The thromboxane analogue U 46619, when locally placed, **increased the rate of OTM**. It suggests that inhibition of thromboxane synthesis by, eg, nonsteroidal anti-inflammatory drugs (NSAIDs) might inhibit the rate of OTM.

Prostacyclins: The effects of prostacyclins are opposite to those of thromboxanes. They act as vasodilators and prevent platelet aggregation. Synthetic prostacyclin (**epoprostenol**) or analogues such as **iloprost increased rate of OTM**. Therefore, administration of the prostacyclin analogue iloprost and the thromboxane analogue U 46619 increases the synthesis of prostaglandins, thereby increasing the rate of OTM. Synthesis of prostacyclins can thus be inhibited by NSAIDs.

Prostaglandins: Prostaglandins play important role in inflammation. Synthetic prostaglandin analogues, e.g. **misoprostol**, are used for various conditions, including prevention of peptic ulcers and induction of labor. The local injections of synthetic exogenous prostaglandin (PGE2) (**dinoprostone**) resulted increased rate of OTM in a **dose-dependent manner** after single or multiple local injections of exogenous PGE2. Exogenous PGE1 (**alprostadil**) and its synthetic analogue misoprostol also resulted in increased rate of OTM in animals. A **diet rich in omega-3 fatty acids** in rats showed decreased arachidonic acid and PGE2 concentrations in alveolar bone and decreased rate of orthodontic incisor separation.

NSAIDs: NSAIDs are the most important class of prostanoid synthesis inhibitors. They have analgesic, antipyretic, and anti-inflammatory effects, and are used for many conditions like rheumatoid arthritis, osteoarthritis, gout, dysmenorrhea, headache, migraine, and postoperative pain, as well as for the prevention of cardiovascular diseases.

Mechanism of action: NSAIDs suppress production of all prostanoids (thromboxanes, prostacyclins, and prostaglandins) by inhibiting COX-1 and COX-2 enzymes required for synthesis of prostanoids. Acetylsalicylic acid inhibits both types of COX, so it effectively inhibits prostaglandin synthesis. A category of NSAIDs called **coxibs** are specific COX-2 inhibitors used for management of osteoarthritis. They decrease the number of osteoclasts, because prostaglandins are involved directly or indirectly in osteoclast differentiation or in stimulating their activity. It also occurs with acetylsalicylic acid, flurbiprofen, indomethacin, and ibuprofen.

Salicylates: Acetylsalicylic acid administration in low doses in guinea pigs did not reduce rate of tooth movement but OTM was found to be reduced at higher dosage **Arylalkanoic acids:** Administration of a single dose of indomethacin has short-lasting inhibitory effect leading reduced bone turnover and thus a decrease in OTM rate. Diclofenac also decreased OTM. **Arylpropionic acids,** e.g. ibuprofen leads to reduction in rate of OTM, but no inhibitory effect was found at a low dose (10 mg per kilogram per day) of flurbiprofen in rabbits. **Oxicams:** No experimental data are available from the literature on the effects of oxicams on the rate of OTM. **Coxibs,** i.e. selective COX-2 inhibitors decrease the OTM, e.g. Rofecoxib, celecoxib, but **Valdecoxib** has no effect on PGE-1 levels and can be safely used in managing orthodontic pain.

Drugs Promoting Rate of OTM

They enhance bone resorption thus increasing the rate of OTM. They affect the synthesis and effects of inflammatory mediators to enhance tooth movement. Some of these drugs are prostaglandins; leucotriens; cytokines; vitamin D; osteocalcin; corticosteroids, etc. The bone turn-over rate in patients taking such drugs will be more, so care should be taken during orthodontic treatment. Low forces are used and the time duration between appointments is prolonged. Orthodontic tooth movement has been described with many theories, e.g. pressure-tension hypothesis; theory of vascular occlusion; concept of periodontal ligament as a hydrostatic mechanism; and piezoelectric or bone bending theory. Osteoclasts are involved in bone-remodeling process, and they originate from monocytes. A combination of mechanical, chemical, and electrical stimuli lead to cellular activations and a more rapid bone turnover and hence faster orthodontic tooth movement. Techniques that can stimulate the formation and activation of osteoclasts include local injections of prostaglandins; the administration of PEMF, pulsed electromagnetic fields to the area; and the use of a local, direct electrical current can increase the rates of tooth movement than that produced by mechanical orthodontic forces alone.

a. Prostaglandings

Prostaglandins especially PGE2 are produced with force application which stimulates osteoclastic bone resorption. Since PGs are produced during inflammation, the OTM is considered an inflammatory process. Thus giving anti-inflammatory drugs during OTM tends to decreases PG synthesis and thus decreases the OTM. Indomethacin, a specific inhibitor of prostaglandin synthesis, reduces the rate of orthodontic tooth movement.

Effect of prostaglandins on tooth movement: Lee 1990 discussed that PGE1 is a promoting factor in bone resorption, which in turn activates enzyme adenyl-cyclase, which induces an increase in intracellular cyclic AMP. This increase stimulates the release of PGs again. The secretion of PGs is regulated by a **feedback mechanism**, since PGs are believed to inhibit adenylcyclase activity above a certain concentration. PGs promote bone resorption, not only by increasing the number and the size of osteoclasts, but also by stimulating the activation of existing osteoclasts.

Local administration of PGE1 or PGE2 in gingiva helps in accelerating the rate of tooth movement as it stimulates bone resorption. PGE1 produces increased resorption, changes in alveolar bone morphology like extensive loss of bone matrix, fibrous replacement, and increased vascularity.

Cyclic-AMP and calcium are intracellular second messengers which help to modulate osteoclasts and bone resorption. PGs cause a significant increase of cyclic-AMP. Intracellular calcium is important in mechanism of bone resorption of PGs and thus increased rate of tooth movement.

Anchorage augmentation: It now is possible in periodontal therapy to place small spheres which release specific antibiotic into gingival sulcus and periodontal pockets. If a prostaglandin inhibitor could be placed in a similar fashion in the sulcus around anchor teeth, thus reducing their movement, it might lead to improved anchorage and thus more effective movement of the teeth.

b. Local Use of Vitamin D to Increase Rate of Tooth Movement

Collins and Sinclair (1988) discussed that vitamin D plays a role in maintenance of calcium homeostasis by stimulating the osteoclastic activity. It is a steroid hormone that has specific receptors in many target organs and tissues. It acts by activating DNA and RNA within the target cell to produce proteins and enzymes which are used in the bone resorption process. Active form of vitamin D, i.e. 1, 25-dihydroxycholecalciferol is one of the most potent stimulators of osteoclastic activity. 1, 25 D acts directly on the nucleus of circulating monocytes and osteoprogenitor cells, which have specific receptors for it. This allows a cellular activation and faster than normal recruitment of resorptive cells and increasing the rate of alveolar resorption.

c. Pulsed Fields PEMF, and Direct Electrical Currents

These are non-invasive methods to activate osteoclasts by increasing the levels of cAMP and cGMP. Various studies have shown that PEMF helps in increasing the rate and amount of OTM by increasing the cellular activity and the number of osteoclasts without changing the ultrastructure of the cells.

d. Effect of Low-Level Laser Therapy (LLLT)

One of the treatment objectives of orthodontic treatment is to provide a pain-free treatment. Laser has helped the dental clinicians to provide various pain-free procedures to the patients, e.g. periodontal surgery, RCT, surgeries, etc. Many patients reject orthodontic treatment due to fear of pain during treatment. Low-level (GaAlAs) diode laser (809 nm, 100 mW) can be used during orthodontic movement and has been found that it can highly accelerate tooth movement during orthodontic treatment and can also effectively reduce pain level. LLLT is used at 4 seconds per point (buccal, palatal, and mesial) with a GaAlAs diode laser source (830 nm, 100 mW, 18 J/cm^2. It has been found that orthodontic forces lead to a reversible hyperemia in the pulp tissues. LLLT leads to a faster repair of the pulpal tissue due to orthodontic movement. Individually, the corticision and low-level laser therapy are known to increase the rate of tooth movement. A study done on dogs to find the combined effects of corticision and LLLT on the tooth movement rate and paradental remodelling found that periodic LLLT after corticision around a moving tooth decreased the tooth movement rate and alveolar remodeling activity.

e. Relaxin

Relaxin is well known for its effects on remodeling soft tissue. It has been found to stimulate collagenase production in human gingival fibroblast cultures. The research has found that relaxin therapy can be used to speed tooth movement and prevent relapse in orthodontic practice.

f. Effects of Corticosteroids on Tooth Movement

Ashcraft, Southard and Tolley (1992) discussed that corticosteroids are widely used in treatment of many medical conditions, but they have osteoporosis as a side effect, due to a disturbance of normal processes of bone remodeling. Thus corticosteroid-induced osteoporosis leads to a more rapid orthodontic tooth movement and subsequent increased relapse as shown in animal models.

Corticosteroids are produced in adrenal cortex. They are involved in many physiologic systems, like stress response, inflammatory and immune responses, carbohydrate metabolism, protein catabolism, and blood electrolyte levels. They are of 2 types. **Glucocorticoids** are mainly involved in control of carbohydrate, fat, and protein metabolism, but also have anti-inflammatory properties. **Mineralocorticoids,** such as aldosterone, control mainly electrolyte and water levels by promoting sodium retention in kidneys. Glucocorticoids are also involved in bone physiology and are prescribed for many inflammatory and autoimmune conditions, like rheumatoid arthritis, dermatitis, allergies, asthma, and as immunosuppressants after organ transplantation. Their anti-inflammatory effect is due to indirect blocking of phospholipase A2 and suppression of synthesis of both COX-1 and COX-2, thus inhibition of synthesis of prostaglandins and leukotrienes. The glucocorticoids, e.g. cortisone, prednisolone, and methylprednisolone lead to an increase in the rate of OTM. Also, the relapse rate has been found to be faster in experimental group than in control animals.

Drugs Reducing the Rate of OTM

These agents reduce bone resorption. PGs are the mediators of inflammatory response during OTM. NSAIDs inhibit PG synthesis and thus can decrease the rate of tooth movement. They interfere with arachidonic acid metabolism, and block the production of primary and/or secondary messengers. Bisphosphonates which are used to treat certain forms of cancers, bind with calcium ions and promote apoptosis of working osteoclasts. Thus they inhibit bone resorption and can literally stop the OTM. On the other hand, some of the suppressor agents can be delivered locally near the anchor unit (i.e. molars) to enhance anchorage and retention by reducing the bone turnover. Wong, Reynolds and West (1992) discussed that nonsteroidal anti-inflammatory drugs (NSAIDs), such as acetylsalicylic acid (aspirin), indomethacin, ibuprofen, acetaminophen, and flurbiprofen, are potent inhibitors of PG synthesis, which affect the rate of orthodontic tooth movement.

a. Leukotrienes in Orthodontic Tooth Movement

Mohammed, Tatakis, and Dziak (1989) discussed that prostaglandins (PGs) and leukotrienes (LTs) are produced by arachidonic acid during inflammatory process. PGs are produced from arachidonic acid through the cyclooxygenase pathway. Leukotrienes (LTs) are produced by conversion of arachidonic acid via the lipoxygenase pathway. **AA861**, the specific 5′lipoxygenase inhibitor, inhibited leukotriene production which results in inhibition of tooth movement.

b. Effect of Cetrizine (H1 Receptor Antagonist)

Meh Alja et al (2011) discussed that cetrizine decreases the amount of OTM due to decreased alveolar bone resorption. It thus increases the time of treatment.

Effect of indomethacin on rate of orthodontic tooth movement: Chumbley and Tuncay (1986) discussed that prostaglandins are mediators of bone resorption. Indomethacin, an aspirin-like drug is a potent inhibitor of PG synthesis. PGs are involved in bone resorption during orthodontic treatment, thus blocking the synthesis of these compounds should result in slower tooth movement. Indomethacin inhibits bone resorption by inhibiting the prostaglandin synthetase enzyme system. Since prostaglandins also lead to the resorption of bone in inflammatory periodontal disease, the patients taking aspirin for treatment of chronic arthritis exhibit less periodontal bone loss.

In addition, the **anticonvalscent** drug phenytoin has been reported to decrease tooth movement in rats, and some tetracyclines (e.g. doxycycline) inhibit osteoclast recruitment, an effect similar to bisphosphonates. It is possible that unusual responses to orthodontic force could be encountered in patients taking any of these medications.

Drugs for Pain Management

Prostaglandins are produced in the tissues on force application and are necessary for orthodontic tooth movement, as they help in bone resorption. PGs are the inflammatory products and lead to pain. Patient feels pain for 3–4 days after activation, which is due to increased level of PGs. Controlling the synthesis of PGs can reduce pain, but on the other hand it also slows down OTM.

Degrees of pain: Orthodontic pain can be divided in following three types according to the degree of pain perceived:

1. First degree: Patient is not aware of pain unless orthodontist manipulates the teeth being moved, e.g. by using band pusher or force gauge.
2. Second degree: Pain or discomfort felt during clenching or heavy biting; it usually occurs within first week of appliance placement. The patient will be able to masticate a normal diet with this pain.
3. Third degree: The patient is unable to masticate food of normal consistency.

Medications for pain control in orthodontics can be used few hours before the activation/force application or after the activation. Some of the medicines used are **NSAIDs**, particularly **aspirin** and **ibuprofen**. These are peripherally acting (non-opioid) analgesics, which function by inhibition of cyclo-oxygenase enzyme system thus reducing the formation of prostaglandins and other inflammatory products. Taking these medicines for prolonged time reduces the levels of PGs and thus decreases bone resoprtion and slows the tooth movement. Ngan et al found ibuprofen to be more effective than asprin.

Paracetamol: Paracetamol (acetaminophen) is a commonly used analgesic. It lacks anti-inflammatory properties. Therefore, it does not belong with NSAIDs. Whereas NSAIDs block COX-1 and/or COX-2, paracetamol blocks a third isoform, COX-3, which is expressed only in brain and spinal cord. Its **mode of action is central** rather than peripheral, and thus has minimal effects on prostaglandin synthesis. Thus paracetamol does not affect the rate of OTM, and it should be the analgesic of choice during orthodontic therapy for pain management. Simmons and Brandt (1992) were the first to recommend the use of acetaminophen for managing orthodontic pain.

Keim (2004) described an anesthetic gel, "**ORAQIX**" which is a combination of lidocaine and prilocaine in 1:1 ratio by weight. It is used locally as a chairside pain control method especially during band placement and cementation, archwire ligation and band/bracket removal. Its delivery method is different that it is simply introduced into the gingival crevices and is entirely painless.

White (1984) found approximately 63% patients reported less discomfort with chewing **Aspergum** after mechanotherapy. Proffit (2000) suggested the use of **chewing gum** and a **plastic wafer** during first few hours of appliance activation to reduce pain. It helps to temporarily displace the teeth during mastication which allows blood flow through compressed areas and prevents build-up of inflammatory metabolites.

Vibratory stimulation: The use of **vibratory stimulation** to reduce orthodontic pain was first reported by Marie, et al (2003) but it was found that most patients were unable to tolerate these vibrations once discomfort sets in. So it was recommended that it should be used prior to onset of pain.

Low-level laser therapy (LLLT): Lim et al (1995) found discouraging results in the efficacy of **low level laser therapy** and found that no immediate relief occurred.

Antianxiety Agents

Benzodiazepine antianxiety agents, e.g. diazepam and chlordiazepoxide have limited application in orthodontics. They help to relieve anxiety and tension, as well as controlling the patient's pain reaction and salivation. Diazepam is contraindicated in patients of glaucoma.

Effects of diazepam in orthodontics: Burrow, et al (1986) discussed cyclic-AMP is a possible intracellular mediator in bone remodeling during tooth movement. Thus, an increase in its level should result in faster tooth movement. Breakdown of cAMP was inhibited by administration of diazepam, thus its level remains at a higher level and thus increased rate of tooth movement. Diazepam has an inhibitory action on cAMP phosphodiesterase.

Polat et al (2005) found **Naproxan sodium** (550 mg) to be more effective than ibuprofen (400 mg), after 2 and 6 hours and even at night, administered preoperatively before archwire placement. They also suggested that at least 1–2 postoperative doses should also be administered in addition to preoperative doses for complete pain control.

Medication for TMD Therapy

Following medications can be used for TMD therapy:

1. **Piroxicam**, an NSAID, is specifically indicated for short- and long-term use for treatment of osteoarthritis and rheumatoid arthritis, and thus can be used in treatment of TMD when inflammation of joint is suspected. It works by inhibiting prostaglandin synthesis, and thus exhibits anti-inflammatory, analgesic and antipyretic properties. Dose of 20 mg/day is used for at least two weeks.
2. **Acetaminophen** with **codeine phosphate** is used for moderate to severe pain. It is a schedule III narcotic and is used only for short-term relief of acute orthodontic or TMJ pain. Codeine has a central action and thus has a better control of psychological aspects of pain.
3. **Cyclobenzaprine HCl** is used for TMD patients having acute symptoms of muscular origin. It is used as an adjunct to rest and physical therapy, and should

not be given for more than two or three weeks. It acts as a muscle relaxant by reducing muscle tone activity at brain stem level, thereby alleviating pain and tenderness, and increasing range of motion. It should not be given with MAO inhibitors, and should also be avoided in patients with cardiovascular problems and hyperthyroidism.

4. **Diazepam,** a benzodiazepine derivative, is used for anxiety disorders. It also relieves skeletal muscle spasm caused by muscle and joint inflammation. Dose is 5 mg at night.
5. **Amitriptyline,** a tricyclic antidepressant, is used for affective disorders, and reduces parafunctional activity in patients having nocturnal bruxism. It inhibits reuptake of norepinephrine and serotonin to produce its effects which include sedation. It is effective in treatment of chronic orofacial pain, migraine, fibromyalgia, psychogenic problems and bruxism. It should not be given with MAO inhibitors, and avoided in cardiovascular problems, hyperthyroidism, and children under 12 years age. The 10 mg dose is used for TMD purposes. Migraine is also treated with **Sumatriptan**.
6. **Chloroxazone:** Muscle relaxants, such as chlorzoxazone with acetaminophen, may reduce the spasms and pain associated with the facial muscles.
7. **Pharmacologic agents for myofacial pain:** Orthodontic myofacial and/or dental pain can be controlled by analgesics, such as aspirin, or acetaminophen, with or without codeine. **Propoxyphene**, and **pentazocine** can also be used. Medications help to reduce stress and tension, and thus relax the facial muscles. Mild tranquilizers as chlordiazepoxide, diazepam, and meprobamate have been used to reduce anxiety-tension; and have combined sedative and muscle relaxant properties.
8. **Ethyl chloride** spray directly on facial muscles is also effective in relieving some of the painful symptoms of MPDS. MPDS has a psychological cause also, thus the placebos are also effective in reducing or eliminating the MPD symptoms in some patients.

Antifungal and Antiviral Drugs

Nystatin ointment is an antifungal antibiotic used for treating angular cheilitis and other mycotic infections caused by *Candida albicans*. It functions by increasing fungal membrane permeability. It can also be used through oral route for systemic effects. It is recommended to extend its use 1week more after symptoms are resolved.

Acyclovir ointment is an antiviral medication used for herpes labialis. The drug inhibits viral DNA replication. It has its best efficacy by oral route in immune-compromised patients, but topical application is better for mild problems as seen in orthodontic patients. Zovirax 5% ointment is applied to the affected area 6 times per day until healed.

Calcium and Calcium Regulators

Calcium is an essential mineral for various physiologic processes, e.g. blood clotting, muscle contraction, regulation of heartbeat, fluid balance, and enzyme activities. Hormones, like parathyroid hormone (PTH), thyroid hormones (thyroxine, calcitonin), sex hormones (estrogens), and vitamins (e.g. vitamin D_3) are important regulators of calcium homeostasis. Dietary intake of calcium is also important. A separate class of drugs that affects calcium homeostasis is the bisphosphonates.

Corticosteroid hormones, parathyroid hormone, and thyroxin have all been shown to increase tooth movement. Estrogens probably reduce tooth movement, although no direct evidence is available. Vitamin D_3 stimulates tooth movement, and dietary calcium seemed to reduce it.

Parathyroid hormone: The effect of PTH on OTM was studied in rats. A significant stimulation of the rate of OTM by exogenous PTH appeared to occur in a dose-dependent manner. PTH is secreted by parathyroid glands. Its main effect is an increase in concentration of calcium in blood, thus, it stimulates bone resorption. Hypoparathyroidism leads to a shortage of active PTH and thus hypocalcemia. The most commonly used therapy is administration of vitamin D or calcium supplementation. In primary hyperparathyroidism, overproduction of hormone stimulates bone resorption, reduces renal clearance of calcium, and increases intestinal calcium absorption; these results in increased serum calcium levels, hypercalcemia. It is treated by surgical removal of glands or medication with bisphosphonates. In secondary hyperparathyroidism, the secretion of PTH is increased because of hypocalcemia, and its treatment involves vitamin D_3 supplementation or phosphate binders. Teriparatide is a recombinant form of active fragment of PTH, and is used to treat advanced osteoporosis. Daily injections of teriparatide stimulate new bone formation, leading to increased bone mineral density.

Thyroid hormones: Thyroid produces 2 hormones: thyroxine and calcitonin. Thyroxine (T4) is a prohormone that can be converted to its active form tri-iodothyronine (T3). This active hormone influences the activity and metabolism of all cells, and it plays an important role in physical development and growth. T4 affects intestinal calcium absorption; thus, it is indirectly involved in bone turnover. Hyperthyroidism or thyroxine medication can lead to osteoporosis. The effect of exogenous thyroxine is a significant increase in the rate of OTM. In many ways, calcitonin has the opposite effects to PTH; calcitonin decreases intestinal calcium absorption, osteoclast activity in bone, and renal calcium reabsorption. It is used to treat post-menopausal osteoporosis, hypocalcemia, and Paget's disease. It might be beneficial in osteoarthritis. Although calcitonin is involved in bone remodeling and calcium homeostasis, but there is no experimental data on the effect of administration of exogenous calcitonin on rate of OTM.

Estrogens: Estrogens are female sex hormones. It was found that the rate of OTM increases with decrease serum–estrogen level, and vice versa. Ovariectomy also leads to increase in the rate of OTM. Specific estrogen receptor modulators such as **raloxifene** have been developed, which have estrogenic effect in bone, but reduce the risk of breast cancer. Therefore, it is considered a good alternative for hormone replacement therapy, HRT, for treatment of osteoporosis. It can be hypothesised that estrogen supplementation might slow OTM. But no experimental studies are available to evaluate the effect of exogenous estrogens on OTM. The same is true for raloxifene. Like estrogen supplementation, it might slow OTM, but experimental studies are lacking.

1,25 dihydroxycholecalciferol (vitamin D_3): It regulates calcium and phosphate serum levels by promoting their intestinal absorption and reabsorption in kidneys. It also promotes bone deposition and inhibits PTH release. It also promotes immunosuppression. Its deficiency can occur from inadequate intake, inadequate sunlight exposure, which leads to impaired bone mineralization, rickets, and osteoporosis. Therapy for its deficiency is diet and supplements. Hypervitaminosis D causes hypocalcemia and might cause anorexia, nausea, polyuria, and eventually renal failure. It can be treated with a low-calcium diet and corticosteroids. Studies on rats showed that vitamin D_3 stimulated the rate of OTM in a dose-dependent manner. Physiologic doses of vitamin D_3 do not stimulate bone resorption; but low supplemental dose leads to bone resorption, possibly by upregulation of receptor activator for nuclear factor B ligand (RANKL) expression in osteoblasts, leading ultimately to osteoclast differentiation through the RANK/RANKL system.

Dietary calcium: Adults need 1,000–1300 mg of calcium per day. It is recommended as a dietary supplement to prevent osteoporosis in post-menopausal women. The effect of dietary calcium on OTM was studied in dogs. The dogs on low-calcium diet showed higher rate of OTM than on high-calcium diet. It supports the bone turnover studies showing increased number of osteoclasts and osteoblasts in rats at a low-calcium diet.

Bisphosphonates: They inhibit bone resorption, are used primarily for the prevention and therapy of osteoporosis, Paget's disease, bone metastases, and bone pain from some types of cancer (e.g., alendronate or risedronate). They get incorporated in bone matrix, and are unique in having an extremely long half-life of 10 years or more. Therefore, they can affect bone metabolism for many years after the patient has completed therapy. Effect of bisphosphonates on the rate of OTM has been a dose-dependent decrease in the rate of OTM, with either topical or systemic administration of bisphosphonates. AHBuBP (a nitrogen-containing bisphosphonate) is more effective than clodronate, whereas risedronate was the most effective in inhibiting OTM. Long-term use of bisphosphonates can cause osteonecrosis, especially in alveolar bones of maxilla and mandible. They literally lead to complete stoppage of OTM by preventing any bone remodelling and thus can be useful for anchorage preparation by locally injecting them around the anchor teeth.

Drugs Controlling Salivary Flow

Antisialogogues: Salivary control is very important for successful bonding of orthodontic appliances especially in mandibular arch and on lingual sides. Proper salivation control with gauge-padding, saliva ejectors, isolation with rubber dam, etc. should be used properly for isolation during bonding. Anticholinergics (antimuscarinics) drugs, like **methantheline** (banthine) and **propantheline bromide** (probanthine) are used to reduce salivary flow. They act by competitively blocking acetylcholine action on the effector cells innervated by **postganglionic parasympathetic fibers**. They also exert effects on other organs, e.g. small doses decrease salivary, lacrimal, bronchial and sweat secretions, while larger doses dilate the pupils, increase heart rate, cause urinary retention and constipation. Low doses stimulate CNS while larger doses lead to CNS depression. They antagonize the parasympathetic **"SLUD" syndrome**, i.e. these drugs decrease or block salivation, lacrimation, urination, and defecation.

Anticholinergics, like **atropine and scopolamine,** also have anti-salivary action, but also have pronounced cardiovascular and central effects; and should not be used. Drugs with more selective action, e.g. methantheline (Banthine) and propantheline (Probanthine) should be used as antisialogogues because they have fewer side effects. Methantheline and propantheline have little or no central action, and have milder cardiovascular effects. A single dose 1 hour prior to any orthodontic bonding procedure is needed, which is 50 mg and 15 mg. for Banthine and probanthine respectively for adults. These are contraindicated in patients with glaucoma, prostate hypertrophy, myasthenia gravis and some cardiovascular disease. Patient's physician should be consulted before prescribing such drugs.

Prevention of Bacterial Endocarditis

Infective endocarditis (also called SABE) can occur in susceptible patients due to bacteremia from oral microorganisms during certain dental procedures. The most common organism implicated in infective endocarditis is alpha-hemolytic Streptococcus (e.g. *Streptococcus viridans*). Pretreatment **antibiotic cover** should be given in patients having certain heart diseases, e.g. (1) most congenital heart diseases, (2) rheumatic valvular heart disease, (3) other acquired valvular disease, (4) idiopathic hypertrophic subaortic stenosis, and (5) mitral valve prolapse. Thus, an antibiotic cover should be given during procedures involving bleeding, e.g. orthodontic placement/removal of bands, tooth separation by using brass wires, any surgical procedures, oral prophylaxis, curettage, gingivectomy, endodontics, extractions, biopsy, etc. in patients with valvular heart disease, valvular prosthesis, and a history of rheumatic fever. Bonding of orthodontic appliances should be used as an ideal method in such patients for prevention of infective endocarditis.

AHA recommendations for antibiotic cover for heart patients as given below should be followed.

Drugs Having Anticaries Effects

Fluorides in orthodontics: Fluoride prevents enamel demineralization; inhibits white spot lesions and caries. It is delivered by fluoridated water, fluoride tablets, topical fluorides, or fluoride mouth rinses. Fluoride provides its greatest benefits during period of tooth development, from infancy to 12–14 years of age, as it gets incorporated in enamel in the form of fluor-apatite, which is more resistant to acids produced by bacteria. Maximal protection from dental caries is obtained by daily ingestion of drinking water containing 1 ppm of fluoride and food containing 1 mg of fluoride. Other preventive measures like oral hygiene and diet restriction should be used. Water having less fluoride needs supplementation with other forms of fluoride, the dosage of which depends on the age of the child. Orthodontic appliances act as a plaque harbouring site, leading to localised enamel demineralisation esp around the brackets, it leads to development of white spot lesions. WSL are the subsurface demineralisation without frank surface discontinuity. They can be remineralised under proper environment. The patients should be prescribed strict oral hygiene regimen, fluoride containing tooth pastes; chlorhexidine 0.12% mouthwash, regular oral prophylaxis, etc. on a regular basis.

Fluorosis is most evident in permanent teeth, and deciduous teeth are affected only at high levels of fluoride intake. Accidental ingestion of excessive fluoride results in salty/soapy taste, tremors, convulsions, shock, and renal failure. Treatment consists of inducing emesis with syrup of ipecac or mustard water, followed by having the patient drink large quantities of milk. 10 c.c. of calcium gluconate 10% is given to form insoluble calcium fluoride (CaF_2). It also provides post-eruptive benefits to teeth when infant drops and sodium fluoride tablets are chewed and swallowed. Topical fluorides also improve periodontal conditions by inhibiting microorganisms and their byproducts. Topical fluoride gels, mouth rinses, etc. may be applied immediately before orthodontic banding. There are three types of office fluoride solution: (1) sodium fluoride (NaF), (2) stannous fluoride (SnF_2), and (3) acidulated phosphate fluoride (APF). Orthodontic bands should be fixed with cements containing fluoride, e.g. GIC, zinc polycarboxylate. The caries lesions should be restored with fluoride-containing cements.

Transcutaneous Electrical Neural Stimulation (TENS) for Pain Control

It is a non-invasive pain control technique. TENS is delivered via surface electrodes placed over the painful area. The current is used in a voltage range of 0 to 90 V (or 60 mA) and a frequency range of 0 to 100 Hz. The pulse width duration ranges from 10 to 200 μsec. It is used in general pain control by physiotherapists for chronic pain and post-surgical pain. In dentistry, it was used first for treatment of myofascial pain dysfunction (MPDS). TENS is a short, low-amplitude electrical impulse between two electrodes placed on the skin. Signals from electrical stimulation of large **beta fibers**, i.e. the fibers for pressure and touch, reach CNS before the signals from smaller **slower A and C fibers**, i.e. nerve fibers for pain. Thus, the beta impulse "closes the gate" to the pain impulses. It also stimulates the production of beta endorphin and/or substance "P" in nerve cells which is a local analgesic; and serotonin in brain, raising the patient's pain tolerance.

Conclusions

Medications, such as anti-inflammatory and anti-asthmatic medications, anti-arthritics, analgesics, corticosteroids, estrogens and other hormones, and calcium regulators, all affect the rate of OTM. Some medications stimulate the rate of OTM, but others have an inhibitory effect. Only paracetamol has been

	Adults	*Children*
Parenteral and oral combined	Aqueous crystalline penicillin G (1,000,000 units I/M) mixed with procaine penicillin G (600,000 units I/M), given 30 minutes to 1 hour preoperatively. Continue with Penicillin V (phenoxymethyl penicillin), 500 mg orally every 6 hours for eight doses.	Children: Aqueous crystalline penicillin G (30,000 units per kg body wt I/M) mixed with procaine penicillin G (600,000 units I/M) given 30 minutes to 1 hour preoperatively. For children who weigh less than 60 pounds, the dose of penicillin V is 250 mg. orally every 6 hours for eight doses.
Oral	Penicillin V (2.0 grams orally 30 minutes to 1 hour preoperatively and then 500 mg. orally every 6 hours for eight doses). A dose of amoxicillin 2 gm is given 1 hour before the surgery in adults (AHA 2007)	Same as for adults. But for children less than 60 pounds weight, give 1.0 grams orally 30 minutes to I hour preoperatively and then 250 mg. orally every 6 hours for eight doses.
For patients allergic to penicillin		
Oral route	Erythromycin (1.0 gram orally 1½ to 2 hours preoperatively and then 500 mg. orally every 6 hours for eight doses).	Erythromycin (20 mg. /kg. orally 1½ to 2 hours preoperatively and then 10 mg. /kg. every 6 hours for eight doses).
	Vancomycin (1 g intravenously over 30 minutes to 1 hour). Start initial vancomycin infusion ½ to 1 hour preoperatively; then erythromycin, 500 mg. orally every 6 hours for eight doses.	Vancomycin (20 mg/kg intravenously over 30 minutes to 1 hour). The total dose of vancomycin should not exceed 44 mg/kg/24 hours. Timing of doses for children is the same as for adults. Erythromycin dose is 10 mg/kg every 6 hours for eight doses.
Regimen B—Penicillin plus streptomycin		
	Aqueous crystalline penicillin G (1,000,000 units I/M) mixed with procaine penicillin G (600,000 units intramuscularly) plus streptomycin (1.0 gram intramuscularly) between 30 minutes and 1 hour preoperatively; then give penicillin V, 500 mg orally every 6 hours for eight doses.	Aqueous crystalline penicillin G (30,000 units per kilogram intramuscularly) mixed with procaine penicillin G (600,000 units intramuscularly) plus streptomycin (20 mg/kg intramuscularly). Timing of doses for children of less than 60 pounds: give penicillin V, 250 mg every 6 hours for eight doses.

found to be having no effect on the rate of OTM. Corticosteroids, especially glucocorticoids, stimulate OTM. Local or systemic use of PTH also increases the rate of OTM. The same effect is seen when endogenous PTH synthesis is stimulated by, for example, a low-calcium diet. Administration of exogenous thyroxine increases the rate of OTM in a dose-dependent manner. An inverse relationship between estrogens and OTM exists. Administration of vitamin D_3 increases the rate of OTM in a dose-dependent manner.

Bisphosphonate decreases the rate of OTM, but they may lead to osteonecrosis in maxilla and mandible. In orthodontic patients, bisphosphonates can be used to prevent relapse. Estrogens used to treat osteoporosis might delay OTM, but on appositive side, it can inhibit alveolar bone loss in periodontitis.

Orthodontists see many patients on such medications; and using over the counter drugs. Medications have an important influence on the rate of tooth movement, and information on their consumption is essential to adequately discuss treatment planning with patients.

64

Evolution of Orthodontics

INTRODUCTION

Orthodontics is the first and the oldest speciality of dentistry. In the last more than 150 years, it has evolved in leaps and bounds due to incessant efforts of the practitioners to provide the best possible and comfortable treatment to the patients. Although it started in middle of the 19th century, but the major thrust to its existence came in late 19th and early 20th century with the untiring efforts and constant innovations of EH Angle. It were his efforts which gave us the standard edgewise appliance in 1920s, which is the main foundation for all the fixed appliances being used today, e.g. SWA, Roth's, MBT, etc. This appliance has been modified by many clinicians to suit the needs of patient and clinicians.

Orthodontics being a vast subject, like an ocean, cannot be discussed in limited space of this book, but we have tried to summarize the most important innovations which we consider as the landmarks in the science of orthodontics. We have divided these innovations in following categories for the sake of convenience.

A. Evolution of Fixed Appliances/Brackets

During the last 150 years or so, the fixed appliance has evolved from its crudest form containing a jargon of wires/acrylic/screws, etc. to most sophisticated computer generated/designed appliances being used today. However, the landmark appliance from a clinical perspective was given by Angle in 1920s in the form of **edgewise appliance** after years of research and modification. For many decades, his edgewise appliance remained at the forefront of orthodontic therapy. His discarded ribbon arch appliance was used by his student Raymond Beggs mostly in Australia, due to its concept of using lighter forces, but it is slipping in oblivion day by day, and is rarely used now a days. Meanwhile, many other authors described some modifications in the Angle's appliance system, e.g. Jarabak, vari simplex, etc. but could not undermine the importance of Angle's edgewise system. Another landmark invention was introduced in the form of **straight wire appliance** (SWA) by Andrews in 1970s where he introduced the tip/torque in the brackets themselves and almost eliminated the need of wire bending. Many other appliances having different values of pre-introduced tip/torque values in brackets followed after that depending on the philosophies of their introducers, e.g. Roth's, Rickett's, MBT, etc. which are just the modifications of SWA. But the word "SWA" is mostly used by most of the clinicians as it has deeply ingrained in their minds. Another landmark came with the introduction of **lingual appliances** in 1990s which has almost eliminated the need of labial wires and is mostly used in esthetic-conscious patients only who can pay huge amount of money for it. Another landmark is evolution of **self-ligating brackets** appliance which eliminates the need of individually tying the arch wire in bracket slots using ligature wires or elastomerics. The computer generated **Orametrix system** is also another landmark where the archwires are prefabricated by a computer program for the whole treatment stages in a special lab-guided by a special software. Although in its nascent stages, it is expected to take a major share of orthodontic practice in future once the clinicians are aware of it, get trained and it becomes economical.

Invisalign

It is a recent removable appliance option using a clear resin, full coverage "invisible" orthodontic appliances (Invisalign, Align Technology). These have acceptable esthetics and thus have increased demand from the adult orthodontic cases. But these clear, full-coverage, removable resin appliances can only be used in simple cases needing simple and minor movements; they cannot be used for all types of cases. Any need of 3D movements of teeth is best controlled with fixed appliances. They are more comfortable and result in less periodontal inflammation than fixed appliances. Invisalign cannot be used for cases needing bicuspid extractions. Invisalign appliance is a series of aligners made from transparent, thin (less than 1 mm) plastic material with CAD-CAM techniques which have to be replaced by the patient after every 2 weeks in a predetermined sequence. These aligners resemble the occlusal splints used in TMD cases, etc. Each aligner is designed to move the teeth a maximum of about 0.25 to 0.3 mm over a 2-week period. Excellent compliance is mandatory since the appliance has to be worn a minimum of 20 to 22 hours a day.

B. Evolution of the Arch Wires

The arch wire materials used in orthodontics have evolved tremendously over the years. It all started with gold wires, but with the invention of stainless steel, the SS replaced gold due to its superior properties and lesser cost, and is still reigning the space. Another landmark in the arch wire materials was the introduction of NiTinol wires, which completely changed the way the orthodontics used to be done previously. Although many types of materials have been used for arch wires, e.g. TMA, Elgiloy, beta-Ti, etc. but in the orthodontic clinic, mainly SS and NiTi wires still hold the major space. Only in rare conditions, the other types of wires are used. Differen[t] types of NiTi wire, e.g. M-NiTi, A-NiTi, Japanese-NiTi, Chinese-NiTi, etc. have been described in literature, but they hold only theoretical significance, while in clinica[l] practice, the clinical refers them as NiTi only. Another milestone can be the introduction o[f] esthetic wires due to increased demand o[f] esthetics and tooth-colored bracket by the consumers. Therefore, the ceramic and plastic brackets were introduced.

C. Material of Brackets

Development of dental material sciences have left its imprints on orthodontics. The first brackets used in orthodontics were made of gold, which were of yellow color, costly, and ductile. But with the invention of SS material, the SS brackets came in the existence and are still used. They are cheaper, stronger, not of very bright color like gold. Continued demand for the esthetic appliances led to development of tooth-colored bracket, i.e. plastic, composite and ceramic brackets. Ceramic brackets are high in demand for esthetic conscious patients, but are brittle, and tend to abrade the opposing tooth if it comes in contact. They also possess a tendency of enamel fracture during debonding.

D. Method of Attachment of Brackets and Wires

All the teeth need to be banded for placing the fixed appliance on the teeth, but the advent of etching and bonding has changed everything in orthodontics. Bonding of brackets is one of the most important milestone in orthodontics, where the brackets are directly placed on the enamel surface of teeth with the help of etching and bonding. Invention of self-etching primers SEP has helped to eliminate one step from the bonding procedure, thus further reducing the time of bracket placement. Introduction of light curing method of bonding is again in mile stone in placement of attachments. Now the plasma arc and argon laser are being tried to bond the brackets with considerable reduction of the time taken. Also, the fixing the archwires to brackets needed brass and gold wires, which were later on replaced by SS ligature wires. Now, the elastomeric modules can be wrapped around the brackets, thus fixing the wires in the slots.

E. Evolution in Diagnosis

Diagnosis is the main step for treatment planning of a case of malocclusion. Initially, the clinicians used their experience and clinical acumen to diagnose and decide the treatment plan. But a milestone was established with the advent of cephalostat in 1930s, which entirely changed the thinking of orthodontists and immensely helped in the research related to growth of the jaws also. It helped to provide tremendous insight in the treatment planning, growth of the jaws, treatment changes, etc. and it still remains the most important, mandatory, and unreplaceable diagnostic record. Computerisation of the world has also infiltrated the medical science and thence the orthodontist's office. The latest diagnostic methods have inbuilt computers, e.g. digital video imaging; MRI, CBCT, 2D and 3D CT scans and computerized cephalometry with the help of digigraph/digitization of landmarks and sophisticated, user friendly softwares. Thus just with clicking the mouse, hundreds of cephalometrics calculations can be done within seconds. But, the manual cephalometry is still widely used worldwide due to high cost pertaining to the computerized equipments.

F. Evolution of Myofunctional Appliances

Concept of myofunctional appliances started almost 100 years ago with the chance experimentation by Andersen which he called activator. But it was a crude, bulky and uncomfortable appliance. Many modifications were introduced in due course of time by different authors, e.g. bionator, Frankel appliances, etc. They were widely used throughout the world and especially in Europe. But they were single-piece appliance which were highly uncomfortable and interfered with speech and mouth opening. A mile stone was achieved by Clarks when he introduce twin block appliance in 1980s and overcame all the discomforts of single-piece myofunctional appliances. Now twin-block and its modifications have become the most widely used appliances. Removable appliances always have a factor of patient's non-cooperation. This factor has been eliminated by invention of fixed functional appliances, FFA, which mainly started with Herbst's appliance. But now, many types of fixed functional appliances have been introduced by many clinicians overcoming the major problems with earlier appliances. These FFAs can be used in uncooperative patients and during later stages of active growth to take advantage of remaining growth.

G. Molar Distalization

Many cases need the distalization of upper first molars to achieve class I relation and to gain some space. In the past, crude removable appliances with many wire components were used without much success. Even, the headgear, being a very good appliance for this purpose, was also used, but both of these appliances lost credibility due to non–cooperative behavior of patients. But clinicians did not lose heart and introduced fixed appliances for molar distalization which overcome the factor of patient's cooperation. Presently, there are more than 20 appliances in use for molar distalization, some of which can be made by the clinicians and some are available as prefabricated.

H. Evolution of Retainers

Retention appliances have also evolved over the years form bulky, crude, acrylic removable appliances having soldered wire components to preformed fixed retainers of different sizes to choose from. The present day removable retainers can be made of different attractive colors with stronger acrylic material having lesser chances of breakage during use. Transparent ESSIX retainers have made the life of patients very comfortable as it is removable, very comfortable, colorless and does not interfere with speech.

I. Shift in Treatment Regimens

Angle believed in non-extraction treatment of the patients with his belief that for proper occlusion, all the teeth are required in the oral cavity. So he used mainly expansion of arches in anterior and lateral dimensions. But such cases showed disturbed esthetics and high rate of relapse. Then, Tweed introduced his concept of extraction of some teeth to achieve better stability of the teeth after treatment. His philosophy was followed for almost 60 years, and still followed today. But now, the concept of non-extraction and the arch development is again emerging. However, it is the clinician who determines the best possible treatment regimen for his patient. Also, previously the hard tissue, i.e. relation of jaws and teeth to each other was considered to be more important for treatment planning and evaluation. But now the soft tissue planning is one of the most important parameter for treatment planning.

J. Paradigm Shift in the Age of the Patient for Starting the Treatment

In the past, the orthodontic treatment was generally started once the child used to reach in late MDP or PDP. But with increased knowledge and experience, the clinicians have deciphered many conditions which need to be corrected as early as they are seen. Thus the concept of "2-phase" treatment has emerged, where one phase is used at an early age, followed by a period of no-treatment/rest/retention of previous problem, and then the phase-2 of active fixed appliance is undertaken. This helps to remove those problems which are expected to create restrictive influence on the proper growth of the jaws.

K. Evolution of Maxillary Expansion

Removable, bulky, crude appliances having crude screws were used in the past during initial days of orthodontics. Angle has also described a heavy labiobuccal wire to which all the teeth were ligated with the help of thick brass wires to expand the arches. But with the advent of material science, the different designs/sizes/types of expansion screws are available. Fixed appliances, like Nitanium palatal expanders, NPE I and II, which get activated themselves once placed intraorally, are very comfortable.

L. Evolution of Surgical Orthodontics

Improved knowledge of surgical principals, anesthesia and surgical procedures has helped clinicians and patients to treat the skeletal discrepancies, asymmetries and many congenital conditions. At the forefront is distraction osteogenesis (DO) which involves the gradual lengthening of the bone using heavy duty expansion screw called as distractor and it uses the natural principles of bone lengthening, repair, soft tissue adaptation, etc. Use of palatal splitting for SARPE has led the expansion of narrow maxilla in many patients. Using the principles of distraction osteogenesis, the alveolodental distraction of canines, accelerated osteogenic orthodontics (AOO) i.e. wilckodontics, regional accelerated phenomenon (RAP) etc. are emerging concepts of tooth movements during orthodontics for reducing the treatment timings.

Dentoalveolar distraction (DAD): It was introduced by Kisnisci et al in 2002 for rapid canine retraction. In this approach, the segment that contains the canine is transported as a bone block. It is different from the Liou and Huang technique that the periodontal ligament is not stretched in it. Here, a bone separation is done using corticotomies which forms a bone block containing the canine to allow the tooth to move alongwith the bone that surrounds it through a distraction osteogenesis process. Distraction osteogenesis for rapid orthodontic tooth movement is a promising technique. With DAD, canines can be fully retracted in 8–14 days, and the anchorage teeth withstand the retraction forces with no anchorage loss and without any clinical or radiographical evidence of complications, like root resorption, periodontal problems, soft tissue dehiscence, etc. It reduces orthodontic treatment duration by 6–9 months in the patients who need extraction, with no need for extraoral or intraoral anchorage devices

Surgery before orthodontics: Another concept of treatment of severe skeletal cases needing orthodontics and jaw surgery is to do surgery first before the orthodontic treatment, as was being done previously. But case selection is of utmost importance in such cases. Here, the orthognathic surgery is performed first to correct the skeletal discrepancy, and then the occlusion is refined with orthodontic appliance. Thus the phases and time of treatment is reduced.

M. Evidence-Based Orthodontics

Latest in the medical science is the concept of evidence based practice, which means that the clinician should use and select the best method for treatment of a particular condition based on the current evidences. However, the systematic reviews published in the literature in last 10–15 years could not find the best practice methods for most of the procedures used in orthodontics, and have recommended that randomised controlled trials (RCTs) should be conducted to find out the best methods. In the mean time, they recommend that the clinicians have to decide the best treatment method for his patients based on his knowledge and experience.

N. Evolution in Concepts of OTM

Forces were considered to lead to some changes in PD and bony tissues which led to tooth movements. But the scientific knowledge has now entered the molecular level and has found the receptors and genes, etc. associated with the bone remodelling. Concepts of RANKL and OPG has come in the forefront of biochemical changes associated with forces. Many drugs and chemicals have been found which can influence the rate of OTM, either increasing or decreasing it, and can be used in various circumstances. LASERs, LLLT, PEMF, TENS, etc. are being tried and improved to be used in the orthodontics. Transcutaneous electrical nerve stimulation (TENS) can also be used for pain control during orthodontic treatment.

O. Nanoparticles

These are also being applied to control pain signalling, and increase nerve branching by using nanospheres filled with factors which induce nervous tissues regeneration. But the nanotechnology is still in a very nascent stage. Dr. Sims has also proposed the use of programmed nanorobots to control the biomechanical response and to achieve dental movement, rather than brackets.

P. Application of Cyclic Forces

Research has found that the use of cyclic forces increases the rate of bone remodeling compared to static forces. A pulsating force has been found to increase the amount and rate of tooth movement. Cyclic forces increase the rate of bone remodeling to levels far greater than static forces or intermittent forces. Cyclic forces, also referred to as pulsatile forces, are different from intermittent forces that are applied for some duration of time, removed, and then reapplied. A static force is applied once and affects the cells once; while an intermittent force is still a static force, the only difference is that it is introduced episodically. In contrast, cyclic forces are oscillatory in nature, which change the magnitude rapidly and repeatedly, affecting the cells with each oscillation of force magnitude. The frequency of cyclic forces is never zero. Cyclic forces cause deformation by changing a structure's length multiple times, whereas intermittent and static forces do so once per application. Thus the cells are impacted multiple times by the frequency of the pulsating force being applied. Frequencies for orthodontic application range up to 100 Hz or more. Cyclic forces impact the tissues and cells multiple times, which leads to dramatic differences in biological response in the bones. Multiple cycles in force are significant because cells respond more readily to rapid oscillation in force magnitude than to constant force. A force passing through biological tissues is transduced as a mechanical stress which induces interstitial flow. Cells are known to respond more readily to oscillatory force (cyclic forces) than to constant forces. Animal studies using cyclic forces have demonstrated increased bone remodeling and increased tooth movement. It also leads to less root resorption. A new device (AcceleDent, OrthoAccel Technologies) utilizes cyclic forces to reduce the duration of orthodontic treatment and to relieve discomfort.

AcceleDent Device

One portion of the device is a mouthpiece, which the patient bites onto during use. It is connected to another piece (activator) that stays outside the mouth; that provide the cyclic forces (vibration). It is used once daily for 20 minutes. The applied force from the device is at 0.2 N (20 gm), which is barely noticeable and not uncomfortable.

Q. Evolution in Anchorage Management

Entrance of microimplants and miniplates, also known as temporary anchorage devices (TADs); onplants, dental implants, etc. have been another milestone which has completely changed the concept of anchorage in orthodontics, and a new concept of absolute anchorage, without any anchorage loss has come up. It is being widely used in clinics worldwide and a lot of research is being dedicated to it. Certain locally injected chemicals and drugs are being tried to prevent anchorage loss by preventing the localized bone absorption.

R. Evolution in Genetic Knowledge

Research of genes controlling various aspects of growth, clefting, biochemical changes, etc. have changed the outlook of clinicians and it is expected that a lot of genetic knowledge will be used in near future to prevent the congenital conditions from developing.

Summary of Orthodontic Evolution

The major milestones in clinical orthodontics which have come up in last many decades can be summarised as follows.

a. Orthodontic appliances: Removable ⟶ Angle's edgewise appliance ⟶ SWA ⟶ self-ligating and lingual appliances
b. Wires: GOLD ⟶ S.S ⟶ NiTi and esthetic wires
c. Bracket materials: GOLD ⟶ S.S. ⟶ ceramic
d. Anchorage: Tooth tissue supported ⟶ TADs
e. Diagnosis: Clinical exam ⟶ cephalometry ⟶ computerized video imaging, CBCT, MRI, 3D-CT, etc
f. FJO: Removable activator ⟶ twin block ⟶ fixed functional appliances
g. Molar distalization: Removable appliances ⟶ headgear ⟶ fixed appliances for molar distalization
h. Philosophy of treatment: Non-extraction ⟶ extraction ⟶ non-extraction
i. One phase treatment ⟶ 2-phase treatment
j. Method of attachment: Banding ⟶ bonding ⟶ SEP (self-etching primers)
k. Soft-tissue importance: Hard tissue evaluation ⟶ soft tissue-evaluation

65

Risk Factors of Root Resorption after Orthodontic Treatment

INTRODUCTION

Root resorption is a common sequela of orthodontic treatment. It is an inflammatory process leading to an ischemic necrosis in a localized area of PDL when the orthodontic force is applied. Certain risk factors are associated with the onset and progression of root resorption, e.g. duration of treatment, magnitude of force applied, direction of tooth movement, method of force application (continuous versus intermittent), type of orthodontic movement. Patient-related risk factors are the individual susceptibility on a genetic basis, some systemic diseases, abnormal root morphology, dental trauma, and previous endodontic treatment. The prevention of root resorption during orthodontic treatment may be done by controlling risk factors. The periodic radiographic examination during the treatment is necessary to detect the occurrence of root damages and thus plan the further treatment.

External apical root resorption (EARR) is an iatrogenic consequence of orthodontic treatment. The root resorption is significantly correlated with treatment duration, fixed appliance treatment, tooth structure, individual susceptibility, type of orthodontic tooth movement. EARR is one of the side effects induced by orthodontic treatment, but sometimes it is diagnosed without any orthodontic treatment. It is usually asymptomatic and is generally detected by routine radiological examination. Some amount of RR always occurs during orthodontic treatment which is considered as clinically non significant. But extensive RR should be taken care of as early as possible. RR can occur at root apex as well as the lateral surfaces of root, but only apical root resorption is seen on radiographs. Usually, orthodontic treatment doesn't cause clinically significant root resorption but only microscopic changes appear on the roots, which are difficult to detect in radiological images. Root resorption is considered as clinically important when 1–2 mm (one-fourth) of the root length is lost. Severe root resorption during orthodontic treatment (>5 mm) occurs rarely, just in 1–5% of patients. There exist certain risk factors for root resorption which should be known to the orthodontist to assess a patient for planning orthodontic treatment and to choose the best method for treatment.

Types of Root Resorption

It is of three types:

1. Microresorption = is confined to cementum; is localized, superficial, and gets repaired.
2. Progressive root resorption = appears at the site of continuous and heavy forces; it may involve entire apex.
3. Idiopathic root resorption = it is seen even before the start of orthodontic treatment. It gets aggravated by the orthodontic treatment.

Degrees of Severity of Root Resorption

There are three degrees of severity of root resorption:

1. Cementum or surface resorption, occurring together with remodeling, when

only outer cementum layer is resorbed, which regenerates or remodels later. This process is similar to trabecular bone remodeling.

2. Dentin resorption with repair (deep resorption), when cementum and outer dentin layer are resorbed; resorption is irreversible because only cementum regenerates. Tooth root form after this resorption and remodeling may stay the same or altered.
3. Surrounding apical root resorption, when hard apical root tissue is fully resorbed and root shortening is observed. Apical tissues under cementum are lost, root tissues do not regenerate. Repair of outer surface occurs in the cementum layer.

The degree of root resorption: A. Irregular root contour, B. Apical root resorption is less than 2 mm, C. Apical root resorption is from 2 mm to one-third of the initial root length, D. Apical root resorption is more that one-third of the initial root length of root resorption.

Root resorption index:

1. Grade I = irregular root contour
2. Grade II = root resorption at the apex; is less than 2 mm.
3. Grade III = root resorption from 2 mm to one-third of the root length.
4. Grade IV = root resorption is more than one-third of the root length.

Mechanism of Root Resorption

Mechanism of root resorption is not completely understood. According to Brudvik and Rygh, inflammatory root resorption induced by orthodontic treatment is a part of process of elimination of hyaline zone. It is considered that occurrence of root resorption can be induced by heavy orthodontic forces and hyalinisation of periodontal ligaments induced by increased activity of cementoclasts and osteoclasts. During removal of hyalined zone, the root surface consisting of layer of cementoblasts may be damaged, exposing the underlying highly dense mineralized cementum. It is possible that a force during orthodontic treatment may damage outer root surface.

Risk Factors for Root Resorption

There are many factors which can induce root resorption during orthodontic treatment. These factors can be divided into biological, mechanical and combined factors and other circumstances.

I. Biological Factors

Individual susceptibility is a main factor determining root resorption, which may be due to a systemic or innate predisposition to occurrence of resorption.

Genetics: Predisposition to root resorption may be related to genes. Genetic factors account for at least 50% of the variation in root resorption.

Systemic factor: Allergic patients are susceptible to increased risk of root resorption. Conditions like asthma also appear to be associated with greater risk of apical root resorption. Lack of estrogens induces quick orthodontic tooth movement, and calcitonin inhibits activity of odontoclasts.

Impacted third molars may also cause root resorption of the second molar. Maxillary canines are the second most commonly impacted teeth; they can induce root resorption of the incisors and first premolars.

Tooth structure: Root resorption most often occurs in the apical part of the root, because forces are concentrated at the root apex because orthodontic tooth movement is never entirely translatory and the fulcrum is usually occlusal to the apical part of the root; the apical third of root is covered with cellular cementum, whereas the coronary third is covered by noncellular cementum. Levander and Malmgren divide root forms to: normal, short, blunt, dilacerated and pipette-shaped. Most authors have shown that roots with abnormal shape have a higher susceptibility to root resorption. According to Sinclaire, normal and blunt tooth roots resorb the least.

Pipette-shaped roots are the most susceptible to root resorption. Short roots have a greater risk for root resorption than average length roots. It was found that small roots resorb almost twice more than other root forms.

Nutrition: Becks has shown that root resorption occurred in the animals lacking calcium and vitamin D in their foods.

Chronological age: Periodontal membrane becomes narrower and less vascularized, aplastic, alveolar bone becomes denser, less vascularized and aplastic, and cementum becomes wider with age. Through these changes adults show higher susceptibility to root resorption. When a patient is older than 11 years, risk for root resorption increases due to closure of apical foramen.

Dental age: Rosenberg has stated that teeth with incomplete root formation undergo less root resorption than those with completely formed roots. Brezniak et al have stated that if tooth roots are not completely formed in the beginning of orthodontic treatment, they are further developing during treatment. Linge and Linge have established that ortodontically treated teeth lose averagely 0.5 mm of the root length.

Sex: No significant relationship between sex and root resorption was found.

Ethnic group: Root resorption more rarely occurs in Asians than in white, Caucasian or Hispanic patients.

Root Resorption Prior to Orthodontic Treatment

Intrusion and Torque are probably the most detrimental to the tooth involved. Using rapid palatal expansion techniques, premolars and molars are pressed in a buccal direction against the thin cortical plate with risk of similar damage.

Root resorption which existed prior to orthodontic treatment increases risk of root resorption during orthodontic treatment.

Habits, such as bruxism, nail biting, tongue thrust associated with open bite and increased tongue pressure are related to increased root resorption.

Anomalies of position and number of teeth: Hypodontia increases risk of root resorption. Impacted teeth may also induce root resorption. Longer roots are more likely to be resorbed than shorter ones because longer roots need stronger forces to be moved and the actual displacement of root apex is greater during tipping or torquing movements. It has been found that a normal root form of central incisors and wide roots are preventive factors of these roots, decreasing risk of root resorption. Slightly increased root resorption is characteristic of narrower roots. Dental trauma may lead to root resorption without orthodontic treatment. Orthodontically moved traumatized teeth with previous root resorption are more sensitive to further loss of root material. The teeth can be treated orthodontically three months after the tooth transplantation or replantation which react as normal tooth to orthodontic force if not ankylosed. Endodontically treated tooth subjected to orthodontic forces is more prone to root resorption. When the root canal filling reaches the root apex, resorption doesn't start, but in case of a shorter filling, the part without the filling may resorb. Denser is alveolar bone, the more root resorption occur during the orthodontic treatment.

Correlation between malocclusion and tooth root resorption was assessed. There is no relation between root resorption and malocclusion. The greater the overjet during the orthodontic treatment, the greater the root resorption for maxillary anterior teeth, because greater tooth movement is necessary in order to decrease overjet. Increased overbite may correlate with more root resorption of maxillary lateral incisors. It was established that the deeper is overbite, the greater is root resorption of a maxillary permanent first molar distal root and maxillary incisor.

Specific tooth vulnerability to root resorption: Maxillary teeth are more sensitive to root resorption than the mandibular teeth and anterior teeth are more susceptible to root resorption than posterior teeth. Maxillary incisors are most affected by root resorption, because the degree of root resorption is correlated with the distance the apex of an incisor moves and the length of time of orthodontic treatment. The most resorbed tooth in lower arch is canine; followed by lateral and central incisors. Root resorption of molars and premolars is very low (less than 1 mm). The most resorbed teeth are the maxillary lateral, maxillary central, lower incisors, maxillary canine, distal root of the first molar, lower second premolar and maxillary second premolar.

II. Mechanical Factors

Orthodontic appliances: Root resorption is more induced with fixed appliances. Heavy, uncontrolled forces applied by removable appliances lead to RR of incisors. Root resorption is less in children who have undergone 2-phase orthodontic treatment, i.e. first with functional appliance and later with fixed appliance, than in children, who have undergone orthodontic treatment with fixed orthodontic appliances. While assessing the influence of metal and aesthetic brackets on root resorption, it was diagnosed more often in patients treated with aesthetic brackets. This is because treatment with aesthetic brackets takes longer time and more friction is involved between wire and slot. Application of an additional upper utility arch for intrusion of maxillary incisors induces root resorption of maxillary central incisors more often than by treating with straight arch.

Intermaxillary elastics: Greater root resorption is found on the tooth/arch where elastics were used. Use of class III elastics increases root resorption of first mandibular molars distal root. Higher root resorption rate (0.43 mm) is seen in patients treated with extraction of teeth than in those treated without extraction (0.31 mm).

Type of orthodontic tooth movement: It may be associated with any type of tooth movement, but most commonly, it is associated with intrusion and torquing of upper incisors. According to Reitan, the force per unit of root surface area (RSA), is less during bodily movement as compared to tipping, where force gets concentrated at the root apex during tipping. Thus the bodily movement induces less risk for root resorption than tipping. Therefore, lighter forces should be used during tipping. Intrusion causes four times more root resorption than extrusion. Resorption areas during the tooth rotation appear in the medial third of root. Harry and Sims found that distribution of resorbed lacunae is directly related to the force magnitude, resorbed lacunae develop more quickly with higher forces. According to Schwartz, forces more than 20–26 g/cm^2 may lead to root resorption. Optimal force for orthodontic tooth movement to avoid root resorption should be 7–26 g/cm^2 of root surface area. Also, the intermittent force causes less root resorption than continuous force because it allows reorganization of periodontal ligaments and restoration of blood circulation, when forces are not active. Continuous force does not provide any resting period when repair of damaged blood vessels and other periodontal tissues may occur, and this may lead to higher rate of root resorption.

III. Combined Biological and Mechanical Factors

Duration of orthodontic treatment is considered an important factor causing root resorption. Goldin has stated that the amount of root resorption during orthodontic treatment is 0.9 mm per year. Patients with longer active fixed appliances therapy see more grade 2 root resorption. Minor root resorption or an irregular root contour detected 6–9 months after the beginning of orthodontic treatment indicates a high risk of further root resorption. Root resorption associated with orthodontic treatment generally stops after completion of active orthodontic treatment. But if sever RR is noted, then all the active forces should be removed for at least 2–3 months. Active root resorption lasts approximately about a week after removal of orthodontic appliances, afterwards cementum repair takes 5–6 weeks. Root resorption after removal of orthodontic appliances is mostly related to causes like occlusal trauma, active retainers, etc.

IV Other Circumstances

Tooth vitality: Tooth vitality and color doesn't change even at extensive root resorption. Orthodontic movement may cause pulp blood flow disturbances, vacuolization and, in rare cases, pulp necrosis, however, it does not relate to root resorption.

Alveolar bone loss and tooth stability: Marginal bone loss is more harmful than the equivalent amount of root length loss because of root resorption. Results indicate that 4 mm of root resorption translate into 20% total attachment loss and 3 mm apical root loss equals only 1mm crestal bone loss. Bone loss leads to decreased stability of a tooth. About 0.2–0.5 mm of alveolar bone height is lost during orthodontic treatment.

Effect of pharmacological agents on root resorption: Several pharmacological agents have been tested to prevent or minimize the incidence of root resorption associated with orthodontics. Drugs which restrict osteoclast activity, e.g. bisphosphonates, have the potential to reduce root resorption, but they also reduce tooth movement. Studies have suggested that local injection of clodronate decreases the number of osteoclasts and thus inhibits root resorption associated with tooth movement. Side effect of bisphosphonates is their association with osteonecrosis of the jaws. It is given to treat certain cancer patients and osteoporosis. The administration of echistatin, an arginineglycine-aspartate acid (RGD)-containing peptide has been found to reduce root resorption in rats. The administration of corticosteroids in doses of 15 mg/kg to rats during orthodontic treatment increased root resorption, whereas low doses of 1 mg/kg decreased root resorption. **Doxycycline**, a potent collagenase inhibitor, has shown to significantly reduce root resorption, the number of odontoclasts, osteoclasts, mononuclear cells on root surface, and TRAP-positive cells on the root and bone in rats. The administration of high doses (50 mg/kg) of celebrex, a cyclogenase-2 inhibitor, during the application of orthodontic forces was reported to reduce root resorption in rats without interfering with the rate of tooth movement.

The administration of very low doses of **L-thyroxin** was shown to decrease RR in both rats and human studies. It is assumed that thyroxin either increases the resistance of the cementum and dentin to clastic activity or increases the rate of alveolar bone resorption. It is well documented that thyroid hormone exerts a biphasic effect on bone formation and resorption. At lower doses, it may increase bone formation, whereas at larger doses bone resorption is enhanced.

Evidence-based knowledge on root resorption: Root resorption has been found to occur in many cases and is associated with multiple factors. It can also be found in patients who are not undergoing orthodontic treatment. Constantinou in a systematic review found that RR can occur in individuals whether they undergo orthodontic treatment or not. During orthodontic treatment, frequency and severity of RR may increase, which in turn is affected by many factors. RR also undergoes certain degree of repair. Whether age, time, and OTM can increase RR remains controversial.

Root resorption associated with orthodontic tooth movement—a systematic review: In an another systematic review, it was found that comprehensive orthodontic treatment causes increased incidence and severity of root resorption, and heavy forces might be particularly harmful. There is not effect of archwire sequencing, bracket prescription, and self-ligation on the root resorption. Previous trauma and tooth morphology are unlikely causative factors. There is some evidence that a 2 to 3 month rest period during treatment decreases total root resorption. In conclusion, the results have been inconclusive in clinical management of root resorption, but evidence supports the use of light forces, especially with incisor intrusion.

In a meta-analysis performed on the treatment-related factors of external apical root resorption, it was found that the total distance the apex had moved and the time it took are also the treatment-related causes of root resorption.

Conclusion

Microscopic root resorption is inevitable during orthodontic treatment. It is clinically insignificant and radiologically invisible. Individual susceptibility is the main risk factor for root resorption during orthodontic treatment; in case of such susceptibility root resorption can start already in the early stage of orthodontic treatment. It is possible to avoid severe root resorption by doing control X-ray images to all orthodontic patients after 6–9 months of orthodontic treatment. Minor root resorption or an irregular tooth root contour detected during this period show that there is a high risk for further root resorption. Optimal force for orthodontic tooth movement but not causing root resorption should be 7–26 g/cm^2 on root surface area.

Selected Further Readings

CLASSIFICATION

Ackerman JL, Proffit WR: The characteristics of malocclusion: a modern approach to classification and diagnosis, Am J Orthod 56:443–454, 1969.

Andrews LF: The six keys to normal occlusion, Am J Orthod 62:296–309, 1972.

Angle EH: Classification of malocclusion, Dental Cosmos 41:248–264; 350–357, 1899.

Begg PR: Begg orthodontic theory and technique, Philadelphia, 1965, WB Saunders.

Koski K: The norm concept in dental orthopedics, Angle Orthod 25:113–117, 1955.

Roth RH (1981): Functional occlusion for the orthodontist. J Cli Orthod, 15: 32–51.

Sampson WJ and Sims MR (1992): Variability of Occlusal Traits in Tropical Populations. In: Prabhu SR, Wilson DF, Daftary DK, Johnson NW (eds.): Oral diseases in the Tropics. Oxford: Oxford University Press, pp. 59–67.

Summers CJ (1971). The Occlusal Index: A System for Identifying and Scoring Occlusal Disoders. Am J Orthod Dentofacial Orthop, 59(6): 553–567.

Tung AW, Kiyak HA: Psychological influences on the timing of orthodontic treatment, Am J Orthod Dentofacial Orthop 113:29–39, 1998.

CAST ANALYSIS AND CEPHALOMETRICS

Ackerman JL, Proffit WR: The characteristics of malocclusion a modern approach to classification and diagnosis. Am J Orthod 56(5): 443–54, 1969.

Afzal A, Ahmed I, Vohra F, Uzair M: Bolton tooth size discrepancies among different malocclusion groups.

Al-Tamimi T, Hashim HA: Bolton tooth-size ratio revisited. World J Orthod 6(3): 289–295, 2005.

Andrews LF: The six keys to normal occlusion. Am J Orthod 62: 296–309, 1972.

Angle EH: Classification of malocclusion. Dental Cosmos 41: 248–264, 1899.

Arya BS, Savara BS, Thomas D, Clarkson Q: Relation of sex and occlusion to mesiodistal tooth size. Am J Orthod 66: 479–486, 1974.

Ballard ML: Assymetry in tooth size a factor in etiology, diagnosis and treatment of malocclusion. Angle orthod 14: 67–71, 1944.

Bolton WA: Clinical application of tooth size analysis. Am J Orthod 48: 504–529, 1962.

Bolton WA: Disharmony in the tooth size and its relation to the analysis and treatment of malocclusion. Angle Orthod 28(1): 113–130, 1958.

Bolton WA: Disharmony in tooth size and its relation to the analysis and treatment of malocclusion. Am J Orthod 1958; 14:67.

Bolton WA: The clinical application of a tooth size analysis. Am J. Orthod 1962; 48:504–29.

Champagne M. Reliability of measurements from photocopies of study models. J Clin Orthod 10: 648–650, 1992.

Crosby DR, Alexander CG: The occurrence of tooth size discrepancies among different malocclusion groups. Am J Orthod Dentofac Orthop 95: 457–461, 1989.

Dalidjan M, Sapmson W, Townsend G: Prediction of dental arch development: an assessment of Pont's Index in three human populations. Am J Orthod Dentofac Orthop 107: 465–475, 1995.

Goyal S: Cephalometric Evaluation of Hypodivergent Facial Types. J. Pierre Fauchard Academy, 2004: 18 (1, 2): 7–17.

Goyal S: Skeletal Characteristics of Hyperdivergent Faces. J. Ind. Orth. Soc. 32:1999: 96–104.

Gupta DS, Sharma VP, Aggarwal SP: Pont's Index as applied on Indians. Angle Orthod 49: 69–71, 1979.

Howes AE: Case analysis and treatment planning based upon the relationship of tooth material to its supporting bone. Am J Orthod Oral Surg 33: 499–511, 1947.

Jacobson A: Introduction to radiographic cephalometry. Philadelphia: Lea and Febiger; 1985.

Neff CW: Tailored occlusion with the anterior coefficient Am J Orthod 35: 309–314, 1949.

Othman SA, Harradine NWD: Tooth size discrepancies and Bolton's ratios–A literature review. Journal of Orthodontics 2006; 33:45–51.

Pont A: Der Zahn-Index in der Orthodontie. Zahnartzliche Orthopadie 3: 306–321, 1909.

Proffit WR, Fields HW, Sarver DM: Contemporary Orthodontics. 4th edition. Elsevier; 2007.

Qu Hong, et al.: Review on Tooth Size and Aarch Width Measurement.

Rakosi TM, Jonas I, Graber T: Color atlas of dental medicine, orthodontic diagnosis. New York: Thieme Publishing, 1993.

Richardson ER, Malhotra SK: Mesiodistal crown dimension of the permanent dentition of American Negroes. Am J Orthod 68: 157–164, 1975.

Steiner C: Cephalometrics in clinical practice, Angle Orthod 29:8, 1959.

Steiner CC: Cephalometric for you and me. Am J Orthod 1953; 39:729–54.

Stifter J: A study of Pont's, Howe's, Rees', Neff's and Bolton's analysis on class 1 Adult dentition. Angle Orthod 28: 215–225, 1958.

Subtelny JD, Sakuda M: Openbite, diagnosis and treatment, Am J Orthod 50:337, 1964.

Tayer BH: The asymmetric extraction decision. Angle Orthod 1992; 62:291–7.

Ten Cate AR, et al: Oral histology: development, structure, and function, St Louis, 1980, Mosby.

Tweed CH: Clinical orthodontics, St Louis, 1966, Mosby.

Tweed CH: The diagnostic facial triangle in the control of treatment objectives, Am J Orthod 55:651, 1969.

Tweed CH: Treatment planning and therapy in the mixed-dentition, Am J Orthod 49:900, 1963.

Uysal T, Sari Z, Basciftci FA, Memili B: Intermaxillary tooth size discrepancy and malocclusion: Is there a relation? Angle Orthod 75(2): 208–213, 2005.

ETIOLOGY

A Rare Case of Multiple Supernumerary Teeth. J. Int. College. Dentist. 46: 1999: 36–37.

Andrews LF: The six keys to normal occlusion. Am J Orthod 1972; 62:296–309.

Angle EH: In Angle. Treatment of malocclusion of the teeth, 7th edition. Philadelphia: S.S. White Dental Manufacturing Co., 1907:167.

Attia Y: Midline diastemas: closure and stability. Angle Orthod 1993; 63:209–12.

Bagga DK, Goyal S: Inheritance of malocclusion: A contemporary overview. The Cusp 2007; 4:12–7.

Baum AT: The midline diastema. J Oral Med 1966; 21:30–9.

Becker A: The median diastema. Dent Clin North Am 1978; 22:685–710.

Bergstrom K, Jensen R, Martensson B: The effect of superior labial frenectomy in cases with midline diastema. Am J Orthod 1973; 63:633–8.

Bishara SE, Andreasen G: Third molars: a review. Am J Orthod 1983; 83:131–7.

Bishara SE: Management of diastemas in orthodontics. Am JOrthod 1972; 61:55–63.

Broadbent BH: Ontogenic development of occlusion. Angle Orthod, 1941; 11: 223–241.

Goyal S, Bagga DK: Inheritance of Malocclusion: A Contemporary Overview (The Cusp).

Goyal S, Gupta D: Cornelia de–Lange Syndrome. J. Ind. Soc. Pedo. Prev. Dent. March 2005, 38–41.

Goyal S: Cleidocranial Dysplasia-A Case Report & Treatment Considerations. J. Pier. Fauch. Acad. 14:L1:2000:27–29.

Goyal S: Macroglossia–A Review. Impressions (an official publication of Yamuna nagar branch of IDA.)

Goyal S: Multidisciplinary Approach To Manage A Case of Partial Anodontia. J. Ind. Prosth. Soc vol. 1 (2): June 2001: 26–28

Goyal S: Transposición del Canino Maxilar en el Espacio del Incisivo Central: Consideraciones y Tratamiento. June, 2010 ORTHDOONTIC CYBERJOURNAL.

Gugnani N, Goyal S: Primary Anterior Tooth Trauma-A Review of Literature. J. Int. College Dentist 48:2000:21–25.

Gupta D, Goyal S: Cornelia de-Lange syndrome. J Indian Soc Pedod Prev Dent. 2005 Mar; 23(1): 38–41.

Gupta ND, Goyal S, Maheshwari S: Neurofibromatosis of Gingiva - A Rare Case.J. Ind. Soc. Perio. 2(3):1999:97.

Haskell BS, Mink JR: An aid to stop thumbsucking: the "Bluegras" appliance. Pediatr Dent 1991; 13:83–5.

Helm S, Prydso U: Prevalence of malocclusion in medieval and modern Danes contrasted. Scand J Dent Res 1979; 87:91–7.

Hobkirk JA, King PA, Goodman JR, Jones SP: Hypodontia: 2.The management of severe hypodontia. Dent Update 1995; 22:8–11.

Huang WJ, Creath CJ: The midline diastema: a review of its etiology and treatment. Pediatr Dent 1995; 17:171–9.

Munjal P, Goyal S, Ragini: Prediction of Third Molar Eruption: J. Ind. Orth. Soc. 2003: 36: 103–112.

Popovich F, Thompson GW: Maxillary diastema: indications for treatment. Am J Orthod 1979; 75:399–404.

Proffit W, Fields H: Contemporary Orthodontics. 3rd ed. St. Louis: CV Mosby, 2000: 170–661.

Rakosi T, Jonas I, Graber TM: Orthodontic Diagnosis. Stuttgart-New York: Theme medical Publishers, 1993: 116–65.

Rakosi T: An Atlas and Manual of Cephalometric Radiography. Great Britain: Thomas Rakosi - Wolfe Medical Publications Ltd., 1982: 96–100.

Treiman SB: Significance of physiological migration of buccal teeth on the development of prognathism. In: Collection of Scientific.

Warren JJ, Slayton RL, Bishara SE, Levy SM, Yonezu T, Kanellis MJ: Effects of nonnutritive sucking habits on occlusal characteristics in the mixed dentition. Pediatr Dent 2005; 27:445–50.

Weiss LS, White JA. Macroglossia: A review. J La State Med Soc 1990; 142:13–6.

Wolford LM, Cottrell DA: Diagnosis of macroglossia and indications for reduction glossectomy. Am J Orthod Dentofacial Orthop 1996; 110:170–7.

SKELETAL MATURITY INDICATORS

Bjork A: Timing of interceptive orthodontic measures based on stages of maturation. Trans Eur Orthod Soc 1972; 48: 61–74.

Demirjian A, Buschang PH, Tanguay R, Patterson DK: Interrelationship among measures of somatic, skeletal, dental and sexual maturity. Am J Orthod 1985; 88: 433–38.

Demirjian A, Goldstein H, Tanner JM: A new system of dental age assessment. Human Biol. 1973; 45:211–227 (s).

Fishman L: Maturational patterns and prediction during adolescence. Angle Orthod 1987; 57: 178–93.

Fishman LS: Chronological versus skeletal age, an evaluation of craniofacial growth. Angle Orthod 1979; 49: 181–9.

Fishman LS: Radiographic evaluation of skeletal maturation; a clinically oriented method based on hand wrist films. Angle Orthod 1982; 52: 88–112.

Hagg U, Taranger J: Maturation indicators and the pubertal growth spurt. Am J Orthod 1982; 82: 299–308.

Hassel B, Farman AG: Skeletal maturation evaluation using cervical vertebrae. Am J Orthod Dent Ofac Orthop 1995; 107:58–66 (s).

Hotz R, Boulanger G, Weisshaupt H: Calcification time of permanent teeth in relation to chronological and skeletal age in children. Helv Odontol Acta. 1959; 3:4–9 (s).

Kamal M, Goyal S, Ragini: Comparative evaluation of hand wrist x-rays with CVMI in 10–12 years old children for skeletal maturation. J. Ind. Soc. Pedo. Prev. Dent. March 2006.

Kamal M; Ragini, Goyal S: Comparative evaluation of hand wrist radiographs with cervical vertebrae for skeletal maturation in 10–12 years old children. J Indian Soc Pedod Prev Dent. 2006 Sep; 24(3):127–35.

Nolla CM: The development of the permanent teeth. J Dent Child. 1960; 27:254–263 (s).

ORTHODONTIC SCARS

Adriaens ML, Dermaut LR, Verbeeck MH: The use of Fluor Protector, a fluoride vernish, as a caries prevention method under orthodontic molar bands. Eur J Orthod 1990; 12:316–319.

Alstad S, Zachrisson BU: Longitudinal study of periodontal condition associated with orthodontic treatment in adolescents. Am J Orthod 1979; 76:277–86.

Bagga DK: Enamel changes with fixed orthodontic therapy: An overview. The Cusp 2007; 4:20–4.

Banks PA, Chadwick SM, Asher-McDade C, Wright JL: Fluoride-releasing elastomerics–a prospective controlled clinical trial. Eur J Orthod 2000; 22:401–407.

Bass JK, Fine H, Cisneros GJ: Nickel hypersensitivity in the orthodontic patient. Am J Orthod Dentofac Orthop 1993; 103:280–285.

Booth-Mason S, Birnie D: Penetrating eye injury from orthodontic headgear–a case report. Eur J Orthod 1988; 10:111–114.

Brite Melson: OVERVIEW Mini-Implants: Where Are We? JCO 2005; 39, 09:539–547.

Dunlap CL, Vincent SK, Barker BF: Allergic reaction to orthodontic wire: report of case. J Am Dent Assoc 1989; 118:449–450.

Geiger AM, Gorelick L, Gwinnett AJ, Benson BJ: Reducing white spot lesions in orthodontic populations with fluoride rinsing. Am J Orthod Dentofac Orthop 1992; 101:403–407.

Gorelick L, Geiger AM, Gwinnett AJ: Incidence of white spot formation after bonding and banding. Am J Orthod 1982; 81:93–98.

Jones M: Enamel loss on bond removal. Br J Orthod 1980; 7:39–44.

Mattick CR, Mitchell L, Chadwick SM, Wright J: Fluoride-releasing elastomeric modules reduce decalcification: a randomized controlled trial. J Orthod 2001; 28:217–219.

McComb JL: Orthodontic treatment and isolated gingival recession: a review. Br J Orthod 1994; 21:151–159.

McGuinness N: Prevention in orthodontics—a review. Dent Update 1992; 19:168–70, 172–75.

Mitchell L: Decalcification during orthodontic treatment with fixed appliances- an overview. Br J Orthod 1992; 19:199–205.

Mizrahi E: Enamel demineralization following orthodontic treatment. Am J Orthod 1982; 82:62–67.

Pamela E: Ellis And Philip E. Benson. Potential Hazards of Orthodontic Treatment–What Your Patient Should Know. Dental Update; December 2002:493–97.

Park HS, Bae SM, Kyung HM, Sungh JH: Microimplant anchorage for treatment of skeletal Class I bialveolar protrusion. J Clin Orthod 2001; 35:417–22.

Paul Yun-Wah Lau, Ricky Wing-Kit Wong: Risks And Complications In Orthodontic Treatment. Hong Kong Dental Journal 2006; 3:15–22.

Poley GE Jr, Slater JE: Latex allergy. J Allergy Clin Immunol 2000; 105(6): 1054–62.

Polson AM, Subtelny JD, Meitner SW, et al: Long-term periodontal status after orthodontic treatment. Am J Orthod Dentofac Orthop 1988; 93:51–58.

Sadowsky C, BeGole EA: Long-term effects of orthodontic treatment on periodontal health. Am J Orthod 1981; 80:156–172.

Samuels RH, Jones ML. Orthodontic facebow injuries and safety equipment. Eur J Orthod 1994; 16:385–94.

Statemann MW, Shannon IL: Control of decalcification in orthodontic patients by daily self-administered application of a water free 0.4% stannous fluoride gel. Am J Orthod 1974; 66:273–279.

Swartz ML: Ceramic brackets. J Clin Orthod 1988; 22:82–8.

Travess H, Roberts-Harry D, Sandy J. Orthodontics. Part 6: Risks in orthodontic treatment. Br Dent J 2004; 196:71–77.

Vanarsdall RL: Complications of orthodontic treatment. Curr Opin Dent 1991; 1:622–33.

WR Proffit, HW Fields, DM Sarver: Contemporary orthodontics. 4th ed; Mosby.

Zachrisson BU, Zachrisson S: Caries incidence and oral hygiene during orthodontic treatment. Scand J Dent Res 1971; 79:394–401.

Zachrisson BU, Zachrisson S: Caries incidence and orthodontic treatment with fixed appliances. Scand J Dent Res 1971; 79:183–192.

Zachrisson BU: Cause and prevention of injuries to teeth and supporting structures during orthodontic treatment. Am J Orthod 1976; 69:285–300.

MOLAR DISTALIZATION

Aldo Giancotti, Paola Cozza: Nickel Titanium double-loop system for simultaneous distalization of first and second molars: J Clin Orthod 1998; 32: 255–260.

Carano A, Testa M: The distal jet appliance for upper molar distalization. J Clin Orthod 1996; 30:374–80.

Ghosh J, Nanda RS: Evaluation of an intraoral maxillary molar distalization technique, Am J Orthod Dentofac Orthop 110:639, 1996.

Gianelly AA, Vaitas AS, Thomas WM: The use of magnets to move molars distally, Am J Orthod 96:161, 1989.

Greenfield RL: Fixed piston appliance for rapid Class II correction, J Clin Orthod 29:174, 1995.

Hilgers J: The pendulum appliance for Class II non-compliant therapy, J Clin Orthod 26:706, 1992.

Hilgers JJ: The pendulum appliance for Class II non-compliance therapy. J Clin Orthod 1992; 26:706–14.

Itoh T, et al: Molar distalization with repelling magnets, J Clin Orthod 25:611, 1991.

Kalra V: The K-loop molar distalizing appliance. J Clin Orthod 1995; 29: 298–301.

Kyu-Rhim Chung: C-Space Regainer for Molar Distalization: J Clin Orthod 2000; 34:32–39.

FUNCTIONAL APPLIANCES

Arvystas, MG: The rationale for early orthodontic treatment, Am. J. Orthod. 113:15–18, 1998.

Bench RW, Gugino CF and Hilgers, JJ: Bioprogressive therapy, Part 8, J. Clin. Orthod. 12:279–298, 1978.

Bishara, SE and Ziaja, RR: Functional appliances: A review, Am. J. Orthod. 95: 250–258, 1989.

Clark WJ: Twin Block functional therapy. Applications in Dentofacial Orthopaedics. Mosby, 2nd edition 2002; 1–10.

Cozza P, De Toffol L: Funtional appliance treatment for Severe classII malocclusion in the early mixed dentition. J. Clin. Orthod.2003; 37(2): 69–74. 2012

Murillo, JC: Mixed-dentition treatment with the selective functional appliance, Am. J. Orthod. 63:596–605, 1973.

White, L: Early Orthodontic intervention, Am. J. Orthod.113:24–28, 1998.

APPLIANCES

Adams CP: The Design and Construction of Removable Appliances, ed 4. Bristol, England: john right & Sons; 1 970.

Adelman, HC: Asphyxial deaths as a result of aspiration of dental appliances: a report of three cases, Journal of Forensic Dentistry, 1988; 33, 389–395.

Adriano G. Crismani, Michael H. Bertl, Ales G. Èelar, Hans-Peter Bantleon, Charles J. Burstone: Miniscrews in orthodontic treatment: Review and analysis of published clinical trials, American Journal of Orthodontics & Dentofacial Orthopedics, January 2010: Vol. 137, Issue 1, Pages 108–113.

American Association of Orthodontists: Special bulletin on extraoral appliance care. Am J Orthod 1975; 68:457.

Bagga DK: An overview of deep bite malocclusion. U P State Dent J 2007; 25:5–9.

Bagga DK: Lingual orthodontics versus labial orthodontics: An overview. J Ind Orth Soc 2007; 41:70–3.

Bhatnagar S, Dhandapani G, Bagga DK: Evaluation of bond failures and shear bond strength in indirect bonding technique using 4 different transfer tray materials: An in vitro study. J Ind Dent Asso 2011; 5(5):595–8.

Bishara SE: Text book of Orthodontics, 2001, WB Saunders company.

Bjork A: Prediction of mandibular growth rotation, Am J Orthod 55:585, 1965.

Booth Mason S, Birnie D: Penetrating eye injury from orthodontic headgear—A case report. Eur J Orthod 1988; 10:111–4.

Brook I: Bacteriology of chronic maxillary sinusitis in adults. Ann Otol Rhinol Laryngol 1989; 98:426–8.

Cameron, SM, Whitlock, WL and Tabor MS: Foreign body aspiration in dentistry: a review, Journal of the American Dental Association, 1996; 127, 1224–1228.

Coco JW, Pankey GA: The use of antimicrobials in dentistry. Compend Contin Educ Dent 1989; 10:664–73.

Costa A, Raffini M, Melsen B: Microscrews as orthodontic anchorage. Int J Adult Orthod Orthogn Surg. 1998; 13:201–209.

Dobson TB, Kaban LB: Diagnosis and management of pediatric facial infections. Oral Maxillofac Surg Clin North Am 1994; 6:13–20.

Edmondson, HD, Frame, JW and Malins, AF: Medical emergencies in dental practice: an update on the drugs and the management of acute airway obstruction, Dental Update, 1989; 16, 254–256.

Graber TM: Orthodontics: Principles and practice. Third Ed. Philadelphia, 1988, WB Saunders company.

Graber TM, Neumann B, Removable orthodontic Appliances, WB Saunders, Philadelphia, 1984.

Graber TM, Vanarsdall RL, eds: Current Orthodontic principles and Techniques, ed 3. St Louis: Mosby; 2000.

Holland GN, Wallace DA, Mondino BY, Cole SH, Ryan SJ. Severe occular injuries from orthodontic headgear. J Clin Orthod 1985; 19:819–25.

Ji GP, Yu Q, Shen G: The relationship between the stability of microimplants and factors of gender and age: Shanghai Kou Qiang Yi Xue. 2008 Aug; 17(4):360–3.

Josephine M. Abelson: The labial arch: its form, progress and adaptability.Am. J.Orthod. and oral surgery; june 1938; 24, issue6, 554–560.

Kanomi R: Mini-implant for orthodontic anchorage. J Clin Orthod. 1997; 31:763–767.

Nazif, MM and Ready, MA: Accidental swallowing of an orthodontic expansion appliance keys: a report of two cases, ASDC Journal of Dentistry for Children, 1983; 50, 126–127.

Oliver RG, Knapman YM: Attitudes to orthodontic treatment. Br J Orthod 1985; 12:179–88.

Padmanabhan R, Deviah S, Suchindran, Kumar P, Singh GD: Treatment of Periodontally Compromised Teeth using Adjunctive Orthodontic Therapy: A Multidisciplinary Approach. J of Ind Ortho Soc 2010; 44(4):115–118

Pancherz H: Treatment of Class II malocclusions by jumping the bite with the Herbst appliance: a cephalometric investigation. Am J Orthod 1979; 76: 423–42.

Parkhouse, RC: Medical complications in orthodontics, British Journal of Orthodontics, 1991: 18, 51–57.

Proffit WR, Fields HW, Sarver DM: Contemporary orthodontics, ed 4, St Louis, 2007, Mosby.

Seel D. Extra-oral hazards of extra-oral traction. Br J Orthod 1980; 7:53.

Sharma P, Jamwal S, Sharma R, Jamwal RS: Molar intrusion with a removable appliance- a case report. Clin Dent, 2010; 4(1):41–44.

Stafford GD, Caputo AA, Turley PK: Characteristics of headgear release mechanisms: Safety implications. Angle Orthod 68:319–326, 1998.

Yan Chen, Hee Moon Kyung, Wen Ting Zhao, Won Jae Yu: Critical factors for the success of orthodontic mini-implants: A systematic review, American Journal of Orthodontics & Dentofacial Orthopedics; March 2009, Vol. 135, Issue 3, Pages 284–291.

ROOT RESORPTION AND OTM

Branemark PI, et al: Osseointegrated implants in the treatment of the edentulous jaw. Experience from a 10-year period, Stockholm, Sweden, 1977, Almqvist & Wiksell Int.

Brezniak N, Wasserstein A: Root resorption after orthodontic treatment. Literature review, Am J Orthod Dentofac Orthop 103(62):138, 1993.

Brudvik P, Rygh P: Multi-nucleated cells remove the main hyalinized tissue and start resorption of adjacent root surfaces, Eur J Orthod 16:265, 1994.

Brudvik P, Rygh P: The initial phase of orthodontic root resorption incident to local compression of the PDL, Eur J Orthod 15:249, 1993.

Brudvik P, Rygh P: The repair of orthodontic root resorption. An ultrastructural study, Eur J Orthod 17:189, 1995.

Davidovitch Z, et al: Neurotransmitters, cytokines and the control of alveolar bone remodeling in orthodontics, Adult Orthod Dent Clin North Am 32:411, 1988.

Dibbets J, van der Weele L: Long-term effects of orthodontic treatment, including extraction, on signs and symptoms attributed to CMD, Eur J Orthod 14:16, 1992.

Droschl H: The effect of heavy orthopedic forces on the suture of the facial bones, Angle Orthod 45:36, 1975.

Edwards J: A surgical procedure to eliminate rotational relapse, Am J Orthod 57:35, 1970.

Roberts WE, et al: Bone physiology: evaluation of bone metabolism, JAm DentAssoc 122:59, 1991.

Roberts WE, Garetto LP, Simmons KE: Endosseous implants for rigid orthodontic anchorage. In Bell WH, editor: Surgical correction of dentofacial deformities, vol 2, Philadelphia, 1992, WB Saunders.

Roberts WE, Goodwin WC, Heiner SR: Cellular response to orthodontic force, Dent Clin North Am 25:3, 1981.

Roberts WE, Hartsfield JK, Jr: Multidisciplinary management of congenital and acquired compensated malocclusions: diagnosis, etiology and treatment planning, Indiana Dent Assoc J 76(2):42, 1997.

EARLY TREATMENT

Baccetti TB, Franchi L, Toth LR, McNamara JA: Treatment timing for twin-block therapy. Am J Orthod Dentofacial Orthop 2000; **118:** 159–170.

Bagga DK: Lip Bumper: A simplified design. U P State Dent J 2006; 4:27–9.

Bagga DK: Serial extraction: An overview. U P State Dent J 2006; 24:144–9.

Battagel JM, Orton HS: A comparative study of the effects of customized facemask therapy or headgear to the lower arch on the developing Class III face. Eur J Orthod 1995; **17:** 467–482.

Bell RA, LeCompte EJ: The effects of maxillary expansion using a quad-helix appliance during the deciduous and mixed dentition. Am J Orthod 1981; **79:** 152–161.

Bishara: The textbook of orthodontics. Orthodontic treatment in primary dentition. 2001; 248.

Brennan MB, Gianelly AA: The use of the lingual arch in the mixed dentition to resolve incisor crowding. Am J Orthod Dentofacial Orthop 2000; **117:** 81–85.

Cetlin NM, Ten Hoeve A: Nonextraction treatment, J Clin Orthod 17:396, 1983.

Da Silva Filho OM, Magro AC, Filho LC: Early treatment of class III malocclusion with rapid maxillary expansion and maxillary protraction. Am J Orthod Dentofacial Orthop 1998; **113:** 196–203.

Dugoni SA: Comprehensive mixed dentition treatment. Am J Orthod Dentofacial Orthop 1998; **113:** 75–84.

Gianelly AA: Crowding: timing of treatment, Angle Orthod 64:415, 1994.

Goyal S, Maheshwari S, Dahiya A: Maxillary Expansion - An Interceptive Modality In Mixed

Dentition. J. Ind. Soc. Pedo. Prev. Dent. 18:1:2000: 24–28.

Goyal S, Sharma A, Gera A: Conservative Management of Malocclusion In Mixed Dentition. J. Ind. Soc. Pedo. Prev. Dent 18:3:2000:103–107.

Goyal S: Early Orthodontics-A Current Perspective. J. Int. College. Dentist. 46:1999:15–21.

Goyal S: Fixed Space Regainer–A New Simplified Appliance. Impressions (an official publication of Yamuna nagar branch of IDA).

Grim SE: Treatment of pseudo class III relationship in primary dention: A case history. ASDC J Dent Child 1991. 58(6):484–88.

Haas AJ: Long-term posttreatment evaluation of rapid palatal expansion, Angle Orthod 50:189, 1980.

Haas AJ: Palatal expansion: just the beginning of dentofacial orthopedics, Am J Orthod 57:219, 1970.

Haas AJ: Rapid expansion of the maxillary dental arch and nasal cavity by opening the mid-palatal suture, Angle Orthod 31:73, 1961.

Haas AJ: The treatment of maxillary deficiency by opening the mid-palatal suture, Angle Orthod 65:200, 1965.

Harrison JE, Ashby D: Orthodontic treatment for posterior crossbites (Cochrane Review). In: The Cochrane Library, 4. Oxford: Update Software, 2001.

Haruki T, Little RM: Early versus late treatment of crowded first premolar extraction cases: postretention evaluation of stability and relapse. Angle Orthod 1998; **68:** 61–68.

Helm S, Kreiborg S, Solow B: Psychosocial implications of malocclusion: a 15-year follow-up study on 30-year-old Danes. Am J Orthod Dentofacial Orthop 1985; **87:** 110–118.

Herold JC: Maxillary expansion: a retrospective study of three methods of expansion and their long term sequelae. Br J Orthod 1989; **16:** 195–200.

Kidner G, DiBiase A, Ball J, DiBiase D: Reverse twin blocks for early treatment of class III. Eur J Orthod 1999; **21:** 631 (Abstr. 189).

Leighton BC: The early signs of malocclusion, Trans Eur Orthod Soc 45:353, 1969.

Little RM, Riedel RA, Stein A: Mandibular arch length during the mixed dentition: postretention evaluation of stability and relapse treatment. Am J Orthod Dentofacial Orthop 1990; **97:** 393–404.

Littlewood SJ, Tait AG, Mandall NA, Lewis DH: The role of removable appliances in contemporary orthodontics. Br Dent J 2001; **161:** 304–310.

Liveratos FA, Johnson LE: A comparison of one-stage and two-stage nonextraction alternatives in matched Class II samples. Am J Orthod Dentofacial Orthop 1995; **108:** 118–131.

Loh MK, Kerr WJS: The Functional Regulator III–effects and indications for use. Br J Orthod 1985; **12:** 153–157.

Malmgren O, Omblus J, Hagg U, Pancherz H: Treatment with an appliance system in relation to treatment intensity and growth periods. Am J Orthod Dentofacial Orthop 1987; **91:** 143–151.

Mckeown H. and Sandler J: The two by four appliance:a versatile appliance. Dent Update 2001; 28: 496–500.

McKeown HF, Sandler J: The two by four appliance: a versatile appliance. Dent Update 2001; **28:** 496–500.

McNamara JA, Brookstein FL, Shaughnessy TG: Skeletal and dental changes following functional regulator therapy on Class II patients. Am J Orthod 1985; **87:** 1–20.

Michael G. Arvystas: The rationale for early orthodontic treatment. AJO DO 1998; 113(1):15–18.

Shaw WC, Meek SC, Jones DS: Nicknames, harassment and the salience of dental features among school children. Br J Orthod 1980; **7:** 75–80.

Sheridan JJ, Hastings J: Air-rotor stripping and lower incisor extraction treatment, J Clin Orthod 26:18, 1992.

Sheridan JJ: Air-rotor stripping update. J Clin Orthod 21:781, 1987.

Sheridan JJ: Air-rotor stripping, J Clin Orthod 19:43, 1985.

Stephens CD. The use of natural spontaneous tooth movement in the treatment of malocclusion. Dent Update 1989; **16:** 337–342.

Tulloch JFC, Philips C, Proffit WR: Benefit of early Class II treatment: Progress report of a two-phase randomized control trial. Am J Orthod Dentofacial Orthop 1998; **113:** 62–72.

Tung AW, Kiyak HA: Psychological influences on the timing of orthodontic treatment. AJO DO 1998; 113: 29–39.

Verma V, Mehrotra A, Sikri A: Early orthodontic treatment. JIDA 2009; 3(12): 423–426.

Wertz RA: Skeletal and dental changes accompanying rapid midpalatal suture opening, Am J Orthod 58:41, 1970.

White L: Early Orthodontic Intervention. American Journal of Orthodontics and Dentofacial Orthopedics 1998; 113(1):24–28.

LASERS

Almeida HC, Vedovello Filho M, Vedovello SA, Young A A A, Ramirez-Yañez GO. ER: YAG laser for composite removal after bracket debonding: a qualitative SEM analysis. Int J Orthod Milwaukee. 2009 Spring; 20(1):9–13.

Bader C, Krejci I: Marginal quality in enamel and dentin after preparation and finishing with an Er:YAG laser. Am J Dent. 2006 Dec; 19(6):337–42.

Coluzzi DJ, Goldstein AJ: Lasers in dentistry. An overview. Dent Today. 2004 Apr; 23(4):120–2, 124–7.

Convissar RA, Goldstein EE: An overview of lasers in dentistry. Gen Dent. 2003 Sep-Oct; 51(5):436–40. Review.

Genovese MD, Olivi G: Use of laser technology in orthodontics: hard and soft tissue laser treatments. Eur J Paediatr Dent. 2010 Mar; 11(1):44–8.

Hilgers JJ, Tracey SG. J: Clinical uses of diode lasers in orthodontics. Clin Orthod. 2004 May; 38(5): 266–73.

Ishida K, Endo T, Shinkai K, Katoh Y: Shear bond strength of rebonded brackets after removal of adhesives with Er, Cr:YSGG laser. Odontology. 2011 May 7.

Roberts-Harry D. Lasers in orthodontics. Br J Orthod. 1994 Aug; 21(3):308–12. Review.

EXPANSION

Arndt, W.V: Nickel titanium palatal expander, J. Clin. Orthod. 27:129–137, 1993.

Bishara SE, Staley RN: Maxillary expansion: clinical implications. Am J Orthod Dentofacial Orthop 1987; 91:3–14.

Cohen M and Silverman E: A new and simple palate splitting device. J Clin Orthod 1973; VII 368–369.

Corbett, MC: Slow and continuous maxillary expansion, molar rotation, and molar distalization, J. Clin. Orthod. 31:253–263, 1997.

Gianelly A: Leeway space and the resolution of crowding in the mixed dentition. Semin Orthod 1995; 1:188–94.

Haas AJ: Just the beginning of dentofacial orthopedics. Am J Orthod 1970; 57:219–55.

Haas AJ: Rapid expansion of the maxillary dental arch and nasal cavity by opening the midpalatal suture. Angle Orthod 1961; 31:73–90.

Haas AJ: The treatment of maxillary deficiency by opening the midpalatal suture. Angle Orthod 1965; 35:200–17.

Mew J: Long-term effect of rapid maxillary expansion. Eur J Orthod 1993; 15:543.

Moss JP: Rapid expansion. Int J Orthod 1976; 14:15–9.

Proffit WR, Fields HW: Orthodontic treatment planning: limitations, controversies and special problems. In: Contemporary orthodontics. 3rd ed. St. Louis: Mosby; 2000:271.

Sharma A, Kaur G, Gera A, Goyal S: Conservative management of malocclusion in mixed dentition. J Indian Soc Pedod Prev Dent. 2000 Sep; 18(3):103–7.

Timms DJ. A study of basal movement with rapid maxillary expansion. Am J Orthod 1980; 77:500–7.

Viazis AD, Vadiaks G, Zelos L and Gallagher R. Designs and applications of palatal expansion appliances. J Clin Orthod 1992; 1 239–243.

BONDING

Boyd RL: Periodontal considerations in the use of bonds or bands on molars in adolescents and adults, Angle Orthod 62:117, 1992.

Brandt S, Servoss JM, Persily KB: Atropine sulphate-an effective antisialagogue, J Clin Orthod 15:629, 1981.

Buonocore MG, Vezin JC: Orthodontic fluoride protection, J Clin Orthod 14:321, 1980.

Buonocore MG: A simple method of increasing the adhesion of acrylic filling materials to enamel surface, J Dent Res 34:849, 1955.

Burapavong V, Marshall GW, Apfel DA: Enamel surface characteristics on removal of bonded orthodontic brackets, Am J Orthod 74:176, 1978.

ADULT ORTHODONTICS

Ackerman JL: The challenge of adult orthodontics, J Clin Orthod 12:43, 1978.

Ahrens DG, Shapira Y, Kuftinec M: An approach to rotational relapse, Am J Orthod 80:83, 1981.

Aimamo J: Relationship between malalignment of teeth and periodontal disease, Scand J Dent Res 80:104, 1972.

Bagga DK, Goyal S: Orthodontics for adults seeking periorestorative treatment: An overview. J Ind Dent Asso 2007; 1:67–9.

Bagga DK: Adult orthodontics versus adolescent orthodontics: An overview. J Oral Health Comm Dent 2010; 4(2):42–7.

Bagga DK: Consideration of age factor in planning orthognathic surgery: A contemporary view. U P State Dent J 2006; 24:93–6.

Bagga DK: Limitations in adult orthodontics: A review. J Oral Health Comm Dent 2009; 3(2):48–51.

Goyal S, Gugnani S: Mouthwashes–A boon or bane. A must know statement for every dental practitioner. J. Ind. Soc. Perio. 5 (2) : 2002 : 73–78.

Kathuria P, Goyal S: Endodontic Miscellany–Endo–Ortho management of subgingivally transversely fractured tooth. Endodontology; 13 (1): 2001: 31–34.

LaSuta EP: Orthodontic considerations in prosthetic and restorative dentistry, DCNA 32:1447, 1988.

Levitt HL: Adult orthodontics, J Clin Orthod 5:1130, 1971.

Machen BE: Developing protocols for adult patients, Am J Orthod Dentofac Orthop 98:476, 1990.

Marks MH: Tooth movement in periodontal therapy. In Goldman HM, Cohen DW editors: Periodontal therapy, ed 6, St Louis, 1980, Mosby.

Mathews DP, Kokich VG: Management treatment for the orthodontic patient with periodontal problems, Semin Orthod 3:21, 1997.

SURGICAL ORTHODONTICS

Codivilla A: On the means of lengthening the lower limbs, the muscles and tissues of which are shortened through deformity, Am J Orthop Surg 2:353, 1905.

Epker BN: Vascular considerations in orthognathic surgery. I. Maxillary osteotomies, Oral Surg Oral Med Oral Pathol 57:467, 1984.

Epker BN: Vascular considerations in orthognathic surgery. II. Maxillary osteotomies, Oral Surg Oral Med Oral Pathol 57:473, 1984.

Proffit WR, Ackerman JL: Diagnosis and treatment planning. In Graber TM, Swain BF, editors: Orthodontics: current concepts and techniques, St Louis, 1985, Mosby.

Proffit WR, Phillips C, Turvey TA: Stability following superior repositioning of the maxilla by Le Fort I osteotomy, Am J Orthod Dentofac Orthop 92:151, 1987.

RETENTION

Bergious M, Kiliaridis S, Berggren U: Pain in orthodontics. A review and discussion of the literature. J Orofac Orthop 2000; 61:125–37.

Bishara SA, Ziaja RR: Functional appliances: A review. Am J Orthod Dentofac Orthop 1989; 95:250–8.

Bolton W: The clinical application of a tooth size analysis, Angle Orthod 28:113, 1958.

Bolton WA: Disharmony in tooth size and its relation to the analysis and treatment of malocclusion, Angle Orthod 28:113, 1958.

Brain WE: The effect of surgical transsection of free gingival fibers on the regression of orthodontically rotated teeth in the dog, Am J Orthod 55:50, 1969.

Fraenkel R, Loeffler U: Functional aspects of mandibular crowding. Eur J Orthod 1990; 12:224–9.

Fraenkel R: A functional approach to orofacial orthopaedics. Br J Orthod 1980; 7:41–51.

Hawley CA: A removable retainer, Dent Cosmos 61:449, 1919.

Hellman M: Fundamental principles and expedient compromises in orthodontic procedures. In Transactions of the American association of orthodontists, St Louis, 1945, Mosby.

Hernandez JL: Mandibular bicanine width relative to overbite, Am J Orthod 36:445, 1969.

Hicks EP: Slow maxillary expansion: a clinical study of the skeletal versus dental response to low-magnitude force, Am J Orthod 73:121, 1978.

Horowitz SL, Hixon EH: Physiologic recovery following orthodontic treatment, Am J Orthod 55:1, 1969.

Kaplan R: Mandibular third molars and postretention crowding, Am J Orthod 66:411, 1974.

Tweed CH: Indications for extraction of teeth in orthodontic procedure, Am J Orthod Oral Surg 30:405, 1944.

CLEFTS

Spilson SV, Kim HJ, Chung KC: Association between maternal diabetes mellitus and newborn oral cleft. Ann Plast Surg 2001; 47(5):477.

Tziafas D: Development of the orofacial region and formation of the dental tissues. In: Tziafas D. Biology of the dental tissues. Development, structure and function. Thessaloniki: University Studio Press, 1999:11–15.

Veau V: Division palatine. Paris: Masson et Cie, 1931.

Vieira AR, Orioli IM, Murray JC: Maternal age and oral clefts: a reappraisal. Oral Surg Oral Med Oral Pathol Oral Radiol Endod 2002; 94(5):530.

Werler MM, Lammer EJ, Rosenberg L, Mitchell AA: Maternal cigarette smoking during pregnancy in relation to oral clefts. Am J Epidemiol 1990; 132(5):926.

IMPLANTS

Baumgaertel S, Mohammad R. Razavi, b and Mark G. Hansc: Mini-implant anchorage for the orthodontic practitioner. Am J Orthod Dentofacial Orthop 2008; 133:621–7.

Critical factors for the success of orthodontic mini-implants: A systematic review. Chen Y, Kyung HM, Zhao WT, and Yud WJ. Am J Orthod Dentofacial Orthop 2009; 135: 284–91.

Eriksson AR, Albrektsson T: Temperature threshold levels for heat-induced bone tissue injury: a vital-microscopic study in the rabbit. J Prosthet Dent 1983; 50:101–7.

Kravitz ND, Kusnoto B: Risks and complications of orthodontic Miniscrews. Am J Orthod Dentofacial Orthop 2007; 131:00.

Ludwig B, Baumgaertel S, Bbhm B: Mini-implants in Orthodontics. Innovative Anchorage Concepts.Quimessence Publishing Co Ltd; 21, 26.

Moon CH, Park HK, Nam JS, Im JS, Baek SH: Relationship between vertical skeletal pattern and success rate of orthodontic mini-implants. Am J Orthod Dentofacial Orthop 2010; 138:51–7.

Nanda R, Uribe FA: Temporary anchorage devices in orthodontics 2009, Mosby Elsevier. 91, 101.

Park HS, Jeong SH, b and Kwon OW: Factors affecting the clinical success of screw implants used as orthodontic anchorage. Am J Orthod Dentofacial Orthop 2006; 130:18–25.

Poggioa PM, Incorvatib C, Stefano Velob S, Aldo Carano A: "Safe Zones" A Guide for Miniscrew Positioning in the Maxillary and Mandibular Arch. Angle Orthod 2006; 76:191–197.

Prasad N, Sharma T, Dabla N, Nandakumar T: Temporary Anchorage Devices Simplified. Indian J Dent Resear. 2010; 6(2):54–57.

Predrilling of the implant site: Is it necessary for orthodontic mini-implants? Am J Orthod Dentofacial Orthop; 2010; 137:825–9.

Wilmes B, Drescher D, Nienkemper M: A Miniplate System for Improved Stability of Skeletal Anchorage. J Clinic Orthod 2009; 43 (8): 494–501.

MEDICAL CONDITIONS

Ashcraft MB, Southa JKA, Tolley EA: The effect of corticosteroid induced osteoporosis on orthodontic tooth movement; Am J Orthod Dentofacial Orthop 1992; 102:310–19.

Baum E, Peters Km: The diagnosis and treatment of primary osteoporosis according to current guidlines; Dtsch Arztebl Int; 2008; 105; 33; 573–582.

Bensch L, Braem M, van Acker K, Willems G: Orthodontic treatment considerations in patients with diabetes mellitus. Am J Orthod Dentofacial Orthop 2003; 123: 74–78.

Burden D, Mullally B, Sandler J: Orthodontic treatment of patients with medical disorders. Eur J Orthod 2001; 23: 363–72.

Burden D, Mullally B, Sandler J: Orthodontic treatment of patients with medical disorders. Eur J Orthod 2001; 23: 363–72.

C.F Hildebolt; Osteoporosis and oral bone loss; Dentomaxillofacial radiology; 1997; Vol 26; Issue 13–15.

Dahllof G, Huggare J: Orthodontic considerations in the pediatric cancer patients: a review. Semin Orthod 2004; 10:266–76.

Danchin N, Duval X, Leport C: Prophylaxis of infective endocarditis: French recommendations 2002. Heart 2005; 91:715–18.

Fatemeh Ezoddini Ardakani; Seyed-Jalil Mirmohamadi; Osteoporosis and oral bone resorption: a review; J Maxillofac Oral Surg; 2009; 8(2):121–126.

Fiona Y. C Leung, A. Bakrm.Rabie; Ricky WK Wong: Osteoporosis, osteonecrosis and orthodontics; World J of Orthod 2009; 10; 261–271.

Fiske J, Boyle C. Epilepsy and oral care; Dent update; 2002; 29; 180–87.

Gowri Sankar Singaraju, et al: Management of The Medically Compromised Cases In Orthodontic Practice; Asian Journal of Medical Sciences 1 (2010) 68–74.

Gupta A, Epstein JB, Cabay RJ: Bleeding disorders of importance in dental care and related patient management.J Canadian Dent Assoc 2007; 73: 77–83.

Jennifer E. Weiss, Norman T. ilowite: Juvenile Idiopathic Arthritis; Pediatr Clin N Am; 52 2005; 413–44.

Leite LP, Bell RA: Adverse hypersensitivity reactions in orthodontics. Semin Orthod 2004; 10: 240–43.

Luc Bensch, Marc Braem and Guy Willems: Orthodontic Considerations in the Diabetic Patient; Semin Orthod 10:252–258.

Marx RE, Sawatri Y, Fortin M, Broumand V: Bisphosphonate induced exposed bone (osteonecrosis / osteopetrosis) of the jaws; risk factors, recognition, prevention and treatment. J Oral Maxillofac Surg 2005; 63; 1567–75.

McCarthy GM, Mamandras AH, MacDonald JK: Infection control in the orthodontic office in Canada. Am J Orthod Dentofacial Orthop 1997; 112: 275–81.

Miller, Chris H: Infection Control and Management of Hazardous Materials for the Dental Team, 3rd Edition. Mosby Elsevier Health Science, 2005; 91, 437.

Miyajima, Nagahara K, Lizuka T: Orthodontic treatment for a patient after menopause; Angle Orthod 1996; 66; 173–180.

Moreillon P, Que Y-A: Infective endocarditis. Lancet 2004; 363: 139–49.

Patricia Vale ria, Milanezi Alves, Daniele Karina M. Alvesb, Margareth Maria Gomes de Souza; Sandra Regina Torres; Orthodontic Treatment of Patients with Sickle-cell Anemia; Angle Orthod 2006; 76:269–273

Pepmueller PH, Cassidy JT, Allen SH, et al: Bone mineralization and bone metabolism in children with juvenile rheumatoid arthritis. Arthritis Rheum 1996; 39(5):746–57.

Rinchuse DJ, Rinchuse DJ, Sosovicka MF, Robison JM, Pendleton R: Orthodontic treatment of patients using bisphosphonates: a report of 2 cases. Am J Orthod Orthop 2007; 131: 321–26.

Sanders BJ, Weddell JA, Dodge NN: Managing patients who have seizure disorders: dental and medical issues. J Am Dent Assoc 126:1641–47, 1995.

Simon HS Pearce and Tim D Cheetham Diagnosis and management of vitamin D deficiency; BMJ 2010; 340:b5664.

Sonis ST: Orthodontic management of selected medically compromised patients: cardiac disease, bleeding disorders, and asthma. Semin Orthod 2004; 10: 277–80.

Stanley F: Malamed Medical Emergencies in the Dental Office, 6thEdition; 225–28.

Van Venrooy JR, Proffit WR: Orthodontics care for medically compromised patients: possibilities and limitation. J Am Dent Assoc 1985; Ill: 262–66.

Verna C, Hartig LE, Kalia S Melsen B: Influence of steroid drugs on orthodontically induced root resorption. Orthod Craniofac Res; 2006; 9; 57–62.

Zahrowski JJ: Bisphosphonate treatment: an orthodontic concern calling for a proactive approach. Am J Orthod Dentofacial Orthop 2007; 131: 311–20.

Zahrowski JJ:. Bisphosphonate treatment: an orthodontic concern calling for a proactive approach. Am J Orthod Dentofacial Orthop 2007; 131: 311–20.

Zahrowski JJ: Bisphosphonates treatment; A preset orthodontic concern calling for a proactive approach.The bulletin; AAO 2006; 24 (5); 4, 8, 9.

EXTRACTIONS IN ORTHODONTICS

Angelis DV: The rationale for maxillary second premolar extractions in adult Class II treatment. J. Clin. Orthod 2007; 41: 445–450.

Arnett GW, Bergman RT: Facial keys to orthodontic diagnosis and treatment planning. Am. J. Orthod Dentofac Orthop 1993; 103:299–312.

Arnett GW, Jelic JS, Kim J, Cummings DR, Beress A, Worley C.M. Jr, Chung B, Bergman R.: Soft tissue cephalometric analysis: Diagnosis and treatment planning of dentofacial deformity. Am. J. Orthod Dentofac Orthop 1999; 116:239–253.

Bahreman AA: Lower incisor extraction in orthodontic treatment. Am. J. Orthod 1977; 72:560–567.

Bernstein. Angle versus Calvin S. Case: Extraction versus non-extraction, Historical revisionsm. Am J Orthod Dentofac Orthop1992; 102: 464–470.

Bishara S.E.Cummins DM, Jakobsen JR, Zaher AR: Dentofacial and soft tissue changes in Class II, division 1 cases treated with and without extractions. Am. J. Orthod Dentofac Orthop 1995; 107:28–37.

Bishara SE, Jakobsen JR, Hession TJ, Treder, JE: Soft tissue profile changes from 5 to 45 years of age. Am. J. Orthod Dentofac Orthop 1998; 114:698–706.

Bishara, Burkey: Second molar extractions: A review. Am. J. Orthod Dentofac Orthop 1986; 89: 415–424.

Björk, A, and Skieller, V: Facial development and tooth eruption: An implant study at the age of puberty. Am. J. Orthod 1972; 62: 339–383.

Björk, A: The face in profile: An anthropological x-ray investigation on Swedish children and conscripts, Sven. Tandläk. Tidskr. 40: No. 5B, 1947.

Bolton WA: Disharmony in tooth size and its relation to the analysis and treatment of malocclusion. Am. J. Orthod 1958; 28:113–130.

Bolton WA: The clinical application of a tooth-size analysis. Am. J. Orthod 1962; 48:504–52.

Brandt S: JCO Interviews Dr. Richard A. Riedel on retention and relapse, J. Clin. Orthod 1976; 10:454–472.

Canut JA: Mandibular incisor extraction: indications and long-term evaluation, Eur. J. Orthod 1996. 18:485–489.

Cassidy KM, Harris EF, Tolley EA, Keim RG: Genetic influence on dental arch form in orthodontic patients. Angle Orthod 1998; 68:445–454.

Celli D: Bimaxillary Protrusion Treated Without Extractions. J. Clin. Orthod 2007; 41: 33–38.

Clark, WJ: Twin Block Functional Therapy: Applications in Dentofacial Orthopaedics. Mosby-Wolfe; London 1995: pp.10–11.

Cummins DM, Bishara SE, Jakobsen JR: A computer assisted photogrammetric analysis of soft tissue changes after orthodontic treatment, Part II: Results. Am. J. Orthod Dentofac Orthop 1995; 108:38–47.

David Birnie: The Damon Passive Self-Ligating Appliance System. Semin Orthod 2008; 14:19–35.

Djeu G, Hayes C, Zawaideh, S: Correlation between mandibular central incisor proclination and gingival recession during fixed appliance therapy. Angle Orthod 2002. 72:238–245.

Faerovig E, Zachrisson, BU: Effects of mandibular incisor extraction on anterior occlusion in adults with Class III malocclusion and reduced overbite. Am. J. Orthod Dentofac Orthop 1999; 115:113–124.

Farrow AL, Zarrinnia K, Azizi, K: Bimaxillary protrusion in black Americans: An esthetic evaluation and treatment considerations. Am. J. Orthod Dentofac Orthop 1993; 104:240–250.

Foley TF, Duncan PG: Soft tissue profile changes in late adolescent males. Angle Orthod 1997; 67:373–380.

Gianelly AA: Arch width after extraction and non-extraction treatment. Am. J. Orthod Dentofac Orthop 2003; 123:25–28.

Johnson DK, Smith RJ: Smile esthetics after orthodontic treatment with and without extraction of four first premolars. Am. J. Orthod Dentofac Orthop 1995; 108:162–167.

Kaplan, RG: Mandibular third molars and post-retention crowding, Am. J. Orthod 1974; 66: 411–430.

Kesling, HD: The philosophy of the Tooth Positioning Appliance, Am. J. Orthod 1945; 31:297–304.

Kirsten Nigul: Factors related to apical root resorption of maxillary incisors in orthodontic patients. Stomatologija, Baltic Dental and Maxillofacial Journal 2006; 8:76–9.

Koch R, Gonzales A, Witt E: Profile and soft tissue changes during and after orthodontic treatment. Eur. J. Orthod 1979; 1:193–199.

Kokich VG, Shapiro PA: Lower incisor extraction in orthodontic treatment: Four clinical reports. Angle Orthod 1984; 54:139–153.

Kurz C, Bennett R: Extraction cases and the lingual appliance. J Am Ling Orthod Assoc. 1998; 3:10–13.

La Mastra SJ: Relationships between changes in skeletal and integumental points A and B following orthodontic treatment. Am. J. Orthod 1981; 79:416–423.

Lew K: Profile changes following orthodontic treatment of bimaxillary protrusion in adults with the Begg appliance. Eur. J. Orthod 1989; 11:375–381.

Luppanapornlap S, Johnston LE Jr: The effects of premolar extraction: A long-term comparison of outcomes in "clear-cut" extraction and non-extraction Class II patients. Angle Orthod 1993; 63:257–272.

Miller RJ, Duong TT, Derakhshan M: Lower incisor extraction treatment with the Invisalign system. J. Clin. Orthod 2002; 36:95–102.

Moore T, Southard KA, Casko JS, Qian F, Southard TE: Buccal corridors and smile esthetics, Am. J. Orthod Dentofac Orthop; 127:206–213, 2005.

Nance, Hays N: The removal of second premolars in orthodontic treatment. Am J Orthod 1949; 35: 685–695.

Nanda, Uribe: Considerations in mandibular incisor extraction cases. J. Clin. Orthod 2009; 43:45–51.

Owen AH: Single lower incisor extractions, J. Clin. Orthod 1993; 27:153–160.

Peck S, Peck L: Selected aspects of the art and science of facial esthetics. Semin. Orthod 1995; 1:105–126.

Pinar Saatçi, Filiz Yukay: The effect of premolar extractions on tooth-size discrepancy. Am. J. Orthod Dentofac Orthop 1997; 111: 428–434.

Proffit WR, Field HW: Orthodontic treatment planning: Limitations, controversies and special problems, in Contemporary Orthodontics. 3rd ed., Mosby; St. Louis 2000.

Proffit WR, White RP. Jr.: Surgical Orthodontic Treatment. Mosby; St. Louis, 1990: pp. 340–349.

Richardson, ME: Late lower arch crowding: Facial growth or forward drift? Eur. J. Orthod. 1979; 1: 219–225.

Riedel RA Little RM, Bui TD: Mandibular incisor extraction—post-retention evaluation of stability and relapse. Angle Orthod 1992; 62:103–116.

Robert L. Boyd, HeeSoo Oh, Mohamed Fallah, Vicki Vlaskalic: An update on present and future considerations of aligners. CDA. Journal 2006; 34:793–805.

Sameshima GT, Sinclair PM: Predicting and preventing root resorption: part I. Diagnostic factors. Am J Orthod Dentofac Orthop 2001; 119: 505–10.

Schulhof, RJ: Third molars and orthodontic diagnosis. J. Clin. Orthod. 1976; 10: 272–281.

Schwarze CW: The influence of third molar germectomia—A comparative long-term study. Trans. Eur. Orthod. Soc. 1975; pp. 551–562.

Sheridan JJ, Hastings J: Air-rotor stripping and lower incisor extraction treatment. J. Clin. Orthod 1992; 26:18–22.

Siatkowski, RE: Incisor uprighting: Mechanism for late secondary crowding in the anterior segments of the dental arches. Am. J. Orthod 1974; 66: 398–410.

Sillman, JH: Dimensional changes of the dental arches: Longitudinal study from birth to 25 years (appendix). Am. J. Orthod 1964; 50: 824–842.

Silvia Geron: Anchorage Loss—A Multifactorial Response. Angle Orthod 2003; 73:730–737.

Tae-Kyung Kim: First or second premolar extraction effects on facial vertical dimension. Angle Orthod 2005; 75: 177–182.

Takemoto K: Anchorage control in lingual orthodontics. In: Romano R. Lingual Orthodontics. Hamilton, Canada: BC Decker; 1998: 75–82.

Urban Hagg: Maxillary second molar extraction in orthodontic treatment. World J Orthod 2008; 9: 52–61.

Valinoti JR: Mandibular incisor extraction therapy. Am. J. Orthod 1994. 105:107–116.

Wiliams R: The effect of different extraction sites upon incisor retraction. Am. J. Orthod Dentofac Orthop 1976; 69: 388–410.

Womack WR: A new approach to correction of crowding. Am. J. Orthod Dentofac Orthop 2002; 122:310–316.

Index

C

D

E

J

K

L

M

T

U

V

W

Z

Reader's Notes

Reader's Notes

Reader's Notes